Meyler's Side Effects of Analgesics and Anti-inflammatory Drugs

Meyler's Side Effects of Analgesics and Anti-inflammatory Drugs

Editor

J K Aronson, MA, DPhil, MBChB, FRCP, FBPharmacolS, FFPM (Hon)
Oxford, United Kingdom

AMSTERDAM • BOSTON • HEIDELBERG • LONDON • NEW YORK • OXFORD
PARIS • SAN DIEGO • SAN FRANCISCO • SINGAPORE • SYDNEY • TOKYO

Elsevier
Radarweg 29, PO Box 211, 1000 AE Amsterdam, The Netherlands
The Boulevard, Langford Lane, Kidlington, Oxford OX5 1GB, UK
525 B Street, Suite 1900, San Diego, CA 92101-4495, USA

Notice
No responsibility is assumed by the publisher for any injury and/or damage to persons
or property as a matter of products liability, negligence or otherwise, or from any use or operation
of any methods, products, instructions or ideas contained in the material herein. Because of rapid
advances in the medical sciences, in particular, independent verification of diagnoses and drug
dosages should be made

Medicine is an ever-changing field. Standard safety precautions must be followed, but as new
research and clinical experience broaden our knowledge, changes in treatment and drug therapy
may become necessary or appropriate. Readers are advised to check the most current product
information provided by the manufacturer of each drug to be administered to verify the
recommended dose, the method and duration of administrations, and contraindications. It is the
responsibility of the treating physician, relying on experience and knowledge of the patient, to
determine dosages and the best treatment for each individual patient. Neither the publisher nor the
authors assume any liability for any injury and/or damage to persons or property arising from this
publication.

British Library Cataloguing in Publication Data
A catalogue record for this book is available from the British Library

Library of Congress Catalog Number
A catalog record for this book is available from the Library of Congress

ISBN: 978-044-453273-2

For information on all Elsevier publications
visit our web site at http://www.elsevierdirect.com

Typeset by Integra Software Services Pvt. Ltd, Pondicherry, India www.integra-india.com
Printed and bound in the USA

08 09 10   10 9 8 7 6 5 4 3 2 1

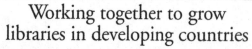

Contents

Contents

Preface

This volume covers the adverse effects of analgesic medicines. The material has been collected from *Meyler's Side Effects of Drugs: The International Encyclopedia of Adverse Drug Reactions and Interactions* (15th edition, 2006, in six volumes), which was itself based on previous editions of *Meyler's Side Effects of Drugs*, and from the *Side Effects of Drugs Annuals* (SEDA) 28, 29, and 30. The main contributors of this material were JK Aronson, PAGM de Smet, E Ernst, and M Pittler.

A brief history of the Meyler series

Leopold Meyler was a physician who was treated for tuberculosis after the end of the Nazi occupation of The Netherlands. According to Professor Wim Lammers, writing a tribute in Volume VIII (1975), Meyler got a fever from para-aminosalicylic acid, but elsewhere Graham Dukes has written, based on information from Meyler's widow, that it was deafness from dihydrostreptomycin; perhaps it was both. Meyler discovered that there was no single text to which medical practitioners could look for information about unwanted effects of drug therapy; Louis Lewin's text "Die Nebenwirkungen der Arzneimittel" ("The Untoward Effects of Drugs") of 1881 had long been out of print (SEDA-27, xxv-xxix). Meyler therefore determined to make such information available and persuaded the Netherlands publishing firm of Van Gorcum to publish a book, in Dutch, entirely devoted to descriptions of the adverse effects that drugs could cause. He went on to agree with the Elsevier Publishing Company, as it was then called, to prepare and issue an English translation. The first edition of 192 pages (*Schadelijke Nevenwerkingen van Geneesmiddelen*) appeared in 1951 and the English version (*Side Effects of Drugs*) a year later.

The book was a great success, and a few years later Meyler started to publish what he called surveys of unwanted effects of drugs. Each survey covered a period of two to four years. They were labelled as volumes rather than editions, and after Volume IV had been published Meyler could no longer handle the task alone. For subsequent volumes he recruited collaborators, such as Andrew Herxheimer. In September 1973 Meyler died unexpectedly, and Elsevier invited Graham Dukes to take over the editing of Volume VIII.

Dukes persuaded Elsevier that the published literature was too large to be comfortably encompassed in a four-yearly cycle, and he suggested that the volumes should be produced annually instead. The four-yearly volume could then concentrate on providing a complementary critical encyclopaedic survey of the entire field. The first *Side Effects of Drugs Annual* was published in 1977. The first encyclopaedic edition of *Meyler's Side Effects of Drugs*, which appeared in 1980, was labelled the ninth edition, and since then a new encyclopaedic edition has appeared every four years. The 15th edition was published in 2006, in both hard and electronic versions.

Monograph structure

The monographs in this volume are arranged in five sections:

- Opioid receptor agonists and antagonists
- Salicylates, paracetamol, and other non-opioid analgesics
- Non-steroidal anti-inflammatory drugs
- Glucocorticoids and disease-modifying antirheumatic drugs
- Drugs used in the treatment of gout

In each monograph in the Meyler series the information is organized into sections as shown below (although not all the sections are covered in each monograph).

Drug names

Drugs have usually been designated by their recommended or proposed International Non-proprietary Names (rINN or pINN); when these are not available, chemical names have been used. In some cases brand names have been used.

Spelling

For indexing purposes, American spelling has been used, e.g. anemia, estrogen rather than anaemia, oestrogen.

Cross-references

The various editions of *Meyler's Side Effects of Drugs* are cited in the text as SED-13, SED-14, etc; the *Side Effects of Drugs Annuals 1–22* are cited as SEDA-1, SEDA-2, etc.

J K Aronson
Oxford May 2008

Organization of material in monographs in the Meyler series (not all sections are included in each monograph)

General information
Drug studies
  Observational studies
  Comparative studies
  Drug-combination studies
  Placebo-controlled studies
  Systematic reviews
Organs and systems
  Cardiovascular
  Respiratory
  Ear, nose, throat
  Nervous system
  Neuromuscular function
  Sensory systems
  Psychological
  Psychiatric
  Endocrine
  Metabolism
  Nutrition
  Electrolyte balance
  Mineral balance
  Metal metabolism
  Acid-base balance
  Fluid balance
  Hematologic
  Mouth
  Teeth
  Salivary glands
  Gastrointestinal
  Liver
  Biliary tract
  Pancreas
  Urinary tract
  Skin
  Hair
  Nails
  Connective tissues
  Sweat glands
  Serosae
  Musculoskeletal
  Sexual function
  Reproductive system
  Breasts
  Immunologic
  Autacoids
  Infection risk
  Body temperature

  Multiorgan failure
  Trauma
  Death
Long-term effects
  Drug abuse
  Drug misuse
  Drug tolerance
  Drug resistance
  Drug dependence
  Drug withdrawal
  Genotoxicity
  Cytotoxicity
  Mutagenicity
  Tumorigenicity
Second-generation effects
  Fertility
  Pregnancy
  Teratogenicity
  Fetotoxicity
  Lactation
  Breast feeding
Susceptibility factors
  Genetic factors
  Age
  Sex
  Physiological factors
  Disease
  Other features of the patient
Drug administration
  Drug formulations
  Drug additives
  Drug contamination and adulteration
  Drug dosage regimens
  Drug administration route
  Drug overdose
Interactions
  Drug-drug interactions
  Food-drug interactions
  Drug-device interactions
  Drug-smoking interactions
  Other environmental interactions
Interference with diagnostic tests
Diagnosis of adverse drug reactions
Management of adverse drug reactions
Monitoring therapy
References

OPIOID RECEPTOR AGONISTS AND ANTAGONISTS

Opioid analgesics (Opioid receptor agonists)

See also individual names

General Information

Receptor nomenclature

Opioid receptors, originally called δ, κ, and μ receptors, then OP$_1$, OP$_2$, and OP$_3$ receptors, are now called DOR, KOR, and MOR receptors respectively

Classes of substances

Opioids are naturally occurring or synthetic substances that have morphine-like activity. The term opiate refers only to substances with morphine-like activity that are derived from opium. Substances that bind to opioid receptors but elicit little agonist activity are known as opioid antagonists. Some drugs have both agonist and antagonist effects (partial agonists). The opioids and their antagonists can be divided into three groups: (a) opioid agonists (morphine and morphine-like opioids); (b) opioid antagonists (for example naloxone and naltrexone); and (c) opioid partial agonists (for example buprenorphine and nalbuphine).

Three separate categories of endogenous substances with morphine-like activity have been identified. These families of neuropeptides are known as enkephalins, endorphins, and dynorphins. Each family is derived from a distinct precursor polypeptide (pro-enkephalin, pro-opiomelanocortin, and prodynorfin) and has a characteristic anatomical distribution. The enkephalins and dynorphins found co-exist with other neurotransmitters, such as serotonin (5-HT) and noradrenaline, but details of how the peptides modulate the activity of co-transmitters await elucidation.

Finally, several molecules with chemical structures similar to morphine have been found in mammalian brain, but it is not certain if these molecules have been derived from dietary sources or if they are synthesized in the brain.

The word narcotic was previously used to describe substances with morphine-like activity and is now largely obsolete, although it is still used in legal parlance.

Opioid receptors

There are three main types of opioid receptor: MOR (OP$_3$, μ), KOR (OP$_2$, κ), and DOR (OP$_1$, δ) receptors. They are mainly found within the central nervous system but also in the periphery. Subtypes of each have been identified. Opioids interact with these receptors to produce their effects, primarily by exerting presynaptic inhibition, which results in reduced release of excitatory transmitters. It is thought that analgesia is primarily mediated via activation of MOR receptors at supraspinal sites and KOR receptors within the spinal cord. The finding that morphine is ineffective as an analgesic

in knock-out mice without μ receptors confirms the importance of this receptor type. However, structural studies in cloned MOR receptors have failed to support pharmacological studies that suggest the existence of separate MOR receptor subtypes that independently mediate analgesia and respiratory depression.

The identification of opioid receptors and the discovery of opioid peptides in the 1970s led to the hope that greater understanding of fundamental mechanisms would lead to the development of new drugs with all the valued properties of known opioids but without their unwanted effects. However, these hopes have remained unrealized, although a synthetic enkephalin (pentapeptide 443C81), which penetrates the blood–brain barrier poorly, produces dose-related analgesia without causing significant miosis or reducing minute volume on rebreathing carbon dioxide in healthy volunteers (SEDA-16, 86).

Understanding of nociceptive processing has progressed in recent years, and the pain mechanisms and opioid effects on various receptors and transmission systems have been elucidated (1–3), as have tolerance and physical dependence and the influence of NMDA receptors (4,5).

The peptides endomorphin 1 and 2 have been identified in human brain and show selectivity and affinity for μ receptors. In mice, endomorphin 1 and 2 produce spinal and supraspinal analgesia. They appear to act through regulation of calcium entry into the target cell via voltage-gated channels and also to inhibit cyclic AMP production in MOR receptor bearing cells. Clinically they mimic the action of other MOR opioids. Their clinical relevance and unique adverse effects profiles await further investigation. Similarly the clinical usefulness of newly discovered receptor systems, such as the orphan opioid receptor for nociceptin (ORL1), which produces analgesia, hyperalgesia, and anti-opioid effects in animals, has yet to be defined.

Differences between individual agents

Morphine remains the gold standard against which all other opioids are compared. Most opioids are used as analgesics, although some are used primarily as antitussives, despite the fact that the cough-suppressing effect of codeine and dextromethorphan has not been demonstrated in children (SEDA-22, 98); others, such as loperamide and diphenoxylate, are used exclusively in the treatment of diarrhea; fentanyl and its congeners are primarily used in anesthesia. Fentanyl, the oldest of the anesthetic opioid agonists, and its derivatives alfentanil and sufentanil, are used either as anesthetic supplements or in appropriate doses as complete anesthetics. Butorphanol and nalbuphine have largely replaced pentazocine in analgesia, because they are less likely to have dysphoric effects and, in contrast to the pure agonists, any respiratory depression that follows their use is not dose-related and reaches a ceiling as the dose increases.

The main characteristics and use of opioid drugs are listed in Table 1. Drugs in widespread clinical use each have a separate monograph.

Table 1 Major characteristics and uses of some opioid drugs

Drug	Typical dose	Route of administration	Half-life (hours)	Usual indication	Main adverse effects
Agonists					
Morphine (active metabolite morphine-6-glucuronide)	10 mg and upwards 3–4 hourly	Oral, subcutaneous, intravenous, intramuscular, intrathecal	2–4	Severe pain, anesthesia	Sedation, constipation, nausea, vomiting, itching, respiratory depression, tolerance and dependence, euphoria
Alfentanil	30–50 µg/kg	Epidural, intravenous	1.6–4	Analgesia, anesthesia	As morphine
Codeine (metabolized to morphine by CYP2D6)	30–60 µg 4-hourly	Oral	3–4	Cough, diarrhea, moderate pain	As morphine; lack of effect in poor metabolizers by CYP2D6
Dextromethorphan	10–30 mg 4–8 hourly	Oral	2.7–3.3	Dry cough	
Dextropropoxyphene(active metabolite norpropoxyphene)	65 mg 6–8 hourly	Oral	6–32 (norpropoxyphene 24–42)	Moderate pain	As morphine; cardiotoxicity, not reversible by naloxone; convulsions possible, due to norpropoxyphene
Fentanyl	50–200 µg	Epidural, intravenous, transdermal patch	2–7	Acute pain, anesthesia	As morphine
Methadone	10 mg 6–8 hourly; 30–80 mg/day	Oral, intravenous, intramuscular	15–60	Severe pain; opioid dependence	As morphine
Pethidine (meperidine)	50–150 mg 3-hourly	Oral, intramuscular	3.2	Moderate/severe pain	As morphine; excitement and convulsions
Sufentanil	Up to 8 µg/kg	Epidural, intravenous	2.7–6	Severe pain, anesthesia	As morphine
Partial agonists					
Buprenorphine	300–600 µg 6–8 hourly; 2–32 µg	Sublingual, intravenous Sublingual	5–12	Moderate/severe pain Opioid dependence	As morphine, but less pronounced; less well reversed by naloxone
Pentazocine	30–60 mg 3–4 hourly	Oral, intravenous, intramuscular	2–4	Acute pain	As morphine; dysphoria
Antagonists					
Naloxone	1.5–3 µg/kg repeated according to response	Intravenous	1.1	Reversal of opioid-induced respiratory depression	Nausea, vomiting, hypertension, cardiac dysrhythmias, rarely seizures
Nalmefene	0.25 µg/kg repeated according to response	Intravenous	10	Reversal of opioid-induced respiratory depression	Nausea, vomiting, tachycardia, hypertension, fever, dizziness
Naltrexone	25–50 mg/day	Oral	2.7	Adjunct to prevent relapse in formerly opioid-dependent patients	Nausea, vomiting, abdominal pain, dysphoria, joint and muscle pains, dizziness

The use of opioid drugs is continuing to increase, mainly because of the development of alternative routes of administration and increasing use in the very young. Pharmacological maneuvres have been made in order to improve analgesic potency and reduce adverse effects. Benzodiazepines have been used to improve analgesic effects (SEDA-17, 78), and methylphenidate has been given to patients in order to reduce drowsiness (SEDA-17, 78). Combinations of opioids with non-steroidal anti-inflammatory drugs have been used to provide analgesia postoperatively, with the aim of reducing the amounts of opioid required, with consequent reduction in adverse effects (SEDA-18, 79).

The more novel routes of administration of opioids, including oral, nasal, rectal, transdermal, spinal, and by patient-controlled methods, have been outlined (SEDA-17, 78). Oral transmucosal fentanyl administration, avoiding first-pass metabolism, produces analgesia and sedation in both adults and children undergoing short, painful outpatient procedures. The quality of analgesia is good, and the adverse effects are those typical of the opioids.

Degrees of risk

When the opioids are used correctly, their adverse effects are usually minimal. However, when they are used illicitly, they are often adulterated with other substances, which can cause adverse effects.

A strategy for controlling pain caused by malignant disease has been outlined and the classic effects that can be associated with opioid administration have been reviewed (6). These include constipation, nausea, sedation, pruritus, urinary retention, myoclonus, and respiratory depression. The latter can be life-threatening. Particular care is needed in opioid-naive individuals, those with compromised respiratory function, and elderly patients.

The use of opioids in very young patients is increasing. In a review of pain management in children, various routes of administration of opioids and their associated adverse effects have been discussed (SEDA-17, 78). Attention has been drawn to the adverse effects of intravenous codeine in children and to the risk of convulsions with pethidine in neonates, because of accumulation of its metabolite norpethidine. The risk of respiratory depression with morphine was also highlighted, and morphine is recommended for use only in neonates who are being ventilated or intensively nursed. Routine use of pulse oximetry has been recommended in all children receiving opioids (SEDA-21, 86).

The use of patient-controlled analgesia (PCA) (SEDA-15, 68) highlights the importance of adequate monitoring, in order to avoid potentially catastrophic adverse effects, such as respiratory depression. With PCA, patients generally use less morphine but still achieve the same degree of pain control (7). This supports the view that self-administration of opioids does not put patients at risk of over-medication or drug dependence.

It has been suggested that the risk of producing opioid dependence in the medical setting is greater in those who prescribe and administer them than in those who receive them (8). The likelihood of dependence in patients treated with opioids has been examined. In the treatment of cancer pain, tolerance and physical dependence occur but psychological dependence (addiction) is rare (9,10). In 11 882 patients who had received at least one opioid, addiction was reasonably well documented only in four (11).

Of 130 patients with chronic malignant and chronic benign pain attending a pain relief unit over 3 years, 9 (18%) were considered to be addicted to analgesics on subjective evaluation (12). Of 71 patients with chronic pain referred to a pain relief center, 86% were taking analgesics, 58% opioids, and 68% psychotropic agents; 49% of those taking opioids were considered to be dependent (13).

These studies emphasize the need to define the meaning of terms such as addiction and dependence correctly and to distinguish between psychological and physical dependence. Failure to do so could lead to unwitting deprivation of opioids in patients for whom they provide undisputed benefit with minimal harm. These results also suggest that patients receiving opioids for less well-defined pain conditions, quite often for longer periods and sometimes along with other drugs with abuse potential, may be at special risk of dependence and abuse. Thus, withdrawal may be important, but may become extremely difficult. The adverse effects encountered during long-term opioid therapy have been reviewed, as well as the evidence that opioids can cause seizures or seizure-like activity (SEDA-22, 97).

Opioid therapy and chronic non-cancer pain has been reviewed by the Canadian Pain Society in a consensus document that states that there is no recorded risk in the medical literature of direct permanent organ damage (including cognitive and psychomotor deficits) due to the appropriate therapeutic use of opioids and that problems are more often due to concurrent use of sedatives, such as benzodiazepines (14,15). Respiratory depression caused by opioid analgesics occurs largely in opioid-naïve patients and is short-lived. Constipation is a common initial adverse effect and is usually more difficult to treat than to prevent. It is therefore important to manage constipation prophylactically, using a stepped approach involving adequate dietary fiber, stool softeners, osmotic agents, and if necessary intermittent stimulant laxatives. Nausea is also a common adverse effect and usually resolves with continued use within days. Patients with a history of addiction should not necessarily be denied a trial of opioid therapy but will require more careful prescribing, closer follow up, and joint clinics between chronic pain and addiction specialists (16,17).

Finally, it must be borne in mind that some of the problems with opioids are treatable: for example, naloxone can reverse respiratory depression, but care must be taken in opioid-dependent individuals, as it may precipitate opioid withdrawal.

General adverse effects

Opioid agonists

Although opioids share many adverse effects, in some respects they are qualitatively and quantitatively different. They all cause constipation by reducing gastrointestinal motility. Respiratory depression, cough suppression, nausea, vomiting, and urinary retention also occur. With the exception of constipation, tolerance to these effects develops. Physical and psychological dependence is also possible. Interaction with monoamine oxidase inhibitors leads to central nervous excitation and hypertension. Hypersusceptibility reactions are rare, although anaphylactic reactions have occurred after intravenous use and skin phenomena can occur. Tumor-inducing effects have not been described in man, but in vitro experiments have suggested a mutagenic effect of papaveretum in mammalian cell lines apparently related to the noscapine content.

The role of opioids in chronic non-malignant pain has been reviewed (18,19), and reports of randomized, double-blind, controlled studies of opioids in chronic non-malignant pain have been identified (19). Opioids appear to be more effective in patients with well-defined nociceptive pain (that is pain associated with clear evidence of tissue damage) than in patients with chronic non-malignant pain of neuropathic origin (i.e. pain associated with injury, disease, or section of the peripheral or central nervous system in the absence of tissue damage) or psychogenic causes (no organic pathology present). Gastrointestinal and CNS adverse effects (sedation, dizziness, cognitive impairment, respiratory depression, myoclonus) were frequent and distressing in most of the studies.

Clinical observations suggest that patients often find adverse effects, particularly nausea and vomiting, more distressing than the postoperative pain for which they are prescribed. Some are even willing to endure pain rather than suffer unpleasant adverse effects. This important aspect of opioid-induced analgesia has been investigated in a randomized, double blind, three-way, crossover study of between- and within-patient variability in response to equianalgesic doses of morphine, pethidine, and fentanyl during postoperative PCA (20). In 82 patients undergoing a variety of surgical procedures, the three opioids were equally efficacious from objective measurements in relieving pain and the subsequent incidence and intensity of adverse effects. However, the responses to the three opioids were highly individual, and there were three types of response. One group of patients tolerated all three opioids, another tolerated none, and a third group was sensitive to one or more of the opioids with no preference for any of the opioids used. The authors suggested that it would be good clinical practice to change from one opioid to another in patients who have intolerable adverse effects during PCA, since there is wide variation in subjective interpretation of pain and adverse effects.

Limitations to the use of opioids in cardiac surgery have been reviewed, highlighting the fact that μ receptor agonists cause dose-related respiratory depression through a reduction in carbon dioxide sensitivity in the respiratory centre (21). This depression, with a reduced respiratory rate and hypoxia, outlasts the analgesic effect of μ receptor agonists. Thoracic muscle rigidity on anesthetic induction with high doses of opioids has also been reported and can further compromise respiration. Hypotension through reduced peripheral vascular resistance occurs, while a negative inotropic effect of opioids acting directly on the heart via κ receptors is proposed, based on evidence from in vitro studies. The above effects have limited the role of opiates in patients with coronary artery disease, although they are of less importance in cardiopulmonary bypass surgery, when the heart is quiescent. In such surgery fentanyl partially blocks the expected tachycardia, hypertension, and release of inflammatory mediators that constitute the stress response, although the block is incomplete, owing to a lack of anesthetic effect.

Opioid partial agonists
There is evidence that in the case of partial opioid agonists, such as buprenorphine, the relative clinical activity of agonist and antagonist actions can differ, depending, among other things, on the dose.

The prevention of opioid-induced adverse effects
Prevention of sedation
The use and possible mechanism of amphetamines to counteract opioid-induced sedation has been reviewed (22). Most studies had methodological problems, including small numbers of patients completing short-term trials (under 1 week) and the small number of randomized, placebo-controlled, crossover trials. The quantitative measure of sedation was highly subjective and no uniform cognitive tests were performed to help compare the results of using amphetamines to reduce opioid-induced sedation. The overall conclusion was that more research is needed to determine the exact role of amphetamines. The use of amphetamine and amphetamine derivatives for the treatment of opioid-induced sedation is not recommended.

Prevention of emesis
Another excellent review has focused on the use of prophylactic antiemetics during PCA (23). A systematic search for relevant randomized controlled trails identified 14 studies involving 1117 adults published between 1992 and 1998. Without antiemetic drugs the incidence of opioid-induced nausea was on average 48% and of vomiting 55%, with a 67% chance of having an emetic episode. The most frequently studied antiemetic was droperidol, which was added to morphine PCA in six placebo-controlled trials in 642 adults and to tramadol in another trial. A wide range of doses of droperidol was used, with a constant degree of antiemetic efficacy. Based on this review, the optimal dose of droperidol is said to be less than 0.1 mg of droperidol per mg of morphine or less than 4 mg/day of droperidol. There were few adverse reactions: 56 in 10 000 patients had extrapyramidal adverse effects when droperidol was added to morphine PCA.

The next most frequently used drugs in the prevention of opioid-induced emesis are the 5-HT$_3$ receptor antagonists (ondansetron and tropisetron). There is no evidence that they prevent nausea, but the effect on vomiting is satisfactory enough for them to be regarded as second-line choices after droperidol. However, in 109 patients undergoing day-case oral surgery there was a higher incidence of nausea with tramadol plus ondansetron compared with three other treatments (fentanyl plus metoclopramide, tramadol plus metoclopramide, and fentanyl plus ondansetron) (24). There was no difference between the groups in analgesic efficacy.

Other prophylactic antiemetic agents include clonidine, promethazine, hyoscine, propofol, and metoclopramide. However, the data on these drugs are either insufficient or non-existent.

In a randomized, double-blind, placebo-controlled study of 80 patients who required epidural morphine after abdominal hysterectomy, 40 received intravenous dexamethasone (8 mg) (25). The incidence of vomiting with dexamethasone group was 5% compared with 25% with placebo; the total incidence of nausea and vomiting was 16% compared with 56%.

Prevention of pruritus

The incidence of opioid-induced pruritus varies widely, and depends on the opioid used and its mode of administration. The highest incidence (up to 80%) is associated with intrathecal morphine. The pruritus is usually localized to the area of the face that is innervated by the trigeminal nerve. A central encephalinergic mechanism has been proposed to explain this localization. The pruritus is often difficult to treat and responds poorly to conventional treatments, except for naloxone and propofol; 10–15% remain unresponsive. Naloxone reversibility of opioid-induced pruritus supports the existence of an opioid-medicated central mechanism. However, naloxone will reverse the analgesic effects of the opioids.

Three studies have suggested the use of ondansetron, a 5-HT$_3$ receptor antagonist, for the treatment of opioid-induced pruritus (26–28). The articles suggested a possible interaction between the opioid and the serotonergic systems. In one prospective, randomized, double-blind, placebo-controlled study, 80 patients undergoing any type of surgery were given intravenous ondansetron 4 mg or 0.9% saline over 1 minute, with alfentanil as the opioid used in the anesthetic technique (26). The study was inconclusive; there was a significant reduction in the incidence of scratching in patients who received ondansetron compared with placebo but a non-significant incidence of itching in the ondansetron group.

In a prospective randomized, double-blind, placebo-controlled study in 100 patients scheduled for elective orthopedic surgery and presenting with pruritus induced by epidural or intrathecal morphine, intravenous ondansetron 8 mg was effective in 70% of cases and placebo in 30% (27). Ondansetron was well tolerated, did not change the degree of analgesia, and was not associated with adverse effects usually associated with ondansetron, such as headache, abdominal pain, and cardiac dysrhythmias.

In a double-blind randomized study of 130 patients given subarachnoid bupivacaine 0.5% with morphine 0.3 mg for surgical and postoperative analgesia, repeated-dose and single-dose ondansetron were compared (28). The overall incidence of pruritus was 73% in the group not given ondansetron, 63% in those who received intravenous ondansetron 4 mg 20 minutes before the spinal analgesia and 2 ml of saline at 12, 24, 26, and 48 hours after surgery, and only 49% in those who received

ondansetron 4 mg 20 minutes before the spinal and 12, 24, 36, and 48 hours after surgery. There were methodological problems—the small number of subjects studied and the lack of an objective scoring system—but these results add to the current discussion of pursuing further studies to determine the effective dose of ondansetron in the treatment of opioid-induced pruritus. Further neurobiological research is needed to determine a "human" model of explaining the role and interactions of the central serotonergic system with the opioid system.

In a prospective, randomized, controlled study, 90 women with moderate to severe pruritus due to intrathecal morphine after cesarean section were given intravenous nalbuphine 2 mg, 3 mg, or 4 mg (29). Nalbuphine 2–3 mg relieved morphine-induced pruritus without increasing pain scores or causing other adverse effects.

Observational studies

Drug-related emergency department visits have been studied in a district hospital in Finland (30). Adverse drug reactions were responsible for 2.3% (n = 167) of all visits over a 6-month period; 102 visits were related to adverse drug reactions without intentional overdoses, and 65 were related to overdose. Opioids were responsible for only four adverse drug reactions; three patients complained of nausea and one of constipation. The opioids involved were fentanyl, oxycodone and tramadol. Two of these patients required admission to hospital.

Systematic reviews

The administration of opioids has been compared with continuous peripheral nerve block for pain control (31). Peripheral nerve catheter analgesia resulted in superior pain control and was associated with fewer adverse effects. Peripheral nerve block was associated with motor block, whereas nausea, vomiting, pruritus, and sedation were associated with opioid administration.

Organs and Systems

Cardiovascular

Orthostatic hypotension can occur and is common after intravenous administration. Histamine release sometimes contributes to this.

Respiratory

Opioids cause respiratory depression by virtue of a direct effect on brain-stem respiratory centers (32). The nadir depends on the route of administration, and occurs at about 7 minutes after intravenous opioids, but not until about 30 minutes after intramuscular and 90 minutes after subcutaneous injection. The mechanisms of the respiratory effects of opioids (with special reference to their postoperative use) have been reviewed (SEDA-20, 76) (SEDA-21, 85). Pulmonary granulomatosis has occurred (33), and asthma after opioid inhalation has been described (34).

Nervous system

Opioids produce analgesia without loss of consciousness, although drowsiness, changes in mood, and mental clouding occur. Responses to painful stimuli are blocked at several locations in the brain, resulting in both an alteration in the sensation of pain and a change in the affective response. The ability of a patient to perceive pain can remain the same while tolerance to pain is markedly increased (35).

Opioids cause nausea and vomiting by stimulating the chemoreceptor trigger zone in the medulla, although tolerance to this effect usually develops within a few days (36).

Patients using chronic opioids tend to have more pain when attempts are made at managing pain by giving larger doses, and pain is probably best managed by withdrawing the opioid medication. In one study higher degrees of pain were experienced with high potency bolus release medications, such as oxycodone modified-release, than with less potent immediate-release medications, such as hydrocodone (37). On the other hand, a study of opiate addicts undergoing detoxification with methadone and/or heroin provided evidence of hyperalgesia (38). Patients and controls were subjected to a cold pressor test and reactions were monitored. Reactions were suggestive of hyperalgesia; however, they also indicated increased pain latency and reduced pain intensity. These phenomena are contradictory and require further research.

Morphine and most opioids cause pupillary constriction, which may be due to an excitatory action on the autonomic segment of the nucleus of the oculomotor nerve. Tolerance to this miotic effect is not usual.

Single therapeutic doses of opioids produce a shift toward increased voltage and lower frequencies in the encephalogram, such as occurs in natural sleep or after very low doses of barbiturates. High doses of morphine can cause sleep disturbances in some children (SEDA-17, 78).

Fentanyl and sufentanil can cause epileptiform activity in patients undergoing coronary artery bypass grafting (SEDA-18, 79).

Catatonia is a rare complication of prolonged epidural opioid administration in cancer pain (SEDA-16, 78). Patients with advanced cancer who were taking opioids had significant but transient cognitive impairment when opioid doses were increased (39). This correlates well with studies of the effects of psychotropic medications on ability to drive (40).

Opioids and hypnotic drugs are often used to prevent increased intracranial pressure and the subsequent reduction in cerebral perfusion pressure. However, it is still uncertain whether opioids can cause increased intracranial pressure. The effects of a bolus injection and infusion of sufentanil, alfentanil, and fentanyl on cerebral hemodynamics and electroencephalographic activity have been studied in a randomized crossover study in six patients with increased intracranial pressure after severe head trauma (41). All three infusions were associated with a significant increase in intracranial pressure (9, 8, and 5.5 mmHg respectively) 3–5 minutes after the bolus opioid injection. Intracranial pressure gradually fell and returned to baseline after 15 minutes. This increase was associated with significant falls in mean arterial pressure and cerebral perfusion pressure throughout the study period. The electroencephalogram changed from a fast to a reduced activity pattern, with an improvement in background activity. It is therefore advisable to avoid using bolus injections of opioids in patients with head injury and to use continuous infusion for sedation.

Psychological

The neuropsychiatric syndrome that results from opioid toxicity consists of cognitive impairment, severe sedation, hallucinations, myoclonic seizures, and hyperalgesia (42). Opioid-induced neurotoxicity is most often seen in patients receiving high doses of opioids for prolonged periods, often in association with psychoactive medications (for example benzodiazepines and tricyclic antidepressants), and in older patients with associated dehydration and renal insufficiency. Strategies for reducing the occurrence of opioid-induced neurotoxicity primarily include opioid rotation and dosage reduction and circadian modulation techniques. Drugs such as amphetamines, amphetamine-like derivatives, and neuroleptic drugs like haloperidol can be used to treat hallucinations and delirium as a result of opioid-induced neurotoxicity and when the minimal dose of opioid that can cause sufficient analgesia also causes excess sedation. Proper assessment of the potential risk factors of opioid-induced neurotoxicity with careful monitoring of early signs is the fundamental principle in prevention.

Delirium and cognitive impairment are common postoperative adverse events, especially in elderly patients. Susceptibility factors and intraoperative and postoperative factors influence the development of postoperative delirium and/or cognitive impairment and are associated with poor functional recovery and increased morbidity. A systematic review including clinical trials and observational studies explored the use of opioids postoperatively in elderly patients and the risk of development of postoperative cognitive impairment and/or delirium (43). Opioids more commonly used postoperatively include morphine, fentanyl, and hydromorphone. When comparing the postoperative use of these opioids with postoperative pethidine, the latter was significantly associated with an increased risk of delirium or cognitive impairment. These studies did not provide sufficient evidence to establish whether there were any differences in the risks of morphine, fentanyl, or hydromorphone. The authors also explored whether the route of administration of opioids made a contribution to the risk of cognitive impairment; there was no significant difference between epidural and parenteral analgesia. They recognized that delirium and/or cognitive impairment are common adverse events that affect morbidity and postoperative recovery, the limitations of the papers reviewed (e.g. small sample sizes and non-standardized measurement of cognitive impairment), and recommended future studies of both the and postoperative cognitive impairment in patients given postoperative opioids.

In another study postoperative cognitive function was assessed after patient controlled analgesia in 30 patients undergoing lower abdominal surgery, who received either fentanyl (n = 17) or tramadol (n = 13) intraoperatively and postoperatively (44). Cognitive function was assessed on days 1 and 2 using the Mini Mental State Examination and the Benton Visual Retention Test. Although the patients in the two groups had similar cognitive abilities, those who received tramadol were motivated to accomplish cognitively demanding tasks.

Dependent drug users, current and former, have impairment of executive and memory function. Executive and memory function has been explored in 25 chronic amphetamine users and 42 chronic opiate users (45). Compared with controls, drug users had impairment of spatial planning, paired associate learning, and visual pattern recognition. Amphetamine users had greater impairment of spatial planning, pattern recognition memory, and attentional set-shifting.

Endocrine

Morphine reduces the response of the hypothalamus to afferent stimulation (46). In many species, opioids alter the equilibrium point of the hypothalamic heat-regulatory mechanisms.

In patients undergoing surgery, opioids inhibit the stress-induced release of ACTH (47).

Secretion of luteinizing hormone (LH) and thyrotropin is suppressed by opioids, whereas the release of prolactin and, in some cases, growth hormone is enhanced (48).

Gastrointestinal

Opioids reduce the secretion of hydrochloric acid and have a marked effect on gastrointestinal motility. Gastric emptying is prolonged and the likelihood of esophageal reflux is increased (49). Tone in the antral part of the stomach and first part of the duodenum is increased. The passage of gastric contents through the duodenum can be delayed by as much as 12 hours, retarding the absorption of orally administered drugs (50). In 260 patients with malignant disease, 23–40% vomited and 8–10% felt nauseated (SEDA-17, 79). Transdermal hyoscine (scopolamine) can reduce these problems (SEDA-17, 79).

Biliary and pancreatic and intestinal secretions are reduced by morphine, and digestion in the small intestine is delayed.

Opioid-induced gastrointestinal dysfunction contributes to patient dissatisfaction and affects quality of life. The pathophysiological mechanisms underlying gastrointestinal dysfunction following opioid use have been reviewed (51). Nausea and vomiting, experienced by a large number of patients who take opioids, are believed to be triggered by both peripheral and central mechanisms. Constipation, experienced by 40–50% of patients, is induced by doses of opioids lower than the doses required for analgesia.

The tone of the anal sphincter is increased and the usual reflex relaxation response to rectal distension is reduced.

Tolerance to constipation does not tend to develop. The authors suggested several options to reduce the incidence of constipation: e.g. administering newer opioid compounds (such as dihydroetorphine hydrochloride); using the transdermal route; opioid-sparing through adjunctive treatment.

Another gastrointestinal effect is ileus, with several potential underlying pathophysiological mechanisms (52).

- A woman on chronic narcotics (oxycodone 5 mg, 2–3 times per week) underwent colonoscopy, during which she was given midazolam 7 mg, pethidine 100 mg, and fentanyl 125 micrograms. She later developed acute colonic pseudo-obstruction necessitating hospital admission.

Ileus is postulated to result from motor inhibition of the gastrointestinal tract by narcotics.

Biliary tract

Therapeutic doses of opioids constrict the sphincter of Oddi, and biliary tract pressure rises ten-fold. Patients with biliary colic can have exacerbation of pain after morphine. Likewise, opioids such as fentanyl, morphine, and dextropropoxyphene can cause bile duct spasm (SEDA-21, 85).

"It is standard teaching that morphine should not be used to treat patients with pancreatitis because it causes a rise in biliary and pancreatic pressure" (53). From this starting point, this comprehensive review discusses current approaches to opioid analgesia in pancreatitis, pointing out that morphine has been reported to cause biliary colic in individuals without biliary tract disease and that pethidine (meperidine) has become the analgesic of choice. Constriction of the sphincter of Oddi and the basal tone of the sphincter and the frequency of phasic contractions have been measured using endoscopic retrograde cholangiopancreatography (ERCP); an increase in basal tone is believed to be the best indication of sphincter dysfunction. Morphine sulfate in intravenous doses of 2.5–5 micrograms/kg caused increased contractions but no change in basal pressure, while doses of 10 micrograms/kg and over caused a rise in basal pressure. Pethidine increased contractions but not basal tone, while tramadol had no effect on basal pressure in a small study. Among mixed opiate agonist/antagonists, pentazocine increased basal pressure. Buprenorphine, a partial opiate agonist, resulted in no pressure changes, while the antagonist naloxone 0.4 mg intravenously had no effect alone on the sphincter basal pressure and did not stop the increase in pressure caused by morphine. However, case reports have suggested that naloxone reduces sphincter spasm in clinical situations.

Urinary tract

The urinary voiding reflex is inhibited by opioids, and both the tone of the external sphincter and the volume of the bladder increase; urinary retention is therefore common.

Skin

Flushing of the face, neck, and upper thorax can follow therapeutic doses of opioids. These effects may be partly due to release of histamine, which is also implicated in the sweating and pruritus seen after opioid administration. Opioid effects on neurons may partly be involved in the pruritus, as pruritus is provoked by opioids that do not release histamine and is abolished by small doses of naloxone.

Urticaria at the site of injection is due to histamine release. It is seen with pethidine and morphine, but not with oxymorphone, methadone, fentanyl, or sufentanil. Wheal and flare responses to various opioids differ (54).

Musculoskeletal

Opioid use results in reduced bone mineral density, probably mediated by suppression of endogenous production of sex hormones. In a large sample of the US population opioid users had a reduced bone mineral density compared with non-users, when adjusting for all co-variates (55). This effect was more evident in long-term users. Owing to lack of data on testosterone and estradiol, the investigators could not prove causality.

A report of bilateral femoral neck stress fractures in a heroin addict has highlighted the importance of early identification of osteopenia (56).

A nationwide case-control study in Denmark established that opiates were associated with an increased risk of fractures (57). The study included all individuals who had sustained a fracture in the year 2000 (n = 124 655). For each case, three controls matched for age and sex were randomly drawn from the general population. A number of opioids (morphine, methadone, fentanyl, ketobemidone, nicomorphine, oxycodone, codeine, and tramadol) were associated with an increased risk of fractures. However, dextropropoxyphene, pethidine, acetylsalicylic acid + codeine combination, and buprenorphine were not associated with an increased risk. With most of the opioids mentioned there was an increased risk at all doses. Fentanyl increased the risk at higher doses, while nicomorphine and ketobemidone increased the risk at lower doses. The increased fracture risk, even at lower doses and even when the opioids had only been taken for a short time, suggested that the most probable underlying primary reason for fractures was falls due to the central nervous system effects of the opioids, as opposed to weakening of the bone structure. The use of alcohol was a significant risk factor in all cases. Although the study had significant limitations and potential confounding factors, the large numbers made the results more reliable.

Sexual function

Although long-term administration of low-dose opioids, especially intrathecally, improves quality of life through improved pain control, it can compromise it by causing impaired sexual function. Low testosterone concentrations have been reported in heroin addicts (58) and subjects in a methadone maintenance program (59).

In prospective non-randomized non-blinded evaluation of the effects of a 12-week course of intrathecal opioids for the control of chronic non-cancer pain on the hypothalamic–pituitary–gonadal axis in 12 men, it was suppressed and serum testosterone concentrations fell (60). This effect not only reduces quality of life through sexual dysfunction but can also increase the risk of spinal osteoporosis in men, with an increased risk of vertebral and hip fractures. Patients receiving long-term intrathecal opioid therapy need to be informed of potential hypothalamic–pituitary–gonadal axis suppression as a result of the treatment, and testosterone replacement after hypothalamic–pituitary–gonadal axis surveillance during treatment should be considered if indicated.

Immunologic

The immunosuppressive effects of morphine, tramadol, and the combination of tramadol + lornoxicam for pain management after elective gastric cancer surgery (n = 45) have been compared (61). Immunosuppression was measured by observing expressions of T lymphocyte subsets, natural-killer cells, and activated T lymphocytes. The combination of tramadol + lornoxicam provided equivalent analgesia but caused less immunosuppression than morphine or tramadol alone.

Infection risk

The immunomodulatory effects of opioids contribute to altered immune responses to injury. In a case-control study patients with burns who developed infections were more likely to be taking high doses of opioids (62). Both burns and opioids induce immunosuppression, and the authors suggested that they act synergistically, increasing the risk of infection, especially in mild to moderate injuries. In those with large burns, opioids had no effect, possibly because of maximal immunosuppression by the burns.

Death

Opiates are widely used all over the world, but recently concerns about opiate use (and deaths from such use) have increased in Australia and the UK (63). The rate of opiate overdose deaths in these countries increased dramatically between 1985 and 1995. Throughout that period, it was four to ten times higher in Australia than the UK, but the rate of increase may have been greater in the UK in the latter half of the period, since the difference in rate narrowed substantially during that time. Methadone maintenance treatment, established in Australia in 1969 and in the UK in 1970, has become the main treatment for opiate dependence in both countries. About half of the opiate deaths in the UK were attributed at least in part to methadone. By contrast, considerably fewer (18%) opiate overdose deaths in Australia were attributed to methadone. The authors suggested that the discrepancy in the rates between the two countries could be artefacts of the differences in (a) the documentation of these deaths, (b) the rate of opiate dependence, (c) the route of opiate administration, (d) opiate purity, and, most importantly, (e) the method of delivery of methadone maintenance treatment.

Methadone-related fatalities have been reported from all countries in which methadone has been used for either detoxification or maintenance treatment of opiate users. These fatalities are often defined as cases of poisoning due to methadone or as polydrug intoxication with methadone as the leading cause of death. Methadone maintenance treatment was introduced in Germany in 1989, and 1396 drug-related deaths were reported from 1990 to 1999 in Hamburg (64). While the absolute numbers of drug-related deaths by poisoning did not change over this period, the rise in methadone-associated deaths paralleled a fall in the number of heroin-associated deaths. From 1990 to 1998, the rate of monovalent heroin intoxication in cases of poisoning fell from 60% to 11%, while the rate of polydrug intoxication increased. Poisoning caused by methadone combined with other substances first gained significance 4 years after methadone maintenance treatment was introduced in Hamburg. Since 1994, methadone-related deaths have increased steadily, and by 1997–1998 the numbers had increased exponentially. In the first 6 months of 1999, 60% of all cases of poisoning among drug addicts showed the presence of methadone. When strict guidelines for describing such poisonings were used, 39 poisonings in 1998 (40%) were predominantly caused by methadone, six of them being monovalent methadone intoxication. About two-thirds of all methadone-related poisonings concerned drug addicts who never stayed in methadone maintenance treatment, implying that they obtained methadone from outside of regular treatment. Almost 10 years after the introduction of methadone maintenance treatment in Hamburg, methadone replaced heroin as the leading cause of death due to poisoning. At the same time, however, the absolute number of drug-related deaths and poisonings fell slightly. While methadone maintenance treatment has clearly reduced overall morbidity and mortality in addicts globally, some issues remain unresolved. There are significant differences in the delivery of methadone maintenance treatment from one country to another. The authors reported that in some patients the starting doses of methadone are quite high and potentially lethal. This is especially so when the patients are also using other drugs and attempting to wean off them. Thus, continued polydrug use in treatment is an important risk factor for mortality. Many patients receive take-home doses for a week at a time. While this is useful in a select group of patients, it is not useful in those who sell methadone to buy heroin and combine the two drugs without knowledge of their half-lives and potential complications. The authors suggested changes in methadone maintenance treatment policy, in order to reduce the chances of accidental overdose/poisoning. Specifically, they recommended: a substantial improvement in quality assurance; a more restrictive methadone take-home policy (at least for patients with evidence for concomitant opiate use); and evaluating heroin or long-acting acetylmethadol as alternatives.

Another report from Australia reviewed all the accidental illicit drug deaths that occurred in the Sydney area in 1995–1997 (65). There were 3559 autopsies, of which 4% were considered accidental illicit drug deaths; of these deaths, 121 were men and 22 were women. While the highest number of male deaths occurred in the 25–35 year age group, female deaths were evenly spread from ages 20–35. Almost half (49%) of the deaths occurred from morphine poisoning, 27% from multiple drug toxicity, and 21% from heroin toxicity combined with alcohol. Methadone was detected in 19 cases (13%); 12 of these people were enrolled in a methadone maintenance program. Methadone intoxication alone was responsible for two deaths (1%) only. Methadone was present in the blood in a potentially fatal concentration in 13 cases, while 113 people (80%) had a heroin concentration in the fatal range and 91% had detectable concentrations of heroin. There were no significant neurological findings in the 143 cases studied. More than 50% of those with methadone detected also had heroin in their blood. Unfortunately, this appears to show that some people who participate in a methadone program may still die from accidental heroin overdose. Thus, the authors emphasized the importance of education of heroin users about the risk of accidental overdose.

There is excess mortality in heroin users compared with the general population. The prevalence and experience of heroin overdose in drug users in a general practice in Ireland were examined during 5 months (66). Of the 33 patients identified, 24 agreed to participate. They had had their first overdose on average 5 years after starting to use heroin. Ten had taken an overdose themselves, 23 had witnessed an overdose, 22 knew a victim of fatal overdose, and 4 had been present at a fatal overdose. However, they reported poor understanding of how to deal with an overdose. Despite maintenance treatment with methadone, a significant proportion continued to inject heroin; 17% admitted to the use of illicit methadone, but methadone was not implicated in overdose in any case. The authors suggested that overdose prevention and management should become a priority for general practitioners who care for opiate-dependent patients. Factors implicated in overdose include too high a dose, use after a period of abstinence, and mixing with other drugs.

Clostridium novyi type A, a bacterium that was associated with serious infection during the two World Wars, killed 35 injecting heroin users in Britain and Ireland (67). *Clostridium novyi* type A is present in soil and dust and is a well-recognized cause of infection in sheep, cattle, and other animals. Contaminated batches of heroin from a common source were believed to be responsible for the recent outbreak. The bacteria were able to survive the process of preparation for injection. All recent cases occurred after intramuscular injection, which provides the requisite anerobic conditions for infection. This was the first time that this organism caused an outbreak of infection in drug injectors. In all, 74 cases with the same clinical features were reported.

An increase in the number of deaths of all body packers in New York has been associated with an increase in deaths among opiate body packers: of 50 deaths among body packers from 1990 to 2001, 42 were due to opiates (68). Four were related to cocaine and four to both opiates and cocaine. In 37 cases, open or leaking drug packets in the gastrointestinal tract resulted in acute intoxication and death. Five cases involved intestinal obstruction or perforation, one a gunshot wound, one an intracerebral hemorrhage due to hypertensive disease, and one was undetermined. The number of packets recovered was 1–111 (average 46).

An unbound morphine blood concentration of 100 ng/ml or more is considered potentially fatal. However, fatal cases of heroin intoxication occur in patients with blood morphine concentrations below 100 ng/ml. In 62 cases of heroin intoxication, death was associated with unbound morphine heart blood concentrations below 100 ng/ml in 21 cases and 100 ng/ml or over in 41 cases (69). In the 21 with low concentrations, respiratory tract infections occurred more often, and plausible causes of death were identified in 19.

Unintentional fatal poisoning in the USA increased by 18% per year from 1990 to 2002, and the majority were attributed to 'narcotics' and 'unspecified drugs' (70). From 1999 to 2002 opioid analgesic poisoning increased by 91% and heroin poisoning increased by 12%, making licit drugs the most common cause of fatal drug poisoning in the USA, replacing illicit drugs. Of the opioid analgesic fatalities 54% were from semisynthetic opioids (e.g. oxycodone and hydrocodone), 32% from methadone, and 13% from other synthetic opioids (for example fentanyl). This increase in fatalities has coincided with a change in prescribing practices amongst physicians. Since 1990, they have increased prescribing of opioids for pain management. This epidemiological study has suggested that the increase in prescribing may have contributed to the increase in opioid-related deaths.

In an epidemiological study in the USA the trends in opioid-related deaths in 1990–2003 were analysed (71). Fatalities increased by 529%, from 1.4 per 100 000 in 1990 to 8.8 per 100 000 in 2003, among both sexes, all age groups, and all racial/ethnic groups. These trends in Massachusetts are consistent with trends of opioid-related deaths elsewhere in the USA.

Epidemiological data from the UK from 1993 to 2004 give the number of heroin/methadone deaths as 7072 and methadone deaths as 3298 (72). Age-standardized mortality rates increased from 5 to 15 per million from 1993 to 1997. Methadone deaths fell from 1997 to 2004. During this period there was an increase in the use of methadone, but the data suggest that this was not associated with an increased number of deaths.

Opiate overdose deaths in England fell by 21% from 2002 to 2003; Brighton had the highest drug-related death rate (73). In 75% of the deaths that involved methadone there was also polydrug use, and in 30% there were toxic concentrations of other substances. The authors highlighted the fact that buprenorphine also carries a significant risk of respiratory depression, is easier to inject, and carries a risk of pulmonary edema. This finding was confirmed in study in Germany (74). One buprenorphine death was reported in 2002–2003, resulting from injection of crushed buprenorphine. Of note is the higher numbers of incidents reported with methadone (35%) and heroin (62%). Buprenorphine appears to be associated with a lower risk of fatal overdoses.

Benzodiazepines, identified through toxicology screening at autopsy, were found in a significant number of buprenorphine-related deaths in Singapore (75). Between September 2003 and 2004 there were 21 cases of buprenorphine-related deaths, in 19 of which benzodiazepines had also been used.

The risk of accidental overdose in those found to be positive for methadone is increased by the concomitant use of tricyclic antidepressants, benzodiazepines, and both (76). In a retrospective epidemiological study in New York City in 2003, there were 500 (8.6%) methadone positive deaths, of which 493 were analysed; tricyclic antidepressants were also found in 19% and benzodiazepine in 32%. The authors advised increased awareness of the risk of such combinations.

In a review of the literature the three main factors that predicted fatal opioid overdoses were injecting heroin, chronic alcohol misuse, and having been arrested more than three times (77).

Long-Term Effects

Drug abuse

The abuse potential and importance of identifying and managing the risks of opioids has been reviewed (78). Abuse of opioids is highly prevalent globally, and the authors discussed strategies for reducing it, such as making tablets 'tamper resistant', providing controlled-release dosage forms, partial agonists, and drug combinations that precipitate withdrawal if misused. Such strategies are linked to a risk of overdose. They suggested a standard procedure for evaluating the abuse potential of substances at various stages of drug development.

Drug tolerance

The clinical significance of opioid tolerance has been extensively reviewed (4) and the evidence for tolerance in acute and prolonged opioid administration has been presented. The former remains controversial while the latter has been adequately demonstrated. Different patterns of opioid use in chronic cancer-related pain are described, these being essentially escalating prescribing, steady-dose prescribing, and opioid withdrawal. The particular pattern followed by any individual is the result of the balance between physical changes in the level of nociceptive activity, psychological processes, such as increased anxiety and depression, and the degree of tolerance itself. While tolerance to an opiate reduces its clinical effectiveness, the tolerance may be beneficial if it mitigates drug adverse effects. Tolerance to respiratory depression and nausea occurs swiftly, sedation takes longer to resolve, and constipation is relatively resistant to the development of tolerance. Cross-tolerance is partial; hence switching from one opioid to another can relieve particular adverse effects without loss of clinical effect.

Physical dependence on opioids appears to occur in patients who use opioids for long-term pain relief, and cases of addiction have been reported. However, rates of addiction are low and occur mainly in individuals who have a history of substance misuse. The role of long-term opioid medication in non-cancer-related chronic pain remains controversial. "Opiophobia," a fear of the legitimate use of opioid analgesics because of the potential for addiction, remains a significant issue for physicians, patients, and relatives alike. The review is illustrated with a report of a 52-year-old man with multiple myeloma who displayed tolerance to oral morphine over 2 years.

Opioid tolerance in neonates

Tolerance to opioids in neonates has been reviewed (79). There are two forms of neonatal opioid exposure. First, in-utero exposure to opioids of neonates with opiate-addicted mothers; secondly, preterm infants requiring prolonged support in intensive care when opioid administration is used to reduce the stress response. The adverse effects of opioids on neonates are similar to those described in adults (sedation, dysphoria, seizures, nausea and vomiting, urinary retention, reduced intestinal motility, biliary tract spasm, histamine release, and chest wall rigidity), but it has been proposed that differences in the densities of the different opioid receptor subtypes lead to an increased theoretical propensity for respiratory depression with given opioid doses compared with older people. However, clinical studies have not confirmed increased sensitivity to respiratory depression in neonates or young infants. Tolerance may occur more swiftly in neonates due to slower opioid metabolism and a more permeable blood–brain barrier. Opioid withdrawal symptoms in neonates are similar to those for other age groups but can be mimicked by hypoxia, hypercarbia, hypoglycemia, hypocalcemia, or hypomagnesemia. Assessment of tolerance and withdrawal is made using the neonatal abstinence score rating scale and the neonatal withdrawal index.

Management of neonatal opioid withdrawal relies on gradually reducing doses of opioids to reduce the severity of withdrawal symptoms. Paregoric was formerly used as a withdrawal aid but is little used now owing to toxic effects. Tincture of opium (10% solution), consisting of 1 ml in 24 ml of sterile water, 0.05 ml/kg 4-hourly is proposed as the most suitable replacement. Speed of reduction depends on the length of neonatal exposure to opioids and a short reducing regimen (over 2–3 days) can be sufficient. A methadone replacement withdrawal regimen is also discussed, while benzodiazepines, phenobarbital, chlorpromazine, and clonidine are all reviewed as having a potential role in symptomatic relief during withdrawal; however, each has its own associated adverse effects, which limit their usefulness.

Mechanism

At micromolar concentrations opioids cause an increase in the cell membrane threshold, shortened action potentials, and inhibition of neurotransmitter release. At nanomolar concentrations opioid agonists are excitatory and prolong the action potential via the stimulatory G proteins, which act on the adenylate cyclase/cAMP system and on protein kinase A-dependent ion channels. Tolerance is proposed to be the result of an increase in the association of opioid receptors to stimulatory G proteins, to an activation of N-methyl-D-aspartate receptors via protein kinase C, and calmodulin-dependent increases in cytosolic calcium, resulting in cellular hyperexcitability.

Drug withdrawal

Chronic administration of opioids produces physical and psychological dependence. A characteristic withdrawal syndrome occurs when the opioid is stopped abruptly or an opioid antagonist is given. In the case of morphine and other OP_3 receptor agonists with a similar duration of action, lacrimation, rhinorrhea, yawning, and sweating occur about 8–12 hours after the last dose. Symptoms peak at about 24–48 hours after withdrawal, with restlessness, irritability, and insomnia, as well as severe sneezing, weakness, anxiety, and depression. Other symptoms include dilated pupils, anorexia, piloerection, nausea, vomiting, diarrhea, pyrexia, hypertension, muscle cramps, dehydration, and weight loss (80).

Treatment of opioid withdrawal

Various regimens were used in the past in an attempt to withdraw patients from opioid addiction (81). The modern scientific basis for the evaluation of opioid withdrawal regimens was established by Kolb and Himmelsbach (82), who concluded that the methods that produced the least discomfort and the best results were either abrupt or rapid withdrawal of the opioid. Rapid withdrawal consisted of gradually reducing doses of morphine over 4–10 days. Such methods were in regular use until the advent of methadone as a heroin substitute in the 1950s.

Antidepressant, anxiolytic, and neuroleptic drugs can allow some patients to participate in treatment programs, especially when drug abuse is associated with psychiatric disorders such as depression, chronic anxiety, or schizophrenia.

Methadone

A widely used technique, pioneered by Isbell and Vogel (83), involves the substitution of methadone for the illicit opioid, followed by a gradual reduction in the amount of methadone taken. Methadone is used to substitute for a variety of opioid drugs. It is well absorbed after oral ingestion, with peak blood concentrations after about 4 hours. Steady-state concentrations are reached after about 5 days. By virtue of its long duration of action (the half-life with regular dosing is about 22 hours), methadone suppresses opioid withdrawal symptoms for 24–36 hours. In the early stages of treatment, patients may report problems such as drowsiness, insomnia, nausea, euphoria, difficulty in micturition, and excessive sweating. With the exception of chronic constipation and excessive sweating, these effects do not generally persist.

British studies have shown that, using methadone, about 80% of inpatients but only 17% of outpatients were successfully withdrawn (84,85). However, the technique is not without problems, one being that the methadone reduces but does not eliminate withdrawal symptoms. The withdrawal response has been described as being akin to a mild case of influenza, objectively mild but subjectively severe (86). The fear of withdrawal symptoms expressed by those dependent on drugs should not be underestimated: these factors are associated with the subsequent severity of withdrawal symptoms, and they are more closely related to symptom severity than drug dosage (87). Methadone substitution can result in a protracted withdrawal response, with patients still experiencing significantly more symptoms than controls 2 weeks after withdrawal (88).

In a study of methadone withdrawal, patients who were withdrawn over 10 days had a withdrawal syndrome that began to increase in severity from day 3, with peak severity of symptoms on day 13; in those who were withdrawn over 21 days, symptoms began to increase about day 10 with a peak on day 20 and abated thereafter, although some patients did not recover fully until 40 days after starting withdrawal (89). Thus, the duration of the withdrawal syndrome is much the same for both treatments in terms of symptom severity. It is possible that an exponential rather than a linear reduction in dosage may improve the withdrawal response. These results may be of clinical significance, in that patients may feel it important that they recover from withdrawal as quickly as possible, in order to participate fully in other aspects of drug withdrawal programs. However, although there was no difference between the 10-day and the 21-day programs regarding completion rates for detoxification (70 and 79% respectively), the dropout rates after detoxification were significantly different. During the 10 days after the last dose of methadone, the dropout rate in the 21-day group was 18% compared with 30% in the 10-day group. These results may also have financial implications in respect of the number of subjects who can be admitted to treatment programs.

In some treatment programs total abstinence is not considered to be a practical objective and treatment may involve the use of drugs such as methadone as maintenance therapy with the expectation of reducing illicit drug consumption (90). Well-organized methadone maintenance treatment can reduce the intake of illicit opioids in many injecting drug users (91,92).

The methadone maintenance treatment was established in 1964 in New York City by Vincent Dole and Marie Nyswander (see the monograph on Methadone). In the initial studies, subjects who were heavily addicted to heroin were evaluated and stabilized on daily methadone doses as inpatients before transfer to an outpatient clinic for continued treatment. With further experience, it was feasible to drop the inpatient phase.

Outcome studies of methadone maintenance treatment have reported favorable results, with high rates of patient retention, reduced criminality, and improved social rehabilitation. However, despite its proved effectiveness, it remains a controversial approach among substance abuse treatment providers, public officials, policy makers, the medical profession, and the public at large. Nevertheless, almost every nation with a significant narcotic addiction problem has established a methadone maintenance treatment program.

For patients entering treatment from an institution where they have been drug-free, initial daily methadone doses should be no more than 20 mg. Otherwise initial daily doses of 30–40 mg should be sufficient to obtain the necessary balance between withdrawal and narcotic symptoms. Thereafter, stabilization is achieved by gradually increasing the dose. When methadone is given in adequate oral doses (usually 60 mg/day or more), a single dose in a stabilized patient lasts 24–36 hours, without creating euphoria and sedation. Tolerance to methadone seems to remain steady, and patients can be maintained on the same dose, in some cases for more than 20 years.

The methadone dose must be determined individually, because of individual variability in pharmacokinetics and pharmacodynamics. Maintenance of appropriate methadone blood concentrations is recommended.

Tolerance to the narcotic properties of methadone develops within 4–6 weeks, but tolerance to the autonomic effects (for example constipation and sweating) develops more slowly.

The major adverse effects during treatment occur during the initial stabilization phase. In addition to constipation and sweating, the most frequently reported adverse effects are transient skin rash, weight gain, and fluid retention. Since the main metabolic pathway of methadone is CYP3A4 numerous drug interactions can be expected. Drugs that interact with methadone and other opioid analgesics are listed in Table 2.

Methadone maintenance treatment is considered to be a medically safe treatment with relatively few and minimal adverse effects. However the danger of serious adverse effects and death with the increasing use of methadone as maintenance therapy in drug addicts has been highlighted. It must be emphasized that a daily maintenance dose of 50–100 mg is toxic in a non-tolerant adult, and as little as 10 mg can be fatal in a child. There is an increasing number of reports of the deaths of children of mothers on maintenance therapy from inadvertent ingestion.

Clonidine

Clonidine appears to ameliorate the opioid withdrawal syndrome by reducing central noradrenergic activity. It has been hypothesized that the opioid withdrawal syndrome is due to increased noradrenergic neuronal activity in areas such as the locus ceruleus, which are regulated by both opioid receptors and α_2-adrenoceptors (93). Opioids and clonidine both act at the locus ceruleus, reducing central noradrenergic function. This common pathway hypothesis is supported by the similarity of clonidine and opioid withdrawal in respect to their effects on vital signs, mood, and noradrenergic hyperactivity (94). Since the actions of clonidine are mediated by α-adrenoceptors they are not antagonized by opioid antagonists.

There have been many reports of the use of clonidine in the treatment of acute opioid withdrawal (95). A dose of 500 micrograms/day for 10 days reduced but did not completely abolish withdrawal symptoms in 50 patients

Table 2 Some drug interactions involving opioid analgesics

Object drug	Precipitant drug	Clinical consequences	Proposed mechanism(s)
Carbamazepine	Dextropropoxyphene	Increased effect of carbamazepine	Reduced metabolism
Codeine	Quinidine	Reduced analgesic effect	Reduced liver metabolism of codeine to morphine
Dextropropoxyphene	Ethanol	Increased effect of dextropropoxyphene	Reduced metabolism
Methadone	Carbamazepine	Reduced effect of methadone	Increased metabolism
Methadone	Cimetidine	Increased effect of methadone	Reduced metabolism
Methadone	Phenobarbital	Reduced effect of methadone	Increased metabolism
Methadone	Fluvoxamine	Increased effect of methadone	Reduced metabolism
Methadone	Phenytoin	Reduced effect of methadone	Increased metabolism
Methadone	Rifampicin	Reduced effect of methadone	Increased metabolism
Morphine	Cimetidine	Increased effect of morphine	Reduced metabolism
Morphine	Amitriptyline	Increased effect of morphine	Increased systemic availability
Morphine	Clomipramine	Increased effect of morphine	Increased systemic availability
Nortriptyline	Dextropropoxyphene	Increased effect of nortriptyline	Reduced metabolism
Pethidine	Cimetidine	Increased effect of pethidine	Reduced metabolism
Pethidine	Chlorpromazine	Increased toxicity of pethidine	Altered metabolism
Pethidine	Moclobemide	Increased effect of pethidine	Serotonin syndrome reported
Pethidine	Selegiline	Increased effect of pethidine	Serotonin syndrome reported
Phenobarbital	Dextropropoxyphene	Increased effect of phenobarbital	Reduced metabolism
Phenytoin	Dextropropoxyphene	Increased effect of phenytoin	Reduced metabolism

dependent on methadone or heroin. The patients still complained of sluggishness, insomnia, and bone pain, but there were none of the usual complaints associated with opioid withdrawal, such as anxiety, abdominal cramps, chills, muscle spasms, irritability, and anger.

Others have reported good results from the use of clonidine (96,97). Of 25 inpatients physically dependent on methadone, 20 were able to withdraw completely from methadone at the end of 2 weeks. In most patients, 10–11 days of clonidine, in a peak dose of 16 micrograms/kg/day, produced a perceived reduction in symptoms compared with previous attempts to become opioid-free. In these dosages, clonidine significantly reduced standing blood pressure without producing clinical problems. Withdrawal symptoms of anxiety, restlessness, insomnia, and muscle aching were still evident.

In a randomized double-blind, placebo-controlled comparison of clonidine with a reducing dose of methadone, there was no difference in success rate: 42% abstinence with clonidine and 39% with methadone (98). However, patients who received clonidine had more self-rated withdrawal symptoms and a higher percentage of days on which symptoms were severe.

Clonidine has been reported to reduce both diastolic and systolic blood pressure by 10–15 mmHg during treatment for opioid withdrawal. Sedation and insomnia have also been noted. However, it is often difficult to distinguish which symptoms are due to the treatment and which are caused by opioid withdrawal. In a comparison of clonidine and methadone, seven of 14 patients in the clonidine group were withdrawn from the study because they had unacceptable adverse effects, compared with one of 11 in the methadone group. Two of those taking clonidine had severe immediate adverse effects that prevented them from continuing beyond 2 days (99).

One of the limitations of clonidine treatment is that it does not appear to reduce the duration of the opioid withdrawal syndrome. In one study, 10 days of clonidine therapy were required to suppress the symptoms of opioid withdrawal from long-acting opioids such as methadone (97).

The effect of clonidine in the management of opioid-dependent individuals undergoing gradual methadone detoxification over 14 days has been studied (100). In those who completed the course, clonidine did not significantly reduce either the symptoms or objective signs of opioid withdrawal. There was a substantial dropout rate, and several subjects were withdrawn from the study because of symptoms related to hypotension. In those who completed detoxification, clonidine did not reduce either the symptoms or the signs of opioid withdrawal. Clonidine therefore seems to have no place as an adjunct to a program of gradual methadone detoxification.

Clonidine plus an opioid antagonist

In a double-blind study using titrated doses of clonidine and naltrexone, combined clonidine and naltrexone treatment allowed 38 out of 40 patients physically dependent on methadone to withdraw completely in 4–5 days (101). For most patients naltrexone was gradually increased from 1 to 50 mg/day over 4 days. The dose of clonidine was 200–600 micrograms every 4 hours. After the first 48 hours the dose was rapidly tapered without recurrence of withdrawal symptoms. Flurazepam was used for night sedation. Although clonidine reduced the intensity of naltrexone-induced withdrawal symptoms, it did not eliminate them completely. On the first day after withdrawal of methadone and initiation of naltrexone and clonidine the frequencies of craving, anxiety, restlessness, insomnia, muscular aching, anorexia, hot and cold flushes, and diarrhea were significantly higher than whilst taking methadone. However, after 4 days of naltrexone, the patients were considerably less symptomatic. Compared with their feelings whilst taking methadone, they complained of significant increases in irritability, unpleasantness, and lethargy during the first 3 days.

The combined use of clonidine and naltrexone appears to allow successful withdrawal from long-term methadone therapy within 4–5 days of its abrupt withdrawal. Although patient selection may be an important consideration, the apparent success rate compares favorably with other methods and is achieved in a much shorter time (97).

Buprenorphine

In a study designed to assess the safety of buprenorphine for the treatment of cocaine and opiate dependence there were no adverse effects or serious interactions with a single dose of intravenous morphine or cocaine during daily maintenance on buprenorphine (SEDA-18, 85).

Second-Generation Effects

Pregnancy

A major review of the problems of drug dependence in pregnancy and the clinical management of mother and child was published in 1979, and its findings remain valid today (SED-11, 138) (102).

Opioids taken in pregnancy by a drug-dependent mother, or administered to the parturient, can cause respiratory depression in the newborn. Abstinence symptoms have been reported in the infants of mothers who are opioid-dependent at term (103).

The adverse consequences for the neonate of drug abuse in pregnancy can be dramatically reduced by comprehensive medical and psychosocial care for the mothers during pregnancy and delivery (SED-11, 138) (104,105). However, without due care during pregnancy problems are likely.

The long-term consequences of maternal opioid dependency on the child have been examined in detail in 89 infants born to mothers addicted to heroin, morphine, and methadone (SED-11, 138) (106); 20% were preterm and 31% were light for gestational age; 85% of the infants had withdrawal symptoms and 12% had convulsions. The somatic and neurobehavioral findings in children in their first 18 months of life, born to methadone-maintained mothers and to a matched drug-free comparison group of mothers, have been reported (SED-11, 138) (107). At 18 months the methadone children had: (a) a significantly higher incidence of otitis media; (b) a significant incidence of head circumference below the third percentile; (c) neurological findings of tone discrepancies, developmental delays, and poor motor co-ordination; (d) a high incidence of abnormal eye findings; and (e) significantly lower scores on the Bayley mental and motor developmental indices. In a study of 72 such children investigated 1–10 years after birth, only 25% were physically, mentally, and behaviorally normal (106).

In 41 children born to methadone-maintained mothers and 23 children from matched controls at 6 months of age, there was delayed motor development in methadone-

exposed infants and greater vulnerability of males to adverse environmental conditions; in adult male rats there was a correlation between early methadone exposure and behavioral abnormalities (SED-11, 138) (108).

Opioid analgesia during the first stage of labor

The 50% and 95% effective doses (ED_{50} and ED_{95}) of intrathecal sufentanil for analgesia in labor have been characterized in several studies (109,110). The same criteria have been applied to fentanyl in 90 women in active early labor (at least 5 cm dilatation), who received a range of doses of intrathecal fentanyl (5–25 micrograms) in a double-blind, randomized study (111). Fentanyl induced rapid and effective dose-dependent analgesia in early labor. Pruritus occurred in 66% of patients and falls in ventilation were dose-related. The ED_{50} and ED_{95} values were 5.5 and 17.4 micrograms respectively.

In 60 women who requested epidural analgesia during labor randomized to sufentanil 10 micrograms, fentanyl 10 µg, or saline in addition to intrathecal bupivacaine 2.5 mg, the combination of sufentanil plus bupivacaine gave a significantly longer duration of analgesia (112). Pruritus was more common in women given sufentanil (80%) and fentanyl (47%) than in those given plain bupivacaine. However, there were no differences in the incidences of gastrointestinal effects, hypotension, or motor blockade between the groups. Adding sufentanil 10 micrograms to intrathecal bupivacaine 2.5 mg provided fast onset, better analgesia for a longer duration than the other treatments.

In another similar study, the adverse effects profile, especially in regard to pruritus, improved if intrathecal sufentanil 2.5 micrograms was added to bupivacaine 1.25 mg and adrenaline 2.5 micrograms, without compromising analgesia in women in the first stage of labor (113).

In 30 women randomized to receive either sufentanil 7.5 micrograms plus bupivacaine 2.5 micrograms, with or without clonidine 50 micrograms, using a combined spinal-epidural technique, analgesia was prolonged in those given clonidine without an increased incidence of adverse effects or worse pain scores (114).

In a prospective, randomized, double-blind comparison of nalbuphine with pethidine in 310 women requiring analgesia during labor, nalbuphine produced a lower incidence of nausea and vomiting (115). There were no differences between the two groups in the other adverse effects of the opioids, and nalbuphine did not afford major analgesic benefits.

Use of opioids in cesarean section

The use of intrathecal or epidural opioids has been recommended for the relief of pain after cesarean section, and there have been several comparisons of intrathecal and epidural opioid use.

In 50 women randomized to intrathecal diamorphine 0.25 mg or epidural diamorphine 5 mg in addition to intrathecal bupivacaine 10 mg, there was no significant difference in the duration or quality of analgesia (116). The incidence of nausea and vomiting was higher in the epidural group (24 versus 4%). There was no difference in the incidence of pruritus, but the incidence was as high as 88% of patients, and it was severe enough to require treatment in 20%.

In a double-blind, randomized study, 55 women undergoing elective cesarean section were allocated to either epidural diamorphine 3 mg or intrathecal morphine 0.2 mg (117). There were no significant differences between the two groups in pain assessed by visual analogue scale or in the incidence of pruritus, sedation, or respiratory depression measured by pulse oximetry during the 28-hour postoperative period. Nausea and vomiting were significantly more common in the intrathecal morphine group (73 versus 41%).

Patient-controlled analgesia with epidural pethidine or a single bolus of epidural morphine 4 mg during the 24 hours after cesarean section has been studied in 78 women (118). There were no differences in the degree of analgesia or opioid adverse effects profiles.

In 66 cesarean section patients the effects of sufentanil (2 micrograms/ml), tramadol (10 mg/ml), or a mixture of the two were compared using patient-controlled extradural analgesia (119). Nausea and vomiting were closely related to the use of tramadol, while pruritus was associated with sufentanil. The combined regimen reduced the dosage requirements of both opioids by 20%. Extradural tramadol cannot be recommended, because of the increased incidence of severe gastrointestinal adverse effects, the high dose required, and inferior analgesia.

Patient-controlled epidural fentanyl (20 micrograms with 10 minute lock-out) has been compared with patient-controlled intravenous morphine (1 mg with a 5-minute lock-out) in 48 women after cesarean section (120). Fentanyl was more efficacious in controlling postoperative pain, with a lower incidence of nausea and drowsiness.

Finally, 60 women undergoing cesarean section were randomly given epidural tramadol 100 mg, epidural tramadol 200 mg, or saline (121). Pain scores and adverse effects were evaluated for 24 hours after surgery. In all three groups there were no opioid-related adverse effects and epidural tramadol 100 mg provided adequate postoperative analgesia.

Fetotoxicity

The pharmacokinetics and effects of various systemically administered analgesics on the uterus, fetus, and neonate have been reviewed (SED-11, 137). Fetal bradycardia lasting up to 7 minutes was reported in 53 of 1910 fetuses (2.7%) after the administration of pethidine (meperidine) 75 mg and promethazine 25 mg intravenously to the mothers during labor (SED-11, 137) (122).

The relation between maternal morphine administration during labor and the Apgar score of the baby at birth has been studied (SED-11, 137) (123). The authors concluded that morphine alone did not seem to cause asphyxia at birth, but that morphine together with other fetal and/or obstetric factors would definitely be a cause for concern with regard to birth asphyxia.

The effect of maternal analgesia on neonatal behavior has been assessed (SED-11, 137) (124). The authors

suggested that neonates respond to pethidine in the same way as adults, but the changes observed were relatively subtle, and comparison of these infants with a control group whose mothers had received no drugs showed no differences in behavior.

Opioid analgesia can cause prolonged reductions in the baseline variability of the fetus during monitoring in labor (SEDA-17, 85). This is thought to occur by a direct effect on the cardiac centers or fetal myocardium. The danger of this is the risk of misinterpretation of the cardiotocogram as being indicative of fetal distress.

Intramuscular tramadol (50 or 100 mg) during labor is associated with fewer adverse effects than pethidine 75 mg (SEDA-18, 83). Pethidine and the higher dose of tramadol had similar analgesic efficacy, but pethidine was associated with a significantly lower neonatal respiratory rate at birth.

Susceptibility Factors

Age

Neonates, infants, and children are at risk of adverse effects of opioids, owing to pharmacokinetic and pharmacodynamic changes (SEDA-17, 78). Routine use of pulse oximetry is recommended in all children receiving opioids (SEDA-21, 85).

Elderly patients are particularly at risk, as a number of other susceptibility factors can co-exist.

Sex

Accumulating evidence suggests that there are sex differences in analgesic responses to opioid agonists (125,126), and there is increasing evidence from both laboratory and clinical studies that women may experience greater MOR (OP$_3$, μ) opioid receptor analgesia than men (127,128,129).The type of pain receptors, pharmacokinetics, and hormone concentrations (estrogens and testosterone) have all been implicated as potential basis for these differences. In a randomized, double-blind, comparison of the MOR receptor agonist morphine sulfate and the KOR (OP$_2$, κ) receptor agonist butorphanol in 94 patients with acute moderate to severe pain following injury showed that women preferred butorphanol (130). Even though the degree of analgesia experienced indicated a sex difference, the adverse effects reported were similar in the two groups. In another study of sex differences in analgesic responses to the KOR receptor partial agonist pentazocine, using an experimentally induced pain model in 41 healthy women and 38 healthy men, there were significant analgesic responses in both sexes, with no sex difference (131). The most likely explanation is that an apparent different occurs when the pain assays used are not objective and standardized.

Renal disease

Renal insufficiency can result in clinically significant accumulation of pharmacologically active opioid metabolites and prolonged narcosis; such patients must be monitored for signs of toxicity (SEDA-17, 79) (SEDA-21, 85)

(132,133). To date, this effect has only been reported with codeine, morphine, and pethidine. Dextropropoxyphene is not recommended in renal insufficiency, as its metabolite norpropoxyphene, which is eliminated by the kidneys, accumulates, causing cardiac depression (SEDA-17, 79) (SEDA-21, 85).

Other features of the patient

In patients with reduced respiratory reserve, such as those with emphysema, severe obesity, cor pulmonale, and kyphoscoliosis, opioids must be used with caution. The relative benefits and harms of using opioids in patients taking monoamine oxidase inhibitors, those with a history of drug abuse, asthma, hepatic impairment, hypotension, raised intracranial pressure, or head injury, and during pregnancy or breast feeding, should be carefully considered. Dextropropoxyphene, pethidine, and methadone should be used with caution (SEDA-21, 85).

Drug Administration

Drug administration route

The usefulness and adverse effects of different administration routes of opioids have been discussed in several articles.

Oral

Oral administration is the method most often used because it is non-invasive, convenient, and easy to titrate. In chronic pain oral opioid formulations that provide longer duration of effect are preferred, because they provide more stable pain control, better tolerability, and increased convenience, patient options, and flexibility.

Modified-release oxymorphone is a new oral tablet formulation aimed to provide a 12-hour dosing interval. In a prospective, open, sequential crossover pilot study patients with cancer with moderate or severe pain, using either modified -release morphine or oxycodone, were safely switched to modified-release oxymorphone at a lower equivalent dosage, with no reduction in pain relief or increase in adverse effects (134). This study was a pilot study with a small sample size. Further studies are required for more robust findings.

In another study oral and rectal tramadol were compared (135). The two routes were equally effective in pain relief and were associated with similar adverse events. However, both patients and physicians preferred the oral route. Nevertheless, rectal administration of tramadol can be safe, reliable, and non-invasive for patients who cannot take oral tramadol.

Sublingual

The combination of naloxone and buprenorphine has been used sublingually, with the aim of reducing the abuse potential of buprenorphine. When crushed and injected, naloxone will exert its opioid receptor antagonist properties. This review reported that the combination drug, when administered parenterally to non-physically dependent individuals, attenuated (but did not block) the effects of buprenorphine (136).

Rectal

Transdermal fentanyl patches typically contain large amounts of fentanyl, thus giving the potential for abuse and toxicity. Fentanyl toxicity has been reported after rectal insertion of fentanyl patches (137).

- A 41 year old man became comatose after inserting three fentanyl patches (100 micrograms/hour) into his rectum. He was given naloxone 6 mg without a response. The patches were removed digitally and he recovered 1 hour later.

This report shows the importance of being aware of the toxic potential of patches. Increased absorption by the rectal mucosa and the relatively high rectal temperature facilitate rapid release and high fentanyl concentrations. The authors pointed out that the low price of the patches could result in more cases of accidental, abusive, or intentional fentanyl toxicity.

Intramuscular and subcutaneous

The intramuscular and subcutaneous routes are most often used in postoperative analgesia (138). The limitations are: discomfort due to repeated injections; large interpersonal variation in dosage requirements; peaks and troughs in blood concentrations, with inconsistent pain relief and incidence of adverse effects; and delayed response times from staff in delivering the analgesic (138).

In patients undergoing posterior lumbar interbody fusion, continuous epidural morphine was compared with continuous subcutaneous morphine as pre-emptive analgesia (139). There were no differences in analgesic effects. However, there more adverse effects were with epidural morphine, despite the fact that subcutaneous doses of morphine were about three times higher. In addition, preoperative epidural catheterization was difficult without seeing the dura mater. Thus, continuous epidural morphine was not suitable for pre-emptive analgesia; continuous subcutaneous morphine was the preferred option because of technical ease and fewer complications.

Inhalation

The pharmacokinetics, pharmacodynamics, safety, and efficacy of therapeutic inhalational opioids have been reviewed (140). Pulmonary delivery of opioids facilitates rapid and increased absorption, making this route suitable for management of acute pain. However, there are very few published data on their safety and efficacy. The literature suggests that this technique is well tolerated and is associated with adverse effects similar to those associated with other routes. The authors highlighted the importance of increased regulatory control of the technique, because of the associated potential for abuse.

Intranasal

Intranasal diamorphine spray has been compared it with injectable diamorphine for maintenance treatment (141).

Intranasal diamorphine was easier of use associated with reduced stigma and a reduced risk of adverse effects due to injection.

Spinal

Compared with conventional routes, spinal opioid administration carries potentially greater morbidity and can only be justified if it produces equal or superior pain relief compared with conventional methods, with fewer unwanted effects (SED-11, 139).

Although the analgesic effect of spinal opioids is largely due to a spinal effect, the opioid can spread rostrally to the brainstem and higher centers, and can cause delayed adverse effects. Lipid solubility affects the rate at which an opioid is absorbed into the spinal cord from the cerebrospinal fluid (CSF), and therefore predicts the likelihood of rostral spread. Hydrophilic drugs, such as morphine, will linger in the CSF and produce prolonged analgesia that may last 12 hours or more. Such drugs can float rostrally, producing more widespread but less intense analgesia. However, if the drug reaches opioid receptors in the respiratory center in the fourth ventricle, delayed respiratory depression can occur. In contrast to morphine, fentanyl is very lipid-soluble but short-acting; a single dose will produce intense highly segmental analgesia lasting 2–3 hours. These properties make it suitable for continuous epidural infusion.

When an opioid is used as the sole agent by the epidural or intrathecal route, the results are disappointing, because of unwanted adverse effects, such as pruritus, nausea, vomiting, respiratory depression, and effects on the neonate, caused by significant systemic absorption (SEDA-17, 85). Hypotension and changes in fetal heart rate are not uncommon (SEDA-21, 91). Combinations of opioids (alfentanil, fentanyl, morphine, sufentanil) with local anesthetics (for example bupivacaine) have therefore been suggested to yield better results (SEDA-18, 83).

The use of alfentanil with bupivacaine via continuous epidural infusion during labor resulted in a significant reduction in motor blockade compared with bupivacaine alone. There was no respiratory depression in the mothers, although shivering and pruritus were more frequent with alfentanil. There were no differences in the neonatal Apgar scores between the groups (SEDA-18, 83).

There has been a comparison of the effects of fentanyl and sufentanil, combined with bupivacaine and adrenaline, given by PCA after cesarean section (SEDA-18, 83). The numbers of requests were greater in the fentanyl group, but there was no difference between the groups with regard to sedation, pruritus, or nausea. However, those who received sufentanil had a significantly higher incidence of vomiting, light-headedness, and dizziness.

It is uncertain whether the addition of adrenaline to intrathecal sufentanil increases the duration of analgesia during labor. In one study, the addition of adrenaline to intrathecal sufentanil did not prolong the duration of analgesia, but reduced the incidence and severity of pruritus (SEDA-18, 83), whereas in another the addition of adrenaline or morphine to intrathecal sufentanil prolonged the duration of analgesia (SEDA-18, 83). However, those given morphine had significantly more nausea and pruritus.

In another comparison of a single dose of epidural morphine with PCA epidural fentanyl after cesarean section, pain relief and the incidence of nausea were similar, but pruritus was significantly less with fentanyl (SEDA-18, 83).

Epidural methadone and diamorphine are useful analgesics during cesarean section, but oxygen desaturation and nausea are more frequent with diamorphine (SEDA-18, 83).

Combined spinal-epidural administration achieves almost instantaneous analgesia with longer pain relief (142). This method gives a faster onset of analgesia and less motor blockade than standard epidural analgesia (143).

Several studies have highlighted the benefits of giving adequate postoperative analgesia in cardiac patients, and the use of intrathecal and epidural anesthesia and analgesia for cardiac surgery has been reviewed (144). Effective postoperative analgesia reduces the risk of postoperative stress and morbidity, hospital stay, and cost, and increases patient satisfaction. There is a role for intravenous opioids in such patients, but those are associated with significant adverse effects. On the other hand, several studies of intrathecal techniques have shown that these provide adequate analgesia although they do not significantly attenuate the stress response associated with cardiac surgery. Despite potentially inducing cardiac sympathectomy, total spinal anesthesia remains unacceptable. Epidural techniques provide adequate analgesia and can attenuate the stress response associated with cardiac surgery, as well as induce thoracic cardiac sympathectomy. There are significant adverse effects associated with the administration of opioids by intrathecal or epidural techniques. The most common is pruritus; nausea and vomiting occur in about 30% of cases and urinary retention occurs mostly in young men. Respiratory depression requiring intervention occurs in about 1% of cases, similar to the incidence after intramuscular or intravenous use. Intrathecal or epidural fentanyl or sufentanil is associated with early respiratory depression (within minutes), whereas morphine is associated with delayed depression (hours). Intrathecal use increases the risk of respiratory depression. Hematoma formation is another complication associated with both intrathecal and epidural techniques. These techniques are therefore associated with significant risks, which make their clinical implementation controversial.

Intrathecal route

Technical problems after intrathecal opioids are rare, although catheter occlusion and leakage of CSF have been reported (SEDA-17, 85) (145–147). In 121 patients with mean follow-up of 68 days (maximum 13 months) there was an incidence of less than 10% (148).

Intrathecal opioids used in obstetrics are well tolerated by mother and child (SED-11, 139, 140) (149–151).

Morphine is the opioid most often chosen for intrathecal administration.

In a comparison of intrathecal morphine and remifentanil in patients undergoing off-pump coronary surgery, opioid related cardiac effects were similar; intrathecal morphine did not produce central neuroaxial hematoma or post-spinal tap headache (152).

The preoperative use of intrathecal morphine 0.5 mg and fentanyl 15 micrograms has been evaluated in 40 patients undergoing major liver resection in a randomized, double-blind, placebo-controlled study (153). Preoperative intrathecal analgesia significantly reduced the need for postoperative morphine for pain management three-fold and was not associated with a significant difference in adverse effects.

Respiratory

Respiratory depression occurs more often after intrathecal than after epidural opioid administration and can be more of a problem in old age or when there is pre-existing respiratory disease (SED-11, 139) (154,155). The time of onset is variable but usually occurs within 6–10 hours of the opioid injection, although delays of up to 11 hours have been reported (156). There have been two cases of prolonged respiratory depression lasting 18 hours after single doses of 3 and 5 mg (156). Repeated doses of naloxone were required, but each incremental dose did not alter the level of analgesia.

It has been suggested that opioid-naive patients may be more susceptible to respiratory depression and that posture may also be important (SED-11, 139) (157).

Return of normal respiration can take up to 23 hours. Peak expiratory flow rate (PEFR) was significantly better in patients who had received intrathecal rather than intravenous morphine after cardiac surgery, but mean $PaCO_2$ was significantly higher in patients given intrathecal morphine 2 mg, rather than intrathecal or intravenous morphine 1 mg (158). The effect was dose-dependent (159).

Nervous system

Central adverse effects are as expected; with the exception of constipation, urinary retention, and respiratory depression, these effects tend to be transient and disappear within a few days of starting therapy.

Drowsiness, miosis, and respiratory depression have been reported after intracerebroventricular administration of morphine in two of 55 patients who received morphine 1–1.5 mg (160). A third patient developed visual hallucinations and behavioral disorders after 1 mg. All effects were rapidly reversed by naloxone.

Myoclonic spasms of the legs have been described after intrathecal morphine, and were abolished by intrathecal bupivacaine (161).

Hyperalgesia and myoclonus were reported after high-dose intrathecal morphine (SEDA-17, 87).

Temporary, totally reversible motor and sensory paralysis has been reported after intrathecal morphine 1.6 mg and was attributed not to a direct spinal action of morphine but to cardiovascular changes occurring as a result of pain relief (162).

Long-term intrathecal administration of pethidine may be associated with toxicity, owing to accumulation of its metabolite norpethidine. This was explored in a study in 10 patients with neuropathic cancer pain, who had not responded sufficiently to recommended regimens (163). There were high plasma concentrations of pethidine and norpethidine in three subjects; however, norpethidine concentrations were still below the concentration reported to induce nervous system toxicity, i.e. under 500 ng/ml, and no patient had evidence of nervous system toxicity. One patient developed a tremor and twitches on day 7; however, these were unlikely to have been due to nervous system excitability, because they resolved spontaneously in 3 hours and further administration of pethidine was not accompanied by further excitation.

Gastrointestinal

There is a high incidence of nausea and vomiting with intrathecal diamorphine, which may not be dose-related (164). Two studies have suggested that the incidence of nausea and vomiting in labor is higher with intrathecal than with epidural opioids (165,166).

Urinary tract

Urinary retention has been described in one of a series of patients who had been given pentazocine 5 mg intrathecally (167); others have since reported similar findings.

Skin

Pruritus is a frequent adverse effect after intrathecal administration, with an incidence of one-third with buprenorphine (168) and diamorphine (169) and over 70% for both diamorphine and morphine (170,171). In one study the incidence of pruritus was higher with morphine than with methadone; analgesia was also superior (170). Pruritus has also been reported with intrathecal pethidine (meperidine). Treatment was not reported to be necessary. This effect is not reported to occur after intrathecal beta-endorphin (172,173). The mechanism of pruritus is not well understood and has been attributed to a disturbance of thiamine metabolism (174) and to a disturbance of afferent input at supraspinal as well as at spinal receptor sites (175).

In a comparison of sufentanil 7.5 micrograms intrathecally and 7.5 micrograms intravenously, intrathecal sufentanil had superior analgesic efficacy (176). There was pruritus in significantly more patients with intrathecal sufentanil (5 versus 0). Peripheral oxygen desaturation was only observed with intravenous sufentanil (n = 6).

Infection risk

Reactivation of *Herpes simplex* infection after epidural administration of opioids is well known. However, there have been reports of reactivation of *Herpes simplex* after intrathecal morphine for cesarean section (SEDA-17, 87) (SEDA-18, 84).

Concern has also been raised about the possible association of pruritus with re-activation of herpes labialis virus type II. Reactivation of oral *Herpes simplex* infection has been explored in patients receiving intrathecal morphine and intravenous morphine (177). More patients had reactivation of *Herpes simplex* with intrathecal morphine than with intravenous morphine (19 versus 8). There was also a significantly higher incidence of pruritus with intrathecal morphine. These results suggest that there is a cause-and-effect relation between pruritus and herpes re-activation.

Susceptibility factors
Knowledge of the use of spinal opioids in children is limited, but adverse effects are similar to those reported in adults (SEDA-18, 85) (178–180). Dysphoria has also been reported, but attributed to systemic absorption (180).

Labor
In a comparison of intrathecal fentanyl and systemic hydromorphone (1mg intramuscularly + 1 mg intravenously) in nulliparous women in spontaneous labor, intrathecal administration was associated with less nausea and vomiting than systemic administration (181). Intrathecal nalbuphine for elective cesarean delivery is associated with fewer adverse effects than other opioids (such as morphine) (138).

Epidural route
The epidural route tends to provide high-quality analgesia and is rational in patients with a short life expectancy when systemic treatment of chronic pain has failed. Fentanyl and morphine are the most common opioids given in this way. Some limitations of this route include: risk of infection; spinal hematoma; reduced mobility due to cumbersome equipment (138). Adverse effects are not infrequent but do not tend to be severe or life-threatening. Again, old age and respiratory disease probably dispose to respiratory depression (182). As can be predicted from pharmacokinetic considerations, delayed respiratory depression is more common with epidural morphine than with fentanyl (183).

All forms of epidural analgesia (both continuous epidural infusion and patient-controlled infusion) provided superior analgesia compared with patient-controlled intravenous analgesia (184,185). Continuous infusion epidural analgesia is superior to patient-controlled epidural analgesia; patients on continuous epidural infusion have a lower incidence of pruritus but higher incidences of nausea, vomiting, and motor block (184).

Epidural administration of opioids has been reviewed (SEDA-21, 92). Morphine causes less respiratory depression and provides better analgesia when it is given by continuous infusion than by intermittent bolus. The authors concluded that epidural fentanyl offers no advantage over the intravenous route and that the mechanism of analgesia is by a systemic effect due to the vascular absorption of this lipophilic drug. However, the administration of lipophilic opioids together with a local anesthetic offers the advantage of using lower doses of both drugs, giving comparable analgesia with a reduction in adverse effects.

Epidural needle or catheter misplacement are complications justifying the need for an epidural test dose. The reliability of the epidural test dose has been reviewed (186).

Postoperative epidural analgesia has been compared with postoperative patient-controlled intravenous analgesia following radical retropubic prostatectomy in 60 patients (187). The epidural techniques gave better pain management. Significantly more patients who received epidural morphine required antiemetics and maximum expiratory pressure was significantly lower at 4 and 24 hours in those whose received it by PCA.

The use of an epidural catheter for liver resection can be associated with adverse events resulting from impaired coagulation related to impaired liver function. In one study continuous naropine epidural analgesia, was compared to single-shot intrathecal morphine in 50 patients undergoing liver resection (188). Both techniques provided adequate pain control. Morphine caused more pruritus (16% versus 0%) and nausea (16% versus 4%), but both groups had the same incidence of vomiting. There were no headaches or hematomas. The authors suggested that the epidural technique was not superior and that the potential associated risks of coagulopathies are worth considering.

Studies of the use of the partial opioid agonist butorphanol to reduce the adverse effects of epidural morphine have not provided evidence of benefit (SEDA-19, 86). Epidural meptazinol has been described as being well tolerated (189).

Respiratory
Respiratory depression occurs less often after epidural than intrathecal opioid administration (154,155). It has been suggested that older patients and those with increased intrathoracic or intra-abdominal pressure are particularly at risk and require reduced dosages (182). In a retrospective study, in which over 6000 patients received epidural morphine, 220 epidural pethidine, and 90 intrathecal morphine, respiratory depression requiring naloxone occurred in about 0.33% after epidural morphine and 5.5% after intrathecal morphine (155). Only two of the patients who received epidural morphine had respiratory depression later than 6 hours after the last dose of opioid. Only three of the 22 patients who had respiratory depression after epidural morphine had not received opioids in addition to epidural morphine during or after the operation. Ten were over 70 years old and 10 had thoracic injections. In another study of 2000 women who received 9000 doses of epidural pethidine 50 mg there was only one case of respiratory depression; this was due to migration of the catheter into the subarachnoid space (190).

The time taken for diffusion of poorly lipid-soluble opioids, such as morphine, from the lumbar subarachnoid space to the fourth ventricle is the most likely explanation for the delayed onset of respiratory depression. It has been suggested that the frequency of respiratory depression can be influenced by the position of the patient and the form of administration, as well as by the dosage of the opioid and the volume of the solution (156).

Doxapram has been used to treat respiratory depression after epidural morphine (191). However, the patient still required endotracheal intubation and mechanical ventilation to correct severe hypercapnia.

Markedly lipid-soluble opioids have also been reported to cause respiratory depression. There was profound respiratory depression 100 minutes after the administration of fentanyl 100 micrograms epidurally (192), whilst epidural sufentanil caused apnea within a couple of minutes, reversed by nalbuphine (193). Epidural buprenorphine 150 micrograms produced prolonged time-dependent biphasic depression of carbon dioxide response in six healthy volunteers. The second maximum occurred at 8–10 hours after injection (194). Similar cases have been reported by others.

Respiratory depression occurred 3.5 hours after a 2.5-year-old child had been given a caudal epidural of 100 micrograms/kg of morphine (195). The effects were successfully reversed by intravenous naloxone.

The efficacy of up to two doses of epidural hydromorphine 1.5 mg has been evaluated in 10 women after cesarean section (196). The mean duration of analgesia was 19.3 hours. Adverse effects were pruritus (56–70%), nausea (11–20%), and vomiting (less than 10%). There was a significant increase in venous PCO_2 3 hours after the second dose of hydromorphine. There was no delayed respiratory depression.

Extradural diamorphine 5 mg, extradural phenoperidine 2 mg, and intramuscular diamorphine 5 mg have been compared (197). Extradural diamorphine produced more prolonged and intense analgesia and there were no serious adverse effects.

Epidural opioids have a much better safety margin in patients who are already tolerant to such drugs (198). Tolerance has also not proven to be a problem (199).

Cardiovascular

Both severe hypotension and severe hypertension have occurred after epidural pethidine (200,201).

There were symptoms of shock lasting 2–3 hours in two women with advanced cancer who were given epidural buprenorphine 300 micrograms after becoming tolerant to epidural morphine (202). The buprenorphine was given 12 hours after the last dose of morphine. Symptoms started within 2 hours of administration and remitted spontaneously.

The use of epidural buprenorphine to treat cancer pain is associated with early respiratory depression (203).

Nervous system

Myoclonic seizures after epidural morphine 25 mg/hour and after intrathecal hydromorphone have been reported (204).

- A 30-year-old known epileptic woman who had undergone cesarean section developed a tonic-clonic seizure 6 hours after epidural morphine (205).

Two cases of Menière-like syndrome (SEDA-16, 83; 206), and vertical nystagmus and blurred vision (SEDA-16, 83; SEDA-17, 86), have been reported after epidural morphine.

Catatonia has been reported after a continuous infusion of epidural morphine (207). Hallucinations were thought to be an important sign of impending intoxication.

Mechanical difficulties, in the form of backflow of solution from epidural catheters, occurred in 31 of 32 patients and there were neurological complications in a further two of eight patients in whom the catheter had been tunnelled and connected to a subcutaneous access port; epidural fibrosis with compression of the spinal cord was presumed to be the cause (198).

Epidural fibrosis is a reported complication after long-term epidural morphine administration (SEDA-17, 85).

Psychological, psychiatric

Psychomotor symptoms have been noted subsequent to epidural buprenorphine (208).

Gastrointestinal

Whereas a high incidence (50%) of delayed (6 hours) nausea and vomiting has been reported in volunteers who received epidural morphine (209), there is a low incidence postoperatively (210). In another series the incidence of nausea (12%) and vomiting (24%) was similar whether morphine was used intramuscularly or epidurally or saline was injected epidurally (211). In labor the incidence of this adverse effect is low with epidural opioids (190,212) compared with intrathecal opioids (165,166). The incidence appears to fall with repeated dosing and is very low in patients with cancer who require long-term opioids (156,213). Nausea and vomiting have also been reported after fentanyl (214,215) and pethidine (216). The effects are abolished by intravenous naloxone without loss of analgesia (217).

Urinary tract

Current evidence suggests that the urodynamic effects of epidural morphine are not dose-related, and the incidence is similar to that reported after intramuscular injections. Urinary retention is more frequent after the use of epidural opioids in volunteers compared with patients (218,221). In one series (209) two patients who had failed to respond to bethanechol 5 mg subcutaneously, responded to intravenous naloxone 400 micrograms, and in other studies all subjects responded to naloxone 800 micrograms (219–222), which suggests that the mechanism involves opioid receptors. There was a 22% incidence of urinary retention in 90 postoperative patients who received epidural morphine (223), and in another series a rate of 39% (157). In a dose–response study of epidural morphine in increments of 0.5–8 mg (224) there was a similar incidence of urinary retention at all doses. These results are similar to those in a volunteer study involving 30 subjects who received 2, 4, or 10 mg of morphine epidurally (219).

Skin

Pruritus has been noted after epidural morphine, pethidine (meperidine), diamorphine (heroin), and fentanyl, with a quoted incidence of 1–100%. Troublesome pruritus occurs in only about 1% of cases (SED-11, 139) (145). In one study of postoperative patients who received morphine 10 mg epidurally, pruritus occurred in 28% of patients (157), but in only 1% of patients in other studies who received 5 and 2 mg morphine (SED-11, 139). With pethidine 50 mg epidurally after cesarean section, there was a 50% incidence of pruritus, but it was troublesome in only one patient (190). Pruritus has been reviewed in relation to parturition (225,226). It occurred in 593 cases (43%) in pregnant women compared with 3050 non-parturients (8.4%). These findings are borne out by other comparative work (191). Pruritus after cesarean section was more common with epidural morphine and fentanyl than with buprenorphine or butorphanol (227).

Suggested mechanisms for the difference in the incidence of pruritus in parturients and non-parturients include high plasma concentrations of maternal endorphins during labor together with more distant spread of morphine within the CSF, competition by estrogens for opioid-binding sites, and hormonal modifications of endogenous opioid concentrations at opioid receptors. It has also been suggested that the incidence of all adverse effects after spinal opioids may be higher in pregnant women, for the reasons stated above.

Various approaches have been used to try to eliminate pruritus with opioids. Substitution of epidural buprenorphine for morphine in combination with bupivacaine relieved severe unremitting pruritus in a single case (228). Injection of 10 mg nalbuphine subcutaneously significantly reduced the pruritus induced by epidural fentanyl within 15 minutes in 24 patients (229). Naltrexone 6 mg by mouth significantly reduced the incidence of pruritus after epidural morphine without affecting analgesia, but a dose of 9 mg was associated with a shorter duration of analgesia (230). Naloxone and propofol can reduce pruritus (SEDA-19, 87) (209), and the addition of droperidol to epidural sufentanil reduced the adverse effects of nausea, vomiting, and pruritus (SEDA-19, 88).

Spinal opioids probably cause widespread alterations in sensory modulation, as it occurs when there is evidence of opioid migration over the entire spinal cord to the brain. The dominant feature of facial pruritus, which is often reported, can be explained by rapid penetration of opioid to the superficially placed caudal portions of the nucleus of the spinal tract of the trigeminal nerve (209).

Pruritus is not due to preservatives in formulations, as it occurs with non-preservative-containing opioid solutions (231). It is unlikely to be due to histamine release, as the effect occurs about 3 hours after spinal or epidural administration (209,232–234) and occurs with fentanyl, which does not cause histamine release, in contrast to morphine (235).

Immunologic

An anaphylactic reaction to epidural fentanyl has been reported (236).

Body temperature

Maternal pyrexia has been reported following epidural opioid analgesia during labor. This may be the result of vascular and thermoregulatory modifications induced by the epidural analgesia (237).

Fetotoxicity

The effect of obstetric epidural administration of a mixture of 8 ml of bupivacaine (0.25%) with fentanyl 50 micrograms has been studied in 40 offspring (238). Fetal distress occurred in 11 babies, five of whom needed resuscitation; there was no correlation between fetal distress and plasma fentanyl concentrations in the neonates.

The use of epidural opioids in labor can pose a risk to the fetus (239), but in a series of 40 parturients who received either epidural morphine 2.0–7.5 mg or bupivacaine (10 patients), the opioid did not produce respiratory depression in the neonate (240).

Labor

Patient-controlled epidural analgesia in labor did not result in increased maternal satisfaction or control compared with conventional epidural blockage in 90 mothers who were randomized to three groups: patient-controlled epidural analgesia with bupivacaine and fentanyl; patient-controlled epidural analgesia with bupivacaine; and intermittent bolus epidural analgesia with bupivacaine and fentanyl (241). The two groups who took fentanyl had significantly more adverse effects, such as vomiting and pruritus.

Drug formulations

In comparisons of lipophilic and hydrophilic opioids, the latter are associated with higher pain scores (184). The epidural method is the preferred route by patients undergoing cesarean section, because often the anesthetic procedure itself is epidural.

Lipid-encapsulated morphine (DepoDur™) has the advantage of sustained release and prolonged analgesia when administered epidurally (138). In a comparison of DepoDur™ (5, 10, 15, 20, or 25 mg) and standard epidural morphine a single dose of DepoDur was well tolerated; 97% of patients rated adverse events (nausea, vomiting, pruritus, and hypotension) as mild to moderate (242). Fewer of the patients who received DepoDur (87%) required intravenous fentanyl for breakthrough pain than those who received standard epidural morphine (98%). The doses of DepoDur were well tolerated and the adverse effects profile was acceptable and predictable. However, further studies are required to determine the optimum dosage and safety in different patient populations.

A similar study of DepoDur up to 48 hours after elective cesarean delivery showed that DepoDur was well tolerated, with mild to moderate adverse events, and was as beneficial as standard morphine (243).

In a study of a low-volume continuous infusion mix (9 ml bupivacaine 0.5%; clonidine 150 micrograms, and diamorphine over 30 hours) in 65 patients, pain relief improved, as did adverse effects, such as drowsiness, confusion, hallucinations, and constipation. Serious adverse reactions were infrequent. More common adverse events were related to the route of administration, such as superficial infections (11%), deep infections (2.1%), paresthesia (4.3%), and line migration/dislocation (32%) (244).

Patient-controlled analgesia

Patient-controlled analgesia (PCA), intravenously, subcutaneously, intramuscularly, epidurally, or transdermally, is the method that patients prefer (245). It gives them increased autonomy, greater control, reduced anxiety, "better pain relief", and "not worrying about receiving too much drug" (138,184,244). The technique's effectiveness depends on appropriate patient alertness, education, and motivation. Methods that require a pump have some disadvantages— well-trained nursing staff are required and pumps can be cumbersome, limiting patient mobility. Potentially life-threatening adverse events can occur through errors in programming (246).

- A 51-year-old man was given postoperative piritramide by perfusor pump. He was found dead a few hours later. Autopsy, histopathology, and toxicology suggested piritramide overdose. Recent servicing of the perfusor pump had resulted in a change in settings from mg/hour to ml/hour. Consequently, he had received 1.5 times the intended dose of piritramide.

Despite its limitations, the technique has the advantage of reducing peaks and troughs and is superior to ordinary intramuscular administration. Recent technology has seen the development of a fentanyl–PCA transdermal patch. This is a needle-free patch that delivers fentanyl on demand through a low-intensity direct electric current, transferring ionizable drug transdermally into the systemic circulation. It is programmed to deliver fixed doses over 10 minutes, to a total of 80 doses or over a total period of 24 hours. This system overcomes the various limitations of PCA outlined above. It reduces programming errors, is non-invasive, does not require patient motivation, and it is not attached to a pump, facilitating early mobility and recovery (244). It is easy to use and produces adequate pain relief. It is also well-tolerated, the most common adverse effect being nausea. It is less sedating and disorienting than intravenous PCA morphine and may therefore be more suitable for elderly patients (244).

Drug overdose

Acute opioid poisoning involves marked CNS depression, with drowsiness, loss of consciousness, and coma. Other prominent features are a reduced respiratory rate, hypotension, and symmetrical pinpoint pupils (unless the patient has been hypoxic for some time, in which case the pupils can be dilated). Reduced urine output, hypothermia, flaccid skeletal muscles, and pulmonary edema can also be present. Convulsions have occurred in children.

Rhabdomyolysis in association with myoglobinuric renal insufficiency and cardiac failure has been reported with a variety of agents (SEDA-8, 76) (247).

Respiratory depression can be rapidly reversed by clearing the airway, ventilating the patient, and giving intravenous naloxone. The duration of action of naloxone is generally shorter than that of opioids, necessitating periodic repeated administration.

Drug–Drug Interactions

General

For various interactions, see Table 2.

Opioids can reduce or prolong the gastrointestinal absorption of other drugs. The partial opioid agonists, for example buprenorphine and pentazocine, can antagonize the effect of poor opioid agonists.

Increased respiratory depression can occur if other respiratory depressant drugs, for example hypnotics, sedatives, or alcohol, are taken concurrently. Muscle relaxants and antihistamines with sedative properties have a similar effect.

Alcohol

The use and abuse of alcohol by individuals taking opioid substitution therapy is common. The effect of opioid substitution therapy on blood alcohol concentration has been studied in compared non-drug-using controls (n = 22) and individuals taking methadone (n = 14), levacetylmethadol (n = 14), or buprenorphine (n = 12) (248). Participants were given alcohol 14.7 g/kg 2–3 hours before opioid therapy and 1–2 hours after. In those taking opioid substitution therapy there was a reduced blood alcohol concentration, especially at peak opiate plasma concentrations. Although the difference was significant the clinical implication is likely to be minimal.

COX-2 inhibitors

Analgesic agents are commonly used in combination, with the aim of benefiting from their additive or synergistic effect on analgesia and from the potential to reduce the prevalence of adverse effects due to lower dosage regimens. There has been a systematic review of opioid-related adverse events in studies of opioid-sparing postoperative pain treatment with COX-2 inhibitors (rofecoxib, celecoxib, parecoxib and valdecoxib) (249). The opioids were hydrocodone, fentanyl, hydromorphone, morphine, tramadol, and pethidine. The results did not support the opinion that opioid-sparing is associated with a reduced frequency of adverse events. Vomiting was significantly reduced in only three of the 18 trials. There was also no evidence to support a reduced risk of other opioid-related adverse events, except for dizziness.

Hormonal contraceptives—oral

Increased glucuronidation may explain the fact that oral contraceptives enhance morphine clearance (252).

Lidocaine

A synergistic interaction of intrathecal fentanyl 100 µg and morphine 0.5 mg, given before induction, with systemically administered lidocaine 200 mg 4 hours later for ventricular tachycardia, resulted in potentiation of opioid effects in a 74-year-old man with major heart disease after coronary artery bypass grafting; during the 5 minutes after lidocaine he had a respiratory arrest with loss of consciousness and miotic pupils, all reversed by naloxone (253). The proposed mechanism was thought to be a reduction in calcium ion concentrations in opioid-sensitive CNS sites.

Monoamine oxidase inhibitors

Opioid analgesics interact with non-selective monoamine oxidase inhibitors, causing nervous system excitation and hypertension (250).

Concomitant use of some opioid analgesics, such as pethidine or dextropropoxyphene, with the selective monoamine oxidase inhibitors selegiline and moclobemide can enhance their nervous system toxicity (251).

Phenothiazines

Hypotensive effects are increased if opioids and phenothiazines are used together (SED-9, 109).

References

1. Grubb BD. Peripheral and central mechanisms of pain. Br J Anaesth 1998;81(1):8–11.
2. Jordan B, Devi LA. Molecular mechanisms of opioid receptor signal transduction. Br J Anaesth 1998;81(1):12–9.
3. Harrison C, Smart D, Lambert DG. Stimulatory effects of opioids. Br J Anaesth 1998;81(1):20–8.
4. Collett BJ. Opioid tolerance: the clinical perspective. Br J Anaesth 1998;81(1):58–68.
5. Elliott K, Kest B, Man A, Kao B, Inturrisi CE. N-methyl-D-aspartate (NMDA) receptors, mu and kappa opioid tolerance, and perspectives on new analgesic drug development. Neuropsychopharmacology 1995;13(4):347–56.
6. Belgrade MJ. Control of pain in cancer patients. Postgrad Med 1989;85(4):319–23326–9.
7. Chapman CR, Hill HF. Prolonged morphine self-administration and addiction liability. Evaluation of two theories in a bone marrow transplant unit. Cancer 1989;63(8):1636–44.
8. Royal College of Surgeons. The College of Anaesthetists Commission on the Provision of Surgical Services. Report on the Working Party on Pain after Surgery. London, 1991:12.
9. Foley KM. The treatment of cancer pain. N Engl J Med 1985;313(2):84–95.
10. Angell M. The quality of mercy. N Engl J Med 1982;306(2):98–9.
11. Porter J, Jick H. Addiction rare in patients treated with narcotics. N Engl J Med 1980;302(2):123.
12. Evans PJ. Narcotic addiction in patients with chronic pain. Anaesthesia 1981;36(6):597–602.
13. Coote JC, Hughes AM, McKane M, et al. Drug consumption in chronic pain patients. Br J Pharm Pract 1986;9:193.
14. Jovey, RD, Ennis J, Gardner-Nix J, Goldman B, Hays H, Lynch M, Moulin M, Moulin D. Use of opioid analgesics for the treatment of chronic non-cancer pain. A consensus statement and guidelines from the Canadian Pain Society, 2002. Pain Res Manage 2003;8 Suppl A:3A–14A.
15. Gilron I, Bailey JM. Trends in opioid use for chronic neuropathic pain: a survey of patients pursuing enrolment in clinical trials. Can J Anesth 2003;50:42–7.
16. Littlejohn C, Baldacchino A, Bannister J. Chronic non-cancer pain and opioid dependence. J R Soc Med 2004;97:62–5.
17. Littlejohn C, Bannister J, Baldacchino S. Comorbid chronic non-cancer pain and opioid use disorders. Hosp Med 2004;65:206–9.
18. Molloy AR. The role of opioids in chronic nonmalignant pain. Mod Med Aust 1999;42:52–61.
19. Bannwarth B. Risk–benefit assessment of opioids in chronic noncancer pain. Drug Saf 1999;21(4):283–96.
20. Symon DN. Twelve cases of analgesic headache. Arch Dis Child 1998;78(6):555–6.
21. Scott BH. Opioids in cardiac surgery: cardiopulmonary bypass and inflammatory response. Int J Cardiol 1998;64(Suppl 1):S35–41.
22. Corey PJ, Heck AM, Weathermon RA. Amphetamines to counteract opioid-induced sedation. Ann Pharmacother 1999;33(12):1362–6.
23. Tramer MR, Walder B. Efficacy and adverse effects of prophylactic antiemetics during patient-controlled analgesia therapy: a quantitative systematic review. Anesth Analg 1999;88(6):1354–61.
24. Broome IJ, Robb HM, Raj N, Girgis Y, Wardall GJ. The use of tramadol following day-case oral surgery. Anaesthesia 1999;54(3):289–92.
25. Wang JJ, Ho ST, Liu YH, Ho CM, Liu K, Chia YY. Dexamethasone decreases epidural morphine-related nausea and vomiting. Anesth Analg 1999;89(1):117–20.
26. Kyriakides K, Hussain SK, Hobbs GJ. Management of opioid-induced pruritus: a role for 5-HT$_3$ antagonists? Br J Anaesth 1999;82(3):439–41.
27. Borgeat A, Stirnemann HR. Ondansetron is effective to treat spinal or epidural morphine-induced pruritus. Anesthesiology 1999;90(2):432–6.
28. Dimitriou V, Voyagis GS, Kyriakides K. Opioid-induced pruritus: repeated vs single dose ondansetron administration in preventing pruritus after intrathecal morphine. Br J Anaesth 1999;83(5):822–3.
29. Somrat C, Oranuch K, Ketchada U, Siriprapa S, Thipawan R. Optimal dose of nalbuphine for treatment of intrathecal-morphine induced pruritus after caesarean section. J Obstet Gynaecol Res 1999;25(3):209–13.
30. Juntti-Patinen L, Kuitunen T, Pere P, Neuvonen PJ. Drug-related visits to a district hospital emergency room. Basic Clin Pharmacol Toxicol 2006;98(2):212–7.
31. Richman JM, Liu SS, Courpas G, Wong R, Rowlingson AJ, McGready J, Cohen SR, Wu CL. Does continuous peripheral nerve block provide superior pain control to opioids? A meta-analysis. Anesth Analg 2006;102:248–57.
32. Snir-Mor I, Weinstock M, Davidson JT, Bahar M. Physostigmine antagonizes morphine-induced respiratory depression in human subjects. Anesthesiology 1983;59(1):6–9.
33. Brashear RE. Effects of heroin, morphine, methadone and propoxyphene on the lung. Semin Respir Med 1980;2:59.
34. Agius R. Opiate inhalation and occupational asthma. BMJ 1989;298(6669):323.
35. Sternbach HA, Annitto W, Pottash AL, Gold MS. Anorexic effects of naltrexone in man. Lancet 1982;1(8268):388–9.
36. Campora E, Merlini L, Pace M, Bruzzone M, Luzzani M, Gottlieb A, Rosso R. The incidence of narcotic-induced emesis. J Pain Symptom Manage 1991;6(7):428–30.
37. Miller NS, Swiney T, Barkin RL. Effects of opioid prescription medication dependence and detoxification on pain perceptions and self-reports. Am J Ther 2006;13(5):436–44.
38. Pud D, Cohen D, Lawental E, Eisenberg E. Opioids and abnormal pain perception: new evidence from a study of chronic opioid addicts and healthy subjects. Drug Alcohol Depend 2006;82:218–23.
39. Bruera E, Macmillan K, Hanson J, MacDonald RN. The cognitive effects of the administration of narcotic analgesics in patients with cancer pain. Pain 1989;39(1):13–6.
40. Nielsen SL, Christensen LQ, Nielsen LM. Analgetika, benzodiazepiner og trafik. [Analgesics, benzodiazepines and traffic.] Ugeskr Laeger 1989;151(28):1822–5.

41. Albanese J, Viviand X, Potie F, Rey M, Alliez B, Martin C. Sufentanil, fentanyl, and alfentanil in head trauma patients: a study on cerebral hemodynamics. Crit Care Med 1999;27(2):407–11.

42. Daeninck PJ, Bruera E. Opioid use in cancer pain. Is a more liberal approach enhancing toxicity? Acta Anaesthesiol Scand 1999;43(9):924–38.

43. Fong HK, Sands LP, Leung JM. The role of postoperative analgesia in delirium and cognitive decline in elderly patients:a systematic review. Anesth Analg 2006;102:1255–66.

44. Ng KFJ, Yuen TST, Ng VMW. A comparison of postoperative cognitive function and pain relief with fentanyl or tramadol patient-controlled analgesia. J Clin Anesth 2006;18(3):205–10.

45. Ersche KD, Clark L, London M, Robbins TW, Sahakian BJ. Profile of executive and memory function associated with amphetamine and opiate dependence. Neuropsychopharmacology 2006;31:1036–47.

46. George R. Hypothalamus: anterior pituitary gland. In: Clonet DH, editor. Narcotic Drugs: Biochemical Pharmacology. New York: Plenum Press, 1971:283.

47. Raff H, Flemma RJ, Findling JW. Fast cortisol-induced inhibition of the adrenocorticotropin response to surgery in humans. J Clin Endocrinol Metab 1988;67(6):1146–8.

48. Pfeiffer A, Herz A. Endocrine actions of opioids. Horm Metab Res 1984;16(8):386–97.

49. Duthie DJ, Nimmo WS. Adverse effects of opioid analgesic drugs. Br J Anaesth 1987;59(1):61–77.

50. In: Goodman Gilman A, Rall TW, Nies AS, Taylor P, editors. Goodman and Gilman's The Pharmacological Basis of Therapeutics. 8th ed.. Oxford: Pergamon Press, 1990:494.

51. Mehendale SR, Yuan C-S. Opioid-induced gastrointestinal dysfunction. Dig Dis 2006;24:105–12.

52. Longacre AV, Aslanian H. Acute colonic pseudo-obstruction after colonoscopy in a young woman on narcotics. J Clin Gastroenterol 2006;40(3):225.

53. Isenhower HL, Mueller BA. Selection of narcotic analgesics for pain associated with pancreatitis. Am J Health Syst Pharm 1998;55(5):480–6.

54. Levy JH, Brister NW, Shearin A, Ziegler J, Hug CC Jr, Adelson DM, Walker BF. Wheal and flare responses to opioids in humans. Anesthesiology 1989;70(5):756–60.

55. Kinjo M, Setoguchi S, Schneeweiss S, Solomon DH. Bone mineral density in subjects using central nervous system-active medications. Am J Med 2005;118(12):1414.e7-1414.e12.

56. Lazarides SP, Varghese D, Nanu AM. Heroin induced osteopenia: a cause of bilateral insufficiency femoral neck fracture in a young adult. Eur J Orthop Surg Traumatol 2005;15(4):322–5.

57. Vestergaard P, Rejnmark L, Mosekilde L. Fracture risk associated with the use of morphine and opiates. J Intern Med 2006;260:76–87.

58. Mendelson JH, Mello NK. Plasma testosterone levels during chronic heroin use and protracted abstinence. A study of Hong Kong addicts. Clin Pharmacol Ther 1975;17(5):529–33.

59. Spring WD Jr, Willenbring ML, Maddux TL. Sexual dysfunction and psychological distress in methadone maintenance. Int J Addict 1992;27(11):1325–34.

60. Roberts LJ, Finch PM, Pullan PT, Bhagat CI, Price LM. Sex hormone suppression by intrathecal opioids: a prospective study. Clin J Pain 2002;18(3):144–8.

61. Wang ZY, Wang CQ, Yang JJ, Sun J, Huang YH, Tang QF, Qian YN. Which has the least immunity depression during postoperative analgesia-morphine, tramadol, or tramadol with lornoxicam? Clin Chim Acta 2006;369(1):40–5.

62. Schwacha MG, McGwin JrG, Hutchinson CB, Cross JM, MacLennan PA, Rue LW. The contribution of opiate analgesics to the development of infectious complications in burn patients. Am J Surg 2006;192(1):82–6.

63. Hall W, Lynskey M, Degenhardt L. Trends in opiate-related deaths in the United Kingdom and Australia, 1985–1995. Drug Alcohol Depend 2000;57(3):247–54.

64. Heinemann A, Iwersen-Bergmann S, Stein S, Schmoldt A, Puschel K. Methadone-related fatalities in Hamburg 1990–1999: implications for quality standards in maintenance treatment? Forensic Sci Int 2000;113(1–3):449–55.

65. Garrick TM, Sheedy D, Abernethy J, Hodda AE, Harper CG. Heroin-related deaths in Sydney, Australia. How common are they? Am J Addict 2000;9(2):172–8.

66. Cullen W, Bury G, Langton D. Experience of heroin overdose among drug users attending general practice. Br J Gen Pract 2000;50(456):546–9.

67. Christie B. Gangrene bug killed 35 heroin users. West J Med 2000;173(2):82–3.

68. Gill JR, Graham SM. Ten years of "body packers" in New York City: 50 deaths. J Forensic Sci 2002;47(4):843–6.

69. Koch A, Reiter A, Meissner C, Oehmichen M. Ursache des Todes von Heroinkonsumenten mit niedrigen Morphin-Konzentrationen im Blut. [Cause of death in heroin users with low blood morphine concentration.] Arch Kriminol 2002;209(3–4):76–87.

70. Paulozzi LJ, Budnitz DS, Xi Y. Increasing deaths from opioid analgesics in the United States. Pharmacoepidemiol Drug Saf 2006;15(9):618–27.

71. Fernandez W, Hackman H, McKeown L, Anderson T, Hume B. Trends in opioid-related fatal overdoses in Massachusetts, 1990-2003. J Subst Abuse Treat 2006;31(2):151–6.

72. Morgan O, Griffiths C, Hickman M. Association between availability of heroin and methadone and fatal poisoning in England and Wales 1993-2004. Int J Epidemiol 2006;35:1579–85.

73. Bakker A, Sibanda V. Is methadone too dangerous for opiate addiction? Issue is one of toxicity v acceptability. BMJ 2006;332:53.

74. Soyka M, Penning R, Wittchen U. Fatal poisoning in methadone and buprenorphine treated patients. Are there differences? Pharmacopsychiatry 2006;39:85–7.

75. Siang Hui Lai, Yi Ju Yaob, Danny Siaw Teck Lo. A survey of buprenorphine related deaths in Singapore. Forensic Sci Int 2006;162:80–6.

76. Chan GM, Stajic M, Marker EK, Hoffman RS, Nelson LS. Testing positive for methadone and either a tricyclic antidepressant or a benzodiazepine is associated with an accidental overdose death: analysis of medical examiner data. Acad Emerg Med 2006;13:543–7.

77. Barrie J, Carley S. Prediction of fatal overdose in opiate addicts. Emerg Med J 2006;23:647–8.

78. Wright IV C, Kramer D, Zalman M, Smith MY, Haddox JD. Risk identification, risk assessment, and risk management of abusable drug formulations. Drug Alcohol Depend 2006;83S:S68–S76.

79. Suresh S, Anand KJ. Opioid tolerance in neonates: mechanisms, diagnosis, assessment, and management. Semin Perinatol 1998;22(5):425–33.

80. Eddy NB, Halbach H, Isbell H, Seevers MH. Drug dependence: its significance and characteristics. Bull World Health Organ 1965;32(5):721–33.

81. Kleber HD, Riordan CE. The treatment of narcotic withdrawal: a historical review. J Clin Psychiatry 1982;43 (6 Pt 2):30–4.

82. Kolb L, Himmelsbach CK. Clinical studies of drug addiction. III. A clinical review of withdrawal treatment with a

method of evaluating abstinence syndromes. Am J Psychiatry 1938;94:759.

83. Isbell H, Vogel VH, Chapman KW. Present status of narcotic addiction with particular reference to medical indications and comparative addiction liability of the newer and older analgesic drugs. JAMA 1948;138:1019.

84. Glossop M, Johns A, Green L. Opiate withdrawal: inpatient vs out-patient programmes and preferred vs random assignment to treatment. BMJ (Clin Res Ed) 1986;293:103.

85. Gossop M, Green L, Phillips G, Bradley B. What happens to opiate addicts immediately after treatment: a prospective follow up study. BMJ (Clin Res Ed) 1987;294(6584):1377–80.

86. Kleber HD. Detoxification from narcotics. In: Lowinson L, Ruiz P, editors. Substance Abuse. Baltimore: Williams and Wilkins, 1981:317.

87. Phillips GT, Gossop M, Bradley B. The influence of psychological factors on the opiate withdrawal syndrome. Br J Psychiatry 1986;149:235–8.

88. Gossop M, Bradley B, Phillips GT. An investigation of withdrawal symptoms shown by opiate addicts during and subsequent to a 21-day in-patient methadone detoxification procedure. Addict Behav 1987;12(1):1–6.

89. Gossop M, Griffiths P, Bradley B, Strang J. Opiate withdrawal symptoms in response to 10-day and 21-day methadone withdrawal programmes. Br J Psychiatry 1989;154:360–3.

90. Newman RG, Whitehill WB. Double-blind comparison of methadone and placebo maintenance treatments of narcotic addicts in Hong Kong. Lancet 1979;2(8141):485–8.

91. Lowinson JH, Marion IJ, Joseph H, Dole VP. Methadone maintenance. In: Lowinson JH, Ruiz P, Millman RB, editors. Substance Abuse: A Comprehensive Textbook. 2nd ed.. Baltimore: Williams and Wilkins, 1992:550.

92. Ball JC, Ross A. The Effectiveness of Methadone Maintenance TreatmentNew York: Springer-Verlag;. 1991.

93. Gold MS, Redmond DE Jr, Kleber HD. Noradrenergic hyperactivity in opiate withdrawal supported by clonidine reversal of opiate withdrawal. Am J Psychiatry 1979;136(1):100–2.

94. Gold MS, Byck R, Sweeney DR, Kleber HD. Endorphin-locus coeruleus connection mediates opiate action and withdrawal. Biomedicine 1979;30(1):1–4.

95. Anonymous. Clonidine treatment for acute opiate withdrawal. Med Lett 1979;21:100.

96. Charney DS, Kleber HD. Iatrogenic opiate addiction: successful detoxification with clonidine. Am J Psychiatry 1980;137(8):989–90.

97. Charney DS, Sternberg DE, Kleber HD, Heninger GR, Redmond DE Jr. The clinical use of clonidine in abrupt withdrawal from methadone. Effects on blood pressure and specific signs and symptoms. Arch Gen Psychiatry 1981;38(11):1273–7.

98. Rounsaville BJ, Kosten T, Kleber H. Success and failure at outpatient opioid detoxification. Evaluating the process of clonidine- and methadone-assisted withdrawal. J Nerv Ment Dis 1985;173(2):103–10.

99. Kleber HD, Riordan CE, Rounsaville B, Kosten T, Charney D, Gaspari J, Hogan I, O'Connor C. Clonidine in outpatient detoxification from methadone maintenance. Arch Gen Psychiatry 1985;42(4):391–4.

100. Ghodse H, Myles J, Smith SE. Clonidine is not a useful adjunct to methadone gradual detoxification in opioid addiction. Br J Psychiatry 1994;165(3):370–4.

101. Charney DS, Heninger GR, Kleber HD. The combined use of clonidine and naltrexone as a rapid, safe, and effective treatment of abrupt withdrawal from methadone. Am J Psychiatry 1986;143(7):831–7.

102. National Institute on Drug Abuse. Drug Dependence in Pregnancy: Clinical Management of Mother and Child. Services Research Monograph Series. NIDA, DHEW Publication, No. ADM 79–678.

103. National Institute on Drug Abuse. Drug Dependence in Pregnancy: Clinical Management of Mother and Child. Services Research Monograph Series NIDA, DHEW Publication, No. ADM 79-678;. 1979 Rockville, MD, 1979.

104. Finnegan LP. Pulmonary problems encountered by the infant of the drug-dependent mother. Clin Chest Med 1980;1(3):311–25.

105. Ghodse AH, Reed JL, Mack JW. The effect of maternal narcotic addiction on the newborn infant. Psychol Med 1977;7(4):667–75.

106. Olofsson M, Buckley W, Andersen GE, Friis-Hansen B. Investigation of 89 children born by drug-dependent mothers. I. Neonatal course. Acta Paediatr Scand 1983;72(3):403–6.

107. Rosen TS, Johnson HL. Children of methadone-maintained mothers: follow-up to 18 months of age. J Pediatr 1982;101(2):192–6.

108. Johnson HL, Rosen TS. Prenatal methadone exposure: effects on behavior in early infancy. Pediatr Pharmacol (New York) 1982;2(2):113–20.

109. Herman NL, Calicott R, Van Decar TK, Conlin G, Tilton J. Determination of the dose–response relationship for intrathecal sufentanil in laboring patients. Anesth Analg 1997;84(6):1256–61.

110. Arkoosh VA, Cooper M, Norris MC, Boxer L, Ferouz F, Silverman NS, Huffnagle HJ, Huffnagle S, Leighton BL. Intrathecal sufentanil dose response in nulliparous patients. Anesthesiology 1998;89(2):364–70.

111. Herman NL, Choi KC, Affleck PJ, Calicott R, Brackin R, Singhal A, Andreasen A, Gadalla F, Fong J, Gomillion MC, Hartman JK, Koff HD, Lee SH, Van Decar TK. Analgesia, pruritus, and ventilation exhibit a dose–response relationship in parturients receiving intrathecal fentanyl during labor. Anesth Analg 1999;89(2):378–83.

112. Lo WK, Chong JL, Chen LH. Combined spinal epidural for labour analgesia—duration, efficacy and side effects of adding sufentanil or fentanyl to bupivacaine intrathecally vs plain bupivacaine. Singapore Med J 1999;40(10):639–43.

113. Mardirosoff C, Dumont L. Two doses of intrathecal sufentanil (2.5 and 5 microgram) combined with bupivacaine and epinephrine for labor analgesia Anesth Analg 1999;89(5):1263–6.

114. D'Angelo R, Evans E, Dean LA, Gaver R, Eisenach JC. Spinal clonidine prolongs labor analgesia from spinal sufentanil and bupivacaine. Anesth Analg 1999;88(3):573–6.

115. Lardizabal JL, Belizan JM, Carroli G, Gonzalez L, Campodonico L, Aguillaume CJ. A randomized trial of nalbuphine vs meperidine for analgesia during labor. Ref Gynecol Obstet 1999;6:245–8.

116. Hallworth SP, Fernando R, Bell R, Parry MG, Lim GH. Comparison of intrathecal and epidural diamorphine for elective caesarean section using a combined spinal-epidural technique. Br J Anaesth 1999;82(2):228–32.

117. Caranza R, Jeyapalan I, Buggy DJ. Central neuraxial opioid analgesia after caesarean section: comparison of

epidural diamorphine and intrathecal morphine. Int J Obstet Anesth 1999;8(2):90–3.

118. Fanshawe MP. A comparison of patient controlled epidural pethidine versus single dose epidural morphine for analgesia after caesarean section. Anaesth Intensive Care 1999;27(6):610–4.

119. Vercauteren MP, Mertens E, Schols G, Mol IV, Adriaensen HA. Patient-controlled extradural analgesia after caesarean section: a comparison between tramadol, sufentanil and a mixture of both. Eur J Pain 1999;3(3): 205–10.

120. Cooper DW, Saleh U, Taylor M, Whyte S, Ryall D, Kokri MS, Desira WR, Day H, McArthur E. Patient-controlled analgesia: epidural fentanyl and i.v. morphine compared after caesarean section Br J Anaesth 1999;82(3):366–70.

121. Siddik-Sayyid S, Aouad-Maroun M, Sleiman D, Sfeir M, Baraka A. Epidural tramadol for postoperative pain after Cesarean section. Can J Anaesth 1999;46(8):731–5.

122. Ron M, Menashe M, Scherer D, Palti Z. Fetal heart rate decelerations following the administration of meperidine-promethazine during labor. Int J Gynaecol Obstet 1982;20(4):301–5.

123. Tejavej A, Siripoonya P, Saungsomboon A, Chiewsilp D. Morphine and birth asphyxia. J Med Assoc Thai 1984;67(Suppl 2):73–9.

124. Belsey EM, Rosenblatt DB, Lieberman BA, Redshaw M, Caldwell J, Notarianni L, Smith RL, Beard RW. The influence of maternal analgesia on neonatal behaviour: I. Pethidine. Br J Obstet Gynaecol 1981;88(4):398–406.

125. Gear RW, Miaskowski C, Gordon NC. K-opioids produce significantly greater analgesia in women than in men. Nature Med 1996;2:1248–50.

126. Gear RW, Miaskowski C, Gordon NC. The κ-opioid nalbuphine produces gender and close-dependent analgesia and antianalgesia in patients with postoperative pain. Pain 1999;83:339–45.

127. Dohan A, Sarton E, Teppema I, Olivier C. Sex-related differences in the influence of morphine on ventilatory controls in humans. Anaesthesiology 1998;88L:903–13.

128. Sarton E, Teppema I, Dohan A. Sex differences in morphine induced ventilatory depression reside in the peripheral chemoreflex loop. Anaesthesiology 1999;90:1329–38.

129. Zacny J P. Gender differences in opioid analgesia in human volunteers: cold pressor and mechanical pain (CPDD abstract). NIDA Research Monograph 2002;182:22–3.

130. Miller PL, Ernst A. Sex differences in analgesia: a randomized trial of μ versus κ opioid agonists. South Med J 2004;97:35–41.

131. Fillingim RB, Ness TJ, Glover TL, Campbell CM, Price DD, Staird R. Experimental pain models reveal no sex differences in pentazocine analgesia in humans. Anaesthesiology 2004;100:1263–70.

132. McQuay H, Moore A. Be aware of renal function when prescribing morphine. Lancet 1984;2(8397):284–5.

133. Sear JW, Hand CW, Moore RA, McQuay HJ. Studies on morphine disposition: influence of renal failure on the kinetics of morphine and its metabolites. Br J Anaesth 1989;62(1):28–32.

134. Sloan P, Slatkin N, Ahdieh H. Effectiveness and safety of oral extended-release oxymorphone for the treatment of cancer pain: a pilot study. Supportive Care Cancer 2005;13(1):57–65.

135. Mercadante S, Arcuri E, Fusco F, Tirelli W, Villari P, Bussolino C, Campa T, De Conno F, Ripamonti C. Randomized double-blind, double-dummy crossover clinical trial of oral tramadol versus rectal tramadol

administration of opioid-naive cancer patients with pain. Supportive Care Cancer 2005;13(9):702–7.

136. Elkader A, Sproule B. Buprenorphine: clinical pharmacokinetics in the treatment of opioid dependence. Clin Pharmacokinet 2005;44(7):661–80.

137. Coon TP, Miller M, Kaylor D, Jones-Spangle K. Rectal insertion of fentanyl patches: a new route of toxicity. Ann Emerg Med 2005;46(5):473.

138. Gadsden J, Hart S, Santos AC. Post-caesarean delivery analgesia. Anesth Analg 2005;101(5 Suppl):S62–9.

139. Yukawa Y, Kato F, Ito K, Terashima T, Horie Y. A prospective randomized study of pre-emptive analgesia for postoperative pain in the patients undergoing posterior lumbar interbody fusion: continuous subcutaneous morphine, continuous epidural morphine, and diclofenac sodium. Spine 2005;30(21):2357–61.

140. Farr SJ, Otulana BA. Pulmonary delivery of opioids as pain therapeutics. Adv Drug Delivery Rev 2006;58:1076–88.

141. Mitchell TB, Lintzeris N, Bond A, Strang J. Feasibility and acceptability of an intranasal diamorphine spray as an alternative to injectable diamorphine for maintenance treatment. Eur Addiction Res 2006;12(2):91–5.

142. Bogod D. Advances in epidural analgesia for labour: progress versus prudence. Lancet 1995;345(8958):1129–30.

143. Collis RE, Davies DW, Aveling W. Randomised comparison of combined spinal-epidural and standard epidural analgesia in labour. Lancet 1995;345(8962):1413–6.

144. Chaney MA. Intrathecal and epidural anesthesia and analgesia for cardiac surgery. Anesth Analg 2006;102:45–64.

145. Cousins MJ, Mather LE. Intrathecal and epidural administration of opioids. Anesthesiology 1984;61(3):276–310.

146. Madrid JL, Fatela LV, Alcorta J, Guillen F, Lobato RD. Intermittent intrathecal morphine by means of an implantable reservoir: a survey of 100 cases. J Pain Symptom Manage 1988;3(2):67–71.

147. Dautheribes M, Guerin J. Analgesie par voie intrathécal Aproposde 50 cas. [Intrathecal analgesia. Apropos of 50 cases.] Neurochirurgie 1988;34(3):194–7.

148. Gestin Y, Pere N, Solassol C. Morphinothérapie isobare intrathécale au long cours. [Long-term intrathecal isobaric morphine therapy.] Ann Fr Anesth Reanim 1986;5(4): 346–50.

149. Blain PG, Lane RJ, Bateman DN, Rawlins MD. Opiate-induced rhabdomyolysis. Hum Toxicol 1985;4(1):71–4.

150. Bonnardot JP, Colau JC, Maillet M, Millot F, Salat-Baroux J. Analgesïe morphinique par voie intrathécalean cours de L'accouchement. [Morphine analgesia by the intrathecal route.] J Gynecol Obstet Biol Reprod (Paris) 1982;11(5):619–23.

151. Schmidt WK, Tam SW, Shotzberger GS, Smith DH Jr, Clark R, Vernier VG. Nalbuphine. Drug Alcohol Depend 1985;14(3–4):339–62.

152. Turker G, Goren S, Sahin S, Korfali G, Sayan E. Combination of intrathecal morphine and remifentanil infusion for fast-track anaesthesia in off-pump coronary artery bypass surgery. J Cardiothorac Vasc Anaesth 2005;19(6):708–13.

153. Roy J-D, Massicotte L, Sassine M-P, Seal RF, Roy A. A comparison of intrathecal morphine/fentanyl and patient-controlled analgesia with patient-controlled analgesia alone for analgesia after liver resection. Anesth Analgesia 2006;103(4):990–4.

154. Kossmann B, Dick W, Bowdler I, et al. The analgesic action and respiratory side effects of epidural morphine. A double-blind trial on patients undergoing vaginal hysterectomy. Reg Anaesth 1984;9:55.

155. Gustafsson LL, Schildt B, Jacobsen K. Adverse effects of extradural and intrathecal opiates: report of a nationwide survey in Sweden. Br J Anaesth 1982;54(5):479–86.

156. Glynn CJ, Mather LE, Cousins MJ, Wilson PR, Graham JR. Spinal narcotics and respiratory depression. Lancet 1979;2(8138):356–7.

157. Eriksen HO, Jensen FM. Bivirkninger ved anvendelse af opiater epidwalt og opinalt. [Adverse effects of epidural and spinal opiates.] Ugeskr Laeger 1982;144(36):2627–30.

158. Fitzpatrick GJ, Moriarty DC. Intrathecal morphine in the management of pain following cardiac surgery. A comparison with morphine i.v Br J Anaesth 1988;60(6): 639–44.

159. Yamaguchi H, Watanabe S, Motokawa K, Ishizawa Y. Intrathecal morphine dose–response data for pain relief after cholecystectomy. Anesth Analg 1990;70(2): 168–71.

160. Lazorthes Y. Intracerebroventricular administration of morphine for control of irreducible cancer pain. Ann NY Acad Sci 1988;531:123–32.

161. Glavina MJ, Robertshaw R. Myoclonic spasms following intrathecal morphine. Anaesthesia 1988;43(5):389–90.

162. Kleiner LI, Krzeminski J, Rosenwasser RH. Temporary motor and sensory paralysis associated with intrathecal administration of morphine. Neurosurgery 1989;24(5): 756–8.

163. Vranken JH, Van Der Vegt MH, Van Kan HJM, Kruis MR. Plasma concentrations of meperidine and normeperidine following continuous intrathecal meperidine in patients with neuropathic cancer pain. Acta Anaesthesiol Scand 2005;49(5):665–70.

164. Barron DW, Strong JE. The safety and efficacy of intrathecal diamorphine. Pain 1984;18(3):279–85.

165. Baraka A, Noueihid R, Hajj S. Intrathecal injection of morphine for obstetric analgesia. Anesthesiology 1981;54(2):136–40.

166. Scott PV, Bowen FE, Cartwright P, Rao BC, Deeley D, Wotherspoon HG, Sumrein IM. Intrathecal morphine as sole analgesic during labour. BMJ 1980;281(6236):351–5.

167. Swaraj, Saxena R, Sabzposh SW, Shakoor A. Effect on intrathecal pentazocine on postoperative pain relief. J Indian Med Assoc 1988;86(4):93–6.

168. Lipp M, Daublander M, Lanz E. Bupremorphin 0.15 mg intratheka Zur Postoperativen Analgesie. Eine Klinische Doppelblind studie. [0.15 mg Intrathecal buprenorphine applied for postoperative analgesia. A clinical double-blind study.] Anaesthesist 1987;36(5):233–8.

169. Reay BA, Semple AJ, Macrae WA, MacKenzie N, Grant IS. Low-dose intrathecal diamorphine analgesia following major orthopaedic surgery. Br J Anaesth 1989;62(3):248–52.

170. Jacobson L, Chabal C, Brody MC, Ward RJ, Ireton RC. Intrathecal methadone and morphine for postoperative analgesia: a comparison of the efficacy, duration, and side effects. Anesthesiology 1989;70(5):742–6.

171. Jacobson L, Kokri MS, Pridie AK. Intrathecal diamorphine: a dose–response study. Ann R Coll Surg Engl 1989;71(5):289–92.

172. Oyama T, Matsuki A, Taneichi T, Ling N, Guillemin R. beta-Endorphin in obstetric analgesia. Am J Obstet Gynecol 1980;137(5):613–6.

173. Oyama T, Jin T, Yamaya R, Ling N, Guillemin R. Profound analgesic effects of beta-endorphin in man. Lancet 1980;1(8160):122–4.

174. Saissy JM. Prurit après rachianesthésie à la péthidine. [Pruritus after spinal anesthesia with pethidine.] Ann Fr Anesth Reanim 1984;3(5):402.

175. Shipton EA. Pruritus—a side-effect of epidural fentanyl for postoperative analgesia. S Afr Med J 1984;66(2):61–2.

176. Fournier R, Weber A, Gamulin Z. Intrathecal sufentanil is more potent than intravenous for postoperative analgesia after total-hip replacement. Reg Anesth Pain Med 2005;30(3):249–54.

177. Davies PW, Vallejo MC, Shannon KT, Amortegui AJ, Ramanathan S. Oral Herpes simplex reactivation after intrathecal morphine: a prospective randomized trial in an obstetric population. Anesth Analg 2005;100(5):1472-6.

178. Tyler DC, Krane EJ. Epidural opioids in children. J Pediatr Surg 1989;24(5):469–73.

179. Tobias JD, Deshpande JK, Wetzel RC, Facker J, Maxwell LG, Solca M. Postoperative analgesia. Use of intrathecal morphine in children. Clin Pediatr (Phila) 1990;29(1):44–8.

180. Krane EJ, Tyler DC, Jacobson LE. The dose response of caudal morphine in children. Anesthesiology 1989;71(1):48–52.

181. Wong CA, Scavone BM, Peaceman AM, McCarthy RJ, Sullivan JT, Diaz NT, Yaghmour E, Marcus RJL, Sherwani SS, Sproviero MT, Yilmaz M, Patel R, Robles C, Grouper S. The risk of caesarean delivery with neuroaxial analgesia given early versus late in labor. N Engl J Med 2005;352:655–65.

182. Von Palitzsch J. Respiratory effects of epidural morphine analgesia. Anaesthesiol Reanim 1982;7:335.

183. Lam AM, Knill RL, Thompson WR, et al. Epidural fentanyl does not cause delayed respiratory depression. Can J Anaesth 1983;30:578.

184. Wu CL, Cohen SR, Richman JM, Rowlingson AJ, Courpas GE, Cheung K, Lin EE, Liu SS. Efficacy of postoperative patient-controlled and continuous infusion epidural analgesia versus intravenous patient-controlled analgesia with opioids: a meta-analysis. Anaesthesiology 2005;103(5):1079–88.

185. Axelsson K, Johanzon E, Essving P, Weckstrom J, Ekback G. Postoperative extradural analgesia with morphine and ropivacaine. A double-blind comparison between placebo and ropivacaine 10 mg/h or 16 mg/h. Acta Anaesthesiol Scand 2005;49(8):1191–9.

186. Guay J. On the epidural test dose: a review. Anesth Analgesia 2006;102(3):921-9.

187. Gupta A, Fant F, Axelsson K, Sandblom D, Rykowski J, Johansson J-E, Andersson S-O. Postoperative analgesia after radical retropubic prostatectomy: a double-blind comparison between low thoracic epidural and patient-controlled intravenous analgesia. Anesthesiology 2006;105(4):784–93.

188. De Pietri L, Siniscalchi A, Reggiani A, Masetti M, Begliomini B, Gazzi M, Gerunda GE, Pasetto A. The use of intrathecal morphine for postoperative pain relief after liver resection: a comparison with epidural analgesia. Anesth Analg 2006;102:1157–63.

189. Budd K, Brown PM, Robson PJ. The treatment of chronic pain by the use of meptazinol administered into the epidural space. Postgrad Med J 1983;59(Suppl 1):68–71.

190. Brownridge P. Epidural and intrathecal opiates for postoperative pain relief. Anaesthesia 1983;38(1):74–6.

191. Thangathurai D, Nelson D, Cheung M. Doxapram for respiratory depression after epidural morphine. Anaesthesia 1990;45(1):64–5.

192. Brockway MS, Noble DW, Sharwood-Smith GH, McClure JH. Profound respiratory depression after extradural fentanyl. Br J Anaesth 1990;64(2):243–5.

193. Cheng EY, May J. Nalbuphine reversal of respiratory depression after epidural sufentanil. Crit Care Med 1989;17(4):378–9.

194. Molke Jensen F, Jensen NH, Holk IK, Ravnborg M. Prolonged and biphasic respiratory depression following epidural buprenorphine. Anaesthesia 1987;42(5):470–5.

195. Krane EJ. Delayed respiratory depression in a child after caudal epidural morphine. Anesth Analg 1988;67(1): 79–82.

196. Dougherty TB, Baysinger CL, Gooding DJ. Epidural hydromorphine for postoperative analgesia after delivery by caesarean section. Reg Anaesth 1986;11:118.

197. Macrae DJ, Munishankrappa S, Burrow LM, Milne MK, Grant IS. Double-blind comparison of the efficacy of extradural diamorphine, extradural phenoperidine and i.m. diamorphine following caesarean section Br J Anaesth 1987;59(3):354–9.

198. Driessen JJ, de Mulder PH, Claessen JJ, van Diejen D, Wobbes T. Epidural administration of morphine for control of cancer pain: long-term efficacy and complications. Clin J Pain 1989;5(3):217–22.

199. Zenz M, Piepenbrock S, Tryba M. Epidural opiates: long-term experiences in cancer pain. Klin Wochenschr 1985;63(5):225–9.

200. Balaban M, Slinger P. Severe hypotension from epidural meperidine in a high-risk patient after thoracotomy. Can J Anaesth 1989;36(4):450–3.

201. Robinson RJ, Metcalf IR. Hypertension after epidural meperidine. Can Anaesth Soc J 1985;32(6):658–9.

202. Christensen FR, Andersen LW. Adverse reaction to extradural buprenorphine. Br J Anaesth 1982;54(4):476.

203. Davis MP. Buprenorphine in cancer pain. Support Care Cancer 2005;13:878–87.

204. Parkinson SK, Bailey SL, Little WL, Mueller JB. Myoclonic seizure activity with chronic high-dose spinal opioid administration. Anesthesiology 1990;72(4):743–5.

205. Borgeat A, Biollaz J, Depierraz B, Neff R. Grand mal seizure after extradural morphine analgesia. Br J Anaesth 1988;60(6):733–5.

206. Linder S, Borgeat A, Biollaz J. Meniére-like syndrome following epidural morphine analgesia. Anesthesiology 1989;71(5):782–3.

207. Engquist A, Jorgensen BC, Andersen HB. Catatonia after epidural morphine. Acta Anaesthesiol Scand 1981;25(5):445–6.

208. MacEvilly M, Carroll CO. Hallucination repression after epidural buprenorphine. BMJ 1989;298:928.

209. Bromage PR, Camporesi EM, Durant PA, Nielsen CH. Nonrespiratory side effects of epidural morphine. Anesth Analg 1982;61(6):490–5.

210. Torda TA, Pybus DA. Clinical experience with epidural morphine. Anaesth Intensive Care 1981;9(2):129–34.

211. Lanz E, Theiss D, Riess W, Sommer U. Epidural morphine for postoperative analgesia: a double-blind study. Anesth Analg 1982;61(3):236–40.

212. Perriss BW, Malins AF. Pain relief in labour using epidural pethidine with adrenaline. Anaesthesia 1981;36(6):631–3.

213. Howard RP, Milne LA, Williams NE. Epidural morphine in terminal care. Anaesthesia 1981;36(1):51–3.

214. Lirzin JD, Jacquinot P, Dailland P, Jorrot JC, Jasson J, Talafre ML, Conseiller C. Controlled trial of extradural bupivacaine with fentanyl, morphine or placebo for pain relief in labour. Br J Anaesth 1989;62(6):641–4.

215. Kreitzer JM, Kirschenbaum LP, Eisenkraft JB. Epidural fentanyl by continuous infusion for relief of postoperative pain. Clin J Pain 1989;5(4):283–90.

216. Perriss BW, Latham BV, Wilson IH. Analgesia following extradural and i.m. pethidine in post-caesarean section patients Br J Anaesth 1990;64(3):355–7.

217. Rawal N, Wattwil M. Respiratory depression after epidural morphine—an experimental and clinical study. Anesth Analg 1984;63(1):8–14.

218. Bromage PR, Camporesi E, Chestnut D. Epidural narcotics for postoperative analgesia. Anesth Analg 1980;59(7): 473–80.

219. Rawal N, Mollefors K, Axelsson K, Lingardh G, Widman B. An experimental study of urodynamic effects of epidural morphine and of naloxone reversal. Anesth Analg 1983;62(7):641–7.

220. Torda TA, Pybus DA, Liberman H, Clark M, Crawford M. Experimental comparison of extradural and i.m. morphine Br J Anaesth 1980;52(9):939–43.

221. Thompson WR, Smith PT, Hirst M, Varkey GP, Knill RL. Regional analgesic effect of epidural morphine in volunteers. Can Anaesth Soc J 1981;28(6):530–6.

222. Rawal N, Mollefors K, Axelsson K, Lingardh G, Widman B. Naloxone reversal of urinary retention after epidural morphine. Lancet 1981;2(8260–1):1411.

223. Rawal N, Sjostrand U, Dahlstrom B. Postoperative pain relief by epidural morphine. Anesth Analg 1981;60(10): 726–31.

224. Martin R, Salbaing J, Blaise G, Tetrault JP, Tetreault L. Epidural morphine for postoperative pain relief: a dose–response curve. Anesthesiology 1982;56(6):423–6.

225. Ballantyne JC, Loach AB, Carr DB. Itching after epidural and spinal opiates. Pain 1988;33(2):149–60.

226. Ballantyne JC, Loach AB, Carr DB. The incidence of pruritus after epidural morphine. Anaesthesia 1989;44(10):863.

227. Ackerman WE, Juneja MM, Kaczorowski DM, Colclough GW. A comparison of the incidence of pruritus following epidural opioid administration in the parturient. Can J Anaesth 1989;36(4):388–91.

228. Keaveny JP, Harper NJ. Treatment of epidural morphine-induced pruritus with buprenorphine. Anaesthesia 1989;44(8):691.

229. Davies GG, From R. A blinded study using nalbuphine for prevention of pruritus induced by epidural fentanyl. Anesthesiology 1988;69(5):763–5.

230. Abboud TK, Afrasiabi A, Davidson J, Zhu J, Reyes A, Khoo N, Steffens Z. Prophylactic oral naltrexone with epidural morphine: effect on adverse reactions and ventilatory responses to carbon dioxide. Anesthesiology 1990;72(2):233–7.

231. Sghirlanzoni S, Sala F, Servadio G, et al. Epidural morphine and pruritus: the role of sodium metabisulphite. Anest Rianim 1983;24:177.

232. Bromage PR, Camporesi EM, Durant PA, Nielsen CH. Rostral spread of epidural morphine. Anesthesiology 1982;56(6):431–6.

233. Bromage PR, Camporesi EM, Durant PA, Nielsen CH. Influence of epinephrine as an adjuvant to epidural morphine. Anesthesiology 1983;58(3):257–62.

234. Bromage PR, Camporesi E, Leslie J. Epidural narcotics in volunteers: sensitivity to pain and to carbon dioxide. Pain 1980;9(2):145–60.

235. Rosow CE, Moss J, Philbin DM, Savarese JJ. Histamine release during morphine and fentanyl anesthesia. Anesthesiology 1982;56(2):93–6.

236. Zucker-Pinchoff B, Ramanathan S. Anaphylactic reaction to epidural fentanyl. Anesthesiology 1989;71(4):599–601.

237. Fusi L, Steer PJ, Maresh MJ, Beard RW. Maternal pyrexia associated with the use of epidural analgesia in labour. Lancet 1989;1(8649):1250–2.

238. Dezeros G, Levron JC, Simon A, Taureau I, Roullier MA. Association bupivacaine-fentanyl dans l'analgésie péridwale de long ue durée au cours du travail. [Combination of bupivacaine and fentanyl in long-term epidural analgesia during labor.] Agressologie 1988;29(1):33–7.

239. Nybell-Lindahl G, Carlsson C, Ingemarsson I, Westgren M, Paalzow L. Maternal and fetal concentrations of morphine

after epidural administration during labor. Am J Obstet Gynecol 1981;139(1):20–1.

240. Hughes SC, Rosen MA, Shnider SM, Abboud TK, Stefani SJ, Norton M. Maternal and neonatal effects of epidural morphine for labor and delivery. Anesth Analg 1984;63(3):319–24.

241. Nikkola E, Läärä A, Hinkka S, Ekblad U, Kero P, Salonen M. Patient-controlled epidural analgesia in labour does not always improve maternal satisfaction. Acta Obstet Gynaecol 2006;85:188–94.

242. Gambling D, Hughes T, Martin G, Horton W, Manvelian G. A comparison of DepoDur(tm), a novel, single-dose extended-release epidural morphine for pain relief after lower abdominal surgery. Anesth Analg 2005;100(4):1065–74.

243. Carvalho B, Riley E, Cohen SE, Gambling D, Palmer C, Huffnagle HJ, Polley L, Muir H, Segal S, Lihou C, Manvelian G. Single-dose, sustained-release epidural morphine in the management of post-operative pain after elective caesarean delivery: results of a multicentre randomized controlled study. Anesth Analg 2005;100(4):1150–8.

244. Linklater GT, Macaulay L. Epidural analgesia in advanced cancer patients. Anesth Analg 2005;100(2):600–1.

245. Sinatra R. The fentanyl HCl patient-controlled transdermal system. Clin Pharmacokinet 2005;44(Suppl 1):1–6.

246. Musshoff F, Padosch SA, Madea B. Death during patient-controlled analgesia: piritramide overdose and tissue distribution of the drug. Forensic Sci Int 2005;154:247–51.

247. Scherrer P, Delaloye-Bischof A, Turini G, Perret C. Participation myocardique à la rhabdomyolyse non traumatique après surdosage aux opiates. [Myocardial involvement in nontraumatic rhabdomyolysis following an opiate overdose.] Schweiz Med Wochenschr 1985;115(34):1166–70.

248. Clark NC, Dietze P, Lenne' MG, Redman JR. Effect of opioid substitution therapy on alcohol metabolism. J Subst Abuse Treat 2006;30:191–6.

249. Romsing J, Moiniche S, Mathiesen O, Dahl JB. Reduction of opioid-related adverse events using opioid-sparing analgesia with COX-2 inhibitors lacks documentation: a systematic review. Acta Anaesthesiol Scand 2005;49(2):133–42.

250. British Medical Association, Royal Pharmaceutical Society of Great Britain. In: British National Formulary. 22nd ed. 1991:458.

251. Bonnet U. Moclobemide: therapeutic use and clinical studies. CNS Drug Rev 2003;9(1):97–140.

252. Watson KJR, Ghabrial H, Mashford ML, Harman PJ, Breen KJ, Desmond PV. The oral contraceptive pill increases morphine clearance but does not increase hepatic blood flow. Gastroenterology 1986;90:1779.

253. Jensen E, Nader ND. Potentiation of narcosis after intravenous lidocaine in a patient given spinal opioids. Anesth Analg 1999;89(3):758–9.

Alfentanil

General Information

Alfentanil is a potent short-acting opioid used in anesthesia. Beside its effects on opioid receptors, there is some evidence that it may affect acetylcholine, since intrathecal neostigmine produced a dose-dependent increase in the effect of alfentanil (SEDA-22, 3). Its rapid onset and short duration of action make alfentanil suitable for use in day care, although it is important to treat adverse effects before discharge.

Alfentanil is an ideal analgesic for focused and ambulatory interventions. In a prospective, uncontrolled study in three consecutive groups of outpatients undergoing shock-wave lithotripsy, group 1 (152 patients) had an induction dose of a combination of propofol 0.8 mg/kg and alfentanil 8 µg/kg; in group 2 (78 patients) and group 3 (250 patients), the induction dose was reduced by 20% (1). For all three groups the maintenance dose was a mixture of propofol 0.25 mg/kg and alfentanil 5 µg/kg given via a PCA device with a lock-out time of 5 minutes. In groups 1 and 2 the lithotripter was equipped with a standard electromagnetic shock-wave emitter (the EMSE 200), while in group 3 an upgraded EMSE F150 was used. Analgesic consumption was lower in the patients treated with the EMSE 150; groups 2 and 3, with a 20% reduction in induction dose, did not compensate by using more PCA. Groups 2 and 3 also had a significant reduction in the incidence of oxygen desaturation. The intravenous administration of a mixture of alfentanil and propofol, using the updated EMSE F150 device as in group 3, was therefore considered to be safe and reliable, with good patient tolerance and rapid recovery.

In a non-comparative study of 24 consecutive outpatients undergoing extracorporeal shock-wave lithotripsy, alfentanil (initial dose 15 µg/kg followed by 0.38 µg/kg/minute) and propofol (initial dose 1 mg/kg followed by 59 µg/kg/minute) were used for sedation (2). Both alfentanil and propofol were effective and safe, provided respiratory and cardiovascular parameters were routinely monitored.

Comparative studies

Alfentanil has been compared with morphine in the attenuation of experimental muscle pain in 28 healthy volunteers (3). The two opioids had similar analgesic effects, with limited effects in attenuating central hypersensitivity, showing that other drugs (in combination or alone) would be required for adequate muscle pain with a central component. The two drugs had similar adverse effects profiles, the main effects being dizziness, tiredness, itching, and flushing. Nausea was more common after morphine. No volunteers withdrew because of adverse effects.

Alfentanil has been compared with fentanyl and remifentanil in 135 patients undergoing stereotactic brain biopsy (4). All regimens (intravenous alfentanil 7.5 micrograms/kg followed by 0.25 micrograms/kg/minute; intravenous fentanyl bolus 1 microgram/kg; and remifentanil 0.05 micrograms/kg/minute) provided similar hemodynamic and respiratory effects; however, fentanyl produced a lower mean heart rate, providing less hemodynamic stability.

Organs and Systems

Cardiovascular

When alfentanil 30 µg/kg was given to six healthy volunteers there were no clinical changes in respiratory or cardiovascular function (SEDA-16, 78).

Bradycardia often occurs with the combination of a potent short-acting opioid with suxamethonium during induction of anesthesia, and alfentanil has been reported to have caused sinus arrest in three patients (SEDA-17, 79; 5).

In one study alfentanil was particularly likely to cause hemodynamic instability and myocardial ischemia; however, drug interactions or the dosage regimen may have been responsible (6).

Respiratory

Significant respiratory depression occurs after alfentanil in doses in excess of 1000 μg and delayed-onset respiratory depression has been reported. Used as a general anesthetic for urgent cesarean section, alfentanil can cause marked neonatal respiratory depression, which is reversible with naloxone (SEDA-16, 78).

- A 35-year-old man developed recurrent respiratory depression after being given alfentanil 0.0125 mg/kg for vitreoretinal surgery (7). General anesthesia was induced with a combination of propofol, rocuronium, and alfentanil, subsequent inhalation of isoflurane, and three additional doses of alfentanil (total 0.04 mg/kg over 2 hours). The pulse oxygen saturation fluctuated and was as low as 89% 180 minutes after extubation.

The severity of respiratory depression with alfentanil has been assessed in 49 patients undergoing abdominal hysterectomy under general anesthetic, who were randomly allocated to three groups (8). Group 1 did not receive alfentanil during surgery, group 2 received alfentanil 30 μg/kg, and group 3 received a bolus dose of alfentanil 10–20 μg/kg and an alfentanil infusion increasing in increments of 0.25–0.5 mg/kg/minute. In this randomized double-blind study alfentanil had respiratory depressant effects (measured by plethysmography and pulse oximetry), in one patient in group 1 and three each in groups 2 and 3, but there were no cases of clear-cut recurrent respiratory depression.

Nervous system

Increased intracranial pressure in normal pressure hydrocephalus patients has been described (SEDA-17, 79). An acute dystonic reaction has been reported in an untreated patient with Parkinson's disease (SEDA-16, 78).

Simultaneous scalp and depth electrode recordings were performed on five patients with complex partial epilepsy who underwent alfentanil anesthesia induction before depth electrode removal (9). Five equal bolus doses of alfentanil 100 μg were given to each patient at 60-second intervals (total dose 500 μg). Epileptiform activity was increased in three of the five, but without clinical evidence of seizure activity.

Gastrointestinal

Alfentanil is associated with a high incidence of nausea and vomiting. Droperidol can reduce emetic symptoms but moclobemide does not (SEDA-17, 79).

- A 30-year-old woman with multiple body injuries required five general anesthetics in under 7 days for reconstructive surgery and dressing changes. In order to avoid further general anesthesia she was given a target-controlled infusion of alfentanil in 50 ml of 0.9% sodium chloride (a total dose of 5 mg over 35 minutes). There was one self-limiting episode of nausea with no vomiting. Oxygen saturation was 93–98% on air. There were no episodes of hypotension, cardiac dysrhythmias, or sedation (10).

Musculoskeletal

Muscular rigidity involving many muscle groups has been described with alfentanil (SEDA-12, 62).

Immunologic

A possible hypersensitivity reaction to alfentanil was reported in an atopic 13-year-old girl who developed life-threatening bronchospasm and confluent urticarial wheals (11).

Second-Generation Effects

Fetotoxicity

Alfentanil 10 μg/kg in normal parturients does not reduce Apgar scores, but a higher dose (15–30 μg/kg) is recommended for attenuation of the "stress" response in nonpregnant patients. In a randomized, placebo-controlled, double-blind study alfentanil was used in 40 patients in a dose of 10 μg/kg 1 minute before induction of anesthesia in 40 uncomplicated cesarean deliveries to determine whether it would reduce the maternal stress response after tracheal intubation without subsequent neonatal depression (12). There was a small but significant improvement in maternal hemodynamic stability in the alfentanil group at the expense of early but transient neonatal depression.

Susceptibility Factors

Age

Care is needed when alfentanil is used in the elderly, in whom the elimination of alfentanil is slower (13).

Other features of the patient

Recovery times were shorter in smokers than in nonsmokers (14).

Alfentanil is 90% protein bound, and variability in protein binding can affect its actions. In 10 patients who received standardized anesthesia and alfentanil to a target concentration of 150 ng/ml for postoperative analgesia interindividual variation in plasma protein binding explained at least 39% of the interindividual variability in alfentanil requirements (15). There was a high incidence of adverse effects: seven patients had emesis and five had urinary retention.

Drug dosage regimens

The combination of alfentanil + propofol is indicated for classic laryngeal mask airway insertion. In 75 adult Chinese patients undergoing minor surgery there was apnea in all subjects, increasing with increasing doses of alfentanil (5, 10, 15, and 20 micrograms/kg) (16). The optimal combination for effective insertion of a laryngeal mask was propofol 2.5 mg/kg + alfentanil 10 micrograms/kg.

Drug administration route

Administration of intranasal alfentanil to 36 children with acute moderate to severe pain provided adequate analgesia with no adverse events (17).

Drug–Drug Interactions

Benzodiazepines

Muscle rigidity after high-dose opioid can be reduced by the benzodiazepines midazolam and diazepam (SEDA-19, 82).

Diltiazem

Diltiazem reduces the elimination of alfentanil and prolongs the time to tracheal extubation (SEDA-21, 86); erythromycin may do the same (18).

Fluconazole

There has been a double-blind randomized control study of the effect of the antifungal drug fluconazole 400 mg on the pharmacokinetics and pharmacodynamics of intravenous alfentanil (19). Fluconazole given either orally or intravenously 1 hour before alfentanil 20 μg/kg intravenously caused a significant doubling of the half-life, by inhibition of CYP3A4, which metabolizes alfentanil. Intravenous and oral fluconazole both increased alfentanil-induced respiratory depression by reducing the respiratory rate by 10–15% compared with alfentanil alone. Alfentanil should therefore be given cautiously to patients taking fluconazole and the authors suggested that such patients require 60% less alfentanil for maintenance of analgesia, irrespective of the mode of administration of the antifungal drug.

In a randomized, double-blind, placebo-controlled, crossover study in nine subjects, fluconazole 400 mg reduced the clearance of alfentanil 20 micrograms/kg by 55% and increased alfentanil-induced subjective effects (19).

Ketamine

Eight healthy men participated in a 2-day study in which alfentanil was given to a constant plasma concentration of 50 ng/ml followed by the addition of ketamine at escalating plasma concentrations of 50, 100, and 200 ng/ml (20). The resting hypoventilation induced by alfentanil was antagonized by ketamine 200 ng/ml, but not 50 ng/ml.

The interaction of ketamine with the respiratory depressant effect of alfentanil has been studied in eight healthy men, who received alfentanil as a continuous computer-controlled infusion aiming at a plasma concentration of 50 ng/ml and either an infusion of racemic ketamine increasing step-wise through 50, 100, and 200 ng/ml or placebo (20). Alfentanil caused hypoventilation by reducing respiratory rate, and this was antagonized by ketamine in a concentration-dependent manner. This combination may be effective in overcoming the adverse effects of either agent individually.

Macrolide antibiotics

The metabolism of alfentanil, a potent short-acting narcotic, is inhibited by macrolide antibiotics, resulting in significant changes in half-life and clearance (21).

Reserpine

The combination of reserpine with alfentanil is reported to cause ventricular dysrhythmias (SEDA-17, 79).

Tranylcypromine

There is no interaction of alfentanil with the monoamine oxidase inhibitor tranylcypromine (SEDA-17, 79).

References

1. Tailly GG, Marcelo JB, Schneider IA, Byttebier G, Daems K. Patient-controlled analgesia during SWL treatments. J Endourol 2001;15(5):465–71.
2. Nociti JR, Zuccolotto SN, Cagnolatl CA, Oliveira ACM, Bastos MM. Propofol and alfentanil sedation for extracorporeal shock wave lithotripsy. Rev Bras Anestesiol 2002;1:74–8.
3. Schulte H, Segerdahl M, Graven-Nielsen T, Grass S. Reduction of human experimental muscle pain by alfentanil and morphine. Eur J Pain 2006;10(8):733–41.
4. Bilgin H, Basagan Mogol E, Bekar A, Iscimen R, Korfali G. A comparison of effects of alfentanil, fentanyl, and remifentanil on hemodynamic and respiratory parameters during stereotactic brain biopsy. J Neurosurg Anesthesiol 2006;18(3):179–84.
5. Ananthanarayan C. Sinus arrest after alfentanil and suxamethonium. Anaesthesia 1989;44(7):614.
6. Nathan HJ. Narcotics and myocardial performance in patients with coronary artery disease. Can J Anaesth 1988;35(3Pt 1):209–13.
7. Calenda E, Muraine M. Recurrent respiratory depression after low doses of alfentanil. Eur J Anaesthesiol 1999;16(3):206.
8. Snijdelaar DG, Katz J, Clairoux M, Sandler AN. Respiratory effects of intraoperative alfentanil infusion in post-abdominal hysterectomy patients: a comparison of high versus low dose. Acute Pain 2000;3:131–9.
9. Ross J, Kearse LA Jr, Barlow MK, Houghton KJ, Cosgrove GR. Alfentanil-induced epileptiform activity: a simultaneous surface and depth electroencephalographic study in complex partial epilepsy. Epilepsia 2001;42(2):220–5.
10. Gallagher G, Rae CP, Watson S, Kinsella J. Target-controlled alfentanil analgesia for dressing change following extensive reconstructive surgery for trauma. J Pain Symptom Manage 2001;21(1):1–2.
11. Coventry DM, Stone P. Hypersensitivity reactions to alfentanil? Anaesthesia 1988;43(10):887–8.
12. Gin T, Ngan-Kee WD, Siu YK, Stuart JC, Tan PE, Lam KK. Alfentanil given immediately before the induction of anesthesia for elective cesarean delivery. Anesth Analg 2000;90(5):1167–72.

13. Kent AP, Dodson ME, Bower S. The pharmacokinetics and clinical effects of a low dose of alfentanil in elderly patients. Acta Anaesthesiol Belg 1988;39(1):25–33.
14. Dechene JP. Alfentanil as an adjunct to thiopentone and nitrous oxide in short surgical procedures. Can Anaesth Soc J 1985;32(4):346–50.
15. van den Nieuwenhuyzen MC, Engbers FH, Burm AG, Vletter AA, van Kleef JW, Bovill JG. Target-controlled infusion of alfentanil for postoperative analgesia: contribution of plasma protein binding to intra-patient and inter-patient variability. Br J Anaesth 1999;82(4):580–5.
16. Yu ALY, Critchley LAH, Lee A, Gin T. Alfentanil dosage when inserting the classic laryngeal mask airway. Anesthesiology 2006;105(4):684–8.
17. Brenchley J, Ramlakhan S. Intranasal alfentanil for acute pain in children. Emerg Med J 2006;23:488.
18. Ahonen J, Olkkola KT, Salmenpera M, Hynynen M, Neuvonen PJ. Effect of diltiazem on midazolam and alfentanil disposition in patients undergoing coronary artery bypass grafting. Anesthesiology 1996;85(6):1246–52.
19. Palkama VJ, Isohanni MH, Neuvonen PJ, Olkkola KT. The effect of intravenous and oral fluconazole on the pharmacokinetics and pharmacodynamics of intravenous alfentanil. Anesth Analg 1998;87(1):190–4.
20. Persson J, Scheinin H, Hellstrom G, Bjorkman S, Gotharson E, Gustafsson LL. Ketamine antagonises alfentanil-induced hypoventilation in healthy male volunteers. Acta Anaesthesiol Scand 1999;43(7):744–52.
21. Bartkowski RR, Goldberg ME, Larijani GE, Boerner T. Inhibition of alfentanil metabolism by erythromycin. Clin Pharmacol Ther 1989;46(1):99–102.

Alphaprodine

General Information

Alphaprodine is a synthetic opioid that is rapidly absorbed after oral submucosal injection (1). It is used in pediatric dentistry, but it has been withdrawn from the market on a number of occasions because of concerns about its safety. Problems include hypoxia, reduced respiratory rate, and generalized venodilatation with local cyanosis.

Reference

1. Currie WR, Biery KA, Campbell RL, Mourino AP. Narcotic sedation: an evaluation of cardiopulmonary parameters and behavior modification in pediatric dental patients. J Pedod 1988;12(3):230–49.

Buprenorphine

General Information

Buprenorphine is a partial agonist at OP_3 (μ) opioid receptors and an antagonist at OP_2 (κ) receptors.

In a double-blind, randomized study of three groups of 18 patients having abdominal surgery who received single doses of either intramuscular pethidine 75 mg, with sublingual buprenorphine 400 µg, or buprenorphine 300 µg alone, sedation and nausea were the most common adverse effects in all three groups. Patients who received sublingual buprenorphine were significantly less sedated in the immediate postoperative period (1).

In a 3-day randomized, placebo-controlled study, 40 patients with acute pancreatitis or acute-on-chronic pancreatitis were given either buprenorphine 2.4 mg/day or procaine hydrochloride 2 g/day by constant intravenous infusion (2). The patients who received buprenorphine had significantly lower pain scores than those given procaine and were significantly less likely to demand additional analgesia. The adverse effect profiles were similar in the two groups, with the exception of a significantly higher rate of sedation in those who were given buprenorphine. The authors suggested that intravenous buprenorphine is more effective and safer than procaine in acute pancreatitis.

Buprenorphine has been suggested to be useful for the treatment of cocaine and opiate dependence. In a study designed to assess its safety for this purpose (SEDA-18, 85) there were no adverse effects or serious interactions with a single dose of intravenous morphine or cocaine during daily maintenance on buprenorphine.

International experience with buprenorphine has been reviewed, highlighting the role of buprenorphine in reducing drug-related harm and curtailing the spread of infection (3). Its effect in reducing drug-related deaths, premature births, and drug abuse by injection is also described.

The adverse effects profile of buprenorphine has been reviewed and suggested to be favorable compared with other opioid agonists (4). The common adverse effects are headache, pain, insomnia, sweating, gastrointestinal discomfort, and the opioid withdrawal syndrome. Although it is rare, respiratory depression has occurred, especially with parenteral use and with concomitant use of benzodiazepines. This risk has also been highlighted elsewhere (5).

Placebo-controlled studies

In a randomized controlled trial the safety of buprenorphine for detoxification from opiates was highlighted (6). There were no withdrawals because of treatment-related adverse events.

Systematic reviews

A systematic review of the role of buprenorphine in the treatment of opioid dependence showed that it has therapeutic efficacy and a high safety profile, but is not necessarily suitable as a replacement to methadone (7). It is an additional treatment option for heroin-dependent patients, especially those who do not want to start or continue taking methadone, or for those who do not seem to benefit from optimal dosages of methadone (8).

Organs and Systems

Cardiovascular

- A 27-year-old man injected a 2 mg suspension of crushed oral buprenorphine into his left ulnar artery, leading to acute ischemia of the hand; he was successfully treated with iloprost and dextran-40 (9).
- A 22-year-old man snorted an 8 mg crushed tablet of buprenorphine and 2 hours later had crushing chest pain, which resolved within a few minutes (10). The symptom recurred 3 weeks later after another inhalation of buprenorphine. An electrocardiogram suggested an acute anterior myocardial infarction caused by buprenorphine-induced coronary artery spasm.

Respiratory

Respiratory depression can occur with buprenorphine. It is not often a clinical problem, except in older and weaker subjects, in whom it can be fatal (11). When it occurs it is often prolonged and can be particularly difficult to reverse (SEDA-16, 87). Norbuprenorphine, a metabolite of buprenorphine via CYP3A4 causes dose-dependent respiratory depression, perhaps mediated by opioid receptors in the lung rather than the brain, and is 10 times more potent than buprenorphine (SEDA-22, 103).

Buprenorphine showed a ceiling effect in its ability to cause respiratory depression in both rats and humans (12). There was a non-linear dose-response relation, due to partial MOR receptor agonism, between buprenorphine and respiratory effect.

Non-cardiogenic pulmonary edema has been reported after a single dose of buprenorphine (SEDA-19, 89).

Nervous system

Sedation and nausea are relatively frequent. When buprenorphine is used for patient-controlled analgesia, minor dysphoria or euphoria has been reported (SEDA-16, 88).

In one of three patients receiving epidural buprenorphine for the relief of pain from head and neck cancers, it was discontinued because of severe dizziness (SEDA-17, 87).

Psychiatric

In a comparison of buprenorphine and methadone in alleviating mood disturbances in conjunction with carbamazepine in 30 patients, buprenorphine was associated with better mood stabilization and short-term relief of depressive symptoms than methadone; both treatments were safe and without unexpected adverse effects (13).

Mouth and teeth

There have been reports of facial and lingual ulcers, the ulceration following repeated injection of buprenorphine into the left superior cervical ganglion for trigeminal neuralgia (14) and the use of sublingual buprenorphine (15).

Gastrointestinal

Impaired gastric emptying and delayed absorption after sublingual buprenorphine have been reported (SEDA-17, 87).

Buprenorphine has a low incidence of constipation compared with other opioids (16).

Liver

Buprenorphine can cause increased liver enzymes at normal doses and at high doses can cause hepatitis (16).

- A 33-year-old man developed severe hepatitis after an oral overdose of buprenorphine tablets 112 mg over 48 hours (17). He presented with an acute confusional state, including disorientation in time and The condition led to anuria and hepatorenal insufficiency. He was successfully treated with hemodialysis.

With increasing use of buprenorphine in the treatment of opioid dependence, it has been confirmed that the use of buprenorphine in opioid-dependent individuals with a history of hepatitis causes significant increases in aspartate transaminase and alanine transaminase activities (18). Liver enzymes should be monitored before giving buprenorphine to patients with hepatitis.

Four former opiate-dependent individuals with confirmed hepatitis C virus were given substitution therapy with sublingual buprenorphine. After injecting buprenorphine together with their sublingual doses, they had a marked increase in serum aspartate transaminase activity (13–50 times the upper limit of the reference range), resulting in jaundice (19). Another patient who was positive for hepatitis C and HIV developed jaundice, with panlobular liver necrosis and microvesicular steatosis, after using sublingual buprenorphine and small doses of paracetamol and aspirin (19).

Intravenous buprenorphine abuse precipitated acute-on-chronic hepatitis in a 25-year-old woman who was hepatitis C positive with a history of chronic diamorphine dependence (20).

Skin

There have been reports of severe pruritus with buprenorphine (21).

Musculoskeletal

Two cases of rhabdomyolysis and compressive neuropathy have been described (22). In both cases there was a history of drug abuse by injection and intravenous administration of crushed buprenorphine. It is not clear whether the adverse effects were due to buprenorphine or impurities.

Sexual function

Buprenorphine causes less sexual dysfunction than other opioids (16).

Immunologic

There have been reports of anaphylactic reactions with buprenorphine (23).

There is some evidence of immune system stimulation by buprenorphine at toxic concentrations (24). However, these results are based on experimental studies in rats and are unlikely to be relevant to humans.

Infection risk

Soft tissue infections due to *Gamella morbillorum* have been reported in patients who had received buprenorphine (25):

- A 38 year old male drug user with hepatitis C developed fever, pain, erythema, and areas of necrosis at the site of intravenous administration of buprenorphine. *Gamella morbillorum* was identified and he was treated with amoxicillin and gentamicin.
- A 39 year old male drug user developed fever and a subcutaneous abscess at the site of intravenous administration of buprenorphine. *Gamella morbillorum* was grown from pus cultures. He was treated with co-amoxiclav and gentamicin followed by amoxicillin.

Although cutaneous infections are frequent in drug addicts, there are not usually due to *Gamella morbillorum*. However, contamination by *Gamella morbillorum*, which forms part of the normal flora of the mouth, is possible, because addicts often use saliva to convert solid forms of drugs into solutions for intravenous administration.

Death

Two series of 39 and 78 deaths attributed to buprenorphine have respectively been reported in Strasbourg and 13 other French forensic centers between 1996 and 2000 (26). The risks incurred by the misuse of buprenorphine seem to arise through a combination of (a) the concomitant use of other psychotropic drugs (especially benzodiazepines and neuroleptic drugs) and (b) the improper use of tablets for intravenous administration and/or massive oral doses. The total recorded number of buprenorphine-related deaths is largely underestimated, because the very low concentrations require sensitive immunoassay techniques, making them difficult to detect; furthermore different cut-off points are used by different forensic pathology laboratories in diagnosing drug-related deaths.

Buprenorphine-related deaths have been reviewed (27). Between 1980 and 2002 43 deaths were identified in which buprenorphine was mentioned either in the death certificate or in the coroner's report. In most cases other drugs (often benzodiazepines) and alcohol had also been used, suggesting that the risk of death increased when buprenorphine was used in combination with other drugs. In seven cases, buprenorphine only was detected, questioning its high safety profile.

Long-Term Effects

Drug abuse

Abuse of buprenorphine has been reported in many countries and it is now widely dealt with under psychotropic drug legislation.

Although sublingual buprenorphine has been used in the management of heroin addiction (SEDA-16, 88), widespread abuse of buprenorphine by addicts is known (SEDA-16, 88), including the snorting of crushed sublingual tablets (SEDA-16, 88).

Buprenorphine is taken in the form of a sublingual tablet, which takes 3–5 minutes to dissolve and be absorbed. In order to reduce the likelihood of intravenous abuse of buprenorphine, it has been combined with naloxone. This combined product is poorly absorbed by mouth and if injected can precipitate unpleasant opioid withdrawal reactions. Further large-scale studies are needed to study the efficacy and safety profile of buprenorphine, with or without naloxone, in different opioid-dependent populations, in order to determine the cumulative effect of repeated administration (28), and to explore alternative delivery systems, such as intravenous (29), intramuscular (30), and depot formulations (31).

Buprenorphine is increasingly being used as a substitute for other opioids in the treatment of opioid abuse and is generally considered to be safe because of the ceiling effect. One report from Vienna described 50 opioid-dependent subjects who received gradual (10-day) detoxification with buprenorphine, contacting the outpatient clinic daily, so that buprenorphine could be administered according to their clinical need in a free dosage scheme (32). The mean daily dosage was 2.3 mg on day 1 and the highest mean daily dose was administered on day 2, followed by daily reduction over the study period. There was 70% compliance with the regimen and withdrawal symptoms during the study period were described as moderate.

Less satisfactory outcomes have been reported from France (33–35), where acute poisoning during buprenorphine substitution has been described in three series of patients. The first included 29 opiate addicts taking high-dosage sublingual buprenorphine with non-fatal poisoning and the second included 20 addicts who died (33). Blood concentrations of buprenorphine in the first group were low (1.0–2.3 ng/ml, mean 1.4 ng/ml), but there was concomitant intake of psychotropic medication, especially benzodiazepines, in 18 cases. Blood concentrations of buprenorphine in the fatal cases were 1.1–29 (mean 8.4) ng/ml, while concentrations of its primary metabolite, norbuprenorphine, were 0.2–13 (mean 2.6) ng/ml, within or slightly over the target range. Extensive tissue distribution buprenorphine was reported (myocardium, kidney, brain, and liver) but the highest concentrations of buprenorphine and norbuprenorphine were found in the bile, and the authors suggested that this may be the sample of choice for postmortem screening. Buprenorphine was also identified in eight of 11 hair samples assayed. Intravenous injection of crushed tablets and the concomitant use of benzodiazepines were identified as the major risk factors in the fatal cases (34).

Drug dependence

Sublingual buprenorphine is an alternative to methadone in treating opiate dependence, but its opioid agonist effects pose the risk of intravenous abuse and subsequent dependence. This abuse potential may be limited by using a combination of buprenorphine with naloxone, which will precipitate opiate withdrawal when given intravenously but not sublingually. The effects of three combinations of intravenous buprenorphine and naloxone on agonist effects and withdrawal signs and symptoms in 12 opiate-dependent patients have been described (36). After stabilization with morphine 60 mg intramuscularly the patients were challenged with intravenous doses of buprenorphine 2 mg, either alone or in combination with naloxone in ratios of 2:1, 4:1, and 8:1, with morphine alone (15 mg), or with placebo. In those given the combination there was a naloxone dose-dependent increase in opiate withdrawal signs and a reduction in the pleasurable effects that might induce abuse liability. The authors suggested that the combination of buprenorphine with naloxone in a ratio of 2:1 or 4:1 can be useful in the treatment of opiate dependence.

There have been three studies of the use of buprenorphine to treat opiate dependence.

The authors of a randomized, multicenter, placebo-controlled, double-blind study of 72 opioid-dependent individuals, who were given either buprenorphine 8 mg/day or methadone 60 mg/day for 6 months, claimed that there were no significant differences in adverse effects during induction or maintenance (37). Buprenorphine provided an alternative to methadone, with equal improvement in quality of life, psychopathology, and compliance. The results of this study should be interpreted with care, because of the unusual experimental design, which did not reflect practices in ordinary methadone maintenance programs. However, similar observations were observed during an open, flexible-dose study involving inpatient induction and outpatient maintenance in 15 opioid-dependent pregnant women (38). Sublingual buprenorphine (1–10 mg/day) was well accepted by the women, and there was a low incidence of neonatal abstinence syndrome. Further controlled and larger studies need to be done to substantiate these observations.

In a double-blind, randomized comparison of sublingual buprenorphine tablets with oral methadone in a 6-week trial in 58 patients using a flexible dosing procedure the retention rate was significantly better in those using methadone (90 versus 50%) (39). Those who completed the study had a similar number of opioid-positive urine samples, with a mean stabilization dose of 11 mg/day of buprenorphine and 70 mg/day of methadone. This study had several limitations: 6 weeks is too short a period to determine any intermediate or long-term treatment outcomes, the sample size was too small, and the comparison of non-equivalent doses makes interpretation difficult.

Drug withdrawal

The effects of buprenorphine (sublingually or by injection) in an opioid-dependent population have been studied (40,41). There was benefit in using buprenorphine to counteract opioid withdrawal effects in patients with chronic heroin use and subsequent dependence. However, the results are limited and the benefits short-term if psychosocial support is not in place as part of an overall treatment package before buprenorphine is prescribed (42).

- A 35-year-old man with a 10-year history of heroin use was given sublingual buprenorphine 24 mg/day (43). Although it was dispensed daily by a pharmacist, he was not adequately supervised: he saved the buprenorphine tablets and continued to use heroin. He then took buprenorphine 40 mg and stopped using heroin; he immediately developed opioid withdrawal symptoms. In an attempt to relieve these symptoms, he took a further 40 or 45 mg buprenorphine in 24 hours. He subsequently came to a drug treatment clinic, where he was given another 16 mg of buprenorphine, with no effect. After 3 days, he was transferred to methadone and his withdrawal symptoms resolved.

In this case buprenorphine precipitated opioid withdrawal symptoms after heroin use. This highlights the importance of regular monitoring and supervision of community-dispensed buprenorphine.

Second-Generation Effects

Pregnancy

In a randomized controlled study, 18 pregnant women in the second trimester were switched from short-acting morphine to buprenorphine without difficulty and minimal withdrawal effects in either mother or fetus (44).

High-dose buprenorphine and methadone have been compared in 259 pregnant women (45). There were no major variations in perinatal outcomes between those taking buprenorphine (n = 159) and those taking methadone (n = 100). Delivery was premature in 10% of those who used buprenorphine and 16% of those who used methadone. Neonatal abstinence syndrome occurred in 75% beginning at a mean age of 40 hours; there were no deaths.

It is inadvisable to use buprenorphine during labor, as its effects on the fetus cannot be reversed.

Lactation

Buprenorphine passes into breast milk in concentrations similar to those in maternal plasma. However, exposure tends to be minimal (46). A mild neonatal abstinence syndrome and secretion of buprenorphine into breast milk, potentially resulting in exposure to the infant, have been reviewed (3).

Susceptibility Factors

Age

Respiratory depression after the use of buprenorphine in adults tends to be associated with parenteral administration. Respiratory depression and central nervous system depression after oral buprenorphine (2 mg in one case and 8 mg in four cases) has been described in five toddlers (47).

Renal impairment

The long-term use of buprenorphine by patients with renal impairment could result in accumulation of metabolites (norbuprenorphine) in the plasma, although this may not be clinically significant (46).

Liver disease

Patients with hepatitis treated with buprenorphine should have liver enzymes monitored (46). HIV-positive patients taking antiretroviral drug therapy are susceptible to increased concentrations of buprenorphine exposure because of drug-drug interactions (46,48).

Drug Administration

Drug formulations

A sublingual formulation that combines buprenorphine and naloxone is thought to be ideal for reducing parental buprenorphine abuse. In a small pilot study in nine opioid-dependent individuals already stabilized on buprenorphine 8 mg/day, naloxone 0, 4, or 8 mg was added (49). The addition of naloxone did not precipitate opiate withdrawal.

A transdermal therapeutic system (TTS) for rate-controlled delivery of buprenorphine is available in three strengths, with release rates of 35, 52.5, and 70 µg/hour for 72 hours. This is equivalent to daily doses of 0.8, 1.2, and 1.6 mg respectively. In a double-blind, randomized, controlled study using one of three dosage strengths of buprenorphine TTS in 445 patients with chronic pain the adverse effects were mild and typical of the opioid analgesics; they included nausea (17%), vomiting (9.3%), dizziness (6.8%), tiredness (5.6%), constipation (5.3%), and sweating (3.7%) (50). There was erythema in 25% and pruritus in 22%. More than half of the cases of erythema and one-third of the cases of pruritus resolved within 24 hours. In a single-blind, randomized study sublingual buprenorphine 0.2 mg provided an effective and convenient alternative in the treatment of acute renal colic compared with pethidine 50 mg intramuscularly (51). There was a slightly but non-significantly higher incidence of nausea, vomiting, and dizziness in those given buprenorphine.

In 151 patients with severe chronic pain of malignant or non-malignant origin in a double-blind, randomized, placebo-controlled study of the efficacy and tolerability of buprenorphine transdermal therapeutic system, three strengths of the formulation were prescribed, 35, 52.5, or 70 micrograms/hour (52). Overall, 23% of patients reported adverse events, with no significant differences between the treatment groups. There were local adverse reactions in 10-20% of patients and about 50% of the symptoms lasted under 24 hours. One patient had severe pruritus and a severe allergic rash with mild vesiculation; another reported moderate swelling, severe pruritus, and

erythema. Both were receiving buprenorphine 52.5 micrograms/hour. Another patient, receiving 70 micrograms/hour, had severe nausea and vomiting with urinary retention. The authors concluded that buprenorphine transdermal therapeutic system is an effective analgesic medication for chronic moderate to severe pain, but there was also a marked placebo effect, which minimized any difference in response rate between buprenorphine and placebo. One should not underestimate the effect of placebo in studies in which patient expectation plays a prominent role, if pain is measured as remembered pain (as in the above study) rather than based on an assessment of current pain. In a similar study from the same research group 79% of patients receiving placebo or buprenorphine transdermal therapeutic system reported at least one adverse event during the study (53). Most of these events were mild or moderate and were typical of those that occur at the start of therapy with a strong opioid.

A review of other double-blind, placebo-controlled trials has confirmed that most of the adverse effects of buprenorphine transdermal therapeutic system are transient and predictably opioid related. All the trials confirmed analgesic efficacy; patients reported that their analgesia was maintained for a mean duration of 4.7 months and that the patch was user-friendly (54,55).

Sublingual buprenorphine is increasingly being used in the treatment of opioid dependence. In several double-blind, randomized, controlled studies buprenorphine has been compared with methadone (56), naltrexone and/or methadone (57), naloxone (58), or placebo (59) in opioid-dependent individuals who are treatment seekers. Most of the results have reiterated the importance of identifying a clear rationale for prescribing sublingual buprenorphine, of adequate psychosocial support, and of adequate dosage (a fixed dose of 12-16 mg of sublingual buprenorphine for 12 months) in order to maximize treatment outcomes in this challenging population. A combined buprenorphine/naloxone formulation was safe, well tolerated, and efficacious, reducing the use of illicit opioids and craving for opioids in dependent individuals (60). Low doses of buprenorphine (5–8 mg) did not have any additional benefits over methadone (61).

Drug dosage regimens

Two doses (8 and 16 mg) of sublingual buprenorphine have been compared in a 6-week double-blind, placebo-controlled inpatient study of the reinforcing effects of intravenous diamorphine (62). Only eight diamorphine-dependent men were recruited and the authors could only postulate that doses over 16 mg might be more effective in blocking the reinforcing effects of diamorphine.

Drug administration route

Adverse effects after parenteral, sublingual, and rectal use have included hypotension, bradycardia, reduced systolic blood pressure, reduced stroke volume, nausea, sweating, vomiting, vertigo, sedation, and a reduction in respiratory rate (63). In some intravenous studies nausea and vomiting have occurred in as many as 20%.

Hypotension occurs in 1–5% of patients, and hypertension, tachycardia, or bradycardia in under 1%.

Drug overdose

The concomitant use of benzodiazepines and intravenous injections of dissolved buprenorphine tablets increases the risk of serious overdose. In a retrospective study of opioid overdose in Helsinki between 1995 and 2002 there were 11 cases of overdose in which buprenorphine was involved (64). Buprenorphine had been used intravenously in seven cases and concomitant benzodiazepines in three, alcohol in four, and heroin in two.

Drug–Drug Interactions

Buprenorphine is mainly metabolized by CYP3A4. Concomitant use of medications that induce CYP3A4 (for example rifampicin, phenytoin) or inhibit it (for example fluoxetine, cimetidine, saquinavir) may increase or inhibit buprenorphine metabolism and caution should be taken when buprenorphine is given with such drugs (46,65).

Antiretroviral drugs

The interaction of buprenorphine with antiretroviral drugs has been reviewed (66,67). Adverse effects due to this interaction have been reported; the interaction of buprenorphine with atazanavir and ritonavir resulted in reduced mental functioning and central nervous system depression (68).

An interaction of buprenorphine + naloxone (Suboxone) with *delavirdine* or *ritonavir*, which inhibit CYP3A4, can prolong the QT interval. In 50 HIV-positive patients taking antiretroviral drugs, buprenorphine + naloxone caused QT interval prolongation which was statistically but not clinically significant; there was no prolongation in opioid-dependent subjects who were taking only buprenorphine + naloxone (69).

Benzodiazepines

Six deaths linked to misuse of buprenorphine plus benzodiazepine combinations have been described (35). The authors emphasized that blood concentrations of buprenorphine were in the target range in three subjects, although higher in three others. Exhaustive screening detected no traces of opiates in postmortem blood, but all subjects had target range concentrations of both desmethyldiazepam and 7-aminoflunitrazepam. The risk of high-dose substitution therapy (2–8 mg), if physicians do not comply with correct practices for the prescription, and use of buprenorphine were emphasized, particularly when there is a large population of patients being treated, as there was in France in 1997 (34 000 patients).

An interaction of therapeutic doses of diazepam (10 and 20 mg) with buprenorphine in 16 subjects resulted in increased subjective measures of sedation and some impairment of psychomotor performance (deterioration in cancellation time) (70). This interaction of was compared with that of methadone and diazepam. The former caused less psychomotor impairment.

HIV-1 protease inhibitors

The metabolism of buprenorphine is inhibited by the HIV-1 protease inhibitors (71).

Ifosfamide

An interaction has been reported between buprenorphine and the chemotherapeutic agent ifosfamide (72).

- A 34-year-old man was given transdermal buprenorphine for pain, initially 35 micrograms/hour, later increased to 52.5 micrograms/hour. He developed respiratory depression, which resolved on withdrawal of the patch.

The authors suggested that respiratory depression had been triggered by the dual action of buprenorphine and ifosfamide on CYP3A4.

Naloxone

Naloxone is of limited use in reversing the effects of buprenorphine, because of its relative inability to displace it from opioid receptors. Naloxone 1 mg had little effect on the respiratory depression caused by buprenorphine 300 µg/70 kg, although both 5 and 10 µg produced consistent reversal, which was more complete with the larger dose (73). Insignificant effects on circulation and respiration have been reported at lower doses of buprenorphine (4.5–10 µg/kg) (74).

Opioid agonists

Under some conditions the antagonist action of buprenorphine can jeopardize the effect of subsequently administered pure opioid agonists, by blocking $MOR(OP_3, \mu)$ opioid receptors so effectively that normal doses of the opioid agonist are ineffective, necessitating the administration of a higher dose, with the attendant risk of respiratory depression, from which deaths have been reported (SEDA-13, 60). Fortunately such instances appear to be rare.

References

1. Carl P, Crawford ME, Madsen NB, Ravlo O, Bach V, Larsen AI. Pain relief after major abdominal surgery: a double-blind controlled comparison of sublingual buprenorphine, intramuscular buprenorphine, and intramuscular meperidine. Anesth Analg 1987;66(2):142–6.
2. Jakobs R, Adamek MU, von Bubnoff AC, Riemann JF. Buprenorphine or procaine for pain relief in acute pancreatitis. A prospective randomized study. Scand J Gastroenterol 2000;35(12):1319–23.
3. Carrieri MP, Amass L, Lucas GM, Vlahov D, Wodak A, Woody GE. Buprenorphine use: the international experience. Clin Infect Dis 2006;43(Suppl 4):S197-215.
4. Sung S, Conry JM. Role of buprenorphine in the management of heroin addiction. Ann Pharmacother 2006;40:501-5.

5. Robinson SE. Buprenorphine-containing treatments. Place in the management of opioid addiction. CNS Drugs 2006;20(9):697–712.

6. Oreskovich MR, Saxon AJ, Ellis MLK, Malte CA, Reoux JP, Knox PC. A double-blind, double-dummy, randomized, prospective pilot study of the partial mu opiate agonist, buprenorphine, for acute detoxification from heroin. Drug Alcohol Depend 2005;77, 71–9.

7. Davids E, Gaspar M. Buprenorphine in the treatment of opioid dependence. Eur Neuropsychopharmacol 2004;14:209–16.

8. Verthein U, Prinzleve M, Farnbacher G, Haasen C, Krausz M. Treatment of opiate addicts with buprenorphine: a prospective naturistic trial. Addict Disord Treat 2004;3:58–70.

9. Gouny P, Gaitz JP, Vayssairat M. Acute hand ischemia secondary to intraarterial buprenorphine injection: treatment with iloprost and dextran-40—a case report. Angiology 1999;50(7):605–6.

10. Cracowski JL, Mallaret M, Vanzetto G. Myocardial infarction associated with buprenorphine. Ann Intern Med 1999;130(6):536–7.

11. Fincham JE. Cardiopulmonary arrest and subsequent death after administration of buprenorphine in an elderly female: a case report. J Geriatr Drug Ther 1989;3:103.

12. Dahan A, Yassen A, Bijl H, Romberg R, Sarton E, Teppema L, Olofsen E, Danhof M. Comparison of the respiratory effects of intravenous buprenorphine and fentanyl in humans and rats. Br J Anesth 2005;94(6):825–34.

13. Martell BA, Arnsten JH, Krantz MJ, Gourevitch MN. Impact of methadone treatment on cardiac repolarisation and conduction in opioid users. Am J Cardiol 2005;95(7):915–8.

14. Schleicher G, Lechner W, Muller E. [Trophic ulcers after intraganglionic injection of buprenorphine and root canal therapy.]Aktuelle Derm 1985;11:90.

15. Lockhart SP, Baron JH. Tongue ulceration after lingual buprenorphine. BMJ (Clin Res Ed) 1984;288:1346.

16. Davis MP. Buprenorphine in cancer pain. Support Care Cancer 2005;13:878–87.

17. Houdret N, Asnar V, Szostak-Talbodec N, Leteurtre E, Humbert L, Lecomte-Houcke M, Lhermitte M, Paris JC. Hépatonéphrite et ingestion massive le buprénorphines. [Hepatonephritis and massive ingestion of buprenorphine.] Acta Clin Belg Suppl 1999;1:29–31.

18. Petry NM, Bickel WK, Piasecki D, Marsch LA, Badger GJ. Elevated liver enzyme levels in opioid-dependent patients with hepatitis treated with buprenorphine. Am J Addict 2000;9(3):265–9.

19. Berson A, Gervais A, Cazals D, Boyer N, Durand F, Bernuau J, Marcellin P, Degott C, Valla D, Pessayre D. Hepatitis after intravenous buprenorphine misuse in heroin addicts. J Hepatol 2001;34(2):346–50.

20. Wisniewski B, Perlemuter G, Buffet C. Hepatite aiguë liée a l'injection intraveineuse de buprenorphine chez une toxicomane substituée. [Acute hepatitis following intravenous buprenorphine injection as a substitute drug in a drug-addict.] Gastroenterol Clin Biol 2001;25(3):328–9.

21. Woodham M. Pruritus with sublingual buprenorphine. Anaesthesia 1988;43(9):806–7.

22. Seet RCS, Lim ECH. Intravenous use of buprenorphine tablets associated with rhabdomyolysis and compressive sciatic neuropathy. Ann Emerg Med 2006;47(4):396–7.

23. Peduto VA, Di Martino M, Tani R, Toscano A, Napoleone M. Reazione anafilattoide da bupreuorfina: descrizione di un caso. [Anaphylactoid reaction to buprenorphine: a case report.] Anaesthesiol Reanim 1988;38:241.

24. Seifert J, Metzner C, Paetzold W, Borsutzky M, Ohlmeier M, Passie T, Hauser U, Becker H, Wiese B, Emrich HM, Schneider U. Mood and affect during detoxification of opiate addicts: a comparison of buprenorphine versus methadone. Addict Biol 2005;10:157–64.

25. Bachmeyer C, Landgraf N, Daumas L. Soft tissue infection caused by Gemella morbillorum in two intravenous drug users. J Am Acad Dermatol 2005;52(4):704–5.

26. Kintz P. Deaths involving buprenorphine: a compendium of French cases. Forensic Sci Int 2001;121(1–2):65–9.

27. Schifano F, Corkery J, Gilvarry E, Deluca P, Oyefeso A, Ghodse AH. Buprenorphine mortality, seizures and prescription data in the UK, 1980–2002. Hum Psychopharmacol Clin Exp 2005;20, 343–8.

28. Mintzer MZ, Correia CJ, Strain EC. A dose-effect study of repeated administration of buprenorphine/naloxone on performance in opioid-dependent volunteers. Drug Alcohol Dep 2004;74:205–9.

29. Umbricht A, Huestis MA, Cone EJ, Preston KL. Effects of high-dose intravenous buprenorphine in experienced opioid abusers. J Clin Psychopharmacol 2004;24:479–87.

30. Assadi MS, Hafezi M, Mokri A, Razzaghi EM, Ghaelc P. Opioid detoxification using high doses of buprenorphine in 24 hours: a randomized double blind, controlled clinical trial. J Substance Abuse Treat 2004;27:75–82.

31. Sobel B-FX, Sigmon SC, Walsh SL, Johnson RE, Liebson IA, Nuwayser ES, Kerrigan JH, Bigelow GE. Open-label trial of an injection depot formulation of buprenorphine in opioid detoxification. Drug Alcohol Depend 2004;73:11–22.

32. Diamant K, Fischer G, Schneider C, Lenzinger E, Pezawas L, Schindler S, Eder H. Outpatient opiate detoxification treatment with buprenorphine. Preliminary investigation. Eur Addict Res 1998;4(4):198–202.

33. Tracqui A, Tournoud C, Flesch F, Kopferschmitt J, Kintz P, Deveaux M, Ghysel MH, Marquet P, Pepin G, Petit G, Jaeger A, Ludes B. Intoxications aiguës par traitement substitutif a base de buprénorphine haut dosage. 29 observations cliniques—20 cas mortels. [Acute poisoning during substitution therapy based on high-dosage buprenorphine. 29 clinical cases—20 fatal cases.] Presse Méd 1998;27(12):557–61.

34. Tracqui A, Kintz P, Ludes B. Buprenorphine-related deaths among drug addicts in France: a report on 20 fatalities. J Anal Toxicol 1998;22(6):430–4.

35. Reynaud M, Tracqui A, Petit G, Potard D, Courty P. Six deaths linked to misuse of buprenorphine–benzodiazepine combinations. Am J Psychiatry 1998;155(3):448–9.

36. Mendelson J, Jones RT, Welm S, Baggott M, Fernandez I, Melby AK, Nath RP. Buprenorphine and naloxone combinations: the effects of three dose ratios in morphine-stabilized, opiate-dependent volunteers. Psychopharmacology (Berl) 1999;141(1):37–46.

37. Pani PP, Maremmani I, Pirastu R, Tagliamonte A, Gessa GL. Buprenorphine: a controlled clinical trial in the treatment of opioid dependence. Drug Alcohol Depend 2000;60(1):39–50.

38. Fischer G, Johnson RE, Eder H, Jagsch R, Peternell A, Weninger M, Langer M, Aschauer HN. Treatment of opioid-dependent pregnant women with buprenorphine. Addiction 2000;95(2):239–44.

39. Petitjean S, Stohler R, Deglon JJ, Livoti S, Waldvogel D, Uehlinger C, Ladewig D. Double-blind randomized trial of buprenorphine and methadone in opiate dependence. Drug Alcohol Depend 2001;62(1):97–104.

40. Welsh CJ, Suman M, Cohen A, Broyles L, Bennett M, Weintraub E. The use of intravenous buprenorphine for

the treatment of opioid withdrawal in medically ill hospitalized patients. Am J Addict 2002;11(2):135–40.

41. Krook AL, Brors O, Dahlberg J, Grouff K, Magnus P, Roysamb E, Waal H. A placebo-controlled study of high dose buprenorphine in opiate dependents waiting for medication-assisted rehabilitation in Oslo, Norway. Addiction 2002;97(5):533–42.

42. Varescon I, Vidal-Trecan G, Nabet N, Boissonnas A. Substitution et mésusage: l'injection intraveineuse de buprénorphine haut dosage. [Buprenorphine abuse: high dose intravenous administration of buprenorphine.] Encephale 2002;28(5 Pt 1):397–402.

43. Clark NC, Lintzeris N, Muhleisen PJ. Severe opiate withdrawal in a heroin user precipitated by a massive buprenorphine dose. Med J Aust 2002;176(4):166–7.

44. Ryle PR. Justification for routine screening of pharmaceutical products in immune function tests: a review of the recommendations of Putman et al. (2003). Fundam Clin Pharmacol 2005;19:317–22.

45. Lejeune C, Simmat-Durand L, Gourarier L, Aubisson S. Prospective multicenter observational study of 260 infants born to 259 opiate dependent mothers on methadone or high dose buprenorphine substitution. Drug Alcohol Depend 2006;82:250–7.

46. Elkader A, Sproule B. Buprenorphine: clinical pharmacokinetics in the treatment of opioid dependence. Clin Pharmacokinet 2005;44(7):661–80.

47. Geib A, Babu K, Ewald MB, Boyer EW. Adverse effects in children after unintentional buprenorphine exposure. Pediatrics 2006;118:1746–51.

48. Sullivan LE, Fiellin Da. Buprenorphine: its role in preventing HIV transmission and improving the care of HIV-infected patients with opioid dependence. Clin Infect Dis 2005;41, 891–6.

49. Harris DS, Jones RT, Welm S, Upton RA, Lin E, Mendelson J. Buprenorphine and naloxone co-administration in opiate-dependent patients stabilized on sublingual buprenorphine. Drug Alcohol Depend 2000;61(1):85–94.

50. Bohme K. Buprenorphine in a transdermal therapeutic system—a new option. Clin Rheumatol 2002;21(Suppl 1): S13–6.

51. Chang CH, Wang CJ, Yen YC, Hsu SJ. Effectiveness of sublingual buprenorphine and intramuscular pethidine in acute renal colic. Formosan J Surg 2002;35:9–13.

52. Bohme K, Likar R. Efficacy and tolerability of a new opioid analgesic formulation, buprenorphine transdermal therapeutic system (TDS) in the treatment of patients with chronic pain. A randomized, double-blind, placebo-controlled study. Pain Clinic 2003;15:193–202.

53. Sear R, Graessinger N, Likar R. Analgesic efficacy and tolerability of transdermal buprenorphine in patients with inadequately controlled chronic pain related to cancer and other disorders: a multicentre, randomized, double-blind, placebo-controlled trial. Clin Ther 2003;25:150–68.

54. Radbruch L. Buprenorphine TDS: use in daily practise, benefits for patients. Int J Clin Pract 2003;Suppl 133:Feb.

55. Radbruch L, Vielgoye-Kerkmeer A. Buprenorphine TDS: the clinical development-rationale and results. Int J Clin Pract 2003;Suppl 133:15-18.

56. Mattick RP, Ali R, White JM, O'Brien S, Wolk S, Danz C. Buprenorphine versus methadone maintenance therapy: a randomized double-blind trial with 405 opioid-dependent patients. Addiction 2003;98:441–52.

57. Ahmedi J, Ahmedi K, Ohalri J. Controlled randomized trial in maintenance treatment of intravenous buprenorphine dependence with naltrexone, methadone or buprenorphine: a novel study. Eur J Clin Invest 2003;33:824–9.

58. Fudala PJ, Bridge TP, Herbert S, Williford WO, Chian CN, Jones K, Collins J, Raisch D, Casadonte P, Goldsmith RJ, Ling W, Malkerneker U, McNicolas L, Renner J, Stine S, Tusel D, for the Buprenorphine/Naloxone Collaborative Study Group. Office-based treatment of opiate addiction with sublingual-tablet formulation of buprenorphine and naloxone N Engl J Med 2003;349:949–58.

59. Kakko J, Svanborg KD, Kreek MJ, Heilig M. 1-year retention and social function after buprenorphine-assisted relapse prevention treatment for heroin dependence in Sweden: a randomized, placebo-controlled trial. Lancet 2003;361:661–72.

60. Bridge TP, Fudala PJ, Herbert S, Leiderman DB. Safety and health policy considerations related to the use of buprenorphine/naloxone as an office-based treatment for opiate dependence. Drugs Alcohol Depend 2003;70:579–85.

61. Scottish Executive Effective Intervention Unit. The Effectiveness of Treatment for Opiate Dependent Drug Users: an International Systematic Review of the Evidence. July 2002 http://www.drugmisuse.isdscotland.org/eiu/pdfs/eiu_opi.pdf.

62. Comer SD, Collins ED, Fischman MW. Buprenorphine sublingual tablets: effects on IV heroin self-administration by humans. Psychopharmacology (Berl) 2001;154(1): 28–37.

63. Weiss P, Ritz R. Analgetische Wirkung und Nebenwirkungen von Buprenorphine bei der akuten koronaren Herzkrankheit. Ein randomisiertes Doppelblindvergleich mit Morphine. [Analgesic effect and side-effects of buprenorphine in acute coronary heart disease. A randomized double-blind comparison with morphine.] Anästh Intensivther Notfallmed 1988;23(6): 309–12.

64. Boyd J, Randell T, Luurila H, Kuisma M. Serious overdoses involving buprenorphine in Helsinki. Acta Anaesthesiol Scand 2003;47:1031–3.

65. Kreek MJ, Bart G, Lilly C, Laforge KS, Nielson DA. Pharmacogenetics and human molecular genetics of opiate and cocaine addictions and their treatments. Pharmacol Rev 2005;57(1):1–26.

66. McCance-Katz EF, Moody DE, Morse GD, Friedland G, Pade P, Baker J, Alvanzo A, Smith P, Ogundele A, Jatlow P, Rainey P. Interactions between buprenorphine and antiretrovirals. 1. The non-nucleotide reverse-transcriptase inhibitors efavirenz and delavirdine. Clin Infect Dis 2006;43(Suppl 4):S224–34.

67. McCance-Katz EF, Moody DE, Smith P, Morse GD, Friedland G, Pade P, Baker J, Alvanzo A, Jatlow P, Rainey P. Interactions between buprenorphine and antiretrovirals. 2. The protease inhibitors nelfinavir, lopinavir/ritonavir, and ritonavir. Clin Infect Dis 2006;43(Suppl 4):S235–46.

68. Douglas Bruce R, Altice FL. Three case reports of a clinical pharmacokinetic interaction with buprenorphine and atazanavir plus ritonavir. AIDS 2006;20:783–4.

69. Baker JR, Best AM, Pade PA, McCance-Katz EF. Effect of buprenorphine and antiretroviral agents on the QT interval in opioid-dependent patients. Ann Pharmacother 2006;40(3):392–6.

70. Ramirez-Cacho WA, Flores S, Schrader RM, McKay J, Rayburn WF. Effect of chronic maternal methadone therapy on intrapartum fetal heart rate patterns. J Soc Gynecol Investig 2006;13:108–11.

71. Iribarne C, Berthou F, Carlhant D, Dreano Y, Picart D, Lohezic F, Riche C. Inhibition of methadone and buprenorphine N-dealkylations by three HIV-1 protease inhibitors. Drug Metab Dispos 1998;26(3):257–60.

72. Moro C, Taino R, Mandalà M, Labianca R. Buprenorphine-induced acute respiratory depression during ifosfamide-based chemotherapy. Annals Oncol 2006;17(9):1466–7.

73. Gal TJ. Naloxone reversal of buprenorphine-induced respiratory depression. Clin Pharmacol Ther 1989;45(1):66–71.
74. Rifat K, Magnin C, Morel D. L'analgésie per et postopératoire à la buprénorphine: effets cardio-circulatoires et respiratoires. [Pre- and postoperative buprenorphine analgesia: cardiocirculatory and respiratory effects.] Cah Anesthesiol 1984;32(1):33–6.

Butorphanol

General Information

Butorphanol is a synthetic 14-hydroxymorphinan analogue with a low dependence potential and a low propensity to cause opioid adverse effects (1). It is a synthetic OP_2 (κ) receptor agonist and OP_3 (μ) receptor antagonist.

General adverse reactions

In some patients, effective doses cause troublesome effects. For example, in a randomized study of patients with sickle-cell crisis who received either butorphanol 2 mg intramuscularly or morphine 6 mg intramuscularly, adverse effects occurred in 23 and 13% respectively (2). On the other hand, a wide range of doses (4–48 mg/day) over 1 month failed to produce scores indicative of euphoric effects, and the withdrawal syndrome resembled a cyclazocine rather than a morphine abstinence effect (1).

Observational studies

Butorphanol is a partial agonist at MOR opioid receptors and an agonist at KOR receptors. Intranasal butorphanol has been used to treat five patients with intractable pruritus due to inflammatory skin disease or systemic disease (3). All had marked improvement, but one had severe nausea and withdrew. No other adverse effects were reported.

Organs and Systems

Cardiovascular

Although cardiovascular toxicity with butorphanol is slight, raised pulmonary wedge pressure has occurred at cardiac catheterization (1).

Respiratory

Respiratory depression occurs minimally at doses of 2–4 mg (1).

Biliary tract

Butorphanol is generally believed to have a much smaller effect on biliary pressure than morphine, fentanyl, or pethidine, but 2 mg has caused biliary spasm (4).

Musculoskeletal

Fibrous myopathy has been reported in a 40-year-old woman who injected butorphanol intramuscularly (SEDA-17, 87).

Second-Generation Effects

Fetotoxicity

Two cases of sinusoidal fetal heart rhythm have been reported in which there was a significant temporal relation between the administration of butorphanol and the onset of the abnormal heart rhythm (5). In both instances the pattern reverted to normal after further analgesia was given.

Drug Administration

Drug administration route

Butorphanol has been used for epidural anesthesia in obstetric practice without adversely affecting the neonate, and no patients had pruritus (SEDA-16, 88).

As butorphanol is not orally active, reports of its transnasal administration are of interest. The most common adverse effects of transnasal butorphanol were dizziness, nausea and/or vomiting, headache, and drowsiness (SEDA-20, 83). Increased cardiac workload can also occur.

After cesarean section, transnasal butorphanol did not work quite as quickly as intravenous butorphanol. The effect lasted longer but the adverse effects were similar (SEDA-16, 88).

References

1. Pachter IJ, Evens RP. Butorphanol. Drug Alcohol Depend 1985;14(3–4):325–38.
2. Gonzalez ER, Ornato JP, Ware D, Bull D, Evens RP. Comparison of intramuscular analgesic activity of butorphanol and morphine in patients with sickle cell disease. Ann Emerg Med 1988;17(8):788–91.
3. Dawn AG, Yosipovitch G. Butorphanol for treatment of intractable pruritus. J Am Acad Dermatol 2006;54(3):527–31.
4. Dolan PF. Butorphanol and biliary spasm. Anesthesiology 1985;63(3):340.
5. Welt SI. Sinusoidal fetal heart rate and butorphanol administration. Am J Obstet Gynecol 1985;152(3):362–3.

Ciramadol

General Information

Ciramadol is a partial agonist at MOR opioid receptors. Data on the incidence of adverse effects after usual doses of oral ciramadol are conflicting. In one study there was a low incidence of mild adverse effects (1), but in another, in which ciramadol 60 mg was more effective than codeine 60 mg or placebo, there was a high incidence of opioid adverse effects (2); some other workers have had the same experience.

References

1. Graf DF, Pandit SK, Kothary SP, Freeland GR. A double-blind comparison of orally administered ciramadol and codeine for relief of postoperative pain. J Clin Pharmacol 1985;25(8):590–5.
2. van Steenberghe D, Verbist D, Quirynen M, Thevissen E. Double-blind comparison of the analgesic potency of ciramadol, codeine and placebo against postsurgical pain in ambulant patients. Eur J Clin Pharmacol 1986;31(3):355–8.

Codeine

General Information

The pharmacodynamic and adverse effects of codeine are mainly due to O-demethylation by CYP2D6 to morphine or a metabolite of morphine (SEDA-21, 86; SEDA-22, 5). Poor metabolizers may lack the analgesic effect of codeine.

In a retrospective study of patients with chronic rheumatological conditions, 290 of 644 clinic patients had received either codeine or oxycodone analgesia, of whom 137 had been given opioids for a continuous period of over 3 months (1). Adverse effects were described in 38% of both long-term and short-term opioid users, of which the most common were constipation, nausea, and sedation. Headache, dizziness, rash or itching, confusion, insomnia, depression, diarrhea, and myoclonic jerking were also reported. No significant differences in the adverse effects profile were reported between the groups and no subjects discontinued medication because of adverse effects. There were opioid abuse behaviors in 3% of the long-term users, but no association with a history of substance misuse was established.

A prospective double-blind, randomized study in 184 patients with cancers involved three treatment regimens (2): diclofenac alone (50 mg qds), diclofenac plus codeine (40 mg qds), or diclofenac plus imipramine (10–25 mg tds). There was no significant difference between the different treatments in terms of their analgesic effects, as measured on a visual analogue scale after 4 days. However, 10 of 61 subjects taking codeine withdrew because of adverse effects, compared with three taking imipramine group and two taking diclofenac alone. Gastrointestinal disturbances, dry mouth, and central nervous system disturbances were all more frequent in those taking codeine. These results suggest that the addition of a low-potency opioid to diclofenac fails to give enhanced analgesia while the frequency of opioid-related adverse effects increases.

Organs and Systems

Nervous system

Patients with migraine who use daily codeine or other opioids can be more susceptible to chronic daily headaches; this is evident in opiate overuse. In a pilot questionnaire study of 32 patients who used codeine or other opioids for control of their bowel motility after colectomy, chronic daily headaches occurred in those who were misusing opioids, but only if they had pre-existing migraine (3). The study had significant limitations, including the small sample size, diagnosis by means of a mailed questionnaire, a short duration of overuse of opioids, and the fact that it was uncontrolled.

Twelve cases of analgesic-related headache have been reported in children aged 6–16 years, half of whom were taking paracetamol in combination with codeine (4). Headaches occurred on at least 4 days per week and analgesic withdrawal led to symptom resolution in 50% and some improvement in the other cases.

Sensory systems

Reduced pupil size has been related to plasma codeine concentration (5).

Pancreas

Acute pancreatitis has been attributed to codeine (SEDA-21, 86), in one case in a patient taking co-codamol (paracetamol plus codeine) (6).

- A 20-year-old woman, who had previously taken paracetamol without adverse effects, took paracetamol 1 g and codeine 60 mg for a headache. After 3 hours she developed severe upper abdominal pain radiating to the back. The abdominal pain resolved within 24 hours of the administration of phloroglucinol and tiemonium. Her serum amylase activity was raised 3-fold and the serum lipase 15-fold. Other biochemical parameters, abdominal ultrasound, and an MRI scan were normal. Contrast-enhanced computed tomography showed pancreatic edema.

The previous use of paracetamol without adverse reactions supports the theory that the reaction was linked to the addition of codeine.

Four other cases of acute pancreatitis related to codeine have been reported (7).

- A 65-year-old man presented with severe abdominal pain 90 minutes after taking codeine and low-dose paracetamol. Serum amylase and lipase were significantly raised. Liver function tests were moderately abnormal. Abdominal ultrasound and CT scan showed edematous pancreatitis. Endoscopic retrograde cholangiography showed a papilla with a spastic appearance and an abnormal bile duct. He recovered completely, but 3 months later took codeine and paracetamol after a hemorrhoidectomy; abdominal pain recurred 1 hour later and acute pancreatitis was confirmed.
- A 26-year-old woman developed abdominal pain 2 days after taking codeine for a respiratory tract infection. Three hours later she complained of epigastric pain

and vomiting. Her serum amylase and lipase were raised. Her symptoms resolved and the diagnosis was mild idiopathic pancreatitis. One week later she took codeine for similar respiratory symptoms. Two hours later she developed similar symptoms and a CT scan showed an enlarged and heterogeneous pancreas, with necrosis of the tail of the pancreas involving the left kidney. She responded to conservative treatment.

- A 53-year-old woman developed severe central abdominal and epigastric pain 90 minutes after taking codeine for migraine. Pancreatic amylase, lipase, and liver function tests were mildly raised. Abdominal ultrasound was consistent with acute pancreatitis.
- A 57-year-old woman developed severe abdominal pain 2 hours after taking codeine. She had had two similar episodes in the past, once with loperamide and once with codeine. An abdominal CT scan showed edematous acute pancreatitis.

In three of these cases unintentional rechallenge with codeine resulted in recurrence of the symptoms, and the diagnosis was confirmed radiologically and biochemically. All the patients had previously had a cholecystectomy, suggesting that this may increase the likelihood of codeine-induced pancreatitis. The authors speculated that codeine could cause a rise in biliary and/or pancreatic sphincter pressure in cholecystectomized patients, either by exacerbating pre-existing disease of the sphincter of Oddi or as a consequence of reduced storage capacity of the biliary tract, initiating acute pancreatitis. They cautioned that codeine-associated acute pancreatitis can be misconstrued—it may seem as if patients are taking codeine for pancreatic pain when in fact the codeine is producing the pain.

Skin

Rashes have been attributed to codeine.

- A 72-year-old man developed a generalized maculopapular rash 12 hours after taking co-codamol (codeine 10 mg plus paracetamol 500 mg) (8). The lesions persisted for 7 days, became scaly, and disappeared. He later reported a similar skin condition after having taken a combination of acetylsalicylic acid, codeine, and caffeine. Patch tests gave a positive result for codeine, suggesting a type IV allergic reaction.
- A 58-year-old man developed a maculopapular rash on the dorsal aspects of the hand and upper body 6 days after taking codeine as an analgesic for hemoptysis secondary to tuberculosis; on withdrawal of codeine, the rash subsided after 48 hours (9).

Two reports have highlighted the importance of using an oral provocation test and not a patch test to determine if codeine is the causative agent in non-urticarial skin lesions (10,11).

- A 58-year-old man developed a pruritic rash on the body and face, with periorbital swelling 3 hours after taking codeine 20 mg, acetylcysteine 600 mg, and acetylsalicylic acid 500 mg. An oral provocation test over 2 hours with codeine phosphate (1 mg, 4 mg, and 8 mg)

precipitated a pruritic scarlatiniform rash for 24 hours, with swelling of the arms, starting 7 hours after the 8 mg dose. A rechallenge test confirmed the effect of codeine. Throughout this period, histamine release tests (CAST-ELISA with codeine) were negative.

- A 57-year-old patient presented with generalized malaise, fever, pruritus, and palpebral and labial angioedema 6 hours after taking a tablet containing paracetamol 500 mg, saccharin 10 mg, and codeine phosphate 30 mg. There was complete resolution in 8 hours, after treatment with prednisolone, hydroxyzine, and metamizole. Later a patch test with 1% codeine and an oral provocation test with paracetamol were both negative. Following an oral provocation test with codeine 5 mg, the patient developed similar symptoms.

Immunologic

True allergy to opioids is extremely rare. However, a near anaphylactic reaction in a patient taking codeine has been reported; the management of true codeine allergy was discussed and agents with different structures, such as phenylpiperidines or methadone-like compounds, are recommended (SEDA-17, 80).

Long-Term Effects

Drug abuse

Recreational use and abuse of codeine cough syrup is becoming more frequent. In a literature search of scientific journals and news media, complemented with in-depth interviews of 12 professionals working in the law enforcement or treatment aspects of drug abuse and 25 adults who reported using codeine syrup in the 30 days before their interview, the information provided useful insights into the different types of cough formulations, the reported reasons for their use, and the various types of administration (12). The effects of cough syrup, including their adverse effects, were reported. The most frequently mentioned negative effects included taste disturbance, prolonged sedation beyond the desired effect, loss of co-ordination, lethargy, constipation, and urinary retention. This qualitative study cannot be described as authoritative or representative, because of its limited nature, involving as it did only a small number of individuals living in the Houston area.

Drug dependence

In an exploratory survey among long-term codeine users recruited via newspaper advertisements in Toronto, Canada, more than 300 individuals who used codeine on at least 3 days per week for a minimum of 6 months and were older than 16 years were studied (13). Those who used codeine for pain related to malignancy were excluded. The mean age of the respondents included in the final analysis ($n = 339$) was 44 years and 51% were women. On average, the total number of years of regular codeine use was 12, with a current mean daily dose of 115 mg. About 60% ($n = 213$) had sought help for mental health problems, most commonly for depression (70%), followed by generalized anxiety (55%) and panic attacks (24%).

One-third of the subjects (*n* = 339) identified at least one family member as having a mental health problem, with depression as the most frequent. Current antidepressant use was reported by 14% of the whole sample. Men used significantly higher doses of codeine than women; they also used the drug for a longer period and more commonly took it for pleasurable effects and under social pressure. Regular codeine users, in addition to having high rates of drug dependence, had raised scores on general measures of psychological distress and depressive symptoms. From the survey it was not clear to what extent these symptoms preceded codeine use and may have initiated the use and to what extent they were caused by codeine. The authors speculated that many respondents used codeine to modulate mood, particularly dysphoria, in the absence of more appropriate interventions. They suggested that understanding long-term codeine use and its relation to dysphoria may be important in designing both preventive and secondary treatment interventions.

The same investigators further analysed the data according to codeine abuse/dependent and non-dependent status (14). There was codeine abuse/dependence in 41% of the subjects. The most common psychological and physical problems attributed to codeine use in the dependent/abuse group (*n* = 124) were depression (23%), anxiety (22%), gastrointestinal disturbances (15%), constipation (6%), and headache/migraine (5%). The codeine-dependent subjects were younger than those who were not dependent. The mean age of the respondents when they first started using codeine was 26 (range 2–78) years. A total of 563 codeine products had been used on a regular basis; the most common combination involved codeine with paracetamol (70%). Codeine was used for headaches (41%), back pain (22%), and other types of pain (25%). Those in the dependent group were more likely to have used codeine initially for other reasons, for example for pleasure and to relax or reduce stress. Most subjects said that they had obtained their codeine from one physician (66%) or by purchasing it over the counter (54%). Subjects in the dependent group also obtained codeine from friends (32%), from family (11%), "off the street" (19%), and through prescriptions from more than one physician (11%). Overall, more subjects in the dependent group considered themselves to have problems with a larger number of substances (3.3: range 0–15) compared with those in the non-dependent group (1.2: range 0–8). In the dependent group, more subjects said that their physical or mental health problems interfered with normal social activities at least "quite a bit." Significantly more subjects in the dependent group had sought help for a mental health problem, had had an inpatient psychiatric admission, or had sought help for a substance-use disorder, especially alcohol and stimulants. A larger number of subjects in the dependent group identified at least one family member (usually male) with substance-use problems compared with those in the non-dependent group.

This study suggests that codeine dependence may be more common in the general population than has been previously thought. The authors suggested that it is important to identify those with codeine abuse or codeine dependence, since

they may be using substantial doses of codeine for apparently little benefit compared to the risks. Furthermore, there are also health risks of associated chronic use of paracetamol and a potential for analgesic rebound headache.

Susceptibility factors

Genetic

There has been a report of opioid toxicity in a breast-fed baby of a mother taking codeine, and a subsequent meta-analysis and a case-control study have supported the view that in a few mothers who are ultraextensive metabolizers of codeine, breast-feeding while taking codeine may not be safe.

Codeine is mainly eliminated by glucuronidation, but 10% is O-demethylated by CYP2D6 to morphine and 10% is N-demethylated to norcodeine; morphine is further metabolized to two glucuronides, morphine-6-glucuronide (via uridine diphosphate-dependent glucuronosyltransferase 2B7), which is active, and morphine-3-glucuronide, which is not. CYP2D6-mediated O-demethylation of codeine is necessary for its pharmacodynamic effects (15), and its adverse effects are mainly due to O-demethylation to morphine or its active metabolite (16). The ability to O-demethylate codeine is polymorphically distributed in the population. There are two major phenotypes, called extensive and poor metabolizers. Most people are extensive metabolizers. Poor metabolizers are unable to metabolize codeine to morphine. However, a few individuals are very extensive (so-called 'ultrarapid', better 'ultraextensive') metabolizers, who form larger amounts of morphine and its metabolites than extensive metabolizers (17). This results from CYP2D6 gene duplication, which occurs with variable frequencies in different populations (Table 1) (18,19,20,21,22,23). In ultraextensive metabolizers even small doses of codeine can cause severe toxicity (24).

An early study of the pharmacokinetics of codeine in 17 samples of breast milk from seven mothers and 24 samples of plasma from 11 healthy full-term neonates showed that milk codeine concentrations were 34–314 ng/ml

Table 1 Population frequencies of ultraextensive metabolizers

Population	Frequency
Korean	0.3%
Scandinavian	1%
Chinese	1%
Nicaraguan	1%
German	1–2%
White British	1–3%
Spanish	1–10%
French	2%
Black American	2%
White American	2–4%
Croatian	4%
Turkish	6–9%
Greek, Portuguese	10%
Saudi Arabian	21%
Ethiopian	29%

20–240 minutes after codeine and morphine concentrations were 1.9–21 ng/ml; infant plasma samples 1–4 hours after feeding had concentrations of codeine < 0.8–4.5 ng/ml and morphine < 0.5–2.2 ng/ml (25). The authors suggested that moderate codeine use during breast-feeding (no more than four doses of 60 mg) is probably safe, and this has been subsequently taken to be so (26).

However, there have been occasionally anecdotal reports of adverse events in breast-fed neonates (27,28,29,30), and a neonate died after being breast-fed by his mother, who had taken codeine (31).

- A neonate developed increasing lethargy and difficulty in breast-feeding at 7 days of age. On day 13 he was cyanotic and lacked vital signs. Resuscitation was unsuccessful. Full postmortem analysis failed to identify an anatomical cause of death. Postmortem toxicology showed a blood morphine concentration of 70 ng/ml and paracetamol 5.9 μg/ml. Immediately after birth the mother had taken Tylenol® 3 (codeine 30 mg + paracetamol 500 mg), initially 2 tablets twice daily then half that dose on postpartum day 2 because of somnolence and constipation. After the neonate started to feed badly, the mother expressed her milk and stored it in a freezer. Analysis of the milk showed a morphine concentration of 87 ng/ml.

Neonates receiving morphine for analgesia have been reported to have serum concentrations of morphine of 10–12 ng/ml (32), and the maximum plasma morphine concentration in breast-fed infants of mothers who had taken codeine 60 mg for postnatal pain was 2.2 ng/ml (24). However, in this case the mother was compound heterozygous for a CYP2D6*2A allele and a CYP2D6*2x2 gene duplication, possibly originating from a homologous, unequal crossover event involving two 29 kb XbaI wild-type alleles(33). She had three functional CYP2D6 genes and was an ultraextensive metabolizer. Both the father and the infant had only two functional CYP2D6 alleles (CYP 2D6*1/*2 genotypes). Both the mother and the infant were homozygous for the UGT2B7*2 (–161TT, 802TT) allele, which has been associated with increased formation of morphine-6-glucuronide compared with the UGT2B7*1 allele (–161C, 802C).

In a systematic review, three abstracts and two full-length studies were found that had reported adverse drug reactions (unexplained episodes of drowsiness, apnea, bradycardia, and cyanosis) in 35 infants exposed to codeine in breast milk (34). In a subsequent case-control study, based mainly on telephone interviews, there were 17 cases in which mothers reported nervous system depression in their breast-fed infants, one of whom died; two mothers each had two rare genotypes: CYP2D6 UM, leading to ultraextensive metabolism of codeine to morphine, and UGT2B7*2/*2, leading to extensive formation of morphine-6-glucuronide (35). The mothers of the 17 symptomatic infants had taken a mean 59% higher codeine dose than the mothers of 55 asymptomatic infants (1.62 versus 1.02 mg/kg/day). There was 71% concordance between maternal and neonatal nervous system depression.

Despite the problems in measuring fluid and tissue concentrations of drugs post mortem (36), this case and the subsequent studies suggest that women with these rare polymorphisms should not breast-feed their babies while taking codeine. Various strategies have therefore been proposed to deal with the use of codeine in breast-feeding mothers (37):

- avoid prescribing codeine and use non-steroidal anti-inflammatory drugs instead; this approach might not be possible in cases of severe pain, although other analgesics may be available;
- prescribe codeine-containing products for no more than 2–3 days, so that neonatal accumulation of morphine does not occur; this strategy would not work if the baby also was an ultraextensive metabolizer;
- genotype all postpartum women about to receive codeine; this is probably not a cost-effective strategy, and in any case the relevant tests are not generally available;
- carefully monitor all breast-feeding women taking codeine;
- carefully monitor all breast-fed infants of codeine-using mothers; measure morphine concentrations whenever there are adverse events consistent with opioid toxicity; give naloxone if you suspect opioid toxicity.

None of these strategies is ideal.

Drug Administration

Drug dosage regimens

In a comparison of the adverse effects of 30, 60, and 90 mg codeine the most frequent adverse effects, headache, drowsiness, nausea, thirst, and a feeling of strangeness, occurred after 60 and 90 mg doses only. Visuomotor co-ordination was altered with 60 and 90 mg and dynamic visual acuity with 90 mg only (38).

Drug–Drug Interactions

Amitriptyline

There were signs of opiate toxicity, reversible with naloxone, in an 80-year-old woman after concomitant treatment with amitriptyline and co-codamol (codeine plus paracetamol) (SEDA-18, 79).

Inhibitors of CYP2D6

Inhibitors of CYP2D6 can reduce or abolish the analgesic effects of codeine (39).

Quinidine

Quinidine inhibits the hepatic metabolism of codeine to morphine. Whether this diminishes or abolishes the analgesic effect of codeine is uncertain (40,41).

Quinidine inhibits the metabolism of codeine by CYP2D6 in extensive but not in poor metabolizers (42).

References

1. Ytterberg SR, Mahowald ML, Woods SR. Codeine and oxycodone use in patients with chronic rheumatic disease pain. Arthritis Rheum 1998;41(9):1603–12.
2. Minotti V, De Angelis V, Righetti E, Celani MG, Rossetti R, Lupatelli M, Tonato M, Pisati R, Monza G, Fumi G, Del Favero A. Double-blind evaluation of short-term analgesic efficacy of orally administered diclofenac, diclofenac plus codeine, and diclofenac plus imipramine in chronic cancer pain. Pain 1998;74(2–3):133–7.
3. Wilkinson SM, Becker WJ, Heine JA. Opiate use to control bowel motility may induce chronic daily headache in patients with migraine. Headache 2001;41(3):303–9.
4. Symon DN. Twelve cases of analgesic headache. Arch Dis Child 1998;78(6):555–6.
5. Peacock JE, Henderson PD, Nimmo WS. Changes in pupil diameter after oral administration of codeine. Br J Anaesth 1988;61(5):598–600.
6. Renkes P, Trechot P. Acetaminophen–codeine combination induced acute pancreatitis. Pancreas 1998;16(4):556–7.
7. Hastier P, Buckley MJ, Peten EP, Demuth N, Dumas R, Demarquay JF, Caroli-Bosc FX, Delmont JP. A new source of drug-induced acute pancreatitis: codeine. Am J Gastroenterol 2000;95(11):3295–8.
8. Estrada JL, Puebla MJ, de Urbina JJ, Matilla B, Prieto MA, Gozalo F. Generalized eczema due to codeine. Contact Dermatitis 2001;44(3):185.
9. Rodriguez Arroyo LA, Ortiz de Saracho J, Pantoja Zarza L, Gonzalez Valle O. Reacción adversa cutánea tras administración de codeina. [Adverse cutaneous side-effect of codeine administration.] Aten Primaria 2001;27(6):444–6.
10. Mohrenschlager M, Glockner A, Jessberger B, Worret WI, Ollert M, Rakoski J, Ring J. Codeine caused pruritic scarlatiniform exanthemata: patch test negative but positive to oral provocation test. Br J Dermatol 2000;143(3):663–4.
11. Vidal C, Perez-Leiros P, Bugarin R, Armisen M. Fever and urticaria to codeine. Allergy 2000;55(4):416–7.
12. Elwood WN. Sticky business: patterns of procurement and misuse of prescription cough syrup in Houston. J Psychoactive Drugs 2001;33(2):121–33.
13. Romach MK, Sproule BA, Sellers EM, Somer G, Busto UE. Long-term codeine use is associated with depressive symptoms. J Clin Psychopharmacol 1999;19(4):373–6.
14. Sproule BA, Busto UE, Somer G, Romach MK, Sellers EM. Characteristics of dependent and nondependent regular users of codeine. J Clin Psychopharmacol 1999;19(4):367–72.
15. Caraco Y, Sheller J, Wood AJJ. Pharmacogenetic determination of the effects of codeine and prediction of drug interactions. J Pharmacol Exp Ther 1996;278:1165–74.
16. Poulsen L, Brøsen K, Arendt-Nielsen L, Gram LF, Elbaek K. Codeine and morphine in extensive and poor metabolizers of sparteine. Pharmacokinetics, analgesic effect and side effects. Eur J Clin Pharmacol 1996;51:289–95.
17. Dalen P, Frengell C, Dahl M-L, Sjøqvist F. Quick onset of severe abdominal pain after codeine in an ultrarapid metabolizer of debrisoquine. Ther Drug Monit 1997;19:543–4.
18. Findlay JWA, DeAngelis RL, Kearney MF, Welch RM, Findlay JM. Analgesic drugs in breast milk and plasma. Clin Pharmacol Ther 1981;29:625–32.
19. Abraham BK, Adithan C. Genetic polymorphism of CYP2D6. Indian J Pharmacol 2001;33:147–69.
20. Bozina N, Tramisak I, Granić P, Puljević D, Stavljenić-Rukavina A. Prevalenza dei metabolizers ultraextensive della droga in popolazione croata—rilevazione basata lungo-PCR del gene amplificato CYP2D6. (Prevalence of ultraextensive drug metabolizers in Croatian population—

21. long-PCR based detection of amplified CYP2D6 gene.) Lijec Vjesn 2002;124(3-4):63–6.
22. Cascorbi I. Pharmacogenetics of cytochrome p94502D6: genetic background and clinical implication. Eur J Clin Invest 2003;33(Suppl 2):17–22.
23. Bernard S, Neville K, Nguyen A, Flockhart D. Interethnic differences in genetic polymorphisms of CYP2D6 in the U.S. population: clinical implications. Oncologist 2006;11:126–35.
24. Münstedt A, Nolan L, Golightly P. Can breastfeeding mothers take codeine? http://www.nelm.nhs.uk/en/Download/?file=MDs1Mzk0OTsvdXBsb2FkL2RvY3VtZW50cy9Fdml-kZW5jZS9NZWRpY2luZXMgUSAmIEEvUUExODhf-M19Db2RlaW5lQk1fZmluYWwuZG9j.doc.
25. Gasche Y, Daali Y, Fathi M, Chiappe A, Cottini S, Dayer P, Desmeules J. Codeine intoxication associated with ultrarapid CYP2D6 metabolism. N Engl J Med 2004;351:2827–31.
26. Meny RG, Naumburg EG, Alger LS, Brill-Miller JL, Brown S. Codeine and the breastfed neonate. J Hum Lact 1993;9(4):237–40.
27. Bar-Oz B, Bulkowstein M, Benyamini L, Greenberg R, Soriano I, Zimmerman D, Bortnik O, Berkovitch M. Use of antibiotic and analgesic drugs during lactation. Drug Saf 2003;26(13):925–35.
28. Ito S, Blajchman A, Stephenson M, Eliopoulos C, Koren G. Prospective follow-up of adverse reactions in breast-fed infants exposed to maternal medication. Am J Obstet Gynecol 1993;168(5):1393–9.
29. Davis JM, Bhutari UK. Neonatal apnea and maternal codeine use. Pediatr Res 1984;19:170A.
30. Naumburg EG, Meny RG. Breast-milk opioids and neonatal apnea. Am J Dis Child 1988;142:11–12.
31. Smith JW. Codeine-induced bradycardia in a breast-fed infant. Clin Res 1982;30:A259.
32. Koren G, Cairns J, Chitayat D, Gaedigk A, Leeder SJ. Pharmacogenetics of morphine poisoning in a breastfed neonate of a codeine-prescribed mother. Lancet 2006;368(9536):704.
33. Bouwmeester NJ, Hop WC, van Dijk M, Anand KJ, van den Anker JN, Tibboel D. Postoperative pain in the neonate: age-related differences in morphine requirements and metabolism. Intensive Care Med 2003;29(11):2009–15.
34. Løvlie R, Daly AK, Molven A, Idle JR, Steen VM. Ultrarapid metabolizers of debrisoquine: characterization and PCR-based detection of alleles with duplication of the CYP2D6 gene. FEBS Lett 1996;392(1):30–4.
35. Madadi P, Shirazi F, Walter FG, Koren G. Establishing causality of CNS depression in breastfed infants following maternal codeine use. Paediatr Drugs 2008;10(6):399–404.
36. Madadi P, Ross CJD, Hayden MR, Carleton BC, Gaedigk A, Leeder JS, Koren G. Pharmacogenetics of neonatal opioid toxicity following maternal use of codeine during breastfeeding: a case-control study. Clin Pharmacol Ther 2009;85(1):31–5.
37. Ferner RE. Did the drug cause death? Codeine and breastfeeding. Lancet 2008;372 (9639):606–8.
38. Madadi P, Koren G, Cairns J, Chitayat D, Gaedigk A, Leeder JS, Teitelbaum R, Karaskov T, Aleksa K. Safety of codeine during breastfeeding: fatal morphine poisoning in the breastfed neonate of a mother prescribed codeine. Can Fam Physician 2007;53(1):33–5.
39. Bradley CM, Nicholson AN. Effects of a mu-opioid receptor agonist (codeine phosphate) on visuo-motor coordination and dynamic visual acuity in man. Br J Clin Pharmacol 1986;22(5):507–12.
40. Sindrup SH, Brosen K, Bjerring P, Arendt-Nielsen L, Larsen U, Angelo HR, Gram LF. Codeine increases pain thresholds to copper vapor laser stimuli in extensive but not

poor metabolizers of sparteine. Clin Pharmacol Ther 1990;48(6):686–93.

40. Desmeules J, Gascon MP, Dayer P, Magistris M. Impact of environmental and genetic factors on codeine analgesia. Eur J Clin Pharmacol 1991;41(1):23–6.
41. Sindrup SH, Arendt-Nielsen L, Brosen K, Bjerring P, Angelo HR, Eriksen B, Gram LF. The effect of quinidine on the analgesic effect of codeine. Eur J Clin Pharmacol 1992;42(6):587–91.
42. Kirkwood LC, Nation RL, Somogyi AA. Characterization of the human cytochrome P450 enzymes involved in the metabolism of dihydrocodeine. Br J Clin Pharmacol 1997;44(6):549–55.

Conorfone

General Information

Conorfone is an opioid analgesic, a codeine derivative, with mixed agonist–antagonist activity (SED-11, 150). It has adverse effects similar to those of codeine, but causes more drowsiness (1).

Reference

1. Dionne RA, Wirdezk PR, Butler DP, Fox PC. Comparison of conorphone, a mixed agonist-antagonist analgesic, to codeine for postoperative dental pain. Anesth Prog 1984;31(2):77–81.

Cyclazocine

General Information

Cyclazocine is an agonist at KOR(OP$_2$, κ) opioid receptors and it is its affinity for these receptors that is thought to account for disruption of the normal sleep pattern, urination, and sustained arousal that it causes (1). Visual disturbances and racing thoughts have also been reported and are subject to tolerance (2).

Long-Term Effects

Drug withdrawal

Abrupt withdrawal resulted in a classical withdrawal syndrome, but without drug-seeking behavior (2). Adverse effects could be minimized by gradual increments in daily dosage over 3 weeks.

References

1. Pickworth WB, Neidert GL, Kay DC. Cyclazocine-induced sleep disruptions in nondependent addicts. Prog Neuropsychopharmacol Biol Psychiatry 1986;10(1):77–85.

2. Resnick RB, Schuyten-Resnick E, Washton AM. Narcotic antagonists in the treatment of opioid dependence: review and commentary. Compr Psychiatry 1979;20(2):116–25.

Dextromethorphan

General Information

Dextromethorphan is the dextrorotatory isomer of the synthetic opioid levorphanol (1). is a non-competitive antagonist at N-methyl-D Aspartate (NMDA) receptors. It also binds to CNS sigma opioid binding sites and increases 5-HT concentrations by inhibiting the uptake of 5-HT and by enhancing its release (SEDA-25, 110). It is antitussive and has antihyperalgesic effects.

Dextromethorphan is metabolized by CYP2D6 to dextrorphan, which binds to phencyclidine receptors and is thought to account for the toxic effects of hallucinations, tachycardia, hypertension, ataxia, and nystagmus (2,3).

Drug studies

Pain relief

The role of dextromethorphan in acute and chronic pain control has been reviewed (4). There is a clear beneficial role of oral dextromethorphan (in doses of 30–90 mg) in acute pain management; it has no or few adverse effects and even reduces the need for analgesic adjuncts.

Three double-blind, crossover, randomized, placebo-controlled studies of the role of dextromethorphan in neurological pain conditions in 40 adults with diabetic neuropathy, postherpetic neuralgia, and non-specific neuropathic pain syndromes have been reviewed (5). Dextromethorphan dosages varied from 13.5 mg tds on alternate days to 120 mg qds. High-dose dextromethorphan significantly reduced pain in diabetic neuropathy with no effect in postherpetic neuralgia. Sedation (58%) and dizziness (25%) were the most commonly reported adverse effects.

In a randomized, placebo-controlled study in 60 patients given dextromethorphan 10, 20, or 40 mg intramuscularly before abdominal surgery, there was a dose-dependent effective postoperative analgesic effect, with lower total consumption of rescue morphine during the 3-day observation period (6). There were no opioid-related adverse effects in those who were given dextromethorphan 40 mg.

The effect of dextromethorphan premedication on postoperative analgesic requirements, pain scores, and adverse effects has been examined in two double-blind, randomized studies (7,8). In the first study, 60 adults scheduled for elective upper abdominal surgery were randomly allocated to three equal groups (7). One group received intramuscular dextromethorphan 120 mg 30 minutes before skin incision (preincisional group); the second group received placebo (intramuscular saline) 30 minutes before skin incision and intramuscular dextromethorphan 120 mg 30 minutes before the end of surgery (postincisional group); and the third group received placebo 30 minutes before skin incision and 30 minutes before the end of surgery (control group). Preincisional intramuscular dextromethorphan 120 mg provided pre-emptive analgesia, reduced the need for postoperative analgesic supplements, and had a minimal and non-significant adverse effects profile. In the second study, oral dextromethorphan 90 mg was compared with placebo given 90 minutes preoperatively to patients undergoing laparoscopic cholecystectomy or inguinal hernioplasty under general anesthesia (8). Pain intensity and sedation were significantly reduced in the experimental group, with sparing of postoperative analgesics for up to 24 hours. Dextromethorphan 90 mg also abolished postoperative thermal-induced hyperalgesia and hyperpathia. No adverse effects were recorded in either group.

A randomized, double-blind, placebo-controlled study of oral dextromethorphan and PCA morphine has been performed in 66 patients undergoing knee surgery (9). The study was in two parts. The first was a dose escalation study in 25 postoperative patients to determine the maximum tolerated oral dose of dextromethorphan. The second involved giving less than the maximum tolerated dose divided into three increments at 8-hour intervals. The maximum tolerated dose of dextromethorphan was 750 mg. One patient, who was given 800 mg of dextromethorphan, had adverse effects, including severe slurred speech and light-headedness followed by deep sedation. In the second part of the study 66 patients were intended to receive dextromethorphan 800 mg in three doses of 400, 200, and 200 mg. The treatment group was subsequently reduced to 22 patients, compared with 34 in the placebo group, because of unexpected nausea and vomiting in five patients given dextromethorphan 400 mg. Dextromethorphan 200 mg 8-hourly caused a significant increase in nausea 2–24 hours after the first dose. One patient given dextromethorphan had mild hallucinations on one occasion only. There was an associated modest reduction in postoperative morphine consumption (29%), with no other benefits. The study failed to provide evidence that the maximum tolerated dose of dextromethorphan 200 mg 8-hourly is useful in the treatment of postoperative pain after knee surgery.

In 25 volunteers intravenous dextromethorphan 0.5 mg/kg significantly reduced areas of established hyperalgesia by 39% and prevented the development of further hyperalgesia (10). There was large inter-subject variability in the timing of this effect, with an average duration of 2 hours in relation to peak serum concentration. Most of the volunteers (n = 22) reported adverse events, such as mild to moderate dizziness and drowsiness. However, attention should be paid to the potential for dextromethorphan to cause phencyclidine-like effects and its potential as a drug of abuse.

In a double-blind, randomized study dextromethorphan and intrathecal morphine were used for analgesia after cesarean section under spinal anesthetic in 120 patients in six groups (11). The groups had differing mixtures of intrathecal morphine (0.05 mg, 0.1 mg, 0.2 mg) and dextromethorphan (60 mg) or placebo. The results suggested that the addition of dextromethorphan reduced postoperative pain and reduced the doses of morphine. The combination reduced the incidence of nausea, vomiting, and pruritus.

Dextromethorphan and pholcodine were equally effective in 129 patients with acute, non-productive cough in a double-blind, randomized, parallel-group, multicenter trial (12).

In 15 patients with chronic neuropathic pain of traumatic origin a single oral dose of dextromethorphan (270 micrograms) produced up to 30% more reduction in analgesia than placebo (13). This was significant for up to 4 hours after medication. Most patients who took dextromethorphan had light-headedness and drowsiness (n = 10) and eight had visual disturbances. None of these adverse effects was considered severe. There was individual variation in the duration of the adverse effects. Four patients were defined as poor metabolizers and four as extensive metabolizers. Even though the analgesic effect was more pronounced in the extensive metabolizers, the intensity of the adverse effects did not exhibit similar categorization and was more related to the dose.

Neuropathic pain

In a double-blind, placebo-controlled, crossover pilot study in three patients with cancer-associated postamputation phantom limb pain, oral dextromethorphan 60–90 mg bd or placebo were given for 1 week each, followed by dextromethorphan or placebo again (14). Dextromethorphan satisfactorily improved phantom limb pain at a dosage of 60 mg bd in two patients and 90 mg bd in the third. Even though a relatively high total dose of dextromethorphan was used, there were no adverse effects.

There have been two randomized, placebo-controlled, double-blind trials in 19 patients with painful diabetic neuropathy and 17 with postherpetic neuralgia (15). In the first trial dextromethorphan was compared with memantine and/or lorazepam. Among the patients with diabetic neuropathy, dextromethorphan (median dose 400 mg/day) reduced pain intensity by a mean of 33% from baseline; memantine reduced pain by a mean of 17% and lorazepam by 16%, showing no significant difference to placebo. Among the patients with postherpetic neuralgia, dextromethorphan (median dose 400 mg/day) reduced pain intensity by a mean of 6.5%, which was not different from the effects of memantine and lorazepam. In the second trial the 10 patients with diabetic neuropathy who had responded to dextromethorphan shared a significant dose–response effect on pain intensity; the highest dose was significantly better than that of lorazepam. The median dose was 520 (range 240–920) mg/day. The adverse effects profiles were uneventful. These results confirm the long-term safety of high-dose dextromethorphan for selected patients with painful diabetic neuropathy (5).

Non-ketotic hyperglycinemia
A review of *N*-methyl-D-aspartic acid (NMDA) antagonist interventions in the treatment of non-ketotic hyperglycinemia included six cases in which dextromethorphan

was used (3). Non-ketotic hyperglycinemia is an autosomal recessive disorder in which there is failure of the glycine cleavage enzyme system, leading to impaired oxidative decarboxylation of glycine and a toxic accumulation of this amino acid. Antagonism at NMDA receptors is hypothesized to offer partial relief to the effects of this inborn error of metabolism. Of the six cases, adverse effects were described in three. Patient 1 had profound sedation in response to a dose of 7.5 mg/kg of dextromethorphan administered as a single dose when the infant was 5 days old. The same daily dosage split into three doses relieved symptoms without sedation, but doses in excess of 7.5 mg/kg resulted in somnolence, agitation, and involuntary movements. Patient 4 developed apnea, hypotonia, nystagmus, and seizures at 38 days of age and was given dextromethorphan 1 mg/kg/day at the age of 10 months, resulting in anorexia. In patient 5 an increase in dextromethorphan dosage to 10 mg/kg/day was associated with lethargy, apnea, and a return of seizure activity. Further trials are required for clarification of the use of dextromethorphan in the treatment of non-ketotic hyperglycinemia.

Parkinson's disease

In a trial of dextromethorphan in Parkinson's disease only one-third of the initial sample entered the double-blind, placebo-controlled phase (16). One-third of the sample had a reduction in the benefits of levodopa when dextromethorphan 30 mg/day was given. A further one-third withdrew because of failure to gain clinical benefit from the highest tolerated dose of dextromethorphan. Adverse effects included drowsiness, increased dystonia, increased impotence, light-headedness, sweating, and nausea.

Huntington's disease

Of 11 patients with Huntington's disease adverse effects were reported in seven. These included eczematoid rash, clumsiness, dysarthria, drowsiness, and worsening rigidity (17).

Systematic reviews

A systematic review of the postoperative effects of perioperative dextromethorphan in 28 randomized, double-blind studies in 1629 patients showed that there was no dosage regimen that could be recommended, but identified its safety as an adjunctive treatment with other opioid analgesics, with potential opioid-sparing effects and reduced opioid-related adverse effects (18). However, the authors reported that constancy of adverse effects was questionable and highlighted the fact that effective dextromethorphan analgesia is route specific, the parenteral route being more effective.

Organs and Systems

Nervous system

Although generally safe, dextromethorphan can in some individuals cause nervous system adverse effects,

including hyperexcitability, increased muscle tone, and ataxia. Respiratory depression can occur with excessive doses.

Dextromethorphan has been implicated in a case of movement disorder (19).

- An 8-year-old boy complained of abnormal facial movements and hallucinations. One day before these symptoms, he had been given his sister's Cordec DM droplets (carbinoxamine maleate 2 mg, pseudoephedrine hydrochloride 25 mg, and dextromethorphan 4 mg) for a cold. He had facial dyskinesia, dilated pupils, pyrexia, tachycardia, and reduced bowel sounds and responded to a benzodiazepine.

Dextromethorphan-induced nervous system impairment has been described in a man with a history of drug abuse (20).

- A 28-year-old man had episodes of tiredness, lightheadiness, headaches, and disorientation, on one occasion associated with psychomotor retardation, apparent intoxication, and profound sleepiness; 9 hours later he developed mild stupor, had reduced attention, and was slow in responding. He had prominent gaze-evoked nystagmus and gait ataxia. Comprehensive urine toxicology was positive for dextromethorphan.

Psychological, psychiatric

Dextromethorphan-induced psychotic and/or manic-like symptoms have been reported.

- A 2-year-old child developed hyperirritability, incoherent babbling, and ataxia after being over-medicated with a pseudoephedrine/dextromethorphan over-the-counter combination cough formulation for upper respiratory symptoms (21). The symptoms abated after withdrawal of the product.

In another three cases (girls aged 10, 13, and 15 years) severe acute psychosis was associated with the use of an over-the-counter formulation containing ephedrine or pseudoephedrine and dextromethorphan combined with other compounds (22). The psychopathology included agitation, depressed mood, flat affect, pressure of speech, visual and auditory hallucinations, and paranoia. All three improved dramatically, with residual symptoms of irritability, 2–4 days after withdrawal of the mixture and treatment with risperidone 0.5–2.0 mg/day.

- An 18-year-old student had dissociative phenomenon, nihilistic and paranoid delusions, vivid visual hallucinations, thought insertion, and broadcasting after having consumed 1–2 bottles of cough syrup (dextromethorphan 711 mg per bottle) every day for several days (23). The psychotic symptoms remitted completely without any treatment 4 days after withdrawal of dextromethorphan. He was hospitalized twice more over the next 2 months with similar symptoms; each time he had consumed large doses of dextromethorphan.

Cautious use of over-the-counter formulations is recommended in patients with a predisposition to affective illness (SEDA-21, 87).

Cognitive deterioration has been reported from prolonged use of dextromethorphan (24).

Endocrine

During a double-blind, placebo-controlled study of the effect of high doses of dextromethorphan in children with bacterial meningitis, two of four patients developed type 1 diabetes mellitus; they had received dextromethorphan and the other two placebo (25).

- A 10-year-old boy received dextromethorphan 36 mg/kg/day by nasogastric tube. He developed hyperglycemia with ketoacidosis after 5 days and required insulin. The dose of dextromethorphan was reduced over the next 4 days and withdrawn. Insulin was withdrawn 4 days later.
- A 14-year-old girl received dextromethorphan 26 mg/kg/day by nasogastric tube. She developed hyperglycemia after 2 days and needed insulin for 6 days. A later glucose tolerance test was normal.

Pancreatic beta cells in rats express NMDA receptors, stimulation of which leads to insulin secretion (26). The authors postulated that dextromethorphan inhibits insulin secretion by blocking NMDA receptors and thus impairs glucose tolerance. Both patients had reduced insulin concentrations, implying that peripheral insulin resistance was unlikely to have been the cause of diabetes.

Skin

On two occasions, a fixed drug eruption occurred on the arm of a 45-year-old woman after using dextromethorphan as an antitussive (SEDA-16, 79). Worsening of urticaria pigmentosa has been attributed to dextromethorphan (SEDA-21, 87).

A multifocal fixed drug eruption has been attributed to dextromethorphan.

- A 64-year-old healthy Japanese woman developed fingertip- to egg-sized erythematous patches surrounded by peripheral pigmentation on the buttocks, back, and thighs after taking an antitussive formulation containing dextromethorphan (27). Histopathological examination confirmed the diagnosis. The lesions were reproduced 2 hours after an oral challenge test with dextromethorphan 15 mg.

Sexual function

Spontaneous ejaculation occurred in a 64-year-old man who took dextromethorphan for a common cold (28). His sexual activity normalized 7 days after stopping the dextromethorphan. He had had a similar episode 5 months before, when spontaneous ejaculation had started 3 days after he took dextromethorphan and abated 4 days after withdrawal of the drug.

Immunologic

Dextromethorphan-induced anaphylactic symptoms have been reported (29).

- A 40-year-old woman suffered repeated hives, lip swelling, and shortness of breath on taking cough suppressants

containing dextromethorphan. None was sufficient to require emergency medical intervention. On challenge with dextromethorphan 1 mg, mild transient pruritus occurred. After dextromethorphan 30 mg, hives and nasal and conjunctival congestion occurred. Vital signs and peak flow remained stable. There was no bronchospasm or angioedema. No reaction occurred to hydrocodone or codeine.

The authors noted that many opioids are potent histamine releasers and most reactions to opioids are anaphylactoid rather than IgE-mediated. It was of particular interest that the patient was able to tolerate the opioids hydrocodone and codeine.

Second-Generation Effects

Teratogenicity

In 184 pregnancies exposed to dextromethorphan (128 exposures in the first trimester) there were 172 live births, 10 spontaneous abortions, one therapeutic abortion, and one stillbirth (30). There were three major malformations and seven minor malformations in the children of women who had used dextromethorphan in the first trimester. In the control group there were 174 live births, 8 spontaneous abortions, and 2 therapeutic abortions; there were 5 major and 18 minor malformations. This small study did not show that dextromethorphan used during pregnancy increases the rates of major malformations above the expected baseline rate of 1–3%.

Susceptibility Factors

Genetic

Dextromethorphan is metabolized by CYP2D6 in the liver to its active metabolite dextrorphan, which contributes to its analgesic and adverse effects (31). The gene locus that codes for CYP2D6 is highly polymorphic, with over 50 variant alleles. Poor metabolizers are defined as carriers of any two non-functional alleles of the CYP2D6 gene.Individuals who are poor CYP2D6 metabolizers are at increased risk of serotonergic adverse effects, as well as the narcotic adverse effects of coma and respiratory depression (32).

When dextromethorphan hydrobromide 80 mg orally (equivalent to 62 mg of dextromethorphan base) was given to 419 healthy subjects, adverse events were experienced by 17%, most being mild (33). Body mass index, weight, female sex, increased CYP2D6 and CYP3A4 metabolic ratios, and CYP2D6 poor metabolizer phenotypes were significantly associated with adverse events, but CYP2D6 extensive metabolizers were not protected against adverse events. Adverse events were more closely associated with CYP2D6 activity than the CYP2D6 phenotype. Investigators found no association between the MOR opioid receptor and the occurrence of adverse events, possibly because dextromethorphan is a weak opioid agonist, binding to sigma rather than MOR receptors.

Neurological disease

The combination of dextromethorphan and quinidine was beneficial in treating pseudobulbar palsy in 150 patients with multiple sclerosis (34). Dizziness was the only significant adverse effect.

Drug Administration

Drug formulations

Individuals who take long-acting dextromethorphan formulations are at increased risk of serotonergic adverse effects, as well as the narcotic adverse effects of coma and respiratory depression (32).

A fixed-dose combination of dextromethorphan 30 mg and quinidine 30 mg has been developed and is undergoing Phase II and Phase III trials in the treatment of emotional lability, neuropathic pain, and chronic cough, and in weaning drug dependent patients from narcotics and antidepressants. The usefulness of the combination results from the ability of quinidine to sustain therapeutic concentrations of dextromethorphan over a 12-hour dosing schedule by inhibiting oxidative first-pass metabolism of dextromethorphan, and hence reducing dosage requirements to only 2.5–5% of the usual therapeutic dose. The combination significantly improved emotional lability in different patient populations, for example those with multiple sclerosis and amyotrophic lateral sclerosis and was well tolerated (35). The most commonly reported adverse events were nausea, constipation, diarrhea, dry mouth, fatigue, dizziness, insomnia, headache, upper respiratory tract infection, and somnolence. In most cases the adverse events were mild to moderate. Of those with diabetic neuropathy 24% withdrew because of adverse events from the combination drug compared with 6% of those taking dextromethorphan alone and 8% of those taking quinidine alone.

Drug dosage regimens

The effects of dextromethorphan on postoperative pain and other parameters have been investigated in a double-blind, randomized study in 60 patients undergoing surgery for bone malignancies (36). They received either placebo (n=30) or dextromethorphan 90 mg preoperatively and 2 days postoperatively (n=30). Those given dextromethorphan had 50% less postoperative pain, required 30–50% less epidural analgesia, and demanded fewer rescue drugs than their placebo counterparts. Those given dextromethorphan were 40-60% less sedated and reported 50% fewer overall adverse effects. The authors recommended that this dextromethorphan protocol is promising and safe for patients with severe orthopedic and oncological disease without affecting the time to discharge.

Drug overdose

Intentional dextromethorphan overdose has caused two deaths (SEDA-17, 210). Dextromethorphan toxicity occurred in a 3-year-old child who ingested up to 270 mg. The effects were reversed by naloxone (2).

Drug–Drug Interactions

Moclobemide

Four healthy volunteers taking moclobemide (600 mg/day for 9 days) had reduced clearance of dextromethorphan, a marker of hepatic CYP2D6 activity (47). These findings suggest that at the higher end of its therapeutic dosage range, moclobemide inhibits the metabolism of drugs that are substrates for CYP2D6, for example antipsychotic drugs and tricyclic antidepressants (SEDA-14, 22).

Monoamine oxidase inhibitors

A possible interaction between dextromethorphan and the monoamine oxidase inhibitor isocarboxazid has been described, with myoclonic jerks, choreoathetoid movements, and marked urinary retention (37).

Individuals who take monoamine oxidase inhibitors are at increased risk of serotonergic adverse effects, as well as the narcotic adverse effects of coma and respiratory depression (37,38)

Four subjects had markedly reduced O-demethylation of dextromethorphan after they had taken moclobemide 300 mg bd for 9 days (39). N-demethylation was not affected. This result supports the hypothesis that moclobemide or a metabolite reduces the activity of the cytochrome enzyme CYP2D6. The clinical implications of this particular interaction remain to be clarified.

Morphine sulfate

Morphi Dex contains morphine sulfate and dextromethorphan in a 1:1 ratio. Double-blind, single-dose analgesic efficacy studies in over 800 patients with post-surgical pain have shown superior analgesic activity for the combination (60:60 mg) than separate doses of the individual components (40,41). In double-blind, multiple-dose studies in 321 patients with chronic pain the combination provided satisfactory pain control with a significantly lower mean daily dose of morphine sulfate. Other studies have shown similar responses (40) and an adverse events profile similar to that of a similar dose of morphine sulfate (42). The most common adverse events seen in a multiple-dose, non-placebo-controlled study in 1400 subjects were nausea, dizziness, vomiting, somnolence, confusion, and pruritus. There was a significant trend toward lower incidence of constipation with the combination than with morphine sulfate alone (43,44).

Quinidine

The effects of quinidine sulfate, 50 mg orally, an inhibitor of cytochrome CYP2D6, on the metabolism of dextromethorphan 50 mg have been studied in seven healthy volunteers in a randomized, double-blind, crossover, placebo-controlled study (32). Quinidine suppressed the conversion of dextromethorphan to dextrorphan in extensive metabolizers to the extent seen in poor metabolizers. The increased concentrations of dextromethorphan increased subjective and objective pain thresholds by 35 and 45% respectively. This result suggests that debrisoquine/sparteine-type polymorphisms account for important differences in the effect of dextromethorphan and the balance between the analgesic effect of dextromethorphan and the hallucinogenic effect of dextrorphan. Concomitant use of quinidine or other inhibitors of CYP2D6 could further affect this balance, increasing the risk of serotonergic- and narcotic-related adverse effects.

Selective serotonin re-uptake inhibitors (SSRIs)

Those who take serotonin reuptake inhibitors are at increased risk of adverse effects because of inhibition of CYP2D6 and pharmacodynamic potentiation; hallucinations and the serotonin syndrome have been reported (45,46).

SSRIs inhibit hepatic CYP isozymes and can thereby increase the activity of co-administered drugs that are metabolized by this route (SEDA-22, 13; SEDA-24, 15). In healthy volunteers randomly allocated to fluoxetine (20 mg/day), sertraline (100 mg/day), or paroxetine (20 mg/day) the activity of CYP2D6 was measured by dextromethorphan testing once steady state had been achieved and the medication was withdrawn (48). Extrapolated calculations showed that the mean time for full CYP2D6 recovery after fluoxetine (63 days) was significantly longer than that for sertraline (25 days) or paroxetine (20 days). Accordingly, even after SSRIs have been withdrawn, the potential for drug interactions persists for substantial periods of time, particularly in the case of fluoxetine.

References

1. Shaul WL, Wandell M, Robertson WO. Dextromethorphan toxicity: reversal by naloxone. Pediatrics 1977;59(1):117–8.
2. Katona B, Wason S. Dextromethorphan danger. N Engl J Med 1986;314(15):993.
3. Deutsch SI, Rosse RB, Mastropaolo J. Current status of NMDA antagonist interventions in the treatment of nonketotic hyperglycinemia. Clin Neuropharmacol 1998;21(2):71–9.
4. Weinbroum AA, Rudick V, Paret G, Ben-Abraham R. The role of dextromethorphan in pain control. Can J Anaesth 2000;47(6):585–96.
5. Generali J, Cada DJ. Dextromethorphan: neuropathy. Hosp Pharm 2001;36:421–5.
6. Wu CT, Yu JC, Liu ST, Yeh CC, Li CY, Wong CS. Preincisional dextromethorphan treatment for postoperative pain management after upper abdominal surgery. World J Surg 2000;24(5):512–7.
7. Helmy SA, Bali A. The effect of the preemptive use of the NMDA receptor antagonist dextromethorphan on postoperative analgesic requirements. Anesth Analg 2001;92(3):739–44.
8. Weinbroum AA, Gorodezky A, Niv D, Ben-Abraham R, Rudick V, Szold A. Dextromethorphan attenuation of postoperative pain and primary and secondary thermal hyperalgesia. Can J Anaesth 2001;48(2):167–74.
9. Wadhwa A, Clarke D, Goodchild CS, Young D. Large-dose oral dextromethorphan as an adjunct to patient-controlled analgesia with morphine after knee surgery. Anesth Analg 2001;92(2):448–54.
10. Duedahl TH, Dirks J, Petersen KB, Romsing J, Larsen NE, Dahl JB. Intravenous dextromethorphan to human volunteers: relationship between pharmacokinetics and antihyperalgesic effect. Pain 2005;113(3):360–8.
11. Choi DMA, Kliffer AP, Douglas MJ. Dextromethorphan and intrathecal morphine for analgesia after Caesarean section under spinal anaesthesia. Br J Anaesth 2003;90:653–8.
12. Equinozzi R, Robuschi M; on behalf of the Italian Investigational Study Group on Pholcodine in Acute Cough. Comparative efficacy and tolerability of pholcodine and dextromethorphan in the management of patients with acute, non-productive cough: a randomized, double-blind, multicentre study. Treat Respir Med 2006;5(6):509–13.
13. Carlsson KC, Hoem NO, Moberg ER, Mathiesen LC. Analgesic effect of dextromethorphan in neuropathic pain. Acta Anaesthesiol Scand 2004;48:328–36.
14. Ben Abraham R, Marouani N, Kollender Y, Meller I, Weinbroum AA. Dextromethorphan for phantom pain attenuation in cancer amputees: a double-blind crossover trial involving three patients. Clin J Pain 2002;18(5):282–5.
15. Sang CN, Booher S, Gilron I, Parada S, Max MB. Dextromethorphan and memantine in painful diabetic neuropathy and postherpetic neuralgia: efficacy and dose-response trials. Anesthesiology 2002;96(5): 1053–61.
16. Verhagen Metman L, Blanchet PJ, van den Munckhof P, Del Dotto P, Natte R, Chase TN. A trial of dextromethorphan in parkinsonian patients with motor response complications. Mov Disord 1998;13(3):414–7.
17. Walker FO, Hunt VP. An open label trial of dextromethorphan in Huntington's disease. Clin Neuropharmacol 1989;12(4):322–30.
18. Duedahl TH, Romsing J, Moiniche S, Dahl JB. A qualitative systematic review of peri-operative dextromethorphan in postoperative pain. Acta Anaesthesiol Scand 2006;50(1):1–13.
19. Nairn SJ, Diaz JE. Cold-syrup induced movement disorder. Pediatr Emerg Care 2001;17(3):191–2.
20. Cherkes JK, Friedman JH. Dextromethorphan-induced neurologic illness in a patient with negative toxicology findings. Neurology 2006;66(12):1952–3.
21. Roberge RJ, Hirani KH, Rowland PL 3rd, Berkeley R, Krenzelok EP. Dextromethorphan- and pseudoephedrine-induced agitated psychosis and ataxia: case report. J Emerg Med 1999;17(2):285–8.
22. Soutullo CA, Cottingham EM, Keck PE Jr. Psychosis associated with pseudoephedrine and dextromethorphan. J Am Acad Child Adolesc Psychiatry 1999;38(12):1471–2.
23. Price LH, Lebel J. Dextromethorphan-induced psychosis. Am J Psychiatry 2000;157(2):304.
24. Hinsberger A, Sharma V, Mazmanian D. Cognitive deterioration from long-term abuse of dextromethorphan: a case report. J Psychiatry Neurosci 1994;19(5):375–7.
25. Konrad D, Sobetzko D, Schmitt B, Schoenle EJ. Insulin-dependent diabetes mellitus induced by the antitussive agent dextromethorphan. Diabetologia 2000;43(2):261–2.
26. Molnar E, Varadi A, McIlhinney RA, Ashcroft SJ. Identification of functional ionotropic glutamate receptor proteins in pancreatic beta-cells and in islets of Langerhans. FEBS Lett 1995;371(3):253–7.
27. Kawarkami A, Nakayama H, Yamada Y, Hirosaki K, Yamashita T, Kondo S, Jimbown K. Dextromethorphan induces multifocal fixed drug eruption. Int J Dermatol 2003;42:501–2.
28. Rafols A, Garcia Vicente JA, Farre M, Mas M. Disfuncion sexual por dextrometorfang. [Dextromethorphan-induced sexual dysfunction.] Aten Primaria 1999;24(8):495–7.
29. Knowles SR, Weber E. Dextromethorphan anaphylaxis. J Allergy Clin Immunol 1998;102(2):316–7.
30. Einarson A, Lyszkiewicz D, Koren G. The safety of dextromethorphan in pregnancy: results of a controlled study. Chest 2001;119(2):466–9.

31. Albers GW, Atkinson RP, Kelley RE, Rosenbaum DM. Safety, tolerability and pharmacokinetics of the N-methyl-D-aspartate antagonist dextromethorphan in patients with acute stroke. Dextromethorphan Study Group. Stroke 1995;26:254–8.

32. Desmeules JA, Oestreicher MK, Piguet V, Allaz AF, Dayer P. Contribution of cytochrome P-450 2D6 phenotype to the neuromodulatory effects of dextromethorphan. J Pharmacol Exp Ther 1999;288(2):607–12.

33. Funck-Brentano C, Boelle PY, Verstuyft C, Bornert C, Becquemont L, Poirier JM. Measurement of CYP2D6 and CYP3A4 activity in vivo with dextromethorphan: sources of variability and predictors of adverse effects in 419 healthy subjects. Eur J Clin Pharmacol 2005;61(11):821–9.

34. Panitch HS, Thisted RA, Smith RA, Wynn DR, Wymer JP, Achiron A, Vollmer TL, Mandler RN, Dietrich DW, Fletcher M, Pope LE, Berg JE, Miller A. Randomized controlled trial of dextromethorphan/quinidine for pseudobulbar affect in multiple sclerosis. Ann Neurol 2006;59(5):780–7.

35. Avis R & D Profile. Dextromethorphan/quinidine AVP 923, dextromethorphan/cytochrome P450-2D6 inhibitor, quinidine/dextromethorphan. Drugs R & D 2005;6(3):174–7.

36. Weinbroum AA, Bender B, Bickels J, Nikkin A, Marounai N, Chazam S, Meller I, Kollender Y. Pre-operative and post-operative dextromethorphan provides sustained reduction in post-operative pain and patient-controlled epidural analfesia. Cancer 2003;97:2334–40.

37. Sovner R, Wolfe J. Interaction between dextromethorphan and monoamine oxidase inhibitor therapy with isocarboxazid. N Engl J Med 1988;319(25):1671.

38. Anonymous. High-dose fentanyl. Lancet 1979;1(8107):81–2.

39. Hartter S, Dingemanse J, Baier D, Ziegler G, Hiemke C. Inhibition of dextromethorphan metabolism by moclobemide. Psychopharmacology (Berl) 1998;135(1):22–6.

40. Caruso FS, Goldblum R. Dextromethorphan, an NMDA receptor antagonist, enhances the analgesic properties of morphine. Inflammopharmacology 2000;8:161–73.

41. Caruso FS. MorphiDex pharmacokinetic studies and single-dose analgesic efficacy studies in patients with postoperative pain. J Pain Symptom Manage 2000;19(Suppl 1):S31–6.

42. Katz NP. MorphiDex (MS:DM) double-blind, multiple-dose studies in chronic pain patients. J Pain Symptom Manage 2000;19(Suppl 1):S37–41.

43. Goldblum R. Long-term safety of MorphiDex. J Pain Symptom Manage 2000;19(Suppl 1):S50–6.

44. Chevlen E. Morphine with dextromethorphan: conversion from other opioid analgesics. J Pain Symptom Manage 2000;19(Suppl 1):S42–9.

45. Achamallah NS. Visual hallucinations after combining fluoxetine and dextromethorphan. Am J Psychiatry 1992;149(10):1406.

46. Skop BP, Finkelstein JA, Mareth TR, Magoon MR, Brown TM. The serotonin syndrome associated with paroxetine, an over-the-counter cold remedy, and vascular disease. Am J Emerg Med 1994;12(6):642–4.

47. Hartter S, Dingemanse J, Baier D, Ziegler G, Hiemke C. Inhibition of dextromethorphan metabolism by moclobemide. Psychopharmacology (Berl) 1998;135(1):22–6.

48. Liston HL, DeVane CL, Boulton DW, Risch SC, Markowitz JS, Goldman J. Differential time course of cytochrome P450 2D6 enzyme inhibition by fluoxetine, sertraline, and paroxetine in healthy volunteers. J Clin Psychopharmacol 2002;22(2):169–73.

Dextropropoxyphene

General Information

The most frequent adverse effects of dextropropoxyphene are dizziness, sedation, and nausea and vomiting. Other reported effects include constipation, abdominal pain, skin rashes, light-headedness, headache, weakness, euphoria, dysphoria, minor reversible visual disturbances, and liver dysfunction (1).

A systematic review of single-dose dextropropoxyphene for postoperative pain identified 130 published articles (2). Of these, 11 placebo-controlled studies met the inclusion criteria for the review, 6 of dextropropoxyphene (65 mg) and five of the same dose of dextropropoxyphene plus paracetamol (650 mg) (co-proxamol). Pooled data from the studies showed that the incidence of nausea, drowsiness, and headache with dextropropoxyphene alone was not significantly different from placebo. Previous reports have suggested that dextropropoxyphene is significantly associated with dizziness, sedation, and nausea and vomiting. However, co-proxamol caused significantly increased dizziness (relative risk 2.2, 95% CI = 1.1, 4.3) and drowsiness (2.1, 1.5, 2.9). The relative risk of headache was reduced to 0.5 (0.3, 0.9). Analgesic effect was greater with co-proxamol than with dextropropoxyphene alone.

Organs and Systems

Cardiovascular

Dextropropoxyphene-induced cardiogenic shock has been described (3).

- A 32-year-old man became deeply comatose, with intraventricular conduction disturbances, after taking dextropropoxyphene 4.6 g. Treatment-resistant seizures lasted for hours. He was treated with an intra-aortic balloon pump and a continuous infusion of milrinone for 7 days and recovered fully.

The mechanism of cardiotoxicity of dextropropoxyphene is unknown, but the membrane-stabilizing effect of its major metabolite, norpropoxyphene, seems to play a central part. The cardiac effects are not reversed by naloxone (4), but dopamine may be effective.

Respiratory

Hypersensitivity pneumonitis has been associated with co-proxamol (paracetamol plus dextropropoxyphene) (5).

- A 61-year-old man, who was taking prednisolone 20 mg and co-proxamol as required for cranial arteritis, presented with a 2-month history of increasing breathlessness. His chest X-ray showed vague shadowing in both lower zones, consistent with an interstitial abnormality, and a lung biopsy confirmed focal interstitial hypersensitivity pneumonitis. After a diffuse rash appeared, the co-proxamol was withdrawn and then reintroduced. The rash recurred and the breathlessness deteriorated. A subsequent challenge with paracetamol did not produce the same symptoms. The dosage of prednisolone was not altered.

Sensory systems

Nerve deafness in a 44-year-old woman, dependent on co-proxamol (dextropropoxyphene plus paracetamol), has been reported (SEDA-17, 80).

Metabolism

Severe hypoglycemia has been reported in the elderly (SEDA-17, 80).

Hematologic

Hemolytic anemia has been attributed to dextropropoxyphene (6).

Gastrointestinal

Four cases each of necrotizing anorectitis and proctitis have been reported after long-term (2–24 months) use of suppositories containing dextropropoxyphene and paracetamol (SEDA-10, 62). Perineal ulceration can also occur (7).

Liver

Various forms of hepatotoxicity, sometimes involving jaundice or mimicking biliary tract disease, have been reported by the UK Committee on Safety of Medicines (8). In most, but not all, cases the drug had been taken with paracetamol. In some cases, rechallenge caused hepatotoxicity within a few hours, and an immunologically based mechanism has been suggested.

Dextropropoxyphene has been implicated in hepatic injury in four patients taking co-proxamol (dextropropoxyphene plus paracetamol) (9). The cases were recorded at the Regional Centre of Pharmacovigilance in St Etienne, France between 1985 and 2000 and were similar to 29 cases published in the international literature between 1971 and 1994. The risk factors identified in the confirmed cases included age over 50 years, female sex, and a history of excessive alcohol consumption or previous pathology that might have caused liver damage. Drug withdrawal produced good outcomes.

Skin

Acute generalized pustulosis attributed to dextropropoxyphene has been reported (10).

- A 43-year-old woman, who had taken antibiotics and analgesics, including dextropropoxyphene, for parotitis, developed generalized erythema with numerous pustules on the trunk followed by a pyrexia. Patch testing was positive with dextropropoxyphene only and negative with paracetamol, spiramycin, aspirin, and tenoxicam.

Musculoskeletal

Fibrous myopathy has been reported after long-term dextropropoxyphene injections (SEDA-18, 85).

Musculoskeletal

In a prospective cohort study of 362 503 patients during a mean follow-up of 464 days, about 10% (37 569) had at least one prescription for propoxyphene and about 1% (5065) had a hip fracture (11).

Long-Term Effects

Drug dependence

In common with other opioids, dextropropoxyphene can produce dependence (12). However, it has also been used to withdraw patients from morphine (13).

Susceptibility Factors

Age

Acute respiratory failure predominated in patients under 30 years of age whilst cardiotoxic effects predominated in the elderly.

Renal disease

Severe hypoglycemia has been reported in a patient with chronic renal insufficiency (14).

Drug Administration

Drug overdose

Dextropropoxyphene is widely prescribed in combination with aspirin or paracetamol. It is particularly dangerous when taken in overdose (15). A mortality rate of 8% was described in a series of 222 self-harm patients (16).

In the UK self-poisoning with co-proxamol (dextropropoxyphene hydrochloride 32.5 mg + paracetamol 325 mg) has accounted in the past for 5% of all cases and was the second most commonly used drug in cases of self-poisoning. When it was marketed in the UK about 1.7 million people received 7.5 million prescriptions annually (17). In a multicenter study based on an examination of coroners' reports in 2000–1, death results from respiratory depression and/or cardiac effects (18). There were 123 deaths from co-proxamol poisoning, of which 42% were in those aged 55 years or more, possibly because of increased prescribing in older age groups, increased vulnerability to toxicity, and higher degrees of suicidal intent. Alcohol was consumed in 59% of cases and most of these were young people with low degrees of suicidal intent. About half had a history of self-harm and one-third were in contact with psychiatric services. Co-proxamol has been withdrawn in the UK.

Drug–Drug Interactions

Alcohol

Cardiorespiratory arrest can occur only 15 minutes after drug ingestion (19). This risk is enhanced if ethanol is taken concomitantly.

Alprazolam

Inhibition of alprazolam metabolism by dextropropoxyphene has been reported (20).

Carbamazepine

Dextropropoxyphene inhibits the oxidative metabolism of carbamazepine, leading to clinically significant rises in carbamazepine concentrations (21).

Severe carbamazepine toxicity can occur if dextropropoxyphene is taken concurrently (22).

Nortriptyline

Inhibition of nortriptyline metabolism by dextropropoxyphene has been reported (23).

Warfarin

Prolongation of the prothrombin time was observed in a patient concurrently taking warfarin and a compound analgesic containing dextropropoxyphene (24).

Smoking

Heavy smoking can increase the elimination of dextropropoxyphene (25).

References

1. Grover H. Propoxyphene. J Indian Med Assoc 1988; 86(1):21–3.
2. Collins SL, Edwards JE, Moore RA, McQuay HJ. Single-dose dextropropoxyphene in post-operative pain: a quantitative systematic review. Eur J Clin Pharmacol 1998;54(2):107–12.
3. Gillard P, Laurent M. Dextropropoxyphene-induced cardiogenic shock: treatment with intra-aortic balloon pump and milrinone. Intensive Care Med 1999;25(3):335.
4. Pickar D, Dubois M, Cohen MR. Behavioral change in a cancer patient following intrathecal beta-endorphin administration. Am J Psychiatry 1984;141(1):103–4.
5. Matusiewicz SP, Wallace WA, Crompton GK. Hypersensitivity pneumonitis associated with co-proxamol (paracetamol + dextropropoxyphene) therapy Postgrad Med J 1999;75(886):475–6.
6. Fulton JD, McGonigal G. Steroid responsive haemolytic anaemia due to dextropropoxyphene paracetamol combination. J R Soc Med 1989;82(4):228.
7. Bosisio OA, Gonzales AU, Bravard JD, et al. Ulcera medicamentosa de ano. Prensa Med Argent 1986;73:437.
8. Committee on Safety of Medicines. Hepatotoxicity with dextropropoxyphene. Curr Probl 1986;17:.
9. Bergeron L, Guy C, Ratrema M, Beyens MN, Mounier G, Ollagnier M. Dextropropoxyphène et atteintes hépatiques: à propos de 4 cas et revue de literature. [Dextropropoxyphene hepatotoxicity: four cases and literature review.] Thérapie 2002;57(5):464–72.
10. Machet L, Martin L, Machet MC, Lorette G, Vaillant L. Acute generalized exanthematous pustulosis induced by dextropropoxyphene and confirmed by patch testing. Acta Derm Venereol 2000;80(3):224–5.
11. Kamal-Bahl SJ, Stuart BC, Beers MH. Propoxyphene use and risk for hip fractures in older adults. Am J Geriatr Pharmacother 2006;4:219–26.
12. Strode SW. Propoxyphene dependence and withdrawal. Am Fam Physician 1985;32(3):105–8.
13. Hasday JD, Weintraub M. Propoxyphene in children with iatrogenic morphine dependence. Am J Dis Child 1983;137(8):745–8.
14. Almirall J, Montoliu J, Torras A, Revert L. Propoxyphene-induced hypoglycemia in a patient with chronic renal failure. Nephron 1989;53(3):273–5.
15. Proudfoot AT. Clinical features and management of Distalgesic overdose. Hum Toxicol 1984;3(Suppl):S85–94.
16. Sloth Madsen P, Strom J, Reiz S, Bredgaard Sorensen M. Acute propoxyphene self-poisoning in 222 consecutive patients. Acta Anaesthesiol Scand 1984;28(6):661–5.
17. Scott DGI. In the days of patients' choice, why is the patient being ignored? Lancet 2005;366(9482):287–8.
18. Hawton K, Simkin S, Gunnell D, Sutton L, Bennewith O, Turnbull P, Kapur N. A multicentre study of coproxamol poisoning suicides based on coroners' records in England. Br J Clin Pharmacol 2005;59(2):207–12.
19. Young RJ. Dextropropoxyphene overdosage. Pharmacological considerations and clinical management. Drugs 1983;26(1):70–9.
20. Abernethy DR, Greenblatt DJ, Morse DS, Shader RI. Interaction of propoxyphene with diazepam, alprazolam and lorazepam. Br J Clin Pharmacol 1985; 19(1):51–7.
21. Hansen BS, Dam M, Brandt J, Hvidberg EF, Angelo H, Christensen JM, Lous P. Influence of dextropropoxyphene on steady state serum levels and protein binding of three anti-epileptic drugs in man. Acta Neurol Scand 1980; 61(6):357–67.
22. Yu YL, Huang CY, Chin D, Woo E, Chang CM. Interaction between carbamazepine and dextropropoxyphene. Postgrad Med J 1986;62(725):231–3.
23. Jerling M, Bertilsson L, Sjoqvist F. The use of therapeutic drug monitoring data to document kinetic drug interactions: an example with amitriptyline and nortriptyline. Ther Drug Monit 1994;16(1):1–12.
24. Smith R, Prudden D, Hawkes C. Propoxyphene and warfarin interaction. Drug Intell Clin Pharm 1984; 18(10):822.
25. D'Arcy PF. Tobacco smoking and drugs: a clinically important interaction? Drug Intell Clin Pharm 1984; 18(4):302–7.

Dezocine

General Information

Dezocine is structurally related to pentazocine (1). It reacts primarily with OP_3 (μ) receptors, but also has some affinity for OP_1 (δ) and OP_2 (κ) receptors. It is slightly more potent than morphine, but with similar adverse effects at effective doses (2.5–10 mg). The most common adverse effects (3–9%) are nausea and vomiting, sedation, or local injection site reactions; dizziness/vertigo have also been reported (1–3%) (SEDA-16, 88). However, in some trials nausea and/or vomiting were reported in 5–22%, while headache was the most common CNS complaint (16–35%). Other adverse effects reported in 1% of patients involve the cardiovascular system, respiratory system, urogenital system, CNS, gastrointestinal system, and visual senses.

Reference

1. O'Brien JJ, Benfield P. Dezocine. A preliminary review of its pharmacodynamic and pharmacokinectic properties, and therapeutic efficacy. Drugs 1989;38(2):226–48.

Diamorphine

General Information

Diamorphine (heroin) is a potent opioid that offers no substantial advantages over morphine. In the UK it is the preferred parenteral opioid for subcutaneous administration to cachectic cancer patients, because of its high solubility.

In a randomized, double-blind study, 14 patients who underwent elective surgery for correction of bilateral arthritic deformities of the feet received 15 ml of 0.9% saline containing diamorphine 2.5 mg into the cannula in one foot and 15 ml of saline into the other foot (1). Intravenous regional diamorphine did not improve postoperative pain relief or secondary hyperalgesia. There were no significant adverse effects.

High-dose diamorphine has been compared with morphine in a double-blind, crossover, randomized study in 39 intravenous opioid users who were allocated to either morphine 3% solution or diamorphine 2% solution, gradually increasing up to an individual maintenance dose adjusted to meet the patient's subjective needs (2). Those who started with diamorphine and subsequently switched to morphine terminated prematurely owing to excessive histamine reactions, all of which occurred during crossover to morphine. Symptoms included severe pruritus, flushing, swelling, urticaria, severe headaches, nausea, general malaise, hypotension, and tachycardia. Only 44% of the original cohort finished the 6-week study (14 getting diamorphine at the end and three getting morphine). Average daily doses were 491 mg for diamorphine and 597 mg for morphine. These results suggest that diamorphine produces fewer adverse effects than morphine and may be preferable for high-dose maintenance prescription. However, the study was very small and the subject selection was biased, as were the variables used to determine a successful outcome. The result was contrary to all the well-established pharmacological facts, and the authors did not mention the risks associated with high doses of short-acting opioids.

In a randomized, double-blind study, 64 patients undergoing total knee arthroplasty received either intrathecal morphine 0.3 mg or intrathecal diamorphine, 0.3 mg in 0.3 ml, with 2–2.5 ml of 0.5% heavy spinal bupivacaine (3). The patients given morphine had significantly greater analgesia at 4, 8, and 12 hours postoperatively. The incidence of opioid-related adverse effects was not significantly different between the groups.

In a single-blind, randomized, controlled study, 70 patients scheduled for elective cesarean section under spinal anesthesia using hyperbaric bupivacaine 0.5% received intrathecal fentanyl 20 µg, intrathecal diamorphine 300 µg, or 0.9% saline (4). Significantly less intraoperative and postoperative "analgesic control" was required in the opioid groups, especially in those given diamorphine. Diamorphine produced longer-lasting analgesia than fentanyl (12 hours versus 1 hour). Nausea, vomiting, and pruritus occurred relatively infrequently, with no differences between the groups; sedation was more frequent with fentanyl.

Observational studies

In two separate open, randomized, controlled but unblinded trials, 549 patients were divided into five treatment groups. In the first study there were 375 patients in three groups

- methadone alone for 12 months (controls);
- methadone plus inhaled heroin for 12 months;
- methadone alone for 6 months followed by methadone plus inhaled heroin for 6 months.

In the second study there were 174 patients in two similar experimental groups in whom injectable rather than inhaled heroin was used (5). A response to treatment was defined as at least a 40% improvement in physical, mental, or social domains of quality of life, if not accompanied by a substantial (over 20%) increase in the use of another illicit drug, such as cocaine or amphetamines. After 12 months those who took methadone and heroin (smoked or injected) had significantly better outcomes. The incidences of adverse effects (constipation and drowsiness) were similar in all the groups. However, owing to the limitations of the study and the complex nature of drug dependence, the therapeutic outcomes could not be justifiably and solely attributed to the specific drug(s).

Organs and Systems

Respiratory

"Chasing the dragon," or inhaling heroin vapor through a straw, is a technique by which heroin users avoid the risks of injection. In Amsterdam, 85% of heroin users smoke or chase the drug. Pulmonary function can be affected by heroin inhalation. It can depress the respiratory center, release histamine (which can trigger asthma), result in septic emboli, and increase susceptibility to infectious diseases, such as tuberculosis and pneumonia. In 100 methadone maintenance users, lung function and shortness of breath were evaluated using spirometry and clinical history (6). Impaired lung function and shortness of breath correlated with chronic heroin smoking.

Heroin-induced pulmonary edema, or "heroin lung" (SEDA-19, 29; SEDA-25, 39), is a serious complication, which may be due to release of histamine, with increased pulmonary lymph flow and capillary permeability. There have been 27 reports of non-fatal heroin overdose associated with non-cardiogenic pulmonary edema (7). In a retrospective case-control study there were 23 heroin fatalities and 12 controls with sudden cardiac deaths (8). The authors tried to verify that defects of the alveolar capillary membranes and/or an acute anaphylactic reaction can lead to pulmonary congestion, edema, and hemorrhages. There were defects of the epithelial and endothelial basal laminae of the alveoli in both groups. There was an insignificant increase in IgE-positive cells in the heroin group. The findings suggested that heroin-associated lung edema is generally not caused by an anaphylactic reaction.

Bilateral pulmonary edema associated with heroin abuse has been reported several times (9). Bronchospasm has been noted following the use of street heroin, perhaps due to contaminants (10).

In a retrospective study of the case notes of patients who had been admitted to hospital with acute attacks of asthma, there was a high prevalence of heroin use.-15% had used only heroin and another 16% had used both heroin and cocaine (11). Heroin users had been intubated more often than non-drug users (17 versus 2.3%). Similarly more heroin users had been admitted to ICU than non-users (21 versus 12%). However, they did not spend more time receiving mechanical ventilation or being in hospital. These findings suggest that heroin induced some degree of bronchoconstriction and respiratory depression, which worsened the initial presentation of asthma.

Nervous system

Delayed onset oculogyric crisis and generalized dystonia occurred in a 19-year-old man after intranasal heroin use, possibly due to bilateral hypoxic infarction of the pallidum and pallidothalamic tracts (12).

There has been one report of mixed transcortical aphasia attributed to heroin (13).

Myoclonic spasm has been reported about 24 hours after withdrawal of an epidural infusion of diamorphine (SEDA-16, 81).

Demyelination has been attributed to diamorphine (14).

- A 41-year-old chronic diamorphine user developed an unsteady gait and dysarthria over 2 weeks, followed by severe cerebellar ataxia and moderate dysmetria of the arms and legs. An MRI scan suggested myelin damage, with symmetrical involvement of the cerebellar hemispheres and decussation of the superior cerebellar peduncles, the corticospinal tracts, and the centrum semiovale, suggesting spongiform leukoencephalopathy. Two years later having taken no more diamorphine he was improved, with minor regression of the MRI lesions, especially the white matter lesions.

Myelopathy has been reported after intranasal insufflation of diamorphine (15).

- A 52-year-old man with a history of diamorphine abuse presented with sudden paraplegia a few hours after intranasal insufflation. He had flaccid paralysis of both legs, acute urinary retention, and reduced rectal tone. Deep tendon reflexes were absent and plantar responses were extensor. An MRI scan of the spine and an immunoglobulin profile supported the conclusion that this was a case of acute myelopathy with an immunopathological cause, involving a protein specific to spinal cord parenchyma, triggering acute local inflammation, ischemia, and tissue damage. Seven weeks later he recovered normal neurological function.

This case of heroin myelopathy is similar to other reported cases, except that this case occurred with intranasal rather than intravenous use. The MRI findings were consistent with a transverse myelitis. The authors suggested that hypersensitivity and an immune-mediated attack on the spinal cord was the likely mechanism of injury.

Reflex sympathetic dystrophy, in which there is an excessive or abnormal sympathetic nervous system response in a limb, has been associated with rhabdomyolysis secondary to heroin abuse (16).

- A 37-year-old male heroin smoker developed tea-colored urine and pain, swelling, and tenderness in both feet. He had acute renal insufficiency and rhabdomyolysis and was treated with hemodialysis. Urine toxicology was negative. He also had persistent, burning pain in both feet, with cool, pale, thin skin on both legs, a mild reduction in sensation on the lateral aspects of the lower legs and diminished bilateral knee and ankle reflexes. Walking was restricted, with limited range of movement owing to the severe pain. His feet would swell and redden after a 5-meter walk, suggesting loss of sympathetic regulation. Nerve conduction velocity studies of the tibial, peroneal, and sural nerves were abnormal. Radiographs showed mildly reduced bone mineralization in the legs. Three-phase bone scintigraphy showed diffusely increased radiotracer accumulation over both feet in all three phases, as found in reflex sympathetic dystrophy. The diagnosis was confirmed by local anesthetic sympathetic blockade. Nasal calcitonin spray led to pain relief 2 months later. A follow-up three-phase bone scintigram showed less radiotracer uptake, consistent with a good response to calcitonin therapy.

Substance-induced polyradiculopathy has been described in a 23-year-old Caucasian man after administration of high doses of heroin and cocaine into the left internal carotid artery (17).

Six patients developed some form of neuropathy following heroin use (18). Four developed a plexopathy and two a symmetric distal axonal sensorimotor neuropathy. Five also had rhabdomyolysis with high creatinine kinase activities.

Progressive spongiform leukoencephalopathy

A rare consequence of inhaling heated heroin ("chasing the dragon") is a progressive spongiform leukoencephalopathy. The first three cases in the USA were reported in 1996 (SEDA-22, 35). The presentation includes apathy, bradyphrenia, motor restlessness, and progressive cerebellar ataxia. Another report has provided more details from physical assessments and laboratory and radiological (MRI and MRS) data, and more information about the course of this heroin-related effect (19). The three cases showed raised concentrations of intracerebral lactate (reflecting mitochondrial dysfunction), which suggests a conversion of aerobic to anaerobic metabolism seen in hypoxic-ischemic conditions, including stroke. One patient recovered quite well after antioxidant therapy, supporting a metabolic effect of the heroin-related toxin; a similar response to co-enzyme Q has been found in other mitochondrial disorders with a high CSF lactate. Thus, the authors recommended that although the role of antioxidant therapy in this condition is unclear, it may be prudent to administer oral co-enzyme Q supplemented with vitamins C and E to patients with this syndrome.

Spongiform leukoencephalopathy has been described in a 26-year-old after inhalation of heroin (20). The diagnosis was confirmed by MRI scan.

- A 46-year-old man with a 26-year history of heroin abuse developed a slowly progressive gait disorder with paresthesia in the legs after he had bought heroin from a different illicit heroin dealer (21). After another few weeks he developed urinary incontinence and impotence. Neurological examination, an MRI scan of the brain and neck, and evoked potentials confirmed a progressive myelopathy affecting only the corticospinal tracts and posterior columns as a result of inhalation of heroin vapor. Prolonged multivitamin supplementation and subsequent high-dose prednisone for 10 days did not improve the symptoms.

Other cases of possible toxic leukoencephalopathy following probable inhalation of heroin vapor have been reported (22).

- A 55-year-old man developed confusion, behavioral change, aggression, poor attention, disorientation in time, and impaired short term memory. He had full ocular movements with no nystagmus, brisk deep tendon reflexes, and bilateral extensor plantar responses. He became progressively drowsy with myoclonic jerks and died 2 weeks later.
- A 36-year-old man with a history of substance abuse became unresponsive, with his eyes in mid-position gaze, with pinpoint pupils, brisk deep tendon reflexes, and bilateral extensor plantar responses. On day 9 he spontaneously opened his eyes. However, he died 1 month later with persistent pyrexia from meticillin-resistant Staphylococcus aureus.Neuroimaging and neuropathology in both cases showed diffuse symmetrical degeneration of white matter, with sparing of subcortical U fibers, cerebellum, and brain stem.

Toxicology was negative, but was done some time after the report of substance use. In these case reports heroin use could not be confirmed. Although the findings suggested the possibility of heroin toxicity due to inhalation, sparing of the cerebellum and brain stem, frontal predominance of degeneration, and the more prominent axonal involvement are not typical of heroin toxicity, throwing speculation on an unidentified impurity.

- Four patients developed acute toxic spongiform leukoencephalopathy after inhaling heroin vapor (23,24). One died and the other three were discharged with residual neurological symptoms.

Intravenous administration of pure heroin did not cause a leukoencephalopathy in a patient in whom inhalation had caused it (25), and toxicity in these cases may have been due to the heating of the heroin. This might have implications for young heroin users who, because of the known increased risk of HIV infection, prefer to "chase" (smoke) the drug, rather than to inject it intravenously.

- A 23-year-old pregnant woman at 39 weeks of gestation developed tonic-clonic seizures and hypothermia after taking excessive heroin intravenously (26). She developed Cheyne-Stokes respiration needing intubation and a cesarean section was performed, after which she developed inappropriate secretion of antidiuretic hormone and acute renal insufficiency. She made a complete recovery.

The etiology of this leukoencephalopathy is unclear. Because cases occur in clusters, even though many others who inhale heroin do not get this effect, there is suspicion about the possible role of contaminants of small batches of drug by an unknown substance. In addition, some have suggested that heating could be important, since leukoencephalopathy has not been reported with other means of heroin use (until this year, as reported in the next case). The authors of the report postulated that there might be a relation between the amount of heroin inhaled and the severity of the illness. Once symptoms develop, progression continues, usually for 2–3 weeks, but in some individuals it progresses for up to 6 months after exposure. "Coasting," or the phenomenon of symptom progression after cessation of exposure to toxins, has been observed with other toxins, and it is proposed to result from the storage of toxin in lipid-rich neural or non-neural body tissues, with subsequent release into the bloodstream. Although the "toxin" involved in this condition is unknown, progression could be due to "coasting." Alternatively, oxidative damage could be initiated by the toxin and produce persistent metabolic changes in the affected white matter. Whatever the mechanism, the illness is extremely grave, with no known treatment and with progression to akinetic mutism and death in about 20% of reported cases.

- A 37-year-old male cocaine abuser was admitted with intoxication, mutism, and substupor (27). His toxicological screening was positive for heroin and cocaine. There was spasticity of all limbs and Babinski reflexes. The CSF contained some erythrocytes. The electroencephalogram showed generalized slowing, and a CT scan showed bifrontal confluent hypodensities in the deep white matter. The cranial MRI scan showed diffuse bihemispheric white matter lesions dominantly in the frontal lobe on T2-weighted images. There were abnormal hyperintense lesions in the pyramidal tracts and the corpus callosum. He gradually improved and made a complete recovery within 6 months, as confirmed by neurological and neuropsychological examination.

The findings of toxic leukoencephalopathy in this patient's brain-imaging studies were similar to those reported in patients who have inhaled impure heroin. However, he had used intravenous heroin and cocaine. This is therefore the first case report of leukoencephalopathy after intravenous use of these drugs. However, it should be noted that the authors did not indicate how the route of drug use was confirmed. They noted that lipophilic substances, such as hexachlorophene or triethyltin, were likely impurities in the abused substances.

- A 53-year-old man with a 7-year history of heroin abuse presented with confused speech and unsteady gait (28). A CT scan showed low attenuation in the white matter tracts and an MRI scan showed increased signal intensity in the white matter tracts extending from the centrum semiovale, corpus callosum, corona radiata, posterior limbs of the internal capsules, cerebral and cerebellar peduncles, and pyramidal tracts, suggestive of spongiform demyelination. He became bed-bound and tetraplegic and died of a chest infection.
- A 37-year-old man, with a short history of heroin and cocaine use, presented with spasticity of all limbs, a confusional state, and mutism (27). The electroencephalogram, CT scan, and MRI scan showed predominantly positive frontal pathology, with other lesions in the pyramidal tracts and corpus callosum. The diagnosis was leukoencephalopathy. The symptoms gradually abated after 4 weeks, and repeat tests after 6 months shown to be normal.

Three cases of toxic and progressive spongiform leukoencephalopathy have also been reported as a result of vapor inhalation of heroin (19). There were generalized white matter abnormalities and pathology in the cerebellum, internal capsule, corpus callosum, and brain stem.

Heroin-induced leuckoencephalopathy has been misdiagnosed as psychiatric illness (29).

- A 47-year-old woman, with a history of amphetamine abuse, depression, and paranoia, smoked heroin for 4 weeks after stopping amphetamines, and 10 days later became drowsy and confused with increased paranoia and depression. She was disoriented and restless. Her speech was garbled. She had frequent non-purposeful movements and an unsteady gait. A CT brain scan was normal. She was given chlorpromazine, doxepin, and diazepam, but her ataxia and incontinence worsened, her speech and all her movements slowed, with increased tone in all limbs and cogwheel rigidity. Her power and sensation were normal. Truncal ataxia

impaired walking. An MRI brain scan showed diffuse high-intensity signals in both cerebral hemispheres, and review of the CT scan showed hypodensities in the same regions. She was treated with co-enzyme Q and regained mobility and continence, but with no improvement in cognitive impairment.

Sensory systems

Profound reversible deafness with vestibular dysfunction has been attributed to heroin abuse (30).

- A 47-year-old intravenous opiate user, after a period of abstinence, injected about 0.25 g of illicit diamorphine during a period of 24 hours and developed bilateral symmetrical sensorineural hearing loss, ear fullness, and loud tinnitus 20 minutes later. His symptoms gradually subsided with no sequelae after 3 weeks.

The authors pointed out that bilateral deafness after heroin relapse after prolonged abstinence had been reported in previous two cases, suggesting resensitization of a tolerized opioid system or prolonged hypersensitization of a system in withdrawal.

Endocrine

The syndrome of inappropriate secretion of antidiuretic hormone (SIADH) has been attributed to heroin (26).

- A 23-year-old pregnant woman developed antepartum bleeding at 35 weeks and a tonic-clonic convulsion and hypothermia at 39 weeks, having used heroin 4 hours before. She had further tonic-clonic seizures, became obtunded, and required intubation. She had occasional runs of ventricular bigeminy. A cesarean section was performed. The neonate had poor respiratory effort and required ventilation. Blood chemistry suggested inappropriate secretion of antidiuretic hormone, acute renal insufficiency, and acute pancreatitis. She and the baby recovered after 2 weeks.

Gastrointestinal

In a small randomized study, 40 women undergoing elective cesarean section received either diamorphine 300 micrograms or 0.9% saline as part of a standard spinal anesthesia (31). Intrathecal diamorphine may contribute to the delay in gastric emptying that occurs immediately after elective spinal cesarean section. This is relevant within the context of other possible compounding variables that might delay the reintroduction of a solid diet postoperatively.

Urinary tract

Following an observation that many patients develop acute renal insufficiency after using heroin, the authors identified 27 patients (mostly men, average age 29 years) who developed renal insufficiency after intravenous heroin use (32). Rhabdomyolysis was the likely cause of renal insufficiency in all cases. Twelve had a history of polydrug abuse and all had a history of intravenous diamorphine use in the 24 hours before presentation. Eight patients required renal dialysis for an average of 14 days. Patients who required dialysis had a higher admission creatine kinase, a higher peak creatine kinase, and a lower urine output in the initial 24 hours. They also had a longer hospital stay. Some had positive tests for hepatitis B (10%), hepatitis C (74%) and HIV (5%); viral infections can compound rhabdomyolysis and subsequent renal impairment through glomerulonephritis. No patient died and all patients recovered normal renal function. Rhabdomyolysis is a recognized cause of renal insufficiency, but its pathogenesis after heroin use is not fully understood.

In most of 19 renal specimens from autopsies of intravenous diamorphine users there was severe lymphomonocytic glomerulonephritis as a result of activation of the classical pathway of the complement binding system (33). This could have been a result of diamorphine itself, adulterants, or active hepatitis B and/or C infection.

Heroin was presumed to be the cause of reversible nephrotic syndrome in patients dependent on heroin (34).

Renal amyloidosis can be a late effect (34).

Skin

A traumatic skin lesion with blisters and sweat gland necrosis was described in a 24-year-old man who was comatose as a result of heroin overdose; immunofluorescence showed deposits of immunoglobulin and C3 in dermal vessels (35).

Musculoskeletal

Focal myopathy has been reported after intramuscular diamorphine (36).

- A 36-year-old man developed progressive, painless stiffness of both knee joints over 3 months. It had started 4 weeks after he began to give himself heroin injections two to three times a day in alternate thigh muscles. He had a broad-based stiff gait, and he walked without bending his knees. Because of contractures of the quadriceps muscles, which were indurated, active and passive knee flexion was limited to an angle of 5–10 degrees. Electromyography of the right quadriceps muscle showed firm fibrous resistance to needling without insertional activity. Ultrasound showed a preserved but enlarged muscle structure and thickening of the connective tissue. A muscle biopsy showed variation in fiber size with scattered collection of atrophic fibers and perivascular and endomysial infiltrates comprised chiefly of lymphocytes and macrophages. The serum creatine kinase activity was normal. After 7 weeks of physiotherapy, MRI of the thighs showed severe fibrosis of the muscle, suggesting a possible inflammatory component. Following treatment with prednisone and D-penicillamine, he was entirely normal, except for slightly limited knee flexion on both sides.

This patient's main symptom was progressive stiffness, due to contractures of the quadriceps muscles induced by chronic heroin injections. The findings made it very likely that heroin caused a primarily vascular lesion leading to non-specific inflammatory changes and subsequent fibrosis. Clinically, weakness was minimal and there was painless contracture. This presumably reflects the predominantly fibrotic process within muscle tissue. Combination therapy with prednisone and D-penicillamine led to significant improvement. The regenerating process was confirmed by the second muscle biopsy, and electromyography showed reinnervation. The second biopsy did not show inflammatory cells, indicating absence of the inflammatory component. Thus, this case suggests that heroin-induced fibrotic myopathy is reversible.

Immunologic

Intrathecal diamorphine 0.5 mg for total hip arthroplasty in a 42-year-old with a history of anaphylaxis resulted in an anaphylactic reaction (37). The reaction was controlled and diamorphine was avoided.

Infection risk

Injection of heroin can cause local infection.

- A 32-year-old man with pyomyositis developed abdominal pain and vomiting, fresh rectal bleeding, hematuria, and a swelling on his lower back (38). Two weeks before, he had accidentally given himself an extravascular injection of heroin into his left groin. A CT scan showed a large left sided gluteal abscess communicating through the left sacroiliac joint with the retroperitoneal space. He needed catheterization and multiple open drainage of the abscess and was discharged after 2 months.

Long-Term Effects

Drug abuse

Smoking heroin by heating the free base over tin foil and inhaling the vapors is known as "chasing the dragon," a method that probably originated in Southeast Asia. Some are using this to reverse the stimulant effects of ecstasy. In 102 patients (55 men and 47 women, mean age 21 years) interviewed at four clinics in Dublin, Ireland, three subgroups of opiate users were identified: (a) those who had ever used opiates to come off ecstasy, who were compared with those who had never used opiates for this purpose, (b) those whose first use of opiates had been to come off ecstasy, and (c) those who had started opiates by "chasing" and then did or did not move to injecting (39). Of the 102 patients, 92 reported having taken ecstasy, 68 of whom reported having taken opiates to come off it, and the remaining 24 of whom had not. The 68 patients who reported taking opiates to come off ecstasy had significantly heavier ecstasy use, in terms of the number of nights per week and number of tablets taken per night. Of 36 who reported that their first ever experience of using opiates was in the context of "chasing" to come off ecstasy, 28 reported this as their main reason for starting to use opiates and the other eight reported that they would probably have tried opiates independent of their ecstasy use. Of the 86 patients whose initial route of using heroin was "chasing," 61 reported changing to injecting, 23 continued to smoke heroin, and two switched to an oral formulation of methadone or morphine. When those who came to inject heroin were compared with those who did not (61 versus 23), the injectors had begun illicit drug use earlier, had started heroin at a younger age, were younger at the time of interview, and had been more likely to have a history of ecstasy use. Despite the younger age of onset of illicit drug use in those who came to inject, they had not been using illicit drugs for longer at the time of interview. This study confirmed the authors' previous findings that heroin smoking was associated with ecstasy use.

The Swiss government has developed a program called PROVE, which provides prescriptions of injectable opioids for the treatment of heroin-dependent patients. This program has generally been viewed to be successful in terms of retention in treatment, morbidity and mortality, legal behavior, and cost-effectiveness. However, during the 26-month observation period, epileptic seizures occurred in 11% of the 186 patients treated. This finding, along with previous reports of reduced regional blood supply to the brains of opioid users, led the authors to study cerebral deoxygenation after intravenous opioid administration in ten opioid-dependent subjects and to compare it with intravenous saline in ten matched controls using Near Infrared Spectroscopy (NIRS) (40). Heroin and methadone produced a rapid and dramatic reduction in both respiratory rate and cortical hemoglobin oxygenation, while saline had no effects. The authors suggested that opioid-induced acute deoxygenation of cortical hemoglobin was probably associated with respiratory depression. In one in three subjects, oxygen saturation after intravenous heroin fell rapidly, a finding that has not previously been described in humans.

The authors suggested two possible mechanisms for this phenomenon. They discounted the possibility that opioids increase the utilization of oxygenated hemoglobin in the CNS, because PET data from other studies suggest decreased utilization of glucose (indicating reduced brain activity) following opioids. They believed that it was more likely that the increase in cortical-reduced hemoglobin was related to opioid-induced respiratory depression, with carbon dioxide retention and resulting vasodilatation. Although preliminary, these data have potential implications for treatment programs involving intravenous opioid maintenance. The authors suggested that intravenous opioids may produce both systemic and cerebral hypoxia, which may at least in part account for the hyperexcitability (as measured by electroencephalography) found after intravenous opioids in other studies. Furthermore, hypoxia may mediate or contribute to the rush sensation, similar to that seen with high altitude or in cases of asphyxiophilia.

The prevalence of heroin as a drug of abuse has been reviewed (41). There are over 1 million heroin addicts in the USA. The lifetime prevalence among those aged 12–25 continues to increase gradually.

Drug withdrawal

The relation between the severity of opiate withdrawal and the dose, duration, and route of administration of heroin has been assessed in a retrospective analysis of heroin withdrawal in 22 patients (42). Abrupt withdrawal from opiates resulted in increased symptom severity, peaking on day 2 and then abating after that until day 7. Both the dose and the route of administration were related to the withdrawal score: intravenous heroin was linked to greater total and maximum withdrawal severity than smoking heroin. The authors speculated that the effect of the route of administration may have been due to lower systemic availability of smoked compared with injected heroin. Their data suggested that even the duration of the withdrawal symptoms seemed to increase with higher doses and intravenous use. However, there were several limitations to this study. It was retrospective and the period of observation lasted only 7 days although the withdrawal symptoms lasted much longer. In addition, many subjects took doxepin and benzodiazepines during the observation phase, which may have reduced or suppressed their withdrawal symptoms.

Opioid withdrawal symptoms should be included as part of the differential diagnosis in young people with restless legs syndrome.

- Restless legs syndrome was a feature of opioid withdrawal on days 3-4 in two heroin-dependent individuals (43). They were treated with levodopa and clonidine.

Second-Generation Effects

Fetotoxicity

A report of death associated with intravenous heroin use has provided insights about the distribution of heroin and its metabolites in the fetus (44).

- A 17-year-old girl with a history of heavy drug abuse for 2 years was found dead in a public restroom, with fresh needle puncture marks. She was 18–20 weeks pregnant with a male fetus, and had massive brain and lung edema from acute intoxication. Analysis of her hair showed that she had used heroin over the previous few months. Drug screening of body fluids showed only opiates (high concentrations of 6-monoacetyl-morphine and morphine) in the maternal and fetal circulation at the time of death. Unexpectedly high amounts of morphine, 6-monoacetyl-morphine, and morphine-3-glucuronide were also found in the amniotic fluid. Only morphine-3-glucuronide was detected in the fetus, whereas both morphine-3-glucuronide and morphine-6-glucuronide were detected in the mother, in the body fluids, and in all investigated organ tissues except the brain.

The authors noted that heroin is considered a "prodrug," with 6-monoacetyl-morphine, morphine, and morphine-6-glucuronide accounting for most of its narcotic activity. In blood, diamorphine is rapidly converted to the active metabolite 6-monoacetyl-morphine, which is presumably converted to morphine in the liver. The majority of the morphine is converted to morphine-3-glucuronide and small amounts are converted to morphine-6-glucuronide, which is pharmacologically active. They concluded that morphine-3-glucuronide can cross the placenta and that high concentrations of heroin and its metabolites can be found in fetal compartments during heroin abuse by the mother. Lastly, heroin and its pharmacologically active metabolites appear to be present in the fetal central nervous system for much longer than in the maternal circulation, because of low fetal drug-metabolizing capacity as well as minimal drug elimination from the amniotic fluid in advancing pregnancy.

Susceptibility Factors

Genetic

In 420 Chinese heroin addicts cravings were significantly higher in carriers of the dopamine D4 receptor gene with a variable number tandem repeat long type allele than non-carriers (45)

Drug Administration

Drug contamination

Atypical reactions after the of use heroin have been attributed to contamination with clenbuterol (46).

- Four patients, aged 21-43 years, all developed chest pain, palpitation, and shortness of breath after inhaling heroin. They had tachycardias, low blood pressures, hypokalemia, and hyperglycemia.

In all the cases the heroin had been adulterated with veterinary clenbuterol.

Drug dosage regimens

High-dose intrathecal diamorphine for analgesia after elective cesarean section has been studied in 40 women who were randomized to diamorphine 0.5 or 1 mg (47). All also received diclofenac 100 mg at the end of the cesarean section and morphine via a patient-controlled analgesia system. Postoperative analgesia was more prolonged and reliable in those who were given diamorphine 1 mg, who needed significantly less morphine. There was postoperative nausea in just under half of the patients in each group, and most of the patients (93%) had mild to moderate pruritus. There were no cases of excessive sedation or oxygen desaturation.

Drug administration route

Nasal
Nasal diamorphine is as effective as intramuscular morphine and is much better tolerated by children, with no apparent increased risk of adverse effects (48,49). In a multicenter, randomized, controlled study, 404 children aged 3–16 years with a fracture of an arm or leg were given either nasal diamorphine 0.1 mg/kg or intramuscular morphine 0.2 mg/kg. The onset of pain relief was faster with nasal diamorphine, and there were no serious adverse effects. The frequencies of opioid-related mild adverse effects were similar in the two groups.

The pharmacokinetic profile of nasal diamorphine has been studied in adults. Diamorphine is rapidly absorbed as a dry powder and has similar pharmacokinetic properties to intramuscular diamorphine, with similar physiological responses (for example reduced pupil diameter, respiration, and temperature) and behavioral measures (for example euphoria, sedation, and dysphoria).

Nasal diamorphine has been evaluated in a multicenter, randomized, controlled trial as an alternative to intramuscular morphine in 404 patients aged 3-16 years with suspected limb fractures (i.e. in acute pain of moderate to severe intensity) (50). They were randomized to either intramuscular morphine sulfate 0.2 mg/kg (n=200) or intranasal diamorphine hydrochloride 0.1 mg/kg (n=204). Intranasal diamorphine was significantly better tolerated: 80% had no obvious discomfort compared with only 9% of those given morphine. There were no serious adverse effects of diamorphine, but the lack of blinding may have introduced bias.

The nasal route of administration is also not without problems when abused. Some non-fatal complications include neurological, acute myelopathy, oculogyric crisis and generalized dystonia, hypersensitivity reactions, pneumonitis, pemphigus, and pancreatitis (50).

Spinal
In a randomized, placebo-controlled, double-blind study of the relative efficacies of patient-controlled analgesia (PCA) regimens (51), 60 patients undergoing elective total hip or knee replacement were randomly allocated to receive epidural diamorphine 2.5 mg followed by a PCA bolus 1 mg with a 20-minute lockout (group 1), subcutaneous diamorphine 2.5 mg followed by a PCA bolus 1 mg with a 10-minute lockout (group 2), or epidural diamorphine 2.5 mg in 4 ml of 0.125% bupivacaine followed by a PCA bolus of 1 mg diamorphine in 4 ml 0.125% bupivacaine with a 20-minute lockout (group 3). Diamorphine demands were significantly higher in group 2 in the first postoperative 24-hour period, but pain scores were only significantly higher in group 2 in the first 3 hours postoperatively compared with group 3 and group 1. There were also fewer opioid-related adverse effects in group 2, and group 3 reported higher incidences of various adverse effects. The conclusion was that PCA diamorphine given with or without bupivacaine provides analgesia of similar efficacy once adequate pain relief has been achieved. Taking the incidences of adverse effect profiles into account, diamorphine subcutaneous PCA was a simple and effective method of providing analgesia.

In 62 women who asked for regional analgesia in labor and who were randomized to an intrathecal injection of either bupivacaine 2.5 mg with fentanyl 25 µg or bupivacaine 2.5 mg with diamorphine 250 µg, the diamorphine provided longer analgesia (52). There were significant differences in adverse effects between the groups. There were no instances of nausea or vomiting, but pruritus was more common in those who received fentanyl. The dose of diamorphine was deliberately low, and more studies are needed to confirm these findings.

Drug overdose

The main life-threatening complications of heroin intoxication include acute pulmonary edema and delayed respiratory depression with coma after successful naloxone treatment. In a prospective study of the management of 160 heroin and heroin mixture intoxication cases treated in an emergency room in Switzerland between 1991 and 1992, there were no rehospitalizations after discharge from the emergency room and there was only one death outside the hospital due to pulmonary edema, which occurred at between 2.25 and 8.25 hours after intoxication (53). A literature review found only two reported cases of delayed pulmonary edema, which occurred 4 and 6 hours after hospitalization. The authors recommended surveillance of a heroin user for at least 8 hours after successful opiate antagonist treatment.

Among heroin users, the annual rate of mortality is 1–4%; overdose and HIV infection being the leading causes. The effect of the frequency and route of heroin administration on the occurrence of non-fatal heroin overdose has been studied (54). Among 2556 subjects with heroin dependence, 10% had taken overdoses requiring emergency care in the prior 12 months. The cumulative risk of overdose increased as the frequency of heroin use fell. Among daily heroin users, the risk was greater with increased frequency of heroin injection, but not among non-daily users. The risk of overdose was greater with injection than with other routes of administration.

Strategies for preventing heroin overdose have been discussed (55).Education, family support groups, and motivational interviews after overdose have been proposed as complementary strategies to reduce morbidity and mortality. The author concluded that methadone maintenance is the most effective method of reducing mortality from overdose, and that home treatment with naloxone by a significant other is a possible future strategy. However, the use of naloxone is regarded as controversial by some health professionals.

Various initiatives have addressed prevention of heroin overdose. Educational programs that aim at harm reduction activities for heroin users are widely accepted. In such programs, heroin users are taught about overdose susceptibility factors and appropriate responses to overdose, such as resuscitation techniques. In a cross-sectional study, 257 heroin overdose survivors recruited by ambulance paramedics in Melbourne between 1999 and 2001 participated in structured interviews within 10 days of the overdose (56). The questionnaire addressed knowledge of overdose risk reduction strategies, behavior in the 12 hours before the overdose, and overdose causality. Most (75%) of the subjects had taken an additional overdose, half of them in the preceding 6 months; 20% had engaged in risky overdose behaviors before the overdose; and 90%

had knowledge of overdose prevention messages. Most overdoses occurred within 5 minutes of purchasing the drug. The heroin user was usually alone at the time of the overdose. Heroin was commonly mixed with other drugs. Paradoxically, subjects who reported awareness of the "don't mix drugs" message were 2.8 times as likely to have mixed alcohol and or benzodiazepines with heroin than those who did not report such awareness. The authors noted that this last finding is contrary to a popular assumption that increased knowledge may reduce risky behavior.

In a retrospective study of outcomes after cardiac arrest caused by heroin overdose the Helsinki Emergency Medical Service in Finland recorded 94 cases of cardiac arrest due to acute drug poisoning (25 heroin-related and 69 overdoses by other agents) during 1997-2000 (57). Resuscitation was attempted in 19 of the heroin-related cases and in 53 of the others. Survival after heroin overdose was poor: only three heroin users and six of the others survived, which is not a statistically significant difference. The survivors had acute renal failure, hypoglycemia, and hypothermia.

Drug–Drug Interactions

Alcohol

Many heroin users use heroin and alcohol together. There has been an evaluation of the pharmacokinetic interaction between heroin and alcohol and the role of that interaction in the cause of 39 heroin-related deaths that were attributed to either heroin or heroin + ethanol (58). The cases were arbitrarily divided into two groups according to blood ethanol concentration (low-ethanol group, under 1000 µg/ml, and high ethanol group, over 1000 µg/ml. The high-ethanol group was associated with reduced hydrolysis of 6-acetylmorphine to morphine, and there was an inverse correlation between blood ethanol concentration and hydrolysis of 6-acetylmorphine to morphine. The concentration of total morphine was lower in the high-ethanol group. High blood ethanol concentrations were also associated with an increased ratio of unbound to total morphine and with reduced excretion of unbound and total morphine. The relative concentrations of conjugated heroin metabolites were reduced in the presence of a high blood ethanol concentration. The authors hypothesized that alcohol inhibits the glucuronidation of morphine, resulting in less conjugated morphine in the blood. Thus, in patients with high blood ethanol concentrations the additional depressant effects of unconjugated heroin metabolites may contribute to a more acute death.

Anticholinergic drugs

Combining opiates with anticholinergic drugs is a common practice in recreational abuse (SEDA-21, 34). Heroin mixed with hyoscine (scopolamine) is nicknamed "polo" and "point on point." Mixed drug toxicity, with atypical signs and symptoms of opiate abuse, has been reported (59).

- A 41-year-old woman who had taken 11 alprazolam tablets and heroin mixed with an unknown substance developed slurred speech and a staggering gait. She was also taking paroxetine. Her pupils were dilated, her skin warm and dry. Electrocardiography showed a sinus bradycardia. She was given intravenous naloxone 2.0 mg and became acutely agitated and combative. She was delirious, agitated, and disoriented, and was given an intravenous sedative and intubated. Her urine contained codeine, morphine, and atropine.

This case exemplifies the difficulty in identifying anticholinergic drugs such as atropine, and unfortunately the finding of dilated pupils did not raise the suspicion of mixed drug toxicity. The use of naloxone uncovered florid agitation due to anticholinergic drug toxicity.

Cocaine

Rhabdomyolysis and ventricular fibrillation has been attributed to cocaine plus diamorphine (heroin) ingestion (62).

- A 28-year-old man went into cardiorespiratory arrest after using intravenous cocaine and diamorphine. He was intubated and ventilated and given adrenaline, naloxone, and sodium bicarbonate. During a thoracotomy he developed ventricular fibrillation and was electrically converted to sinus rhythm. He had hyperkalemia and myoglobinuria. He developed acute renal insufficiency, disseminated intravascular coagulopathy, and a right leg compartment syndrome. There were cocaine metabolites and opioids in his urine. Hemodialysis and fasciotomy were performed, but he died 2 months later with a complicating bronchopneumonia.

The authors discussed the possibility that naloxone, an effective opioid antidote, may have been harmful in this case.

Interference with Diagnostic Tests

Blood glucose

Diamorphine flattens the glucose tolerance curve and increases glycosylation of HbA$_1$ (60).

Antithrombin III

Diamorphine depresses the biological activity of antithrombin III (61).

References

1. Serpell MG, Anderson E, Wilson D, Dawson N. I.v. regional diamorphine for analgesia after foot surgery Br J Anaesth 2000;84(1):95–6.
2. Haemmig RB, Tschacher W. Effects of high-dose heroin versus morphine in intravenous drug users: a randomised double-blind crossover study. J Psychoactive Drugs 2001;33(2):105–10.
3. Riad T, Williams B, Musson J, Wheatley B. Intrathecal morphine compared with diamorphine for postoperative analgesia following unilateral knee arthroplasty. Acute Pain 2002;4:5–8.
4. Cowan CM, Kendall JB, Barclay PM, Wilkes RG. Comparison of intrathecal fentanyl and diamorphine in addition to bupivacaine for caesarean section under spinal anaesthesia. Br J Anaesth 2002;89(3):452–8.
5. Van den Brink W, Hendricks VM, Blanken P, Koeter WJM, Van Zureten JB, Van Ree JM. Medical prescription of heroin to treatment resistant heroin addicts: two randomized controlled trials. BMJ 2003;327:310–2.
6. Buster M, Rook L, van Brussel GH, van Ree J, van den Brink W. Chasing the dragon, related to the impaired lung function among heroin users. Drug Alcohol Depend 2002;68(2):221–8.
7. Servin FS, Raeder JC, Merle JC, Wattwil M, Hanson AL, Lauwers MH, Aitkenhead A, Marty J, Reite K, Martisson S, Wostyn L. Remifentanil sedation compared with propofol during regional anaesthesia. Acta Anaesthesiol Scand 2002;46(3):309–15.
8. Dettmeyer R, Schmidt P, Musshoff F, Dreisvogt C, Madea B. Pulmonary edema in fatal heroin overdose: immunohistological investigations with IgE, collagen IV and laminin— no increase of defects of alveolar-capillary membranes. Forensic Sci Int 2000;110(2):87–96.
9. Reynes AN, Pujol JA, Baixeras RP, Fernandez B. Edema agudo de pulmon unilateral en paciente con sobredosis do heroina y tratado con naloxona intravenosa. Med Clin (Barc) 1990;94:637.
10. Anderson K. Bronchospasm and intravenous street heroin. Lancet 1986;1(8491):1208.
11. Levine M, Iliescu ME, Margellos-Anast H, Estarziau M, Ansell DA. The effects of cocaine and heroin use on intubation rates and hospital utilization in patients with acute asthma exacerbations. Chest 2005;128(4):1951–7.
12. Schoser BG, Groden C. Subacute onset of oculogyric crises and generalized dystonia following intranasal administration of heroin. Addiction 1999;94(3):431–4.
13. Chenery HJ, Murdoch BE. A case of mixed transcortical aphasia following drug overdose. Br J Disord Commun 1986;21(3):381–91.
14. Koussa S, Tamraz J, Nasnas R. Leucoencephalopathy after heroin inhalation. A case with partial regression of MRI lesions. J Neuroradiol 2001;28(4):268–71.
15. McCreary M, Emerman C, Hanna J, Simon J. Acute myelopathy following intranasal insufflation of heroin: a case report. Neurology 2000;55(2):316–7.
16. Lee BF, Chiu NT, Chen WH, Liu GC, Yu HS. Heroin-induced rhabdomyolysis as a cause of reflex sympathetic dystrophy. Clin Nucl Med 2001;26(4):289–92.
17. Kraus J, Baumeier A, Boentert M, Husstedt IW, Nabavi DG, Bernd Ringelstein E, Schäbitz W. Acute toxic polyradiculopathy after exorbitant intracarotid substance abuse. J Neurol 2006;253:815–6.
18. Dabby R, Djaldetti R, Gilad R, Herman O, Frand J, Sadeh M, Watemberg N. Acute heroin-related neuropathy. J Peripheral Nerv Syst 2006;11(4):304–9.
19. Kriegstein AR, Shungu DC, Millar WS, Armitage BA, Brust JC, Chillrud S, Goldman J, Lynch T. Leukoencephalopathy and raised brain lactate from heroin vapor inhalation ("chasing the dragon"). Neurology 1999; 53(8):1765–73.
20. Chang W-C, Lo C-P, Kao H-W, Chen C-Y. MRI features of spongiform leukoencephalopathy following heroin inhalation. Neurology 2006;67(3):504.
21. Nyffeler T, Stabba A, Sturzenegger M. Progressive myelopathy with selective involvement of the lateral and posterior

columns after inhalation of heroin vapour. J Neurol 2003;250:496–8.

22. Ryan A, Molloy FM, Farrell MA, Hutchinson M. Fatal toxic leukoencephalopathy: clinical, radiological, and necropsy findings in two patients. J Neurol Neurosurg Psychiatry 2005;76(7):1014–6.

23. Vella S, Kreis R, Lovbled KO, Steinlin M. Acute leukoencephalopathy after inhalation of a single dose of heroin. Neuropediatrics 2003;34:100–4.

24. Keogh CF, Andrews GT, Spacey SD, Forkheim KE, Graeb DA. Neuroimaging features of heroin inhalation toxicity. Am J Roentgenol 2003;180:547–59.

25. Wolters EC, van Wijngaarden GK, Stam FC, Rengelink H, Lousberg RJ, Schipper ME, Verbeeten B. Leucoencephalopathy after inhaling "heroin" pyrolysate. Lancet 1982;2(8310):1233–7.

26. Cooley S, Lalchandani S, Keane D. Heroin overdose in pregnancy: an unusual case report. J Obstet Gynaecol 2002;22(2):219–20.

27. Maschke M, Fehlings T, Kastrup O, Wilhelm HW, Leonhardt G. Toxic leukoencephalopathy after intravenous consumption of heroin and cocaine with unexpected clinical recovery. J Neurol 1999;246(9):850–1.

28. Au-Yeung K, Lai C. Toxic leucoencephalopathy after heroin inhalation. Australas Radiol 2002;46(3):306–8.

29. Sayers GM, Green MC, Shaffer RE. Heroin-induced leucoencephalopathy misdiagnosed as psychiatric illness. Int J Psychiatry Clin Pract 2002;6:53–5.

30. Ishiyama A, Ishiyama G, Baloh RW, Evans CJ. Heroin-induced reversible profound deafness and vestibular dysfunction. Addiction 2001;96(9):1363–4.

31. King H, Barclay P. The effects of intrathecal diamorphine on gastric emptying after elective Caesarian section. Anaesthesia 2004;59:565–9.

32. Rice EK, Isbel NM, Becker GJ, Atkins RC, McMahon LP. Heroin overdose and myoglobinuric acute renal failure. Clin Nephrol 2000;54(6):449–54.

33. Dettmeyer R, Stojanovski G, Madea B. Pathogenesis of heroin-associated glomerulonephritis. Correlation between the inflammatory activity and renal deposits of immunoglobulin and complement? Forensic Sci Int 2000;113(1–3):227–31.

34. Llach F, Descoeudres C, Massry SG. Heroin associated nephropathy: clinical and histological studies in 19 patients. Clin Nephrol 1979;11(1):7–12.

35. Rocamora A, Matarredona J, Sendagorta E, Ledo A. Sweat gland necrosis in drug-induced coma: a light and direct immunofluorescence study. J Dermatol 1986;13(1):49–53.

36. Weber M, Diener HC, Voit T, Neuen-Jacob E. Focal myopathy induced by chronic heroin injection is reversible. Muscle Nerve 2000;23(2):274–7.

37. Gooch I, Gwinnutt C. Anaphylaxis to intrathecal diamorphine. Resuscitation 2006;70(3):470–3.

38. Crossley A. Temperature pyomyositis in an injecting drug misuser. A difficult diagnosis in a difficult patient. J Accid Emerg Med 2003;20:299–300.

39. Gervin M, Hughes R, Bamford L, Smyth BP, Keenan E. Heroin smoking by "chasing the dragon" in young opiate users in Ireland: stability and associations with use to "come down" off "Ecstasy". J Subst Abuse Treat 2001;20(4): 297–300.

40. Stohler R, Dursteler KM, Stormer R, Seifritz E, Hug I, Sattler-Mayr J, Muller-Spahn F, Ladewig D, Hock C. Rapid cortical hemoglobin deoxygenation after heroin and methadone injection in humans: a preliminary report. Drug Alcohol Depend 1999;57(1):23–8.

41. Kreek MJ, Bart G, Lilly C, Laforge KS, Nielson DA. Pharmacogenetics and human molecular genetics of opiate and cocaine addictions and their treatments. Pharmacol Rev 2005;57(1):1–26.

42. Smolka M, Schmidt LG. The influence of heroin dose and route of administration on the severity of the opiate withdrawal syndrome. Addiction 1999;94(8):1191–8.

43. Scherbaum N, Stüper B, Bonnet U, Gastpar M. Transient restless-leg-like syndrome as a complication of opiate withdrawal. Pharmacopsychiatry 2003;36:70–2.

44. Potsch L, Skopp G, Emmerich TP, Becker J, Ogbuhui S. Report on intrauterine drug exposure during second trimester of pregnancy in a heroin-associated death. Ther Drug Monit 1999;21(6):593–7.

45. Shao C, Li Y, Jiang K, Zhang D, Xu Y, Lin L, Wang Q, Zhao M, Jin L. Dopamine D4 receptor polymorphism modulates cue-elicited heroin craving in Chinese. Psychopharmacology 2006;186:185–90.

46. Hoffman RS, Nelson LS, Chan GM, Halcomb SE, Bouchard NC, Ginsberg BY, Cone J, Jea-Francois Y, Voit S, Marcus S, Ford M, Sanford C, Michels JE, Richardson WH, Bertous LM, Johnson-Arbor K, Thomas J, Belson M, Patel M, Schier J, Wolkin A, Rubin C, Duprey Z. Atypical reactions associated with heroin use—Five States, January–April 2005. JAMA 2005;294(19):2424–7.

47. Stacey R, Jones R, Kar G, Poon A. High-dose intrathecal diamorphine for analgesia after Caesarean section. Anaesthesia 2001;56(1):54–60.

48. Davies M, Crawford I. Towards evidence based emergency medicine: best BETs from the Manchester Royal Infirmary. Nasal diamorphine for acute pain relief in children. Emerg Med J 2001;18(4):271.

49. Kendall JM, Reeves BC, Latter VSNasal Diamorphine Trial Group. Multicentre randomised controlled trial of nasal diamorphine for analgesia in children and teenagers with clinical fractures. BMJ 2001;322(7281):261–5.

50. Kendall JM, Latter VS. Intranasal diamorphine as an alternative to intramuscular morphine. Clin Pharmacokinet 2003;42:501–3.

51. Gopinathan C, Sockalingham I, Fung MA, Peat S, Hanna MH. A comparative study of patient-controlled epidural diamorphine, subcutaneous diamorphine and an epidural diamorphine/bupivacaine combination for postoperative pain. Eur J Anaesthesiol 2000;17(3):189–96.

52. Vaughan DJ, Ahmad N, Lillywhite NK, Lewis N, Thomas D, Robinson PN. Choice of opioid for initiation of combined spinal epidural analgesia in labour—fentanyl or diamorphine. Br J Anaesth 2001;86(4):567–9.

53. Osterwalder JJ. Patients intoxicated with heroin or heroin mixtures: how long should they be monitored? Eur J Emerg Med 1995;2(2):97–101.

54. Brugal MT, Barrio G, De LF, Regidor E, Royuela L, Suelves JM. Factors associated with non-fatal heroin overdose: assessing the effect of frequency and route of heroin administration. Addiction 2002;97(3):319–27.

55. Sporer KA. Strategies for preventing heroin overdose. BMJ 2003;326:442–4.

56. Dietze P, Jolley D, Fry CL, Bammer G, Moore D. When is a little knowledge dangerous? Circumstances of recent heroin overdose and links to knowledge of overdose risk factors. Drug Alcohol Dep 2006;84:223–30.

57. Boyd JJ, Kuisma MJ, Alaspaa AO, Vuori E, Repo JV, Randell TT. Outcome after heroin overdose and cardiopulmonary resuscitation. Acta Anaesthesiol Scand 2006;50:1120–4.

58. Polettini A, Groppi A, Montagna M. The role of alcohol abuse in the etiology of heroin-related deaths. Evidence for pharmacokinetic interactions between heroin and alcohol. J Anal Toxicol 1999;23(7):570–6.

59. Wang HE. Street drug toxicity resulting from opiates combined with anticholinergics. Prehosp Emerg Care 2002;6(3):351–4.

60. Ceriello A, Giugliano D, Dello Russo P, Sgambato S, D'Onofrio F. Increased glycosylated haemoglobin A_1 in opiate addicts: evidence for a hyperglycaemic effect of morphine. Diabetologia 1982;22(5):379.

61. Ceriello A, Dello Russo P, Curcio F, Tirelli A, Giugliano D. Depressed antithrombin III biological activity in opiate addicts. J Clin Pathol 1984;37(9):1040–2.

62. Cann B, Hunter R, McCann J. Cocaine/heroin induced rhabdomyolysis and ventricular fibrillation. Emerg Med J 2002;19(3):264–5.

Dihydrocodeine

General Information

Dihydrocodeine is an opioid analgesic related to codeine, in which the double bond in the 7th position is saturated. It is about one-tenth as potent as morphine and 2–3 times more potent than codeine. It is similar to codeine in other respects. The most common adverse effects are nausea, vomiting, and drowsiness (SEDA-16, 79) (SEDA-17, 80) (SEDA-18, 79).

In a randomized, double-blind comparison of the antitussive effect of dihydrocodeine 10 mg tds with levodropropizine 75 mg tds in 140 adults with primary lung cancer or metastatic cancer there was no significant difference between the two drugs as far as cough severity and the numbers of night wakings were concerned, both drugs leading to significant improvement (1). However, dihydrocodeine caused significantly more somnolence, which was reported by 11% and in some cases was continuous. Other adverse effects reported by those taking dihydrocodeine included erythema of the abdomen and epigastric pain, although constipation, a potential adverse effect of codeine derivatives, was not reported.

Organs and Systems

Sensory systems

Severe narcosis after therapeutic doses (2) has been reported.

Urinary tract

Acute renal insufficiency after therapeutic doses (2) has been reported.

Dihydrocodeine was implicated in cases of granulomatous interstitial nephritis (3).

Immunologic

Anaphylaxis has been reported with dihydrocodeine (4).

Susceptibility Factors

Age

There is a risk in giving dihydrocodeine to the elderly (2).

Renal disease

There is a risk in giving dihydrocodeine to those with renal insufficiency (2).

Drug Administration

Drug formulations

A modified-release formulation extends the duration of action of dihydrocodeine from 2–4 hours to 12 hours. In 12 volunteers who took modified-release dihydrocodeine 60 mg or 120 mg and 120 minutes later lactulose 40 mg diluted in 100 mg of water, the orocecal transit time was significantly prolonged by dihydrocodeine compared with placebo (5). Dihydrocodeine also significantly suppressed the pupillary light reflex. Both dosages caused similar adverse effects. Tiredness and dry mouth were reported in 80%, vertigo in 5%, and headache in 1%.

References

1. Luporini G, Barni S, Marchi E, Daffonchio L. Efficacy and safety of levodropropizine and dihydrocodeine on nonproductive cough in primary and metastatic lung cancer. Eur Respir J 1998;12(1):97–101.

2. Park GR, Shelly MP, Quinn K, Roberts P. Dihydrocodeine— a reversible cause of renal failure? Eur J Anaesthesiol 1989;6(4):303–14.

3. Singer DR, Simpson JG, Catto GR, Johnston AW. Drug hypersensitivity causing granulomatous interstitial nephritis. Am J Kidney Dis 1988;11(4):357–9.

4. Panos MZ, Burnett S, Gazzard BG. Use of naloxone in opioid-induced anaphylactoid reaction. Br J Anaesth 1988;61(3):371.

5. Freye E, Baranowski J, Latasch L. Dose-related effects of controlled release dihydrocodeine on oro-cecal transit and pupillary light reflex. A study in human volunteers. Arzneimittelforschung 2001;51(1):60–6.

Enadoline

General Information

Enadoline is an opioid agonist at KOR(OP$_2$, κ) receptors and has no effects attributable to MOR(OP$_3$, μ) receptor actions, such as respiratory depression. However, enadoline does not offer any benefits over other currently available opioids (1).

Reference

1. Pande AC, Pyke RE, Greiner M, Wideman GL, Benjamin R, Pierce MW. Analgesic efficacy of enadoline versus placebo or morphine in postsurgical pain. Clin Neuropharmacol 1996;19(5):451–6.

Fentanyl

General Information

Fentanyl citrate is a synthetic opioid 1000 times more potent than pethidine. It has a relatively short duration of action, and its effects are rapidly reversed by opioid antagonists (1). It is useful (2) but has typical opioid adverse effects.

The analgesic effect of fentanyl 1.5 µg/kg has been compared with that of tramadol 1.5 mg/kg in 61 patients receiving standardized anesthetics for day-case arthroscopic knee surgery (3). Opioid adverse effects and analgesia were similar in the two groups.

The analgesic effects and adverse effects profiles of subcutaneous fentanyl and subcutaneous morphine have been compared in a double-blind, crossover, 6-day study in 23 patients with cancer pain (4). There were no significant differences in pain scores between the two drugs and no changes in the level of acute confusion (using the Saskatoon Delirium Checklist) or cognitive impairment (in tests of semantic fluency and trail-making tests). Fentanyl caused significantly less constipation. The patients in this study were highly stable and compliant, and the results cannot be generalized.

Observational studies

In a small open study, in which patients using transdermal fentanyl were switched to an intravenous infusion of fentanyl for acute cancer-related pain relief, there was no excessive sedation or opioid adverse effects (5).

The safety of intrathecal fentanyl was demonstrated In 31 patients undergoing transurethral resection of the prostate fentanyl (n = 15) or saline (n = 16) was added to ropivacaine for subarachnoid block; the only significant adverse effect was pruritus (6).

Transdermal fentanyl 25 micrograms/hour has been assessed in 22 patients with painful oral mucositis induced by high-dose chemotherapy after stem cell transplantation (7). Three had severe dizziness, severe vomiting, and extensive rashes. These patients were subsequently withdrawn from the analysis. Mild nausea (in 32%) and dizziness (in 11%) were the two most common adverse events. There was no respiratory depression, constipation, or withdrawal symptoms.

The incidence of adverse events in 14 386 patients receiving fentanyl has been studied after implementation of the Joint Commission on Accreditation of Healthcare Organization guidelines for procedural sedation and analgesia in an urban tertiary-care children's hospital (8). The combination of fentanyl + midazolam was the regimen with the highest incidence (9.7%) of adverse events compared with other regimens involving opioids. The most common adverse event was hypoxemia (7.1%), followed by hypotension (1.0%), prolonged sedation (0.7%), vomiting (0.4%), airway obstruction (0.4%), bradycardia (0.1%), pain-related agitation (0.1%), and agitation (not pain-related) (0.04%).

Comparative studies

Bupivacaine + clonidine as an alternative to bupivacaine + fentanyl has similar analgesic efficacy and is associated with fewer adverse effects, as reported in a study of 47 children undergoing the Nuss procedure (9). The children were randomized to bupivacaine + clonidine, bupivacaine + fentanyl, or bupivacaine + fentanyl + clonidine. Vomiting and pruritus were significantly more common in those who received fentanyl. Vomiting occurred in 27% of those who received bupivacaine + clonidine, compared with 69% of those who received bupivacaine + fentanyl and 55% of those who received bupivacaine + fentanyl + clonidine. Pruritus occurred in 85% of those who received bupivacaine + fentanyl and 54% of those who received bupivacaine + fentanyl + clonidine, but in none of those who received bupivacaine + clonidine,.

Placebo-controlled studies

In a double-blind, randomized, placebo-controlled study 29 boys undergoing day-case penile surgery were allocated to either intravenous fentanyl 1 microgram/kg intraoperatively or intravenous saline (10). Pain and opioid-related adverse effects were monitored for the first 24 hours after surgery. The authors concluded that intraoperative intravenous fentanyl is associated with an increased incidence of nausea and vomiting, without any significant contribution to postoperative pain relief.

In a placebo-controlled study in 399 patients with moderate to severe osteoarthritis transdermal fentanyl produced better pain management (11). The most common adverse effects were nausea, vomiting, and somnolence.

Organs and Systems

Cardiovascular

A hypertensive crisis occurred in a patient with a previously unknown pheochromocytoma (12).

Bolus intravenous fentanyl 1 micrograms/kg in stereotactic brain biopsy for intracranial mass lesions in 135 patients was well tolerated but provided less hemodynamic stability than alfentanil and remifentanil (13).

Fentanyl failed to produce adequate protection of the myocardium from ischemic injury following cardiopulmonary bypass in a comparative study with morphine in 46 patients (14). Global cardiac function was assessed by the myocardial performance index. Fentanyl significantly improved left ventricular function, but morphine improved global ventricular function.

Midazolam + fentanyl has been compared with dexmedetomidine during carotid endarterectomy in 56 patients (15). Those who received fentanyl required more interventions to control hypertension and/or tachycardia (72% versus 40%), and in the post-anesthesia care unit fewer interventions were required for hypotension (11% versus 28%). Many more of the patients who were given dexmedetomidine required additional pain relief (72% versus 38%).

Heart rate variability during anesthesia has been studied in patients who received sevoflurane + fentanyl; in two cases there was *reduced heart rate variability* associated with junctional rhythm (16). In a 9-year-old girl with hereditary sensory autonomic neuropathy type 2 there was altered heart rate variability with improved hemodynamic stability after the administration of propofol + fentanyl (17).

A 68-year-old man with Brugada syndrome developed *ventricular tachycardia* during general anesthesia and thoracic paravertebral block using anesthetic agents + fentanyl (18). Is not clear how fentanyl contributed to the cardiac rhythm changes in this case.

Respiratory

Even small doses of fentanyl can cause respiratory depression. Delayed respiratory depression can be a particular problem in the elderly, in whom the half-life is approximately three times longer than in younger patients (19). Respiratory depression has been reversed with nalbuphine; doxapram could only antagonize this effect for 2–5 minutes (20). However, the need for prolonged treatment of respiratory depression with naloxone, because of pharmacokinetic variability and/or transdermal drug reservoir, has been emphasized by several authors (SEDA-16, 80) (SEDA-17, 80).

The respiratory effects of fentanyl have been demonstrated in 21 volunteers who were given a high-dose infusion (21). Four of them developed apnea shortly after the infusion, thought to be due to rapid crossing of the blood–brain barrier and rapid depression of respiratory neurons.

Fentanyl can evoke the pulmonary chemoreflex, as evidenced by 50% of patients in one study and 28% in another, who coughed after the administration of fentanyl through a central line (SEDA-16, 79) (22). The coughing caused by fentanyl is inhibited by terbutaline (SEDA-21, 88).

Intravenous fentanyl is associated with coughing in 28-45% of patients. Coughing due to fentanyl may not always be benign and brief; it can sometimes be explosive, requiring immediate intervention on the operating table. Coughing occurs because fentanyl constricts the tracheal smooth muscle, stimulating the irritant receptors. Other possible factors are release of histamine, leukotrienes, interleukins, and other inflammatory mediators from mast cells. In 200 patients scheduled for elective laparoscopic cholecystectomy under general anesthesia and given intravenous fentanyl 2 micrograms/kg, pretreatment with salbutamol, beclomethasone, or sodium cromoglicate by aerosol before the fentanyl bolus reduced the incidence of cough (23).

- A 7-year-old boy with trisomy 21 (Down syndrome) had explosive coughing, 30 seconds after fentanyl 50 μg (2 μg/kg) had been injected and flushed through

an intravenous cannula(24). The cough was unproductive and persisted in spasmodic bursts for a further 2–3 minutes until anesthesia was induced with propofol 60 mg and atracurium 15 mg intravenously. The coughing immediately ceased. A petechial rash in the conjunctivae and periorbital regions was subsequently noted and disappeared by the end of the first postoperative day.

The incidence of fentanyl-induced cough has been studied in patients undergoing surgery (25). Fentanyl (100 micrograms for those weighing 40–69 kg; 150 micrograms for those weighing 70–90 kg) was given intravenously at three different rates, over 2, 15, or 30 seconds. A longer injection time resulted in a reduced incidence of cough. Light smoking was associated with a reduced incidence of cough.

The addition of intrathecal fentanyl 20 micrograms to hyperbaric bupivacaine in 40 women undergoing cesarean section improved the quality of subarachnoid blockade but did not result in worsening of respiratory function (26).

A method of estimating analgesic fentanyl requirements after surgery, while avoiding respiratory depression, has been evaluated prospectively (27). The method was based on a fentanyl challenge before surgery. The patients required only very small adjustments to the settings that were based on estimates from the challenge. There was no evidence of respiratory depression.

Nervous system

Movement disorders after withdrawal of continuous infusion, without the characteristic autonomic signs of opioid withdrawal, have been reported in children (SEDA-17, 80).

Fentanyl-induced seizures have been reported (28).

Life-threatening complications have included raised intracranial pressure and critically reducing cerebral perfusion (29).

- A 55-year-old man was given fentanyl 0.05 mg for treatment of left chest pain and immediately developed an acute confusional state and fluctuating tetraparesis (30). The symptoms abated 12 hours after withdrawal. A provocation test confirmed that fentanyl 0.1 mg was enough to cause myoclonic and dystonic reactions with increased agitation. Administration of intravenous naloxone 0.8 mg improved the condition.
- A 14-year-old girl developed a dystonic reaction to fentanyl 50 μg given as a general anesthesia for dental extraction; her abnormal movements stopped completely after 3 days (31).

Fentanyl can displace bilirubin from albumin in neonates, with a risk of kernicterus; other drugs should be used (SEDA-17, 81).

Psychological, psychiatric

Mood alteration during patient-controlled epidural anesthesia with either morphine or fentanyl was compared in a randomized, double-blind study of 52 patients undergoing elective hip or knee joint arthroplasty under general anesthesia (32). Mood was assessed preoperatively and at 24, 48, and 72 hours, using the bipolar version of the Profile of Mood States. Pain intensity postoperatively did not vary with morphine or fentanyl and, as expected, both fentanyl and morphine users had significant somnolence, pruritus, and nausea compared with baseline. With morphine, the mean score for measures of composure/anxiety, elation/depression and clearheadedness/confusion increased, indicating a change toward the more positive pole, but there were negative changes for the fentanyl users' scores for five of the six components of the Profile of Mood States. The difference in test scores between morphine and fentanyl was significant at 48 hours of patient-controlled anesthesia and 24 hours after withdrawal. There was no correlation between mood scores and pain scores, and mood scores with fentanyl fell with increasing plasma concentrations. Previous investigations have shown transient positive feelings with intravenous fentanyl, followed by more negative feelings in the longer term. The authors suggested that the differences in mood between the two groups may have been explained by differences in the lipid solubility and pharmacokinetics of epidural morphine and fentanyl.

Endocrine

Hypothalamic–pituitary–adrenal (HPA) axis suppression has been attributed to chronic administration of fentanyl (33).

- A 64-year-old man with chronic sciatic pain had taking transdermal fentanyl 200 micrograms/hour for 2 years. He developed back pain, miosis, somnolence, and a blood pressure of 70/40 mmHg. Adrenocortical insufficiency was diagnosed, but the cause was unclear, and he was given hydrocortisone 25 mg/day. After poor compliance with hydrocortisone he again presented in adrenal crisis. On re-stabilization, opiate-induced suppression of the HPA axis was suspected. On gradual reduction of the dose of fentanyl, HPA axis function improved markedly.

Gastrointestinal

In a retrospective cohort study, 1836 patients using long-term opioids for chronic malignant and non-malignant pain were analysed to compare the incidence of constipation; 601 used transdermal fentanyl, 514 used morphine CR, and 721 used oxycodone CR) (34). Crude (unadjusted) rates of constipation were 3.7% for transdermal fentanyl, 5.1% for morphine, and 6.1% for oxycodone CR. Transdermal fentanyl had a lower annual incidence density and risk of constipation than the other two medications. The adjusted risk of constipation was estimated as 78% greater with oxycodone CR and 44% greater with morphine CR than with transdermal fentanyl.

Constipation is a common adverse effect of opioids. In a 13-month, open, parallel-group comparison of a fentanyl transdermal reservoir and oral modified-release morphine in 677 patients with chronic low back pain who were given transdermal fentanyl or oral modified-release morphine there was less severe constipation with fentanyl (35). The Patient Assessment of Constipation Symptoms 12-item questionnaire was a reliable measure of the severity of opioid-induced constipation.

Ileus occurred more commonly in 30 mechanically ventilated patients receiving co-sedation with midazolam + fentanyl (two episodes) than in those who received midazolam alone (no episodes) (36). However, the combination provided more reliable sedation.

Fentanyl and remifentanil have been compared in patients undergoing plastic surgery, anesthetized with propofol (37). There was a higher incidence of postoperative nausea and vomiting in those who received fentanyl. Despite this, patient satisfaction was the same in the two groups.

In a comparison of transdermal fentanyl (n = 299) and modified-release oral morphine (n = 298) in patients with chronic low back pain, transdermal fentanyl was associated with significantly less constipation (31 versus 48%); a smaller proportion of those who received transdermal fentanyl needed to use laxatives (38). In both groups, the most common adverse events leading to treatment withdrawal were nausea, vomiting, and constipation.

Urinary tract

There have been two cases of urinary retention leading to renal pelvocalyceal dilatation as a result of continuous infusion of fentanyl (3 µg/kg/hour) in premature neonates (39). In both cases the problem was resolved by inserting an indwelling catheter.

Skin

A rash has been attributed to fentanyl (40).

- A 70-year-old man with metastatic cancer of the colon was given transdermal fentanyl 50 mg for analgesia. After 10 days he developed an itchy pustular eruption on the trunk and limbs. The lesions subsided on withdrawal of fentanyl. When he restarted transdermal fentanyl 2 months later, the skin lesions reappeared and became more generalized. The pustules were scattered, sparse, and superficial, and included the tongue and buccal mucosa, but not the conjunctivae or genitalia. A history of eosinophilia suggested an immunoallergic origin.

Like other opioids, fentanyl can cause pruritus. Prophylactic intravenous ondansetron 8 mg with hyperbaric bupivacaine 7–10 mg and fentanyl 25 µg significantly reduced the incidence of intrathecal fentanyl-induced pruritus in 125 patients undergoing knee arthroscopy or urological surgery in a randomized, double-blind, placebo-controlled trial (41). The incidence of pruritus was 39% with ondansetron and 68% with placebo.

Musculoskeletal

There have been three reports and a prospective study of muscle rigidity after fentanyl administration in neonates (42,43).

- Two neonates had transient (0.5–2 minutes) chest wall rigidity after intravenous boluses of fentanyl 2 and 4 μg/kg. They were already compromised, one with a respiratory distress syndrome and one with a diaphragmatic hernia.
- A premature male infant of 28 weeks gestation was given an intravenous bolus of fentanyl 3 μg/kg before intubation and this was followed by isolated rigidity of the tongue lasting 20 seconds (42).

In a prospective case series study of 89 preterm and term infants who received fentanyl out of a total of 404 neonatal intensive care patients in one year, eight neonates (9%) had chest wall rigidity (43). The spectrum of neuromuscular activity extends from mild muscle rigidity through abnormal muscle movements (chewing) to tonic-clonic movements. In two cases there was laryngospasm with chest wall rigidity. In all cases low-dose fentanyl (3–6 μg/kg) had been given for analgesia or sedation.

Chest wall rigidity, sometimes lasting for more than 24 hours and causing hypoxia, can occur postoperatively; it can be attenuated with naloxone or neuromuscular blockers (SEDA-22, 98) (44).

Autacoids

Surgical procedures generally cause perioperative stress, with release of cortisol, cytokines (interleukin-6 and tumor necrosis factor alfa) and acute phase proteins (C-reactive protein and leptin). Opioids are believed to have an inhibitory effect on cortisol release, reducing the neuroendocrine perioperative response. This has been studied in 14 patients undergoing hemorrhoidectomy, who were given either general anesthesia with thiopental 5–7 mg/kg (n = 7) or fentanyl 0.5 micrograms/kg (n = 7) (45). There were higher leptin concentrations in the general anesthesia group, but this was not clinically significant. There were no other differences between the two groups.

Death

Four deaths have been attributed to intravenous injection of fentanyl extracted from transdermal patches (46).

- A 35-year old man, with no history of drug abuse was found by his wife on the floor of his workshop. The police recovered a fentanyl patch, needle, and syringe on the scene and toxicological analysis of the aortic blood established fentanyl poisoning.
- A 38-year old man, with a history of polydrug abuse, undergoing a treatment program using "morphine patches", was found by his brother dead in bed. The police found evidence of recent intravenous injection. Toxicological analysis established fentanyl poisoning.
- A 42-year old man, with a history of polydrug abuse, was found dead in his house with evidence of having injected substantial amounts of fentanyl from several fentanyl patches, and having taken cocaine and oral diazepam. Fentanyl overdose was listed as the main cause of death due to suicide.
- A 39-year old man, with a history of drug and alcohol abuse, died from fentanyl toxicity from illicitly procured fentanyl patches. Hydrocodone and oxycodone were listed as significant contributing factors in his death.

Long-Term Effects

Drug abuse

Abuse of fentanyl-containing analgesics is increasing. In the USA, reports of fentanyl abuse increased to over 6000% (1506 cases) from 1995 to 2002 (47).

Drug withdrawal

In a prospective interventional cohort study in 19 neonates who received fentanyl by continuous infusion for a minimum of 24 hours, those who received fentanyl in a total dose of at least 415 micrograms/kg or as an infusion for more than 8 days were at risk of developing opioid withdrawal symptoms on stopping fentanyl (48). Having identified patients who are at risk of developing withdrawal symptoms, one needs to be able to monitor withdrawal signs and symptoms adequately and objectively, reduce the dose of fentanyl gradually, or even use methadone.

Second-Generation Effects

Pregnancy

The efficacy of intrathecal fentanyl and sufentanil for labor analgesia has been studied in 75 nulliparous women in a two-part comparison (49). In the first phase, 20 subjects received varying doses of fentanyl; the ED_{50} of intrathecal fentanyl for 60 minutes of labor analgesia was 18 μg, with a potency ratio of intrathecal sufentanil to intrathecal fentanyl of 4.4. In the second phase, 55 subjects participated in a double-blind, randomized comparison of the efficacy and safety of either intrathecal fentanyl 36 μg or sufentanil 8 μg. Sufentanil gave 25 minutes longer analgesia than fentanyl. There were no significant differences in adverse effects between the two groups: 83% had pruritus and 27% of those given sufentanil and 10% of those given fentanyl had nausea.

In a randomized, double-blind, placebo-controlled study of whether patient-controlled epidural fentanyl could produce effective and safe postoperative analgesia following 25 μg of spinal fentanyl at cesarean section in 36 patients, the fentanyl group used a mean of 23 μg/hour of fentanyl compared with 27 μg/hour in the control group (50). There was pruritus in 15 patients given fentanyl compared with one control; 9 given fentanyl had mild or moderate drowsiness during the operation compared with 8 controls. Postoperative nausea, pruritus, and drowsiness did not differ between the two groups.

In a randomized, controlled trial, 52 patients in labor were randomly given either intrathecal fentanyl 25 μg with saline or fentanyl 25 μg with magnesium sulfate 50 mg as part of a combined spinal-epidural technique (49). The incidence of pruritus with fentanyl alone was 65%, significantly lower than with fentanyl plus magnesium sulfate (77%). However, fentanyl plus magnesium sulfate produced significantly better and longer-lasting pain control, potentially reducing postoperative opioid requirements.

Breast feeding

The method by which infants were fed at discharge from hospital has been studied in a random sample of 425 healthy primiparae who delivered health singleton babies at term (51). The main determinants of bottle feeding were: maternal age (OR = 0.90; 95% CI = 0.85, 0.95); occupation (OR = 0.63; 95% CI = 0.40, 0.99 for each category, unemployed, manual, non-manual); antenatal feeding (OR = 0.12; 95% CI = 0.08, 0.19 for each category, bottle feeding, undecided, breast feeding); cesarean section (OR = 0.25; 95% CI = 0.13, 0.47, cesarean or vaginal delivery); and the dose of fentanyl administered intrapartum (OR = 1.004; 95% CI = 1.000, 1.008). The authors suggested that intrapartum fentanyl, particularly at higher doses, may impede the establishment of breast feeding by impairing suckling.

Susceptibility Factors

Genetic

A study (52) explored whether beta 2-adrenoceptor genotype affects vasopressor requirements to manage opioid-induced hypotension. Spinal anesthesia with 12 micrograms hyperbaric bupivacaine, 25 micrograms fentanyl and 200 micrograms morphine was administered to 170 women undergoing elective caesarean section. Vasopressor treatment was required in 90%, but those with glycine at position 16 and/or glutamate at position 27 of the beta 2-adrenoceptor required lower vasopressor doses for opioid-induced hypotension.

Age

In children aged 2–16 years with chronic malignant and non-malignant pain, the adverse effects of transdermal fentanyl were those of a potent opioid, with no specific risks in this group of patients (53).

Impaired protein binding

When the concentration of α_1-acid glycoprotein is reduced, with reduced binding, highly protein-bound basic drugs, such as fentanyl, should be given with caution in order to avoid high unbound concentrations and unwanted effects (SEDA-17, 81).

Drug Administration

Drug formulations

- A woman suffered sedation, localized erythematous lesions on the hands, and reduced appetite with weight loss after removing transdermal fentanyl patches from her daughter's skin and replacing them without wearing protective gloves (54). She had severe headaches, night sweats, irritability, nausea, and insomnia. When she

used gloves, her weight gradually increased and the sedation abated.
- A 57-year-old woman using transdermal fentanyl (75 µg/hour) developed a reduced respiratory rate and bilateral pinpoint pupils when an upper body warming blanket was used as a normal postoperative procedure (55). The resultant increase in skin temperature significantly enhanced skin perfusion, and increased the systemic absorption of fentanyl from the intracutaneous fentanyl depot, leading to symptoms of opioid overdose. She recovered after removal of the fentanyl patch and the intravenous administration of naloxone 60 µg.

Oral transmucosal fentanyl administration, avoiding first-pass metabolism, produces analgesia and sedation in both adults and children undergoing short painful outpatient procedures. The quality of analgesia is good, and the adverse effects are those typical of the opioids. However, an unusual reaction, with agitation and hyperactivity, progressing over a week to delirium, has been reported. Mild impairment of hepatic and renal function, with accumulation of norfentanyl, has been postulated as a possible mechanism (SEDA-20, 77).

The bioequivalence of four 100-microgram fentanyl buccal tablets given simultaneously has been compared with that of one 400-microgram tablet. Fentanyl C_{max} was higher in those receiving four tablets possibly because of an increased surface area exposure; however, there was no significant difference in adverse events (56).

The fentanyl HCl patient-controlled iontophoretic transdermal system (IONSYS) uses low-level electrical energy to transport fentanyl across the skin, providing adequate analgesia with minimal drug-related adverse effects (57).

The fentanyl HCL iontophoretic transdermal system has been compared with patient-controlled intravenous morphine after total hip replacement in a multicentre study in 799 patients (58). Patient global assessment of the route of administration, pain intensity, and adverse events were recorded for the first 24 hours. There were no significant differences, suggesting that transdermal fentanyl was suitable for acute pain after total hip replacement.

Drug additives

Bupivacaine and/or adrenaline
The addition of bupivacaine and/or adrenaline to epidural fentanyl analgesia has also been studied in 100 women after elective cesarean section. All received fentanyl (3 µg/ml) by patient-controlled analgesia (PCA) for 48 hours and were randomly assigned double-blind to receive either bupivacaine 0.01%, ephedrine 0.5 µg/ml, both, or neither (59). Patients who received fentanyl alone made more attempts at PCA than the other groups, suggesting that this regimen was less effective and the higher dose of fentanyl used perhaps contributed to a higher incidence of nausea and urinary retention and to a higher frequency of severe pruritus. The authors suggested that with lower doses of fentanyl there was less rostral spread of the drug and lower concentrations at the brain stem, thus reducing adverse effects. Breast-fed

neonates were neurologically assessed at 2 and 48 hours by a pediatrician and, despite the different fentanyl requirements of mothers, neurobehavioral scores were equally high in the different groups.

Bupivacaine

Effective postoperative pain relief can be obtained with a mixture of fentanyl and bupivacaine, which not only provides better analgesia than either drug alone, but also fewer adverse effects. There have been several studies of the efficacy of this mixture, using different doses and routes of administration, the addition of clonidine, and in comparison with morphine.

In a randomized, double-blind study in 56 patients, continuous infusion of fentanyl (1 µg/kg/hour or 0.5 µg/kg/hour) and bupivacaine 0.1 mg/kg/hour, with intravenous morphine PCA as rescue analgesia, produced better pain relief after knee ligament operations than epidural saline combined with intravenous morphine PCA (60). There was a non-significant increase in nausea in the fentanyl group.

In another randomized, double-blind study, 84 parturients requesting epidural analgesia were given either bupivacaine 20 ml only, followed by intravenous fentanyl 60 µg or bupivacaine 20 ml with fentanyl 60 µg followed by intravenous saline (61). The minimum local analgesia concentration (MLAC) of bupivacaine + intravenous fentanyl was 0.064% w/v and the MLAC of bupivacaine + epidural fentanyl was 0.034% w/v. The epidural fentanyl solution significantly increased the analgesic potency of bupivacaine by a factor of 1.88 compared with intravenous fentanyl. This was associated with increased pruritus with epidural fentanyl.

Women scheduled for cesarean section ($n = 32$) were given spinal bupivacaine 10 mg (0.5%) or spinal bupivacaine 5 mg (0.5%) plus fentanyl 25 µg (62). Those given fentanyl had adequate spinal anesthesia for cesarean section with fewer adverse effects (nausea and hypotension). This observation was reproduced by spinal anesthesia with bupivacaine 4 mg plus fentanyl 20 µg, which provided adequate spinal anesthesia for surgical repair of hip fracture in elderly patients, with fewer adverse effects than bupivacaine 10 mg (63).

Bupivacaine, clonidine

Different combinations of fentanyl, bupivacaine, and clonidine were investigated in a multicenter (6 sites) trial of 78 women undergoing elective cesarean section under "spinal block" (64). In some cases, this appeared to imply intrathecal administration, and in others combined intrathecal and epidural administration. Patients received hyperbaric bupivacaine alone, or with 75 µg of clonidine, or with 75 µg of clonidine and 12.5 µg of fentanyl. There were no reported hemodynamic differences between the groups, but sedation and pruritus were significantly more common in those who received fentanyl, occurring in 65% and 25% of subjects respectively. Apgar scores and umbilical artery blood pH were unaffected by the drug regimens.

Bupivacaine or ropivacaine

The addition of fentanyl 1 µg/ml to ropivacaine 7.5 mg/ml did not improve nerve blockade by axillary brachial plexus anesthesia in a double-blind, randomized study in 30 patients undergoing orthopedic procedures (65). In another double-blind, randomized study, 60 patients receiving axillary brachial plexus blockade were given 0.25% bupivacaine 40 mg, 0.25% bupivacaine 40 mg plus fentanyl 2.5 µg/ml, or 0.125% bupivacaine 40 mg plus fentanyl 2.5 µg/ml (66). The addition of fentanyl 2.5 µg/ml prolonged sensory and motor blockade without any improvement in the onset of anesthesia and no significant increase in adverse effects. These two studies have reaffirmed the current position of conflicting results in studies of the benefits of adding fentanyl to local anesthetics for peripheral nerve blockade.

Bupivacaine or lidocaine

The addition of clonidine or fentanyl to local anesthetics for single shot caudal blocks has been studied in 64 children undergoing bilateral correction of vesicoureteral reflux randomized into four groups (67). The control group received a mixture of 0.25% bupivacaine with adrenaline plus 1% lidocaine; other groups received the same combination plus 1.5 µg/kg of clonidine, or the control combination plus 1 µg/kg of fentanyl, or the control combination plus 0.5 µg/kg of fentanyl plus 0.75 µg/kg of clonidine. The addition of either clonidine or fentanyl significantly prolonged anesthesia, and during recovery the groups receiving local anesthetics alone or with the addition of fentanyl alone had significantly increased heart rates. Two of the children who received extradural fentanyl had a transient reduction in oxygen of saturation to 92% in the first hour of recovery. One of these was from those who received fentanyl alone, while one had received fentanyl plus clonidine. Vomiting occurred only in children exposed to fentanyl (nine of 29 subjects). This is the first report of respiratory depression in children after the caudal administration of fentanyl or clonidine, this adverse effect having been previously described with extradural opioids and clonidine in adults.

Lidocaine

In 100 patients undergoing arthroscopic outpatient surgery minidose spinal lidocaine plus fentanyl (0.5% lidocaine 20 mg plus fentanyl 20 µg) has been compared with traditional spinal anesthesia (1% lidocaine 30 ml with titrated intravenous propofol infusion) (68). The study was randomized and prospective but unblinded. Whereas those given local anesthesia were more likely to have pain requiring analgesic medication before discharge (44 versus 20%), those given spinal anesthesia group were more likely to have nausea (8 versus 22%) or pruritus (8 versus 68%). Both techniques provided a high degree of patient satisfaction, with comparable efficacy both intraoperatively and postoperatively.

Ropivacaine

In a randomized, placebo-controlled study, a mixture of ropivacaine 0.2% and fentanyl 2 µg/ml plus a background infusion of 5 ml/hour was given to 20 patients for postoperative patient-controlled epidural analgesia after gynecological surgery. Another 21 patients were given the same mixture without the background infusion. Both groups were monitored hourly for arterial blood pressure, heart rate, and respiratory rate, and pain, sedation, motor blockade, and sensory levels were monitored every 6 hours (69). There was no difference in pain scores or patient satisfaction scores between the two groups, but the patients who received the background infusion had a higher incidence of adverse effects (71 versus 30%). The authors suggested that there was no additional benefit in using a background infusion.

Fentanyl 2 µg/ml has been used in combination with ropivacaine 2 mg/ml to determine its impact on the quality of postoperative analgesia and the incidence of adverse effects after colonic surgery in 155 patients scheduled for elective colonic surgery in a multicenter, double-blind, randomized study (70). The incidences of hypotension and pruritus in those given fentanyl were significantly increased, although they had better analgesic control. They also had an increased incidence of serious adverse effects affecting the respiratory, cardiovascular, and genitourinary systems.

The ideal combination strength of ropivacaine with fentanyl for postoperative epidural analgesia has been investigated in two studies. In a double-blind, randomized study, 30 patients undergoing lower abdominal surgery received one of three solutions for PCA after a standardized combined epidural and general anesthetic: ropivacaine 0.2% plus fentanyl 4 µg, ropivacaine 0.1% plus fentanyl 2 µg, or ropivacaine 0.05% plus fentanyl 1 µg (71). All three solutions produced equivalent analgesia. Motor block secondary to the ropivacaine was significantly more frequent and intense with ropivacaine 0.2% plus fentanyl 4 µg. Pruritus, nausea, sedation, and hypotension occurred equally often in the three groups and were mild. It was therefore inferred that ropivacaine 0.2% plus fentanyl 4 µg is preferable for analgesia after lower abdominal surgery.

Sufentanil

There was no difference in analgesic efficacy or the incidence of adverse effects when fentanyl 100 µg was compared with sufentanil 20 µg in women in labor who requested epidural analgesia (72).

Drug dosage regimens

Fentanyl is widely used for obstetric analgesia and the dose–response relation for intrathecal fentanyl has been examined in a randomized study of 84 nulliparous full-term parturients in labor (73). They received intrathecal doses of fentanyl of 5–45 µg and visual analogue scales were used to measure analgesia and adverse effects. The mean duration of anesthesia increased in the dose range 5–25 µg of fentanyl and then reached a plateau. Adequate analgesia was obtained with all doses of fentanyl above 10 µg. Maternal systolic blood pressure was not significantly affected at any dose, although diastolic blood pressure fell significantly at 10–30 minutes after fentanyl. Nausea and vomiting were uncommon, but pruritus was

common in all groups and was more severe with higher doses of fentanyl. Fetal heart rate did not change significantly with fentanyl at any dose, although the authors acknowledged that they did not undertake continuous fetal heart tracing. They concluded that there is no benefit in using doses of intrathecal fentanyl above 25 µg when fentanyl is used as the sole analgesic agent in labor.

Continuous epidural infusion during labor in 40 women has been compared with regular intermittent bolus administration of ropivacaine and fentanyl (74). Intermittent administration resulted in the use of less ropivacaine and fentanyl, less requirement for rescue analgesia, equivalent pain relief, and less potential compromise of cardiovascular stability.

Co-administration of propofol 3 mg/kg + fentanyl 3 micrograms/kg was the optimal regimen for tracheal intubation in 60 children aged 3–10 years (75). This regimen facilitated tracheal intubation with effective blunting of pressor response, but without triggering a fall in cardiac output (as observed in high dose regimens, e.g. propofol 3.5 mg/kg + fentanyl 3 micrograms/kg).

Drug administration route

Opioids have traditionally been given intramuscularly and intravenously. Other methods of administration are oral, subcutaneous, rectal, intrathecal, and extradural. Novel routes include intranasal, inhalational, intra-articular, and transdermal.

Buccal

Oral transmucosal fentanyl citrate has two advantages: it is more acceptable as a flavored lozenge than an oral elixir or tablet would be, especially in children, and 25% goes directly into the systemic circulation without first-pass metabolism (SEDA-20, 77). Its main adverse effect is dose-dependent nausea and/or vomiting, which occurs in 25–50% of patients. In a double-blind, placebo-controlled comparison of oral transmucosal fentanyl citrate (10 µg/kg) and oral oxycodone (0.2 mg/kg) in outpatient wound care procedures in 22 children, there were similar outcomes and no adverse effects in either group (76).

Transdermal

Fentanyl can be used transdermally because of its high solubility in both fat and water, low molecular weight, high analgesic potency, and fewer adverse effects, especially gastrointestinal symptoms (77). It is easy to administer and can be given at 3-day intervals. Transdermal fentanyl has been extensively reviewed in patients with chronic cancer pain (50) and in a review in which the possibilities and techniques available for acute and/or chronic pain relief were considered (78).

Transdermal fentanyl has an adverse effects profile similar to that associated with parenteral administration (SEDA-20, 77). Local erythema and rash have been reported (79), as well as the usual opioid adverse effects. However, an unusual reaction, with progressive agitation to acute delirium, has occurred (SEDA-20, 79).

Local heating and cutaneous hyperthermia of the patch area can cause lethal problems of overdose, owing to increased release and absorption (SEDA-18, 80; SEDA-19, 83).

Transdermal administration of fentanyl has been extensively reviewed (80). In systemic availability studies, 92% of the fentanyl dose delivered from the transdermal therapeutic system into the skin reached the systemic circulation as unchanged unmetabolized fentanyl (77). Morphine, codeine, and hydromorphone are not good candidates for transdermal administration. Pethidine has a high transdermal permeability but poor analgesic potency. Besides fentanyl, only sufentanil and buprenorphine would be suitable opioids for transdermal administration (81).

There are three techniques used for the transdermal administration of fentanyl. The transdermal therapeutic system (TTS) is a membrane-controlled system designed to release fentanyl at a constant rate for up to 3 days, and is useful in patients with chronic cancer pain (82). There are still limited and predominantly uncontrolled studies that show that TTS fentanyl is useful in chronic pain of neuropathic or somatic origin. An open randomized, crossover trial in 18 patients with painful chronic pancreatitis concluded that TTS fentanyl should not be the first-choice analgesic, because of a high incidence of skin adverse effects and low analgesic effects compared with morphine (83).

TTS fentanyl is not useful in acute or postoperative pain, because of the risk of respiratory depression due to the long delay and decay time, which do not allow adequate dose finding (80). Some patients have acute symptoms of morphine withdrawal, in spite of adequate pain control, when they are converted from morphine to transdermal fentanyl. The mechanism has not yet been determined (84,85).

Transdermal fentanyl was the cause of an opioid overdose when a 77-year-old man with a history of severe arthritis developed respiratory failure after starting epidural diamorphine–bupivacaine mixture for postoperative pain (86). The fentanyl patch was removed, the epidural infusion was stopped, and naloxone was given to counteract the excessive opioid effects.

Fentanyl transdermal delivery systems (FTDS) use an unsealed multilaminate system containing a solid matrix, in which fentanyl is embedded instead of the reservoir designed in the TTS. FTDS is not to be recommended for routine postoperative pain treatment, even though it has a faster onset of action (4–6 hours) after cases of fentanyl toxicity, especially respiratory depression. FTDS has not been investigated adequately in chronic pain and is not expected to be superior to the TTS technique.

Iontophoretic transdermal application of opioids is another technique that is currently being tested. The factors that affect the delivery of opioids like fentanyl and sufentanil by this technique include the physicochemical nature of the drug solution, the voltage used, and the duration and nature of the current used (87,88).

An electrotransport therapeutic system (ETS) for fentanyl has been developed. Preliminary studies show that ETS of fentanyl may be useful for the treatment of acute pain (89).

Transdermal fentanyl has been compared with modified-release oral formulations of morphine among 504 patients with advanced cancer in a multicenter, cross-sectional quality-of-life study using four widely validated scales plus original scales, generated and validated for this study (90). The authors used conversion rates "often reported in the literature" to calculate that the fentanyl group used significantly more opiate (200–300 mg of morphine-equivalent units/day) than the oral morphine users (195 mg/day). Despite this, transdermal fentanyl patients reported fewer and less bothersome adverse effects, although these were not separately identified; 50% reported never having any adverse effects compared with 36% of morphine users without adverse effects, although measures of pain intensity showed no significant difference between the two groups. Subgroup analysis by sex showed that the difference in adverse effects between the two modes of administration was significant only in men. However, it should be noted that the mean ages of the two treatment groups were significantly different, a fact that may qualify the reported results.

Transdermal fentanyl avoids the discomfort of injections and reduces fluctuations in drug concentrations. In an open study of transdermal fentanyl patches 50 µg for postoperative pain management in 15 thoracotomy patients, two patients had nausea and one had erythema over the site of application of the patch (91).

Transdermal fentanyl in chronic cancer pain control has been extensively reviewed (50). Data from non-blinded, randomized trials suggest that it is as effective as modified-release oral morphine and that the most common adverse effects include nausea, vomiting, and constipation. The most serious adverse effect reported was hypoventilation, which occurred in about 2% of patients. Skin reactions occurred in 1–3%. A number of non-comparative trials have described the use of transdermal fentanyl for periods of at least a year without serious adverse effects.

In a follow-up study of 78 patients with cancer who participated in a crossover, randomized study of transdermal fentanyl (mean final dose 100 µg/hour) and oral morphine for 4 weeks, the incidences of skin reactions and gastrointestinal symptoms were low (92). Other adverse effects reported were breakthrough pain, light-headedness, and diarrhea. In the original randomized study, which lasted 15 days, there was significantly less constipation with fentanyl than with morphine (93). These results suggest that many patients have stable analgesic requirements with transdermal fentanyl up to the time of death, with no need for additional medication.

In a questionnaire survey of 1005 patients, only 11 had chronic pain from non-malignant disease while taking transdermal fentanyl (94). Their physicians were asked to provide information about their reasons for switching to transdermal fentanyl and were then surveyed until withdrawal of fentanyl because of death, change in analgesic regimen, or serious adverse effects. Modified-release morphine (median dose 90 mg/day) was used in 72% of patients before switching to fentanyl. More than 20% of the cohort had received no continuous opioid medication before the start of transdermal therapy. Most of the patients were switched to fentanyl because of inadequate analgesia or opioid-induced gastrointestinal symptoms. The simplicity of administration and patients' wishes were also contributory factors. Transdermal fentanyl was discontinued primarily because patients died (46%); other reasons included inadequate pain relief (10%), pain relief with another analgesic regimen (10%), adverse effects (5%), rejection of transdermal therapy by the patient (6%), and other unspecified causes, such as pathological fractures and anemia (16%). There were opioid-related adverse effects in 26% of the patients. Serious neurotoxic effects, such as hallucinations (0.2%), withdrawal symptoms (0.1%), or convulsions (0.1%), were rare.

Under controlled conditions, transdermal fentanyl is a useful option for direct conversion from mild to strong opioids in cancer patients. In addition, 25 µg/hour daily incremental steps of transdermal fentanyl can be made by palliative care specialists, if it is required for cancer pain management (95).

Transdermal fentanyl for chronic non-cancer pain control has been studied in two open trials (96,97). In a multicenter, open, randomized study of 256 patients with a history of chronic non-cancer pain, 65% preferred transdermal fentanyl, whereas 28% preferred modified-release oral morphine. Subjective pain control and quality of life were significantly better in the patients who used transdermal fentanyl. Despite a preference for transdermal fentanyl, more patients withdrew because of adverse effects in the first fentanyl period (16%) than in the first morphine period (9%). The difference could have been related to patients' previous experience of morphine, with enhanced tolerance of its adverse effects.

In the second study, 35 patients with severe AIDS-related chronic pain were recruited in a prospective, open, before/after comparison of the analgesic efficacy and adverse effects profile of a stable dose of transdermal fentanyl (25–300 µg/hour) or oral morphine (less than 45 mg/day) for 15 consecutive days (97). Transdermal fentanyl alleviated chronic pain and those who were already dependent on an opioid needed less fentanyl for the same analgesic result.

The long-term use of transdermal fentanyl in patients with chronic non-cancer pain (back pain, leg pain, arthritic pain, trigeminal neuralgia, and intestinal cystitis), which is controversial, has been discussed (98). Transdermal fentanyl was effective and safe and improved quality of life and independent living. However, these case reports were collected by authors closely associated with the company that manufactures transdermal fentanyl patches; a degree of case selectivity and bias might have occurred.

In a prospective study, 64 patients with a recent history of at least one vertebral fracture caused by primary and secondary osteoporosis were recruited from six osteoporosis centers in Germany between December 1999 and April 2001 (99). Transdermal fentanyl 25 µg/hour was the recommended starting dose, with incremental steps of 25 µg/hour if there was insufficient analgesia.

Treatment was stopped after less than 28 days in 15 patients (23%). In 10 of these, fentanyl was stopped because of nausea and/or vomiting and/or dizziness. In 49 patients, pain at rest (55% reduction) and on motion (47% reduction) abated significantly from baseline. The starting dose of 25 µg/hour of fentanyl was sufficient in most patients (70%).

The use of transdermal fentanyl in 113 patients with undertreated chronic cancer pain was studied in a non-randomized, uncontrolled, open study for 42 days (100). The mean dose of fentanyl increased from 25 µg/hour to 117 µg/hour between the start and end of the study. By day 3, six patients reported sleepiness and two reported dizziness; five reported nausea and two had vomiting, and by days 21–42 four of the 100 patients who completed the study had severe nausea and vomiting. Non-compliance was not related to the adverse effects of fentanyl, but to insufficient pain control (nine patients) and/or death (three patients).

Transdermal administration of fentanyl has been evaluated in a placebo-controlled study in 484 adults admitted to the post-anesthesia care unit after major surgery (101). They were given supplementary intravenous fentanyl as required. Pain was better controlled by transdermal fentanyl and fewer of these patients withdrew because of dissatisfaction. There were no differences in treatment-related adverse effects.

A patient-controlled transdermal system (PCTS) consists of a preprogrammed, self-contained drug-delivery system that uses electrotransport technology to deliver 40 micrograms of fentanyl hydrochloride over 10 minutes on demand for patient-controlled analgesia. In an open study of the psychiatric effects of transdermal fentanyl there was an improvement in depressive and anxiety symptoms with time (102). In a pharmaceutical company-sponsored randomized, double-blind, placebo-controlled trial, this non-invasive delivery of parenteral opioids for the management of postoperative pain was considered to be superior to placebo and well tolerated (103). At least one adverse event was experienced by 64% of those who used fentanyl compared to 51% of those who used placebo. These included opioid-related events, such as nausea, vomiting, gastrointestinal disorders, and urinary retention; 13 patients withdrew because of adverse events, eight in the fentanyl group. The main limitation of this study is that disproportionately more patients (5:1) were randomized to the fentanyl group with pain intensity scores of >75 relative to placebo.

The rate of absorption of fentanyl by transdermal administration can be increased by increasing the local temperature.

- A 42-year-old woman with cervical carcinoma had a fentanyl patch delivering 100 micrograms/hour applied to her chest and at the same time started using a heated pad on her abdomen (104). Two hours later she developed pinpoint pupils and shallow respiration, which was reversed with intravenous naloxone hydrochloride 0.4 mg. The heating pad had covered the fentanyl patch and had presumably increased the rate of absorption of the drug.

- A 57-year-old woman developed opioid toxicity after thick blankets were used during surgery because her nasopharyngeal temperature was low, inadvertently covering her fentanyl patch (104). Naloxone was used to reverse opioid toxicity.

These two cases highlight the need to inform patients that fever and even participation in outdoor activities in hot climates and in hot tubs/saunas can cause an increase in fentanyl absorption, with a risk of opioid toxicity.

Epidural
In view of the popularity of fentanyl as an epidural analgesic in labor, its site of action is of some interest, and this has been examined in a randomized study in 55 parturients who received 0.125% bupivacaine plus one of three treatments: epidural saline plus intravenous saline; epidural fentanyl (20 µg/hour) plus intravenous saline; epidural saline plus intravenous fentanyl (20 µg/hour) (105). Study treatments were continuously infused, while epidural bupivacaine was patient-controlled. There was a significant reduction (28%) in bupivacaine use with epidural but not intravenous fentanyl, but there was no significant difference in the incidence of adverse effects. This result suggested that the analgesic effects of epidural fentanyl in labor are due to a spinal mechanism, rather than to systemic absorption and a supraspinal effect. However, the authors acknowledged various limitations of their study and commented that they were able to use low doses of fentanyl because of the concomitant use of bupivacaine, which acts synergistically. It is possible that this synergy allows effective analgesia of the visceral afferents at a spinal level without the need for the higher doses that are required for analgesia with fentanyl alone. Higher doses of fentanyl may mask this spinal effect.

In a prospective study of 1030 mixed surgical patients receiving patient-controlled epidural analgesia with 0.05% bupivacaine and fentanyl 4 µg/ml, the incidence of adverse effects was broadly as expected (106): 17% had pruritus, 15% nausea, 13% sedation, 6.8% hypotension, 2% motor block, and 0.3% respiratory depression. Two patients required naloxone for respiratory depression and sedation. Analgesia was terminated electively in 82%, 12% of cases were terminated owing to a displaced catheter, and 3% of cases required anticoagulation, while infection, adverse effects, and inadequate analgesia each accounted for termination of epidural analgesia in 1% of cases. Risk factors for adverse effects were identified as: patient age under 58 years, weight under 73 kg, being female, high fentanyl consumption (over 9 ml/hour), and lumbar placement of the epidural catheter. There was a significant association between patient age and pruritus, and between female sex and nausea, hypotension, and sedation.

The relations between fentanyl and local anesthetics and their adverse effects profiles in epidural analgesia (107) further demonstrate the need for well-controlled, double-blind studies (108,109).

The use of a continuous epidural infusion of lidocaine 0.4% plus fentanyl 1 µg/ml in combination with intravenous metamizol 40 mg/kg provided significantly better analgesia than epidural morphine 20 µg/kg plus intravenous metamizol 40 mg/kg during the first 3 postoperative days in 30 children undergoing orthopedic surgery, without increasing the incidence of adverse effects; however, the difference in beneficial effect was small (110).

Prophylactic nalbuphine 4 mg and droperidol 0.625 mg with minidose lidocaine + fentanyl spinal anesthesia in a randomized, double-blinded, controlled study in 62 patients having outpatient knee arthroscopy provided significantly better analgesia and reduced nausea and pruritus than in another 62 patients who received only nalbuphine 4 mg with minidose lidocaine + fentanyl spinal anesthesia (111).

Cervical epidural and intravenous patient-controlled analgesia with fentanyl have been compared in 42 patients undergoing pharyngolaryngeal surgery (112). The cervical epidural route provided better analgesia at rest in the first 6 hours postoperatively, but this was not accompanied by a reduction in fentanyl dosage requirements. There were no differences in adverse effects and there were no episodes of clinical respiratory depression or severe sedation. Although the results were favorable, there were no clinical benefits from the cervical epidural technique.

Epidural anesthesia in 43 patients undergoing lumbar microdiscectomy has been compared with general anesthesia (113). Fentanyl 5 micrograms/kg + propofol + vecuronium was used for induction of general anesthesia, followed by 1.2 micrograms/kg/hr + N2O/O2 + isoflurane as maintenance anesthesia. The epidural group received fentanyl 100 micrograms + lidocaine + adrenaline. Nausea, vomiting, and headaches were more common in those who received general anesthesia.

Intravenous patient-controlled analgesia
In a randomized, double-blind, multicenter trial, 150 postoperative patients who had undergone major surgery received demand doses of fentanyl 20, 40, or 60 µg delivered intravenously by PCA (114); higher doses of fentanyl were associated with improved analgesic effect. Adverse effects were reported in 70 patients; the most commonly reported were nausea and vomiting and most adverse effects were described as mild to moderate. Bradypnea occurred in 6% of patients who received fentanyl 60 µg, in one case sufficiently severe to warrant temporary withdrawal of treatment; respiratory depression and moderate hypoxia occurred in one patient on 40 µg and in one on 60 µg, again requiring withdrawal. Overall, mean respiratory rates in the 60 µg group were significantly lower than in the 20 µg group throughout the study, and at 6 hours after initiation compared with the 40 µg group. One patient developed acute confusion and aggression while receiving fentanyl 40 µg. The authors concluded that 40 µg of fentanyl is an appropriate dose for PCA, as this balances analgesic efficacy against the incidence of adverse effects.

Patient-controlled analgesia with intravenous fentanyl was as effective as subacromial ropivacaine with minimal adverse effects and high patient satisfaction in 48 patients undergoing open acromioplasty surgery (115). In contrast, those who received subacromial fentanyl did not have adequate analgesia and required rescue doses of tramadol. In all cases, nausea and vomiting were the most common adverse effects.

Drug overdose

Accidental overdose can be caused by fentanyl patches.

- A 71-year-old woman was found unconscious, with reduced respiration and miotic pupils, having previously had nausea, dizziness, and drowsiness (116). She had inappropriately applied a fentanyl patch 100 μg/hour a day before the symptoms occurred. She recovered fully after treatment with intravenous naloxone 0.4 mg.
- A 24-year-old woman, with a history of polysubstance abuse and extensive psychiatric history, presented with acute opioid overdose caused by the intentional oral ingestion of a fentanyl patch (Duragesic) (117).

Drug–Drug Interactions

Bupivacaine

Bupivacaine is increasingly being used in combination with fentanyl for obstetric analgesia and has been reported to reduce the incidence of pruritus. In a prospective study, 65 parturients in labor were randomly assigned to receive intrathecal fentanyl (25 μg), intrathecal bupivacaine (2.5 mg), or both as part of epidural anesthesia (118). The group that received both drugs had more prolonged analgesia and significantly less pruritus than those who received fentanyl alone (36 versus 95%). However, the incidence of facial pruritus was not significantly different. The type of analgesia did not affect the outcome of labor, although one patient in the combined treatment group required ephedrine for reduced blood pressure. It was proposed that pruritus is the result of stimulation of mu receptors supraspinally and in the dorsal horn of the spinal cord, and that facial itching is associated with mu receptor activation in the medullary dorsal horn, affecting the trigeminal nerve. Local anesthetics may alter this adverse effect by local neuronal blockade or by direct modulation of mu-opioid receptors. Bupivacaine also promotes opioid binding to kappa-opioid receptors, which reduce pruritus. The failure to relieve facial pruritus suggests a direct effect of fentanyl in the brain stem.

Cimetidine

The hepatic metabolism of fentanyl can be inhibited by cimetidine, leading to respiratory depression and sedation (119,120).

Desflurane

The MAC of desflurane was significantly reduced 25 minutes after a single dose of fentanyl (130).

Droperidol

The addition of droperidol 2.5 mg to fentanyl 0.4 mg in 40 ml of 0.125% bupivacaine lowered the incidence of postoperative nausea and vomiting compared with a solution without droperidol or with butorphanol added instead in patients undergoing anorectal surgery in a prospective randomized, single-blind study (121).

Fentanyl plus droperidol (neuroleptanalgesia) was more effective than morphine in relieving anginal pain during unstable angina. However, the patients who received the neuroleptanalgesia also had longer hospital stays, because of significantly more cardiac instability and anginal episodes, and a higher total mortality (122).

An exception to the relatively safe use of high-potency agents has been noted in the combination of droperidol with the narcotic fentanyl, which can cause marked hypotension (131).

Etodimate

Used as a pretreatment for anesthetic induction with etomidate, fentanyl 500 μg produced apnea in all patients, with a 67% incidence of nausea and a 47% incidence of postoperative vomiting (123).

Fluconazole

Death from respiratory depression and circulatory failure due to fentanyl intoxication after the addition of fluconazole has been reported (124).

- A 64-year-old man received transdermal fentanyl 150 micrograms/hour for pain in the mouth following radiation therapy for tonsillar cancer. He developed an oral fungal infection and was given fluconazole 50 mg/day. Three days later he died in his sleep. Post-mortem blood concentrations of fentanyl were high.

Although the blood concentration of fentanyl before fluconazole was given was not known, the authors believed that fluconazole had increased the concentration of fentanyl by inhibition of CYP3A4, which metabolizes fentanyl.

Itraconazole

Oral itraconazole 200 mg did not alter the pharmacokinetics of intravenous fentanyl 3 μg/kg, despite being a strong inhibitor of CYP3A4 in vitro (125). In vitro research suggests that itraconazole should inhibit the elimination of fentanyl, as it has been shown to do to alfentanil. This difference can be accounted for by the higher hepatic extraction ratio of fentanyl (0.8–1.0) compared with alfentanil (0.3–0.5), so that even large changes in the activity of enzymes that metabolize fentanyl significantly affect its pharmacokinetics.

Fentanyl is a substrate of CYP3A4, CYP2C9, and CYP2C19. However, in one study, the pharmacokinetics and pharmacodynamics of fentanyl 3 micrograms/kg were similar after itraconazole 200 mg and placebo in 10 healthy volunteers (125).

• An interaction of itraconazole with fentanyl has been reported in a 67-year-old man with cancer on a stable dose of transdermal fentanyl 50 micrograms/hour (132). He took itraconazole 200 mg bd for oropharyngeal candidiasis, and 24 hours later developed signs of opioid toxicity, which was reversed by withdrawal of fentanyl and replacement with short-acting opioids.

This may be an interaction to which only some individuals are susceptible.

Lopinavir and ritonavir

By inhibiting CYP3A4, ritonavir can significantly inhibit the metabolism of fentanyl, and considerable caution is needed (133).

Midazolam

Several adverse effects have been reported with the combined use of fentanyl and midazolam, including chest wall rigidity, making ventilation with a bag and mask impossible (SEDA-16, 79).

In neonates, hypotension can occur (SEDA-16, 80), and respiratory arrest in a child and sudden cardiac arrest have been reported (SEDA-16, 80). However, in one study there were no cardiac electrophysiological effects of midazolam combined with fentanyl in subjects undergoing cardiac electrophysiological studies (SEDA-18, 80).

Monoamine oxidase inhibitors

There is a risk of hypertension, tachycardia, hyperpyrexia, and coma with the concurrent administration of opioids and monoamine oxidase inhibitors (SEDA-19, 83).

Prilocaine

The addition of fentanyl to the local anesthetic prilocaine does not seem to cause major analgesic benefits, but increases the incidence of adverse effects, particularly affecting the nervous system (126).

Propofol

The interaction between propofol and fentanyl has been studied in relation to suppressing the somatic or hemodynamic responses to three types of surgical event—skin incision, peritoneum incision, and abdominal retraction (127). Three of ninety-nine subjects were withdrawn from the study after bradycardia of under 50/minute occurred when intravenous fentanyl (dose not stated) was given to those already anesthetized with propofol. Propofol and fentanyl (concentration range 0.5–9 ng/ml maintained by computer-assisted continuous infusion for at least 30 minutes) had a predictable synergistic effect and caused a fall in systolic blood pressure. After stimulation, the different concentrations of fentanyl required to block somatic responses to surgery in 50% of subjects were 9.7 ng/ml, 15 ng/ml, and 28 ng/ml respectively for skin incision, peritoneum incision, and abdominal retraction. Concentrations required to give a 15% or less increase in post-incision systolic blood pressure were 5.3 ng/ml, 9.7 ng/ml, and 12 ng/ml respectively. At doses of less than 3 ng/ml of fentanyl the hemodynamic response to peritoneal incision or abdominal retraction was inadequate, even when sufficient propofol was present to suppress somatic responses. Somatic response suppression correlated with fentanyl for skin incision, fentanyl and propofol for peritoneal incision, and propofol for abdominal retraction. Prestimulation propofol reduced systolic blood pressure in a concentration-dependent fashion, while post-stimulation fentanyl significantly suppressed increases in systolic blood pressure. This difference in effect was attributed to propofol's mainly sedative and hypnotic effects, while fentanyl is primarily analgesic.

Ritonavir

Ritonavir is an inhibitor of HIV protease and a potent inhibitor of CYP3A4 and CYP2D6. The interaction between ritonavir and intravenous fentanyl has been investigated in 12 healthy volunteers in a double-blind, placebo-controlled, crossover study (128). The volunteers took ritonavir 600 mg on day 1, ritonavir 900 mg and intravenous fentanyl 5 μg/kg on day 2, and ritonavir 300 mg or placebo on day 3. Ritonavir reduced the clearance of fentanyl by 67% by inhibiting its metabolism. This could result in prolongation of fentanyl-induced respiratory depression in a patient with an already compromised cardiorespiratory system.

Ropivacaine

In a prospective, randomized, double-blind study, the analgesic effect and adverse effects profile of epidural ropivacaine (2 mg/ml) alone was compared with three different fentanyl/ropivacaine combinations (fentanyl 1, 2, and 4 μg/ml) for up to 72 hours of postoperative analgesia in 244 patients after major abdominal surgery, most commonly colorectal surgery (129). Hypotension was significantly more common with fentanyl 4 μg (52%) compared with the other three groups (31–34%) in the first 24 hours, but not later. Nausea was not significantly different among the groups, although there was more antiemetic drug use in patients given fentanyl 2 and 4 μg by day 3. Pruritus was significantly more common in patients who received fentanyl 4 μg throughout the whole 72 hours. Ropivacaine 2 μg/ml plus fentanyl 4 μg/ml provided the most effective pain relief over the 3 days.

Sevoflurane

The minimum alveolar concentrations of sevoflurane required to suppress movements and adrenergic responses to surgery in the presence of the potent opioid fentanyl have been quantified in 226 adults (134). Fentanyl 3 ng/ml and 6 ng/ml reduced sevoflurane requirements to suppress movement to pain by 61% and 74%, respectively, and requirements to suppress the adrenergic responses to pain by 83% and 91%, respectively.

There was no further reduction in sevoflurane requirements at concentrations of fentanyl above 6 ng/ml. The degree of interaction was similar to that seen in previous studies of other volatile anesthetic + opioid combinations.

Management of Adverse Drug Reactions

Pruritus is a common cause of patient dissatisfaction after opioid administration for post-operative pain control. In 98 parturients undergoing elective cesarean section who were given morphine 160 micrograms and fentanyl 15 micrograms postoperatively, ondansetron or tropisetron did not prevent itching caused by intrathecal morphine and fentanyl (135). The incidences of pruritus were 87% with ondansetron, 79% with tropisetron, and 76% with placebo. Medication for pruritus was required in all three groups (in 23%, 39%, and 31% respectively). In five prospective randomized controlled studies in 483 outpatients who were given fentanyl for selective spinal anesthesia, pruritus occurred in 75% and was not prevented by ondansetron (136).

The management of pseudoallergic reactions to opioids using continuous intravenous infusion is well exemplified in a case report (137).

- A 22-year-old woman, with a history of repeated neurosurgical procedures for meningomyelocele and hydrocephalus, developed opioid intolerance. General measures such as substitution with non-opioid medications, a well tolerated opioid, or antihistamines were not effective. She was then given escalating doses of intravenous fentanyl, and tolerated 0.5 micrograms/kg, with a cumulative dose of 50 micrograms. Postoperatively she was given and of infusion fentanyl 0.25 micrograms/kg/hour. A continuous infusion was chosen, given that the total dose of opioid required for pain control was significantly less than the amount required through intermittent administration. This regimen was better tolerated. A similar regimen was used at a later operation, this time by gradually escalating the dose of hydromorphone. A starting infusion rate of 0.2 mg/hour was inadequate and she required 1 mg bolus doses for pain control, which produced severe dyspnea. Increasing the infusion rate by 0.05 mg/hour as required, up to a maximum of 0.35 mg/hour, provided adequate pain control, with no need for further bolus doses and no further allergic reactions.

This case shows that continuous opioid infusion is better tolerated than bolus doses, because the total dose requirements with continuous infusions are significantly less.

References

1. Anonymous. High-dose fentanyl. Lancet 1979;1(8107):81–2.

2. Chudnofsky CR, Wright SW, Dronen SC, Borron SW, Wright MB. The safety of fentanyl use in the emergency department. Ann Emerg Med 1989;18(6):635–9.

3. Cagney B, Williams O, Jennings L, Buggy D. Tramadol or fentanyl analgesia for ambulatory knee arthroscopy. Eur J Anaesthesiol 1999;16(3):182–5.

4. Hunt R, Fazekas B, Thorne D, Brooksbank M. A comparison of subcutaneous morphine and fentanyl in hospice cancer patients. J Pain Symptom Manage 1999;18(2):111–9.

5. Kornick CA, Santiago-Palma J, Schulman G, O'Brien PC, Weigard S, Payne R, Manfredi PL. A safe and effective method for converting patients from transdermal to intravenous fentanyl for the treatment of acute cancer related pain. Cancer 2003;97:3121–4.

6. Yegin A, Sanli S, Hadimioglu N, Akbas M, Karsli B. Intrathecal fentanyl added to hyperbaric ropivacaine for transurethral resection of the prostate. Acta Anaesthesiol Scand 2005;49(3):401–5.

7. Kim JG, Sohn SK, Kim DH, Baek JH, Chae YS, Bae NY, Kim SY, Lee KB. Effectiveness of transdermal fentanyl patch for treatment of acute pain due to oral mucositis in patients receiving stem cell transplantation. Transplant Proc 2005;37(10):4488–91.

8. Pitetti R, Davis PJ, Redlinger R, White J, Wiener E, Calhoun KH. Effect on hospital-wide sedation practices after implementation of the 2001 JCAHO procedural sedation and analgesia guidelines. Arch Pediatr Adolesc Med. 2006;160:211–6.

9. Cucchiaro G, Adzick SN, Rose JB, Maxwell L, Watcha M. A comparison of epidural bupivacaine–fentanyl and bupivacaine–clonidine in children undergoing the Nuss procedure. Anesth Analg 2006;103:322–7.

10. Kokinsky E, Nilsson K, Larsson LE. Increased incidence of postoperative nausea and vomiting without additional analgesic effects when a low dose of intravenous fentanyl is combined with a cardial block. Paediatr Anaesth 2003;13:334–8.

11. Langford R, McKenna F, Ratcliffe S, Vojtassak J, Richarz U. Transdermal fentanyl for improvement of pain and functioning in osteoarthritis: a randomized placebo-controlled trial. Arth Rheum 2006;54(6):1829–37.

12. Barancik M. Inadvertent diagnosis of pheochromocytoma after endoscopic premedication. Dig Dis Sci 1989;34(1):136–8.

13. Bilgin H, Basagan Mogol E, Bekar A, Iscimen R, Korfali G. A comparison of effects of alfentanil, fentanyl, and remifentanil on hemodynamic and respiratory parameters during stereotactic brain biopsy. J Neurosurg Anesthesiol 2006;18(3):179–84.

14. Murphy GS, Szokol JW, Marymont JH, Avram MJ, Vender JS. Opioids and cardioprotection: the impact of morphine and fentanyl on recovery of ventricular function after cardiopulmonary bypass. J Cardiothorac Vasc Anesth 2006;20(4):493–502.

15. McCutcheon CA, Orme RM, Scott DA, Davies MJ, McGlade DP. A comparison of dexmedetomidine versus conventional therapy for sedation and hemodynamic control during carotid endarterectomy performed under regional anesthesia. Anesth Analg 2006;102(3):668–75.

16. Fujiwara Y, Asakura Y, Shibata Y, Nishiwaki K, Komatsu T. A marked decrease in heart rate variability associated with junctional rhythm during anesthesia with sevoflurane and fentanyl. Acta Anaesthesiol Scand 2006;50(4):509–11.

17. Fujiwara Y, Hirokawa M, Wakao Y, Itou H, Komatsu T. Heart rate variability in a child with hereditary sensory autonomic neuropathy 2 (HSAN 2) during general

anesthesia with propofol and fentanyl. Paediatr Anaesth 2006;16(3):363–6.

18. Fujiwara Y, Shibata Y, Kurokawa S, Satou Y, Komatsu T. Ventricular tachycardia in a patient with Brugada syndrome during general anesthesia combined with thoracic paravertebral block. Anesth Analg 2006;102:1590–1.

19. Chung F, Evans D. Low-dose fentanyl: haemodynamic response during induction and intubation in geriatric patients. Can Anaesth Soc J 1985;32(6):622–8.

20. Grote B, Kugler J, Gutzeit M, Doenicke A. Einfluss von Doxapram auf eine fentanylinduzierte Atemdepression bein Menshen. [The influence of doxapram in human on the respiratory depression by fentanyl.] Anaesthesist 1978;27(6):287–90.

21. Dahan A, Yassen A, Bijl H, Romberg R, Sarton E, Teppema L, Olofsen E, Danhof M. Comparison of the respiratory effects of intravenous buprenorphine and fentanyl in humans and rats. Br J Anesth 2005;94(6):825–34.

22. Bohrer H, Fleischer F, Werning P. Tussive effect of a fentanyl bolus administered through a central venous catheter. Anaesthesia 1990;45(1):18–21.

23. Agarwal A, Azim A, Ambesh S. Bose N, Dhiraj S, Sahu D, Singh U. Salbutamol beclomethasone or sodium chromoglycate suppress coughing induced by IV fentanyl. Can J Anesth 2003;50:297–300.

24. Tweed WA, Dakin D. Explosive coughing after bolus fentanyl injection. Anesth Analg 2001;92(6):1442–3.

25. Lin JA, Yeh CC, Lee MS, Wu CT, Lin SL, Wong CS. Prolonged injection time and light smoking decrease the incidence of fentanyl-induced cough. Anesth Analg 2005;101(3):670–4.

26. Arai Y-CP, Ogata J, Fukunaga K, Shimazu A, Fujioka A, Uchida T. The effect of intrathecal fentanyl added to hyperbaric bupivacaine on maternal respiratory function during cesarean section. Acta Anaesthesiol Scand 2006;50(3):364–7.

27. Davis JJ, Swenson JD, Hall RH, Dillon JD, Johnson KB, Egan TD, Pace NL, Niu SY. Pre-operative 'fentanyl challenge' as a tool to estimate postoperative opioid dosing in chronic opioid-consuming patients. Anesth Analg 2005;101(2):389–95.

28. Scott JC, Sarnquist FH. Seizure-like movements during a fentanyl infusion with absence of seizure activity in a simultaneous EEG recording. Anesthesiology 1985;62(6):812–4.

29. Knuttgen D, Doehn M, Eymer D, Muller MR. Hirudrucksteigerung nach Fentanyl. [An increase in intracranial pressure following fentanyl.] Anaesthesist 1989;38(2):73–5.

30. Stuerenburg HJ, Claassen J, Eggers C, Hansen HC. Acute adverse reaction to fentanyl in a 55 year old man. J Neurol Neurosurg Psychiatry 2000;69(2):281–2.

31. Bragonier R, Bartle D, Langton-Hewer S. Acute dystonia in a 14-yr-old following propofol and fentanyl anaesthesia. Br J Anaesth 2000;84(6):828–9.

32. Tsueda K, Mosca PJ, Heine MF, Loyd GE, Durkis DA, Malkani AL, Hurst HE. Mood during epidural patient-controlled analgesia with morphine or fentanyl. Anesthesiology 1998;88(4):885–91.

33. Oltmanns KM, Fehm HL, Peters A. Chronic fentanyl application induces adrenocortical insufficiency. J Int Med 2005;257(5):478–80.

34. Staats PS, Markowitz J, Schein J. Incidence of constipation associated with long acting opioid therapy: a comparative study. Southern Med J 2004;97:129–34.

35. Slappendel R, Simpson K, Dubois D, Keininger DL. Validation of the PAC-SYM questionnaire for opioid-induced constipation in patients with chronic low back pain. Eur J Pain 2006;10(3):209–17.

36. Richman PS, Baram D, Varela M, Glass PS. Sedation during mechanical ventilation: a trial of benzodiazepine and opiate in combination. Crit Care Med 2006;34(5):1395–401.

37. Rama-Maceiras P, Ferreira TA, Molins N, Sanduende Y, Bautista AP, Rey T. Less postoperative nausea and vomiting after propofol + remifentanil versus propofol + fentanyl anaesthesia during plastic surgery. Acta Anaesthesiol Scand 2005;49(3):305–11.

38. Allan L, Richarz U, Simpson K, Slappendel R. Transdermal fentanyl versus sustained release oral morphine in strong-opioid naive patients with chronic low back pain. Spine 2005;30(22):2484–90.

39. Das UG, Sasidharan P. Bladder retention of urine as a result of continuous intravenous infusion of fentanyl: 2 case reports. Pediatrics 2001;108(4):1012–5.

40. Mancuso G, Berdondini RM, Passarini B. Eosinophilic pustular eruption associated with transdermal fentanyl. J Eur Acad Dermatol Venereol 2001;15(1):70–2.

41. Gurkan Y, Toker K. Prophylactic ondansetron reduces the incidence of intrathecal fentanyl-induced pruritus. Anesth Analg 2002;95(6):1763–6.

42. Muller P, Vogtmann C. Three cases with different presentation of fentanyl-induced muscle rigidity—a rare problem in intensive care of neonates. Am J Perinatol 2000;17(1):23–6.

43. Fahnenstich H, Steffan J, Kau N, Bartmann P. Fentanyl-induced chest wall rigidity and laryngospasm in preterm and term infants. Crit Care Med 2000;28(3):836–9.

44. Christian CM 2nd, Waller JL, Moldenhauer CC. Postoperative rigidity following fentanyl anesthesia. Anesthesiology 1983;58(3):275–7.

45. Buyukkocak U, Caglayan O, Daphan C, Aydinuraz K, Saygun O, Kaya T, Agalar F. Similar effects of general and spinal anaesthesia on perioperative stress response in patients undergoing haemorrhoidectomy. Mediators Inflam 2006;2006(1):97257.

46. Tharp AM, Winecker RE, Winston DC. Fatal intravenous fentanyl abuse. Four cases involving extraction of fentanyl from transdermal patches. Am J Med Pathol 2004;25:178–81.

47. Kreek MJ, Bart G, Lilly C, Laforge KS, Nielson DA. Pharmacogenetics and human molecular genetics of opiate and cocaine addictions and their treatments. Pharmacol Rev 2005;57(1):1–26.

48. Dominguez KD, Lomako DM, Katz RW, Kelly HW. Opioid withdrawal in critically ill neonates. Ann Pharmacother 2003;37:473–7.

49. Buvanendran A, McCarthy RJ, Kroin JS, Leong W, Perry P, Tuman KJ. Intrathecal magnesium prolongs fentanyl analgesia: a prospective, randomized, controlled trial. Anesth Analg 2002;95(3):661–6.

50. Muijsers RB, Wagstaff AJ. Transdermal fentanyl: an updated review of its pharmacological properties and therapeutic efficacy in chronic cancer pain control. Drugs 2001;61(15):2289–307.

51. Jordan S, Emery S, Bradshaw C, Watkins A, Friswell W. The impact of intrapartum analgesia on infant feeding. BJOG 2005;112(7):927–34.

52. Smiley RM, Blouin J-L, Negron M, Landau R. Beta-2-adrenoceptor genotype affects vasopressor requirements during spinal anesthesia for cesarean delivery. Anesthesiology 2006;104(4):644–50.

53. Finkel JC, Finley A, Greco C, Weisman SJ, Zeltzer L. Transdermal fentanyl in the management of children with

chronic severe pain: results from an international study. Cancer 2005;104(12):2847–57.

54. Gardner-Nix J. Caregiver toxicity from transdermal fentanyl. J Pain Symptom Manage 2001;21(6):447–8.

55. Frolich MA, Giannotti A, Modell JH, Frolich M. Opioid overdose in a patient using a fentanyl patch during treatment with a warming blanket. Anesth Analg 2001;93(3):647–8.

56. Darwish M, Kirby M, Robertson P Jr, Hellriegel E, Jiang JG. Comparison of equivalent doses of fentanyl buccal tablets and ateriovenous differences in fentanyl pharmacokinetics. Clin Pharmacokin 2006;45(8):843–50.

57. Mayes S, Ferrone M. Fentanyl HCl patient-controlled iontophoretic transdermal systems for the management of acute postoperative pain. Ann Pharmacother 2006;40(12):2178–85.

58. Hartrick CT, Bourne MH, Gargiulo K, Damaraju CV, Vallow S, Hewitt DJ. Fentanyl Iontophoretic transdermal system for acute pain management after orthopedic surgery: a comparative study with morphine intravenous patient-controlled analgesia. Reg Anesth Pain Med 2006;31(6):546–54.

59. Cohen S, Lowenwirt I, Pantuck CB, Amar D, Pantuck EJ. Bupivacaine 0.01% and/or epinephrine 0.5 microg/ml improve epidural fentanyl analgesia after cesarean section Anesthesiology 1998;89(6):1354–61.

60. Silvasti M, Pitkanen M. Continuous epidural analgesia with bupivacaine–fentanyl versus patient-controlled analgesia with i.v. morphine for postoperative pain relief after knee ligament surgery Acta Anaesthesiol Scand 2000;44(1):37–42.

61. Polley LS, Columb MO, Naughton NN, Wagner DS, Dorantes DM, van de Ven CJ. Effect of intravenous versus epidural fentanyl on the minimum local analgesic concentration of epidural bupivacaine in labor. Anesthesiology 2000;93(1):122–8.

62. Ben-David B, Miller G, Gavriel R, Gurevitch A. Low-dose bupivacaine-fentanyl spinal anesthesia for cesarean delivery. Reg Anesth Pain Med 2000;25(3):235–9.

63. Ben-David B, Frankel R, Arzumonov T, Marchevsky Y, Volpin G. Minidose bupivacaine–fentanyl spinal anesthesia for surgical repair of hip fracture in the aged. Anesthesiology 2000;92(1):6–10.

64. Benhamou D, Thorin D, Brichant JF, Dailland P, Milon D, Schneider M. Intrathecal clonidine and fentanyl with hyperbaric bupivacaine improves analgesia during cesarean section. Anesth Analg 1998;87(3):609–13.

65. Fanelli G, Casati A, Magistris L, Berti M, Albertin A, Scarioni M, Torri G. Fentanyl does not improve the nerve block characteristics of axillary brachial plexus anaesthesia performed with ropivacaine. Acta Anaesthesiol Scand 2001;45(5):590–4.

66. Karakaya D, Buyukgoz F, Baris S, Guldogus F, Tur A. Addition of fentanyl to bupivacaine prolongs anesthesia and analgesia in axillary brachial plexus block. Reg Anesth Pain Med 2001;26(5):434–8.

67. Constant I, Gall O, Gouyet L, Chauvin M, Murat I. Addition of clonidine or fentanyl to local anaesthetics prolongs the duration of surgical analgesia after single shot caudal block in children. Br J Anaesth 1998;80(3):294–8.

68. Ben-David B, DeMeo PJ, Lucyk C, Solosko D. A comparison of minidose lidocaine–fentanyl spinal anesthesia and local anesthesia/propofol infusion for outpatient knee arthroscopy. Anesth Analg 2001;93(2):319–25.

69. Wong K, Chong JL, Lo WK, Sia AT. A comparison of patient-controlled epidural analgesia following gynaecological surgery with and without a background infusion. Anaesthesia 2000;55(3):212–6.

70. Finucane BT, Ganapathy S, Carli F, Pridham JN, Ong BY, Shukla RC, Kristoffersson AH, Huizar KM, Nevin K, Ahlen KGCanadian Ropivacaine Research Group. Prolonged epidural infusions of ropivacaine (2 mg/ml) after colonic surgery: the impact of adding fentanyl Anesth Analg 2001;92(5):1276–85.

71. Liu SS, Moore JM, Luo AM, Trautman WJ, Carpenter RL. Comparison of three solutions of ropivacaine/fentanyl for postoperative patient-controlled epidural analgesia. Anesthesiology 1999;90(3):727–33.

72. Connelly NR, Parker RK, Vallurupalli V, Bhopatkar S, Dunn S. Comparison of epidural fentanyl versus epidural sufentanil for analgesia in ambulatory patients in early labor. Anesth Analg 2000;91(2):374–8.

73. Palmer CM, Cork RC, Hays R, Van Maren G, Alves D. The dose–response relation of intrathecal fentanyl for labor analgesia. Anesthesiology 1998;88(2):355–61.

74. Fettes PDW, Moore CS, Whiteside JB, Mcleod GA, Wildsmith JAW. Intermittent vs continuous administration of epidural ropivacaine with fentanyl for analgesia during labour. Br J Anaesth 2006;97(3):359–64.

75. Gupta A, Kaur R, Malhotra R, Kale S. Comparative evaluation of different doses of propofol preceded by fentanyl on intubating conditions and pressor response during tracheal intubation without muscle relaxants. Paediatr Anesth 2006;16(4):399–405.

76. Sharar SR, Carrougher GJ, Selzer K, O'Donnell F, Vavilala MS, Lee LA. A comparison of oral transmucosal fentanyl citrate and oral oxycodone for pediatric outpatient wound care. J Burn Care Rehabil 2002;23(1):27–31.

77. Varvel JR, Shafer SL, Hwang SS, Coen PA, Stanski DR. Absorption characteristics of transdermally administered fentanyl. Anesthesiology 1989;70(6):928–34.

78. Alexander-Williams JM, Rowbotham DJ. Novel routes of opioid administration. Br J Anaesth 1998;81(1):3–7.

79. Caplan RA, Ready LB, Oden RV, Matsen FA 3rd, Nessly ML, Olsson GL. Transdermal fentanyl for postoperative pain management. A double-blind placebo study. JAMA 1989;261(7):1036–9.

80. Grond S, Radbruch L, Lehmann KA. Clinical pharmacokinetics of transdermal opioids: focus on transdermal fentanyl. Clin Pharmacokinet 2000;38(1):59–89.

81. Roy SD, Flynn GL. Transdermal delivery of narcotic analgesics: comparative permeabilities of narcotic analgesics through human cadaver skin. Pharm Res 1989;6(10):825–32.

82. Vielvoye-Kerkmeer AP, Mattern C, Uitendaal MP. Transdermal fentanyl in opioid-naive cancer pain patients: an open trial using transdermal fentanyl for the treatment of chronic cancer pain in opioid-naive patients and a group using codeine. J Pain Symptom Manage 2000;19(3):185–92.

83. Niemann T, Madsen LG, Larsen S, Thorsgaard N. Opioid treatment of painful chronic pancreatitis. Int J Pancreatol 2000;27(3):235–40.

84. Davies AN, Bond C. Transdermal fentanyl and the opioid withdrawal syndrome. Palliat Med 1996;10(4):348.

85. Zenz M, Donner B, Strumpf M. Withdrawal symptoms during therapy with transdermal fentanyl (fentanyl TTS)? J Pain Symptom Manage 1994;9(1):54–5.

86. Alsahaf MH, Stockwell M. Respiratory failure due to the combined effects of transdermal fentanyl and epidural bupivacaine/diamorphine following radical nephrectomy. J Pain Symptom Manage 2000;20(3):210–3.

87. Vanbever R, LeBoulenge E, Preat V. Transdermal delivery of fentanyl by electroporation. I. Influence of electrical factors. Pharm Res 1996;13(4):559–65.

88. Vanbever R, Morre ND, Preat V. Transdermal delivery of fentanyl by electroporation. II. Mechanisms involved in drug transport. Pharm Res 1996;13(9):1360–6.

89. Dunn C. "Touch of a button" delivers transdermal fentanyl. In Pharm 1997;1087:19–20.

90. Payne R, Mathias SD, Pasta DJ, Wanke LA, Williams R, Mahmoud R. Quality of life and cancer pain: satisfaction and side effects with transdermal fentanyl versus oral morphine. J Clin Oncol 1998;16(4):1588–93.

91. Pereira B, Jain PN, Kakhandki V, Dasgupta D. Transdermal fentanyl in post-thoracotomy pain. J Anaesthesiol Clin Pharmacol 1999;115:169–72.

92. Nugent M, Davis C, Brooks D, Ahmedzai SH. Long-term observations of patients receiving transdermal fentanyl after a randomized trial. J Pain Symptom Manage 2001;21(5):385–91.

93. Ahmedzai S, Brooks D. Transdermal fentanyl versus sustained-release oral morphine in cancer pain: preference, efficacy, and quality of life. The TTS–Fentanyl Comparative Trial Group. J Pain Symptom Manage 1997;13(5):254–61.

94. Radbruch L, Sabatowski R, Petzke F, Brunsch-Radbruch A, Grond S, Lehmann KA. Transdermal fentanyl for the management of cancer pain: a survey of 1005 patients. Palliat Med 2001;15(4):309–21.

95. Mystakidou K, Befon S, Kouskouni E, Gerolymatos K, Georgaki S, Tsilika E, Vlahos L. From codeine to transdermal fentanyl for cancer pain control: a safety and efficacy clinical trial. Anticancer Res 2001;21(3C):2225–30.

96. Allan L, Hays H, Jensen NH, de Waroux BL, Bolt M, Donald R, Kalso E. Randomised crossover trial of transdermal fentanyl and sustained release oral morphine for treating chronic non-cancer pain. BMJ 2001;322(7295):1154–8.

97. Newshan G, Lefkowitz M. Transdermal fentanyl for chronic pain in AIDS: a pilot study. J Pain Symptom Manage 2001;21(1):69–77.

98. Libretto SE. Use of transdermal fentanyl in patients with continuous non-malignant pain: a case report series. Clin Drug Invest 2002;22:473–83.

99. Ringe JD, Faber H, Bock O, Valentine S, Felsenberg D, Pfeifer M, Minne HW, Schwalen S. Transdermal fentanyl for the treatment of back pain caused by vertebral osteoporosis. Rheumatol Int 2002;22(5):199–203.

100. Mystakidou K, Befon S, Tsilika E, Dardoufas K, Georgaki S, Vlahos L. Use of TTS fentanyl as a single opioid for cancer pain relief: a safety and efficacy clinical trial in patients naive to mild or strong opioids. Oncology 2002;62(1):9–16.

101. Viscusi ER, Reynolds L, Tait S, Melson T, Atkinson LE. An iontophoretic fentanyl patient-activated analgesic delivery system for postoperative pain: a double-blind, placebo-controlled trial. Anesth Analg 2006;102(1):188–94.

102. Mystakidou K, Tsilika E, Paepa E, Papageorgiou C, Georgaki S, Vlahos L. Investigating the effects of TTS-fentanyl for cancer pain on the psychological status of patients naïve to strong opioids. Cancer Nursing 2004;27:127–33.

103. Chelly JE, Grass J, Houseman TW, Minkowitz H, Pue A. The safety and efficacy of a fentanyl patient-controlled transdermal system for acute postoperative analgesia: a multi-centre, placebo-controlled trial. Anesth Analg 2004;98:427–33.

104. Carter KA. Heat-associated increase in transdermal fentanyl absorption. Am J Health-Syst Pharm 2003;60:191–2.

105. D'Angelo R, Gerancher JC, Eisenach JC, Raphael BL. Epidural fentanyl produces labor analgesia by a spinal mechanism. Anesthesiology 1998;88(6):1519–23.

106. Liu SS, Allen HW, Olsson GL. Patient-controlled epidural analgesia with bupivacaine and fentanyl on hospital wards: prospective experience with 1030 surgical patients. Anesthesiology 1998;88(3):688–95.

107. Niemi G, Breivik H. Epidural fentanyl markedly improves thoracic epidural analgesia in a low-dose infusion of bupivacaine, adrenaline and fentanyl. A randomized, double-blind crossover study with and without fentanyl. Acta Anaesthesiol Scand 2001;45(2):221–32.

108. Wigfull J, Welchew E. Survey of 1057 patients receiving postoperative patient-controlled epidural analgesia. Anaesthesia 2001;56(1):70–5.

109. Lovstad RZ, Stoen R. Postoperative epidural analgesia in children after major orthopaedic surgery. A randomised study of the effect on PONV of two anaesthetic techniques: low and high dose i.v. fentanyl and epidural infusions with and without fentanyl Acta Anaesthesiol Scand 2001;45(4):482–8.

110. Reinoso-Barbero F, Saavedra B, Hervilla S, de Vicente J, Tabares B, Gomez-Criado MS. Lidocaine with fentanyl, compared to morphine, marginally improves postoperative epidural analgesia in children. Can J Anaesth 2002;49(1):67–71.

111. Mendelson JH, Mello NK. Plasma testosterone levels during chronic heroin use and protracted abstinence. A study of Hong Kong addicts. Clin Pharmacol Ther 1975;17(5):529–33.

112. Roussier M, Mahul P, Pascal J, Baylot D, Prades JM, Auboyer C, Molliex S. Patient-controlled cervical epidural fentanyl compared with patient-controlled i.v. fentanyl for pain after pharyngolaryngeal surgery. Br J Anaesth 2006;96(4):492–6.

113. Papadopoulos EC, Girardi FP, Sama A, Pappou IP, Urban MK. Lumbar microdiscectomy under epidural anesthesia: a comparison study. Spine J 2006;6(5):561–4.

114. Camu F, Van Aken H, Bovill JG. Postoperative analgesic effects of three demand-dose sizes of fentanyl administered by patient-controlled analgesia. Anesth Analg 1998;87(4):890–5.

115. Eroglu A. A comparison of patient-controlled subacromial and i.v. analgesia after open acromioplasty surgery. Br J Anesth 2006;96(4):497–501.

116. Klockgether-Radke AP, Gaus P, Neumann P. Opioidintoxikation durch transdermales Fentanyl. [Opioid intoxication following transdermal administration of fentanyl.] Anaesthesist 2002;51(4):269–71.

117. Purucker M, Swann W. Potential for Duragesic patch abuse. Ann Emerg Med 2000;35(3):314.

118. Asokumar B, Newman LM, McCarthy RJ, Ivankovich AD, Tuman KJ. Intrathecal bupivacaine reduces pruritus and prolongs duration of fentanyl analgesia during labor: a prospective, randomized controlled trial. Anesth Analg 1998;87(6):1309–15.

119. Knodell RG, Holtzman JL, Crankshaw DL, Steele NM, Stanley LN. Drug metabolism by rat and human hepatic microsomes in response to interaction with H_2-receptor antagonists. Gastroenterology 1982;82(1):84–8.

120. Lee HR, et al. Effect of histamine H_2-receptors on fentanyl metabolism. Pharmacology 1982;24:145.

121. Kotake Y, Matsumoto M, Ai K, Morisaki H, Takeda J. Additional droperidol, not butorphanol, augments epidural fentanyl analgesia following anorectal surgery. J Clin Anesth 2000;12(1):9–13.

122. Burduk P, Guzik P, Piechocka M, Bronisz M, Rozek A, Jazdon M, Jordan MR. Comparison of fentanyl and droperidol mixture (neuroleptanalgesia II) with morphine on clinical outcomes in unstable angina patients. Cardiovasc Drugs Ther 2000;14(3):259–69.

123. Stockham RJ, Stanley TH, Pace NL, Gillmor S, Groen F, Hilkens P. Fentanyl pretreatment modifies anaesthetic induction with etomidate. Anaesth Intensive Care 1988;16(2):171–6.

124. Hallberg P, Marten L, Wadelius M. Possible fluconazole-fentanyl interaction: a case report. Eur J Clin Pharmacol 2006;62(6):491–2.

125. Palkama VJ, Neuvonen PJ, Olkkola KT. The CYP 3A4 inhibitor itraconazole has no effect on the pharmacokinetics of i.v. fentanyl Br J Anaesth 1998;81(4):598–600.

126. Pitkanen MT, Rosenberg PH, Pere PJ, Tuominen MK, Seppala TA. Fentanyl–prilocaine mixture for intravenous regional anaesthesia in patients undergoing surgery. Anaesthesia 1992;47(5):395–8.

127. Kazama T, Ikeda K, Morita K. The pharmacodynamic interaction between propofol and fentanyl with respect to the suppression of somatic or hemodynamic responses to skin incision, peritoneum incision, and abdominal wall retraction. Anesthesiology 1998;89(4):894–906.

128. Olkkola KT, Palkama VJ, Neuvonen PJ. Ritonavir's role in reducing fentanyl clearance and prolonging its half-life. Anesthesiology 1999;91(3):681–5.

129. Scott DA, Blake D, Buckland M, Etches R, Halliwell R, Marsland C, Merridew G, Murphy D, Paech M, Schug SA, Turner G, Walker S, Huizar K, Gustafsson U, Deam RK, Blyth C, Wallace M, Buckland M, Downey G, Etches R, Bignell S, Pavy T, Orlikowski C, Ryan C, Eugster D, Lim W, Dillenbeck C, Sidebotham D. A comparison of epidural ropivacaine infusion alone and in combination with 1, 2, and 4 microgram/ml fentanyl for seventy-two hours of postoperative analgesia after major abdominal surgery. Anesth Analg 1999;88(4):857–64.

130. Sebel PS, Glass PS, Fletcher JE, Murphy MR, Gallagher C, Quill T. Reduction of the MAC of desflurane with fentanyl. Anesthesiology 1992;76(1):52–9.

131. Mandelstam JP. An inquiry into the use of Innovar for pediatric premedication. Anesth Analg 1970;49(5):746–50.

132. Mercadante S, Villari P, Ferrera P. Itraconazole–fentanyl interaction in a cancer patient. J Pain Symptom Manage 2002;24(3):284–6.

133. Olkkola KT, Palkama VJ, Neuvonen PJ. Ritonavir's role in reducing fentanyl clearance and prolonging its half-life. Anesthesiology 1999;91(3):681–5.

134. Katoh T, Kobayashi S, Suzuki A, Iwamoto T, Bito H, Ikeda K. The effect of fentanyl on sevoflurane requirements for somatic and sympathetic responses to surgical incision. Anesthesiology 1999;90(2):398–405.

135. Sarvela PJ, Halonen PM, Soikkeli AI, Kainu JP, Korttila KT. Ondansetron and tropisetron do not prevent intraspinal morphine- and fentanyl-induced pruritus in elective cesarean delivery. Acta Anaesthesiol Scand 2006;50(2):239–44.

136. Korhonen A-M. Discharge home in 3 hours after selective spinal anesthesia: studies on the quality of anesthesia with

hyperbaric bupivacaine for ambulatory knee arthroscopy. Acta Anaesthesiol Scand 2006;50(5):627.

137. Tcheurekdjian H, Gundling K. Continuous hydromorphone infusion for opioid intolerance. J Allergy Clin Immunol 2006;118:282–4.

Frakefamide

General Information

Frakefamide is a peripherally acting opioid MOR receptor agonist. It has restricted penetration of the blood-brain barrier into the central nervous system and has selective MOR receptor agonist activity. It is a large molecule (molar mass 600 Da), a fluorinated tetrapeptide, H-Tyr-(D)Ala-(pF)Phe-Phe-NH2 hydrochloride, with potent analgesic activity in both rats and humans.

Placebo-controlled studies

In a randomized placebo-controlled comparison with morphine in 12 healthy volunteers, frakefamide (like placebo) did not impair responses to hypercarbic or hypoxic challenges, demonstrating its peripheral activity with no effects on central breathing mechanisms [1]. On the other hand, morphine impaired responses to both hypercarbic and hypoxic challenges. All those who were given frakefamide had transient myalgia (mild to severe) which started within 15 minutes after administration and disappeared after 15-20 minutes. Six of the subjects also had rhinitis.

Reference

1. Modalen AO, Quiding H, Frey J, Westman L, Lindahl S. A novel molecule with peripheral opioid properties: the effects on hypercarbic and hypoxic ventilation at steady-state compared with morphine and placebo. Anesth Analg 2006;102(1):104–9.

Hydrocodone

General Information

Hydrocodone is a semisynthetic narcotic analgesic and a cough suppressant, similar to codeine. It is metabolized to the *O*- and *N*-demethylated products, hydromorphone and norhydrocodone (1).

Comparative studies

Hydrocodone is effective in the management of pain after augmentation mammoplasty but is associated with opioid-related adverse effects. In a study of the potential opioid-sparing effect of a combination of hydrocodone + celecoxib one group of 50 patients had postoperative pain managed by hydrocodone and another 50 received celecoxib + hydrocodone (2). The hydrocodone group required hydrocodone 110 mg (mean dose) in the 7-day postoperative period. The combination group required celecoxib 400 mg/day + hydrocodone 34 mg. The latter also achieved superior pain relief and caused 53% less nausea.

Long-Term Effects

Drug dependence

Dependence on hydrocodone has been described (3).

A specialist physician in practice for several years became addicted after self-medicating with a cough syrup containing hydrocodone to alleviate an upper respiratory tract infection. The hydrocodone not only improved his cough but also his mood, with perceived improvements and increases in work performance. This led him to take hydrocodone on a regular basis and he subsequently became dependent physically and psychologically.

This case was used as an introduction to the issue of the "sick and addicted doctor" and the need, not only to easily recognize signs, but also to provide an effective and supportive environment to help such individuals.

Drug Administration

Drug administration route

Five patients who abused prescribed opioids intranasally have been described (4). All took hydrocodone bitartrate plus cocaine ($n = 2$), codeine phosphate ($n = 2$), oxycodone hydrochloride ($n = 2$), or methadone hydrochloride ($n = 1$). The symptoms included nasal obstruction and congestion, foul smelling nasal crusting and discharge, headaches and nasal pain, and in one case dysphagia with odynophagia. Physical findings included a perforated septum, soft palate erosion, and a mucopurulent exudate. All except one patient had positive fungal cultures and two had invasive rhinitis. Not only can intranasal opioids cause septal perforation, commonly associated with intranasal cocaine, but it is also possible that intranasal abuse of opioids, especially hydrocodone, can cause localized immunosuppression, supporting the growth of fungal organisms.

References

1. Hutchinson MR, Menelaou A, Foster DJ, Coller JK, Somogyi AA. CYP2D6 and CYP3A4 involvement in the primary oxidative metabolism of hydrocodone by human liver microsomes. Br J Clin Pharmacol 2004;57(3):287–97.
2. Freedman BM, Balakrishan TP, O'Hara EL. Celecoxib reduces narcotic use and pain following augmentation mammoplasty. Aesthetic Surg J 2006;26(1):24–8.
3. Knight JR. A 35-year old physician with opioid dependence. JAMA 2004;292:1351–7.
4. Yewell J, Haydon R, Archer S, Manaligod JM. Complications of intranasal prescription narcotic abuse. Ann Otol Rhinol Laryngol 2002;111(2):174–7.

Hydromorphone

General Information

Intolerable adverse effects or inadequate analgesia occur in 10–15% of patients with chronic pain given continuous intrathecal morphine. Hydromorphone is a semisynthetic derivative of morphine used extensively in the management of cancer pain. It is more soluble than morphine, has a slightly shorter duration of action, and is about five times more potent when given systemically.

In a retrospective review of 37 patients with chronic non-malignant pain (mostly from failed lumbosacral spine surgery) treated with intrathecal hydromorphone there was an analgesic response in six of the 16 patients who were switched from morphine to hydromorphone because of poor pain relief (1). Opioid-related adverse effects, such as nausea, vomiting, pruritus, and sedation, were also reduced by hydromorphone in the 21 patients who were switched to hydromorphone because of morphine-related adverse effects, especially 1 month after use. These results should be treated cautiously, because of the limitations of a retrospective study that lacks strict inclusion criteria, with obvious population bias and under-reporting, and without standardized procedures for rotation to hydromorphone.

Three randomized, double-blind comparisons of morphine and hydromorphone have been reported. Modified-release hydromorphone hydrochloride 4 mg bd was compared with modified-release morphine sulfate 30 mg bd in 89 patients with cancer pain (2). In all, 88 adverse effects were thought to be directly related to the study medication. Other adverse events were related to the disease process, the re-emergence of pain, or not specified.

In a comparison of hydromorphone and morphine delivered by continuous subcutaneous infusion in 74 patients with severe cancer pain, the number of adverse effects was small and comparable in both groups (3).

When epidural morphine (Duramorph 10 micrograms/kg/hour) was compared with epidural fentanyl (1 microgram/kg/hour) and epidural hydromorphone (1 microgram/kg/hour) in 90 children undergoing orthopedic procedures, hydromorphone was considered to be safe and efficacious (4). The combined incidences of pruritus, nausea, and vomiting were 25, 20, and 10% respectively and for pruritus alone 35, 15, and 8% respectively.

Observational studies

In an open, single and multiple dose study, intranasal hydromorphone hydrochloride 1 and 2 micrograms were evaluated for tolerability and safety in 24 healthy volunteers (5). Repeated intranasal administration of hydromorphone every 6 hours was well tolerated and adverse effects were generally mild to moderate and as expected for this drug.

Comparative studies

Hydromorphone 0.015 mg/kg intravenously has been compared with intravenous morphine 0.1 mg/kg in 198 patients attending the emergency department for acute severe pain (6). There was adequate pain relief in the two groups and the adverse effects were similar, except for pruritus, which was not experienced in those who received hydromorphone.

Systematic reviews

The efficacy of hydromorphone in 43 studies in acute and chronic pain published between 1966 and 2000 has been reviewed (7). There was little difference between hydromorphone and other opioids in terms of analgesic efficacy, adverse effects, and patient preference. However, most of the studies were of poor quality, low statistical power, and non-standardized, making it difficult to determine real differences between interventions.

Organs and Systems

Neuromuscular function

Long-term and high-dose opioid administration can cause *myoclonus*. However, there have been two reports of myoclonus after low doses of short-term hydromorphone.

- A 75-year-old man with multiple system atrophy fractured a hip and was given intravenous hydromorphone 1 mg over 20 minutes (8). His developed severe generalized myoclonus and rigidity and reduced consciousness. His symptoms were relieved by naloxone.

- A 55-year-old man with non-obstructive hypertrophic cardiomyopathy was given intravenous hydromorphone + ondansetron for pain and vomiting (9). On day 1 he was given a total of 4 mg hydromorphone, which was increased on day 2. He developed myoclonus involving the head, neck, and limbs. The contractions continued even when ondansetron was withdrawn, but the symptoms abated within hours of hydromorphone withdrawal.

These cases suggest that opioid-induced myoclonus can occur after low doses of opioids given for short periods and that neuroexcitotoxicity can be caused by opioids themselves rather than by accumulation of metabolites. Multiple system atrophy in the first case is likely to have increased the individual's susceptibility to opioid-induced myoclonus.

Sensory systems

In a retrospective review in a specialized otological center, 12 patients were identified with rapidly progressive hearing loss and a concurrent history of hydrocodone overuse with paracetamol (10). These patients were helped by cochlear implantation.

Drug Administration

Drug administration route

The use of intrathecal hydromorphone in the management of chronic non-malignant pain has been described (1).

References

1. Yeh HM, Chen LK, Shyu MK, Lin CJ, Sun WZ, Wang MJ, Mok MS, Tsai SK. The addition of morphine prolongs fentanyl-bupivacaine spinal analgesia for the relief of labor pain. Anesth Analg 2001;92(3):665–8.
2. Moriarty M, McDonald CJ, Miller AJ. A randomised cross-over comparison of controlled release hydromorphone tablets with controlled release morphine tablets in patients with cancer pain. J Clin Res 1999;2:1–8.
3. Miller MG, McCarthy N, O'Boyle CA, Kearney M. Continuous subcutaneous infusion of morphine vs. hydromorphone: a controlled trial. J Pain Symptom Manage 1999;18(1):9–16.
4. Goodarzi M. Comparison of epidural morphine, hydromorphone and fentanyl for postoperative pain control in children undergoing orthopaedic surgery. Paediatr Anaesth 1999;9(5):419–22.
5. Rudy AC, Coda BA, Archer SM, Wermeling DP. A multiple close phase 1 study of intranasal hydromorphone hydrochloride in healthy volunteers. Anesth Analg 2004;99:1379–86.
6. Chang AK, Bijur PE, Meyer RH, Kenny MK, Solorzano C, Gallagher EJ. Safety and efficacy of hydromorphone as an analgesic alternative to morphine in acute pain: a randomized clinical trial. Ann Emerg Med 2006;48(2):164–72.
7. Quigley C. A systematic review of hyrdomorphone in acute and chronic pain. J Pain Symptom Manage 2003;25:169–78.

8. Hofmann A, Tangri N, Lafontaine A-L, Postuma RB. Myoclonus as an acute complication of low-dose hydromorphone in multiple system atrophy. J Neurol Neurosurg Psychiatry 2006;77:994–5.
9. Patel S, Roshan VR, Lee KC, Cheung RJ. A myoclonic reaction with low dose hydromorphone. Ann Pharmacother 2006;40(11):2068–70.
10. Friedman RA, House JW, Luxford WM, Gherini S, Mills D. Profound hearing loss associated with hydrocodone/acetaminophen abuse. Am J Otol 2000;21(2):188–91.

References

1. Janiri L, Mannelli P, Pirrongelli C, Lo Monaco M, Tempesta E. Lephetamine abuse and dependence: clinical effects and withdrawal syndrome. Br J Addict 1989;84(1):89–95.
2. Mannelli P, Janiri L, De Marinis M, Tempesta E. Lefetamine: new abuse of an old drug—clinical evaluation of opioid activity. Drug Alcohol Depend 1989;24(2):95–101.
3. De Angelis L. Lefetamine hydrochloride. Drugs Today 1983;19:82.

Ketobemidone

General Information

Ketobemidone is an opioid receptor agonist, with pharmacokinetics and potency similar to morphine. Combined with the antispasmodic drug, N,N-dimethyl-3,3-diphenyl-1-methylallylamine chloride, ketobemidone is often used in Scandinavia.

In a study of postoperative pain relief, ketobemidone equalled morphine and pethidine with respect to efficacy of analgesia and adverse effects, such as shivering, nausea, and vomiting (SEDA-16, 81).

Organs and Systems

Respiratory

Early cough in 40 of 121 patients given ketobemidone for postoperative analgesia has been reported. Four of the patients found it severe and distressing. The lower frequency of cough in patients previously exposed to ketobemidone in the premedication may reflect tachyphylaxis (SEDA-17, 81).

Lefetamine

General Information

Lefetamine is an opioid receptor partial agonist, which combines the actions of amphetamines with opioid-like effects. It was a drug of abuse in Japan in the 1950s and later also in Italy (1). In 10 opiate addicts, lefetamine relieved acute opiate withdrawal symptoms and did not precipitate withdrawal symptoms in stable addicts (2).

During ordinary use sedation, tiredness, gastrointestinal disturbances, headache, sweating, and flushing have been observed with lefetamine (3).

Levacetylmethadol (levo-α-acetylmethadol, LAAM)

General Information

Levacetylmethadol, an MOR receptor agonist, is a congener of methadone with a longer half-life. It was developed as an alternative to methadone for the management of opioid withdrawal (1). However, it was removed from the market throughout the European Union in 2001 because of reports of prolongation of the QT interval and 10 cases of life-threatening cardiac disorders, including torsade de pointes (2). At the same time, in the USA the Food and Drug Administration (FDA) required the addition of a black box warning to the drug labelling in 2001. Electrocardiographic monitoring before and periodically during therapy was made compulsory and there was a consequent marked drop in the use of the drug. The manufacturers therefore decided to stop marketing the drug in the USA in 2003, although it is still approved by the FDA (3,4).

During levacetylmethadol induction there is a delay in opioid activity as the long-acting metabolites are formed; withdrawal medication must therefore usually be given during the first 96 hours of treatment to suppress opioid withdrawal symptoms adequately and prevent self-administration by the patient.

Comparative studies

In a randomized comparison of levacetylmethadol three doses per week and daily methadone maintenance therapy for 26 weeks in 315 patients those taking levacetylmethadol were less likely to test positive for opioid use, both during treatment and at 26-weeks (40% versus 60%) (5). There were no adverse events, cardiological or otherwise.

In a randomized, crossover trial 62 patients stable on methadone received levacetylmethadol on alternate days and daily methadone for 3 months each, followed by a further 6 months, during which they were free to choose between the two drugs (6). Levacetylmethadol maintenance was associated with a lower rate of heroin use than methadone maintenance. Most of the subjects preferred levacetylmethadol rather than methadone (27 versus 12). Their main reasons were that it produced less withdrawal, fewer adverse effects, and less craving for heroin, and entailed fewer pick-up days.

Systematic reviews

In a meta-analysis of 18 comparisons of levacetylmethadol and methadone, (15 randomized controlled trials and three controlled prospective studies), three were excluded because of lack of data on retention, heroin use, or mortality (7). Opioid withdrawal (11 studies, 1473 participants) was better with levacetylmethadol (RR = 1.36; 95% CI = 1.07, 1.73; NNT = 8). Non-abstinence was less with levacetylmethadol (5 studies, 983 participants; RR = 0.81, 95% CI = 0.72, 0.91; NNT = 9). In 10 studies (1441 participants) there were six deaths from a range of causes, five in participants assigned to levacetylmethadol (RR = 2.28; 95% CI = 0.59, 8.9).

Organs and Systems

Cardiovascular

Reports of torsade de pointes attributed to levacetylmethadol started to appear in 2001 (8).

- A patient whose heroin dependency was being managed with high doses of levacetylmethadol developed a prolonged QT interval and polymorphic QRS complexes on consistent with torsade de pointes. The patient was taking other drugs that prolong the QT interval (fluoxetine and intravenous cocaine), and others that inhibit the P450 enzymes that metabolize levacetylmethadol and its active metabolite (fluoxetine, cocaine and marijuana).

In a 17-week randomized, controlled trial of equally effective doses of levacetylmethadol, methadone, and buprenorphine in 154 opioid-addicted subjects with normal baseline QT_c intervals, 12-lead electrocardiograms were collected at baseline and every 4 weeks (9). Levacetylmethadol and methadone were significantly more likely to prolong the QT_c interval to over 470 or 490 milliseconds or to increase the QT_c interval from baseline by more than 60 milliseconds.

In a randomized, controlled comparison of levacetylmethadol with racemic methadone in 53 patients, electrocardiographic recordings were made during a run-in period when all the patients were taking methadone and 24 weeks after randomization to methadone or levacetylmethadol (10). After 24 weeks, the patients taking levacetylmethadol had a significant increase in QT interval (409 versus 418 msec), whereas there were no significant changes in patients taking methadone.

The effects of levacetylmethadol on the cloned human cardiac potassium channels HERG (human ether-a-go-go-related gene), KvLQT1/mink, and Kv4.3 have been studied using patch clamp electrophysiology (11). Levacetylmethadol inhibited HERG channel currents in a voltage-dependent manner, with an IC_{50} value of 3 μmol/l. Its major active metabolite, noracetylmethadol, inhibited HERG channels with an estimated IC_{50} of 12 μmol/l. Levacetylmethadol had little or no effect on Kv4.3 or KvLQT1/minK channel currents at concentrations up to 10 μmol/l. The authors concluded that the prodysrhythmic effects of levacetylmethadol are due to blockade of the HERG cardiac potassium channel and suggested that noracetylmethadol might be a safer alternative in the treatment of opioid addiction.

Respiratory

Five occasional opioid users took once weekly doses of either placebo, levacetylmethadol, or methadone (15, 30, or 60 mg/70 kg) and then received naloxone (1.0 mg/70 kg intramuscularly) 24, 72, and 144 hours after agonist exposure (12). Three subjects were withdrawn because of greater than anticipated and clinically relevant respiratory depression after levacetylmethadol 60 mg. Naloxone did not fully reverse the pupillary constriction produced by levacetylmethadol 60 mg.

Psychiatric

Of 28 heroin addicts who received levacetylmethadol instead of methadone over 6 weeks in an out-patient detoxification programme, nine withdrew early and crossed over to methadone (13). They had a variety of complaints, ranging from anxiety about possibly receiving an experimental drug to withdrawal symptoms and dysphoria, which they had not experienced while taking methadone.

Endocrine

In nine male heroin addicts who took levacetylmethadol for 5 months there was no change in plasma concentrations of testosterone and luteinizing hormone 72 hours after a dose and during 2 weeks after abrupt withdrawal of levacetylmethadol (14).

Liver

In 959 opioid addicts treated with levacetylmethadol for up to 36 months, there was no evidence of long-term hepatic toxicity or tumor formation as studied by liver function studies and liver–spleen imaging (15).

Long-Term Effects

Genotoxicity

Levacetylmethadol was genotoxic in the ad-3 forward-mutation test in *Neurospora crassa* and weakly mutagenic in the mouse lymphoma forward-mutation assay (16). Analysis of the ad-3 mutants showed that they were the result of a parasexual phenomenon rather than forward mutation. There was one confirmed translocation carrier in the heritable translocation study, which by conservative interpretation might imply some germ-cell risk associated with exposure to LAAM.

Drug Administration

Drug dosage regimens

In a randomized, double-blind trial, 180male and female opioid-dependent patients were assigned to one of three doses of levacetylmethadol. Low-dose induction (25 mg) was constant from the start of treatment (n = 62), medium-dose induction (50 mg) lasted 7 days (n = 59), and high-dose induction (100 mg) lasted 17 days (n = 59) (17). There were more agonist-related adverse effects in the high-dose group. All those who dropped out because of levacetylmethadol-related adverse effects were in the high-dose group (5 women and 3 men). The adverse effects reported included anorexia, feeling overmedicated, sedated/drowsy, nausea, and vomiting. The 31 patients who dropped out averaged 14 days in treatment and had a mean dose of 53 mg. One woman in the high-dose group died during the second week of treatment and toxicological analysis showed the presence of multiple drugs, although the concentrations of levacetylmethadol, norlevacetylmethadol, and dinorlevacetylmethadol were within the expected ranges.

Drug-Drug Interactions

Levacetylmethadol is metabolized by CYP3A4-mediated N-demethylation and CYP3A-mediated inactivation. Its metabolites are norlevacetylmethadol and dinorlevacetylmethadol. Patients who take CYP3A4 inducers (for example. rifampicin) are susceptible to increased metabolism, reduced plasma concentrations, and withdrawal. Those taking CYP3A inhibitors (for example troleandomycin) are susceptible to reduced metabolism, increased plasma concentrations and toxicity (18). However, unexpectedly, CYP3A induction reduced and inhibition increased the concentrations and clinical effects of the active metabolites, which suggests that there is a CYP3A-mediated metabolic pathway that leads to inactive metabolites, which predominates over CYP3A-dependent conversion to the active metabolites.

Antiretroviral drugs

In a study in 40 patients taking methadone or levacetylmethadol, delavirdine significantly reduced methadone clearance and increased methadone half-life, with a resultant increase in AUC of 19% and C_{min} of 29% (19). Delavirdine significantly increased the AUC of the total concentration of levacetylmethadol and its active metabolites, norlevacetylmethadol and dinorlevacetylmethadol by 43%, the C_{max} by 30%, and the C_{min} by 59% and reduced the t_{max}. There were no changes in cognitive function over the 7-day study period, measured by the Mini-Mental State Examination, no opioid withdrawal symptoms, measured by the Objective Opioid Withdrawal Scale, and no complaints of adverse symptoms. Neither methadone nor levacetylmethadol altered delavirdine concentrations.

Ketoconazole

In vivo inhibition of CYP3A by ketoconazole altered the pharmacokinetics and pharmacodynamics of levacetylmethadol 5 mg/70 kg in a single-blind, crossover, randomized study in 13 opioid-naive subjects (6 women and 7 men) (20). Co-administration of ketoconazole resulted in 3.22-fold and 5.29-fold increases in the C_{max} and AUC of levacetylmethadol. The t_{max} of norlevacetylmethadol and dinorlevacetylmethadol increased 2.43 and 11.6 times respectively, and their C_{max} values were reduced to 77 and 55%. The AUCs of norlevacetylmethadol and dinorlevacetylmethadol were increased 2.25 and 1.21 times respectively. Pupil diameter was significantly reduced by levacetylmethadol after both placebo and ketoconazole pretreatment; ketoconazole increased the t_{max} for miosis 2.92 times.

References

1. Eissenberg T, Bigelow GE, Strain EC, Walsh SL, Brooner RK, Stitzer ML, Johnson RE. Dose-related efficacy of levo-methadyl acetate for treatment of opioid dependence. JAMA 1997;277:1945–51.
2. European Medicines Agency (EMEA). Public statement on the recommendation to suspend the marketing authorisation for Orlaam (levacetylmethadol) in the European Union. 2001. http://www.emea.europa.eu/pdfs/human/press/pus/877601en.pdf.
3. Jaffe JH. Can LAAM, like Lazarus, come back from the dead? Addiction 2007;102:1342–3.
4. Guay DRP. Cardiotoxicity of oral methadone as an analgesic—recommendations for safe use. Clin Med Ther 2009;1:1073–101.
5. Longshore D, Annon J, Anglin MD, Rawson RA. Levo-alpha-acetylmethadol (LAAM) versus methadone: treatment retention and opiate use. Addiction 2005;100(8):1131–9.
6. White JM, Danz C, Kneebone J, La Vincente SF, Newcombe DA, Ali RL. Relationship between LAAM–

methadone preference and treatment outcomes. Drug Alcohol Depend 2002;66(3):295–301.

7. Clark N, Lintzeris N, Gijsbers A, Whelan G, Dunlop A, Ritter A, Ling W. LAAM maintenance vs methadone maintenance for heroin dependence. Cochrane Database Syst Rev 2002;(2):CD002210.

8. Deamer RL, Wilson DR, Clark DS, Prichard JG. Torsades de pointes associated with high dose levomethadyl acetate (ORLAAM). J Addict Dis 2001;20:7–14.

9. Wedam EF, Bigelow GE, Johnson RE, Nuzzo PA, Haigney MC. QT-interval effects of methadone, levomethadyl, and buprenorphine in a randomized trial. Arch Intern Med 2007;167(22):2469–75.

10. Wieneke H, Conrads H, Wolstein J, Breuckmann F, Gastpar M, Erbel R, Scherbaum N. Levo-alpha-acetylmethadol (LAAM) induced QTc-prolongation—results from a controlled clinical trial. Eur J Med Res 2009;14(1):7–12.

11. Kang J, Chen XL, Wang H, Rampe D. Interactions of the narcotic l-alpha-acetylmethadol with human cardiac K+ channels. Eur J Pharmacol 2003;458(1-2):25–9.

12. Eissenberg T, Stitzer ML, Bigelow GE, Buchhalter AR, Walsh SL. Relative potency of levo-alpha-acetylmethadol and methadone in humans under acute dosing conditions. J Pharmacol Exp Ther 1999;289(2):936–45.

13. Sorensen JL, Hargreaves WA, Weinberg JA. Heroin addict responses to six weeks of detoxification with LAAM. Drug Alcohol Depend 1982;9(1):79–87.

14. Mendelson JH, Ellingboe J, Judson BA, Goldstein A. Plasma testosterone and luteinizing hormone levels during levo-alpha-acetylmethadol maintenance and withdrawal. Clin Pharmacol Ther 1984;35(4):545–7.

15. Tennant FS Jr, Rawson RA, Pumphrey E, Seecof R. Clinical experiences with 959 opioid-dependent patients treated with levo-alpha-acetylmethadol (LAAM). J Subst Abuse Treat 1986;3(3):195–202.

16. Brusick D, Matheson D, Jagannath D, Braude M, Brockman H, Hung C. Genetic screening of compounds used in drug abuse treatment. III. LAAM. Drug Chem Toxicol 1981;4(1):19–35.

17. Jones HE, Strain EC, Bigelow GE, Walsh SL, Stitzer ML, Eissenberg T, Johnson RE. Induction with levomethadyl acetate: safety and efficacy. Arch Gen Psychiatry 1998;55(8):729–36.

18. Kharasch ED, Whittington D, Hoffer C, Krudys K, Craig K, Vicini P, Sheffels P, Lalovic B. Paradoxical role of cytochrome P4503A in the bioactivation and clinical effects of levo-α-acetylmethadol: importance of clinical investigations to validate in vitro drug metabolism studies. Clin Pharmacokinet 2005;44(7):731–51.

19. McCance-Katz EF, Rainey PM, Smith P, Morse GD, Friedland G, Boyarsky B, Gourevitch M, Jatlow P. Drug interactions between opioids and antiretroviral medications: interaction between methadone, LAAM, and delavirdine. Am J Addict 2006;15(1):23–34.

20. Moody DE, Walsh SL, Rollins DE, Neff JA, Huang W. Ketoconazole, a cytochrome P450 3A4 inhibitor, markedly increases concentrations of levo-acetyl-alpha-methadol in opioid-naive individuals. Clin Pharmacol Ther 2004;76(2):154–66.

Meptazinol

General Information

Meptazinol is a centrally-acting opioid analgesic with an affinity for MOR(OP$_3$, μ) receptors (1). Common adverse effects are typically opioid in character; vomiting seems to be a problem and abdominal pain can occur in some patients. Euphoria and hallucinations are uncommon.

Organs and Systems

Respiratory

Clinically and statistically significant respiratory depression can occur within 1 minute of the start of a meptazinol infusion 1 mg/kg. Respiratory depression was less than after pethidine 1 mg/kg, but more than after 0.5 mg/kg (2). Other studies have confirmed these effects. In 49 patients who received either PCA with meptazinol (20 mg bolus, maximum 120 mg/hour) or morphine (2 mg bolus, maximum 12 mg/hour) after major orthopedic surgery, there was a tendency for more patients receiving meptazinol to have obstructive apnea and central apnea.

Drug Administration

Drug administration route

Prophylactic administration of intramuscular prochlorperazine 12.5 mg did not prevent meptazinol-induced emesis; in fact, the incidence of vomiting with this combination was twice the expected frequency; cyclizine was an effective antiemetic (3). Prolonged vomiting has followed the use of intravenous meptazinol 50 mg (4).

References

1. Holmes B, Ward A. Meptazinol. A review of its pharmacodynamic and pharmacokinetic properties and therapeutic efficacy. Drugs 1985;30(4):285–312.

2. Kay NH, Allen MC, Bullingham RE, Baldwin D, McQuay RJ, Moore HA, Price RK, Sear JW. Influence of meptazinol on metabolic and hormonal responses following major surgery. A comparison with morphine. Anaesthesia 1985;40(3):223–8.

3. Westconbe RE, Price RKJ. Meptazinol in the casualty department: a comparison against morphine. Curr Ther Res 1985;37:969.

4. Barnes PR, Williams CB, Davies RL, Childs CS, Hedges A, Graham D. The use of intravenous meptazinol for analgesia in colonoscopy. Postgrad Med J 1985;61(713):221–4.

Methadone

General Information

Methadone is an MOR(OP$_3$, μ) receptor agonist with pharmacological properties similar to those of morphine. It is an attractive alternative OP$_3$ opioid receptor analgesic, because of its lack of neuroactive metabolites, a clearance that is independent of renal function, good oral systemic availability, a longer half-life with fewer doses needed per day, and extremely low cost. It is mainly metabolized by CYP3A4.

Drug studies

Pain relief
Experience with methadone in cancer pain is limited. Its long half-life tends to produce delayed toxicity, especially in older patients, but in chronic renal insufficiency and stable liver disease methadone is safe, unlike morphine.

Methadone is being used increasingly for treating chronic pain and cancer pain (neuropathic and somatic) that is non-responsive or has lost responsiveness because of tolerance to high-dose μ opioid receptor agonists (for example morphine, fentanyl, oxycodone) (1). There are several protocols for converting from morphine to methadone and for initiating and stabilizing maintenance dosages.

In a prospective uncontrolled study, 45 patients with advanced cancer were given 0.1% methadone 2–3 times a day as required (2). Ten had nausea and vomiting, none had drowsiness, and 17 had constipation. In another study, nine of 29 patients in a tertiary level cancer pain clinic could not take opioid analgesics owing to uncomfortable adverse effects: nausea, vomiting, and drowsiness in four and other adverse effects in five (3). The average daily dose of methadone at the end of the titration phase (range 1–79 days) was 208 (range 15–1520) mg. Twenty patients had methadone toxicity during titration. In 12 patients mild drowsiness was a problem, six patients had nausea, and one patient each had confusion and severe headaches. In a third cross-sectional prospective study, 24 patients with advanced cancer pain were rapidly switched form oral morphine to oral methadone using a fixed ratio of 1:5 (4). There was a significant reduction in pain intensity and adverse effects intensity within 24 hours of substitution, although five patients required alternative treatments.

In a prospective, open, uncontrolled study 50 patients with a history of cancer taking daily oral morphine (90–800 mg) but with uncontrolled pain with or without severe opioid adverse effects were switched to oral 8-hourly methadone in a dose ratio of 1:4 for patients receiving less than 90 mg of morphine daily, 1:8 for patients receiving 90–300 mg daily, and 1:12 for patients receiving more than 300 mg daily (5). Methadone was effective in 80% of the patients when comparing analgesic response with opioid-related adverse effects. Ten patients were switched because of uncontrolled pain, eight because of moderate or severe adverse effects in the presence of acceptable pain control, and 32 because of uncontrolled pain with morphine-related adverse effects. In the last 32 there were significant improvements in pain intensity, nausea and vomiting, constipation, and drowsiness, with a 20% increase in methadone dose over and above the recommended starting dose.

In a prospective uncontrolled study of intrathecal methadone in 24 patients with a history of intractable chronic non-malignant pain, methadone was a better analgesic than morphine, with improved quality of life and no adverse effects in 13 patients (6). The final rates of methadone infusion were 20% higher than the preceding morphine rates.

In 60 patients who enrolled in a methadone programme tailored to meet the needs of the patient with pain, the most common causes of pain were: low back pain (n = 12), neuralgia (n = 8), idiopathic (n = 8), and musculoskeletal (n = 7) (7). The oral opioids most commonly misused were ketobemidone and codeine. Patients took methadone 100 (range 10–350) mg/day for a mean duration of 34 months. Meticulous dose titration was required to achieve optimal dosages for adequate pain control. Most of the patients (75%) achieved good pain relief, and 50% reported a good quality of life. The incidence of adverse effects was significant: 40–60% had sedation, anergia, increased weight, sweating, and sexual dysfunction. There was dyspnea in 30% and edema in 19%. Other serious events include: pulmonary embolism (n = 4), cerebral thromboembolic events (n = 2), and torsade de pointes (n = 1). Although methadone can provide effective pain control in such patients, careful monitoring for adverse effects is necessary. In-patient treatment with a multiprofessional approach is recommended.

Opioid dependence
An analysis of the balance of benefit to harm during methadone maintenance treatment for diamorphine dependence has shown lower mortality and morbidity with improvement in quality of life (8). The risks of methadone treatment include an increased risk of opiate overdosage during induction into treatment, and adverse effects of methadone in some patients. However, with careful management the benefits of prescribing methadone outweigh the risks.

The validity of self-reported opiate and cocaine use has been studied in 175 veterans enrolled in a methadone treatment program (9). Urine analysis showed higher rates of substance use than the patients themselves reported. The authors encouraged the development of more objective measures for assessing patient progress and the performance of the methadone program.

Restless legs syndrome

Methadone 16 mg/day was effective in 29 patients with restless legs syndrome that had not responded to dopamine receptor agonists (10). Most (n = 17) were still taking methadone at follow-up and reported a 75% reduction in symptoms. Of 27 patients, 17 reported at least one adverse event while taking methadone, including constipation (n = 11), fatigue (n = 2), and insomnia, sedation, rash, reduced libido, confusion, and hypertension (one each). Five patients stopped treatment because of adverse events.

Mood disturbances

The combinations of methadone + carbamazepine and buprenorphine + carbamazepine have been compared in the treatment of mood disturbances during the detoxification of 26 patients with co-morbidities (11). The buprenorphine combination had more of an effect. More patients taking the methadone combination dropped out of the study (58 versus 36%). However, both regimens were considered safe and without unexpected adverse effects. The results of this study need to be interpreted with caution because of the small sample size.

Organs and Systems

Cardiovascular

A variety of complications following parenteral self-administration of oral methadone were noted, including regional thrombosis, often associated with shock and multiorgan failure (12).

The use of methadone/dihydrocodeine has been linked to an acute myocardial infarction (13).

- A 22-year-old man with a 6-year history of intravenous heroin use was maintained on methadone 60 mg/day and dihydrocodeine 0.5 g/day. He had an extensive anterior myocardial infarction as a result of occlusion of the left anterior descending coronary artery, which was reopened by percutaneous transluminal coronary angioplasty.

This case presents circumstantial evidence only, and the association was probably not a true one.

QT interval prolongation and torsade de pointes can occur after intravenous or high-dose methadone. There is a linear relation between QT interval prolongation and the dose of methadone (14). It is prudent to avoid concomitant use of other drugs that prolong the QT interval. This is of significance in individuals infected with HIV, who might have not only viral cardiomyopathies or autonomic neuropathies but also be taking macrolides, quinolones, clindamycin, trimethoprim, fluconazole, pentamidine, and other drugs that are closely associated with torsade de pointes and other cardiac dysrhythmias (15). Several case have been described in which methadone in a dose of more than 300 mg/day was associated with an increased risk of cardiac dysrhythmias, especially if prescribed with other drugs that inhibit CYP3A4 (16).

QT interval prolongation has been studied retrospectively in 167 patients taking methadone maintenance and 80 controls (17). There was QT_c prolongation in 16% of the methadone group compared to none of the controls. Torsade de pointes also occurred in six patients the methadone group. The risk of QT_c prolongation correlated positively with methadone dosage, hepatic impairment, potassium depletion, and the use of inhibitors of CYP3A4. However, it was also found at low doses of methadone, even as low as 30 mg/day, raising the question of cardiac monitoring, even for patients not believed to be at risk.

In 78 patients taking methadone QT_c prolongation was associated with higher doses of methadone (18). The (R)-enantiomer was found to be responsible.

The association between methadone treatment and QT_c interval prolongation, QRS widening, and bradycardia has been explored in 160 patients with at least a 1-year history of opioid misuse (19). The QT_c interval increased significantly from baseline at 6 months (n = 149) and 12 months (n = 108). The QRS duration and heart rate did not change. There were no cases of torsade de pointes, cardiac dysrhythmias, syncope, or sudden death. There was a positive correlation between methadone concentration and the QT_c interval.

Methadone has been associated with cardiac dysrhythmias (20).

- A 6-month old infant who received methadone 0.1 mg/kg on three occasions to counteract opiate withdrawal symptoms following treatment with fentanyl for sedation during mechanical ventilation developed a sinus bradycardia, which responded to tactile stimulation. Methadone was withdrawn and 10 hours later sinus rhythm returned.

There have been another 11 cases showing a direct link between QT interval prolongation and oral methadone maintenance treatment at doses of 14–360 micrograms/day (21,22). QT interval prolongation can lead to arrhythmias such as torsade de pointes, especially when high doses of methadone are given intravenously and associated with concomitant use of cocaine and/or medications that inhibit the hepatic clearance of methadone (for example antidepressants and antihistamines).

Methadone-related torsade de pointes has been reported in a patient with chronic bone and vaso-occlusive pain due to sickle cell disease (23).

- A 40-year-old man with sickle cell disease, hypertension, congestive heart failure, and a past history of cocaine and marihuana abuse, was given a large dose of oral methadone 560 mg/day, following hydromorphone 170 mg intravenously and by PCA for progressive back and leg pain. On day 2, he developed asymptomatic bradycardia and QT_c prolongation (454–522 msec). On day 3, he developed profuse sweating and non-sustained polymorphous ventricular tachycardia consistent with torsade de pointes. He had hypokalemia and hypocalcemia. Echocardiography showed normal bilateral ventricular function, mild pulmonary hypertension, and trivial four-valve regurgitation. Methadone was replaced by modified-release morphine and a continuous epidural infusion of hydromorphone + bupivacaine. Daily electrocardiography showed a heart rate of 50–69/minute, a QT_c interval of 375–463 msec and no further dysrhythmias.

This case highlights the importance of very careful monitoring, especially when prescribing such large doses of methadone. The effects of methadone on cardiac function are potentially fatal.

Another report has highlighted the potential risks of combining prodysrhythmic drugs on cardiovascular function (24).

- A 39-year-old was had recurrent episodes of sinus tachycardia at 115/minute, with no other abnormalities. He was taking methadone 120 mg/day for opioid dependency and doxepin 100 mg/day for anxiety, and was given metoprolol 50 mg/day. During the next few weeks he developed episodes of recurrent syncope with sinus bradycardia (47/minute) and prolongation of the QT interval (542 ms). The QT interval and heart rate normalized after withdrawal of all treatment.

In this case it is likely that the myocardial repolarization potential of methadone and doxepin may have been influenced or triggered by bradycardia induced by metoprolol. This shows the importance of cardiac monitoring in patients receiving combination therapy with potential adverse cardiac effects. Patients with co-morbidities are at high risk.

There has been a report of five cases of episodes of syncope and an electrocardiogram showing ventricular tachydysrhythmias with prolonged QT intervals and episodes of torsade de pointes; all the patients were taking high doses of methadone (270–660 mg/day) with no previous history of cardiac disease (25). Torsade de pointes also occurred when high doses (3 mg/kg) of the long-acting methadone derivative, levomethadyl acetate HCl (LAAM), were given to a 41-year-old woman with a history of heroin dependence (26). She was also taking fluoxetine and intravenous cocaine, which can prolong the QT interval, and fluoxetine and marijuana, which inhibit the activity of CYP3A4, which is responsible for the metabolism of LAAM and its active metabolite.

In a retrospective case study in methadone maintenance treatment programs in the USA and a pain management center in Canada, 17 methadone-treated patients developed torsade de pointes during 5 years (27). The dose of methadone was 65–1000 mg/day. Six patients had had an increase in methadone dose in the months just before the onset of torsade de pointes. One patient had taken nelfinavir, a potent inhibitor of CYP3A4, begun just before the development of torsade de pointes. The above two risk factors (increased drug dosage and drug interactions) are important when eliciting the cause of torsade de pointes in patients taking methadone.

Respiratory

In 10 stable methadone-maintained patients (50–120 mg/day) and nine healthy subjects assessed using polysomnography, the methadone-maintained patients had more abnormalities of sleep architecture, with a higher prevalence of central sleep apnea (28). Methadone depresses respiration, probably by acting on μ opioid receptors in the ventral surface of the medulla and possibly on other receptor sites in the lung and spinal cord. All the patients taking methadone also used benzodiazepines and cannabis, which may have influenced the above findings.

Nervous system

Reversible choreic movements of the upper limbs, torso, and speech mechanism developed in a 25-year-old man taking methadone as a heroin substitute (29).

Spastic paraparesis has been attributed to methadone (30).

- A 43-year-old patient taking methadone for pain secondary to a squamous cell carcinoma of the larynx, which progressed despite surgery and radiation therapy, developed reversible spastic paraparesis with prominent extensor spasms in the legs while receiving an infusion of high-dose intravenous methadone 100 mg/hour. On the second day, after 5 hours on 100 mg/hour, he noted weakness in both legs, uncontrollable trembling, bilateral tinnitus, and generalized anxiety. Dexamethasone 6 mg intravenously every 6 hours was started and the methadone was reduced to 60 mg/hour. Dexamethasone was withdrawn when an MRI scan confirmed the absence of metastases in the thoracic and cervical spinal cord. Because of persistent spastic paraparesis, methadone was switched to levorphanol 40 mg/hour intravenously, and there was complete resolution of symptoms 24 hours later.

Methadone can cause movement disorders characterized by tremor, choreiform movements, and a gait abnormality (31).

- A 41-year-old woman with a 15-year history of chronic neuropathic pain was given methadone 5 mg tds and then qds. One month after the final increase she had bilateral tremor spreading from her arm up to her neck, followed by choreiform movements of the torso, a broad-based gait, and staccato-like speech. She was switched from methadone to modified-release oxycodone 60 mg/day, with complete resolution after 3 weeks.

Toxic encephalopathy has been reported after accidental ingestion of methadone in a 3-year-old boy, who developed coma and acute obstructive hydrocephalus due to massive cerebellar edema and supratentorial lesions (32).

Psychological, psychiatric

In a randomized, double-blind, crossover study of 20 patients on a stable methadone regimen, a single dose of methadone caused episodic memory deficits (33). This was significant in patients with a history of diamorphine use averaging more than 10 years duration. Such deficits can be avoided by giving methadone in divided doses.

Psychomotor and cognitive performance has been studied in 18 opioid-dependent methadone maintenance patients and 21 non-substance abusers (34). Abstinence from heroin and cocaine for the previous 24 hours was verified by urine testing. The methadone maintenance patients had a wide range of impaired functions, including psychomotor speed, working memory, decision making, and metamemory. There was also possible impairment of inhibitory mechanisms. In the areas of time estimation, conceptual flexibility, and long-term memory, the groups performed similarly.

Endocrine

Prolonged therapy with methadone causes increases in serum thyroid hormone-binding globulin, triiodothyronine, and thyroxine, as well as albumin, globulin, and prolactin, and these must be monitored (SEDA-15, 71) (SEDA-17, 81).

Metabolism

Accidental use of methadone caused acute non-ketotic hyperglycemia in three young children, all of whom developed central nervous system depression or coma (35). The first child had a methadone blood concentration of 0.36 mg/l and the second had taken 20 mg of methadone.

Fluid balance

Methadone-induced edema soon after start of treatment is recognized, and distal leg edema after 7 years of treatment has been described (SEDA-17, 81).

Gastrointestinal

In a randomized, double-blind, placebo-controlled trial of the efficacy of intravenous methylnaltrexone (0.015–0.095 mg/kg) in treating chronic methadone-induced constipation in 22 patients attending a methadone maintenance program (oral methadone linctus 30–100 mg/day), methylnaltrexone induced immediate bowel movements in all subjects (36). There were no opioid withdrawal symptoms or significant adverse effects.

Skin

Subcutaneous administration can cause skin erythema and induration at the injection site (SEDA-16, 81).

Parenteral self-administration of oral methadone can cause cellulitis, abscess formation, and necrosis of the skin and deeper tissues (12).

Musculoskeletal

In 92 patients taking methadone maintenance treatment there was low bone mineral density in about 83%; the risk was positively correlated with lower weight and heavy alcohol use and was more common in men (37).

Immunologic

The immunotoxic potential of methadone has been studied in rats that were given methadone 20–40 mg/kg/day for 6 weeks (38). The higher dose increased serum IgG concentrations but had no effect on functioning of the immune system. This suggests that methadone is not associated with immunotoxicity, even at dosages that were very high compared with usual clinical doses. The author advised caution in extrapolating animal data to humans.

Infection risk

Anterior uveitis and lens abscess due to infection with *Candida albicans* has been attributed to methadone by injection (39).

- A 31-year-old woman who injected methadone mixed with orange juice, developed a painful red eye and impaired vision. *Candida albicans* was isolated from the anterior chamber and lens.

This patient probably developed the infection from spread of blood-borne fungal spores from the mixture of orange juice and methadone.

Death

There has been a cross-sectional survey of 238 patients in New South Wales who died during a methadone maintenance program in a 5-year period (40). There were 50 deaths (21%) in the first week of methadone maintenance treatment, 88% of which were drug-related. These findings reinforce the importance of a thorough drug and alcohol assessment of people seeking methadone maintenance treatment, cautious prescribing of methadone, frequent clinical review of patients, and tolerance to methadone during stabilization.

In a retrospective study of cases from the Jefferson County Coroner/Medical Examiners Office, Alabama, USA between January 1982 and December 2000 there were 101 deaths in patients in whom methadone was detected in the blood (41). Methadone was the sole intoxicant in 15 cases, with a mean concentration of 0.27 µg/ml. A benzodiazepine was the most frequently detected co-intoxicant in 60 of the 101 cases and the only co-intoxicant in another 30 cases. In 26 cases methadone had been taken with a range of non-benzodiazepine substances, including antidepressants, antipsychotic drugs, antiepileptic drugs, and cocaine. The high incidence of benzodiazepine + methadone related deaths can be explained by synergistic respiratory depression. Higher concentrations of methadone can occur with chronic abuse of methadone plus benzodiazepines, because over time benzodiazepines inhibit the hepatic enzymes that metabolize methadone. This might explain why the mean methadone concentration in the 30 deaths attributed to methadone plus a benzodiazepine was only 0.6 µg/ml.

There have been two retrospective studies of drug-related deaths, investigating the role of methadone. In one, there were 605 deaths from 1989 to 2000 registered in Cologne (42) and in the other 398 deaths from 1997 to 2001 registered in Bonn (43). The most common agents in drug-related deaths were combinations of substances, especially opioids (morphine or heroin), benzodiazepines, antidepressants, and alcohol. Methadone played a minor role, and most methadone-related deaths occurred in individuals who were not participating in a methadone maintenance programme. The rate of methadone-related deaths has risen, but not significantly when other variables are taken into account. Similar conclusions were reached in another extensive retrospective study of all drug-related deaths between 1992 and 2002 in Minnesota (44).

Long-Term Effects

Drug tolerance

Several methadone studies have focused on opioid-dependent or opioid-abusing subjects. For example, six opioid-dependent individuals maintained on methadone subsequently developed cancer and continued to use methadone, but in a higher dose as an analgesic (30,45). The first five were partly refractory to the analgesic effects of opioids other than methadone, but all six achieved adequate analgesia without sedation or respiratory depression from aggressive upward intravenous methadone titration using an infusion of 100 mg/hour. Methadone was given in divided doses every 6–12 hours rather than once daily, as is customary in maintenance therapy for opioid dependence. The reasons for increasing the methadone dosage and frequency of administration are cross-tolerance to other opioids and the presence in methadone-maintained individuals of hyperalgesia to pain (a low pain tolerance to pain detection ratio) (46). These issues are also relevant to determining whether other drugs are more effective than morphine in managing acute pain in these patients.

In 37 children who had been given a continuous intravenous opioid infusion for at least 120 hours, tolerance was managed by weaning off oral methadone (47). The children were randomized to two groups. One group was weaned off over 5 days (n = 16) and the other over 10 days (n = 21). There were minimal differences between the groups.

Drug withdrawal

Four patients with methadone withdrawal psychosis have been described (SEDA-20, 79).

The neonatal abstinence syndrome occurs in 30–80% of infants whose mothers have taken opiates during pregnancy. The incidence is higher in those whose mothers have a history of opioid dependence and are taking methadone maintenance than in those who are taking methadone for chronic pain (48). The methadone blood concentration may be a useful predictor of the likelihood of severe withdrawal requiring treatment, but clinical assessment by a standardized scoring system is still required to determine the need to treat the neonatal abstinence syndrome (49).

Second-Generation Effects

Pregnancy

Methadone is extensively used in opioid withdrawal and maintenance programs (see Drug tolerance in this monograph), and has been safely used for this purpose in pregnancy, with only mild effects on the offspring (50). However, fetal exposure to methadone in utero can cause a neonatal abstinence syndrome after delivery.

The outcomes in 100 chronic opiate-dependent pregnant women who received levomethadone substitution treatment have been reported (51). The average gestational age at delivery was 38 weeks and the mean birth weight was 2869 g. The rate of premature labor was 19% and the risk of premature delivery 11%. There were withdrawal symptoms in 74% of the neonates at a mean of 39 hours and all responded well to levomethadone.

In a randomized controlled trial in 18 pregnant women in the second trimesters, a change from short-acting morphine to methadone or buprenorphine was explored (52). The transition was accomplished without any adverse events in mother or fetus and with minimal withdrawal discomfort.

Fetotoxicity

A newborn girl born of an HIV-positive mother who took antiretroviral drugs and methadone during pregnancy developed a methadone abstinence syndrome at day 7 (53). She was HIV-negative and was treated symptomatically for 15 days with chlorpromazine. The platelet count was $1049 \times 10^9/l$ on day 17 and fell progressively to $290 \times 10^9/l$ at 8 weeks. The authors suggested that the thrombocytosis had been secondary to intrauterine methadone exposure.

In 42 methadone-maintained women methadone had profound effects on fetal neurobehavioral functioning, implying a disruption of or threat to fetal neural development (54). At peak concentrations, the fetuses had slower heart rates, less heart rate variability, fewer heart rate accelerations, reduced duration of movements, reduced motor activity, and a lower degree of coupling between fetal movement and fetal heart rate. The long-term effects of such daily changes in the fetus are not known. There were very few effects on maternal physiology.

The effect of chronic maternal methadone use on intrapartum fetal heart rate has been investigated in 56 mothers using methadone, median dose 70 mg/day, and 51 controls (pregnant women attending the general obstetric clinic) (55). Fetuses who were exposed to methadone had lower fetal heart rate scores, with less marked variability, a lower proportion of accelerations, and a lower baseline. More troublesome fetal heart rate decelerations were also observed in exposed fetuses during the second stage of labor. These findings were not thought to be compatible with hypoxia or acidosis and did not affect outcomes in the neonates.

Lactation

- A 3.8-kg infant girl had irritability recurrent episodes of apnea requiring endotracheal intubation (56). The mother had taken methadone and Vicodin® (hydrocodone + paracetamol) before breastfeeding. The infant's urine drug screen was positive for opioids and she improved with naloxone.

Susceptibility Factors

From a literature search and subsequent analysis of data on the relation between methadone prescribing and mortality, it was concluded that (57):

(a) 69% of deaths attributed to methadone occurred in subjects who had not previously received methadone;
(b) 51% of deaths attributed to methadone occurred during the dose-stabilizing period of methadone maintenance treatment;
(c) the dose of illicit methadone exceeded that prescribed for methadone maintenance therapy;
(d) deaths were attributed to discharge from prison and immediate intravenous injection of methadone in people who had lost their tolerance to high doses of methadone when incarcerated.

Subsequent advice related to the above identifiable susceptibility factors included:

(a) restriction of take-home prescriptions with daily supervised consumption of methadone in pharmacy premises;
(b) meticulous evaluation of substance abuse history;
(c) slowing down of increases and tolerance testing during the stabilization period of methadone maintenance; enhanced psychosocial assistance during the first months out of prison;
(d) use of naloxone as an adjunct to methadone syrup.

Drug Administration

Drug dosage regimens

The role of opioid rotation in cancer pain management has been described, highlighting the limitations of equianalgesic tablets and the need for monitoring and individualization of dose. This is particularly important when methadone is used as the opioid for conversion. The authors referred to a greater than expected potency of methadone, with excessive sedation and opioid-related adverse effects, if the switch is done on a one-to-one basis. They suggested that the calculated equianalgesic dose of methadone should be reduced by 75–90% and the dose then titrated upwards if necessary (58,59).

As methadone is being increasingly used for analgesia in chronic pain, investigators are looking at how to make conversion from other opioids to methadone pain-free and effective in a short period of time without producing toxicity. In a prospective study 10 consecutive patients with cancer taking oral morphine successfully converted to methadone using a fixed ratio of 5:1. There were significant improvements in pain intensity and adverse effects over an average of 1-2 days, because methadone rapidly achieved a stable concentration in the first 2 days of conversion as morphine was rapidly withdrawn (60).

In a similar study methadone in 1/12 of the total daily dose of morphine, up to a maximum of 30 mg/day, achieved good pain control 7 days after conversion (61).

Drug administration route

Methadone has been used for intrathecal administration. Although this route can provide prolonged analgesia, the adverse effects have been reported to be unacceptable (SEDA-16, 81).

Of 90 patients undergoing abdominal or lower limb surgery randomly assigned double-blind to two groups, 60 received racemic methadone in initial doses of 3–6 mg followed by 6–12 mg by continuous infusion over 24 hours, and 30 received repeated boluses of 3–6 mg every 8 hours (62). In both groups the highest visual analogue score occurred 2 hours after surgery. From then on the pain diminished gradually and significantly at each recording. Opioid-related adverse effects were not different between the two groups, except for miosis, which was significantly more common in the bolus group. The results suggested that both epidural methadone protocols used in this study provide effective and safe postoperative analgesia. However, the infusion method should be preferred, as the doses of methadone can be reduced after the first day of treatment.

Drug–Drug Interactions

Antiretroviral drugs

Methadone is often used for opioid replacement therapy in intravenous drug abusers. The incidence of HIV infection is significantly higher in this population than in the general public, and interactions with drugs used for the treatment of AIDS are therefore important.

Methadone is predominantly metabolized by CYP3A4. Antiretroviral therapy with a non-nucleoside reverse transcriptase inhibitor (for example efavirenz, abacavir, and nevirapine) and/or a protease inhibitor (for example amprenavir) will induce the metabolism of methadone. This therapeutic combination is becoming increasingly common in HIV-positive substance misusers. Two studies have explicitly shown a significant reduction of methadone concentration by 28–87%. In the first study, 11 patients taking methadone maintenance therapy were given efavirenz and had a mean increase in methadone dosage requirement of 22% (63). In the second study, five methadone-maintained opioid-dependent individuals were given a combination of abacavir and amprenavir; the methadone concentration fell to 35% of the original concentration within 14 days (64).

In a prospective study of 54 patients taking antiretroviral drugs who also took methadone and a further 154 patients who did not take methadone there were similar clinical, virological, and immunological outcomes after 12 months (65). These results support the usefulness of methadone in the management of intravenous drug users with HIV infection.

Ritonavir, indinavir, saquinavir

In an in vitro study of the effects of the HIV-1 protease inhibitors, ritonavir, indinavir, and saquinavir, which are metabolized by the liver CYP3A4, all three protease inhibitors inhibited methadone demethylation and buprenorphine dealkylation in rank order of potency ritonavir > indinavir > saquinavir (66). Clinical studies are required to establish the further relevance of these observations.

Ropinavir + ritonavir

In 20 HIV-infected patients starting therapy with ropinavir + ritonavir while taking part in a methadone maintenance programme, there were no opioid withdrawal symptoms over 28 days (67).

Zidovudine

The metabolism of the antiviral nucleoside zidovudine to the inactive glucuronide form in vitro was inhibited by methadone (68). The concentration of methadone required for 50% inhibition was over 8 μg/ml, a supratherapeutic concentration, thus raising questions about the clinical significance of the effect. However, in eight recently detoxified heroin addicts, acute methadone treatment increased the AUC of oral zidovudine by 41% and of intravenous zidovudine by 19%, following the start of oral methadone (50 mg/day) (69). These effects resulted primarily from inhibition of zidovudine glucuronidation, but also from reduced renal clearance of zidovudine, and methadone concentrations remained in the target range throughout. It is recommended that increased toxicity surveillance, and possibly reduction in zidovudine dose, are indicated when the two drugs are co-administered.

Cimetidine

Cimetidine increases the effects of methadone, probably by inhibition of methadone metabolism (70).

Clusiaceae (St John's wort)

Methadone is a substrate of both CYP3A4 and P glycoprotein. Caution should be taken when patients on methadone maintenance treatment take St John's wort, which induces CYP3A4 and P glycoprotein. Four patients taking both methadone and St John's wort had a median reduction in methadone concentration of 47%; two also had opioid withdrawal symptoms (71).

Diazepam

The concomitant use of diazepam with methadone in individuals with substance misuse problems is common. The effects of single doses of diazepam 10 and 20 mg in patients stable on either methadone or buprenorphine did not result in changes in physiological parameters, but the interaction produced changes in subjective effects and psychomotor performance (72). More methadone-treated patients given diazepam than those given placebo experienced euphoria, drug liking, and strength of drug effects. Similarly, more patients had worse psychomotor performance, reflected in measures of reaction time, cancellation time, and digit symbol substitution task. The effects peaked at 1–2 hours after dosing. The extent of impairment in reaction time (324 milliseconds versus 274 milliseconds) suggests risks in the performance of tasks such as driving or operating machinery.

Enzyme inducers

Enzyme-inducing drugs, such as carbamazepine, phenobarbital, phenytoin, and rifampicin, enhance the metabolism of methadone, leading to lower serum methadone concentrations (73).

Fluconazole

In a randomized, double-blind, placebo-controlled trial, oral fluconazole increased the serum methadone AUC by 35% (74). Although renal clearance was not significantly affected, mean serum methadone peak and trough concentrations rose significantly, while renal clearance was not significantly altered.

Grapefruit juice

In an unblinded study, the effect of grapefruit juice on the steady-state pharmacokinetics of methadone was evaluated for 5 days in eight patients taking methadone (mean dose 107, range 63–150, micrograms/day) (75). Grapefruit juice was associated with a modest increase in methadone availability that would not normally enhance its adverse effects. Only 6–8 glasses of grapefruit juice per day can lead to inhibition of hepatic CYP3A. Further studies need to be done to clarify to what extent intestinal and/or hepatic metabolic activities play a part in methadone availability and the subsequent risk of overdosage in individuals taking high maintenance doses of methadone. Since the therapeutic effect of methadone is mainly mediated by the R-enantiomer, monitoring plasma concentrations of R-methadone could be recommended, but it is an imprecise indicator of therapeutic activity (76).

Phenytoin

Phenytoin enhances the metabolism of methadone (74).

Rifampicin

Enzyme-inducing drugs, such as rifampicin, enhance the metabolism of methadone, leading to lower serum methadone concentrations (74). This interaction is thought to have caused acute methadone withdrawal symptoms in two patients with AIDS (SEDA-16, 81).

In a randomized four-way crossover study in healthy subjects, the effects of intravenous and oral methadone were measured after pre-treatment with rifampicin (hepatic/intestinal CYP3A induction), troleandomycin (hepatic/intestinal CYP3A inhibition), grapefruit juice (selective intestinal CYP3A inhibition), or nothing (77). Intestinal and hepatic CYP3A activity affected methadone N-demethylation only slightly and had no significant effects on methadone concentrations, clearance, or clinical effects. There was a significant correlation between methadone oral availability and intestinal availability, since only rifampicin altered oral methadone availability. This suggests a role of intestinal metabolism and in first-pass extraction of methadone. This study used a single, relatively low dose of methadone (15 micrograms) rather than a therapeutic dose at steady state (80–100 micrograms/day), when tolerance will be taken into consideration.

Selective serotonin re-uptake inhibitors

Fluvoxamine

Fluvoxamine increases the effects of methadone, probably by inhibition of methadone metabolism (78).

Fluvoxamine inhibits CYP3A4 and has been used to achieve higher and more effective serum methadone concentrations in three patients (79). Fluvoxamine should not be withdrawn suddenly in such cases, since it can precipitate an acute opioid withdrawal syndrome. Equally, the introduction of fluvoxamine should be slow and gradual, giving time to monitor for potential oversedation or intoxication with methadone.

Paroxetine

Paroxetine 20 mg/day, a selective CYP2D6 inhibitor, was given for 12 days to 10 patients on methadone maintenance (80). Eight were genotyped as CYP2D6 homozygous extensive metabolizers and two as poor metabolizers. Paroxetine increased the steady-state concentrations of *R*-methadone and *S*-methadone, especially in the extensive metabolizers.

Use of methadone in opioid withdrawal

A widely used technique for opioid detoxification, pioneered by Isbell and Vogel (81), involves the substitution of methadone for the illicit opioid, followed by a gradual reduction in the amount of methadone taken.

Methadone maintenance treatment was established in 1964 in New York City by Vincent Dole and Marie Nyswander. In the initial studies, subjects who were heavily addicted to heroin were evaluated and stabilized on daily methadone doses as inpatients before transfer to an outpatient clinic for continued treatment. With further experience, it was feasible to drop the inpatient phase (82).

Methadone is used to substitute for a variety of opioid drugs. It is well absorbed after oral ingestion, with peak blood concentrations after about 4 hours. Steady-state concentrations are reached after about 5 days. By virtue of its long duration of action (the half-life with regular dosing is about 22 hours), methadone suppresses opioid withdrawal symptoms for 24–36 hours. In the early stages of treatment patients may report problems such as drowsiness, insomnia, nausea, euphoria, difficulty in micturition, and excessive sweating. With the exception of chronic constipation and excessive sweating, these effects do not generally persist.

Methadone maintenance treatment is considered to be a medically safe treatment with relatively few and minimal adverse effects. However, the danger of serious adverse effects and death with the increasing use of methadone as maintenance therapy in drug addicts has been highlighted. It must be emphasized that a daily maintenance dose of 50–100 mg is toxic in a non-tolerant adult and as little as 10 mg can be fatal in a child. There is an increasing number of reports of the deaths of children of mothers on maintenance therapy from inadvertent ingestion.

British studies have shown that, using methadone, about 80% of inpatients, but only 17% of outpatients, were successfully withdrawn (83,84). However, the technique is not without problems, one being that the methadone reduces but does not eliminate withdrawal symptoms. The withdrawal response has been described as being akin to a mild case of influenza, objectively mild but subjectively severe (85). The fear of withdrawal symptoms expressed by those dependent on drugs should not be underestimated: these factors are associated with the subsequent severity of withdrawal symptoms, and they are more closely related to symptom severity than drug dosage (86). Methadone substitution can result in a protracted withdrawal response, with patients still experiencing significantly more symptoms than controls 2 weeks after withdrawal (87).

In a study of methadone withdrawal, patients who were withdrawn over 10 days had a withdrawal syndrome that began to increase in severity from day 3, with peak severity of symptoms on day 13; in those who were withdrawn over 21 days, symptoms began to increase about day 10 with a peak on day 20 and abated thereafter, although some patients did not recover fully until 40 days after starting withdrawal (88). Thus, the duration of the withdrawal syndrome is much the same for both treatments in terms of symptom severity. It is possible that an exponential rather than linear reduction in dosage may improve the withdrawal response. These results may be of clinical significance, in that patients may feel it important that they recover from withdrawal as quickly as possible, in order to participate fully in other aspects of drug withdrawal programs. However, although there was no difference between the 10-day and 21-day programs regarding completion rates for detoxification (70 and 79% respectively), the dropout rates after detoxification were significantly different. During the 10 days after the last dose of methadone, the dropout rate in the 21-day group was 18% compared with 30% in the 10-day group. These results may also have financial implications in respect of the number of subjects who can be admitted to treatment programs.

In some treatment programs, total abstinence is not considered to be a practical objective and treatment may involve the use of drugs such as methadone as maintenance therapy with the expectation of reducing illicit drug consumption (89). Well-organized methadone maintenance treatment can reduce the intake of illicit opioids in many injecting drug users (90,91).

Outcome studies of methadone maintenance treatment have reported favorable results. High rates of patient retention, reduced criminality, and improved social rehabilitation are reported. Despite its proved effectiveness, it remains a controversial approach among substance abuse treatment providers, public officials, policy makers, the medical profession, and the public at large. Nevertheless, almost every nation with a significant narcotic addiction problem has established a methadone maintenance treatment program.

For patients entering treatment from an institution where they have been drug-free, initial daily methadone doses should be no more than 20 mg. Otherwise initial daily doses of 30–40 mg should be sufficient to obtain the necessary balance between withdrawal and narcotic symptoms. Thereafter, stabilization is achieved by gradually increasing the dose. When methadone is given in adequate oral doses (usually 60 mg/day or more), a single dose in a stabilized patient lasts 24–36 hours, without creating euphoria and sedation. Tolerance to methadone seems to remain steady, and patients can be maintained on the same dose, in some cases for more than 20 years. The methadone dose must be determined individually, owing to individual variability in pharmacokinetics and pharmacodynamics. Maintenance of appropriate methadone blood concentrations is recommended.

Tolerance to the narcotic properties of methadone develops within 4–6 weeks, but tolerance to the autonomic effects (for example constipation and sweating) develops more slowly.

The major adverse effects during treatment occur during the initial stabilization phase. In addition to constipation and sweating, the most frequently reported adverse effects are transient skin rash, weight gain, and fluid retention. Since the main metabolic pathway of methadone is CYP3A4, numerous drug interactions can be expected. Drugs that interact with methadone are listed in the table in the monograph on opioids.

References

1. Ayonrinde OT, Bridge DT. The rediscovery of methadone for cancer pain management. Med J Aust 2000;173(10):536–40.
2. Mercadante S, Casuccio A, Agnello A, Barresi L. Methadone response in advanced cancer patients with pain followed at home. J Pain Symptom Manage 1999;18(3):188–92.
3. Hagen NA, Wasylenko E. Methadone: outpatient titration and monitoring strategies in cancer patients. J Pain Symptom Manage 1999;18(5):369–75.
4. Mercadante S, Casuccio A, Calderone L. Rapid switching from morphine to methadone in cancer patients with poor response to morphine. J Clin Oncol 1999;17(10):3307–12.
5. Mercadante S, Casuccio A, Fulfaro F, Groff L, Boffi R, Villari P, Gebbia V, Ripamonti C. Switching from morphine to methadone to improve analgesia and tolerability in cancer patients: a prospective study. J Clin Oncol 2001;19(11):2898–904.
6. Mironer YE, Tollison CD. Methadone in the intrathecal treatment of chronic nonmalignant pain resistant to other neuraxial agents: the first experience. Neuromodulation 2001;4:25–31.
7. Rhodin A, Gronbladh L, Nilsson L-H, Gordh T. Methadone treatment of chronic non-malignant pain and opioid dependence. A long term follow-up. Eur J Pain 2006;10(3):271–8.
8. Bell J, Zador D. A risk-benefit analysis of methadone maintenance treatment. Drug Saf 2000;22(3):179–90.
9. Chermack ST, Roll J, Reilly M, Davis L, Kilaru U, Grabowski J. Comparison of patient self-reports and urinalysis results obtained under naturalistic methadone treatment conditions. Drug Alcohol Depend 2000;59(1):43–9.
10. Ondo WG. Methadone for refractory restless legs syndrome. Movement Disord 2005;20(3):345–8.
11. Seifert J, Metzner C, Paetzold W, Borsutzky M, Ohlmeier M, Passie T, Hauser U, Becker H, Wiese B, Emrich HM, Schneider U. Mood and affect during detoxification of opiate addicts: a comparison of buprenorphine versus methadone. Addict Biol 2005;10:157–64.
12. Nathan HJ. Narcotics and myocardial performance in patients with coronary artery disease. Can J Anaesth 1988;35(3 Pt 1):209–13.
13. Backmund M, Meyer K, Zwehl W, Nagengast O, Eichenlaub D. Myocardial Infarction associated with methadone and/or dihydrocodeine. Eur Addict Res 2001;7(1):37–9.
14. Kornick CA, Kilborn MJ, Santiago-Palma J, Schulman G, Thaler HT, Keefe DL, Katchman AN, Pezzullo JC, Ebert SN, Woosley RL, Payne R, Manfredi PL. QTc interval prolongation associated with intravenous methadone. Pain 2003;105:499–506.
15. Gil M, Sola M, Anguera I, Chapinal O, Cervantes M, Guma JR, Sequra F. QT prolongation and torsades de pointes in patients infected with human immunodeficiency virus and treated with methadone. Am J Cardiol 2003;8:995–7.
16. Walker PW, Klein D, Kasza L. High dose methadone and ventricular arrhythmia: a report of three cases. Pain 2003;103:321–4.
17. Ehret GB, Voide C, Gex-Fabry M, Chabert J, Shah D, Broers B, Piguet V, Musset T, Gaspoz J, Perrier A, Dayer P, Desmeules JA. Drug-induced long QT syndrome in injection drug users receiving methadone. High frequency in hospitalized patients and risk factors. Arch Intern Med 2006;166:1280–7.
18. Skjervold B, Bathen J, Spigset O. Methadone and the QT interval: relations to the serum concentrations of methadone and its enantiomers (R)-methadone and (S)-methadone. J Clin Psychopharmacol 2006;26(6):687–9.
19. Martell BA, Arnsten JH, Krantz MJ, Gourevitch MN. Impact of methadone treatment on cardiac repolarisation and conduction in opioid users. Am J Cardiol 2005;95(7):915–8.
20. Wheeler AD, Tobias JD. Bradycardia during methadone therapy in an infant. Pediatr Crit Care Med 2006;7(1):83–5.
21. Piquet V, Desmeules J, Enret G, Stoller R, Dayer P. QT interval prolongation in patients on methadone with concomitant drugs. J Clin Psychopharmacol 2004;24:446–8.
22. Decerf JA, Gressens B, Brohet C, Liolios A, Hantson P. Can methadone prolong the QT interval? Intensive Care Med 2004;30:1690–1.
23. Porter BO, Coyn PJ, Smith WR. Methadone-related torsade de pointes in a sickle cell patient treated for chronic pain. Am J Hematol 2005;78(4):316–7.
24. Rademacher S, Dietz R, Haverkamp W. QT prolongation and syncope with methadone, doxepin, and a beta-blocker. Ann Pharmacother 2005;39(10):1762–3.
25. Hays H, Woodroffe MA. High dosing methadone and a possible relationship to serious cardia arrhythmias. Pain Res Manag 2001;6(2):64.
26. Deamer RL, Wilson DR, Clark DS, Prichard JG. Torsades de pointes associated with high dose levomethadyl acetate (ORLAAM). J Addict Dis 2001;20(4):7–14.
27. Krantz MJ, Lewkowiez L, Hays H, Woodroffe MA, Robertson AD, Mehler PS. Torsade de pointes associated with very-high-dose methadone. Ann Intern Med 2002;137(6):501–4.
28. Teichtahl H, Prodromidis A, Miller B, Cherry G, Kronborg I. Sleep-disordered breathing in stable methadone programme patients: a pilot study. Addiction 2001;96(3):395–403.
29. Wasserman S, Yahr MD. Choreic movements induced by the use of methadone. Arch Neurol 1980;37(11):727–8.
30. Manfredi PL, Gonzales GR, Payne R. Reversible spastic paraparesis induced by high-dose intravenous methadone. J Pain 2001;2(1):77–9.
31. Clark JD, Elliott J. A case of a methadone-induced movement disorder. Clin J Pain 2001;17(4):375–7.
32. Anselmo M, Campos Rainho A, de Carme Vale M, Estrada J, Valente R, Correia M, Viera JP, Barata D. Methadone intoxication in a child: toxic encephalopathy? J Child Neurol 2006;21(7):618–20.
33. Curran HV, Kleckham J, Bearn J, Strang J, Wanigaratne S. Effects of methadone on cognition, mood and craving in

detoxifying opiate addicts: a dose-response study. Psychopharmacology (Berl) 2001;154(2):153–60.

34. Mintzer MZ, Stitzer ML. Cognitive impairment in methadone maintenance patients. Drug Alcohol Depend 2002;67(1):41–51.

35. Tiras S, Haas V, Chevret L, Decobert M, Buisine A, Devictor D, Durand P, Tissières P. Nonketotic hyperglycemic coma in toddlers after unintentional methadone ingestion. Ann Emerg Med 2006;48:448–51.

36. Yuan CS, Foss JF, O'Connor M, Osinski J, Karrison T, Moss J, Roizen MF. Methylnaltrexone for reversal of constipation due to chronic methadone use: a randomized controlled trial. JAMA 2000;283(3):367–72.

37. Kim TW, Alford DP, Malabanan A, Holick MF, Samet JH. Low bone density in patients receiving methadone maintenance treatment. Drug Alcohol Depend 2006;85(3):258–62.

38. Ryle PR. Justification for routine screening of pharmaceutical products in immune function tests: a review of the recommendations of Putman et al. (2003). Fundam Clin Pharmacol 2005;19:317–22.

39. Trpin S, Gracner T, Pahor D, Gracner B. Phacoemulsification in isolated endogenous Candida albicans anterior uveitis with lens abscess in an intravenous methadone user. J Cataract Refract Surg 2006;32(9):1581–3.

40. Zador D, Sunjic S. Deaths in methadone maintenance treatment in New South Wales, Australia 1990–1995. Addiction 2000;95(1):77–84.

41. Mikolaenko I, Robinson CA Jr, Davis GG. A review of methadone deaths in Jefferson County, Alabama. Am J Forensic Med Pathol 2002;23(3):299–304.

42. Grab H, Behnsen S, Kimont HG, Staak M, Käferstein H. Methadone and its role in drug-related fatalities in Cologne 1989-2000. Forensic Sci Int 2003;132:195–200.

43. Musshoff F, Lachenmeier DW, Medea B. Methadone substitution: medicological problems in Germany. Forensic Sci Int 2003;133:118–24.

44. Gagajewski A, Apple FS. Methadone related deaths in Hennepin County, Minnesota: 1992-2002. J Forensic Sci 2003;48:668–71.

45. Manfredi PL, Gonzales GR, Cheville AL, Kornick C, Payne R. Methadone analgesia in cancer pain patients on chronic methadone maintenance therapy. J Pain Symptom Manage 2001;21(2):169–74.

46. Doverty M, Somogyi AA, White JM, Bochner F, Beare CH, Menelaou A, Ling W. Methadone maintenance patients are cross-tolerant to the antinociceptive effects of morphine. Pain 2001;93(2):155–63.

47. Berens RJ, Meyer MT, Mikhailov TA, Colpaert KD, Czarnecki ML, Ghanayem NS, Hoffman GM, Soetenga DJ, Nelson TJ, Weisman SJ. A prospective evaluation of opioid weaning in opioid-dependent pediatric critical care patients. Anesth Analg 2006;102:1045–50.

48. Sharpe C, Kuschel C. Outcomes of infants born to mothers receiving methadone for pain management in pregnancy. Arch Dis Child Fetal Neonatal Ed 2004;89:F33–F36.

49. Kuschel CA, Austerberry L, Cornwell M, Couch R, Rowley RSH. Can methadone concentrations predict the severity of withdrawal in infants at risk of neonatal abstinence syndrome? Arch Dis Child Fetal Neonatal Ed 2004;89:F390–F393.

50. Pinto F, Torrioli MG, Casella G, Tempesta E, Fundaro C. Sleep in babies born to chronically heroin addicted mothers. A follow up study. Drug Alcohol Depend 1988;21(1):43–7.

51. Kastner R, Hartl K, Lieber A, Hahlweg BC, Knobbe A, Grubert T. Substitutionsbehandlung von opiatabhängigen schwangeren'—Analyse der Behandlungverläufe an der 1. Ufk München. [Maintenance therapy in opiate-dependent pregnant patients—analysis of the course of therapy at the clinic of the University of Munich.] Geburtschilfe Frauenheilkd 2002;62:32–6.

52. Jones HE, Johnson RE, Jasinski DR, Milio L. Randomized controlled study transitioning opioid-dependent pregnant women from short-acting morphine to buprenorphine or methadone. Drug Alcohol Depend 2005;78:33–8.

53. Garcia-Algar O, Brichs LF, Garcia ES, Fabrega DM, Torne EE, Sierra AM. Methadone and neonatal thrombocytosis. Pediatr Hematol Oncol 2002;19(3):193–5.

54. Jannson LM, DiPietro J, Elko A. Fetal response to maternal methadone administration. Am J Obstet Gynecol 2005;193(3):611–7.

55. Ramirez-Cacho WA, Flores S, Schrader RM, McKay J, Rayburn WF. Effect of chronic maternal methadone therapy on intrapartum fetal heart rate patterns. J Soc Gynecol Investig 2006;13:108–11.

56. Meyer D, Tobias JD. Adverse effects following the inadvertent administration of opioids to infants and children. Clin Pediatr (Phila) 2005;44(6):499–503.

57. Vormfelde SV, Poser W. Death attributed to methadone. Pharmacopsychiatry 2001;34(6):217–22.

58. Indelicato RA, Portenoy RK. Opioid rotation in the management of refractory cancer pain. J Clin Oncol 2002;20(1):348–52.

59. Watanabe S, Tarumi Y, Oneschuk D, Lawlor P. Opioid rotation to methadone: proceed with caution. J Clin Oncol 2002;20(9):2409–10.

60. Mercadante S, Bianche M, Villari P, Ferera P, Casuccia A, Fulfera F, Gebbie V. Opioid plasma concentration during switching from morphine to methadone: preliminary data. Support Care Cancer 2003;11:326–31.

61. Tse DMW, Sham MMK, Ng DKH, Ma HM. An ad libitum schedule for conversion of morphine to methadone in advanced cancer patients: an open uncontrolled prospective study in a Chinese population. Palliative Med 2003;17:206–11.

62. Prieto-Alvarez P, Tello-Galindo I, Cuenca-Pena J, Rull-Bartomeu M, Gomar-Sancho C. Continuous epidural infusion of racemic methadone results in effective postoperative analgesia and low plasma concentrations. Can J Anaesth 2002;49(1):25–31.

63. Bart PA, Rizzardi PG, Gallant S, Golay KP, Baumann P, Pantaleo G, Eap CB. Methadone blood concentrations are decreased by the administration of abacavir plus amprenavir. Ther Drug Monit 2001;23(5):553–5.

64. Clarke SM, Mulcahy FM, Tjia J, Reynolds HE, Gibbons SE, Barry MG, Back DJ. The pharmacokinetics of methadone in HIV-positive patients receiving the non-nucleoside reverse transcriptase inhibitor efavirenz. Br J Clin Pharmacol 2001;51(3):213–7.

65. Moreno A, Perez-Elias MJ, Casado JL, Munoz V, Antela A, Dronda F, Navas E, Moreno S. Long-term outcomes of protease inhibitor-based therapy in antiretroviral treatment-naive HIV-infected injection drug users on methadone maintenance programmes. AIDS 2001;15(8):1068–70.

66. Iribarne C, Berthou F, Carlhant D, Dreano Y, Picart D, Lohezic F, Riche C. Inhibition of methadone and buprenorphine N-dealkylations by three HIV-1 protease inhibitors. Drug Metab Dispos 1998;26(3):257–60.

67. Stevens RC, Rapaport S, Marolodo-Connelly L, Patterson JB, Bertz R. Lack of methadone dose alterations or withdrawal symptoms during therapy with lopinavir/ritonavir J AIDS 2003;33:650–1.

68. Trapnell CB, Klecker RW, Jamis-Dow C, Collins JM. Glucuronidation of 3′-azido-3′-deoxythymidine (zidovudine) by human liver microsomes: relevance to clinical

pharmacokinetic interactions with atovaquone, fluconazole, methadone, and valproic acid. Antimicrob Agents Chemother 1998;42(7):1592–6.

69. McCance-Katz EF, Rainey PM, Jatlow P, Friedland G. Methadone effects on zidovudine disposition (AIDS Clinical Trials Group 262). J Acquir Immune Defic Syndr Hum Retrovirol 1998;18(5):435–43.

70. Dawson GW, Vestal RE. Cimetidine inhibits the in vitro N-demethylation of methadone. Res Commun Chem Pathol Pharmacol 1984;46(2):301–4.

71. Elich-Höchli D, Oppliger R, Powell Golay K, Bowmann P, Eap CB. Methadone maintenance treatment and St John's wort. Pharmacopsychiatry 2003;36:35–7.

72. Lintzeris N, Mitchell TB, Bond A, Nestor L, Strang J. Interactions on mixing diazepam with methadone or buprenorphine in maintenance patients. J Clin Psychopharmacol 2006;26(3):274–83.

73. Finelli PF. Letter: Phenytoin and methadone tolerance. N Engl J Med 1976;294(4):227.

74. Cobb MN, Desai J, Brown LS Jr, Zannikos PN, Rainey PM. The effect of fluconazole on the clinical pharmacokinetics of methadone. Clin Pharmacol Ther 1998;63(6):655–62.

75. Benmerbarek M, Devaud C, Gex-Fabry M, Powell Golay K, Brogli C, Baumann P, Gravier B, Eap C B. Effects of grapefruit juice on the pharmacokinetics of the enantiomers of methadone. Clin Pharmacol Ther 2004;76:55–63.

76. Esteban J, de la Cruz Pellin M, Gimeno C, Barril J, Mora E, Gimenez J, Vilenova E. Detection of clinical interactions between methadone and anti-retroviral compounds using an enantioselective capillary electrophoresis for methadone analysis. Toxicol Lett 2004;151:243–9.

77. Kharasch ED, Hoffer C, Whittington D, Sheffels P. Role of hepatic and intestinal cytochrome P450 3A and 2B6 in the metabolism, disposition and mioitic effects of methadone. Clin Pharmacol Ther 2004;76:250–69.

78. Iribarne C, Picart D, Dreano Y, Berthou F. In vitro interactions between fluoxetine or fluvoxamine and methadone or buprenorphine. Fundam Clin Pharmacol 1998;12(2):194–9.

79. De Maria PA, Patlear AA, Vassos K. Fluvoxamine as an adjunct to promote methadone dose optimization. Addict Disord Treatment 2003;2:85–9.

80. Begre S, von Bardeleben U, Ladewig D, Jaquet-Rochat S, Cosendai-Savary L, Golay KP, Kosel M, Baumann P, Eap CB. Paroxetine increases steady-state concentrations of (R)-methadone in CYP2D6 extensive but not poor metabolizers. J Clin Psychopharmacol 2002;22(2):211–5.

81. Isbell H, Vogel VH, Chapman KW. Present status of narcotic addiction with particular reference to medical indications and comparative addiction liability of the newer and older analgesic drugs. JAMA 1948;138:1019.

82. Dole VP, Nyswander M. A medical treatment for diacetyl-morphine (heroin) addiction. A clinical trial with methadone hydrochloride. JAMA 1965;193:646–50.

83. Glossop M, Johns A, Green L. Opiate withdrawal: in-patient vs out-patient programmes and preferred vs random assignment to treatment. BMJ (Clin Res Ed) 1986;293:103.

84. Gossop M, Green L, Phillips G, Bradley B. What happens to opiate addicts immediately after treatment: a prospective follow up study. BMJ (Clin Res Ed) 1987;294(6584):1377–80.

85. Kleber HD. Detoxification from narcotics. In: Lowinson L, Ruiz P, editors. Substance Abuse. Baltimore: Williams and Wilkins, 1981:317.

86. Phillips GT, Gossop M, Bradley B. The influence of psychological factors on the opiate withdrawal syndrome. Br J Psychiatry 1986;149:235–8.

87. Gossop M, Bradley B, Phillips GT. An investigation of withdrawal symptoms shown by opiate addicts during and subsequent to a 21-day in-patient methadone detoxification procedure. Addict Behav 1987;12(1):1–6.

88. Gossop M, Griffiths P, Bradley B, Strang J. Opiate withdrawal symptoms in response to 10-day and 21-day methadone withdrawal programmes. Br J Psychiatry 1989;154:360–3.

89. Newman RG, Whitehill WB. Double-blind comparison of methadone and placebo maintenance treatments of narcotic addicts in Hong Kong. Lancet 1979;2(8141):485–8.

90. Lowinson JH, Marion IJ, Joseph H, Dole VP. Methadone maintenance. In: Lowinson JH, Ruiz P, Millman RB, editors. Substance Abuse. A Comprehensive Textbook. 2nd ed.. Baltimore: Williams and Wilkins, 1992:550.

91. Ball JC, Ross A. The Effectiveness of Methadone Maintenance TreatmentNew York: Springer-Verlag;. 1991.

Methylnaltrexone

General Information

Methylnaltrexone is an opioid receptor antagonist that acts peripherally and can be of value in preventing the unwanted effects of opioids while maintaining their central analgesic effects (SEDA-21, 92; 1).

Reference

1. Yuan CS. Clinical status of methylnaltrexone, a new agent to prevent and manage opioid-induced side effects. J Support Oncol 2004;2(2):111–7.

Morphine

General Information

Morphine and its two glucuronides may have neuroexcitatory effects and affinity for non-opioid receptors (glycine and/or N-methyl-D-aspartate), effects that will not be antagonized by naloxone. Furthermore, these other opioid effects may be related to the mechanism of some adverse effects, including hyperalgesia, allodynia, and myoclonus, which are increasingly being reported after high doses of morphine, but which do not seem to occur after methadone, fentanyl, sufentanil, or ketobemidone (1).

Morphine is the benchmark "step 3" opioid analgesic based on the WHO's concept of an analgesic ladder (2). Revised recommendations for the use of morphine in cancer pain have been published by the European Association for Palliative Care's Expert Working Group on Opioid Analgesics (3). In summary, oral morphine is still the opioid of first choice for moderate to severe cancer pain, every 4 hours for normal-release morphine and 12- or 24-hourly for modified-release morphine. If patients are not able to take morphine orally the preferred alternative is subcutaneous infusion, especially in patients who require continuous parenteral morphine. A small proportion of patients develop intolerable adverse effects with oral morphine, and a change to an alternative opioid (for example hydromorphone, oxycodone, methadone, transdermal fentanyl) or a change in the rate of administration should be considered. If despite optimal use of systemic opioids and non-opioids a patient still has intolerable adverse effects or inadequate analgesia, spinal (epidural or intrathecal) administration of an opioid analgesic in combination with a local anesthetic or clonidine should be considered.

In a randomized, double-blind study in 94 patients with acute renal colic, morphine had equal analgesic efficacy to pethidine and a similar adverse effects profile (4).

Morphine-6-glucuronide is the main active metabolite of morphine, and its formation accounts for the fact that the effects of morphine are increased in renal insufficiency (5,6). It is less potent than morphine and is slower in exerting its analgesic effect. However, it produces adequate and long-lasting analgesia. Its activity and adverse effects profile have been reviewed (7). It is better tolerated than morphine, causing significantly less nausea and vomiting and less depression of the hypoxic ventilator response.

Observational studies

In a prospective non-randomized comparison of epidural analgesia and intravenous morphine after major surgery in 2696 patients, epidural morphine was used in 1670 patients and intravenous morphine in 1026 patients (8). The epidural group had overall less pain both at rest and during mobilization, but also more dosage adjustment and pruritus. Those given intravenous morphine had significantly more opioid adverse effects, such as respiratory depression. Sedation and hallucinations or confusion were also significantly more common after intravenous morphine.

In 20 individuals with heroin dependency attending an addiction out-patient centre a mean dose of modified-release morphine 760 mg/day was reached over 2 weeks (9). There were no serious adverse events, including deaths or withdrawal from study. Mild to moderate events included constipation (5 episodes) and sweating (1 episode).

The incidence of adverse events associated with sedation and analgesia in 14 386 children attending a tertiary care children's hospital has been described after implementation of procedural guidelines (10). A regimen of morphine + midazolam was associated with hypoxia (5.5%), prolonged sedation (0.5%), and hypotension (0.5%). No vomiting, bradycardia, airway obstruction, or agitation was reported.

In a prospective study in 186 patients, 75% achieved adequate pain control with morphine, 20% responded to a switch to oxycodone, and 2% responded after switching to more than one alternative opioid (11). The main reasons for switching included inadequate pain control, confusion and drowsiness, nausea, and nightmares.

Comparative studies

There has been a prospective, randomized, double-blind comparison of the adverse effects of morphine (n=250)

and piritramide 1.5 mg (n=250) with a lockout period of 10 minutes both by patient-controlled analgesia and in patients undergoing abdominal orthopedic or obstetric surgery (12). On postoperative day 1 there were no significant differences in the overall incidences of vomiting (15% with morphine and 19% with piritramide) or nausea (27% versus 30%). Even though the pain scores and adverse effects profiles did not differ between the groups or between day 1 and day 4, the patients still thought that morphine was the better analgesic. The authors suggested that consumption of specific opioids during patient-controlled analgesia may not only depend on analgesic potency and requirements for analgesia but also on euphoric effects or adverse effects.

Morphine via a patient-controlled device for analgesia after cesarean section was associated with more adverse effects than oral oxycodone + paracetamol (13). Morphine caused more nausea and drowsiness 6 hours after delivery, but slightly less nausea 24 hours after delivery.

In a prospective study (14) 130 patients with acute renal colic were randomized to intravenous. morphine 5 mg followed by 5 mg at 20 minutes, intravenous ketorolac 15 mg followed by 15 mg at 20 minutes) or both. The combination regimen gave superior analgesia. Morphine was associated with more adverse effects than ketorolac alone or the combination: nausea in 16% (versus 2% and 4% respectively); vomiting 5% (0% and 2%); itching 2% (0% and 0%); and dizziness 9% (0% and 2%).

The combination of morphine 0.1 mg/kg + ketamine 0.15 mg/kg has been compared with morphine 0.1 mg/kg alone and ketamine 0.15 mg/kg alone in the management of pain after lumbar disk surgery in 68 patients (15). Postoperative analgesia was more effective with the combination regimen and the incidence of nausea and vomiting was less.

Morphine and tramadol have been compared in 40 children undergoing cardiac surgery (16). Morphine was given as an initial dose of 0.2 mg/kg followed by 0.02 mg/kg boluses as nurse-controlled analgesia on a background infusion of 0.015 mg/kg/hour. Tramadol was given as an initial dose of 2 mg/kg followed by 0.2 mg/kg boluses as nurse-controlled analgesia on a background infusion of 0.15 mg/kg/hour. Those who received tramadol recovered earlier, had earlier tracheal extubation, and were less sedated.

Epidural morphine and sufentanil have been compared in 60 patients undergoing major abdominal surgery (17). They were randomized to sufentanil 250 micrograms or morphine 10 mg, both with ropivacaine 0.2%. Those who received morphine had more adverse effects: hypotension (two versus one), pruritus (11 versus three), nausea and vomiting (11 versus one), and problems with micturition (12 versus none).

Opioids are often combined with other analgesics to reduce the need for larger doses of opioids, which is often accompanied by a reduction in adverse effects. In a study of the effect of adding ketamine and nefopam to morphine for postoperative analgesia, ketamine (n = 22) caused more intense sedation and nefopam (n = 22) more tachycardia and profuse sweating than morphine (n = 21); other adverse effects did not differ (18).

Drug combination studies

Morphine + droperidol

A morphine-sparing effect is produced when droperidol is given in combination with morphine (19). However, this combination therapy is also associated with a greater frequency of postoperative nausea and vomiting.

Morphine + gabapentin

Gabapentin and morphine are often used for neuropathic pain. In 57 patients the combination of gabapentin and morphine (20) was more effective in managing pain, than either tablet alone. At the maximum tolerated dose, the combination gave a similar frequency of adverse effects as either drug alone. However, there was an increased frequency of mouth compared with morphine alone and an increased frequency of constipation compared with gabapentin.

Morphine + ketamine

In a large observational study in more than 1000 patients of the combination of morphine + ketamine the combination was safe but was associated with frequent treatable adverse effects (21). Therapy had to be withdrawn in 72 patients because of adverse effects. The most common reasons were nausea, vivid dreams or hallucinations, and pruritus. Respiratory depression and sedation not responding to naloxone occurred in three patients (two of whom had undiagnosed renal insufficiency, resulting in reduced elimination morphine-6-glucuronide, the active metabolite of morphine). A substantial proportion experienced vivid dreams and/or hallucinations (6.2%), not unpleasant dreams (3.3%), and unpleasant dreams (0.8%). Two patients had confusion (one had brain metastases and another had a history of alcohol abuse) and one patient had an anxiety attack. Pain was still not adequately controlled in one-third of patients. Thus, although the combination therapy was overall beneficial, adverse effects were frequent. In another study intravenous ketamine 20 ng/ml or more enhanced morphine analgesia without causing intolerable adverse effects (22).

Morphine + ketorolac

In a study of the combination of ketorolac + morphine as intravenous PCA for postoperative ileus after colorectal resection, the combination resulted in 29% less morphine consumption and a reduction in the duration of recovery of bowel movement and ambulation (23). Opioid-induced adverse effects were similar with morphine and morphine + ketorolac. In another study, of pain relief after anterior cruciate ligament reconstruction, the combination of ketorolac + morphine was associated with morphine sparing and patient satisfaction was similar in the two groups (24).

Morphine + physostigmine

The addition of physostigmine to morphine postoperatively enhances opioid analgesia. In adults undergoing open lower abdominal surgery who were randomly assigned to either morphine-based patient-controlled analgesia (n = 25) or morphine-based patient-controlled analgesia + a continuous infusion of physostigmine (n = 25), those who received the combination had an enhanced analgesic response and required significantly less morphine (25). Physostigmine has antinociceptive properties, attenuates the production of proinflammatory cytokines (IL-1β) that cause pain, attenuates morphine-induced respiratory depression; antagonizes the depressant effect of morphine on the apneic threshold; reverses postoperative somnolence and loss of consciousness through enhancing cholinergic muscarinic transmission, and reduces the postoperative anticholinergic syndrome, which is characterized by agitation, restlessness, disorientation, and respiratory depression. Physostigmine increased nausea and vomiting, especially in the early postoperative period, and the authors suggest that aggressive antiemetic treatment be added to the physostigmine-morphine regimen.

Placebo-controlled studies

The effectiveness of epidural local anesthetics, morphine, or placebo in postoperative pain relief after lumbar disc and other spinal operations has been reviewed (26). The authors suggested that epidural morphine (3-5 mg) rather than intrathecal morphine at the end of surgery significantly reduces postoperative pain with no major adverse effects and should be a routine procedure. Epidural administration of glucocorticoids does not increase effectiveness when combined with epidural morphine.

In a randomized, single-blind study of the analgesic effect and safety of intrathecal morphine 20 micrograms/kg for postoperative pain control in 71 children after heart surgery, even though total intravenous morphine analgesic consumption over the mean 19 postoperative hours was significantly lower in those given morphine, it did not result in earlier extubation or earlier discharge from intensive care (27). Adverse effects were infrequent in both groups (five events with morphine versus four with placebo). This study was limited by the heterogeneous nature of the cohort studied, with wide variations in age, cardiac pathology, and surgical procedures and duration.

Managing the adverse effects of morphine

The strategies used in managing the adverse effects of oral morphine have been reassessed in another special article compiled by the Expert Working Group of the European Association of Palliative Care Network (28). Factors that predict opioid adverse effects include:

(1) *Drug-related factors* There is little evidence suggesting that any one opioid agonist has a substantially better adverse effects profile than any other.
(2) *Route-related factors* There is limited evidence to suggest differences in adverse effects associated with specific routes of systemic administration.
(3) *Patient-related factors* There is evidence to suggest that there is interindividual variability in sensitivity to opioid-related adverse effects; the variables include genetic susceptibility, the presence of co-morbidity, and age.

(4) *Dose-related factors* A dose-response relation is most evident with the CNS adverse effects of sedation, cognitive impairment, hallucinations, myoclonus, and respiratory depression, although there is still interindividual variability in dose responsiveness to these effects; nausea and vomiting are common at the start of therapy but are then unpredictable.

(5) *Starting doses and escalation* The adverse effects of morphine, especially cognitive impairment, occur transiently and abate spontaneously; there are no reports of a relation between the starting dose of morphine or dose escalation and the occurrence of nausea, vomiting, or delirium.

(6) *Drug interactions* Adverse effects of concurrent medications may be synergistic or cumulative with those associated with opioids.

The reviewers also stressed the importance of differentiating opioid-related adverse effects from other causes of co-morbidity that might mimic opioid-induced adverse effects. Examples include cerebral metastases, stroke, metabolic changes, septicemia, bowel obstruction, and iatrogenic factors (other drugs or radiotherapy).

Four different approaches to the management of opioid adverse effects were described in the review:

(1) *Dosage reduction* A reduction in the dosage of the systemic opioid is usually enough to relieve adverse effects. If dosage reduction is accompanied by loss of pain control, a non-opioid analgesic (for example an NSAID) can be added. Specific therapy, such as radiotherapy, chemotherapy, or surgery, that targets the cause of the pain can be helpful, as can a regional anesthetic or neuroablative intervention (for example celiac plexus blockade in patients with pancreatic cancer).

(2) *Symptomatic management of the adverse effects.*

(3) *Opioid rotation.*

(4) *Switching the route of administration.*

The reviewers also examined the symptomatic management of specific adverse effects and commented that most approaches are based on cumulative anecdotal evidence and that there have been few prospective evaluations of the efficacy and toxicity of these approaches over a long period of use. Polypharmacy adds to the burden of adverse effects and drug interactions.

Nausea and vomiting

The authors of two related double-blind, randomized, placebo-controlled studies of the use of dexamethasone prophylaxis for nausea and vomiting after epidural morphine for postcesarean or posthysterectomy analgesia concluded that 5 mg of dexamethasone is an effective dose (29,30). Meanwhile, ADL 8-2698, a trans-3-4-dimethyl-4 piperidine that is a novel opioid antagonist, produced improved gastrointestinal transit time (peripherally mediated opioid activity) without affecting centrally mediated opioid analgesia (31). This contrasts with naloxone or nalmefene, which tend to antagonize central opioid effects, resulting in withdrawal symptoms in up to 50% of patients when used to treat constipation.

Intravenous droperidol 1.25 mg and intravenous dexamethasone 8 mg, given at the end of cesarean section, have been compared in reducing the incidence of nausea and vomiting caused by epidural morphine 3 mg in 120 women in a randomized, double-blind, placebo-controlled study (32). The incidence of nausea and vomiting was 18% with dexamethasone, 21% with droperidol, and 51% with saline. About 11–13% of the women who were given dexamethasone or droperidol required rescue antiemetic therapy compared with 41% in the saline group. The incidence of pruritus was similar among the three groups (26–42%). Six women (16%) given droperidol reported restlessness compared with none in the other two groups.

Pruritus

The effectiveness of intravenous ondansetron in preventing intrathecal morphine-induced pruritus has been investigated in a randomized, double-blind, placebo-controlled study in 60 consecutive women undergoing cesarean section (33). All were given spinal anesthesia with bupivacaine and intrathecal morphine 0.15 mg and then randomly divided into three groups. Group 1 received intravenous saline injections as placebo, group 2 received diphenhydramine 30 mg intravenously, and group 3 received ondansetron 0.1 mg/kg intravenously. Group 3 had a significantly lower incidence of pruritus (25%) than both group 1 (85%) and group 2 (80%), with no difference in postoperative pain scores between the groups.

In another randomized, double-blind study, 140 patients undergoing cesarean section had anesthesia with epidural bupivacaine 100 mg and adrenaline to which was added morphine 2 mg and droperidol 0, 1.25, 2.5, or 5.0 mg (34). Previous evidence had suggested that intravenous droperidol reduces morphine-induced pruritus, but that the effect disappeared when the dose was increased from 2.5 mg to 5.0 mg (35). However, in this study, epidural droperidol caused a dose-dependent reduction in morphine-induced pruritus even at a dose of 5 mg.

Myoclonus

Gabapentin has been used to treat morphine-induced myoclonus in a 54-year-old patient with gallbladder cancer (36). Effective pain control was maintained with morphine 300 mg, but after 24 hours the patient developed generalized muscular movements while asleep. Gabapentin 300 mg bd produced complete resolution of symptoms after 12 hours. In another case gabapentin 600 mg/day was used to treat a 1-month history of spontaneous jerking of both wrists after an increase in the dose of morphine to 120 mg/day; the myoclonus disappeared over the next 24 hours (31,36).

Organs and Systems

Cardiovascular

Adverse cardiac effects due to morphine are rare. They comprise inappropriate heart rate responses to hypotension, rather than conduction defects. They are not especially associated with inferior myocardial infarction, as was previously thought (SED-11, 142) (37).

The hemodynamic effects of morphine have been studied in 144 ventilated neonates, who were randomly allocated to morphine or saline (38). A loading dose of morphine 100 micrograms/kg was followed by a continuous infusion at a rate of 10 micrograms/kg/hour. There were no significant differences in blood pressure or the use of volume expanders and vasopressor drugs, suggesting that recommended morphine dosages in neonates were not associated with major adverse effects. On the other hand, in 11 ventilated premature infants morphine reduced cerebral blood oxygenation and increased cerebral blood volume (39). Furthermore, it has been suggested that morphine may contribute to intraventricular hemorrhage in ventilated preterm infants (40).

Respiratory

Non-cardiogenic pulmonary edema occurred in three cancer patients, all of whom had received rapidly escalating doses of morphine over a short period (41).

Intravenous morphine 0.1 mg/kg caused mild respiratory depression in 38 neonates undergoing central line placement (42). Hypotension developed in 5% and there was a slight increase in ventilator requirements.

In another study in 22 preterm ventilated neonates, those who received morphine by infusion had poor respiratory drive and hypotension (43).

Intrathecal morphine can cause long-term respiratory depression (44).

- A 41-year-old man with chronic pain after a motorcycle accident 6 years before used regular morphine via an intrathecal drug delivery system. The dose was altered according to needs, and was receiving 4 mg/day. He complained of severe tiredness, low mood, and reduced respiratory function. He was weaned off morphine and was eventually switched to oral hydromorphone 12 mg/day. This was followed by considerable improvement in his symptoms, suggesting chronic morphine intoxication.

In 91 preterm neonates low-dose morphine was not associated with apnea, the incidence of which increased at doses above 0.03 mg/kg; increased apnea was only evident after 3 hours (45). The authors suggested that further evidence is required before morphine can be recommended preterm infants.

- A 26-year-old woman with postoperative pain after anterior cruciate ligament reconstruction and bilateral meniscal repair received four consecutive intravenous doses (total 35 mg) (46). This produced adequate pain relief, but she developed fatal respiratory depression.

Nervous system

A patient with Guillain–Barré syndrome experienced shock with morphine sulfate (47).

- A 69-year-old woman developed interscapular pain after a mild respiratory infection. Non-opioid analgesics were ineffective, so she was given modified-release morphine 10 mg. On day 4 she had rapidly progressive weakness in her legs and on day 5 she was found unconscious with no detectable blood pressure. She recovered with naloxone 0.8 intravenously. Her paralysis persisted. Nerve conduction studies confirmed slowed neurotransmission. Further investigation excluded other potential causes and Guillain–Barré syndrome was diagnosed.

The episode of unconsciousness was attributed to opioid toxicity in a patient in whom autonomic dysfunction may already have been present. It was suggested that opioid analgesics should be used with caution in patients with Guillain–Barré syndrome, because of the risk of hypotension consequent on autonomic dysfunction.

High doses of chronic morphine can cause hyperalgesia or allodynia (pain caused by a stimulus that does not normally provoke pain) (48).

- A 9-month-old girl with an inoperable and partially resected astrocytoma of the hypothalamus had morphine-induced allodynia, and became extremely distressed during routine care, such as nappy changing, feeding, and washing. The allodynia resolved after the dosage of morphine was reduced from 6950 μg/kg/hour to 280 μg/kg/hour.

Allodynia in the dermatomes close to the level of injury has been reported in a patient with spinal cord injury who was given a single relatively small dose of intrathecal morphine (49).

- A 66-year-old man with a T8 complete paraplegia after an accident 12 years before was admitted for a trial of intrathecal morphine and clonidine in an attempt to relieve his neuropathic pain, after repeated splanchnic and sympathetic blocks, transcutaneous electrical nerve stimulation, fentanyl, and other medications had produced only transient effects. He received morphine 0.5 mg, which did not relieve his pain but 2 hours later caused mechanical allodynia in a band over dermatomes T6 and T7. The allodynia was a painful sensation after light touch with clothes or sheets. He also had drowsiness, nystagmus, and severe pruritus 30 minutes after the injection. Naloxone 50 micrograms/hour relieved the pruritus but not the allodynia. Another dose of morphine 2 days later produced the same symptoms. The episodes of allodynia resolved spontaneously after about 24 hours.

Intravenous patient-controlled administration of morphine (total 56 mg in 9 hours) was associated with downbeat nystagmus in a 61-year-old man with a Grade 3 adenocarcinoma of the gastro-esophageal junction and a previous small cerebellar infarct (50). Withdrawal of the analgesia led to complete resolution of all signs and symptoms within 12 hours.

Reversible delayed posthypoxic leukoencephalopathy has been reported after morphine overdose (51).

- A 40-year-old woman took an accidental overdose of morphine 360 mg, from which she had been resuscitated for 15 minutes followed by intubation and ventilation. On day 17 she developed a non-specific headache and visual disturbance, echolalia, perseveration, and severe global cognitive impairment, especially in memory and verbal fluency. Electroencephalography showed a significant encephalopathy, with excess delta activity. T2-weighted MR images on day 22 showed diffuse subcortical and supraventricular white matter changes with sparing of the gray matter. She improved with conservative management, but at day 34 still had deficits in orientation and memory. Repeat MR imaging at 6 months showed improvement in the white matter. At 9 months she had recovered cognitive function.

Neuromuscular function

- A 7-year-old girl with L5/S1 spondylolisthesis was given a caudal injection of morphine 2.5 mg in 10 ml of saline during surgery for repeat posterior spinal fusion (52). This technique was used instead of intrathecal morphine, since the usual site of intrathecal administration was close to her spondylolisthesis. After 20 minutes she developed reduced compound muscle action potentials and vigorous electromyographic spontaneous firing. The authors suggested that the temporary loss of motor function and nerve root irritation had been caused by the caudal injection into a narrowed caudal epidural space, causing persistent pressure on the cauda equina from the volume of injectate.

Psychological, psychiatric

Hallucinations have been described after the use of morphine in various dosage forms; in one series, patients experienced adequate pain relief and no further hallucinations or nightmares when changed to oxycodone (53). Delusions and hallucinations have been reported in a patient who was also taking dosulepin (54). Restlessness, vomiting, and disorientation were described in two male patients over 60 years of age taking modified-release morphine for relief of pain in advanced cancer (55).

The impact of adverse effects on mood and quality of life were secondary outcome measures in a clinical trial in 41 patients who received morphine or gabapentin, alone or in combination (56). The most common adverse events were sedation, constipation, and dry mouth. The severity of the adverse effects did not correlate significantly with mood or quality of life, but the study sample size may have been a limiting factor.

In a double-blind, crossover, randomized, placebo-controlled study of the acute effects of immediate-release morphine on everyday cognitive functioning in 14 patients who were also taking modified-release opioids, immediate-release morphine on top of modified-release morphine produced discrete impairment of cognitive functioning (57). Both immediate and delayed memory recall were affected. Impairment in delayed recall was more pronounced. Retrograde amnesia suggested that morphine produces additional difficulties in retrieval of information. Simple tracking tasks were enhanced in the morphine group; however, more demanding tasks and set shifting were impaired. There was no effect on backwards digit span. These findings suggest that morphine produces discrete impairment that is likely to affect quality of life.

Endocrine

Morphine can cause prolactin release (58); this effect is not antagonized by naloxone.

Mouth and teeth

There is a clear association between the administration of morphine and dry mouth (59).

Gastrointestinal

Nausea and vomiting are frequent adverse effects associated with the use of PCA opioids. Droperidol and tropisetron may reduce the incidence and severity of nausea and vomiting caused by morphine (SEDA-19, 84).

In an epidemiological study of pain management in 1540 patients in a University Hospital in Thailand, the majority (80%) were satisfied with their treatment; severe nausea and vomiting were two of the main reasons for dissatisfaction (60).

In a study of intrathecal morphine 50 micrograms after postpartum bilateral tubal ligation, those who received morphine had significantly more vomiting than the controls (21 versus 3.5%) (61).

Morphine reduces the rate of transient lower esophageal sphincter relaxation in patients with reflux disease, thus reducing the number of reflux episodes; the effect was reversed by naloxone (SEDA-22, 12).

Biliary tract

Morphine can cause choledochal sphincter spasm, especially if there is a previous history of cholecystectomy (62).

- A 60-year-old man received intramuscular morphine 10 mg with scopolamine 0.4 mg as premedication and 40 minutes later complained of sharp right upper quadrant pain radiating to the back. The symptoms were identical to the gallbladder pain he had experienced in the past and for which he had had a cholecystectomy 25 years before. He had complete relief from intravenous naloxone 0.9 mg.

Urinary tract

The mechanism by which opioids cause *urinary retention* is incompletely understood. In a randomized double-blind study in 45 healthy volunteers, urodynamic evaluation was performed after the administration of sufentanil 10 or 30 micrograms or morphine 0.1 or 0.3 micrograms (63). Intrathecal opioid administration causes dose-related suppression of detrusor muscle contraction and a reduced sensation of urge. Mean times to recovery of normal lower urinary tract function were respectively 5 and 8 hours after sufentanil 10 and 30 micrograms and 14 and 20 hours after morphine 0.2 and 0.3 micrograms.

In another prospective, double-blind, placebo-controlled study, 60 patients undergoing arthroscopic knee surgery were randomized to bupivacaine 6 micrograms + morphine 50 micrograms, bupivacaine 6 micrograms + fentanyl 25 micrograms, or bupivacaine 6 micrograms + saline; the primary outcome measure was time of voiding (64). Those given bupivacaine + morphine took significantly longer to void urine (422 minutes) than the two other groups (244 and 183 respectively). The incidence of pruritus was significantly greater in those given morphine (80%) and fentanyl (65%) compared with bupivacaine only (no pruritus). The incidence of *nausea* was also significantly higher in those given morphine (35%), than in those given fentanyl (10%) or bupivacaine alone. Minidoses of intrathecal morphine are not acceptable for outpatient surgery because of adverse effects, especially a severely prolonged time to urination.

Skin

A purpuric rash has been reported in a patient taking morphine (65).

Acute generalized exanthematous pustulosis has been attributed to morphine (66).

- A 27-year-old man was given postoperative analgesia, including intravenous morphine 10 mg. He developed itching, burning erythema, and a widespread rash with non-follicular pustules, associated with fever. A few months later patch testing and a lymphocyte transformation test identified morphine as the cause of the eruption. He was generally healthy and had no family history of skin conditions.

Pruritus was common among 98 parturients undergoing elective cesarean section who received postoperative morphine 160 micrograms and fentanyl 15 micrograms; neither ondansetron nor tropisetron was effective in preventing pruritus (67).

In contrast, in a randomized study ondansetron and dolasetron were given 30 minutes before anesthesia to prevent pruritus induced by morphine both treatments were effective (68). One theory of the cause of morphine-induced pruritus is direct stimulation of 5-HT$_3$ receptors, at which ondansetron and dolasetron are antagonists. The results supported this hypothesis, because the frequency of pruritus in the first 8 hours after the operation was reduced by 48% by ondansetron and 70% by dolasetron. Pruritus was still present in a significant number of patients (34% of the ondansetron group and 20% of the dolasetron group), suggesting that several mechanisms are involved in morphine-induced pruritus. The study was methodologically sound but lacked statistical power owing to a small sample size.

Immunologic

The immunotoxic potential of morphine 25 or 50 mg/kg/day has been explored in a 6-week study in rats (69). Morphine had no effect on serum immunoglobulin concentrations, the antibody response to sheep erythrocytes, or host resistance to *Listeria monocytogenes*. However, it was associated with an increase in muscle larvae count after *T spiralis* infection. These findings suggest that morphine has a marginal effect on the immune system. However, these results cannot be extrapolated to effects in humans except with caution.

Death

In 57 039 patients with non-ST segment elevation acute coronary syndromes—the CRUSADE study (Can Rapid Risk Stratification of Unstable Angina Patients Suppress Adverse Outcomes With Early Implementation of the ACC/AHA Guidelines)—patients taking morphine had a higher risk of death (70,71). These findings were consistent even when baseline characteristics and concomitant use of nitroglycerine were accounted for.

- A 14-year-old boy with infectious mononucleosis was given intravenous morphine 10 mg for pain relief with good effect, but 2 hours later was found unresponsive, lying on his back, and not breathing (72). An autopsy showed marked bilateral tonsillar enlargement with considerable narrowing of the upper airway. The blood morphine concentration was 0.08 µg/ml.

The coroner concluded that the morphine had contributed to respiratory compromise and death.

Long-Term Effects

Drug abuse

Abuse of morphine-containing analgesics reported by emergency departments in the USA increased to 116% (2775 cases) from 1995 to 2002 (73).

Drug withdrawal

Acute opioid withdrawal syndrome apparently precipitated by naloxone following epidural morphine has been reported (74).

- A 28-year-old nulliparous woman with no history of opioid exposure underwent elective cesarean section with epidural anesthesia. On delivery she received morphine 2 mg epidurally. At 8 hours after delivery she complained of pruritus and received naloxone 0.14 mg intravenously in fractional doses. After 2 minutes she felt warm in her legs, trunk, and face. Pruritus resolved and analgesia was maintained. After 5 minutes she began to shiver in a waxing and waning pattern every 2 minutes. She was restless and agitated and had tachypnea, lacrimation, and rhinorrhea. Her symptoms resolved in 40 minutes.

Previous reports of opioid withdrawal on single exposure have been described after the administration of intramuscular morphine in healthy individuals. This case suggests that opioid dependence can occur after acute exposure to morphine by the epidural route too. An alternative explanation (75) is that the stress of labor may have led to increased endogenous opioid activity, particularly B-endorphin, and that the antagonistic effect of naloxone on the endogenous opioid system contributed to the clinical effects in this patient. Moreover, the authors pointed out that many symptoms characteristic of the classic opioid withdrawal syndrome were not present in the patient.

Second-Generation Effects

Pregnancy

In a double-blind, randomized, controlled study of analgesia in labor, the addition of morphine 150 µg to an intrathecal combination of fentanyl (25 µg) and bupivacaine (2.5 mg) significantly prolonged analgesia to more than 4 hours without increasing opioid-related adverse effects (76).

Susceptibility Factors

Genetic

Accumulation of morphine-6-glucuronide is a risk factor for opioid toxicity during morphine treatment. However, it does not occur in all patients with renal insufficiency, which is the most common reason for accumulation of morphine-6-glucuronide; this suggests that other risk factors can contribute to morphine-6-glucuronide toxicity.

- Two men, aged 87 and 65 years, both with renal insufficiency, took oral morphine 30 mg/day for pain management (77). While the 65-year-old tolerated morphine well despite a high plasma morphine-6-glucuronide concentration of 1735 nmol/l, the 87-year-old had severe sleepiness and drowsiness, even though the plasma morphine-6-glucuronide concentration was only 941 nmol/l.

The patients were screened for genetic polymorphisms in the OPRM1-gene (coding for MOR receptors), P glycoprotein, and other candidate genes that code for transporters that may play an important role in determining the central nervous system concentration of morphine or morphine-6-glucuronide. The 65-year-old patient was a homozygous carrier of the mutated G118 allele of the µ opioid receptor gene, which has previously been related to reduced glucuromorphine potency (a protector gene). In contrast, the 87-year-old patient was a homozygous carrier of the wild-type allele A118. This observation implies that a single nucleotide polymorphism, the G118 allele, has a protective effect against morphine-6-glucuronide toxicity.

UGT2B7 (UDP-glucuronosyltransferase 2B7) is the predominant enzyme responsible for the glucuronidation of morphine to M6G (morphine-6-glucuronide) and M3G (morphine-3-glucuronide). The analgesic properties of morphine are enhanced by M6G and reduced by M3G. Mutations in the UGT2B7 gene may therefore have pharmacological, toxicological, and physiological significance. A genetic polymorphism of UGT2B7 has been reported in two patients with cancer pain who had different responses to morphine (78).

- A 78-year-old man who was extremely sensitive to the adverse effects of morphine had a rare ATTGAT2C sequence and reference alleles at almost all SNPs.
- A 46-year-old woman who needed more than 2000 mg of morphine a day and still complained of mild to moderate pain had a predominant GCCAGC1G sequence.

Both genotype–phenotype studies in large groups of patients and controls and in vitro studies are needed to establish and interpret results that can have clinical relevance to varying responses to morphine.

The role of single nucleotide polymorphisms at nucleotide position 118 at exon 1 of the MOR gene in the effects of morphine has been explored in two studies. In one study patients undergoing total knee arthroplasty) were divided into three groups: A118 homozygotes (n = 74), A118 heterozygotes (n = 33), and G118 homozygotes (n = 13) (79). The G118 homozygotes required significantly more morphine for analgesic control, suggesting that this genotype confers a reduced response to morphine. There were no differences in adverse reactions in the three groups. In a second study G118 homozygotes required more morphine for adequate analgesia after total hysterectomy (80).

Age

Children

Of 44 children undergoing major genitourinary or lower abdominal surgery in a randomized, single-blind study, 24 were given morphine 0.1 mg/kg epidurally and 20 were given the same dose intravenously immediately after intubation (81). Postoperatively PCA boluses were administered to both groups. Both techniques provided sufficient pain relief. Of the children given epidural morphine, one required treatment for pruritus and seven vomited more than once, compared to none in those given intravenous morphine.

A study of PCA in children suggested that the pharmacokinetics of morphine are similar to those in adults, with the exception of young infants (82).

Neonates with reduced capacity for glucuronidation may have reduced efficacy of morphine, because of reduced renal excretion of morphine-6-glucuronide.

In a 7-year, retrospective, multicenter, observational study, 95 children aged 1–19 years with cancer pain and treated with long-acting morphine were investigated for adverse effects and age-dependent analgesic effects (83). The adverse effects most frequently reported were constipation (10 patients at the beginning of treatment, 20 patients during the course of therapy, and 3 patients at the end of data collection), followed by vomiting (five, eight, and two patients), and nausea (two, six, and three patients), especially in children aged 7 years or more. Some of the children repeatedly complained of pruritus (five, eleven, and two patients). There were no cases of respiratory depression. Oral long-acting morphine proved to be safe and effective, even in very young patients with a history of malignancy.

There have been another two studies of the analgesic effect of intrathecal morphine in children (84,85). In a prospective, double-blind study, 30 children (aged 9–19 years) scheduled for spinal fusion were randomly allocated to a single dose of saline or intrathecal morphine 2 or 5 µg/kg; after surgery, a PCA device provided access to additional intravenous morphine (84). The doses of 2 and 5 µg/kg had similar analgesic effectiveness and adverse effects profiles (nausea, vomiting, pruritus). There were no episodes of severe respiratory depression. Low-dose intrathecal morphine supplemented with PCA morphine provides better analgesia than PCA morphine alone.

In a smaller prospective, open, uncontrolled study, 12 children (3–6 years of age) were given either intermittent intrathecal morphine 5 µg/kg qds or a continuous infusion of a mixture of bupivacaine (40 µg/kg/hour) and morphine (0.6 µg/kg/hour) for intense postoperative pain after selective dorsal rhizotomy (85). The bupivacaine/morphine mixture provided better analgesia with fewer adverse effects. The incidence of pruritus was 83% with morphine compared with 33% with bupivacaine/morphine. Otherwise the adverse effects were similar.

Elderly people
Morphine, as an intravenous bolus of 2 or 3 mg every 5 minutes until pain relief or adverse effects occurred, was given to 875 patients who were under 70 years old and 175 patients who were over 70 years old in a prospective, uncontrolled, non-blinded study (86). The total dose of morphine was not significantly different between the groups. There was no significant difference in the incidence of morphine-related adverse effects, the number of sedated patients, and the number of patients in whom dose titration had to be stopped. The results only applied to the immediate and short-term postoperative periods and the patients studied had a variety of surgical procedures unrelated to age. The results suggested that intravenous morphine can be safely given to elderly patients using the same protocol that is used in younger ones. The generalizability of this study is limited because the sample size was small.

Sex

In a study of sex differences in the experience of pain in 4317 patients (54% men), the women had more postoperative pain and required a higher dosage of morphine (+11%) than men in the immediate postoperative period; these differences disappeared in elderly patients (87).

Renal disease

There was a higher incidence of adverse effects of morphine in patients with renal insufficiency who receive opioids for some time (88), and in patients with hemolytic uremic syndrome who were given ketamine with subcutaneous morphine postoperatively (89).

Patients with renal insufficiency may experience a stronger and more prolonged effect, because of reduced renal excretion of morphine-6-glucuronide.

Hepatic disease

Morphine is extensively metabolized. Its main metabolite, morphine-3-glucuronide is without analgesic effects, while morphine-6-glucuronide (also called morphine glucuronide) is supposed to be more potent than morphine. In patients with cirrhosis, morphine clearance may be reduced and the half-life prolonged, and dosages should be reduced (SEDA-22, 101).

Other features of the patient

Myoclonus is more likely in patients taking psychotropic or non-steroidal anti-inflammatory drugs as adjunct analgesia (90).

Drug Administration

Drug additives

Low-dose intrathecal morphine (0.3 mg) plus 0.5% spinal bupivacaine and patient-controlled intravenous morphine (given as a 1 mg bolus with a 5-minute lockout period) has been compared with patient-controlled intravenous morphine alone in 38 patients undergoing knee surgery in a randomized, double-blind study (91). The former combination provided effective analgesia with a low and non-significant incidence of emesis, pruritus, and respiratory depression.

Drug dosage regimens

Oral morphine is more effective after repeated rather than single doses. This is probably due to penetration into the central nervous system of morphine-6-glucuronide, the active metabolite (92).

In a dose-response study of the effects of epidural morphine after cesarean section the quality of analgesia increased with the dose of morphine to a ceiling dose of 3.75 mg (93). Adverse effects were not dose-related.

Perioperative administration of morphine is another way of enhancing its analgesic properties during the transition from total remifentanil-based anesthesia to the postoperative period, when adequate analgesia is sometimes difficult.

In a randomized study in 245 patients undergoing abdominal or urological surgery the effect of perioperative morphine was evaluated (94). Patients were given a bolus of 0.15 or 0.25 mg/kg 30 minutes before the end of surgery. The results suggested that intraoperative morphine administration did not preclude the need for more morphine in the immediate postoperative period. The 0.25 mg/kg dose was slightly more effective but caused more respiratory depression.

Low-dose and high-dose regimens of intrathecal morphine and bupivacaine have been compared after selective dorsal rhizotomy in 26 children; 11 received a continuous infusion of morphine 0.4 micrograms/kg/hour + bupivacaine 40 micrograms/kg/hour, and 15 received morphine 0.6 micrograms/kg/hour + bupivacaine 40 micrograms/kg/hour (95). Both groups received ketobemidone for breakthrough pain. The high-dose regimen was association with better pain control and seven times less ketobemidone. There were no significant differences in the adverse effects profiles of the two regimens.

Three different dosage regimens for epidural morphine have been compared in a double-blind study in women undergoing postpartum tubal ligation (96). The patients were randomized to receive epidural saline and epidural morphine 2, 3, or 4 mg after epidural anesthesia with lidocaine. Postoperatively they received oral ibuprofen every 6 hours and paracetamol 325 mg + hydrocodone

10 mg on request. Pain was better controlled by epidural morphine. Those who received morphine had opioid-related adverse effects, namely nausea, vomiting, and pruritus. Those who received morphine 4 mg required treatment for nausea/vomiting, and pruritus, more often than those who received 2 mg, without analgesic benefit. Thus morphine 2 mg caused the least "analgesic burden" and is probably the ideal regimen in women undergoing postpartum tubal ligation. There was no respiratory depression. The study did not explore options of smaller dosage regimens and may have lacked power to detect analgesic benefits between the various regimens.

In 45 children aged 1–15 years undergoing hip ortho-pedic surgery with 0.25% bupivacaine, three different dosage regimens of morphine 11.2, 15, or 20 micro-grams/kg were used for caudal or epidural administration that would produce at least 8 hours of postoperative analgesia (97). The adverse effects of morphine were dose-related: 11.2 micrograms/kg produced the lowest frequency of sleeping and vomiting. However, the fre-quency of vomiting was unacceptably high: almost 50% of children given the lowest dose of morphine had vomit-ing. This high frequency was unlikely to be due to the adverse effects of morphine alone, and the authors sug-gested possible contributory factors, such as the adminis-tration of oxygen via a facemask with gastric distension and prolonged preoperative fasting. Morphine was not associated with urinary retention or pruritus.

Drug administration route

The practical administration of morphine has been reviewed in relation to dose (initial dose with titration and rescue), formulations (indication and costs), routes of administration, and adverse effects (98).

There is a similar frequency of adverse effects between buccal and intramuscular morphine, as well as intramus-cular and intravenous infusions.

Two novel routes for the administration of morphine or bupivacaine (intraperitoneal and interpleural) have been studied for the provision of analgesia after laparoscopic cholecystectomy (SEDA-20, 79).

Some patients developed severe local toxicity during the subcutaneous administration of morphine sulfate (and of hydromorphone) via portable pumps (SEDA-16, 82).

Intramuscular morphine has been compared with epi-dural morphine or epidural sufentanil, both with bupiva-caine, in 90 patients undergoing major abdominal surgery (99). Both epidural regimens gave significantly better post-operative analgesia at rest and during movement. The inci-dence of adverse effects did not differ significantly between the groups, although the intraoperative requirement for ephedrine or dopamine was higher for the epidural group. Itching was significantly less in the intramuscular morphine group than the epidural groups (7 versus 69%) but nausea and vomiting were equally common.

The systemic availability of morphine from an aerosol is low (about 10%). A nasal solution containing morphine and chitosan, a linear polysaccharide, has been tested in a pilot study in healthy volunteers and patients with cancer

(100). The formulation was well tolerated and could be a useful delivery system for morphine.

In a double-blind, randomized, uncontrolled study in 150 women to compare intrathecal morphine 100 micro-grams plus ketoprofen, intrathecal morphine 200 micro-grams, or epidural morphine 3 mg, postoperative nausea or vomiting occurred in 16, 28, and 26% respectively (101). The incidence of itching was least in those given intrathecal morphine 100 micrograms. The results were unequivocal and did not justify preferring any one of the techniques as better or safer.

In a double-blind, randomized study in 60 patients undergoing elective knee arthroscopy, direct intrasyno-vial injection of morphine 1 mg provided better long-term analgesia (12–24 hours) than intra-articular mor-phine 1 mg, with no adverse effects (102).

Intrathecal

Intrathecal morphine provides adequate postoperative analgesia in orthopedic surgery, but commonly causes urinary retention, pruritus, and nausea and vomiting. Finding the optimal dose of analgesic effect with minimal adverse effects is still the main objective of most papers published on morphine (103,104).

In a randomized, double-blind study in 143 patients scheduled for total hip surgery the optimal dose of intrathecal morphine was as low as 0.1 mg (105). The patients were allocated to four groups depending on the dose of morphine used (0.025, 0.05, 0.1, and 0.2 mg). The incidence of pruritus, nausea and vomiting, and urinary retention, and the consumption of antiemetics did not differ among the groups.

The use of intrathecal morphine (106) in the manage-ment of chronic non-malignant pain has been reported. Eighty-eight patients were originally evaluated followed by 67 patients 6 months later. At the time of follow-up, mean pain relief was 60%, with 74% of respondents reporting increased activity. There were frequent reports of opioid adverse effects, including sexual dys-function and menstrual disturbances. The reported adverse effects in descending order of frequency were: excessive sweating (62%), weight gain (52%), difficulty in concentrating, thinking, and memory (48%), nausea and vomiting (42%), arthralgia (25%), peripheral edema (25%), and pruritus (21%). Despite these adverse effects, most of the patients expressed satisfac-tion with intrathecal opioid therapy. The results were limited owing to the retrospective nature of the study, differing rates of response to specific questions, and the lack of objective measures.

Intrathecal morphine 0.3 mg preoperatively + intrave-nous patient-controlled morphine postoperatively has been compared with intravenous patient-controlled mor-phine in 78 elderly patients undergoing major colorectal surgery (107). Intrathecal morphine caused more seda-tion, delaying recovery, but immediate postoperative pain was better controlled. All other adverse events (mental function, delirium/confusion, timing of ileus, and ambulation) were similar in the two groups.

Epidural

Epidural morphine gave better postoperative pain control than intravenous morphine after pectoralis major myocutaneous flap reconstruction in 60 patients (108). There were no differences between the two groups in terms of drug-specific adverse effects. The epidural technique is associated with procedural risk and its benefits do not outweigh the risks.

Drug–Drug Interactions

Diclofenac

Although spinal morphine provides effective analgesia, different ways of managing and minimizing its troubling adverse effects are constantly sought. Diclofenac, a non-steroidal anti-inflammatory drug, improves the analgesia provided by epidural morphine and may allow dosage reduction. In an investigation of this drug combination, intrathecal morphine was administered either regularly or on demand to 120 women undergoing cesarean section in doses of 0.1 mg, 0.05 mg, or 0.025 mg with diclofenac 75 mg intramuscularly (109). Severe pruritus was significantly more common in those who received morphine 0.1 mg and there was a trend toward less vomiting with smaller doses. There was no respiratory depression. The results suggested that the adverse effects of intrathecal morphine are dose-dependent and that there was no advantage in using doses of morphine larger than 0.25 mg.

Droperidol

A prospective, randomized, double-blind study of 97 women investigated whether droperidol alleviated the adverse effects of epidural morphine after cesarean section (110). All groups received morphine 5 mg epidurally on delivery, accompanied by no droperidol, or droperidol 2.5 mg epidurally, or droperidol 2.5 mg intravenously. Pruritus occurred in 70% of patients, starting at 6 hours after epidural morphine, peaking at 17 hours, and with no significant difference between the different treatment regimens. Nausea and vomiting were significantly reduced by intravenous droperidol, but not by epidural droperidol. The authors concluded that droperidol acts systemically to counter the adverse effects of epidural morphine but is not entirely effective, and they suggested that its failure to alleviate pruritus may have been due to the fact that they used larger doses of morphine than some other investigators.

Esmolol

Co-administration of esmolol with morphine resulted in increased steady-state concentrations of esmolol (117).

Metamfetamine

Two deaths involving the concurrent abuse of metamfetamine and morphine have been reported (111). The blood concentrations of both drugs were sublethal, and synergism between morphine and metamfetamine, especially in causing hyperthermia, seemed to be the mechanism.

Propofol

Subhypnotic doses of propofol (20 mg) given to 120 women receiving intrathecal morphine after cesarean section had no significant effect on pruritus (112). Higher success rates have been reported for propofol with non-obstetric patients, suggesting that labor-related factors may perpetuate this adverse effect.

Rifampicin

The metabolism of morphine is enhanced by rifampicin, resulting in loss of analgesic effects of morphine (113).

Somatostatin and analogues

Somatostatin and its analogues have been reported to be OP_3 (μ) opioid receptor antagonists (118). Somatostatin infusions significantly reduced the effectiveness of morphine analgesia in a case report of three patients with cancer.

Tricyclic antidepressants

Clomipramine, amitriptyline, and probably other antidepressants that potentiate the serotonergic system, enhance the analgesic effect of morphine.

Interference with Diagnostic Tests

Therapeutic doses of morphine can alter the blood activities of amylase, lipase, lactate dehydrogenase, creatine phosphokinase, and leucine aminopeptidase, BSP retention, and urine glucose concentration (Benedict's) (114–116).

References

1. Jacobsen LS, Olsen AK, Sjogren P, Jensen NH. Morfininduceret hyperalgesi, allodyni og myoklonus—nye morfinbivir-Kninger?. [Morphine-induced hyperalgesia, allodynia and myoclonus—new side-effects of morphine?.] Ugeskr Laeger 1995;157(23):3307–10.
2. World Heath Organization. Cancer Pain Relief. 2nd ed.. Geneva: WHO;. 1996.
3. Hanks GW, Conno F, Cherny N, Hanna M, Kalso E, McQuay HJ, Mercadante S, Meynadier J, Poulain P, Ripamonti C, Radbruch L, Casas JR, Sawe J, Twycross RG, Ventafridda VExpert Working Group of the Research Network of the European Association for Palliative Care. Morphine and alternative opioids in cancer pain: the EAPC recommendations. Br J Cancer 2001;84(5):587–93.
4. O'Connor A, Schug SA, Cardwell H. A comparison of the efficacy and safety of morphine and pethidine as analgesia for suspected renal colic in the emergency setting. J Accid Emerg Med 2000;17(4):261–4.
5. Lötsch J, Geisslinger G. Morphine-6-glucuronide: an analgesic of the future? Clin Pharmacokinet 2001;40(7):485–99.
6. Coller JK, Christrup LL, Somogyi AA. Role of active metabolites in the use of opioids. Eur J Clin Pharmacol 2009;65(2):121–39.
7. Van Dorp ELA, Romberg R, Sarton E, Bovill JG, Dahan A. Morphine-6-glucuronide: morphine's successor for

postoperative pain relief? Anesth Analgesia 2006;102(6):1789–97.

8. Flisberg P, Rudin A, Linner R, Lundberg CJ. Pain relief and safety after major surgery. A prospective study of epidural and intravenous analgesia in 2696 patients. Acta Anaesthesiol Scand 2003;47:457–65.

9. Vasilev GN, Alexieva DZ, Pavlova RZ. Safety and efficacy of oral slow release morphine for maintenance treatment of heroin addicts: a 6-month open noncomparative study. Eur Addict Res 2006;12(2):53–60.

10. Boyd JJ, Kuisma MJ, Alaspaa AO, Vuori E, Repo JV, Randell TT. Outcome after heroin overdose and cardiopulmonary resuscitation. Acta Anaesthesiol Scand 2006;50:1120–4.

11. Riley J, Ross JR, Rutter D, Wells AU, Goller K, du Bois R, Welsh K. No pain relief from morphine? Individual variation in sensitivity to morphine and the need to switch to an alternative opioid in cancer patients. Support Care Cancer 2006;14:56–64.

12. Breitfeld C, Peters J, Vockel T, Lovenz C, Eikermann M. Emetic effects of morphine and pirctramide. Br J Anaesth 2003;91:218–23.

13. Davis KM, Esposito MA, Meyer BA. Oral analgesia compared with intravenous patient-controlled analgesia for pain after cesarean delivery: a randomized controlled trial. Am J Obstet Gynaecol 2006;194(4):967–71.

14. Safdar B, Degutis LC, Landry K, Vedere SR, Moscovitz HC, D'Onofrio G. Intravenous morphine plus ketorolac is superior to either drug alone for treatment of acute renal colic. Ann Emerg Med. 2006;48:173–81.

15. Aveline C, Hetet HL, Vautier P, Gautier JF, Bonnet F. Peroperative ketamine and morphine for postoperative pain control after lumbar disc surgery. Eur J Pain 2006;10(7):653–8.

16. Chu Y-C, Lin S-M, Hsieh Y-C, Chan K-H, Tsou M-Y. Intraoperative administration of tramadol for postoperative nurse-controlled analgesia resulted in earlier awakening and less sedation than morphine in children after cardiac surgery. Anesth Analg 2006;102(6):1668–73.

17. Kim JY, Lee SJ, Koo BN, Noh SH, Kil HK, Kim HS, Ban SY. The effect of epidural sufentanil in ropivacaine on urinary retention in patients undergoing gastrectomy. Br J Anaesth 2006;97(3):414–8.

18. Kapfer B, Alfonsi P, Guignard B, Sessler DI, Chauvin M. Nefopam and ketamine comparably enhance postoperative analgesia. Anesth Analg 2005;100(1):169–74.

19. Lo Y, Chia YY, Liu K, Ko NH. Morphine sparing with droperidol in patient-controlled analgesia. J Clin Anesth 2005;17(4):271–5.

20. Gilron I, Bailey JM, Tu D, Holden RR, weaver DF, Houlden RL. Morphine, gabapentin, or their combination for neuropathic pain. N Engl J Med 2005;352(13):1324–34.

21. Sveticic G, Eichenberger U, Curatolo M. Safety of mixture of morphine with ketamine for post-operative patient-controlled analgesia: an audit with 1026 patients. Acta Anaesthesiol Scand 2005;49(6):870–5.

22. Suzuki M, Kinoshita T, Kikutani T, Yokoyama K, Inagi T, Sugimoto K, Haraguchi S, Hisayoshi T, Shimada Y. Determining the plasma concentration of ketamine that enhances epidural bupivacaine-and-morphine-induced analgesia. Anesth Analg 2005;101(3):777–84.

23. Chen JY, Wu GJ, Mok Ms, Chou YH, Sun WZ, Chen PL, Chan WS, Yien HW, Wen YR. Effect of adding ketorolac to intravenous morphine patient-controlled analgesia on bowel function in colorectal surgery patients – a prospective, randomized, double-blind study. Acta Anaesthesiol Scand 2005;49(4):546–51.

24. Vintar N, Rawal N, Veselko M. Intra-articular patient-controlled regional anesthesia after arthroscopically assisted anterior cruciate ligament reconstruction: ropivacaine/morphine/ketorolac versus ropivacaine/morphine. Anesth Analg 2005;101(2):573–8.

25. Beilin B, Bessler H, Papismedov L, Weinstock M, Shavit Y. Continuous physostigmine combined with morphine-based patient-controlled analgesia in the postoperative period. Acta Anaesthesiol Scand 2005;49(1):78–84.

26. Al-Khalaf B, Loew F, Fichtl M, Donaver E. Prospective comparative study of the effectiveness of epidural morphine and ropivacaine for management of pain after spinal operations. Acta Neurochirurg 2003;145:11–16.

27. Suominen PK, Ragg PG, McKinley DF, Frawley G, But WW, Eyres RL. Intrathecal morphine provides effective and safe analgesia in children after cardiac surgery. Acta Anaesthesiol Scand 2004;48:875–82.

28. Cherny N, Ripamonti C, Pereira J, Davis C, Fallon M, McQuay H, Mercadante S, Pasternak G, Ventafridda VExpert Working Group of the European Association of Palliative Care Network. Strategies to manage the adverse effects of oral morphine: an evidence-based report. J Clin Oncol 2001;19(9):2542–54.

29. Wang JJ, Ho ST, Wong CS, Tzeng JI, Liu HS, Ger LP. Dexamethasone prophylaxis of nausea and vomiting after epidural morphine for post-Cesarean analgesia. Can J Anaesth 2001;48(2):185–90.

30. Ho ST, Wang JJ, Tzeng JI, Liu HS, Ger LP, Liaw WJ. Dexamethasone for preventing nausea and vomiting associated with epidural morphine: a dose-ranging study. Anesth Analg 2001;92(3):745–8.

31. Liu SS, Hodgson PS, Carpenter RL, Fricke JR Jr. ADL 8-2698, a trans-3,4-dimethyl-4-(3-hydroxyphenyl) piperidine, prevents gastrointestinal effects of intravenous morphine without affecting analgesia. Clin Pharmacol Ther 2001;69(1):66–71.

32. Tzeng JI, Wang JJ, Ho ST, Tang CS, Liu YC, Lee SC. Dexamethasone for prophylaxis of nausea and vomiting after epidural morphine for post-Caesarean section analgesia: comparison of droperidol and saline. Br J Anaesth 2000;85(6):865–8.

33. Yeh HM, Chen LK, Lin CJ, Chan WH, Chen YP, Lin CS, Sun WZ, Wang MJ, Tsai SK. Prophylactic intravenous ondansetron reduces the incidence of intrathecal morphine-induced pruritus in patients undergoing cesarean delivery. Anesth Analg 2000;91(1):172–5.

34. Horta ML, Ramos L, Goncalves ZR. The inhibition of epidural morphine-induced pruritus by epidural droperidol. Anesth Analg 2000;90(3):638–41.

35. Horta ML, Ramos L, Goncalves Zda R, de Oliveira MA, Tonellotto D, Teixeira JP, de Melo PR. Inhibition of epidural morphine-induced pruritus by intravenous droperidol. The effect of increasing the doses of morphine and of droperidol. Reg Anesth 1996;21(4):312–7.

36. Mercadante S, Villari P, Fulfaro F. Gabapentin for opioid-related myoclonus in cancer patients. Support Care Cancer 2001;9(3):205–6.

37. Semenkovich CF, Jaffe AS. Adverse effects due to morphine sulfate. Challenge to previous clinical doctrine. Am J Med 1985;79(3):325–30.

38. Simons SHP, Roofthooft DWE, van Dijk M, van Lingen RA, Duivenvoorden HJ, van den Anker JN, Tibboel D. Morphine in ventilated neonates: its effects on arterial blood pressure. Arch Dis Child Fetal Neonatal Ed 2006;91:46–51.

39. Van Alfen-Van Der Velden AAEM, Hopman JCW, Klaessens JHGM, Feuth T, Sengers RCA, Liem KD.

Effects of midazolam and morphine on cerebral oxygenation and hemodynamics in ventilated premature infants. Biol Neonate 2006;90(3):197–202.

40. Anand KJS, Whit Hall R. Morphine, hypotension, and intraventricular hemorrhage. Pediatrics 2006;117:250–2.

41. Bruera E, Miller MJ. Non-cardiogenic pulmonary edema after narcotic treatment for cancer pain. Pain 1989;39(3):297–300.

42. Taddio A, Lee C, Yip A, Parvez B, McNamara PJ, Shah V. Intravenous morphine and topical tetracaine for treatment of pain in preterm neonates undergoing central line placement. JAMA 2006;295(7):793–800.

43. Boyle EM, Freer Y, Wong CM, McIntosh N, Anand KJS. Assessment of persistent pain or distress and adequacy of analgesia in preterm ventilated infants. Pain 2006;124:87–91.

44. Scherens A, Kagel T, Zenz M, Maier C. Long-term respiratory depression induced by intrathecal morphine treatment for chronic neuropathic pain. Anesthesiology 2006;105:431–3.

45. Enders J, Gebauer C, Pulzer F, Robel-Tillig E, Knupfer M. Morphine-related apnoea in CPAP-treated preterm neonates. Acta Paediatr Int J Paediatr 2006;95(9):1087–92.

46. Lotsch J, Dudziak R, Freynhagen R, Marschner J, Geisslinger G. Fatal respiratory depression after multiple intravenous morphine injections. Clin Pharmacokin 2006;45(11):1051–60.

47. Roca B, Mentero A, Simon E, Moulin DE, Hahn A, Hagen N. Pain and opioid analgesics in Guillain—Barré syndrome. Neurology 1998;51(3):924.

48. Heger S, Maier C, Otter K, Helwig U, Suttorp M. Morphine induced allodynia in a child with brain tumour. BMJ 1999;319(7210):627–9.

49. Parisod E, Siddall PJ, Viney M, McClelland JM, Cousins MJ. Allodynia after acute intrathecal morphine administration in a patient with neuropathic pain after spinal cord injury. Anesth Analg 2003;97:183–6.

50. Henderson RD, Wijdicks EF. Downbeat nystagmus associated with intravenous patient-controlled administration of morphine. Anesth Analg 2000;91(3):691–2.

51. Molloy S, Soh, C, Williams TL. Reversible delayed posthypoxic leukoencephalopathy. Am J Neuroradiol 2006;27:1763–65.

52. Gibson PRJ, Johnston S, Lagopoulos J, Cummine JL. Transient loss of motor-evoked responses associated with caudal injection of morphine in a patient with spondylolisthesis undergoing spinal fusion. Paediatr Anesth 2006;16(5):568–72.

53. Kalso E, Vainio A. Hallucinations during morphine but not during oxycodone treatment. Lancet 1988;2(8616):912.

54. D'Souza M. Unusual reaction to morphine. Lancet 1987;2(8550):98.

55. Jellema JG. Hallucination during sustained-release morphine and methadone administration. Lancet 1987;2(8555):392.

56. Deshpande MA, Holden RR, Gilron I. The impact of therapy on quality of life and mood in neuropathic pain: what is the effect of pain reduction? Anesth Analg 2006;102:1473–9.

57. Kamboj SK, Tookman A, Jones L, Curran HV. The effects of immediate-release morphine on cognitive functioning in patients receiving chronic opioid therapy in palliative care. Pain 2005;117(3):388–95.

58. Zis AP, Haskett RF, Albala AA, Carroll BJ, Lohr NE. Prolactin response to morphine in depression. Biol Psychiatry 1985;20(3):287–92.

59. White ID, Hoskin PJ, Hanks GW, Bliss JM. Morphine and dryness of the mouth. BMJ 1989;298(6682):1222–3.

60. Yimyaem PR, Kritsanaprakornkit W, Thienthong S, Horatanaruang D, Palachewa K, Tantanatewin W, Simajareuk S, Theerapongpakdee S. Postoperative pain management by acute pain service in a University hospital, Thailand. Acute Pain 2006;8(4):161–7.

61. Habib AS, Muir HA, White WD, Spahn TE, Olufolabi AJ, Breen TW. Intrathecal morphine for analgesia after postpartum bilateral tubal ligation. Anesth Analg 2005;100(1):239–43.

62. Ho AM. Previous cholecystectomy and choledochal sphincter spasm after morphine sedation. Can J Anaesth 2000;47(1):50–2.

63. Kuipers PW, Kamphuis EdT, Venroorj Ger E, Van Roy John P, Ionescu TI, Knape JT, Kalkman CJ. Intrathecal opioids and lower urinary tract functions: a urodynamic evaluation. Anesthesiology 2004;100:1497–503.

64. Gurken Y, Canatay H, Ozdamar D, Solek M, Toker K. Spinal anesthesia for arthroscopic knee surgery. Acta Anaesthesiol Scand 2004;48:513–7.

65. Whiston RJ, Griffith CD, Hopkinson BR. Purpuric rash associated with slow release morphine. BMJ (Clin Res Ed) 1988;296(6631):1262.

66. Kardaun SH, de Monchy JG. Acute generalized exanthematous pustulosis caused by morphine, confirmed by positive patch test and lymphocyte transformation test. J Am Acad Dermatol 2006;55:S21–3.

67. Eroglu A. A comparison of patient-controlled subacromial and i.v. analgesia after open acromioplasty surgery. Br J Anesth 2006;96(4):497–501.

68. Iatrou CA, Dragoumanis CK, Vogiatzaki TD, Vretzakis GI, Simpoulos CE, Dimitriou VK. Prophylactic intravenous ondansetron and dolasetron in intrathecal morphine-induced pruritus: a randomized, double-blinded, placebo-controlled study. Anesth Analg 2005;101(5):1516–20.

69. Seifert J, Metzner C, Paetzold W, Borsutzky M, Ohlmeier M, Passie T, Hauser U, Becker H, Wiese B, Emrich HM, Schneider U. Mood and affect during detoxification of opiate addicts: a comparison of buprenorphine versus methadone. Addict Biol 2005;10:157–64.

70. Meine TJ, Roe MT, Chen AY, Patel MR, Washam JB, Ohman EM, Peacock WF, Pollack JrCV, Gibler WB, Peterson ED. Association of intravenous morphine use and outcomes in acute coronary syndromes: results from the CRUSADE Quality Improvement Initiative. Am Heart J 2005;149(6):1043–9.

71. Verheugt FWA. Morpheus, god of sleep or god of death? Am Heart J 2005;149(6):945–6.

72. Byard RW. Unexpected death due to infectious mononucleosis. J Forensic Sci 2002;47(1):202–4.

73. Kreek MJ, Bart G, Lilly C, Laforge KS, Nielson DA. Pharmacogenetics and human molecular genetics of opiate and cocaine addictions and their treatments. Pharmacol Rev 2005;57(1):1–26.

74. Sun HL. Naloxone-precipitated acute opioid withdrawal syndrome after epidural morphine. Anesth Analg 1998;86(3):544–5.

75. Eriator II, Sun HL. Naloxone: acute opioid withdrawal syndrome or side effects? Anesth Analg 1998;87(5):1214.

76. Roberts LJ, Finch PM, Goucke CR, Price LM. Outcome of intrathecal opioids in chronic non-cancer pain. Eur J Pain 2001;5(4):353–61.

77. Lotsch J, Zimmermann M, Darimont J, Marx C, Dudziak R, Skarke C, Geisslinger G. Does the A118G polymorphism at the mu-opioid receptor gene protect against morphine-6-glucuronide toxicity? Anesthesiology 2002;97(4):814–9.

78. Hirota T, Leiki I, Takana H, Sano H, Kawamoto K, Aono H, Yamasaki A, Takeuchi H, Masadam M, Shimizu E, Hiquche S, Otsubo K. Sequence variability and candidate gene analysis in two cancer patients with complex clinical outcomes during morphine therapy. Drug Metab Dispos 2003;31:671–80.

79. Chou W-Y, Yang L-C, Lu H-F, Ko J-Y, Wang C-H, Lin S-H, Lee T-H, Concejero A, Hsu C-J. Association of mu-opioid receptor gene polymorphism (A118G) with variations in morphine consumption for analgesia after total knee arthroplasty. Acta Anaesthesiol Scand 2006;50(7):787–92.

80. Chou W-Y, Wang C-H, Liu C-C, Tseng C-C, Jawan B. Human opioid receptor A118G polymorphism affects intravenous patient-controlled analgesia morphine consumption after total abdominal hysterectomy. Anesthesiology 2006;105(2):334–7.

81. Bozkurt P. The analgesic efficacy and neuroendocrine response in paediatric patients treated with two analgesic techniques: using morphine-epidural and patient-controlled analgesia. Paediatr Anaesth 2002;12(3):248–54.

82. Olkkola KT, Maunuksela EL, Korpela R, Rosenberg PH. Kinetics and dynamics of postoperative intravenous morphine in children. Clin Pharmacol Ther 1988;44(2):128–36.

83. Zernikow B, Lindena G. Long-acting morphine for pain control in paediatric oncology. Med Pediatr Oncol 2001;36(4):451–8.

84. Gall O, Aubineau JV, Berniere J, Desjeux L, Murat I. Analgesic effect of low-dose intrathecal morphine after spinal fusion in children. Anesthesiology 2001;94(3):447–52.

85. Hesselgard K, Stromblad LG, Reinstrup P. Morphine with or without a local anaesthetic for postoperative intrathecal pain treatment after selective dorsal rhizotomy in children. Paediatr Anaesth 2001;11(1):75–9.

86. Aubrun F, Salvi N, Coriat P, Riou B. Sex- and age-related differences in morphine requirements for postoperative pain relief. Anesthesiology 2005;103(1):156–60.

87. Aubrun F, Monsel S, Langeron O, Coriat P, Riou B. Postoperative titration of intravenous morphine in the elderly patient. Anesthesiology 2002;96(1):17–23.

88. Sear JW, Hand CW, Moore RA, McQuay HJ. Studies on morphine disposition: influence of renal failure on the kinetics of morphine and its metabolites. Br J Anaesth 1989;62(1):28–32.

89. Bristow A, Orlikowski C. Subcutaneous ketamine analgesia: postoperative analgesia using subcutaneous infusions of ketamine and morphine. Ann R Coll Surg Engl 1989;71(1):64–6.

90. Potter JM, Reid DB, Shaw RJ, Hackett P, Hickman PE. Myoclonus associated with treatment with high doses of morphine: the role of supplemental drugs. BMJ 1989;299(6692):150–3.

91. Cole PJ, Craske DA, Wheatley RG. Efficacy and respiratory effects of low-dose spinal morphine for postoperative analgesia following knee arthroplasty. Br J Anaesth 2000;85(2):233–7.

92. Hanks GW, Twycross RG, Bliss JM. Controlled release morphine tablets: a double-blind trial in patients with advanced cancer. Anaesthesia 1987;42(8):840–4.

93. Palmer CM, Nogami WM, Van Maren G, Alves DM. Postcesarean epidural morphine: a dose-response study. Anesth Analg 2000;90(4):887–91.

94. Fletcher D, Pinaud M, Scherpereel P, Clyti N, Chauvin M. The efficacy of intravenous 0.15 versus 0.25 mg/kg intraoperative morphine for immediate postoperative analgesia after remifentanil-based anesthesia for major surgery Anesth Analg 2000;90(3):666–71.

95. Hesselgard K, Stromblad L-G, Romner B, Reinstrup P. Postoperative continuous intrathecal pain treatment in children after selective dorsal rhizotomy with bupivacaine and two different morphine doses. Paediatr Anesth 2006;16(4):436–43.

96. Marcus RJL, Wong CA, Lehor A, McCarthy RJ, Yaghmour E, Yilmaz M. Postoperative epidural morphine for postpartum tubal ligation analgesia. Anesth Analg 2005;101(3):876–81.

97. Castillo-Zamora C, Castillo-Peralta LA, Nava-Ocampo AA. Dose minimization study of single-dose epidural morphine in patients undergoing hip surgery under regional anesthesia with bupivacaine. Paediatr Anaesth 2005;15(1):29–36.

98. Donnelly S, Davis MP, Walsh D, Naughton MWorld Health Organization. Morphine in cancer pain management: a practical guide. Support Care Cancer 2002;10(1):13–35.

99. Broekema AA, Veen A, Fidler V, Gielen MJ, Hennis PJ. Postoperative analgesia with intramuscular morphine at fixed rate versus epidural morphine or sufentanil and bupivacaine in patients undergoing major abdominal surgery. Anesth Analg 1998;87(6):1346–53.

100. Illum L, Watts P, Fisher AN, Hinchcliffe M, Norbury H, Jabbal-Gill I, Nankervis R, Davis SS. Intranasal delivery of morphine. J Pharmacol Exp Ther 2002;301(1):391–400.

101. Sarvela J, Halonen P, Soikkeli A, Korttila K. A double-blinded, randomized comparison of intrathecal and epidural morphine for elective cesarean delivery. Anesth Analg 2002;95(2):436–40.

102. Kligman M, Bruskin A, Sckliamser J, Vered R, Roffman M. Intra-synovial, compared to intra-articular morphine provides better pain relief following knee arthroscopy meniscectomy. Can J Anaesth 2002;49(4):380–3.

103. Gwirtz KH, Young JV, Byers RS, Alley C, Levin K, Walker SG, Stoelting RK. The safety and efficacy of intrathecal opioid analgesia for acute postoperative pain: seven years' experience with 5969 surgical patients at Indiana University Hospital. Anesth Analg 1999;88(3):599–604.

104. Palmer CM, Emerson S, Volgoropolous D, Alves D. Dose-response relationship of intrathecal morphine for postcesarean analgesia. Anesthesiology 1999;90(2):437–44.

105. Slappendel R, Weber EW, Dirksen R, Gielen MJ, van Limbeek J. Optimization of the dose of intrathecal morphine in total hip surgery: a dose-finding study. Anesth Analg 1999;88(4):822–6.

106. Anderson VC, Cooke B, Burchiel KJ. Intrathecal hydromorphone for chronic nonmalignant pain: a retrospective study. Pain Med 2001;2(4):287–97.

107. Beaussier M, Weickmans H, Parc Y, Delpierre E, Camus Y, Funck-Brentano C, Schiffer E, Delva E, Lienhart A. Postoperative analgesia and recovery course after major colorectal surgery in elderly patients: a randomized comparison between intrathecal morphine and intravenous PCA morphine. Reg Anesth Pain Med 2006;31(6):531–8.

108. Singhal AK, Mishra S, Bhatnagar S, Singh R. Epidural morphine analgesia compared with intravenous morphine for oral cancer surgery with pectoralis major myocutaneous flap reconstruction. Acta Anaesthesiol Scand 2006;50(1):234–8.

109. Cardoso MM, Carvalho JC, Amaro AR, Prado AA, Cappelli EL. Small doses of intrathecal morphine combined with systemic diclofenac for postoperative pain control after cesarean delivery. Anesth Analg 1998;86(3):538–541.

110. Sanansilp V, Areewatana S, Tonsukchai N. Droperidol and the side effects of epidural morphine after cesarean section. Anesth Analg 1998;86(3):532–7.

111. Vemura K, Sorimache Y, Yashiki M, Yoshida K. Two fatal cases involving concurrent use of methamphetamine and morphine. J Forensic Sci 2003;48:1179–81.

112. Beilin Y, Bernstein HH, Zucker-Pinchoff B, Zahn J, Zenzen WJ. Subhypnotic doses of propofol do not relieve pruritus induced by intrathecal morphine after cesarean section. Anesth Analg 1998;86(2):310–3.

113. Fromm MF, Eckhardt K, Li S, Schanzle G, Hofmann U, Mikus G, Eichelbaum M. Loss of analgesic effect of morphine due to coadministration of rifampin. Pain 1997;72(1–2):261–7.

114. Garb S. Undesirable Drug InteractionsLondon: Henry Miller and Medcalf;. 1973.

115. Viars P. Actions périphériques des morphino-mimétiques. In: Utilisation des Morphinomimétiques en Anesthésiologie et Réanimation 1974:149.

116. Hansten PD. Drug Interactions. 4th ed.. Philadelphia: Lea and Febiger;. 1979.

117. Lowenthal DT, Porter RS, Saris SD, Bies CM, Slegowski MB, Staudacher A. Clinical pharmacology, pharmacodynamics and interactions with esmolol. Am J Cardiol 1985;56(11):F14–8.

118. Ripamonti C, De Conno F, Boffi R, Ascani L, Bianchi M. Can somatostatin be administered in association with morphine in advanced cancer patients with pain? Ann Oncol 1998;9(8):921–3.

Nalbuphine

General Information

Nalbuphine is a partial opioid agonist structurally similar to naloxone. Like naloxone it is an antagonist at MOR (OP$_3$, μ) receptors, whilst achieving analgesia via an agonist effect at KOR(OP$_2$, κ) receptors.

Nalbuphine was approximately equianalgesic with morphine (1) and its hemodynamic and respiratory effects were not statistically significantly different from those of morphine (SEDA-14, 69). Other studies have shown that this also applies to other organ systems. However, unlike morphine, nalbuphine has a "ceiling" effect on respiratory depression, a low incidence of dysphoric effects, and a low addiction potential. Ten patients with a history of cardiac or orthopedic problems who received intravenous nalbuphine (6–20 mg) required additional doses of morphine (15–70 mg) to relieve pain (2). However, this report was not supported by objective physiological measures or recognized pain scores.

Nalbuphine has similar efficacy and incidence of adverse effects to tramadol and paracetamol (acetaminophen) (3). Dysrhythmias and coughing occurred more often with nalbuphine than fentanyl (4).

Cardiac dysrhythmias, hypertension, agitation, nausea, and vomiting occurred when nalbuphine was given to four patients to reverse fentanyl-induced respiratory depression (SEDA-16, 89).

In a double-blind, placebo-controlled study in 24 elderly patients scheduled for elective total hip replacement who were randomized to either intrathecal morphine 160 μg or nalbuphine 400 μg postoperatively, when the pain score was greater than 3 cm on a visual analogue scale, nalbuphine produced significantly faster onset and shorter duration of analgesia (5). Both opioids produced adequate maximal pain relief in all patients. The adverse effects profile was unremarkable in both groups.

Intravenous nalbuphine 3 mg (n = 101) has been compared with intravenous propofol 20 mg (n = 90) in a double-blind, randomized study, to determine efficacy in the treatment of intrathecal morphine-induced pruritus after cesarean delivery 10 minutes after the drug was administered (6). Nalbuphine was significantly more effective, especially in cases of moderate but not severe pruritus. Adverse effects such as reduced analgesia and increased nausea, vomiting, sedation, and dizziness were not significantly different between the two groups.

Comparative studies

A randomized, controlled study compared two different regimens of nalbuphine in 175 patients with chest pain or trauma: 5 micrograms over 2 minutes, repeated at 3-minute intervals if pain scores remained above 3, to a maximum dose of 20 micrograms (n = 86); and 10 micrograms over 30 seconds, repeated once after 3 minutes, if the pain score remained above 3 (n = 90) (7). The rapid dosing regimen was more effective but caused significantly more adverse effects (drowsiness, dizziness, and nausea or vomiting).

Organs and Systems

Cardiovascular

The effects of nalbuphine on the cardiovascular and subjective effects of cocaine have been studied in a randomized controlled trial in seven patients (8). The combination of nalbuphine and cocaine was safe and did not have synergistic effects on heart rate and blood pressure or subjective effects. Nalbuphine was safe and well tolerated and its acute administration moderately attenuated the abuse-related effects of cocaine.

Respiratory

Although similar respiratory depression occurs with morphine and nalbuphine after single doses, on cumulative dosing there appears to be a ceiling effect with nalbuphine, which may also occur with respect to analgesic efficacy (9). Considerable respiratory depression requiring prolonged monitoring has been reported in children (SEDA-16, 89).

Neuromuscular function

Psychomotor performance and subjective effects seems to be dose-related (SEDA-22, 104).

Psychological, psychiatric

- A 53-year-old man with no past psychiatric history was found by the police walking aimlessly, unclothed, and responding to auditory hallucinations (10). He had slurred speech and generalized tremors. Lumbar puncture, a CT head scan, and urine drug screen were all normal. He responded to risperidone 1 mg bd with dramatic improvement after 2 days. He reported chronic use of nalbuphine, with recent increased use.

Gastrointestinal

The effects of nalbuphine and morphine on gastrointestinal function have been compared in 17 volunteers. Nalbuphine 10 mg prolonged gastric emptying to a greater extent than nalbuphine 5 mg or morphine 5 mg, which were about equal in their effects (11). However, another study (12) showed that nalbuphine produced significantly less inhibition of gastrointestinal activity than morphine.

Biliary tract

The effect of nalbuphine 20 mg intravenously on biliary tract pressure was examined in 10 patients undergoing surgery for symptomatic cholelithiasis. There was a statistically significant rise in pressure 30 minutes after the administration of nalbuphine, but this did not have any apparent deleterious effects (13). Others have suggested that nalbuphine reverses opioid-induced spasm of the sphincter of Oddi (SEDA-17, 88).

Long-Term Effects

Drug dependence

The development of dependence is unlikely at doses within the usual analgesic range (14).

Second-Generation Effects

Fetotoxicity

Transplacental transfer of nalbuphine was measured in eight mothers who underwent cesarean section and were given nalbuphine 200 µg/kg intravenously along with thiopental and suxamethonium. The umbilical cord/maternal vein ratio was 1.4:1 at delivery, which occurred at 2–10 minutes after nalbuphine injection. Mean Apgar scores at 1 minute were 6.6 and 8.5 at 5 minutes and did not correlate with either the serum nalbuphine concentration or the time between injection of nalbuphine and delivery (15).

Three neonates, whose mothers who had received nalbuphine during labor, developed apnea and cyanosis, which required ventilation within 3 minutes of birth (16,17).

Bradycardia and bradypnea have been reported in babies whose mothers were given nalbuphine a few hours before delivery (SEDA-16, 89).

A case of fetal sinusoidal rate pattern with nalbuphine has been reported (SEDA-17, 87).

Drug Administration

Drug dosage regimens

In a randomized, double-blind, multicenter comparison of three different intrathecal doses of nalbuphine (0.2, 0.8, or 1.6 mg) and a single intrathecal dose of morphine (0.2 mg) for postoperative pain relief after cesarean section in 90 parturients, intrathecal nalbuphine 0.8 mg provided rapid and effective analgesia, with minimal adverse effects but a shorter duration of action, reinforcing morphine's position as an analgesic that provides long-lasting analgesia (18).

References

1. Kururattapun SA, Prakanrattana U. Intravenous dezocine for postoperative pain: a double-blind, placebo controlled comparison with morphine. J Clin Pharmacol 1986;26:275.
2. Houlihan KP, Mitchell RG, Flapan AD, Steedman DJ. Excessive morphine requirements after pre-hospital nalbuphine analgesia. J Accid Emerg Med 1999;16(1):29–31.
3. Jain AK, Ryan JR, McMahon FG, Smith G. Comparison of oral nalbuphine, acetaminophen, and their combination in postoperative pain. Clin Pharmacol Ther 1986;39(3):295–9.
4. Heintz-Bamberg D, Muller H, Dick W, Reiter G. Vergleichende Klinische Untersuchungen zum Verhalten hämodynamischer Parameter be kombinationsnarkosen mit Nalbuphin (Nubain) und Fentanyl. [Comparative clinical studies of the hemodynamic parameters by anesthesia combination with nalbuphine (Nubain) and fentanyl.] Anaesthesist 1987;36(5):217–22.
5. Fournier R, Van Gessel E, Macksay M, Gamulin Z. Onset and offset of intrathecal morphine versus nalbuphine for postoperative pain relief after total hip replacement. Acta Anaesthesiol Scand 2000;44(8):940–5.
6. Charuluxananan S, Kyokong O, Somboonviboon W, Lertmaharit S, Ngamprasertwong P, Nimcharoendee K. Nalbuphine versus propofol for treatment of intrathecal morphine-induced pruritus after cesarean delivery. Anesth Analg 2001;93(1):162–5.
7. Woollard M, Whitfield R, Smith K, Jones T, Thomas G, Thomas G, Hinton C. Less is less: a randomized controlled trial comparing cautious and rapid nalbuphine dosing regimens. Emerg Med J 2004;21:362–4.
8. Mello NK, Mendelson JH, Sholar MB, Jaszyna-Gasior M, Goletiani N, Siegel AJ. Effects of the mixed mu/kappa opioid nalbuphine on cocaine-induced changes in subjective and cardiovascular responses in men. Neuropsychopharmacology 2005;30, 618–32.
9. Gannon R. Drug information update: Hartford Hospital. Nalbuphine. Conn Med 1985;49(10):681–2.
10. Camacho A, Matthews SC, Dimsdale JE. "Invisible" synthetic opiates and acute psychosis. N Engl J Med 2001;345(6):469.
11. Yukioka H, Rosen M, Evans KT, Leach KG, Hayward MW, Saggu GS. Gastric emptying and small bowel transit times in volunteers after intravenous morphine and nalbuphine. Anaesthesia 1987;42(7):704–10.

12. Shah M, Rosen M, Vickers MD. Effect of premedication with diazepam, morphine or nalbuphine on gastrointestinal motility after surgery. Br J Anaesth 1984;56(11):1235–8.

13. Butsch JL, Okoli JA. The effect of nalbuphine on the common bile duct pressure. Am Surg 1988;54(5):253–5.

14. Schmidt WK, Tam SW, Shotzberger GS, Smith DH Jr, Clark R, Vernier VG. Nalbuphine. Drug Alcohol Depend 1985;14(3–4):339–62.

15. Dadabhoy ZP, Tapia DP, Zsigmond EK. Transplacental transfer of nalbuphine in patients undergoing caesarean section. Acta Anaesthesiol Ital 1988;39:227.

16. Guillonneau M, Jacqz-Aigrain E, de Crepy A, Zeggout H. Perinatal adverse effects of nalbuphine given during parturition. Lancet 1990;335(8705):1588.

17. Sgro C, Escousse A, Tennenbaum D, Gouyon JB. Perinatal adverse effects of nalbuphine given during labour. Lancet 1990;336(8722):1070.

18. Culebras X, Gaggero G, Zatloukal J, Kern C, Marti RA. Advantages of intrathecal nalbuphine, compared with intrathecal morphine, after cesarean delivery: an evaluation of postoperative analgesia and adverse effects. Anesth Analg 2000;91(3):601–5.

Nalmefene

General Information

Nalmefene is a pure opioid antagonist, which is structurally similar to naloxone and naltrexone.

Drug studies

Reversal of opioid-induced adverse effects

In a comparison of the efficacy of naloxone and nalmefene in reversing opioid-induced sedation, vertigo and nausea were observed with nalmefene (1). Three of six healthy male volunteers given nalmefene 0.4 mg/70 kg complained of paresthesia in the midthoracic region (2).

In a randomized, placebo-controlled, double-blind study 120 women undergoing lower abdominal surgery were randomized to receive nalmefene 15 micrograms, nalmefene 25 micrograms, or saline intravenously at the end of surgery (3). The total consumption of morphine and the subsequent adverse effects profiles were recorded. Those given nalmefene used significantly less antiemetic and antipruritus medications during the subsequent 24-hours without a change in the quality of analgesia.

Stroke

The Cervene Stroke Study Investigation Group conducted a phase III study to assess the efficacy and safety of nalmefene (Cervene) in patients with acute ischemic strokes and also the safety of combined recombinant tissue plasminogen activator and nalmefene in a subset of patients (4). It was a randomized, placebo-controlled, double-blind study of a 24-hour infusion of nalmefene on 368 patients who received 60 mg nalmefene administered as 10 mg bolus over 15 minutes and then a 50 mg infusion over 24 hours or placebo. Even though nalmefene appeared safe and well tolerated, the study failed to find any benefit in stroke patients treated with nalmefene within six hours.

Pruritus

The role of opioid antagonists in the treatment of pruritus in cholestatic liver disease has been reviewed (5). Their use is based on the theory that implicates opioid neurotransmission as the cause of itching in this condition, and it has been observed that opioid antagonists, while providing relief from itching in patients with cholestasis, also cause symptoms similar to those seen in the opioid withdrawal syndrome. It has therefore been suggested that patients with cirrhosis are chronically exposed to increased concentrations of endogenous opiate receptor agonists.

In 11 patients with cirrhosis-induced pruritus, nalmefene led to relief of itching within 1 month, sustained at 3 and 6 months. However, the first two patients had severe withdrawal reactions that took 3 days to subside. In the light of this experience, the trial was modified so that patients received oral nalmefene 5 mg bd with a gradual increase in dosage over 7–10 days to 20–40 mg/day, and clonidine was administered simultaneously for the first 7 days of nalmefene therapy. Despite these precautions, all patients had withdrawal reactions, including anorexia, nausea, colicky abdominal pain, sweating, tremor, and occasionally visual or auditory hallucinations. These developed within 1 hour of nalmefene therapy and diminished within 2–3 days, despite continuation of nalmefene. This review included reports of two other studies, available in abstract form only, but which appear to have reported a lower incidence of withdrawal symptoms precipitated by nalmefene, although the dose of drug used also appeared to have been lower.

In 14 patients with cholestatic liver disease, oral nalmefene was started at a dose of 2 mg bd and increased until symptomatic relief of pruritus was obtained (6). Five patients were reported to have a transient opioid withdrawal-like reaction that did not preclude continuing with treatment. Other adverse events associated with nalmefene therapy included: perception of pins and needles ($n = 4$), anxiety and depression ($n = 2$), abdominal cramps and nausea ($n = 2$), insomnia ($n = 3$), depersonalization ($n = 2$), and changes in mood ($n = 2$); difficulties in visual focusing, dizziness, chronic goose bumps, mental "fuzziness," anorexia, and nightmares were each reported by one patient only. Of the cases of depersonalization, one occurred after the first dose while the other occurred in the first 2 weeks of therapy. There were no consistent changes in biochemistry with nalmefene. Several patients had a "breakthrough" of pruritus, which was managed by upward adjustment of dose. The authors suggested that this can be explained if nalmefene initially displaced pruritus-mediating ligands from opioid receptors, but then induced an increased density of receptors because of reduced agonist–receptor interactions, allowing further binding of pruritus-mediating ligands to receptors. In a few other patients, exacerbations of pruritus after long-term control on maintenance therapy may have been attributable to the development of tolerance toward nalmefene.

Alcohol dependence

Nalmefene (5, 20, and 40 micrograms/day) has been evaluated in a randomized, double-blind, controlled study over 12 weeks in 270 recently abstinent out-patient alcohol-dependent individuals (7). All concomitantly underwent four sessions of motivational enhancement therapy. Although they all had a reduction in heavy drinking days, craving, and gamma-glutamyl transferase activity, there was no difference between the active medication and placebo. Those who took 20 micrograms/day had more insomnia, dizziness, and confusion and those who took 40 micrograms/day had more nausea than the placebo group.

Organs and Systems

Cardiovascular

Pulmonary edema has been described after nalmefene (SEDA-22, 104).

Reproductive system

The hypothesis that endogenous opioids have a role in the premenstrual dysphoric disorder has been explored in 22 subjects, who received either placebo or nalmefene during the follicular phase and the rest of their cycles (8). Of those who received nalmefene, one complained of insomnia throughout the study. Withdrawal was required in one of those who received nalmefene but none of those who took placebo. Nalmefene did not beneficially influence the symptoms of premenstrual dysphoric disorder.

Long-Term Effects

Drug abuse

When nalmefene was given to six men with history of drug abuse, the adverse effects reported were agitation, irritability, muscle tension, and a feeling of hangover (SEDA-17, 88).

Susceptibility Factors

Age

The efficacy and safety of intravenous nalmefene 0.1 mg/ml has been studied in an open trial in 115 children given fentanyl (9). An initial dose of 0.25 microgram/kg (maximum 10 microgram) was infused over 15 seconds, and another dose of 0.25 microgram/kg (maximum 10 micrograms) was given if there was no response after 1.75 minutes. Further doses were given every 2 minutes until a response occurred or a maximum dose of 1 micrograms/kg (maximum 40 micrograms) was reached. Nalmefene was effective and safe, especially in a mean dose of 0.55 microgram/kg; the median number of doses was two. The limitations of this study included the small study sample and the use of a short-acting opioid,

fentanyl, so that re-sedation was unlikely even without the use of an antagonist.

References

1. Barsan WG, Seger D, Danzl DF, Ling LJ, Bartlett R, Buncher R, Bryan C. Duration of antagonistic effects of nalmefene and naloxone in opiate-induced sedation for emergency department procedures. Am J Emerg Med 1989;7(2):155–61.
2. Konieczko KM, Jones JG, Barrowcliffe MP, Jordan C, Altman DG. Antagonism of morphine-induced respiratory depression with nalmefene. Br J Anaesth 1988;61(3):318–23.
3. Joshi GP, Duffy L, Chehade J, Wesevich J, Gajraj N, Johnson ER. Effects of prophylactic nalmefene on the incidence of morphine-related side effects in patients receiving intravenous patient-controlled analgesia. Anesthesiology 1999;90(4):1007–11.
4. Clark WM, Raps EC, Tong DC, Kelly RE. Cervene (Nalmefene) in acute ischemic stroke: final results of a phase III efficacy study. The Cervene Stroke Study Investigators. Stroke 2000;31(6):1234–9.
5. Terra SG, Tsunoda SM. Opioid antagonists in the treatment of pruritus from cholestatic liver disease. Ann Pharmacother 1998;32(11):1228–30.
6. Bergasa NV, Schmitt JM, Talbot TL, Alling DW, Swain MG, Turner ML, Jenkins JB, Jones EA. Open-label trial of oral nalmefene therapy for the pruritus of cholestasis. Hepatology 1998;27(3):679–84.
7. Anton RF, Pettinati H, Zweben A, Kranzler HR, Johnson B, Bohn MJ, McCaul ME, Anthenelli R, Salloum I, Galloway G, Garbutt J, Swift R, Gastfriend D, Kallio A, Karhuvaara S. A multi-site dose ranging study of nalmefene in the treatment of alcohol dependence. J Clin Psychopharmacol 2004;24:421–8.
8. Van Ree JM, Schagen Van Leeuwen JH, Koppeschaar HP, Te Velde ER. Unexpected placebo response in premenstrual dysphoric disorder: implication of endogenous opioids. Psychopharmacology 2005;182:318–9.
9. Chumpa A, Kaplan RL, Burns MM, Shannon MW. Nalmefene for elective reversal of procedural sedation in children. Am J Emerg Med 2001;19(7):545–8.

Naloxone

General Information

Naloxone is an opioid antagonist devoid of pharmacological activity, except for its reversal of opioid effects.

As naloxone is widely believed to be innocuous, large maintenance doses of opioids are commonly used, in the belief that reversal can be safely achieved at the end of anesthesia.

The adverse effects of naloxone have been reviewed (1). Its potential long-term effects include increased neuronal damage in asphyxia, altered pain responsiveness, and seizures. It also potentially increases sympathetic nervous system activity, resulting in dysrhythmias, hypertension, and pulmonary edema, in those given high doses of naloxone, whether licit or illicit.

Drug studies

Reversal of opioid adverse effects

According to the results of one study, it might be expected that in every 1000 patients with drug overdose treated with naloxone, 4–30 serious complications, such as convulsions, asystole, pulmonary edema, and violent behavior, can be expected (SEDA-21, 92).

The use of naloxone has been studied in an open study in 43 patients having combined thoracic epidural and general anesthesia for subtotal gastrectomy, who were randomly assigned to receive a bolus dose of epidural morphine 3 mg followed by a continuous infusion of 3 mg in 0.125% bupivacaine 100 mg with either no naloxone ($n = 18$) or naloxone 0.208 µg/kg/hour ($n = 25$) for 48 hours (2). The time to the first postoperative passage of flatus and feces (indicating restoration of bowel function) and pain intensity (using a visual analogue scale) were assessed. The results suggested that naloxone 0.208 µg/kg/hour adequately reverses hypomotility induced by epidural morphine.

The preliminary results of two pilot schemes to provide take-home naloxone to opiate users have suggested that this provision can save lives (3). This observation needs corroboration by a prospective case-control study of adequate sample size and response rate, with the ability to collate objective data robust enough for analysis (4).

There was complete resolution of a unilateral neurological deficit associated with anesthesia along with complete resolution of postoperative unilateral EEG evidence of ischemia when naloxone was given to reverse residual opioid effects (5).

The effects of naloxone 0.25 micrograms/kg on the adverse effects of intravenous morphine have been explored in a randomized, double-blind, placebo-controlled trial in 131 patients in pain (6). Naloxone failed to improve nausea, pruritus, and vomiting and failed to reduce the need for rescue antiemetics. Naloxone did not affect pain reduction.

In a postoperative placebo-controlled study in 46 children and adolescents, average age 14 years, naloxone 0.25 micrograms/kg significantly reduced the incidence and severity of opioid-induced adverse effects (pruritus and nausea), without affecting opioid-induced analgesia (7).

Pruritus

In a randomized, double-blind, controlled trial in pruritus in cholestatic liver disease, naloxone was effective in most patients, but five had an increase in mean scratching activity during naloxone therapy, three patients had anxiety, and one developed withdrawal symptoms (8).

Stroke

The efficacy and toxicity of a naloxone loading dose of 4 mg/kg followed by 2 mg/kg per day was evaluated in 36 patients with acute stroke (9). The most common adverse effects were nausea and vomiting, which were easily controlled. The most serious effects were bradycardia and hypotension, which occurred in response to the loading dose. One patient developed hypotension and two developed focal seizures, which were ipsilateral to the affected hemisphere; one had myoclonus.

In another study, the safety of naloxone in much higher doses was studied in 38 patients with acute ischemic stroke (SEDA-16, 87). They were given a loading dose of 160 mg/m^2 over 15 minutes followed by a 24-hour infusion at a rate of 80 mg/m^2/hour. There was nausea and/or vomiting in 26 patients, 3 patients had behavioral changes, and in 7 patients naloxone was withdrawn because of adverse effects. The authors concluded that although naloxone is relatively safe in the dosage used, its efficacy in ischemic stroke is unproven.

In a randomized, double-blind study in 40 patients with moderate to severe acute traumatic brain injury, intravenous naloxone, 0.3–4.8 mg/kg/day for 10 days, reduced morbidity and mortality (10).

Tension headaches

Mild adverse effects, such as dizziness, nausea, coolness of the head, and abdominal pain, were reported when moderate doses of naloxone were given to patients with tension headaches (11).

Organs and Systems

Cardiovascular

Doses of naloxone over 1 pg/kg should be given with caution, especially to patients with hypertension. Massive release of catecholamines in response to pain after administration of naloxone can trigger left ventricular failure, partly by causing a shift in fluid from the intravascular to the interstitial Thus, alpha-blockers such as phentolamine have been postulated to be beneficial in its management (SEDA-17, 88). A fatal case of pulmonary edema followed the use of naloxone in a young man (12), although the causal link was disputed (13).

Severe hypertension and multiple atrial extra beats have been reported after the administration of naloxone, especially in patients with coronary heart disease (14).

Psychological, psychiatric

Behavioral effects have been noted after high doses of naloxone (2 and 4 mg/kg) in volunteers. Most subjects experienced an initial rush or buzz, tingling or numbness in the extremities, dizziness, a heavy head, and reluctance to move or initiate activities, which usually subsided within 15–30 minutes of administration. Transient sweating and yawning occurred later. Nausea and stomachache were often experienced and in two subjects persisted throughout the day, although in mild form. There were no pupillary changes or sleepiness. Increasing doses of naloxone were associated with increasingly impaired cognitive performance. Violent behavior has been reported after the use of naloxone to reverse sedation (SEDA-17, 88).

Endocrine

Marked changes in physiological functions can occur if naloxone is given when the endorphin system has been modified by opioids. Following the use of naloxone, a reduced plasma prolactin concentration was noted (15).

Second-Generation Effects

Fetotoxicity

Convulsions occurred in a baby born to an opioid-dependent mother. This case is unusual, as convulsions due to neonatal opioid withdrawal do not usually occur in the first 24 hours after delivery; it suggests that naloxone should be used with great caution in children born to opioid-dependent mothers (16).

Susceptibility Factors

Patients with pre-existing cardiac abnormalities are particularly susceptible to effects such as hypertension, pulmonary edema, atrial and ventricular dysrhythmias, and cardiac arrest, which can occur when naloxone is given to reverse opioid effects.

Drug Administration

Drug administration route

Age

In a systematic review of nine trials that specifically studied the use of naloxone in treating neonates with respiratory depression due to transplacentally acquired opioids the infants who received naloxone had increased alveolar ventilation compared with control infants, but this was not considered clinically relevant (17). Since naloxone can interfere with the effects of endogenous opioids in neuroendocrine programming and subsequent behavior, its therapeutic role is not clear and there has been no large randomized trial that would justify its use in these cases.

Cardiac disease

The authors of two review papers both concluded that there is no evidence that subcutaneous or intramuscular administration of naloxone is less effective in restoring respiration in patients with opioid overdose than the intravenous route (18,19).

Nasal naloxone in opioid overdose is generally safe and effective. However, lack of effectiveness has been reported in patients with nasal abnormalities, impairing administration (20).

Drug–Drug Interactions

Buprenorphine

Naloxone is of limited use in reversing the effects of buprenorphine, because of its relative inability to displace it from opioid receptors. Naloxone 1 mg had little effect on the respiratory depression caused by buprenorphine 300 µg/70 kg, although both 5 and 10 µg produced

consistent reversal, which was more complete with the larger dose (21). Insignificant effects on circulation and respiration have been reported at lower doses of buprenorphine (4.5–10 µg/kg) (22).

Captopril

Following the use of naloxone the hypotensive effect of captopril was abolished (23).

References

1. Guinsburg R, Wyckoff MH. Naloxone during neonatal resuscitation: acknowledging the unknown. Clin Perinatol 2006;33:121–32.
2. Lee J, Shim JY, Choi JH, Kim ES, Kwon OK, Moon DE, Choi JH, Bishop MJ. Epidural naloxone reduces intestinal hypomotility but not analgesia of epidural morphine. Can J Anaesth 2001;48(1):54–8.
3. Dettmer K, Saunders B, Strang J. Take home naloxone and the prevention of deaths from opiate overdose: two pilot schemes. BMJ 2001;322(7291):895–6.
4. Mountain D. Take home naloxone for opiate addicts. Big conclusions are drawn from little evidence. BMJ 2001;323(7318):934–5.
5. Krechel SW, Orr RM, Couper NB, Gupta N, Eggers GW Jr. Naloxone: report of a beneficial side effect. J Neurosurg Anesthesiol 1989;1(4):346–51.
6. Greenwald PW, Provataris J, Coffey J, Bijur P, Gallagher EJ. Low-dose naloxone does not improve morphine-induced nausea, vomiting or pruritus. Am J Emerg Med 2005;23(1):35–9.
7. Maxwell LG, Kaufmann SC, Bitzer S, Jackson Jr EV, McGready J, Kost-Byerly S, Kozlowski L, Rothman SK, Yaster M. The effects of a small-dose naloxone infusion on opioid-induced side effects and analgesia in children and adolescents treated with intravenous patient-controlled analgesia: a double-blind, prospective, randomized, controlled study. Anesth Analg 2005;100(4):953–8.
8. Terra SG, Tsunoda SM. Opioid antagonists in the treatment of pruritus from cholestatic liver disease. Ann Pharmacother 1998;32(11):1228–30.
9. Barsan WG, Olinger CP, Adams HP Jr, Brott TG, Eberle R, Biller J, Biros M, Marler J. Use of high dose naloxone in acute stroke: possible side-effects. Crit Care Med 1989;17(8):762–7.
10. Bing C, Yun-sheng L. Randomised double-blind clinical trial of moderate dosage naloxone in acute moderate and severe traumatic brain injury. Bull Hunan Med Univ 2002;27:58–60.
11. Langemark M. Naloxone in moderate dose does not aggravate chronic tension headache. Pain 1989;39(1):85–93.
12. Wride SR, Smith RE, Courtney PG. A fatal case of pulmonary oedema in a healthy young male following naloxone administration. Anaesth Intensive Care 1989;17(3):374–7.
13. Allen T. No adverse reaction. Ann Emerg Med 1989;18(1):116.
14. Pallasch TJ, Gill CJ. Naloxone-associated morbidity and mortality. Oral Surg Oral Med Oral Pathol 1981;52(6):602–3.
15. Rubin P, Swezey S, Blaschke T. Naloxone lowers plasma-prolactin in man. Lancet 1979;1(8129):1293.
16. Gibbs J, Newson T, Williams J, Davidson DC. Naloxone hazard in infant of opioid abuser. Lancet 1989;2(8655):159–60.
17. McGuire W, Fowler PW. Naloxone for narcotic exposed newborn infants: systematic review. Arch Dis Child Fetal Neonatal Ed 2003;88:308–11.

18. Clarke S, Dargan P. Towards evidence based emergency medicine: best BETs from the Manchester Royal Infirmary. Intravenous or intramuscular/subcutaneous naloxone in opioid overdose. Emerg Med J 2002;19(3):249.

19. Wasiak J, Clavisi O. Is subcutaneous or intramuscular naloxone as effective as intravenous naloxone in the treatment of life-threatening heroin overdose? Med J Aust 2002;176(10):495.

20. Ashton H, Hassan Z. Intranasal naloxone in suspected opioid overdose. Emerg Med J 2006;23:221–3.

21. Gal TJ. Naloxone reversal of buprenorphine-induced respiratory depression. Clin Pharmacol Ther 1989;45(1):66–71.

22. Rifat K, Magnin C, Morel D. L'analgésie per et postopératoire à la buprénorphine: effets cardio-circulatoires et respiratoires. [Pre- and postoperative buprenorphine analgesia: cardiocirculatory and respiratory effects.] Cah Anesthesiol 1984;32(1):33–6.

23. Ajayi AA, Campbell BC, Rubin PC, Reid JL. Effect of naloxone on the actions of captopril. Clin Pharmacol Ther 1985;38(5):560–5.

Naltrexone

General Information

Naltrexone is an orally-active long-acting pure opioid antagonist with no significant actions of its own. It antagonizes the actions of morphine-like drugs by preferentially binding to opioid receptors in the brain and other tissues, thereby displacing any opioid present and preventing the binding of any pure opioid agonist subsequently administered.

Naltrexone can be used on its own in detoxified individuals to discourage relapse.

The neurotoxic adverse effects of interferon alfa may be mediated by an action at opioid receptors, and naltrexone may antagonize some of this (SEDA-20, 83). Pruritus, probably mediated via enkephalins and opioids, may also be antagonized by naltrexone (SEDA-22, 104).

Gastrointestinal irritation and clinically insignificant increases in blood pressure are commonly reported. Fatigue, irritability, and reduced food intake are also reported.

Drug studies

Opioid dependence

Behavioral disturbances and aversive effects in particular have been observed when naltrexone has been used for treatment of opioid dependence; symptoms noted were loss of energy, gastrointestinal disturbances, and mental depression.

Naltrexone is the only licensed agent approved for the treatment of heroin addiction in Russia (1). In a randomized, placebo-controlled study in 52 opioid-dependent individuals, naltrexone improved outcomes. Five of those who took naltrexone reported abdominal discomfort and nausea and one had an allergic skin rash.

Alcohol dependence

When naltrexone was used in the treatment of alcohol dependence, 5–10% of patients discontinued treatment because of adverse effects (SEDA-20, 83).

The use of naltrexone in alcoholism has been reviewed, highlighting its favorable safety profile (2). It is associated with nausea, vomiting, headaches, anergia, reduced alertness, anxiety, depression, and rashes. Of these, nausea and vomiting are the most common.

Naltrexone 50 mg/day has been studied in early problem drinkers (3) and in people with severe alcohol dependence (4), with or without cognitive behavioral therapy (5,6). In other studies naltrexone and acamprosate have been compared and combined (7,8,9). All of these studies have confirmed the efficacy of naltrexone in reducing drinking and also the risk of relapse into excessive alcohol consumption and dependence. However, these effects are not maintained after 8-10 weeks, unless psychosocial therapeutic techniques and support are also in place. The combination of naltrexone and acamprosate together with behavioral interventions seems promising without causing unacceptable physical symptoms. More patients taking naltrexone plus acamprosate reported fatigue, reduced libido, and diarrhea compared with placebo. The preliminary data suggested that patients taking the combined medication had no more adverse reactions than the other groups, including the placebo-treated group (5). One needs to be cautious in patients with compromised liver function and liver function tests should be checked regularly for any 3- to 5-fold rise in liver enzymes when medication (naltrexone alone or in combination with acamprosate) needs to be withdrawn. Hepatitis status is also important, since one needs to determine if the patient is positive for hepatitis B and/or C due to previous high-risk behavior (for example polydrug intravenous use) since this will further compromise liver function.

Naltrexone significantly improved drinking outcomes in well-targeted alcohol-dependent individuals in a well-structured behavioral program (10,11). The potential of using long acting injectable naltrexone (400 micrograms) was evaluated in a multicenter, randomized, double-blind placebo-controlled, pilot study in 25 alcohol-dependent individuals (12). The reported adverse effects (nausea, dry mouth, vomiting, headache), were mild to moderate, and only two participants withdrew, because of injection site induration and angioedema, both of which were moderate and occurred after the second dose of naltrexone. Large-scale placebo-controlled studies are needed to determine whether injectable naltrexone is more effective and better tolerated than placebo and/or oral naltrexone in improving outcomes in alcohol-dependent individuals (13) and individuals with co-morbid schizophrenia and alcohol dependence (14,15).

A systematic review and meta-analysis of seven double-blind, randomized, placebo-controlled outpatient studies of naltrexone used in the treatment of alcohol dependence between 1976 and 2001 has shown that naltrexone was no more toxic than placebo and was not associated with a significantly greater number of withdrawals because of adverse effects (16). Naltrexone was more effective than placebo in reducing relapses to heavy drinking and improving alcohol abstinence in the short term, considering that the studies lasted for only 12 weeks. Additional long-term follow-up studies, with the possibility of studying outcomes of naltrexone treatment programs after stopping the drug and with suitable comparison groups, are necessary. Similar results with similar conclusions were seen in a 12-week randomized controlled trial in 55 alcohol-dependent men treated with naltrexone 50 mg or placebo (17).

To examine the relation between adverse effects profiles, study retention, and treatment outcomes in alcohol-dependent individuals receiving naltrexone for relapse prevention, 92 subjects had their adverse effects monitored weekly and categorized as either neuropsychiatric or gastrointestinal (18). The neuropsychiatric adverse effects had little effect on medication compliance but reduced the length of study retention. In contrast, the gastrointestinal adverse effects significantly affected medication compliance but not study retention.

In an open, single-blind, randomized study, naltrexone (50 mg/day) and acamprosate (1665–1998 mg/day) were used for 1 year by 157 recently detoxified alcohol-dependent men with moderate dependence (19). The time to first relapse was 63 days (naltrexone) and 42 days (acamprosate); after 1 year, 41% of those given naltrexone and 17% of those given acamprosate had not relapsed. Adverse effects were more common with naltrexone and were worse during the first 2 weeks of treatment. They included nausea (25 versus 4%), abdominal pain (23 versus 4%), drowsiness (35 versus 2%), headache (13 versus 6%), and nasal congestion (23 versus 7%).

The Health Technology Board of Scotland has concluded that in people with alcohol dependence, naltrexone reduces drinking (20). In a multicenter, double-blind, placebo-controlled, 12-week study of naltrexone 50 mg/day in 202 patients with alcohol dependence naltrexone was well tolerated, with few adverse effects: abdominal pain (8.6%), headache (7.5%), nausea (6.5%), and dizziness (5.4%); there were no changes in liver function tests (21). However, those who took naltrexone did not have significant improvements in drinking history or fewer relapses.

Smoking cessation

The effects of Community Reinforcement Approach and naltrexone have been compared for smoking cessation in 25 subjects (22). Naltrexone was well tolerated, but 18 complained of an unpleasant taste sensation. Those taking 50 mg/day (compared with 25 mg/day) had more headaches, nausea, dizziness, insomnia, sleepiness, and impaired taste perception.

The effectiveness of naltrexone (25 mg increased to 50 mg) in smoking cessation has been studied in a placebo-controlled study in 110 subjects (23). In the first week, naltrexone was associated with nausea, light-headedness, sedation, and flushing. After 4 weeks only light-headedness was significantly more common with naltrexone. One patient withdrew because of gastrointestinal distress.

Pruritus

Naltrexone 50 mg/day has been used to relieve pruritus in cholestatic liver disease in five patients (24). Pruritus scores fell, but two patients developed severe nausea, vomiting, light-headedness, or tremor, requiring withdrawal of treatment. The reviewers commented that these reactions may or may not have been related to opioid withdrawal and that the trial had had several design limitations. They pointed out that one concern relating to the chronic use of high-dose naltrexone is an asymptomatic rise in serum transaminases, although the doses used in this study have not been reported to produce liver function abnormalities.

Systematic reviews

The effectiveness of naltrexone in maintenance treatment of opioid and alcohol dependence has been systematically reviewed (25). There is no evidence to support the suggestion that naltrexone causes or exacerbates hepatocellular injury. There are reports of serious adverse events and even deaths after rapid detoxification procedures, and the authors suggested that naltrexone should not be used in this way. The risk of overdose and death from naltrexone withdrawal or receptor hypersensitivity has also been reported.

Organs and Systems

Nervous system

Headache occurred in two children, and an opioid withdrawal syndrome occurred in one child during the first 3 days of treatment when naltrexone was given for protracted apnea in children with increased beta-endorphin concentrations in the cerebrospinal fluid (26).

The literature on the efficacy and safety of naltrexone in children with autistic disorders has been critically reviewed (27). The most common reported adverse effect was transient sedation.

Naltrexone 15 mg was given to eight frequent tanners with the aim of establishing whether opioid blockade induces withdrawal symptoms (28). Nausea and jitteriness occurred in 50%, and in half of those the severity was such that they withdrew. These effects were considered to be consistent with symptoms of opiate withdrawal.

Psychological, psychiatric

Panic attacks precipitated by naltrexone have been reported (29).

- A 29-year-old woman with bulimia nervosa and a family history of anxiety was enrolled in a trial of naltrexone (100 mg/day). She had no history of opioid use. Within hours of her first dose she experienced alarm, anxiety, chest discomfort, shortness of breath, a fear of dying, sweating, nausea, and derealization. She was unable to remain at home or to go out alone. For 3 days she continued to take naltrexone, with an increasing frequency of panic attacks. On day 4 she was treated with alprazolam (0.5 mg) but relapsed after further naltrexone. Withdrawal of naltrexone led to complete remission of symptoms.

This effect was attributed to an action of naltrexone in removing the endogenous opioid effect at OP_3 (μ) opioid receptors in the locus ceruleus and thus resulting in unchecked noradrenergic hyperactivity.

Acute psychosis secondary to the use of naltrexone has been reported (30).

- A 44-year-old physically healthy woman developed auditory and visual hallucinations and persecutory delusions. She had been given naltrexone hydrochloride 50 mg/day 3 days before the acute psychotic incident in order to prevent relapse of alcohol dependence. Her psychotic symptoms completely resolved 48 hours after withdrawal of naltrexone.

In studies of its use in treating alcohol, opioid, and nicotine dependence, naltrexone has not been reported to cause depression or dysphoria. Patients who complain of naltrexone-associated dysphoria often have co-morbid depressive disorders or depression resulting from opioid or alcohol withdrawal states (31). Co-morbid depression is not a contraindication to naltrexone. Small pilot studies have supported the use of naltrexone in combination with antidepressants for the treatment of patients with co-morbid depression. The risk of non-fatal overdose is significantly increased after naltrexone treatment, as a result of reduced tolerance, compared with patients taking substitution methadone (32).

Hematologic

Idiopathic thrombocytopenic purpura has been attributed to naltrexone (33).

Gastrointestinal

The risk factors for naltrexone-induced nausea have been studied in 120 alcohol-dependent patients in an open trial (34). After 5–30 days of abstinence, they received a bolus dose of naltrexone 25 mg followed by 50 mg/day for 10 weeks. Moderate to severe nausea was reported in 15%. The risk of nausea was significantly predicted by poor medication compliance, intensity of drinking during treatment, short duration of abstinence, young age, and female sex.

Gastrointestinal adverse effects of naltrexone were also observed in 183 alcohol-dependent individuals who received either naltrexone or nefazodone (35). These adverse effects predicated early termination of naltrexone used to treat alcohol dependence (36).

Liver

Reversible hepatocellular injury has been reported with naltrexone in doses of up to 300 mg/day, which is five times that usually used for opioid blockade (SED-11, 147) (37). Five of twenty-six patients treated with naltrexone for obesity developed raised serum transaminase activities after 3–8 weeks of treatment. In another study in which 60 obese subjects received naltrexone for 8 weeks, there were abnormal liver function tests in six patients. Three patients failed to complete the course. Nausea and vomiting occurred within the first 24 hours of treatment but responded to a reduction in dose. There were also changes in mentation such as decreased mental acuity, depression, and anxiety, all of which resolved after withdrawal. This is significant, as adverse effects from naltrexone have previously been attributed to mild physical withdrawal syndromes.

Biliary tract

A woman with chronic cholestasis and disabling pruritus had severe but transient opioid withdrawal-like reactions after oral naltrexone 12.5 mg and 2 mg (38). This observation suggests the hypothesis that increased central opioidergic tone is a component of the pathophysiology of cholestasis.

Skin

Skin rashes have been attributed to naltrexone (SEDA-21, 92).

Musculoskeletal

Rhabdomyolysis has been attributed to naltrexone (39).

- A 28-year-old alcoholic was given naltrexone 50 mg/day on the eighth day of a detoxification regimen. On day 17 there was a marked rise in creatine kinase activity (2654 U/l) but no accompanying symptoms of myalgia, weakness, or chest pain. Naltrexone was withheld immediately. The creatine kinase peaked at over 18 000 U/l on day 19 and then fell to within the reference range by day 25. A diagnosis of rhabdomyolysis without accompanying renal insufficiency was suggested.

Long-Term Effects

Drug abuse

Three opiate-dependent individuals abused intravenous naltrexone, believing it to be diamorphine, and developed acute opiate withdrawal symptoms; they were managed with a combined regimen of diazepam, prochlorperazine, and hyoscine (40,41).

Inappropriate use of naltrexone with heroin in an opioid-dependent individual has been reported (42).

- A 39-year-old man took naltrexone 150 mg with an unknown quantity of smoked heroin. He was extremely agitated, disoriented, and sweating, with episodes of profuse projectile vomiting and diarrhea. His pupils were dilated but reactive to light, his heart rate was regular at 180/minute, and his respiration was 40/minute. He was given midazolam 20 mg and droperidol 15 mg but remained acutely confused and became increasingly violent. A lumbar puncture and a CT scan of the brain were normal. He became less agitated over the next 12 hours and took his own discharge.

Drug dependence

The use of naltrexone as constraint therapy in addicted physicians has been reviewed (43). Drug-free retention rates were less than 20%, suggesting that naltrexone was not very effective.

Susceptibility Factors

Alcohol dependence

The safety and effectiveness of naltrexone in alcohol-dependent populations with comorbid axis 1 disorders has been explored in a 12-week multicenter randomized trial (44). The results suggested that naltrexone can be used safely in this group of individuals. Naltrexone was associated with more reported nervousness and restlessness than disulfiram or placebo. Other adverse effects, including after-taste, blurred vision, confusion, constipation, drowsiness, dry mouth, loss of appetite, nausea, and tremor, were more likely to be experienced by subjects taking any medication, i.e. naltrexone (n = 59), disulfiram (n = 66), or naltrexone + disulfiram (n = 65), than subjects taking placebo (n = 64). The combination of Naltrexone + disulfiram was associated with significantly more abdominal pain, nausea, vomiting, numb limbs, pins and needles, irregular heartbeat, restlessness, and higher degrees of depression and general distress, than those taking either medication alone.

Drug Administration

Drug formulations

An alternative way of delivering naltrexone is in a sustained-release form, such as implants or other depot formulations. Adverse effects from naltrexone implants are probably associated with high plasma naltrexone concentrations (45). The adverse effects include irritability, dysphoria, nausea, and muscle discomfort during the first week after insertion of the implant. Individuals can develop local tissue reactions after repeated implantation and they can lead to local necrosis.

Parenteral modified-release naltrexone in two doses (190 and 380 mg) together with a low-intensity psychoso-

Table 3 Frequency of adverse effects of modified-release naltrexone

Adverse event	Dose	Frequency (n)
Nausea	190 mg	25% (53)
	380 mg	33% (68)
Headache	190 mg	16% (33)
	380 mg	22% (45)
Fatigue	190 mg	16% (34)
	380 mg	20% (41)
Discontinuation	Placebo	6.7%(14)
because	190 mg	6.7%(14)
of adverse events	380 mg	14% (29)

cial intervention has been studied in a randomized placebo-controlled trial in 627 individuals with alcohol dependence (46). There were few adverse events, the most common being nausea (mostly mild or moderate and during only the first month of treatment), headache, and fatigue (Table 1). There was no hepatotoxicity. Other adverse events included insomnia, vomiting, reduced appetite, diarrhea, dizziness, nasopharyngitis, upper respiratory tract infection, and pain at the injection-site.

In 42 healthy subjects a long-acting intramuscular naltrexone formulation was well tolerated and there were no serious adverse events (47).

Naltrexone implants were well tolerated in an open study in 13 opioid-dependent patients, with minimal adverse effects (48).

Drug administration route

Six cases of complications loosely related to the use of naltrexone pellet implantation during the highly controversial rapid and ultra-rapid opioid detoxification procedures have been reported (49). These included pulmonary edema, prolonged opioid withdrawal states, drug toxicity, withdrawal from cross-dependence to alcohol and benzodiazepines, aspiration pneumonia, and death. The risk of these controversial procedures and of naltrexone in this novel delivery system are high; a robust scientifically validated program of research is needed to justify such treatment packages.

Drug–Drug Interactions

Clonidine
When naltrexone was given to a group of clonidine-detoxified opioid-dependent subjects, several complained of anorexia and weight loss (50).

Diazepam
The effects of naltrexone on diazepam intoxication were investigated in 26 non-drug-abusing subjects who received either naltrexone 50 mg or placebo and 90 minutes later oral diazepam 10 mg in a double-blind crossover trial (51). Naltrexone was significantly associated with negative mood states, such as sedation, fatigue, and anxiety, compared with placebo, while positive states (friendliness, vigor, liking the effects of diazepam, feeling high from diazepam) were significantly more common with placebo. Naltrexone significantly delayed the time to peak diazepam concentrations (135 minutes) compared with placebo (75 minutes), but there were no significant differences in the concentrations of nordiazepam, the main metabolite of diazepam, at any stage in the study.

References

1. Krupitsky EM, Zvartau EE, Masalov DV, Tsoi MV, Burakov AM, Egorova V Y, Didenko TY, Romanova TN, Ivanova EB, Bespalov AY, Verbitskaya EV, Neznanov NG, Grinenko AY, O'Brien CP, Woody GE. Naltrexone for heroin dependence treatment in St Petersburg, Russia. J Substance Abuse Treat 2004;26:285–94.

2. Pettinati HM, O'Brien CP, Rabinowitz AR, Wortman SM, Oslin DW, Kampman KM, Dackis CA. The status of naltrexone in the treatment of alcohol dependence: specific effects on heavy drinking. J Clin Psychopharmacol 2006;26(6):610–25.

3. Kranzler HR, Armeli S, Tennen H, Blomquist D, Oncken C, Detry N, Feinn R. Targeted naltrexone for early problem drinkers. J Clin Psychopharmacol 2003;23:294–304.

4. Froehlich J, O'Malley S, Hyytiä P, Davidson D, Farren C. Preclinical and clinical studies on naltrexone: what have they taught each other? Alcoholism: Clin Exp Res 2003;27:533–9.

5. Balldin J, Berglund M, Borg S, Mansson M, Berndtsen P, Franck J, Gustafsson L, Halidin J, Nilsson L-H, Stolt G, Willender A. A 6-month controlled naltrexone study: combined effect with cognitive behavioural therapy in outpatient treatment of alcohol dependence. Alcoholism: Clin Exp Res 2003;27:1142–9.

6. O'Malley S, Rovinsaville BJ, Farren C, Namkoong K, Wu R, Robinson J, O'Connor PQ. Initial and maintenance naltrexone treatment for alcohol dependence using primary care vs speciality care. Arch Intern Med 2003;163:1695–704.

7. Kiefer F, Jahn H, Tarnaske T, Helwig H, Briken P, Holzbach R, Kampf P, Stracke R, Baehr M, Naber D, Wiedermons K. Comparing and combining naltrexone and acamprosate in relapse prevention of alcoholism. Arch Gen Psychiatry 2003;60:92–9.

8. COMBINE Study Research Group. Testing combined pharmacotherapies and behavioural interventions for alcohol dependence (The COMBINE Study). A pilot feasibility study. Alcohol Clin Exp Res 2003;27:1123–31.

9. Johnston BA, O'Malley SS, Ciravlo DA, Roache JD, Chambers RA, Sarid-Segal O, Couper D. Dose-ranging kinetics and behavioural pharmacology of naltrexone and acamprosate, both alone and combined, in alcohol-dependent subjects. J Clin Psychopharmacol 2003;23:281–93.

10. Rohsenov DJ. What place does naltrexone have in the treatment of alcoholism? CNS Drugs 2004;18:547–60.

11. Anton RF, Drobes DJ, Voronin K, Durazo-Avizu R, Moak D. Naltrexone effects on alcohol consumption in a clinical laboratory paradigm: temporal effects of drining. Psychopharamacology 2004;173:32.40.

12. Johnson BA, Art-Daoud N, Aubin H-J, van den Brink W, Guzzetta R, Loewy J, Silverman B, Ehrich E. A pilot evaluation of the safety and tolerability of repeat dose administration of long-acting injectable naltrexone (Vivitrex®) in patients with alcohol dependence. Alcohol Clin Exp Res 2004;28:1356–61.

13. Kranzler HR, Wesson DR, Billot E. Naltrexone depot for treatment of alcohol dependence: a multi-centre, randomized, placebo-controlled clinical trial. Alcohol Clin Exp Res 2004;28:1051–9.

14. Petrakis IL, O'Malley S, Rounsaville B, Poling J, McHugh-Strong C, Krystal J H. Naltrexone augmentation of neuroleptic treatment in alcohol abusing patients with schizophrenia. Psychopharmacology 2004;172:291–7.

15. Worrodi I, Adami H, Sherr J, Avila M, Hong E, Thaker G K. Naltrexone treatment of tardive dyskinesia in patients with schizophrenia. J Clin Psychopharmacol 2004;24:441–5.

16. Streeton C, Whelan G. Naltrexone, a relapse prevention maintenance treatment of alcohol dependence: a meta-analysis of randomized controlled trials. Alcohol Alcohol 2001;36(6):544–52.

17. Morris PL, Hopwood M, Whelan G, Gardiner J, Drummond E. Naltrexone for alcohol dependence: a randomized controlled trial. Addiction 2001;96(11):1565–73.

18. Oncken C, Van Kirk J, Kranzler HR. Adverse effects of oral naltrexone: analysis of data from two clinical trials. Psychopharmacology (Berl) 2001;154(4):397–402.

19. Rubio G, Jimenez-Arriero MA, Ponce G, Palomo T. Naltrexone versus acamprosate: one year follow-up of alcohol dependence treatment. Alcohol Alcohol 2001;36(5):419–25.

20. Slattery J, Chick J, Cochrane M, Craig J, Godfrey C, Macpherson K, Parrott S, Quinn S, Tochel C, Watson H. Prevention of relapse in alcohol dependenceGlasgow: Health Technology Board for Scotland;. 2003 Health Technology Assessment Report 3.

21. Guardia J, Caso C, Arias F, Gual A, Sanahuja J, Ramirez M, Mengual I, Gonzalvo B, Segura L, Trujols J, Casas M. A double-blind, placebo-controlled study of naltrexone in the treatment of alcohol-dependence disorder: results from a multicenter clinical trial. Alcohol Clin Exp Res 2002;26(9):1381–7.

22. Roozen HG, Van Beers SEC, Weevers HJA, Breteler MHM, Willemsen MC, Postmus PE, Kerkhof AJFM. Effects on smoking cessation: naltrexone combined with cognitive behavioural treatment based on the community reinforcement approach. Substance Use Misuse 2006;41:45–60.

23. King A, de Wit H, Riley RC, Cao D, Niaura R, Hatsukami D. Efficacy of naltrexone in smoking cessation: a preliminary study and an examination of sex differences. Nicotine Tobacco Res 2006;8(5):671–82.

24. Terra SG, Tsunoda SM. Opioid antagonists in the treatment of pruritus from cholestatic liver disease. Ann Pharmacother 1998;32(11):1228–30.

25. Roozen HG, de Waart R, van der Windt DAWM, van den Brink W, de Jong CAJ, Kerkhof AJFM. A systematic review of the effectiveness of naltrexone in the maintenance treatment of opioid and alcohol dependence. Eur Neuropsychopharmacol 2006;16:311–23.

26. Myer EC, Morris DL, Brase DA, Dewey WL, Zimmerman AW. Naltrexone therapy of apnea in children with elevated cerebrospinal fluid beta-endorphin. Ann Neurol 1990;27(1):75–80.

27. Elchaar GM, Maisch NM, Gianni Augusto LM, Wehring HJ. Efficacy and safety of naltrexone use in pediatric patients with autistic disorder. Ann Pharmacother 2006;40(6):1086–95.

28. Kaur M, Liguori A, Lang W, Rapp SR, Fleischer AB, Feldman SR. Induction of withdrawal-like symptoms in a small randomized, controlled trial of opioid blockade in frequent tanners. J Am Acad Dermatol 2006;54:709–11.

29. Maremmani I, Marini G, Fornai F. Naltrexone-induced panic attacks. Am J Psychiatry 1998;155(3):447.

30. Amraoui A, Burgos V, Baron P, Alexandre JY. Psychose delirante aiguë au cours d'un traitement par chlorhydrate de naltrexone. [Acute delirium psychosis induced by naltrexone chlorhydrate.] Presse Méd 1999;28(25):1361–2.

31. Miotto K, McCann M, Basch J, Rawson R, Ling W. Naltrexone and dysphoria: fact or myth? Am J Addict 2002;11(2):151–60.

32. Ritter AJ. Naltrexone in the treatment of heroin dependence: relationship with depression and risk of overdose. Aust NZ J Psychiatry 2002;36(2):224–8.

33. Atkinson RL, Berke LK, Drake CR, Bibbs ML, Williams FL, Kaiser DL. Effects of long-term therapy with naltrexone on body weight in obesity. Clin Pharmacol Ther 1985;38(4):419–22.

34. O'Malley SS, Krishnan-Sarin S, Farren C, O'Connor PG. Naltrexone-induced nausea in patients treated for alcohol dependence: clinical predictors and evidence for opioid-mediated effects. J Clin Psychopharmacol 2000;20(1):69–76.

35. Kranzler HR, Modesto-Lowe V, Van Kirk J. Naltrexone vs. nefazodone for treatment of alcohol dependence. A placebo-controlled trial. Neuropsychopharmacology 2000;22(5):493–503.

36. Rohsenow DJ, Colby SM, Monti PM, Swift RM, Martin RA, Mueller TI, Gordon A, Eaton CA. Predictors of compliance with naltrexone among alcoholics. Alcohol Clin Exp Res 2000;24(10):1542–9.

37. Anonymous. Naltrexone hydrochloride. Drugs Today 1985;21:257.

38. Jones EA, Dekker LR. Florid opioid withdrawal-like reaction precipitated by naltrexone in a patient with chronic cholestasis. Gastroenterology 2000;118(2):431–2.

39. Zaim S, Wiley DB, Albano SA. Rhabdomyolysis associated with naltrexone. Ann Pharmacother 1999;33(3):312–3.

40. Bristow K, Meek R, Clark N. Acute opioid withdrawal in the emergency department: inadvertent naltrexone abuse? Emerg Med (Fremantle) 2001;13(3):359–63.

41. Quigley MA, Boyce SH. Unintentional rapid opioid detoxification. Emerg Med J 2001;18(6):494–5.

42. Boyce SH, Armstrong PAR, Stevenson J. Effect of inappropriate naltrexone use in a heroin misuser. Emerg Med J 2003;20:381–2.

43. Kreek MJ, Bart G, Lilly C, Laforge KS, Nielson DA. Pharmacogenetics and human molecular genetics of opiate and cocaine addictions and their treatments. Pharmacol Rev 2005;57(1):1–26.

44. Petrakis IL, Poling J, Levinson C, Nich C, Carroll K, Rounsaville B. Naltrexone and disulfiram in patients with alcohol dependence and comorbid psychiatric disorders. Biol Psychiatry 2005;57(10):1128–37.

45. Olsen L, Christophersen AS, Frogopsahl G, Waal H, Morland J. Plasma concentrations during naltrexone implant treatment of opiate-dependent patients. Br J Clin Pharmacol 2004;58:219–22.

46. Garbutt JC, Kranzler HR, O'Malley SS, Gastfriend DR, Pettinati HM, Silverman BL, Loewy JW, Ehrich EW. Efficacy and tolerability of long-acting injectable naltrexone for alcohol dependence. JAMA 2005;293(13):1617–25.

47. Dunbar JL, Turncliff RZ, Dong Q, Silverman BL, Ehrich EW, Lasseter KC. Single- and multiple-dose pharmacokinetics of long-acting injectable naltrexone. Alcoholism Clin Exp Res 2006;30:480–90.

48. Waal H, Frogopsahl G, Olsen L, Christophersen AS, Morland J. Naltrexone implants—duration, tolerability and clinical usefulness: a pilot study. Eur Addict Res 2006;12(3):138–44.

49. Hamilton RJ, Olmedo RE, Shah S, Hung OL, Howland MA, Perrone J, Nelson LS, Lewin NL, Hoffman RS. Complications of ultrarapid opioid detoxification with subcutaneous naltrexone pellets. Acad Emerg Med 2002;9(1):63–8.

50. Sternbach HA, Annitto W, Pottash AL, Gold MS. Anorexic effects of naltrexone in man. Lancet 1982;1(8268):388–9.

51. Swift R, Davidson D, Rosen S, Fitz E, Camara P. Naltrexone effects on diazepam intoxication and pharmacokinetics in humans. Psychopharmacology (Berl) 1998;135(3):256–62.

Oxycodone

General Information

Oxycodone is an opioid analgesic that is 1.5 times as potent as morphine and has a longer duration of action.

Drug studies

Pain relief

The postoperative analgesic effects of intravenous ketamine 10 mg and oxycodone 2 mg have been compared in a randomized, double-blind study in 40 tonsillectomized men (1). There were no significant differences between the two analgesics. The patients found ketamine more acceptable than oxycodone. Oxycodone was associated with more skin problems, especially pruritus. Oxycodone also caused a significantly lower respiratory rate with lower oxygen saturation throughout the recovery period and increased sedation throughout the study.

The effects of modified-release oxycodone in osteoarthritic pain have been evaluated in a placebo-controlled, double-blind trial in 133 patients (2). Oxycodone was effective, and although opioid-related adverse effects were frequent they were considered acceptable by the authors.

In a double-blind, randomized, crossover comparison of the efficacy and safety of modified-release oxycodone bd and immediate-release oxycodone qds in 57 patients with intervertebral disc disease or osteoarthritis, eleven patients withdrew: eight with nausea and constipation while taking modified-release oxycodone and three (one with migraine and two with nausea, vomiting, and headaches) while taking immediate-release oxycodone (3). There were no statistically significant differences in the adverse effects profiles between the two formulations. The overall incidence of adverse effects fell over the three phases of the study: from 89% (51/57 patients) during titration to 77% (36/47 patients) in stage 1 and 62% (29/47 patients) in stage 2. The most common adverse effects were constipation, nausea, pruritus, somnolence, and dizziness, the frequency of which fell with time; the incidence of constipation remained constant.

In a randomized, double-blind, crossover study, previous findings on the adverse effects of oxycodone among sufferers of postherpetic neuralgia were confirmed (4). Oxycodone was analgesic in this group, although 76% of the sample reported adverse effects compared with 49% of the placebo group. Constipation, nausea, and sedation were the most frequently reported adverse effects.

Two studies of oxycodone in patients with cancer pain have been carried out. In the first, modified-release and immediate-release oxycodone were compared (5) in a multicenter, double-blind trial in 180 patients who were given either modified-release oxycodone, mean dose 114 mg bd, or immediate-release oxycodone 127 mg qds, four times a day for cancer-related pain.

A 5-day comparison showed no significant difference in the analgesic effects of the two formulations, both of which provided effective relief of pain. However, of the 160 patients who received at least one dose of medication, 104 reported a total of 295 adverse events, significantly fewer being reported with modified-release oxycodone (109) than immediate-release oxycodone (186). Reported adverse effects included: nausea (18 versus 26%), vomiting (11 versus 23%), and constipation (9 versus 17%). With immediate-release oxycodone headache was reported by 7% and anxiety by 5%; neither was reported with modified-release oxycodone. Altogether, 7% of the modified-release group and 11% of the immediate-release group discontinued medication because of adverse effects. It is suggested that the equianalgesic effect is likely to be a factor of the rapid initial release of the modified-release formulation, allowing adequate drug concentrations to establish sufficient receptor activation, followed by a slower release of the remaining drug, which may be responsible for the reduction in adverse effects. Alternatively the peaks achieved with each administration of medication may account for the observed difference in the rates of adverse effects between the two formulations.

The second study was a randomized, double-blind, crossover comparison of the safety and efficacy of oral modified-release oxycodone with modified-release morphine in 32 patients with cancer pain, nine of whom completed the trial (6). The average dose of oxycodone was 47 mg bd compared with 73 mg bd of morphine. There were no significant differences in the degrees of sedation, nausea, or pain intensity experienced by the subjects on the different regimens and the results suggested that oxycodone may be used as an alternative to morphine.

Organs and Systems

Death

The involvement of oxycodone in drug-related deaths has been reviewed in 1243 confirmed drug-related deaths in 23 states in the USA during August 1999 to January 2002 (7). Each case was evaluated to determine the role of oxycodone and especially the controlled-release formulation. Only 30 (3.3%) cases involved oxycodone as the single reported pharmacological agent, and of these 12 were linked to the controlled-release formulation (OxyContin®). Of the other cases 96-97% were multiple drug deaths in which there was at least one other contributory drug in addition to oxycodone. The drugs that were most commonly combined with oxycodone were a benzodiazepine (8), alcohol, cocaine, other opioids (9), cannabinoids, or antidepressants. This highlights the increased risk of oxycodone abuse and its contribution to either drug-induced or drug-related deaths.

Long-Term Effects

Drug abuse

In 2002 an estimated 1.9 million people were using oxycodone illicitly in the USA; emergency room reports of oxycodone abuse increased to 560% (22 397 cases) from 1995 to 2002 (10).

Drug withdrawal

A patient with atypical oxycodone withdrawal had restlessness and delusions (11).

Susceptibility Factors

Genetic

A 60-year-old man, who was taking rifampicin, had negative urine drug screens for oxycodone, despite using a combination of immediate- and modified-release oxycodone for chronic pain (12). He had an intermediate CYP2D6 genotype, and the authors suggested that rifampicin induced CYP3A4 and CYP2D6, causing increased metabolism of oxycodone, inadequate pain control, and negative drug urine screening. This falsely increased the physician's confidence that the patient was not diverting his medication.

Age

Children may have a faster rate of clearance of oxycodone than adults, and ventilatory depression may be greater than with comparable opioids in children (SEDA-19, 85).

Hepatic disease

In end-stage cirrhosis, reduced clearance and prolonged half-life of oxycodone may necessitate dosage reduction (SEDA-22, 101).

Drug Administration

Drug formulations

Modified-release oxycodone has been reviewed comprehensively in relation to its pharmacokinetics and pharmacodynamics, impact on health economics, addiction potential, and use in palliative care (13).

A double-blind, randomized, crossover comparison of modified-release or immediate-release oxycodone has been carried out in 30 patients with cancer pain (14). There were no significant differences between the two groups with respect to pain intensity or acceptability of therapy. More than 80% of the patients did not require rescue medication. Adverse effects were similar with the two formulations and occurred in relatively low numbers compared with previous morphine studies. The greatest difference in adverse effects was in the incidence of vomiting, which occurred in 6% of those given immediate-release morphine, and none of those given modified-release morphine. The modified-release formulation provided equal analgesia with the benefit of less frequent dosing.

In a systematic review of the safety and efficacy of modified-release oxycodone 16 trials were identified; 7 addressed the safety and efficacy of oxycodone for the treatment of non-cancer pain (15). In these studies, modified-release oxycodone offered no significant advantage over immediate-release oxycodone. There was no consistent beneficial effect on quality of life, despite adequate analgesia. Opioid adverse effects, such as constipation, nausea, vomiting, and drowsiness, were more frequent and severe with oxycodone than with placebo. In six studies, modified-release oxycodone was compared with immediate-release oxycodone in cancer and non-cancer pain. In only one study was modified-release oxycodone superior; in the other five there were no significant differences in analgesic effect. In five randomized, double-blind comparisons there was no advantage in analgesic efficacy nor a consistent reduction in adverse effects with modified-release oxycodone compared with modified-release morphine, hydromorphone, or methadone.

In a multicenter, randomized, double-blind, placebo-controlled, parallel-group, 6-week study in 159 patients with moderate to severe pain due to diabetic neuropathy, controlled-release oxycodone 10 mg was effective at a relatively low average daily dose (52 mg), which was 33% of the maximum dose allowed (16). The adverse effects were predictably opioid-related, but there were no significant differences between placebo and oxycodone in the number of patients who withdrew because of adverse events.

In a randomized, double-blind, crossover comparison in 36 patients the mean dose of controlled-release oxycodone was 40 mg/day (17). Oxycodone was a significantly better analgesic than benzatropine, which was used as a comparator. The incidence of adverse effects was the same with the two treatments (n=131 with oxycodone and n=107 with benzatropine). Four patients had serious adverse effects, three with benzatropine. Only one patient who took oxycodone had a serious adverse reaction, severe opioid withdrawal symptoms during the washout period.

These results contrast with those of similarly constructed studies 1 year before in patients with chronic cancer and non-cancer pain (SEDA-27, 93). Similarly, in a randomized, double-blind, placebo-controlled, parallel-group comparison of oxycodone 10 mg plus paracetamol 325 mg and controlled-release oxycodone 20 mg in post-surgical acute pain, the combination therapy was significantly better in four out of the five outcome measures of pain intensity and pain relief (18).

Drug administration route

Oxycodone has been available in oral form for at least 70 years and is rarely given by other routes. In a study of subcutaneous oxycodone hydrochloride 100 mg/ml for opioid rotation in 63 patients with cancer pain (maximum dose 4.5–660 mg in 24 hours for 1–49 days) there was local toxicity in only two cases, and this included central pallor of the skin at the needle site with surrounding erythema and bruising; there was no necrosis (19). The design of the study made it difficult to compare the adverse effects profile of subcutaneous oxycodone with oral oxycodone or other opioids. Randomized controlled trials are needed to support the conclusions that subcutaneous oxycodone is free from adverse effects and is a better vehicle for analgesia in terminal cancer.

Drug overdose

- A 47-year-old man with a history of drug abuse and suicide attempts was found dead at home, with evidence of cocaine abuse and multiple drug ingestion (20). The concentration of citalopram in the femoral blood was 0.88 mg/l and the heart blood concentration 1.16 mg/l. Femoral blood concentrations of the other drugs were as follows: cocaine 30 µg/l; oxycodone 60 µg/l; promethazine 20 µg/l; propoxyphene 20 µg/l; and norpropoxyphene 70 µg/l.

Drug-Drug Interactions

The involvement of oxycodone in drug-related deaths has been studied by evaluating 1014 deaths in the USA during the period August 1999 to January 2002. The cases were only those in which oxycodone was proven to have been a contributory factor (21). Deaths involving oxycodone abuse in combination with other drugs increased significantly with time. The most frequently cited combinations were oxycodone with benzodiazepines, alcohol, cocaine, other opioids, marijuana, and/or antidepressants. Oxycodone blood concentrations in those cases were about 50% lower than in oxycodone-only drug-related deaths.

Selective serotonin reuptake inhibitors

Serotonin syndrome has been reported in a few patients taking oxycodone and an SSRI.

- A 70-year-old woman developed the serotonin syndrome after taking oxycodone 40 mg bd in addition to fluvoxamine 200 mg/day (22).
- A 34 year-old man had visual hallucinations and severe tremor after dramatically increasing his dosage of oxycodone while taking stable doses of sertraline and ciclosporin. Withdrawal of ciclosporin did not resolve his symptoms, but withdrawal of sertraline did (23).

Oxycodone in a substrate for CYP2D6 (24) and might inhibit the metabolism of SSRIs that are also metabolized by this isoenzyme.

References

1. Levanen J. Ketamine and oxycodone in the management of postoperative pain. Mil Med 2000;165(6):450–5.
2. Roth SH, Fleischmann RM, Burch FX, Dietz F, Bockow B, Rapoport RJ, Rutstein J, Lacouture PG. Around-the-clock, controlled-release oxycodone therapy for osteoarthritis-

related pain: placebo-controlled trial and long-term evaluation. Arch Intern Med 2000;160(6):853–60.

3. Hale ME, Fleischmann R, Salzman R, Wild J, Iwan T, Swanton RE, Kaiko RF, Lacouture PG. Efficacy and safety of controlled-release versus immediate-release oxycodone: randomized, double-blind evaluation in patients with chronic back pain. Clin J Pain 1999;15(3):179–83.

4. Watson CP, Babul N. Efficacy of oxycodone in neuropathic pain: a randomized trial in postherpetic neuralgia. Neurology 1998;50(6):1837–41.

5. Kaplan R, Parris WC, Citron ML, Zhukovsky D, Reder RF, Buckley BJ, Kaiko RF. Comparison of controlled-release and immediate-release oxycodone tablets in patients with cancer pain. J Clin Oncol 1998;16(10):3230–7.

6. Bruera E, Belzile M, Pituskin E, Fainsinger R, Darke A, Harsanyi Z, Babul N, Ford I. Randomized, double-blind, cross-over trial comparing safety and efficacy of oral controlled-release oxycodone with controlled-release morphine in patients with cancer pain. J Clin Oncol 1998;16(10):3222–9.

7. Cone EJ, Fant RV, Rohey JM, Caplan YH, Ballina M, Reder RF, Spyker D, Haddox JD. Oxycodone involvement in drug abuse deaths: a DAWN-based classification scheme applied to an oxycodone postmorten database containing over 1000 cases. J Anal Toxicol 2003;27:57–67.

8. Burrows DL, Hagardorn AN, Harlan GC, Wallen EDB, Ferslew KE. A fatal drug interaction between oxycodone and clonazepam. J Forensic Sci 2003;48:683–6.

9. Spiller HA. Postmorten oxycodone and hydrocodone blood concentrations. J Forensic Sci 2003;48:429–31.

10. Kreek MJ, Bart G, Lilly C, Laforge KS, Nielson DA. Pharmacogenetics and human molecular genetics of opiate and cocaine addictions and their treatments. Pharmacol Rev 2005;57(1):1–26.

11. Fishbain DA, Goldberg M, Rosomoff RS, Rosomoff H. Atypical oxycodone withdrawal syndrome. Pain Management 1989;76Mar/Apr.

12. Lee H, Lewis LD, Tsongalis GJ, McMullin M, Schur BC, Wong SH, Yeo KJ. Negative urine opioid screening caused by rifampin-mediated induction of oxycodone hepatic metabolism. Clin Chim Acta 2006;367:196–200.

13. Davis MP, Varga J, Dickerson D, Walsh D, LeGrantd SB, Lagman R. Normal-release and controlled-release oxycodone: pharmacokinetics, pharmacodynamics, and controversy. Support Care Cancer 2003;11:84–92.

14. Stambaugh JE, Reder RF, Stambaugh MD, Stambaugh H, Davis M. Double-blind, randomized comparison of the analgesic and pharmacokinetic profiles of controlled- and immediate-release oral oxycodone in cancer pain patients. J Clin Pharmacol 2001;41(5):500–6.

15. Rischitelli DG, Karbowicz SH. Safety and efficacy of controlled-release oxycodone: a systematic literature review. Pharmacotherapy 2002;22(7):898–904.

16. Gimbel JS, Richards P, Portenoy RK. Controlled-release oxycodone for pain in diabetic neuropathy. Neurology 2003;60:927–34.

17. Watson CPN, Moulin D, Watt-Watson J, Gordon A, Eisenhoffer J. Controlled-release oxycodone relieves neuropathic pain: a randomized controlled trial in painful diabetic neuropathy. Pain 2003;105:71–8.

18. Gammaitoni AR, Gater BS, Bulloch S, Lacouture P, Caruso F, Ma T, Schlagneck T. Randomised, double-blind, placebo-controlled comparison of the analgesic efficacy of oxycodone 10mg/acetaminophen 325 mg versus controlled-release oxycodone 20 mg in postsurgical pain. J Clin Pharmacol 2003;43:296–304.

19. Gagnon B, Bielech M, Watanabe S, Walker P, Hanson J, Bruera E. The use of intermittent subcutaneous injections of oxycodone for opioid rotation in patients with cancer pain. Support Care Cancer 1999;7(4):265–70.

20. Fu K, Konrad RJ, Hardy RW, Brissie RM, Robinson CA. An unusual multiple drug intoxication case involving citalopram. J Anal Toxicol 2000;24(7):648–50.

21. Cone EJ, Fant RV, Rohay JM, Caplan YH, Ballina M, Reder RF, Haddox JD. Oxycodone involvement in drug abuse deaths. Evidence for toxic multiple drug-drug interactions. J Anal Toxicol 2004;28:616–24.

22. Karunatilake H, Buckley NA. Serotonin syndrome induced by fluvoxamine and oxycodone. Ann Pharmacother 2006;40(1):155–7.

23. Rosebraugh CJ, Flockhart DA, Yasuda SU, Woosley RL. Visual hallucination and tremor induced by sertraline and oxycodone in a bone marrow transplant patient. J Clin Pharmacol 2001;41(2):224–7.

24. Otton SV, Wu D, Joffe RT, Cheung SW, Sellers EM. Inhibition by fluoxetine of cytochrome P450 2D6 activity. Clin Pharmacol Ther 1993;53(4):401–9.

Oxymorphone

General Information

Oxymorphone is a pyridine-ring unsubstituted pyridomorphinan, with greater analgesic potency than morphine, whose antinociceptive effects are mediated predominantly through DOR and MOR opioid receptors. Formulations include oral immediate-release tablets and modified-release tablets (1), parenteral solutions, and suppositories. The pharmacology, clinical pharmacology, efficacy, and adverse effects of oxymorphone have been reviewed (2,3,4). It has a similar adverse effects profile to other potent MOR receptor agonists, although in some studies it caused more nausea and vomiting than morphine when given by patient-controlled devices. There were no differences in nausea and vomiting with the oral modified-release forms of oxymorphone and morphine, but oxymorphone caused more flatulence. Oxymorphone was also reported to provide a better quality of life.

Observational studies

In a 52-week, multicenter, open study of a modified-release formulation of oxymorphone in 153 patients with moderate to severe chronic osteoarthritis-related pain, only 61 patients completed the study (5). Common opioid-related non-serious adverse events caused most of the withdrawals, and about one-half occurred in opioid-naive patients who had received placebo in a previous trial and were given an initial dose of 20 mg every 12 hours. The authors suggested that tolerability could be improved by titrating from a lower initial dose.

Comparative studies

In 39 patients undergoing elective gynecological surgery of at least 2 hours duration, fentanyl 6.5 micrograms/kg or oxymorphone 65 micrograms/kg were given before induction (6). Blood pressure and heart rate were well controlled with both agents, but those who received oxymorphone needed less analgesia postoperatively and more naloxone.

Morphine and oxymorphone have been compared in 32 patients who received traditional patient-controlled analgesia (PCA) after cesarean delivery and 32 who received the same agents plus a basal infusion of the opioid (7). Oxymorphone produced greater reduction in resting pain scores and both opioids reduced pain during movement.

Placebo-controlled studies

In a double-blind, multicenter, randomized placebo-controlled, parallel group, dose-ranging study, three doses of immediate-release (IR) oxymorphone (10, 20, or 30 micrograms) were compared with placebo or oxycodone IR (10 micrograms) in 300 patients receiving total hip or knee replacements (8). All the doses of oxymorphone IR were better at providing pain relief for 8 hours, with a significant analgesic dose response that was maintained over several days, and a safety profile comparable to that of oxycodone IR. The most common adverse events in those who took oxymorphone IR were mild to moderate opioid adverse effects.

In a placebo-controlled study of the effects of modified-release oxymorphone in 126 patients with moderate or severe pain after knee arthroplasty, oxymorphone was more effective than placebo (9). Adverse events such as nausea and constipation were typical of opioids.

In a multicenter, double-blind, placebo-controlled, parallel-group, dose-ranging study of different doses of two different modified-release formulations of oxymorphone in 491 patients, the adverse events in all the opioid groups included mild to moderate nausea, constipation, and somnolence (10).

In a 2-week, multicenter, randomized, double-blind, placebo-controlled, dose-ranging, phase III trial in 370 patients with osteoarthritis of the hip or knee with chronic moderate to severe pain, the most frequently reported adverse events, occurring in at least 5% of patients, were nausea (39%), vomiting (24%), dizziness (23%), constipation (22%), somnolence (18%), pruritus (17%), and headache (15%); most were mild or moderate in intensity (11). There were three serious events (urinary retention, nervous system depression, and pancreatitis) that were considered possibly or probably related to the medication.

In 250 patients with chronic moderate to severe low back pain who were taking an opioid analgesic, an equianalgesic dose of modified-release oxymorphone was substituted, with slow dose titration (12). Withdrawals because of adverse events were similar in the two groups (10% with placebo and 11% with oxymorphone). Opioid-related adverse events included constipation (6%), somnolence (3%), and nausea (3%).

In two combined double-blind placebo-controlled trials of a modified-release formulation of oxymorphone in 347 adults with chronic low back pain, the proportion of patients who had adverse events was significantly greater with oxymorphone than with placebo (26 versus 16%) (13). The most frequent treatment-related adverse events in those taking oxymorphone were nausea (8.0%), constipation (6.3%), vomiting (4.6%), and diarrhea (4.0%); the adverse events in those who took placebo were nausea (5.8%), diarrhea (4.7%), and increased sweating (2.3%).

Organs and Systems

Respiratory

Delayed postoperative respiratory depression has been associated with oxymorphone (14).

Susceptibility Factors

Age

The pharmacodynamics, pharmacokinetics, efficacy, and tolerability of oxymorphone in elderly patients have been reviewed in a systematic review (15). Dosage adjustment is recommended in elderly people.

Renal disease

Oxymorphone should be used with caution in people with renal insufficiency, since it is renally excreted.

Liver disease

Oral oxymorphone is contraindicated in patients with moderate-to-severe hepatic impairment because it is extensively metabolized in the liver to oxymorphone-3-glucuronide and the active metabolite 6-hydroxyoxymorphone (16).

Drug administration

Drug formulations

The pharmacokinetics and dose-proportionality of four dose strengths (5, 10, 20, and 40 mg) of a modified-release formulation of oxymorphone after a single dose and at steady state have been studied in a randomized, three-period, four-sequence, crossover study in 24 healthy adults (17). The kinetics were linear over the doses studied.

Two different types of modified-release formulations of oxymorphone have been compared in 47 adults with moderate to severe cancer pain (18). There were no significant differences in opioid-related adverse events between the groups.

In a similar comparison in a multicenter, randomized, double-blind, placebo-controlled study in 213 ambulatory patients with moderate to severe chronic low back pain, adverse events in those who took the active drugs were similar, the most frequent being constipation and sedation (19).

Drug administration route

Oral oxymorphone is about 1/6 as potent as intramuscular oxymorphone. In terms of peak effect, however, oral oxymorphone was only 1/14 as potent (20). Intramuscular oxymorphone is 8.7 times as potent as morphine in terms of total analgesic effect and 13 times as potent in terms of peak effect.

In a double-blind, twin-crossover comparison single doses of oxymorphone by rectal suppository and intramuscular injection were evaluated in 136 patients with postoperative pain (21). Rectal administration resulted in lower and more delayed peak analgesia and a longer duration of action than intramuscular administration. For duration and intensity of analgesia rectal oxymorphone was 1/10 as potent as the intramuscular form; in peak effect, it was only 1/16 to 1/20 as potent. However, because intramuscular oxymorphone is 9–10 times as potent as intramuscular morphine, oxymorphone 5–10 mg by suppository provides analgesia comparable to that provided by the usually used doses of parenteral narcotics.

The intrathecal route of administration has been associated with edema of the legs and feet, owing to vasodilatation.

References

1. Sloan PA, Barkin RL. Oxymorphone and oxymorphone extended release: a pharmacotherapeutic review. J Opioid Manag 2008;4(3):131–44.
2. Prommer E. Oxymorphone: a review. Support Care Cancer 2006;14:109–15.
3. Gimbel JS. Oxymorphone: a mature molecule with new life. Drugs Today (Barc) 2008;44(10):767–82.
4. Sloan P. Review of oral oxymorphone in the management of pain. Ther Clin Risk Manag 2008;4(4):777–87.
5. McIlwain H, Ahdieh H. Safety, tolerability, and effectiveness of oxymorphone extended release for moderate to severe osteoarthritis pain: a one-year study. Am J Ther 2005;12(2):106–12.
6. Sinatra RS, Harrison DM. A comparison of oxymorphone and fentanyl as narcotic supplements in general anesthesia. J Clin Anesth 1989;1(4):253–8.
7. Sinatra R, Chung KS, Silverman DG, Brull SJ, Chung J, Harrison DM, Donielson D, Weinstock A. An evaluation of morphine and oxymorphone administered via patient-controlled analgesia (PCA) or PCA plus basal infusion in post-cesarean-delivery patients. Anesthesiology 1989;71(4):502–7.
8. Gimbel J, Ahdieh H. The efficacy and safety of oral immediate release oxymorphone for postsurgical pain. Anesth Analg 2004;99:1472–7.
9. Ahdieh H, Ma T, Babul N, Lee D. Efficacy of oxymorphone extended release in postsurgical pain: a randomized clinical trial in knee arthroplasty. J Clin Pharmacol 2004;44(7):767–76.
10. Matsumoto AK, Babul N, Ahdieh H. Oxymorphone extended-release tablets relieve moderate to severe pain and improve physical function in osteoarthritis: results of a randomized, double-blind, placebo- and active-controlled phase III trial. Pain Med 2005;6(5):357–66.
11. Kivitz A, Ma C, Ahdieh H, Galer BS. A 2-week, multicenter, randomized, double-blind, placebo-controlled, dose-ranging, phase III trial comparing the efficacy of oxymorphone extended release and placebo in adults with pain associated with osteoarthritis of the hip or knee. Clin Ther 2006;28(3):352–64.
12. Hale ME, Ahdieh H, Ma T, Rauck R; Oxymorphone ER Study Group 1. Efficacy and safety of OPANA ER (oxymorphone extended release) for relief of moderate to severe chronic low back pain in opioid-experienced patients: a 12-week, randomized, double-blind, placebo-controlled study. J Pain 2007;8(2):175–84.
13. Peniston JH, Gould E. Oxymorphone extended release for the treatment of chronic low back pain: a retrospective pooled analysis of enriched-enrollment clinical trial data stratified according to age, sex, and prior opioid use. Clin Ther 2009;31(2):347–59.
14. Patt RB. Delayed postoperative respiratory depression associated with oxymorphone. Anesth Analg 1988;67(4):403–4.
15. Guay DR. Use of oral oxymorphone in the elderly. Consult Pharm 2007;22(5):417–30.
16. Chamberlin KW, Cottle M, Neville R, Tan J. Oral oxymorphone for pain management. Ann Pharmacother 2007;41(7):1144–52.
17. Adams MP, Ahdieh H. Pharmacokinetics and dose-proportionality of oxymorphone extended release and its metabolites: results of a randomized crossover study. Pharmacotherapy 2004;24(4):468–76.
18. Gabrail NY, Dvergsten C, Ahdieh H. Establishing the dosage equivalency of oxymorphone extended release and oxycodone controlled release in patients with cancer pain: a randomized controlled study. Curr Med Res Opin 2004;20(6):911–8.
19. Hale ME, Dvergsten C, Gimbel J. Efficacy and safety of oxymorphone extended release in chronic low back pain: results of a randomized, double-blind, placebo- and active-controlled phase III study. J Pain 2005;6(1):21–8.
20. Beaver WT, Wallenstein SL, Houde RW, Rogers A. Comparisons of the analgesic effects of oral and intramuscular oxymorphone and of intramuscular oxymorphone and morphine in patients with cancer. J Clin Pharmacol 1977;17(4):186–98.
21. Beaver WT, Feise GA. A comparison of the analgesic effect of oxymorphone by rectal suppository and intramuscular injection in patients with postoperative pain. J Clin Pharmacol 1977;17(5-6):276–91.

Papaveretum

General Information

Papaveretum (Omnopon, Pantopon) is a mixture of several opium alkaloids.

Organs and Systems

Urinary tract

Renal insufficiency has been reported in a 60-year-old patient after the use of papaveretum for perioperative analgesia (SEDA-17, 83).

Second-Generation Effects

Teratogenicity

Because of possible teratogenicity, papaveretum is no longer recommended for women of child-bearing age (SEDA-17, 83).

Susceptibility Factors

Age

There was a 56% incidence of nausea and vomiting with papaveretum in 129 children 24 hours after circumcision with caudal epidural blockade (1).

Reference

1. Wilton NC, Burn JM. Delayed vomiting after papaveretum in paediatric outpatient surgery. Can Anaesth Soc J 1986;33(6):741–4.

Pentamorphone

General Information

Pentamorphone is a potent opiate with a rapid onset and short duration of action, similar to that of fentanyl, which has been reported to produce analgesia with limited depression of ventilation (1).

Subjective symptoms in 23 male volunteers who received pentamorphone were pain on injection, headache, tiredness, euphoria, dizziness, visual disturbances, and nausea (2).

Organs and Systems

Cardiovascular

There was no effect on blood pressure or heart rate with pentamorphone doses of 0.015–0.48 micrograms/kg (2).

References

1. Rudo FG, Wynn RL, Ossipov M, Ford RD, Kutcher BA, Carter A, Spaulding TC. Antinociceptive activity of pentamorphone, a 14-beta-aminomorphinone derivative, compared to fentanyl and morphine. Anesth Analg 1989;69(4):450–6.
2. Glass PS, Camporesi EM, Shafron D, Quill T, Reves JG. Evaluation of pentamorphone in humans: a new potent opiate. Anesth Analg 1989;68(3):302–7.

Pentazocine

General Information

The adverse effects of pentazocine in effective doses are largely typical of its class (1,2), with some quantitative exceptions.

Pentazocine 30 mg had no effect on motor skills but impaired sensory processing and extraocular muscle imbalance (3). Other effects reported in this study were slight respiratory depression (enhanced by concurrent amitriptyline) and feelings of clumsiness, drowsiness, friendliness, and contentedness, and a muzzy head.

The effects of pentazocine were studied in 16 non-abusing volunteers recruited via posters and local newspaper advertisements and were compared with the effects of morphine (4). Pentazocine had dose-related effects on subjective, psychomotor, and physiological variables, and the clinically relevant dose of 30 mg produced a greater magnitude of dysphoric subjective effects than morphine 10 mg and, unlike morphine, impaired psychomotor performance. With pentazocine, peak ratings from the adjective checklist were significantly increased for "dry mouth," "sweating," and "turning of stomach." Compared with morphine, pentazocine led to higher ratings for "drunk," "feel bad," "having pleasant bodily sensations," and "having unpleasant bodily sensations."

Organs and Systems

Psychological, psychiatric

Perceptual disturbances are generally thought to occur more often with pentazocine than with other opioids. Objective definition of such phenomena is difficult, but in a study of postoperative dreaming after the use of pentazocine and morphine as premedicants there was no statistically significant difference between the two drugs (SED-11, 148; 5).

Hematologic

There have been reports of pentazocine-induced agranulocytosis in the absence of other predisposing factors (SED-11, 148) (6).

Skin

Two distinct types of skin lesions have been described in patients taking pentazocine: scleroderma-like changes, subcutaneous abscesses, cellulitis, ulceration, muscle atrophy and granulomas (all of which are well-recognized consequences of pentazocine abuse), and a generalized erythematous desquamative rash.

Severe renal insufficiency associated with toxic epidermal necrolysis has been reported (7).

Long-Term Effects

Drug abuse

Abusers sometimes adulterate the pentazocine with tripelennamine (T's and blues). Medical and psychiatric complications can include seizures, abscesses, depression, psychosis, dysphoria, confusion, and hallucinations (8,9).

Drug dependence

Pentazocine dependence is associated with a mild opioid–like withdrawal syndrome (8,9).

Drug withdrawal

A neonatal withdrawal syndrome has been described, with verification by the detection of pentazocine and its metabolites in the urine of both mother and baby. Within 4 hours of birth the child was irritable, jittery, and hypertonic, with a high-pitched cry, a voracious appetite, and frequent bowel movements. The symptoms improved over 3 days. The mother had abused parenteral pentazocine (23–46 mg) for the previous 10 years and injected the last dose of 46 mg some 10 hours before delivery (10).

Susceptibility Factors

Renal disease

A fatal nephrotic syndrome occurred in a 33-year-old man with renal glomerular disease dependent on pentazocine (SEDA-17, 88).

Other features of the patient

There is evidence that heavy smoking can increase the elimination of pentazocine; thus heavy smokers may require larger doses than non-smokers.

Drug Administration

Drug administration route

Fibrous myopathy and necrotic ulceration can occur at the injection site after repeated parenteral administration (1). Myocutaneous sclerosis and extensive calcinosis at the injection site have also been reported (SEDA-17, 88).

- A 58-year-old nurse who was given parenteral pentazocine developed large sclerotic and infected areas with multiple depressed atrophic scars at sites of prior ulceration; unsterile injection technique could not be excluded as a cause (11).
- A 47-year old woman with a 4-year history of injections of pentazocine into the legs developed very hard thigh and buttock muscles with hard, shiny, hairless overlying skin (12). Imaging showed fibrosis and calcification of the muscles and biopsy showed fibromyopathy. There were associated clinical and electrophysiological polyradiculopathy and multiple mononeuropathy of the lower extremities.
- A 26-year-old woman presented with progressive thickening and tightening of the skin over both her shoulders

and buttocks, with resulting movement restrictions (13). She had a 5-year history of multiple intramuscular pentazocine injections for abdominal pain. The site of skin tightening was initially localized to the injection site. The affected areas increased progressively. There was an ill-defined area of hyperpigmented, indurated, "woody hard" skin bound to underlying structures and over her shoulders and buttocks. The diagnosis was pentazocine-induced widespread cutaneous fibrosis and myofibrosis. There was no evidence of scleroderma or dermatomyositis.

- A 38-year-old man, with a painless progressive restriction of flexion around both knee joints for 4 years, had been injecting pentazocine 1–2 ml intramuscularly for 18–20 years (14). The diagnosis was pentazocine-induced fibromyositis and contracture.

Drug overdose

Pentazocine in overdose can cause generalized tonic-clonic seizures, hypertension, hypotonia, dysphoria, hallucinations, delusions, and agitation, with a poor response to naloxone (15). Others have reported status epilepticus, coma, respiratory depression, acidosis, severe hypotension, and ventricular dysrhythmias.

Drug–Drug Interactions

Alcohol

There is increased toxicity in patients who take pentazocine with alcohol, antihistamines, or CNS depressants; one patient developed opioid pulmonary edema and one died (15).

Rhabdomyolysis and acute renal necrosis occurred in a 26-year-old man after concomitant use of pentazocine and alcohol (16).

Methylphenidate

Intravenous injection of a mixture of methylphenidate and pentazocine intended for oral use resulted in death due to granulomatosis associated with pulmonary hypertension (17).

Monoamine oxidase inhibitors

Opioids interact with monoamine oxidase inhibitors, causing CNS excitation and hypertension (18).

Selective serotonin re-uptake inhibitors

A serious excitatory interaction between fluoxetine and pentazocine has been reported (SEDA-16, 89). The authors commented on the similarity of this syndrome to the reported dangerous interactions between monoamine oxidase inhibitors and narcotic analgesics, and suggested that increased central 5-HT activity may be the basis of the observed interaction.

References

1. Goldstein G. Pentazocine. Drug Alcohol Depend 1985;14(3-4):313–23.
2. Rudra A. Comparison of buprenorphine, morphine, pethidine, and pentazocine as postoperative analgesic after upper abdominal surgery. Calcutta Med J 1989;86:1.
3. Saarialho-Kere U, Mattila MJ, Seppala T. Parenteral pentazocine: effects on psychomotor skills and respiration, and interactions with amitriptyline. Eur J Clin Pharmacol 1988;35(5):483–9.
4. Zacny JP, Hill JL, Black ML, Sadeghi P. Comparing the subjective, psychomotor and physiological effects of intravenous pentazocine and morphine in normal volunteers. J Pharmacol Exp Ther 1998;286(3):1197–207.
5. Heaney RM, Gotlieb N. Granulocytopenia after intravenous abuse of pentazocine and tripelennamine ("Ts and blues"). South Med J 1983;76(5):654–6.
6. Haibach H, Yesus YW, Doggett JJ. Pentazocine-induced agranulocytosis. Can Med Assoc J 1984;130(9):1165–6.
7. Pedragosa R, Vidal J, Fuentes R, Huguet P. Tricotropism by pentazocine. Arch Dermatol 1987;123(3):297–8.
8. Showalter CV. T's and blues. Abuse of pentazocine and tripelennamine. JAMA 1980;244(11):1224–5.
9. Lahmeyer HW, Steingold RG. Medical and psychiatric complications of pentazocine and tripelennamine abuse. J Clin Psychiatry 1980;41(8):275–8.
10. Wu WH, Teng RJ, Shin HY. Neonatal pentazocine withdrawal syndrome—a case report of conservative treatment. Zhonghua Yi Xue Za Zhi (Taipei) 1988;42(3):229–32.
11. Furner BB. Parenteral pentazocine: cutaneous complications revisited. J Am Acad Dermatol 1990;22(4):694–705.
12. Sinsawaiwong S, Phanthumchinda K. Pentazocine-induced fibrous myopathy and localized neuropathy. J Med Assoc Thai 1998;81(9):717–21.
13. Jain A, Bhattacharya SN, Singal A, Baruah MC, Bhatia A. Pentazocine induced widespread cutaneous and myo-fibrosis. J Dermatol 1999;26(6):368–70.
14. Das CP, Thussu A, Prabhakar S, Banerjee AK. Pentazocine-induced fibromyositis and contracture. Postgrad Med J 1999;75(884):361–2.
15. Challoner KR, McCarron MM, Newton EJ. Pentazocine (Talwin) intoxication: report of 57 cases. J Emerg Med 1990;8(1):67–74.
16. Tsai JC, Lai YH, Shin SJ, Chen JH, Torng JK, Tasi JH. Rhabdomyolysis-induced acute tubular necrosis after the concomitant use of alcohol and pentazocine—a case report. Gaoxiong Yi Xue Ke Xue Za Zhi 1987;3(4):299–305.
17. Lundquest DE, Young WK, Edland JF. Maternal death associated with intravenous methylphenidate (Ritalin) and pentazocine (Talwin) abuse. J Forensic Sci 1987;32(3): 798–801.
18. Rossiter A, Souney PF. Interaction between MAOIs and opioids: pharmacologic and clinical considerations. Hosp Formul 1993;28(8):692–8.

Pethidine (meperidine)

General Information

Pethidine (meperidine) is about one-tenth as potent as morphine in terms of analgesia. It is metabolized in the liver by hydrolysis and conjugation, either directly or via N-demethylation to norpethidine. Norpethidine (normeperidine) is significantly less analgesic, with a longer half-life (15–20 hours).

There has been a systematic review of the postoperative analgesic efficacy and adverse effects of pethidine and ketorolac compared with placebo in published randomized, controlled, double-blind studies (1). The authors reviewed studies of moderate to severe postoperative pain relief and the use of single doses by injection (intravenously or intramuscularly) or orally. Studies of epidural, intrathecal, or intravenous administration using patient-controlled analgesia were excluded. Of the 24 placebo-controlled pethidine studies, only 8 met the inclusion criteria and these generated 10 pethidine versus placebo comparisons and 254 patients given pethidine 50 mg or 100 mg intramuscularly. No studies of oral or intravenous pethidine at any dose met the inclusion criteria. Only the eight comparisons of pethidine 100 mg versus placebo ($n = 203$) had sufficient information available for analysis of adverse effects. The overall conclusion was that opioids carry a small but finite risk of serious adverse effects, such as respiratory depression, and a greater risk of minor adverse effects than single-dose injected or oral NSAIDs like ketorolac. Analgesia from the injected opioid or NSAID was equivalent to that achieved with oral NSAIDs. For those who cannot swallow, the choice is injected opioids like pethidine.

In a double-blind, randomized, placebo-controlled study, 40 patients who were scheduled for elective cesarean section under spinal anesthesia were given intrathecal 0.5% hyperbaric bupivacaine 2 ml together with either 5% pethidine 0.2 ml or isotonic saline (2). The pethidine group had a significantly greater incidence of intraoperative nausea or vomiting, with significantly better immediate postoperative analgesia, which was not sustained 4 hours after surgery.

In a randomized, controlled study in 611 mothers, 310 were randomized to intramuscular pethidine up to 300 mg and 301 to epidural 0.25% bupivacaine 10 ml with an infusion of 0.125–0.25% bupivacaine (3). There were no significant differences in analgesic efficacy, adverse effects, or the incidence of backaches.

Pethidine (meperidine)

Observational studies

Hypotension, hypoxemia, and pain-related agitation were adverse events reported after co-administration of pethidine and midazolam for sedation and analgesia in children; no other events were reported (4).

Placebo-controlled studies

The analgesic and adverse effects of pethidine, metoclopramide, and the combination have been compared in a randomized, double-blind, controlled study in the emergency treatment of acute primary vascular and tension-type headaches in 366 patients (5). The drug regimens were:

- intravenous metoclopramide 10 micrograms + intramuscular placebo;
- intramuscular pethidine 50 micrograms + intravenous placebo;
- intravenous metoclopramide 10 micrograms + intramuscular pethidine 50 micrograms;
- intravenous placebo + intramuscular placebo.

Pethidine was more effective than placebo, but metoclopramide was the most effective. There were adverse effects in 126 patients (38%); the most common were drowsiness or light sedation (20%). The adverse effects profile was significantly worse in those given pethidine.

Organs and Systems

Cardiovascular

- A 70-year-old patient with a metastatic carcinoid tumor of the liver presented with a hypertensive crisis after being given pethidine 10 mg/hour by continuous intravenous infusion (6). The patient remained hypertensive with a systolic blood pressure of 210 mmHg, even after chemoembolization of the tumor. The blood pressure fell when pethidine was withdrawn and nitroprusside was given. The serum 5-HT concentration was 15 µmol/l (reference range 0.17–0.26) and the urine 5-hydroxyindoleacetic acid concentration was 1311 mg/g of creatinine (reference range less than 10).

The authors postulated that the hypertensive crisis had occurred from the release of 5-HT from the tumor and blockade by pethidine of 5-HT re-uptake.

When used for sedation in children undergoing esophagogastroduodenoscopy, hypoxia with dysrhythmias was more likely to occur with a combination of pethidine and diazepam than with pethidine and midazolam (SEDA-18, 81).

Nervous system

Cases of severe reversible neurotoxicity and parkinsonism are on record (SED-11, 143; SEDA-18, 82; 7,8). Severe nervous system syndromes may also result from interactions (see the monograph on Opioid analgesics).

Although seizures are uncommon, several cases have been reported, including when pethidine was used in PCA. The metabolite norpethidine is considered to be of significant importance in provoking seizures. Risk factors are renal insufficiency, sickle-cell anemia, high doses of pethidine, and concurrent administration of phenothiazines or drugs that induce hepatic enzymes (SEDA-16, 85; SEDA-18, 82; SEDA-19, 85). Myoclonus can occur (9). Norpethidine is twice as likely as pethidine to cause convulsions. The seizures occur at a norpethidine concentration range of 0.38–9.9 µg/ml, and only few reports have described convulsions within the first 24 hours of pethidine treatment.

- A 35-year-old woman, who was admitted for elective laparotomy and ileostomy formation was given patient-controlled analgesic with pethidine for postoperative

analgesia (10). The device was set to deliver 20 mg of pethidine with a 5-minute lock-out period and no hourly limit. At 4 hours postoperatively she did not have pethidine-related neurotoxicity, but at 23 hours she had myoclonic jerks and facial twitching followed by a brief generalized tonic-clonic seizure and postictal sequelae. The pethidine was withdrawn and there was no further seizure activity. She had self administered a total of 2700 mg. The norpethidine concentration was 1.8 µg/ml.

- A 55-year-old woman developed severe abdominal pain, vomiting, diarrhea, and dysuria. A provisional diagnosis of pyelonephritis was made, and she was given intravenous pethidine in gradually increasing doses until day 4 (cumulative dose 2125 mg), when she had a seizure lasting 1 minute (11). The pethidine was withdrawn and replaced with buprenorphine, with no further complications.
- A 34-year old woman who had undergone left hip revision surgery was first given patient-controlled hydromorphone, which was changed to pethidine 15 micrograms every 6 minutes as needed on the third postoperative day and received 1500 micrograms of pethidine over the first 36 hours (12). On day five she had a witnessed generalized tonic–clonic seizure. Pethidine was withdrawn and no further seizures were witnessed.

Two of three patients with seizures due to norpethidine toxicity (13–15) had renal disease.

- A 46-year-old woman with previous extensive urological problems, including ureteric stricture and recurrent urinary tract infections, was given pethidine in a total cumulative dose of 1500 mg postoperatively over 12 hours when she presented with a single tonic-clonic seizure that lasted 30 seconds. The pethidine concentration was 1200 ng/ml and the norpethidine concentration 2100 ng/ml.
- A 72-year-old patient with end-stage renal insufficiency undergoing peritoneal dialysis developed myoclonic contractions and a generalized tonic-clonic seizure 48 hours after having been given pethidine in a total cumulative dose of 250 mg intravenously and 600 mg orally. The neurotoxicity resolved after withdrawal of pethidine and 4 hours of hemodialysis.
- A 2-month-old boy presented with muscle rigidity of the arms and legs, catatonia, and an exaggerated startle reflex after being erroneously given a single dose of pethidine 1 mg/kg. The symptoms subsided without any active intervention.

Two case reports have highlighted the potential danger of injecting pethidine into the lateral thigh region, which can cause injury to the femoral nerve branch to the vastus lateralis, causing muscle atrophy (16).

In a retrospective survey of 355 medical records of patients who received intravenous PCA pethidine between 1988 and 1994 the mean consumption by patients who had used over 600 mg/day of pethidine was 13.3 mg/kg/day in asymptomatic patients and 16.9 mg/kg/day in the 2% of patients who presented with central nervous system excitatory signs and symptoms (muscle twitches, jitteriness, agitation, and hallucinations) (17). The authors recommended a maximum safe dose of pethidine by PCA of 10 mg/kg/day for no more than 3 days.

Gastrointestinal

A study in which it was intended to recruit 90 women in labor for a comparison of intrathecal bupivacaine 2.5 mg, fentanyl 25 microgram, pethidine 15 mg, and pethidine 25 mg was stopped prematurely after only 34 had been recruited, because of a significant increase in the incidence of nausea and vomiting in the patients who received the two doses of pethidine (18).

The prevalence of nausea after parenteral morphine (n = 37) and pethidine (n = 156) was measured in a prospective study in two groups matched for age, sex, weight, and potency of the opioid administered (19). The average total dose of morphine was 8.4 mg and of pethidine 96 mg. None of those given morphine had nausea, compared with two of those given pethidine. This was a pilot study and a more rigid randomized double-blind study would be helpful. Equally, a more objective study endpoint needs to be considered in future studies rather than "nausea", which is subjective and may not be interpreted similarly by all patients.

Non-steroidal anti-inflammatory drugs have been compared with opioids in the treatment of acute renal colic in a meta-analysis of 20 studies (20). Seven different opioids were studied. In most of the studies there was a higher incidence of adverse events in patients who took opioids. Pooled analysis showed significantly more vomiting in those who took opioids, particularly pethidine. No serious adverse events were reported and adverse event rates did not vary with dosage.

Musculoskeletal

Muscle rigidity after spinal anesthesia occurred in a 17-year-old man admitted for emergency appendicectomy (21). During the operation, he developed shivering and was given intravenous diazepam 5 mg and pethidine 50 mg. Minutes later he developed severe rigidity in the neck, masseters, arms, thoracoabdominal region, and thighs.

Immunologic

Pethidine causes histamine release (9). Of 16 patients given pethidine (mean dose 4.3 mg/kg), 5 had signs of the effects of histamine (hypotension, tachycardia, erythema) and raised histamine concentrations (9).

- A 42-year-old patient presented with generalized pruritus, erythema, urticaria, facial angioedema, dysphagia, dysphonia, and dizziness 15 minutes after a single intramuscular dose of pethidine 100 mg for severe renal colic (22). Prick tests and intradermal tests with pethidine and other compounds confirmed an allergic reaction to pethidine.

Long-Term Effects

Drug dependence

The interaction between the drug-dependent patient and health professional has been investigated in a retrospective study of the medical records of 20 patients with chronic organic pain and perceived as being dependent on pethidine (23). The fact that the patients were perceived as being addicted may have influenced the adequate management of their chronic intractable pain, precipitated poor staff–patient relationships, created a lower pain threshold or tolerance due to anxiety and depression, and led to overuse of placebo, leading to inadequate analgesia. All of these factors may then have led to craving-like behavior and demands for more analgesics, further fuelling the negative stereotyped perception of the addicted personality. The authors suggested that people with dependence-related problems should be evaluated for suicidal intent; concurrent psychiatric illnesses should be treated; and precipitating factors that make pain worse should be identified. Medical and other staff should be educated about the use of opiate analgesics and concepts of dependence, in order to reduce negative judgmental attitudes and misconceptions.

Second-Generation Effects

Pregnancy

In 407 women in labor with dystocia, pethidine, contrary to the belief that it has oxytocic properties, did not reduce the duration of labor and was not useful in the management of first stage dystocia (24). More of those who received pethidine than the controls required augmentation of labor with oxytocic agents. Also, more women in the pethidine group had nausea, vomiting, and dizziness. The fetuses that had been exposed to pethidine were more likely to have an Apgar score under 7 at 1 minute, to have an umbilical cord blood pH under 7.10, and to be admitted to the neonatal intensive care unit.

In 383 singleton pregnancies with dystocia pethidine caused a higher incidence of acidosis than placebo (25).

Fetotoxicity

Pethidine is commonly used in some countries as an analgesic in maternal labor. The analgesic and adverse effects of intramuscular pethidine 5 mg plus diamorphine 100 mg in labor have been studied in a randomized, double-blind, controlled study in 64 multiparous and 69 nulliparous women (26). There was a significantly higher incidence of low Apgar scores at 1 minute after pethidine compared with diamorphine. The study also confirmed that for women who requested intramuscular narcotic analgesia, neither diamorphine nor pethidine provided good pain relief, suggesting that there is a need to consider alternatives.

Pethidine 50 mg plus promethazine 25 mg given intravenously to 14 mothers in labor caused a significant change in fetal heart rate indices 40 minutes after administration (27). There were significant changes in fetal heart rate acceleration of at least 10 beats/minute, acceleration of at least 15 beats/minute, time spent in episodes of high variation, and short-term variation.

Lactation

Pethidine is not often used in post-cesarean analgesia because its active metabolite, norpethidine, can accumulate in breast milk, resulting in reduced scores on neonatal behavior assessment scales (28).

Susceptibility Factors

Renal disease

Norpethidine (normeperidine) accumulates in cases of renal insufficiency (29), leading to symptoms of overdosage.

Hepatic disease

Patients with cirrhosis and acute viral hepatitis can have a 50% reduction in pethidine clearance (SEDA-19, 85).

Drug Administration

Drug dosage regimens

In a double-blind study of 60 patients undergoing elective carpal tunnel release given pethidine 0, 10, 20, 30, 40, or 50 mg in addition to intravenous regional anesthesia with lidocaine 0.5%, the duration of analgesia increased dose-dependently with 0, 10, 20, and 30 µg (30). In those given pethidine 30, 40, and 50 µg there was a significantly higher incidence of sedation, pruritus, nausea, vomiting, and respiratory depression with no increase in analgesic effect. These results support an optimal dose of pethidine 30 mg when used with 0.5% lidocaine for postoperative analgesia.

In a prospective, randomized, single-blind study in 45 men undergoing lower abdominal surgery using one of three doses of intrathecal pethidine (1.2, 1.5, or 1.8 mg/kg) there was no difference in the incidence of adverse effects among the three groups (31). The authors postulated that increasing the dose of pethidine from 1.2 to 1.5 mg/kg increased the duration of analgesia but not the level of sensory block, without an increase in adverse effects.

In 40 patients undergoing prostatectomy with spinal anesthesia with lidocaine 5% (75 mg) intrathecally, either alone or co-administered with pethidine 0.15 or 0.30 mg/kg, the higher dose of pethidine reduced the requirement for parenteral analgesics with a non-significant incidence of pethidine-related adverse effects (32).

Drug administration route

Epidural versus intravenous
In a double-blind, randomized, controlled study, 17 patients undergoing gastrectomy were given epidural PCA pethidine (10 mg bolus and a 4-hourly maximum dose of 3 mg/kg) and were compared with 20 patients

after gastrectomy who were given the same regimen intravenously (33). The mean pethidine consumption in the first 24 hours was 33% less in the epidural group than in the intravenous group. Pain scores, adverse effects profiles, patient satisfaction, and patient outcome were similar. However, the sample size was small, and even though the study was intended to be double-blind, the route of pethidine administration and the patient's perception of an intravenous and epidural injection might have caused bias.

Rectal
Rectal pethidine is not advised in children, owing to enormous variability in systemic availability (SEDA-18, 82).

Drug overdose

Cardiac arrest occurred after pethidine overdose (34).

- A 2-month-old boy had a cardiac arrest when he was given a combination of pethidine, promethazine, and chlorpromazine in 10 times the recommended dose by the wrong route (intravenously rather than intramuscularly). Within seconds he became apneic and stiff. Cardiopulmonary resuscitation was instituted, including two intravenous doses of adrenaline 0.06 mg and naloxone 0.6 mg, with recovery 7 minutes after the incident and complete resolution 24 hours later.

Drug–Drug Interactions

Bupivacaine

Pethidine displaces bupivacaine from plasma proteins (40). However, this interaction is probably not of clinical importance (41).

Cimetidine

The hepatic metabolism of pethidine can be inhibited by cimetidine, leading to respiratory depression and sedation (35,36).

Fluoxetine

Serotonin syndrome has been reported in a patient taking fluoxetine and pethidine (37).

- A 43-year-old man scheduled for endoscopic retrograde cholangiopancreatography to evaluate chronic recurrent episodes of pancreatitis was given pethidine 50 mg intravenously plus midazolam 2 mg. He immediately became agitated and restless, with widely dilated pupils, hyper-reflexia, increased heart rate and blood pressure, and diarrhea. He recovered after 20 minutes without treatment. He subsequently confirmed that he had been taking unspecified doses of fluoxetine irregularly but frequently.

The authors suggested that this presentation was due to serotonin syndrome, but offered no mechanistic explanation.

Midazolam

Rectal pethidine is not advised in children, owing to enormous variability in systemic availability (SEDA-18, 82). When used for sedation in children undergoing esophagogastroduodenoscopy, hypoxia with dysrhythmias was more likely to occur with a combination of pethidine and diazepam than with pethidine and midazolam (SEDA-18, 81).

Phenytoin

Phenytoin enhances the metabolism of pethidine (38).

Selegiline

A syndrome resembling the serotonin syndrome has been reported in a patient taking pethidine plus selegiline (39).

- A woman with Parkinson's disease, taking selegiline 5 mg bd, pergolide 0.75 mg bd, co-careldopa 440 mg qds, imipramine 175 mg qds, and desipramine 25 mg qds, was given pethidine, 325 mg over 3 days, and hydroxyzine for pain. After 2 days she became restless and irritable, and after 4 days she developed delirium, muscle rigidity, sweating, and fever. The symptoms resolved when selegiline was withdrawn.

The authors did not discuss the role of the tricyclic antidepressants in this presentation.

References

1. Smith LA, Carroll D, Edwards JE, Moore RA, McQuay HJ. Single-dose ketorolac and pethidine in acute postoperative pain: systematic review with meta-analysis. Br J Anaesth 2000;84(1):48–58.
2. Yu SC, Ngan Kee WD, Kwan AS. Addition of meperidine to bupivacaine for spinal anaesthesia for Caesarean section. Br J Anaesth 2002;88(3):379–83.
3. Simopoulos TT, Smith HS, Peeters-Asdourian C, Stevens DS. Use of meperidine in patient-controlled analgesia and the development of a normeperidine toxic reaction. Arch Surg 2002;137(1):84–8.
4. Boyd JJ, Kuisma MJ, Alaspaa AO, Vuori E, Repo JV, Randell TT. Outcome after heroin overdose and cardiopulmonary resuscitation. Acta Anaesthesiol Scand 2006;50:1120–4.
5. Cicek M, Karcioglu O, Parlek I, Ozturk V, Duman O, Sirinken M, Guryay M. Prospective, randomized, double blind, controlled comparison of metoclopramide and pethidine in the emergency treatment of acute primary vascular and tension type headache episodes. Emerg Med J 2004;21:323–6.
6. Balestrero LM, Beaver CR, Rigas JR. Hypertensive crisis following meperidine administration and chemoembolization of a carcinoid tumor. Arch Intern Med 2000;160(15):2394–5.
7. Lieberman AN, Goldstein M. Reversible parkinsonism related to meperidine. N Engl J Med 1985;312(8):509.
8. Goetting MG, Thirman MJ. Neurotoxicity of meperidine. Ann Emerg Med 1985;14(10):1007–9.
9. Flacke JW, Flacke WE, Bloor BC, Van Etten AP, Kripke BJ. Histamine release by four narcotics: a double-blind study in humans. Anesth Analg 1987;66(8): 723–30.
10. McHugh GJ. Norpethidine accumulation and generalized seizure during pethidine patient-controlled analgesia. Anaesth Intensive Care 1999;27(3):289–91.
11. Hubbard GP, Wolfe KR. Meperidine misuse in a patient with sphincter of Oddi dysfunction. Ann Pharmacother 2003;37:534–7.
12. Beaul PE, Smith IM, Nguyen VN. Meperidine induced seizure after revision hip arthroplasty. J Arthroplasty 2004;19:516–9.
13. Knight B, Thomson N, Perry G. Seizures due to norpethidine toxicity. Aust NZ J Med 2000;30(4):513.
14. Hassan H, Bastani B, Gellens M. Successful treatment of normeperidine neurotoxicity by hemodialysis. Am J Kidney Dis 2000;35(1):146–9.
15. Baris S, Karakaya D, Sarihasan B. A dose of 1 mg.kg^{-1} meperidine causes muscle rigidity in infants? Paediatr Anaesth 2000;10(6):684.
16. Haber M, Kovan E, Andary M, Honet J. Postinjection vastus lateralis atrophy: 2 case reports. Arch Phys Med Rehabil 2000;81(9):1229–33.
17. Loughnan BA, Carli F, Romney M, Dore CJ, Gordon H. Epidural analgesia and backache: a randomized controlled comparison with intramuscular meperidine for analgesia during labour. Br J Anaesth 2002;89(3):466–72.
18. Booth JV, Lindsay DR, Olufolabi AJ, El-Moalem HE, Penning DH, Reynolds JD. Subarachnoid meperidine (pethidine) causes significant nausea and vomiting during labor. The Duke Women's Anesthesia Research Group. Anesthesiology 2000;93(2):418–21.
19. Silverman ME, Shih RD, Allegra J. Morphine induces less nausea than meperidine when administered parenterally. J Emerg Med 2004;27:241–3.
20. Holdgate A, Pollock T. Systematic review of the relative efficacy of non-steroidal anti-inflammatory drugs and opioids in the treatment of acute renal colic. BMJ 2004;328:1401–9.
21. Kitagawa N, Oda M, Totoki T. Meperidine-induced muscular rigidity during spinal anesthesia? Anesth Analgesia 2006;103:490–1.
22. Anibarro B, Vila C, Seoane FJ. Urticaria induced by meperidine allergy. Allergy 2000;55(3):305–6.
23. Hung CI, Liu CY, Chen CY, Yang CH, Yeh EK. Meperidine addiction or treatment frustration? Gen Hosp Psychiatry 2001;23(1):31–5.
24. Sosa CG, Balaguer E, Alonso JG, Panizza R, Laborde A, Berrondo C, Singh U, Moodley J. Meperidine for dystocia did not reduce the duration of labour and had harmful effects on mother and baby. Evidence-based Obstet Gynecol 2005;7(3):120–1.
25. Sosa CG, Buekens P, Hughes JM, Balaguer E, Sotero G, Panizza R, Piriz H, Alonso JG. Effect of pethidine administered during the first stage of labor on the acid-base status at birth. Eur J Obstet Gynecol Reprod Biol 2006;129(2):135–9.
26. Fairlie FM, Marshall L, Walker JJ, Elbourne D. Intramuscular opioids for maternal pain relief in labour: a randomised controlled trial comparing pethidine with diamorphine. Br J Obstet Gynaecol 1999;106(11): 1181–7.
27. Solt I, Ganadry S, Weiner Z. The effect of meperidine and promethazine on fetal heart rate indices during the active phase of labor. Isr Med Assoc J 2002;4(3):178–80.
28. Gadsden J, Hart S, Santos AC. Post-caesarean delivery analgesia. Anesth Analg 2005;101(5 Suppl):S62–9.
29. Kaiko RF, Foley KM, Grabinski PY, Heidrich G, Rogers AG, Inturrisi CE, Reidenberg MM. Central nervous system excitatory effects of meperidine in cancer patients. Ann Neurol 1983;13(2):180–5.

30. Reuben SS, Steinberg RB, Lurie SD, Gibson CS. A dose-response study of intravenous regional anesthesia with meperidine. Anesth Analg 1999;88(4):831–5.

31. Hansen D, Hansen S. The effects of three graded doses of meperidine for spinal anesthesia in African men. Anesth Analg 1999;88(4):827–30.

32. Murto K, Lui AC, Cicutti N. Adding low dose meperidine to spinal lidocaine prolongs postoperative analgesia. Can J Anaesth 1999;46(4):327–34.

33. Chen PP, Cheam EW, Ma M, Lam KK, Ngan Kee WD, Gin T. Patient-controlled pethidine after major upper abdominal surgery: comparison of the epidural and intravenous routes. Anaesthesia 2001;56(11):1106–12.

34. Brown ET, Corbett SW, Green SM. Iatrogenic cardiopulmonary arrest during pediatric sedation with meperidine, promethazine, and chlorpromazine. Pediatr Emerg Care 2001;17(5):351–3.

35. Knodell RG, Holtzman JL, Crankshaw DL, Steele NM, Stanley LN. Drug metabolism by rat and human hepatic microsomes in response to interaction with H_2-receptor antagonists. Gastroenterology 1982;82(1):84–8.

36. Lee HR, et al. Effect of histamine H_2-receptors on fentanyl metabolism. Pharmacology 1982;24:145.

37. Tissot TA. Probable meperidine-induced serotonin syndrome in a patient with a history of fluoxetine use. Anesthesiology 2003;98:1511–2.

38. Pond SM, Kretschzmar KM. Effect of phenytoin on meperidine clearance and normeperidine formation. Clin Pharmacol Ther 1981;30(5):680–6.

39. Zornberg GL, Bodkin JA, Cohen BM. Severe adverse interaction between pethidine and selegiline. Lancet 1991;337(8735):246.

40. Ghoneim MM, Pandya H. Plasma protein binding of bupivacaine and its interaction with other drugs in man. Br J Anaesth 1974;46(6):435–8.

41. Denson DD, Myers JA, Coyle DE. The clinical relevance of the drug displacement interaction between meperidine and bupivacaine. Res Commun Chem Pathol Pharmacol 1984;45(3):323–30.

Phenoperidine

General Information

Phenoperidine is a potent opioid analgesic often used in neuroleptanalgesia and as a respiratory depressant in ventilated patients.

Organs and Systems

Cardiovascular

Intracranial hypertension occurred within 1 minute in a patient with a severe head injury who received phenoperidine 1 mg intravenously. It was associated with a reduction in arterial blood pressure. A similar reaction occurred when a second 1 mg bolus was given 8 hours later (SED-11, 146; 1).

Reference

1. Grummitt RM, Goat VA. Intracranial pressure after phenoperidine. Anaesthesia 1984;39(6):565–7.

Pholcodine

General Information

Pholcodine, (3-morpholinoethylmorphine), a semi-synthetic alkaloid, is an MOR receptor agonist with similar antitussive properties to codeine (1). It is metabolized to norpholcodine and pholcodine-N-oxide, its main metabolite, but not to morphine, which may explain its lack of analgexic effect (2). In healthy volunteers who took single oral doses of 20 and 60 mg, pholcodine was absorbed rapidly (t_{max} 1.6 hours) and eliminated slowly with a mean half-life of 50 hours. Its renal clearance was 137 ml/min and correlated inversely with urine pH but not with urine flow rate; plasma protein binding was 24%; 26% of the dose was excreted as unchanged pholcodine (3). The concentration of pholcodine in saliva was 3.6 times higher than in plasma. After long-term administration, the pharmacokinetics of pholcodine were not statistically different.

Organs and Systems

Immunologic

Hypersensitivity has been attributed to pholcodine (4).

- A 33-year-old woman developed facial angioedema 8 hours after taking Respilène® syrup (which contains pholcodine, domperidone, tixocortol, and bacitracin). The symptoms resolved with an intravenous corticosteroid. An intradermal test was positive for pholcodine but negative for domperidone, tixocortol, and bacitracin. Open oral challenge with pholcodine 20 mg was positive.

This is believed to have been the first report of allergy to pholcodine.

Anaphylaxis due to drugs can be mediated by immunoglobulin E (IgE) antibodies that bind quaternary ammonium ion epitopes, which are present in many drugs, including pholcodine. Pholcodine can cause an increase in serum IgE concentrations (5). In 17 patients who were randomized to cough syrup containing either pholcodine or guaifenesin for 1 week, pholcodine increased IgE antibodies to pholcodine, morphine, and suxamethonium, the median proportional increases 4 weeks after exposure being 39, 39, and 93 times baseline respectively. The median proportional increase in IgE was 19-fold. Guaifenesin had no such effect.

Drug–Drug Interactions

Activated charcoal

In a randomized study of the effects of single and multiple doses of activated charcoal on the absorption and elimination of pholcodine 100 mg administered in a cough syrup, charcoal 25 g given immediately after the pholcodine significantly reduced the absorption of pholcodine; the $AUC_{0\to96}$ was reduced by 91%, the C_{max} by 77%, and the amount of pholcodine excreted in the urine by 85% (6). When charcoal was given 2 hours after pholcodine, the $AUC_{0\to96}$ was reduced by 26%, the C_{max} by 23%, and the urinary excretion by 28%. When it was given 5 hours after pholcodine, charcoal produced only a 17% reduction in the $AUC_{0?96}$, but reduced the further absorption of pholcodine still present in the gastrointestinal tract at the time of charcoal administration, as measured by the $AUC_{5\to96}$.

References

1. Findlay JW. Pholcodine. J Clin Pharm Ther 1988;13(1):5–17.
2. Jairaj M, Watson DG, Grant MH, Gray AI, Skellern GG. Comparative biotransformation of morphine, codeine and pholcodine in rat hepatocytes: identification of a novel metabolite of pholcodine. Xenobiotica 2002;32(12):1093–107.
3. Chen ZR, Bochner F, Somogyi A. Pharmacokinetics of pholcodine in healthy volunteers: single and chronic dosing studies. Br J Clin Pharmacol 1988;26(4):445–53.
4. Codreanu F, Morisset M, Kanny G, Moneret-Vautrin DA. Allergy to pholcodine: first case documented by oral challenge. Allergy: Eur J Allergy Clin Immunol 2005;60(4):544–5.
5. Harboe T, Johansson SG, Florvaag E, Oman H. Pholcodine exposure raises serum IgE in patients with previous anaphylaxis to neuromuscular blocking agents. Allergy 2007;62(12):1445–50.
6. Laine K, Kivist KT, Ojala-Karlsson P, Neuvonen PJ. Effect of activated charcoal on the pharmacokinetics of pholcodine, with special reference to delayed charcoal ingestion. Ther Drug Monit 1997;19(1):46–50.

Picenadol

General Information

Picenadol is a racemic mixture of an N-methyl-4-phenylpiperidine derivative. It has mixed agonist–antagonist properties, because the dextrorotatory isomer is a potent opioid agonist and the levorotatory isomer is an opioid antagonist. Picenadol also has anticholinergic activity. Its adverse effects include drowsiness, dizziness, and light-headedness (SEDA-16, 90). In a double-blind comparison of the analgesic potency and adverse effects profiles of a single oral dose of picenadol 25 mg with codeine 60 mg and placebo, few adverse effects were reported. Drowsiness was the most frequent, with an incidence of 16% (1).

Picenadol 75 mg was reportedly distinguishable from morphine by sedation, dysphoria, and hallucinatory activity, probably due to anticholinergic activity; at lower doses it was morphine-like (SEDA-16, 90).

Reference

1. Brunelle RL, George RE, Sunshine A, Hammonds WD. Analgesic effect of picenadol, codeine, and placebo in patients with postoperative pain. Clin Pharmacol Ther 1988;43(6):663–7.

Propiram

General Information

Propiram is an orally active opioid analgesic with weak antagonist activity and effects typical of its class (SED-11, 150; 1,2).

References

1. Desjardins PJ, Cooper SA, Gallegos TL, Allwein JB, Reynolds DC, Kruger GO, Beaver WT. The relative analgesic efficacy of propiram fumarate, codeine, aspirin, and placebo in post-impaction dental pain. J Clin Pharmacol 1984;24(1):35–42.
2. Goa KL, Brogden RN. Propiram. A review of its pharmacodynamic and pharmacokinetic properties, and clinical use as an analgesic. Drugs 1993;46(3):428–45.

Remifentanil

General Information

Remifentanil is a pure, MOR ($OP_3\mu$) opioid receptor agonist with a very short duration of action. It therefore has to be given by continuous intravenous infusion and is used as a supplement to general anesthesia during induction and as an analgesic during maintenance of anesthesia. It has the familiar adverse effects of opioids: respiratory depression, sedation, nausea and vomiting, muscle rigidity, bradycardia, and pruritus. These are short-lived and are antagonized by naloxone. The onset of muscle rigidity and apnea can be alarmingly rapid. Bradycardia occurred more often with remifentanil than alfentanil in patients undergoing abdominal surgery and in children undergoing strabismus surgery; the oculocardiac response was more marked with remifentanil than alfentanil (1).

The literature on remifentanil has been reviewed (2). In cardiac anesthesia, remifentanil provides better hemodynamic control intraoperatively and postoperatively than other opioids and is a good anesthetic agent together with propofol for total intravenous cardiac anesthesia. The recommended intraoperative infusion rate is 0.05-0.5 micrograms/kg/minute, changing to 0.05 micrograms/kg/

minute to treat postoperative pain with a view to changing short-acting remifentanil to a longer-acting morphine derivative (3).

Drug studies

Pain relief

Three studies have focused on the analgesic use of remifentanil (4–6). In a double-blind, crossover, randomized study 20 healthy volunteers received an infusion of either remifentanil or saline (4). Thermal sensory testing of the heat pain threshold was performed every 5 minutes and the dose of remifentanil was increased by 0.01 micrograms/kg/minute every 5 minutes. Remifentanil produced a dose-dependent increase in the heat pain threshold, and a dose of 0.05 micrograms/kg/minute was suggested as an effective and safe increment in healthy volunteers. The rate of adverse effects (nausea, vomiting, and pruritus) was comparable with previous reports; there were no cardiovascular adverse effects.

General surgery

Mixtures of remifentanil and sevoflurane have been used in two prospective, open, randomized studies (7,8), which showed that adding remifentanil results in a reduced requirement for sevoflurane for maintenance of anesthesia, leading to faster and easier recovery.

In a double-blind, randomized study a continuous infusion of remifentanil (1 microgram/kg followed by 0.5 micrograms/kg/minute) was compared with alfentanil (25 micrograms/kg followed by 1 microgram/kg/minute) during anesthesia in patients undergoing major abdominal surgery (9). Both systolic pressure and heart rate were significantly lower with remifentanil, with a higher incidence of hypotension (53 versus 39%) and bradycardia (10 versus 3%).

Bronchoscopy

In a randomized study, remifentanil 0.5 micrograms/kg/minute was compared with fentanyl 2 micrograms/kg in 22 patients undergoing rigid bronchoscopy (10). The results suggested that remifentanil attenuated the hemodynamic response to bronchoscopy without significantly increasing the incidences of hypotension or bradycardia. Four patients given remifentanil developed ST segment depression compared with eight patients given fentanyl.

Colonoscopy

Remifentanil by infusion ($n = 49$) has been compared with titrated boluses of pethidine ($n = 51$) in a randomized, double-blind study in 100 patients undergoing outpatient colonoscopy (11). The incidences of tachycardia, hypotension, and nausea were significantly less with remifentanil than with pethidine, but there were higher anxiety and pain scores with remifentanil. However, the study was a comparison of two opioids with different pharmacokinetic profiles, which makes it very difficult to achieve equipotent doses for the purpose of comparison.

Lithotripsy

In two randomized, double-blind, controlled comparisons of anesthetic techniques for extracorporeal shock wave lithotripsy remifentanil infusion had no advantage over the combination of fentanyl bolus plus propofol infusion, but caused more adverse effects (nausea and vomiting) (12). In another study remifentanil infusion provided comparable analgesia and caused less respiratory depression and fewer gastrointestinal symptoms than intravenous boluses of sufentanil (13).

In a double-blind, randomized, placebo-controlled study, 40 patients undergoing extracorporeal shock-wave lithotripsy were given prophylactic dolasetron 12.5 mg before remifentanil (0.15 micrograms/kg/minute) (14). Dolasetron produced a significant reduction in the incidence of nausea and vomiting and significantly earlier discharge.

Cardiac surgery

In a prospective multicenter, double-blind, randomized study in 297 patients undergoing elective coronary artery bypass surgery, remifentanil infusion 1 microgram/kg/minute was compared with a loading dose of fentanyl 15 micrograms/kg (15). The most common adverse effects were nausea and vomiting, which occurred equally often in the two groups. Hypertension and shivering were significantly more common with remifentanil (15).

Remifentanil 0.054 micrograms/kg/minute for postoperative pain after cardiac surgery produced adequate analgesia in 73% of tracheally extubated patients without causing respiratory compromise (16,17). However, the investigators suggested careful monitoring by trained personnel (18).

In infants and children undergoing cardiac surgery, spinal anesthetic blockade with remifentanil significantly reduced postoperative pain and reduced the requirement for fentanyl without significant adverse effects (16).

In a multicenter double-blind randomized, dose-comparison study in 149 patients undergoing first-time elective coronary artery bypass grafting, the recommended remifentanil infusion rate was not more than 1 microgram/kg/minute without any adverse effects that necessitated withdrawal (19).

Obstetrics and gynecology

The role of remifentanil-based anesthesia in gynecological and obstetric procedures has been reviewed (20).

In a double-blind, randomized comparison of remifentanil (0.25/0.5 micrograms/kg/minute) and alfentanil (50 micrograms and 0.5 micrograms/kg/minute) in 35 patients undergoing total abdominal hysterectomy, remifentanil provided more stable analgesia during anesthesia but caused significantly more hypotension (21).

Orthopedic surgery

Intravenous remifentanil 0.3 micrograms/kg with propofol 2 micrograms/ml has been compared with propofol 2 micrograms/ml alone in a double-blind, randomized study in 86 day-case adults undergoing elective orthopedic surgery (22). The study was designed to assess whether remifentanil improves conditions for laryngeal mask airway insertion. Those given remifentanil had a better quality of airway patency, with minimal cardiorespiratory changes.

Orthopedic and urological surgery

The respiratory depressant and gastrointestinal adverse effects of remifentanil have been observed in a randomized, single-blind study of 125 patients undergoing elective orthopedic and urological surgery under spinal or brachial plexus anesthesia (23). They were randomized to either remifentanil (a bolus of 0.5 micrograms/kg plus an infusion of 0.1 micrograms/kg/minute) or propofol (a bolus of 500 micrograms/kg plus an infusion of 50 micrograms/kg/minute). Owing to a significantly higher rate of respiratory depression with remifentanil (46%) than with propofol (19%), the mean remifentanil infusion rate was reduced to 0.078 ± 0.028 micrograms/kg/minute. The incidence of intraoperative nausea and vomiting with remifentanil was 27% compared with 2% with propofol. Postoperatively there was no significant difference in the incidence of gastrointestinal symptoms. Remifentanil may be considered as an alternative if propofol is contraindicated (for example because of amnesic episodes).

Remifentanil + propofol and fentanyl + desflurane have been compared in 49 patients undergoing prolonged surgery (elective abdominal prostatectomy lasting more than 150 minutes) (24). The fentanyl + desflurane combination was associated with faster recovery and extubation, at a significantly lower cost. Significantly more patients had postoperative nausea and vomiting with desflurane.

Vascular surgery

In a double-blind, randomized, placebo-controlled study in 28 adults undergoing carotid endarterectomy, remifentanil provided adequate analgesia, and supplementary local anesthetics were not needed (25). The remifentanil infusion rate was as low as 0.04 micrograms/kg/minute and there were no episodes of respiratory depression or hemodynamic instability.

In 60 patients receiving cervical plexus block during carotid endarterectomy who were given either remifentanil 3 micrograms/kg/hour or propofol 1 mg/kg/hour there was a higher incidence of adverse respiratory effects with remifentanil and a similar sedative effect (26). The authors suggested that when using remifentanil for sedation in patients undergoing carotid endarterectomy, the initial dose of remifentanil should be reduced to 1.5–2 micrograms/kg/hour to minimize cardiovascular and respiratory adverse effects.

Ophthalmological surgery

The analgesic effects of remifentanil and alfentanil have been compared during ophthalmological nerve block in a randomized, double-blind, parallel-group study in 79 patients (27). Remifentanil (as a single dose of 1 microgram/kg or as a loading dose of 1 microgram/kg followed by an infusion of 0.2 micrograms/kg/minute) was more effective than alfentanil (as a single dose of 7 micrograms/kg). Of the patients given remifentanil, three had mild nausea and three had transient muscle rigidity that resolved spontaneously within 1 minute. There were no adverse effects of alfentanil. The authors suggested that remifentanil 1 microgram/kg given over 30 seconds is a useful alternative to alfentanil 7 micrograms/kg as an analgesic before ophthalmological nerve block.

Anesthesia in ischemic heart disease

In a prospective randomized comparison of combined sevoflurane plus remifentanil with combined fentanyl plus etomidate for induction of anesthesia in 10 patients with ischemic heart disease, 3 of the 20 patients given sevoflurane plus remifentanil developed severe bradycardia (heart rate less than 40) and one developed asystole, but the difference between the two groups did not reach statistical significance (28). Therefore, in patients with ischemic heart disease remifentanil should be used with caution, and concurrent administration of glycopyrrolate 0.2 mg is advisable to reduce the incidence of bradycardia, hypotension, or both, without increasing the heart rate.

Radiological procedures

Remifentanil 0.25 micrograms/kg by continuous infusion has been compared with placebo in 62 women undergoing hysterosalpingography (29). Remifentanil afforded better analgesia with minimal opioid adverse effects.

Organs and Systems

Cardiovascular

Three groups of 20 women due to undergo elective surgery were recruited into a randomized, double-blind study (30). Group 1 received a bolus dose of remifentanil 1 microgram/kg and an infusion of remifentanil (0.5 micrograms/kg/minute); groups 2 and 3 received remifentanil 0.5 micrograms/kg and an infusion of 0.25 micrograms/kg/minute. Groups 1 and 2 received pretreatment with glycopyrrolate 200 micrograms whilst group 3 did not. Cardiovascular responses to laryngoscopy and orotracheal intubation were measured. There were no significant differences in the three groups, except that there was a significantly lower heart rate in group 3 after induction of anesthesia and after intubation.

The hemodynamic effects of bolus intravenous remifentanil 0.2, 0.33, and 1 microgram/kg/minute have been studied in patients scheduled for coronary artery bypass grafting (31). The study was terminated after only eight patients had been recruited, because of severe hypotension, bradycardia, and/or evidence of myocardial ischemia. The authors concluded that remifentanil should not be given as a bolus dose of 1 microgram/kg but as an infusion at a low rate. An editorial response to this article suggested that the hemodynamic instability reported may have resulted from other contributing factors, such as hypovolemia, impairment of venous return, or excessive anesthesia due to remifentanil toxicity (32).

In a prospective study in 12 men undergoing elective coronary artery bypass grafting, remifentanil 0.5 and 2.0 micrograms/kg/minute combined with propofol preserved hemodynamic stability and reduced myocardial blood flow and metabolism to a similar extent (33).

Asystole has been attributed to remifentanil (34).

- A 78-year-old man with laryngeal cancer developed asystole 1 minute after an intravenous bolus of remifentanil 0.5 micrograms/kg followed by a continuous infusion of 0.5 micrograms/kg/hour. The asystole was unresponsive to intravenous atropine 1 mg. The remifentanil infusion was stopped and cardiac sinus rhythm resumed after two precordial thumps.

The authors postulated that rapid-sequence induction of anesthesia with sevoflurane had blunted sympathetic tone and allowed uncompensated parasympathetic activation by remifentanil.

Remifentanil-induced bradycardia and asystole may be useful as a protective effect in patients with atrial fibrillation (35).

- A 90-year-old woman with atrial fibrillation was given digoxin for 3 days before surgery for a pelvic mass. Following anesthesia, induced with thiopental and atracurium, her heart rate rose to 105/minute and her electrocardiogram showed fast atrial fibrillation and ST segment depression. She was given remifentanil 0.25 micrograms/kg/minute and her heart rate fell to 95/minute.

Remifentanil was used in a double-blind, randomized trial in 49 infants and children under 5 years old, who were given one of four infusion rates (0.25, 1.0, 2.5, or 5.0 micrograms/kg/minute) (36). Blood glucose, cortisol, and neuropeptide Y concentrations were used as indicators of stress. An infusion rate of 1 microgram/kg/minute was considered a suitable starting rate. Of the 49 patients, nine had significant bradycardia or hypotension requiring intervention. Four of these were neonates with complex cardiac anatomy, and remifentanil should be used with caution in these cases.

In another randomized, double-blind, placebo-controlled study, 25 cardiac surgical patients aged 55–70 years received either remifentanil 0.5 micrograms/kg/minute or placebo during surgery (37). The patients who were given remifentanil had a lower cardiac output, a lower left ventricular stroke work index (LVSWI), and lower mixed venous oxygen saturation (SvO_2) in the early postoperative phase, suggesting postoperative cardiac depression. This occurred within the first 2 hours after termination of the remifentanil infusion, rather than during remifentanil administration. A possible explanation of this unexpected result is an opioid-related alteration in cardiac responsiveness to sympathetic discharge.

In 40 children, cardiac effects were monitored after the administration of remifentanil with or without atropine (38). Remifentanil reduced blood pressure, heart rate, and cardiac index, even when atropine was added (39). Glycopyrrolate 6 micrograms/kg prevented the bradycardia caused by remifentanil + sevoflurane anesthesia for cardiac catheterization in children with congenital heart disease (40). Remifentanil attenuated the rapid rise in systolic blood pressure after electroconvulsive therapy. This sympathetic response can be harmful to patients who already have cardiac problems. Thus, the cardiac effects of remifentanil may be beneficial in patients with compromised cardiac function.

Remifentanil 0.05 micrograms/kg/minute by infusion has been compared with alfentanil and fentanyl during stereotactic brain biopsy in 135 subjects (41). Remifentanil (together with alfentanil) had less hemodynamic effect than fentanyl.

Similarly, the combination of remifentanil + propofol in reduction of anterior glenohumoral dislocation in 22 subjects provided adequate sedation and analgesia, without hemodynamic and/or respiratory complications (42).

Respiratory

In contrast to the studies above, three case reports have highlighted the potential for remifentanil 2–5 micrograms to cause serious respiratory depression, even at moderate doses, possibly due to rapid onset of effect (43). All recovered without incident.

In a randomized, double-blind, two-period, crossover, placebo-controlled, dose-escalation study, 64 patients were given either remifentanil or placebo by bolus injections in a fixed unit dose, separated by an 8-hour washout period (44). There were 48 younger patients (<60 years) and 16 older patients (>60 years). The younger patients who received 75 micrograms or less had minimal respiratory depression, while higher doses (100–200 micrograms) produced mild and easily managed respiratory depression. The older patients had more significant respiratory depression, which occurred at lower doses and more often. However, the most serious respiratory events were episodes of apnea, which occurred in four patients of all age groups (a 68-year old man who was given 75 micrograms, a 36-year old man who was given 150 micrograms, a 27-year old woman who was given 75 micrograms, and a 21-year old man who was given 200 micrograms). There were no other opioid-related adverse effects.

In 11 volunteers remifentanil 0.035 micrograms/kg/minute reduced normoxic and hypoxic ventilation (45). In children who were breathing spontaneously and received inhalational anesthesia, large variations in dosages of remifentanil (0.053–0.3 micrograms/kg/minute) were well tolerated (46). A dose of 0.05 micrograms/kg/minute allowed spontaneous respiration in over 90% of children and 0.3 micrograms/kg/minute prevented spontaneous respiration in 90%. Although this study provided useful indication on the respiratory effects of increasing infusion rates of remifentanil in children, it had several limitations, including not comparing respiratory parameters with blood concentrations.

Nervous system

Intraoperative administration of large doses of remifentanil produces postoperative peri-incisional hyperalgesia. In a randomized study (47) 75 patients undergoing major abdominal surgery were given one of two doses of remifentanil (0.05 and 0.4 micrograms/kg/minute) or remifentanil + ketamine (ketamine: 0.5 mg/kg; remifentanil 0.4 micrograms/kg/minute after induction, 5 micrograms/kg/minute intraoperatively up to skin closure, and 2 micrograms/kg/minute for 48 hours thereafter). High-dose remifentanil was associated with hyperalgesia. The addition of ketamine prevented this, implying involvement of NMDA receptors. There were similar results in a smaller study in patients undergoing major abdominal surgery, in which high-dose remifentanil added to epidural anesthesia resulted in acute opioid tolerance and hyperalgesia immediately after surgery (48).

Pain sensitization induced by remifentanil 3 and 8 ng/ml has been the subject of a randomized controlled study (49). Those who were given the larger dose needed earlier and more postoperative morphine. Nefopam given intraoperatively reversed this effect.

Seizures have been attributed to remifentanil (50).

- A 42-year-old woman asked for an intravenous opioid as analgesia during paracervical block and was given an intravenous infusion of remifentanil 1.0 microgram/minute. After 3 minutes she became unresponsive, with upward deviation of gaze and tonic-clonic contractions of the arms. The infusion was discontinued and after another 3 minutes of generalized seizure activity she was given intravenous propofol 80 mg and intravenous suxamethonium 60 mg; she recovered completely 15 minutes later.
- A 77-year-old woman with long standing hypertension was given a bolus dose of remifentanil 50 micrograms as part of general anesthesia, and 30 seconds later, before any other drugs had been given, developed a generalized tonic–clonic seizure, which lasted 1–2 minutes (51). She was given 100% oxygen and within 10 minutes was wide awake with no neurological sequence.

Psychological, psychiatric

In 201 patients scheduled for day-case surgery, those who received remifentanil had significantly fewer responses to surgical stimulation and had better psychomotor and psychometric function during the recovery period, although there was no significant difference in time to recovery room or hospital discharge (52).

Gastrointestinal

Remifentanil produced less postoperative nausea and vomiting than fentanyl in a prospective, randomized, double-blind study in patients anesthetized with propofol, undergoing plastic surgery (53). The incidence of nausea and vomiting 2–12 hours postoperatively was less if remifentanil was used intraoperatively rather than fentanyl. The need for antiemetic rescue drugs was also less with remifentanil. Known susceptibility factors for postoperative nausea and vomiting were accounted for through exclusion criteria. The patients who received remifentanil also required less postoperative opioid analgesia. Despite

these benefits, the degree of patient satisfaction was the same in the two groups.

Sexual function

Remifentanil by infusion caused *penile erection* in 5.5% of children undergoing cystoscopy (54). The authors reported this as an unusual adverse effect, which could be alleviated by reduction or complete withdrawal of remifentanil infusion and/or deepening the level of anesthesia.

Second-Generation Effects

Pregnancy

Six patients admitted at 36 weeks pregnancy with preeclampsia received patient-controlled intravenous analgesia with remifentanil for labor (5). Remifentanil was delivered as continuous background infusion of 0.05 micrograms/kg/minute and boluses of 25 micrograms with a 5-minute lockout period. The procedure did not cause adverse maternal or neonatal adverse effects and this small uncontrolled study suggests that patient-controlled intravenous analgesia with remifentanil might be an effective alternative when epidural analgesia is contraindicated.

In a dose-finding study in 17 healthy pregnant women in the first stage of labor, the PCA bolus of remifentanil was increased from 0.2 micrograms/kg in 0.2 micrograms/kg increments during 60 minutes until analgesia was considered adequate (55). The median effective dose of remifentanil was 0.4 (range 0.2–0.8) micrograms/kg and consumption was 0.066 (range 0.027–0.207) micrograms/kg/minute. All the women reported slight sedation; five had slight to moderate nausea throughout the study. Supplementary oxygen 2 l/minute via nasal cannula was given to three women who had repeated episodes of oxygen desaturation. Two women reported difficulties in reading and visual focusing and one woman had difficulty in swallowing toward the end of remifentanil administration. In five cases there were changes in fetal heart rate indices within 30 minutes of the first dose. The neonates had Apgar scores of 8–10. The authors concluded that remifentanil is a potentially effective obstetric analgesic but that adverse effects will limit its use.

A similar observation was made in an open pilot study in 36 women randomized during the early stages of labor to either intramuscular pethidine 100 mg or remifentanil given as patient-controlled analgesia (20-microgram bolus over 20 seconds) (56). Remifentanil provided better pain relief but a higher risk of lower oxygen saturation compared with pethidine. Remifentanil was given only a cautious welcome by the authors, owing to its respiratory depressant effects.

In 20 women in labor remifentanil gave better analgesia than nitrous oxide (57). Adverse effects were similar in the two groups, with some exceptions—sedation was more profound with remifentanil and two subjects reported slight itching. The effects on the fetus were similar in the two groups, including reduced beat-to-beat variability in fetal heart rate. The neonates did not suffer from depression; however, there were withdrawals in the remifentanil group because of a requirement for respiratory support or fetal compromise.

Remifentanil has been compared with diazepam during fetoscopic surgery in 54 women in the second trimester, who were randomly assigned to either incremental doses of diazepam or a continuous infusion of remifentanil after combined spinal epidural anesthesia (58). Remifentanil produced adequate maternal sedation, with mild clinically irrelevant respiratory depression and faster and more pronounced fetal immobilization, resulting in better surgical conditions. No respiratory depression was observed with diazepam and sedation was more pronounced.

Fetotoxicity

Opioid-related rigidity in a neonate delivered by a parturient who had received intraoperative remifentanil has been reported (59).

- A 27-year-old primagravida with autoimmune hepatitis complicated by cirrhosis, esophageal varices, and thrombocytopenia had a planned cesarean section. To maintain hemodynamic stability during induction, she was given a remifentanil infusion 0.1 micrograms/kg/minute together with remifentanil boluses up to a total of 2.5 micrograms/kg over 1 minute. The infusion of remifentanil was reduced before delivery, in order to minimize transplacental fetal exposure. On delivery, the baby developed apnea and generalized rigidity and required oxygen. Apgar scores were 7 and 9 at 1 and 5 minutes respectively.

In this case, the possibly higher unbound fraction of remifentanil due to liver dysfunction may have resulted in higher remifentanil blood concentrations and more placental transfer of remifentanil. In addition, fetal prematurity with reduced glycoprotein concentrations and potentially immature metabolic pathways, may have contributed to a susceptibility to respiratory depression and muscle rigidity.

Susceptibility Factors

Age

In maintenance of anesthesia in 62 children vomiting occurred in 31% (60). However, the dose of remifentanil was twice the ED_{50} in adults and may have been much larger than required.

The effects of remifentanil on vomiting and the quality of emergence from anesthesia have been studied in children undergoing dental restoration and extraction (61). The children received desflurane with or without remifentanil 0.2 micrograms/kg/minute. The two groups did not differ in adverse effects profile or quality of recovery.

Seven randomized controlled trials and one descriptive trial using infused remifentanil as part of an anesthetic

technique in children between 1997 and 2000 have been reviewed (62). The general consensus is that a bolus dose of remifentanil 0.5–1 microgram/kg appears to be well tolerated when it is given over at least 60 seconds. However, a loading dose is not required if the infusion can be started at least 10 minutes before the skin incision is made. Infusion rates of 0.25–0.5 micrograms/kg/minute provide hemodynamic stability when propofol or a volatile agent is also given. The authors advised that infants who receive remifentanil should be paralysed and mechanically ventilated, because of the possible risk of respiratory depression due to chest wall rigidity in non-paralysed patients.

Remifentanil is liable to cause respiratory depression in children (62,63), as well as muscle rigidity, hypotension, and bradycardia, without increasing the incidence of gastrointestinal symptoms (64).

The adverse effects profiles of remifentanil in neonates and infants undergoing pyloromyotomy have been investigated (65,66).

The hemodynamic responses, recovery profiles, and perioperative and postoperative respiratory patterns in 38 children given remifentanil plus nitrous oxide and 22 given halothane plus nitrous oxide have been studied in a multicenter, open, randomized comparison (65). There were no cases of bradycardia or dysrhythmias. There were hypertensive responses at the time of incision in 24% of those given remifentanil and 18% of those given halothane and vomiting in 34 and 45% respectively. None of those who were given remifentanil developed new-onset postoperative apnea compared with three of those who were given halothane. All other adverse effects had similar incidences in the two groups.

Remifentanil 0.1 micrograms/kg/minute by infusion was safe and efficacious in 55 patients (aged 2 months to 12 years) undergoing cardiac catheterization (67).

Remifentanil and remifentanil + midazolam provided safe and effective analgesia for bone marrow aspiration in 80 children aged 5–16 years (68). There were no cases of deep sedation, hypotension, bradycardia, hypoxemia, or respiratory depression.

Physiological factors

When remifentanil 5.7 micrograms/kg/hour was given to a 66-year-old woman during treatment for self-poisoning with tranylcypromine, trifluoperazine, lorazepam, and fluoxetine, she developed agitation, sweating, oxygen desaturation, facial myoclonus, generalized hypertension, hyper-reflexia, conjugate ocular movements, and poorly reactive pupils; she did not respond to painful stimuli (69). Withdrawal of remifentanil resulted in improved level of consciousness, reduced rigidity, and disappearance of the abnormal ocular movements. The authors suggested that muscle rigidity due to remifentanil had been caused by an interaction with serotonergic hyperactivity.

Drug Administration

Drug dosage regimens

In a double-blind, randomized study of 178 patients scheduled for major thoracic, intra-abdominal, and orthopedic surgery, a high dose of remifentanil (bolus dose of 1 microgram/kg followed by 1 microgram/kg/minute) was compared with a low dose (bolus dose 1 microgram/kg followed by 0.5 micrograms/kg/minute) (70). In this study, intraoperative hypotension (30% and 27% respectively) and bradycardia (9% and 7% respectively) were equally frequent in the two groups. The authors proposed that infusion rates of remifentanil over 0.4 micrograms/kg/minute provide satisfactory analgesia throughout surgery but can cause significant hypotension. Prolonged infusion of remifentanil for several hours of surgery does not delay recovery or cause respiratory depression.

The postoperative analgesic efficacy and safety of two continuous constant-dose intravenous remifentanil infusions have been investigated in a double-blind, randomized study in 30 patients scheduled to undergo elective abdominal or thoracic surgery (6). The patients were randomly assigned to intravenous remifentanil 0.05 micrograms/kg/minute or 0.1 micrograms/kg/minute. There were no cases of respiratory depression, and nausea and vomiting occurred in one patient in each group. There was adequate analgesia in 75% and 78% of the patients in the low-dose and high-dose groups respectively and pethidine rescue analgesia was required in 26% and 6% respectively. Remifentanil 0.1 micrograms/kg/minute was therefore effective and safe for postoperative pain.

Drug overdose

A nurse was found dead at home with a syringe and empty vials of remifentanil (2 mg) and midazolam (1 mg/ml); toxicological studies showed that she had not been a chronic user of remifentanil (71).

Drug–Drug Interactions

Magnesium

The added analgesic effect of magnesium after on-pump cardiac surgery has been studied in a placebo-controlled study in 40 patients (72). The dose of either magnesium gluconate was 0.21 mmol/kg by intravenous bolus followed by a continuous infusion of 0.03 mmol/kg/hour for 12 hours after extubation. After surgery, remifentanil was reduced to 0.05 micrograms/kg/minute and titrated according to needs. Magnesium reduced the dosage requirements of remifentanil without serious adverse effects. The results suggested that the opioid-sparing effect of magnesium may be greater at higher pain intensities and with increased dosages.

Neostigmine

The addition of neostigmine after anesthesia with propofol + remifentanil alters the state of anesthesia and may enhance recovery (73).

Propofol

In eight subjects the concentration of remifentanil was significantly increased when therapeutic concentrations of propofol were present in the body (74). The combination of propofol and remifentanil can cause cardiovascular depression. As with other opioids, remifentanil competes with propofol for hydrophobic binding in the lungs and heart.

The effects of two doses of remifentanil by intravenous infusion (7.5 micrograms/kg/hour, n = 15, and 30 micrograms/kg/minute. n = 15) have been compared with the effects of equal volumes of saline (n = 15) before induction of anesthesia with propofol (75). Remifentanil significantly reduced propofol requirements and accelerated its hypnotic effects.

In 21 children, mean age 6.5 years, with lymphoblastic leukemia or lymphoma undergoing intrathecal chemotherapy, the combination of propofol and remifentanil achieved earlier recovery (76). Similarly, in 20 children, the addition of remifentanil resulted in reduced propofol consumption and faster emergence times, as measured by the composite auditory evoked potential index (77).

For intracranial surgery, the combination of propofol + remifentanil produced fewer hypotensive events than the combination of sevoflurane + remifentanil (78).

Co-administration of propofol with remifentanil in 45 subjects caused loss of consciousness and affected middle latency auditory provoked potentials, although the contribution of remifentanil to the latter was questionable (79).

References

1. Duthie DJ. Remifentanil and tramadol. Br J Anaesth 1998;81(1):51–7.
2. Servin FS. Remifentanil: an update. Curr Opin Anaesthesiol 2003;16:367–72.
3. Barvais L, Sutcliffe N. Remifentanil for cardiac anaesthesia. In: Vuyk J, Schraag S (editors). Advances in Modelling and Clinical Application of Intravenous Anaesthesia. New York: Kluwer Academic/Plenum Publishers, 2003:171–87.
4. Gustorff B, Felleiter P, Nahlik G, Brannath W, Hoerauf KH, Spacek A, Kress HG. The effect of remifentanil on the heat pain threshold in volunteers. Anesth Analg 2001;92(2):369–74.
5. Roelants F, De Franceschi E, Veyckemans F, Lavand'homme P. Patient-controlled intravenous analgesia using remifentanil in the parturient. Can J Anaesth 2001;48(2):175–8.
6. Calderon E, Pernia A, De Antonio P, Calderon-Pla E, Torres LM. A comparison of two constant-dose continuous infusions of remifentanil for severe postoperative pain. Anesth Analg 2001;92(3):715–9.
7. Breslin DS, Reid JE, Mirakhur RK, Hayes AH, McBrien ME. Sevoflurane–nitrous oxide anaesthesia

supplemented with remifentanil: effect on recovery and cognitive function. Anaesthesia 2001;56(2):114–9.

8. Joo HS, Perks WJ, Belo SE. Sevoflurane with remifentanil allows rapid tracheal intubation without neuromuscular blocking agents. Can J Anaesth 2001;48(7):646–50.

9. Camu F, Royston D. Inpatient experience with remifentanil. Anesth Analg 1999;89(Suppl 4):S15–21.

10. Prakash N, McLeod T, Gao Smith F. The effects of remifentanil on haemodynamic stability during rigid bronchoscopy. Anaesthesia 2001;56(6):576–80.

11. Greilich PE, Virella CD, Rich JM, Kurada M, Roberts K, Warren JF, Harford WV. Remifentanil versus meperidine for monitored anesthesia care: a comparison study in older patients undergoing ambulatory colonoscopy. Anesth Analg 2001;92(1):80–4.

12. Burmeister MA, Brauer P, Wintruff M, Graefen M, Blanc I, Standl TG. A comparison of anaesthetic techniques for shock wave lithotripsy: the use of a remifentanil infusion alone compared to intermittent fentanyl boluses combined with a low dose propofol infusion. Anaesthesia 2002;57(9):877–81.

13. Beloeil H, Corsia G, Coriat P, Riou B. Remifentanil compared with sufentanil during extra-corporeal shock wave lithotripsy with spontaneous ventilation: a double-blind, randomized study. Br J Anaesth 2002;89(4):567–70.

14. Burmeiser MA, Standl TG, Wintruff M, Braver P, Blanc I. Schulte am Esch J. Dolestron prophylaxis reduces nausea and postanaesthesia recovery time after remifentanil infusion during monitored anaesthesia care for extra corporeal shock wave lithotripsy. Br J Anaesth 2003;90:194–8.

15. Mollhoff T, Herregods L, Moerman A, Blake D, MacAdams C, Demeyere R, Kirno K, Dybvik T, Shaikh SRemifentanil Study Group. Comparative efficacy and safety of remifentanil and fentanyl in 'fast track' coronary artery bypass graft surgery: a randomized, double-blind study. Br J Anaesth 2001;87(5):718–26.

16. Steinlechner B, Koinig H, Grubhofer G, Ponschab M, Eislmeir S, Dworschak M, Rajek A. Postoperative analgesia with remifentanil in patients undergoing cardiac surgery. Anesth Analg 2005;100(5):1230–5.

17. Hammer GB, Ramamoorthy C, Cao H, Williams GD, Boltz MG, Kamra K, Drover DR. Postoperative analgesia after spinal blockade in infants and children undergoing cardiac surgery. Anesth Analg 2005;100(5):1283–8.

18. Codreanu F, Morisset M, Kanny G, Moneret-Vautrin DA. Allergy to pholcodine: first case documented by oral challenge. Allergy: Eur J Allergy Clin Immunol 2005;60(4):544–5.

19. Geisler FEA, De Lange S, Royston D, Demeyer R, Duthie DJR, Lehot J-J, Adt M, Dupeyron J-P, Mansfield M, Kirkhem AJT. Efficacy and safety of remifentanil in coronary artery bypass graft surgery: a randomized, double-blind dose comparison study. J Cardiothorac Vasc Anaesth 2003;17:60–8.

20. Buerkle H, Wilhelm W. Remifentanil for gynaecological and obstetric procedures. Curr Opin Anaesthesiol 2000;13:271–5.

21. Kovac AL, Azad SS, Steer P, Witkowski T, Batenhorst R, McNeal S. Remifentanil versus alfentanil in a balanced anesthetic technique for total abdominal hysterectomy. J Clin Anesth 1997;9(7):532–41.

22. Grewal K, Samsoon G. Facilitation of laryngeal mask airway insertion: effects of remifentanil administered before induction with target-controlled propofol infusion. Anaesthesia 2001;56(9):897–901.

23. Servin FS, Raeder JC, Merle JC, Wattwil M, Hanson AL, Lauwers MH, Aitkenhead A, Marty J, Reite K, Martisson S, Wostyn L. Remifentanil sedation compared with propofol during regional anaesthesia. Acta Anaesthesiol Scand 2002;46(3):309–15.

24. Rohm KD, Piper SN, Suttner S, Schuler S, Boldt J. Early recovery, cognitive function and costs of a desflurane inhalational vs. a total intravenous anesthesia regimen in long-term surgery. Acta Anaesthesiol Scand 2006;50(1):14–18.

25. Marrocco-Trischitta MM, Bandiera G, Camilli S, Stillo F, Cirielli C, Guerrini P. Remifentanil conscious sedation during regional anaesthesia for carotid endarterectomy: rationale and safety. Eur J Vasc Endovasc Surg 2001;22(5): 405–9.

26. Krenn H, Deusch E, Jellinek H, Oczenski W, Fitzgerald RD. Remifentanil or propofol for sedation during carotid endarterectomy under cervical plexus block. Br J Anaesth 2002;89(4):637–40.

27. Ahmad S, Leavell ME, Fragen RJ, Jenkins W, Roland CL. Remifentanil versus alfentanil as analgesic adjuncts during placement of ophthalmologic nerve blocks. Reg Anesth Pain Med 1999;24(4):331–6.

28. Wang JY, Winship SM, Thomas SD, Gin T, Russell GN. Induction of anaesthesia in patients with coronary artery disease: a comparison between sevoflurane-remifentanil and fentanyl–etomidate. Anaesth Intensive Care 1999;27(4):363–8.

29. Cengiz M, Kafali H, Artuc H, Baysal Z. Opioid analgesia for hysterosalpingography: controlled double-blind prospective trial with remifentanil and placebo. Gynecol Obstet Investig 2006;62(3):168–72.

30. Hall AP, Thompson JP, Leslie NA, Fox AJ, Kumar N, Rowbotham DJ. Comparison of different doses of remifentanil on the cardiovascular response to laryngoscopy and tracheal intubation. Br J Anaesth 2000;84(1):100–2.

31. Elliott P, O'Hare R, Bill KM, Phillips AS, Gibson FM, Mirakhur RK. Severe cardiovascular depression with remifentanil. Anesth Analg 2000;91(1):58–61.

32. Michelsen LG. Hemodynamic effects of remifentanil in patients undergoing cardiac surgery. Anesth Analg 2000;91(6):1563.

33. Kazmaier S, Hanekop GG, Buhre W, Weyland A, Busch T, Radke OC, Zoelffel R, Sonntag H. Myocardial consequences of remifentanil in patients with coronary artery disease. Br J Anaesth 2000;84(5):578–83.

34. Kurdi O, Deleuze A, Marret E, Bonnet F. Asystole during anaesthetic induction with remifentanil and sevoflurane. Br J Anaesth 2001;87(6):943.

35. Williams H, Spoelstra C. Use of remifentanil in fast atrial fibrillation. Br J Anaesth 2002;88(4):614.

36. Weale NK, Rogers CA, Cooper R, Nolan J, Wolf AR. Effect of remifentanil infusion rate on stress response to the pre-bypass phase of paediatric cardiac surgery. Br J Anaesth 2004;92:187–94.

37. Pleym H, Stenseth R, Wilseth R, Karevola A, Dale O. Supplemental remifentanil during coronary artery bypass grafting is followed by a transient post-operative cardiac depression. Acta Anaesthesiol Scand 2004;48:1155–62.

38. Van Zijl DH, Gordon PC, James MF. The comparative effects of remifentanil or magnesium sulphate versus placebo on attenuating the hemodynamic responses after electroconvulsive therapy. Anesth Analg 2005;101(6):1651–5.

39. Chanavaz C, Tirel O, Wodey E, Bansard JY, Senhadji L, Robert JC, Ecoffey C. Haemodynamic effects of remifentanil in children with and without intravenous atropine. An echocardiographic study. Br J Anaesth 2005;94(1):74–9.

40. Reyntjens K, Foubert L, De Wolf D, Vanlerberghe G, Mortier E. Glycopyrrolate during sevoflurane-remifentanil-based anaesthesia for cardiac catheterization of children with congenital heart disease. Br J Anaesth 2005;95(5):680–4.

41. Bilgin H, Basagan Mogol E, Bekar A, Iscimen R, Korfali G. A comparison of effects of alfentanil, fentanyl, and remifentanil on hemodynamic and respiratory parameters during stereotactic brain biopsy. J Neurosurg Anesthesiol 2006;18(3):179–84.

42. Dunn MJG, Mitchell R, De Souza C, Drummond G. Evaluation of propofol and remifentanil for intravenous sedation for reducing shoulder dislocations in the emergency department. Emerg Med J 2006;23(1):57–8.

43. Koo B-N, Choi SH, Chun DH, Kil HK, Kim KJ, Min KT, Lee SJ. Respiratory depression caused by remifentanil infusion for postoperative pain control. Int Anesth Res Soc 2006;103(6):1627.

44. Egan TD, Kern SE, Muir KT, White J. Remifentanil by bolus injection: a safety, pharmacokinetic, pharmacodynamic, and age effect investigation in human volunteers. Br J Anaesth 2004;92:335–43.

45. Karan S, Voter W, Palmer L, Ward DS. Effects of pain and audiovisual stimulation on the opioid-induced depression of the hypoxic ventilator response. Anesthesiology 2005;103(2):384–90.

46. Ansermino JM, Brooks P, Rosen D, Vandebeek CA, Reichert C. Spontaneous ventilation with remifentanil in children. Pediat Anesth 2005;15(2):115–21.

47. Joly V, Richebe P, Guignard B, Fletcher D, Maurette P, Sessler DI, Chauvin M. Remifentanil-induced postoperative hyperalgesia and its prevention with small-dose ketamine. Anesthesiology 2005;103(1):147–55.

48. Hansen EG, Duedahl TH, Romsing J, Hilsted KL, Dahl JB. Intra-operative remifentanil might influence pain levels in the immediate post-operative period after major abdominal surgery. Acta Anaesthesiol Scand 2005;49(10):1464–70.

49. Tirault M, Derrode N, Clevenot D, Rolland D, Fletcher D, Debaene B. The effect of Nefopam on morphine overconsumption induced by large dose remifentanil during propofol anesthesia for major abdominal surgery. Anesth Analg 2006;102(1):110–7.

50. Haber GW, Litman RS. Generalized tonic-clonic activity after remifentanil administration. Anesth Analg 2001;93(6):1532–3.

51. Neilsen J, Kroigaard M. Seizures in a 77-year old woman after a bolus dose of remifentanil. Acta Anaesthesiol Scand 2004;48:253–4.

52. Cartwright DP, Kvalsvik O, Cassuto J, Jansen JP, Wall C, Remy B, Knape JT, Noronha D, Upadhyaya BK. A randomized, blind comparison of remifentanil and alfentanil during anesthesia for outpatient surgery. Anesth Analg 1997;85(5):1014–9.

53. Kreek MJ, Bart G, Lilly C, Laforge KS, Nielson DA. Pharmacogenetics and human molecular genetics of opiate and cocaine addictions and their treatments. Pharmacol Rev 2005;57(1):1–26.

54. Bakan M, Elicevik M, Bozkurt P, Kaya G. Penile erection during remifentanil anesthesia in children. Paediatr Anesth 2006;16(12):1294–5.

55. Volmanen P, Akural EI, Raudaskoski T, Alahuhta S. Remifentanil in obstetric analgesia: a dose-finding study. Anesth Analg 2002;94(4):913–7.

56. Thurlow JA, Laxton CH, Dick A, Waterhouse P, Sherman L, Goodman NW. Remifentanil by patient-controlled analgesia compared with intramuscular meperidine for pain relief in labour. Br J Anaesth 2002;88(3):374–8.

57. Volmanen P, Akural E, Raudaskoski T, Ohtonen P, Alahuhta S. Comparison of remifentanil and nitrous oxide in labour analgesia. Acta Anaesthesiol Scand 2005;49(4):453–8.

58. Van de Velde M, Van Schoubroeck D, Lewi LE, Marcus MAE, Jani JC, Missant C, Teunkens A, Deprest JA. Remifentanil for fetal immobilization and maternal sedation during fetoscopic surgery: a randomized, double-blind comparison with diazepam. Anesth Analg 2005;101(1):251–8.

59. Carvalho B, Mirikitoni EJ, Lyell D, Evans DA, Druzen M, Riley ET. Neonatal chest wall rigidity following the use of remifentanil for Caesarian delivery in a patient with autoimmune hepatitis and thrombocytopenia. Int J Obstet Anaesth 2004;13:53–6.

60. Davis PJ, Lerman J, Suresh S, McGowan FX, Cote CJ, Landsman I, Henson LG. A randomized multicenter study of remifentanil compared with alfentanil, isoflurane, or propofol in anesthetized pediatric patients undergoing elective strabismus surgery. Anesth Analg 1997;84(5):982–9.

61. Pinsker MC, Carroll NV. Quality of emergence from anesthesia and incidence of vomiting with remifentanil in a pediatric population. Anesth Analg 1999;89(1):71–4.

62. Booker PD, Whyte SD. Paediatric applications of concentration-oriented anaesthesia. Best Pract Res Clin Anaesthesiol 2001;15:97–111.

63. Keidan I, Berkenstadt H, Sidi A, Perel A. Propofol/remifentanil versus propofol alone for bone marrow aspiration in paediatric haemato-oncological patients. Paediatr Anaesth 2001;11(3):297–301.

64. Thees Ch, Frenkel Ch, Hoeft A. Remifentanil in der Neuroanästhesie—eine multizentrische Anwendungsbeobachtung. [Remifentanil in neuroanesthesia – a multicenter study.] Anästhesiol Intensivmed 2001;42:205–11.

65. Davis PJ, Galinkin J, McGowan FX, Lynn AM, Yaster M, Rabb MF, Krane EJ, Kurth CD, Blum RH, Maxwell L, Orr R, Szmuk P, Hechtman D, Edwards S, Henson LG. A randomized multicenter study of remifentanil compared with halothane in neonates and infants undergoing pyloromyotomy. I. Emergence and recovery profiles. Anesth Analg 2001;93(6):1380–6.

66. Galinkin JL, Davis PJ, McGowan FX, Lynn AM, Rabb MF, Yaster M, Henson LG, Blum R, Hechtman D, Maxwell L, Szmuk P, Orr R, Krane EJ, Edwards S, Kurth CD. A randomized multicenter study of remifentanil compared with halothane in neonates and infants undergoing pyloromyotomy. II. Perioperative breathing patterns in neonates and infants with pyloric stenosis. Anesth Analg 2001;93(6):1387–92.

67. Donmez A, Kizilkan A, Berksun H, Varan B, Tokel K. One center's experience with remifentanil infusions for pediatric cardiac catheterization. J Cardiothorac Vasc Anesth 2001;15(6):736–9.

68. Antmen B, Sasmaz I, Birbicer H, Ozbek H, Burgut R, Isik G, Kilinc Y. Safe and effective sedation and analgesia for bone marrow aspiration procedures in children with alfentanil, remifentanil and combinations with midazolam. Paediatr Anaesth 2005;15(3):214–9.

69. Hunter B, Mercedes Kleinert M, Osatnik J, Soria E. Serotonergic syndrome and abnormal ocular movements: worsening of rigidity by remifentanil? Anesth Analg 2006;102:1589.

70. Hogue CW Jr, Bowdle TA, O'Leary C, Duncalf D, Miguel R, Pitts M, Streisand J, Kirvassilis G, Jamerson B, McNeal S, Batenhorst R. A multicenter evaluation of total intravenous anesthesia with remifentanil and propofol for elective inpatient surgery. Anesth Analg 1996;83(2):279–85.

71. Asselborn G, Yegles M, Wennig R. Suicide with remifentanil and midazolam: a case report. Acta Clin Belg Suppl 2002;(1):54–7.

72. Steinlechner B, Dworschak M, Birkenberg B, Grubhofer G, Weigl M, Schiferer A, Lang T, Rajek A. Magnesium moderately decreases remifentanil dosage required for pain management after cardiac surgery. Br J Anaesth 2006;96(4):444–9.

73. Vasella FC, Frascarolo P, Spahn DR, Magnusson L. Antagonism of neuromuscular blockade but not muscle relaxation affects depth of anaesthesia. Br J Anaesth 2005;94(6):742–7.

74. Crankshaw DP, Chan C, Leslie K, Bjorksten AR. Remifentanil concentration during target-controlled infusion of propofol. Anaesth Intensive Care 2002;30(5):578–83.

75. Mustola S, Baer GA, Neuvonen PJ, Toivonen KJ. Requirements of propofol at different end-points without adjuvant and during two different steady infusions of remifentanil. Acta Anaesthesiol Scand 2005;49(2):215–21.

76. Glaisyer HR, Sury MRJ. Recovery after anesthesia for short pediatric oncology procedures: propofol and remifentanil compared with propofol, nitrous oxide and sevoflurane. Anesth Analg 2005;100(4):959–63.

77. Weber F, Seidl M, Bein T. Impact of the AEP-Monitor/2-derived composite auditory-evoked potential index on propofol consumption and emergence times during total intravenous anaesthesia with propofol and remifentanil in children. Acta Anaesthesiol Scand 2005;49(3):277–83.

78. Sneyd JR, Andrews CJH, Tsubokawa T. Comparison of propofol/remifentanil and sevoflurane/remifentanil for maintenance of anaesthesia for elective intracranial surgery. Br J Anaesth 2005;94(6):778–83.

79. Schraag S, Flaschar J, Schleyer M, Georgieff M, Kenny GNC. The contribution of remifentanil to middle latency auditory evoked potentials during induction of propofol anesthesia. Anesth Analg 2006;103(4):902–7.

Sufentanil

General Information

Sufentanil, a fentanyl analogue, is a highly lipid-soluble synthetic opioid with high affinity for OP_3 (μ) opioid receptors and a potency some 5–10 times that of fentanyl. It is a short-acting analgesic.

Its adverse effects include pruritus, sedation, nausea and vomiting, dizziness, urinary retention, light-headedness, miosis, and shivering (SEDA-16, 86). Respiratory depression also occurs (SEDA-21, 89). Motor neuron blockade, acute hypotension, and muscle weakness are rare, affecting under 1% of patients (SEDA-16, 86).

Drug studies

Placebo-controlled studies

In 41 patients undergoing abdominal hysterectomy randomly allocated in a double-blind, controlled study to sufentanil 50 micrograms for 8–16 hours via a lumbar epidural catheter before or at the end of surgery, the pre-emptive group ($n = 20$) used less sufentanil than the control group ($n = 21$) (1). The frequency of adverse effects was similar in the two groups; nine patients in the pre-emptive group and ten in the control group complained of nausea or vomiting and four patients in the pre-emptive group and five patients in the control group complained of mild pruritus.

Comparative studies
Bupivacaine
Intrathecal sufentanil and epidural bupivacaine were compared individually and in combination to establish dose-responsiveness for analgesia in labor in 100 women (2). There was no dose-responsiveness for doses of sufentanil between 2 and 10 micrograms. The ED_{50} for sufentanil was 2.3 micrograms alone (higher than that reported above (3)) and 0.85 micrograms in combination with epidural bupivacaine. Adverse effects included pruritus (incidence 70–90%), nausea, and mild somnolence (10–30%). Transient fetal bradycardia was reported in two cases.

In a double-blind, randomized, placebo-controlled study in 80 patients of the analgesic efficacy of different subarachnoid applications of sufentanil and/or bupivacaine using a microcatheter for easy postoperative pain relief, sufentanil 10 micrograms, bupivacaine 5 mg, or a combination of sufentanil 2.5 micrograms and bupivacaine 2.5 mg provided immediate and adequate postoperative analgesia for 2–3 hours (4). The group who received only sufentanil had the highest incidence of pruritus and respiratory depression. The limitations of this study were highlighted in a letter, which questioned the value of the above procedure when other tried and tested perioperative pain management methods are available (5).

Clonidine
In a double-blind study of the effect of clonidine on intrathecal sufentanil, 53 nulliparous women received sufentanil 5 micrograms intrathecally either alone or with clonidine 30 micrograms (6). The addition of clonidine increased the incidence of hypotension (12% with sufentanil alone, 63% with clonidine) and sedation (23% with sufentanil alone and 46% with clonidine). There was no significant difference in the incidence of pruritus (88%). Again, no motor blockade was observed.

In another randomized, double-blind study in 40 primiparous women in labor at less than 5 cm cervical dilatation who requested epidural analgesia, the addition of clonidine 75 micrograms to epidural sufentanil 20 micrograms did not provide any advantages in analgesic efficacy or adverse effects (7).

Dextrose
The addition of 3.5% dextrose to sufentanil 10 micrograms given intrathecally in a randomized, double-blind study of 48 women in early labor produced a significant reduction in the incidence of clinically important pruritus (8). Dextrose did not compromise the quality and duration of analgesia.

Lidocaine
The analgesic efficacy of intrathecal sufentanil with or without lidocaine has been examined in two groups of outpatients undergoing lithotripsy or gynecological

laparoscopy in order to determine optimal analgesia with rapid recovery and discharge (9,10). In a retrospective case-record study of 62 shock-wave lithotripsy procedures, the 25 cases performed using intrathecal sufentanil alone had better outcomes, significantly shorter postanesthesia care unit time, and time for ambulation compared with 37 procedures performed with intrathecal lidocaine; pruritus was significantly more common with sufentanil (9). A double-blind, randomized study in 13 patients undergoing gynecological laparoscopy, who received either lidocaine 10 mg with sufentanil 10 micrograms or intrathecal sufentanil 20 micrograms, was terminated early owing to unacceptably frequent adverse effects and inferior analgesia in those given intrathecal sufentanil (10).

Piritramide
Sufentanil 1 microgram/ml plus 0.1% ropivacaine by epidural infusion has been compared with intravenous patient-controlled analgesia with piritramide in a double-blind, randomized study in 24 patients undergoing elective total hip replacement (11). The PCA group had significantly more adverse effects than the epidural group, including hypotension, nausea, and vomiting. There were no cases of respiratory depression, pruritus, hypertension, or dysrhythmias in either group. Epidural sufentanil was a better analgesic.

Combination studies
Adrenaline
In a randomized, double-blind, controlled study, the addition of adrenaline (100 micrograms/ml) significantly reduced the incidence of sedation and light-headedness after epidural sufentanil (40 micrograms) in 43 women who received epidural analgesia during early labor (12). However, adrenaline did not help in preventing maternal oxygen desaturation.

Bupivacaine
In a prospective dose-finding study, 170 women with cervical dilatation of 3–5 cm were randomized to receive intrathecal sufentanil 0, 2.5, 5.0, 7.5, or 10 micrograms combined with bupivacaine 5 mg (13). Bupivacaine combined with 2.5 micrograms sufentanil provided analgesia comparable to higher doses with a lower incidence of nausea and vomiting and less severe pruritus.

Bupivacaine and adrenaline
In a randomized, double-blind study in 243 parturients who received three doses of sufentanil (0.5, 0.75, and 1 microgram/ml) in combination with bupivacaine 0.625 mg/ml and adrenaline 1.25 micrograms/ml by continuous epidural infusion there were no differences in analgesic effects, but there was significantly more pruritus in those who received the highest dose of sufentanil (14). The authors suggested using the lowest dose of sufentanil (0.5 micrograms/ml) with bupivacaine solution to minimize the risk of adverse effects on the mother and neonate, with optimal analgesia.

Ropivacaine
In a randomized, double-blind study in 120 patients undergoing major abdominal surgery the combination of sufentanil 0.75 micrograms/ml with ropivacaine 0.2% provided optimal postoperative patient-controlled epidural analgesia with the fewest adverse effects of the regimens used (ropivacaine alone, ropivacaine and sufentanil 0.5, 0.75, or 1.00 microgram/ml) (15).

Organs and Systems

Cardiovascular

The incidence of hypotension with sufentanil is 7% and that of hypertension 3%. In a double-blind comparison of morphine, pethidine, fentanyl, and sufentanil in balanced anesthesia, patients who received sufentanil had the least hemodynamic disturbances. In high doses, adverse effects such as bradycardia and hypotension can lead to complications in some patients (SEDA-16, 85). Sudden hypotension occurred on induction of anesthesia with sufentanil in four patients, in whom the dose was 8.4–22.7 micrograms/kg (16). Other workers noted similar findings at doses of 1 and 1.5 micrograms/kg.

Clinically significant bradycardia or asystole occurred on induction when sufentanil was used in conjunction with vecuronium (17,18).

The effect of sufentanil was examined in 10 healthy men to find out whether it has the same hemodynamic and sensory effects as when it is used in women in labor. Details of the method of recruitment of volunteers for this double-blind study were not provided, but they received either saline or sufentanil 10 micrograms intrathecally (19), and blood pressure, heart rates, oxyhemoglobin saturation, cold and pinprick sensation, motor block, and visual analogue scales for sedation pruritus and nausea were all measured. Pruritus and sensory changes to pinprick and cold occurred only in the sufentanil group and there were no significant hemodynamic changes in either group. In view of the frequency and severity of pruritus when sufentanil is used in labor, it is interesting that all five of the male volunteers experienced this symptom, three of them severely. These findings suggested that the hypotension observed with the use of intrathecal sufentanil during labor and the sensory changes may not be mediated by the same pathway. The authors proposed that the hypotension observed in such studies is a direct result of pain relief, which is not an issue in the pain-free men in this investigation.

Respiratory

Apneic episodes have been reported in patients given sufentanil (SEDA-20, 81; SEDA-21, 89). Respiratory arrest occurred 55 minutes after epidural and intrathecal sufentanil and bupivacaine (SEDA-18, 82).

• A healthy 22-year-old woman at 41 weeks gestation presented for urgent cesarean section following fetal heart rate deceleration (20). She was given sufentanil 10 micrograms plus 0.1% bupivacaine 10 mg intrathecally and 8 minutes later became unrousable and apneic. After 3 minutes spontaneous ventilation resumed.

The authors suggested that giving the local anesthesia first and then the sufentanil later might have contributed to this presentation of spontaneous reversal of short-lived early-onset respiratory arrest.

When nasal sufentanil was used to induce anesthesia in children, ventilatory compliance was mildly or markedly reduced and one child required suxamethonium, oxygen, and positive pressure ventilation (SEDA-16, 86).

Respiratory depression has been attributed to sufentanil (21).

- A 28-year old man, who was scheduled for knee arthroscopy, was given intrathecal injection of sufentanil 5 micrograms, together with bupivacaine 10 micrograms. About 20 minutes after this injection, he complained of mild pruritus and 3 minutes later stated that he felt sleepy; 25 minutes after the intrathecal injection, he became unresponsive and apathetic. Intravenous naloxone 0.4 micrograms was given about 2 minutes after positive pressure ventilation. About 5 minutes later he regained consciousness with normal respiration.

This event may have been due to a supraspinal reflex, to direct cephalic migration in the cerebrospinal fluid, or to a systemic effect after vascular absorption of this very highly lipid-soluble drug.

Respiratory depression has also been described after intrathecal sufentanil 5 micrograms (22).

- An 83-year-old woman scheduled for bilateral knee replacement surgery received midazolam 7.5 mg preoperatively. Continuous spinal anesthesia was planned, with combined general anesthesia. Anesthesia was maintained with 0.3–0.5% of inspired isoflurane in 36% oxygen and 70% nitrous oxide while 5 mg of 0.5% bupivacaine was introduced into the subarachnoid space via an insertion at L3–4. Anesthesia extended to T11. During the procedure two top-up doses of bupivacaine 2.5 mg were administered. Postoperatively she was extubated immediately and was fully conscious on transfer to the recovery room, but 75 minutes later she had violent pain in both knees and received sufentanil 5 micrograms intrathecally. Analgesia was achieved in 10 minutes. At 15 minutes pruritus occurred and at 30 minutes she became unresponsive to verbal and painful stimuli and stopped breathing. Blood pressure was 120/60 mmHg, heart rate 72/minute, and oxygen saturation 97%. Ventilation with 100% oxygen via a facemask started immediately and naloxone 160 micrograms was injected intravenously, with full recovery of consciousness and respiration in 10 minutes.

This report is the first of respiratory depression after intrathecal sufentanil in a non-obstetric patient. Previous obstetric cases had occurred earlier and with larger doses of sufentanil. The site of action of sufentanil in this case is likely to have been supraspinal, by either direct cephalad migration in the CSF or through a systemic effect after vascular absorption.

Respiratory arrest has been reported in labor (23).

- A 20-year-old parturient received sufentanil 10 micrograms and bupivacaine 2.5 mg intrathecally as part of combined spinal-epidural analgesia and developed pruritus 15 minutes after the injection, followed by a sleepy feeling at 20 minutes. After 25 minutes she became unresponsive and apneic; her systolic blood pressure was 130 mmHg and her heart rate 60. The fetal heart rate was 86. She was ventilated manually with 100% oxygen and naloxone 0.4 mg was given with prompt recovery of consciousness and respiratory effort. Drowsiness persisted, and a naloxone infusion was initiated after top-up doses of naloxone had failed to relieve it. Subsequent analgesia was with bupivacaine alone. A vacuum-assisted vaginal delivery was performed after 3 hours. The infant's Apgar score was 8 at 1 minute and 9 at 5 minutes. The mother and baby were subsequently well.

This case highlights the low doses at which arrest may occur.

Violent coughing in young children and adolescents exposed to small doses of sufentanil (1 microgram/kg or less) has been reported (24). Specific cases were not alluded to and the literature remains divided on the significance and mechanism of this age-related effect.

Nervous system

An unexpected transient neurological deficit has been described in neurosurgical patients (SEDA-16, 85).

There have been three reports of neurological changes after the intrathecal administration of sufentanil plus bupivacaine (25,26).

- A 40-year-old pregnant woman developed acute confusion, aphasia, increased salivation, and difficulty in swallowing 15 minutes after intrathecal administration of sufentanil 10 micrograms with bupivacaine 2.5 mg (26). There was spontaneous resolution 1 hour later with no need for pharmacological intervention.
- An 18-year-old nulliparous woman with an uncomplicated pregnancy developed difficulty in swallowing, respiratory abnormalities, and excessive tiredness 13 minutes after receiving sufentanil 5 micrograms with bupivacaine 1.25 mg as a spinal analgesic and disappearing over 20 minutes (25).
- A 36-year-old nulliparous woman complained of dyspnea and sensory block extending to the face 15 minutes after an intrathecal injection of sufentanil 5 micrograms with bupivacaine 1.25 mg (25).

In neither of the last two cases was there motor blockade or neonatal sequelae. Such adverse effects can be caused by sufentanil, bupivacaine, or both. Regardless of which drug caused these events, the intrathecal administration of a hypobaric solution to a patient in the sitting position might have contributed, since rostral spread of intrathecal drugs is accelerated in this setting. The use of smaller doses of sufentanil (2.5 or 5 micrograms) will also prevent such adverse effects.

Musculoskeletal

There have been isolated reports of chest wall rigidity after sufentanil (27).

Second-Generation Effects

Pregnancy

The effects of intrathecal and epidural sufentanil as an analgesic during labor have been described in 50 nulliparous patients in a randomized double-blind study, in which they received sufentanil 1–10 micrograms in preservative-free saline (28). The ED_{50} was 1.8 micrograms, based on those who requested further analgesia after 30 minutes. The incidence of adverse effects was similar in all groups (that is was not dose-related in this dosage range) and included pruritus of a similar intensity in all groups. There was no respiratory depression, but blood pressure and oxygen saturation fell. Other adverse effects included changes in temperature sensitivity at 30 minutes in 19 of the 50 subjects. One woman who received 5 micrograms of sufentanil had a fall in oxygen saturation to 90–92% with a respiratory rate of 16 breaths/minute 10–15 minutes after injection, but recovered spontaneously at 20 minutes. Fetal monitoring showed no significant bradycardia and there were no significant differences in 5-minute Apgar scores. It was suggested that hypotension was due to the effect of intrathecal opioid rather than to an effect on the autonomic nervous system and that the temperature sensitivity changes were due to a concentration-dependent local anesthetic effect of opioids. A drop in oxygen saturation in one subject indicated the need for observation for respiratory changes when sufentanil is given intrathecally.

Combined spinal epidural analgesia has been associated with reports of increased operative deliveries, possibly due to reduced perineal sensation and motor weakness. In a comparison of combined spinal epidural analgesia (intrathecal sufentanil 10 micrograms followed by epidural bupivacaine and fentanyl at their next request for analgesia) with intravenous pethidine analgesia (50 mg intravenously on demand up to a maximum of 200 mg in 4 hours) in 1223 randomly assigned healthy parturients there was no significant difference in the rates of cesarean delivery for dystocia (29). Maternal hypotension and pruritus requiring treatment occurred in 14% and 17% respectively of patients who received combined spinal epidural analgesia. Fetal heart rate deceleration occurred in 21% of patients who received pethidine compared with 18% of patients who received combined spinal epidural analgesia, and in each group most cases resolved spontaneously. However, profound fetal bradycardia (fetal heart rate of less than 60/minute, lasting 60 seconds or more), necessitating emergency cesarean section, occurred within 1 hour of administration of sufentanil in 8 of 400 mothers, while no such events occurred with pethidine. None of the cases responded to conservative management and none was associated with maternal hypotension. Immediate postnatal neonatal outcomes were similar between the two groups, as judged by Apgar scores and umbilical artery blood gases. These findings are significant, in that an increase in cesarean deliveries due to fetal bradycardia has not previously been reported, but findings in this study must be regarded with an element of caution, as fetal monitoring was more extensive in those given combined spinal epidural analgesia. The authors suggested that fetal bradycardia might have been due to uterine hyperstimulation, associated with intrathecal opioids (although they did not consistently monitor for this), and that fetal bradycardia resulted from reduced placental perfusion secondary to uterine tetany. Alternatively, since sufentanil is highly lipid soluble, it can be detectable in plasma within 39 minutes of intrathecal administration of 15 micrograms. Once in the plasma, transplacental transfer can occur and the drug can have a direct vagotonic effect on the fetus. However, they believed that the most probable explanation for the bradycardia was a direct consequence of hypoperfusion of the placenta secondary to maternal hypotension, although they pointed out that none of their cases was associated with this hemodynamic change in the mother.

In a double-blind, randomized study the analgesic efficacy of sufentanil 0.25 micrograms/ml with 0.125% bupivacaine was compared with fentanyl 2 micrograms/ml with 0.125% bupivacaine in 226 patients in labor with a patient-controlled epidural analgesic device (30). Overall analgesia was good, with no observed difference between the two groups. There was a significant difference in the occurrence of mild pruritus, with 10 cases in the fentanyl group ($n = 105$) and only two in the sufentanil group ($n = 101$). There were no gastrointestinal adverse effects. Sufentanil was deemed preferable owing to a lower incidence of adverse effects for equal analgesic potency.

An epidural mixture of sufentanil with ropivacaine has been used in a double-blind, randomized study in 100 women in the first stage of labor (31). They were randomized to receive 0.2% ropivacaine 12 mg either alone or with sufentanil 5, 10, or 15 micrograms. With combined sufentanil plus ropivacaine the duration of analgesia was about 40 minutes longer than with ropivacaine alone. There were no differences in analgesic efficacy or the incidence of opioid-related adverse effects in the three sufentanil groups. Sufentanil 5 micrograms plus ropivacaine 0.2% was therefore recommended.

Fetotoxicity

When epidural sufentanil is used for labor and delivery, the neonates can have subtle neurological signs of drug depression, including mild hypotonia, poor primary reflexes, and poor habituation to repeated stimuli at 1 and 4 hours of life (SEDA-16, 86).

The absence of motor block associated with combined spinal epidural analgesia using sufentanil has also been reported in an investigation in which intrathecal sufentanil 10 micrograms was compared with epidural lidocaine, adrenaline, and sufentanil 40 micrograms in early labor (32). Adverse effects were not significantly different between the groups, except for more frequent and severe pruritus in the intrathecal group. Although three subjects in each group had transient changes in fetal heart rate within 30 minutes of medication, no intervention was necessary.

In a randomized, double-blind, placebo-controlled study, 300 parturients were given intrathecal sufentanil 1.5

micrograms, or a small dose of spinal sufentanil (7.5 micrograms), or epidural analgesia (7.5 micrograms/ml) (33). Fetal heart abnormalities developed during the first hour after initiation of analgesia in 25% of the patients whose mothers were given spinal sufentanil, compared with 12% of those whose mothers were given intrathecal sufentanil and 11% of those whose mothers were given epidural analgesia. There was uterine hyperactivity in 12% of those given spinal sufentanil, but in only 2% in the other groups. These results confirm that a smaller dose of intrathecal sufentanil did not result in more frequent fetal heart abnormalities, despite equally rapid analgesia.

Susceptibility Factors

Genetic

A 7-year-old boy with laminin α2 (merosin) deficiency and severe congenital muscular dystrophy developed suspected malignant hyperthermia after total intravenous general anesthesia with sufentanil 0.004 micrograms/kg/minute and propofol 100 micrograms/kg/minute (34). He developed total body rigidity, increased body temperature, low blood pressure, and an increased heart rate. It is not clear whether sufentanil served as a trigger for malignant hyperthermia, but the authors suggested that laminin α2 (merosin) deficiency may increase susceptibility.

Drug Administration

Drug dosage regimens

In a dose-finding, prospective, double-blind study, 60 men scheduled for unilateral extracorporeal shock-wave lithotripsy were randomized to receive 12.5, 15, 17.5, or 20 micrograms of intrathecal sufentanil (35). The results suggested that 15 micrograms of sufentanil may be the optimal intrathecal dose, since 20 micrograms produced significantly more pruritus than the lower doses and those who were given 12.5 micrograms needed significantly more supplementary analgesia.

Drug administration route

Serious consequences (respiratory arrest and hypotension) related to the use of intrathecal sufentanil have been described in parturients (SEDA-22, 101).

References

1. Akural EI, Salomaki TE, Tekay AH, Bloigu AH, Alahuhta SM. Pre-emptive effect of epidural sufentanil in abdominal hysterectomy. Br J Anaesth 2002;88(6):803–8.
2. Camann W, Abouleish A, Eisenach J, Hood D, Datta S. Intrathecal sufentanil and epidural bupivacaine for labor analgesia: dose-response of individual agents and in combination. Reg Anesth Pain Med 1998;23(5):457–62.
3. Duthie DJ. Remifentanil and tramadol. Br J Anaesth 1998;81(1):51–7.
4. Standl TG, Horn E, Luckmann M, Burmeister M, Wilhelm S, Schulte am Esch J. Subarachnoid sufentanil for early postoperative pain management in orthopedic patients: a placebo-controlled, double-blind study using spinal microcatheters. Anesthesiology 2001;94(2):230–8.
5. Gebhard RE, Fanelli G, Matuszczak M, Doehn M. Subarachnoid sufentanil for early postoperative pain management in orthopedic patients: more disadvantages than benefits? Anesthesiology 2001;95(6):1531–3.
6. Mercier FJ, Dounas M, Bouaziz H, Des Mesnards-Smaja V, Foiret C, Vestermann MN, Fischler M, Benhamou D. The effect of adding a minidose of clonidine to intrathecal sufentanil for labor analgesia. Anesthesiology 1998;89(3): 594–601.
7. Connelly NR, Mainkar T, El-Mansouri M, Manikantan P, Venkata RR, Dunn S, Parker RK. Effect of epidural clonidine added to epidural sufentanil for labor pain management. Int J Obstet Anesth 2000;9(2):94–8.
8. Abouleish AE, Portnoy D, Abouleish EI. Addition of dextrose 3.5% to intrathecal sufentanil for labour analgesia reduces pruritis Can J Anaesth 2000;47(12):1171–5.
9. Nelson CP, Francis TA, Wolf JS Jr. Comparison of shockwave lithotripsy outcomes in patients receiving sufentanil or lidocaine spinal anesthesia. J Endourol 2001;15(5):473–7.
10. Henderson CL, Schmid J, Vaghadia H, Fowler C, Mitchell GW. Selective spinal anesthesia for outpatient laparoscopy. III: sufentanil vs lidocaine–sufentanil. Can J Anaesth 2001;48(3):267–72.
11. Kampe S, Randebrock G, Kiencke P, Hunseler U, Cranfield K, Konig DP, Diefenbach C. Comparison of continuous epidural infusion of ropivacaine and sufentanil with intravenous patient-controlled analgesia after total hip replacement. Anaesthesia 2001;56(12):1189–93.
12. Armstrong KP, Kennedy B, Watson JT, Morley-Forster PK, Yee I, Butler R. Epinephrine reduces the sedative side effects of epidural sufentanil for labour analgesia. Can J Anaesth 2002;49(1):72–80.
13. Wong CA, Scavone BM, Loffredi M, Wang WY, Peaceman AM, Ganchiff JN. The dose-response of intrathecal sufentanil added to bupivacaine for labor analgesia. Anesthesiology 2000;92(6):1553–8.
14. Eriksson SL, Frykholm P, Stenlund PM, Olofsson C. A comparison of three doses of sufentanil in combination with bupivacaine–adrenaline in continuous epidural analgesia during labour. Acta Anaesthesiol Scand 2000;44(8):919–23.
15. Brodner G, Mertes N, Van Aken H, Mollhoff T, Zahl M, Wirtz S, Marcus MA, Buerkle H. What concentration of sufentanil should be combined with ropivacaine 0.2% wt/vol for postoperative patient-controlled epidural analgesia? Anesth Analg 2000;90(3):649–57.
16. Spiess BD, Sathoff RH, el-Ganzouri AR, Ivankovich AD. High-dose sufentanil: four cases of sudden hypotension on induction. Anesth Analg 1986;65(6):703–5.
17. Starr NJ, Sethna DH, Estafanous FG. Bradycardia and asystole following the rapid administration of sufentanil with vecuronium. Anesthesiology 1986;64(4):521–3.
18. Dobson JAR, Davies JM, Hodgson GH. Bradycardia after sufentanil and vecuronium. Can J Anaesth 1988;35:S121.
19. Riley ET, Hamilton CL, Cohen SE. Intrathecal sufentanil produces sensory changes without hypotension in male volunteers. Anesthesiology 1998;89(1):73–8.

20. Kehl F, Erfkamp S, Roewer N. Respiratory arrest during caesarean section after intrathecal administration of sufentanil in combination with 0.1% bupivacaine 10 ml Anaesth Intensive Care 2002;30(5):698–9.

21. Celik JB, Reisli R, Sarkilar G, Okesli S. Respiratory arrest after intrathecal injection of sufentanil and bupivacaine. Acta Anaesthesiol Scand 2004;48:793–4.

22. Fournier R, Gamulin Z, Van Gessel E. Respiratory depression after 5 micrograms of intrathecal sufentanil. Anesth Analg 1998;87(6):1377–8.

23. Katsiris S, Williams S, Leighton BL, Halpern S. Respiratory arrest following intrathecal injection of sufentanil and bupivacaine in a parturient. Can J Anaesth 1998;45(9):880–3.

24. Yemen TA, Bennet JA, Abrams J, Van Riper DF, Horrow JC. Small doses of sufentanil will produce violent coughing in young children. Anesthesiology 1998;89(1): 271–2.

25. Abdou WA, Aveline C, Bonnet F. Two additional cases of excessive extension of sensory blockade after intrathecal sufentanil for labor analgesia. Int J Obstet Anesth 2000;9(1):48–50.

26. Fragneto RY, Fisher A. Mental status change and aphasia after labor analgesia with intrathecal sufentanil/bupivacaine. Anesth Analg 2000;90(5):1175–6.

27. Goldberg M, Ishak S, Garcia C, McKenna J. Postoperative rigidity following sufentanil administration. Anesthesiology 1985;63(2):199–201.

28. Arkoosh VA, Cooper M, Norris MC, Boxer L, Ferouz F, Silverman NS, Huffnagle HJ, Huffnagle S, Leighton BL. Intrathecal sufentanil dose response in nulliparous patients. Anesthesiology 1998;89(2):364–70.

29. Gambling DR, Sharma SK, Ramin SM, Lucas MJ, Leveno KJ, Wiley J, Sidawi JE. A randomized study of combined spinal-epidural analgesia versus intravenous meperidine during labor: impact on cesarean delivery rate. Anesthesiology 1998;89(6):1336–44.

30. Le Guen H, Roy D, Branger B, Ecoffey C. Comparison of fentanyl and sufentanil in combination with bupivacaine for patient-controlled epidural analgesia during labor. J Clin Anesth 2001;13(2):98–102.

31. Debon R, Allaouchiche B, Duflo F, Boselli E, Chassard D. The analgesic effect of sufentanil combined with ropivacaine 0.2% for labor analgesia: a comparison of three sufentanil doses Anesth Analg 2001;92(1):180–3.

32. Dunn SM, Connelly NR, Steinberg RB, Lewis TJ, Bazzell CM, Klatt JL, Parker RK. Intrathecal sufentanil versus epidural lidocaine with epinephrine and sufentanil for early labor analgesia. Anesth Analg 1998;87(2):331–5.

33. Van de Velde M, Teunkens A, Hanskens M, Vandermeersch E, Verhaaghe J. Intrathecal sufentanil and fetal heart abnormalities. A double blind, double placebo controlled trial comparing two forms of combined spinal epidural analgesia with epidural analgesia in labour. Anesth Analg 2004;98:1153–9.

34. Shukry M, Guruli ZV, Ramadhyani U. Suspected malignant hyperthermia in a child with lamin alpha 2 (merosin) deficiency in the absence of a triggering agent. Paediatr Anesth 2006;16(4):462–5.

35. Lau WC, Green CR, Faerber GJ, Tait AR, Golembiewski JA. Determination of the effective therapeutic dose of intrathecal sufentanil for extracorporeal shock wave lithotripsy. Anesth Analg 1999;89(4):889–92.

Tonazocine

General Information

Tonazocine is a partial opioid receptor agonist that has not been reported to have adverse effects on the cardiovascular system or to cause clinically significant respiratory depression. When single doses of tonazocine 2, 4, and 8 mg were compared in 150 adults postoperatively, drowsiness was the most frequent adverse effect and visual hallucinations occurred in two patients (1).

Reference

1. Lippmann M, Mok MS, Farinacci JV, Lee JC. Tonazocine mesylate in postoperative pain patients: a double-blind placebo controlled analgesic study. J Clin Pharmacol 1989;29(4):373–8.

Tramadol

General Information

Tramadol is a synthetic opioid analgesic with activity at MOR(OP$_3$, μ) opioid receptors, but it also inhibits the re-uptake of both 5-HT and noradrenaline and stimulates the presynaptic release of 5-HT. It produces a similar analgesic effect to pethidine and is about one-tenth as potent as morphine.

The reported adverse effects of tramadol are nausea, vomiting, sweating, dry mouth, dizziness, sedation, headache, and hypertension (SEDA-17, 84; SEDA-20, 81). The atypical analgesic effects of tramadol and its associated adverse effects profile have been reviewed (1).

The metabolism of tramadol by CYP2D6 is important for its analgesic effect; tramadol may therefore be a poor analgesic in poor metabolizers by CYP2D6, while extensive metabolizers may have better analgesia and more adverse effects (SEDA-21, 90).

In a review of the use of tramadol in musculoskeletal pain the authors concluded that tramadol can be used at Step 2 of the analgesic ladder, since its efficacy, alone or in conjunction with NSAIDs, in the management of chronic musculoskeletal pain without increasing the frequency of adverse effects has been confirmed (2,3).

Observational studies

In randomized, uncontrolled study caudal tramadol 2 micrograms/kg provided better and longer-lasting postoperative analgesia than the same dose of intravenous tramadol in boys having hypospadias repaired (4).

The combination of paracetamol + tramadol is synergistic and combines the rapid onset of analgesia of paracetamol with prolonged analgesia from tramadol. When this combination is used for acute, subacute, or chronic pain it is associated with a marked reduction in adverse events compared with either drug alone (5).

Tramadol 75 mg + paracetamol 650 mg + lidocaine 1% provided adequate pain control in 60 men for biopsy of the prostate but was associated with light-headedness, dizziness, and itching (6).

Comparative studies

Bupivacaine

In a randomized, controlled study in 60 boys (aged 1–7 years) undergoing unilateral herniorrhaphy, caudal 0.25% bupivacaine 1 mg/kg plus tramadol 1.5 mg/kg resulted in superior analgesia (quality and duration) with no significant increase in opioid-related adverse effects compared with children who received 0.25% bupivacaine 1 mg/kg alone or caudal tramadol 1.5 mg/kg in 0.9% saline alone (7).

Thirty children (1–5 years old) in an open, controlled study were randomly given caudal block with 0.25% bupivacaine 0.8 mg/kg or tramadol 0.8 or 2 mg/kg (8). The duration of analgesia was longer (9.1 hours) in those given tramadol but the incidences of opioid-related adverse effects (gastrointestinal effects and sweating) were significantly higher.

Clomipramine + levomepromazine

Since the monoamine effects of tramadol resemble the effect of antidepressants, it has been compared with clomipramine + levomepromazine in patients with post-herpetic neuralgia. The incidence of adverse effects was 77% with tramadol and 83% with clomipramine (SEDA-20, 81).

Codeine

In a 4-week, double-blind, multicenter, randomized study, tramadol plus paracetamol (37.5/325 mg) was as effective as codeine plus paracetamol (co-codamol 30/300 mg) in chronic non-malignant low back pain and osteoarthritis pain, with acceptable tolerability (9).

When tramadol was compared with codeine in 65 patients undergoing elective intracranial surgery, there was a significantly higher incidence of postoperative nausea, vomiting, and sedation with tramadol 75 mg (10). The patients given codeine had significantly lower pain scores over the first 48 hours postoperatively.

Electro-acupuncture

In a comparison of tramadol + midazolam and electro-acupuncture in relieving pain during shockwave litho-tripsy, electro-acupuncture was more effective (11). There were no adverse effects of electro-acupuncture, but tramadol + midazolam caused mild orthostatic hypotension and dizziness.

Fentanyl

Tramadol + midazolam has been compared with fentanyl + midazolam in 150 patients undergoing colonoscopy (12). Colonoscopy was performed smoothly, although the procedure took significantly longer in those who received tramadol. Pain scores were higher with tramadol, requiring additional doses of fentanyl for effective management. Those who received tramadol had significantly more adverse effects, *nausea and vomiting* being the most common. The incidence was also higher in those who received more tramadol (24% compared with 12%), suggesting that these effects were dose-related. These results suggest that tramadol, even in combination with midazolam, is not as well tolerated as fentanyl and is not the optimal analgesic for colonoscopy.

Lidocaine

Tramadol + ketamine 0.25 mg/kg has been compared with lidocaine + ketamine in 62 children undergoing surgery for hypospadias (13). Lidocaine provided better analgesia and sedation than tramadol, but both were effective and the incidences of *nausea and vomiting* were similar.

Local anesthesia

In another study, intravenous tramadol 1.5 mg/kg was compared with ilioinguinal and iliohypogastric nerve blocks in 60 children undergoing herniorrhaphy (14). Tramadol provided adequate analgesia but was associated with nausea and vomiting. None of the patients had respiratory depression.

Non-steroidal anti-inflammatory drugs

Tramadol and non-steroidal anti-inflammatory drugs have been compared in two studies of patients with joint pain associated with osteoarthritis (15,16). In an open, randomized study 60 patients with osteoarthritis taking NSAIDs were given either modified-release tramadol 100 mg 8-hourly or modified-release dihydrocodeine 60 mg 8-hourly for 4 days; the controls were 30 patients who took an NSAID alone (15). Both opioids provided adequate analgesic adjuncts to NSAIDs, but tramadol caused significantly more minor initial adverse effects.

Diclofenac

In a double-blind, randomized, crossover study in 60 patients with osteoarthritis of the hip or knee, tramadol 50–100 mg up to three times daily was compared with diclofenac (25–50 mg up to three times daily) over 4 weeks (17). Both regimens gave modest pain relief, with no significant differences between the two groups, although within individual patients there were marked differences in analgesic effectiveness. Tramadol was associated with a significantly higher rate of adverse effects (20 versus 3.3%), notably headaches, nausea, constipation, tiredness, and vomiting, but there was no significant difference in adverse events that required withdrawal.

In a comparison of intramuscular tramadol and intramuscular diclofenac sodium in acute migraine, the two treatments were equally effective (18). The adverse effects profiles were also similar and were not considered to be severe. Nausea and vomiting were not associated with tramadol.

Ketorolac

Intravenous tramadol 1.5 mg/kg has been compared with a single dose of intravenous ketorolac 10 ng in 60 patients scheduled to undergo day-case laparoscopic sterilization in a prospective, randomized, double-blind comparison (19). Tramadol was associated with significantly less postoperative pain. There was no difference in the incidence or severity of nausea and vomiting between the two groups. Dry mouth was significantly more common with tramadol (60 versus 27%).

Valdecoxib

Valdecoxib 20 mg daily or bd has been compared with tramadol 50 mg qds in 829 patients with acute first- or second-degree ankle sprain (20). The number of withdrawals due to adverse events in the tramadol group was higher (12% versus 3.4%).

Opioid analgesics
Fentanyl

In a comparison of tramadol (1 or 2 mg/kg) and fentanyl (2 µg/kg) for postoperative analgesia after pediatric anesthesia, the two drugs had equal analgesic potency and produced similar hemodynamic stability and a similar incidence of adverse effects (21).

Hydrocodone

A randomized, double-blind comparison of the effectiveness of a single dose of tramadol 100 mg with a single dose of hydrocodone 5 mg plus paracetamol 500 mg in acute musculoskeletal pain in 68 subjects after minor trauma has been published (22). Tramadol gave significantly worse analgesia. Adverse effects (nausea and vomiting, drowsiness and dizziness, and anxiety) were uncommon and there was no significant difference between the two drugs.

Morphine

In a comparison of the analgesic effects of intermittent boluses of tramadol or morphine after abdominal surgery in 523 patients, tramadol caused more adverse effects (43 versus 34%), although the difference was not statistically significant. The commonest adverse effects were nausea (32 and 22%), vomiting (4.9 and 3.8%), urinary retention (3.0 and 2.7%), and sweating (3.8 and 0.4%) (SEDA-20, 81).

Tramadol and morphine have been compared in 40 women undergoing hysterectomy (23). At the start of wound closure, patients received either tramadol 3 mg/kg or morphine 0.2 mg/kg intravenously, which did not cause changes in arterial pressure or heart rate. There were no differences in times to spontaneous respiration, awakening, or orientation between the two groups, and ventilation frequency and pain scores were similar throughout 90 minutes. Similar numbers in each group required supplementary analgesia. Performance of the p-deletion test, a measure of psychomotor function, was

more rapid in the tramadol group, but the performance of all subjects was impaired at 90 minutes compared with their preoperative scores.

In a randomized, double-blind study in 20 patients with severe postoperative pain given either intravenous tramadol 1 mg/kg or morphine 0.1 mg/kg, both drugs were effective analgesics but higher dosages than those usually administered were necessary (24). Tramadol did not cause any severe adverse effects, but with morphine there was one case each of severe sedation and respiratory depression.

A comparison of tramadol and morphine for subcutaneous patient-controlled analgesia after orthopedic surgery showed that tramadol 40 mg subcutaneously and morphine 2 mg subcutaneously were equally effective in providing analgesia (25). Drug use in the first 24 hours averaged 800 mg for tramadol and 40 mg for morphine. However, mean arterial blood pressure fell significantly in both groups after 24 hours, with a 17% mean maximal fall from baseline concentrations for tramadol and 20% for morphine; heart rate increased by 17 and 15% respectively. Oxygen saturation also fell significantly in both groups, but was not associated with changes in respiratory rate. Nausea and vomiting were more common with tramadol (65%). In this study, patients required significantly more tramadol than had been predicted, and the authors commented that at this dosage, the adverse effects profile was similar to that of morphine.

In a double-blind study 150 patients with post-traumatic musculoskeletal pain were allocated to either tramadol 100 mg, with possible increases to a total of 200 mg, or morphine 5 mg or 10 mg with a total increase to 20 mg (26). Analgesic efficacy and adverse effect profiles were similar in the two groups.

Non-opioid analgesics

In a double-blind, randomized study in 120 patients scheduled to undergo outpatient hand surgery with intravenous regional anesthesia, tramadol 100 mg was compared with either metamizol 1 g or paracetamol 1 g, all 6-hourly (27). Seven patients given tramadol withdrew because of severe nausea and dizziness. Tramadol was the most effective analgesic, but none of the drugs alone provided effective analgesia in all patients and 40% needed rescue analgesia.

Tramadol has been compared with a paracetamol derivative in a double-blind, randomized, controlled study in 80 patients undergoing elective thyroidectomy (28). They were randomly assigned to propacetamol (an injectable prodrug of paracetamol) 2 g or intravenous tramadol 1.5 mg/kg. A single dose of tramadol provided better analgesia than propacetamol during the first 6 hours after surgery, but failed to ensure optimal analgesia subsequently. The incidences of nausea, vomiting, and sedation were comparable in the two groups.

Placebo-controlled studies

In two randomized, double-blind studies tramadol provided effective and safe long-term relief of pain in diabetic neuropathy (29) and fibromyalgia (30). The adverse effects (constipation, nausea, and headache) were well tolerated.

The postoperative analgesic efficacy of tramadol 2 mg/kg has been studied in 80 children (aged 1–3 years) undergoing day-case adenoidectomy without pre-medication in a double-blind, randomized, placebo-controlled study (31). General anesthesia was induced with intravenous alfentanil 10 µg/kg plus lidocaine followed by propofol and mivacurium. The children received intravenous tramadol 2 mg/kg or placebo immediately after induction of anesthesia. Those given tramadol required fewer pethidine rescue medication doses than those given placebo. In fact, 45% of the children who were given tramadol did not require postoperative analgesia at all, compared with 15% of the children who were given placebo. The incidences of adverse effects were similar in the two groups.

The use or addition of tramadol in children undergoing lower abdominal surgery has been examined in three studies (7,8,32). In a double-blind, randomized, controlled study, 125 children undergoing inguinal herniorrhaphy were allocated to receive tramadol 2 mg/kg or morphine sulfate 0.03 mg/kg before surgery; the control group received morphine sulfate 0.03 mg/kg at the end of surgery (32). Caudal tramadol 2 mg/kg provided reliable postoperative analgesia and there were no inter-group differences in postoperative adverse effects or quality and duration of pain relief.

In 129 patients with severe joint pain associated with osteoarthritis, tramadol was significantly more effective than placebo, but 26 patients taking tramadol and 43 taking placebo withdrew because of ineffectiveness or adverse effects; the main adverse effects of tramadol were nausea and constipation (16).

Tramadol has been used in the treatment of shivering after anesthesia. In one study, 150 patients scheduled for general anesthesia and surgery were randomly allocated to intravenous tramadol 1 or 2 mg/kg or 0.9% saline given at the time of wound closure (33). The authors concluded that both doses of tramadol were effective and safe. Of the patients in the higher-dose group, 2% had shivering, compared with 4% in the lower-dose group and 48% in the control group. In a similar study in 96 patients, the optimal dose of tramadol in preventing shivering after anesthesia was 0.5–1 mg/kg intravenously (34).

In a placebo-controlled study in the treatment of idiopathic detrusor overactivity (35) more patients had adverse events while taking tramadol (34% versus 16%). Nausea was the most common (18% of all patients) and was responsible for two withdrawals. Nausea was also reported by 5.3% of patients taking placebo. Other adverse events include vomiting (7.9%), constipation (2.6%), and dizziness (5.3%).

Tramadol 50 mg was beneficial in treating premature ejaculation in a placebo-controlled study in 64 men when given about 2 hours before planned sexual activity (36). There were more adverse events with tramadol group but no drug withdrawals.

Combination studies

Tramadol has been combined with various drugs in order to enhance efficacy or reduce adverse effects.

Aspirin

The analgesic efficacy of tramadol can be further enhanced by adding injectable lysine acetyl salicylate (aspirin) after orthopedic surgery with no significant increase in adverse effects (37).

Dexamethasone

In a randomized, placebo-controlled study, the addition of an intravenous bolus of dexamethasone 150 micrograms/kg with a PCA system programmed to deliver tramadol 20 mg in a 1 ml solution on demand in 50 patients after major abdominal surgery significantly reduced the incidence of nausea, vomiting, and subsequent administration of rescue antiemetic therapy (38).

Droperidol

The use of tramadol for postoperative analgesia by intravenous patient-controlled analgesia (PCA) has gained popularity, mostly because it is less likely to cause sedation and respiratory depression (39). However, it is associated with nausea, vomiting, dry mouth, and sweating. The addition of droperidol to tramadol PCA reduced the incidence of gastrointestinal symptoms without significantly increasing sedation (40). In a double-blind, randomized study, 40 patients undergoing coronary artery bypass grafting and/or valve replacement surgery were given droperidol 0.1 mg/ml plus either tramadol 10 mg/ml or morphine 1 mg/ml. The results in the two groups were comparable in efficacy, adverse effects profiles, and dose requirements, and the authors argued that there may be no advantage in using tramadol rather than morphine in conjunction with droperidol (41).

Ketamine

In 44 patients the addition of ketamine 1 mg/ml to PCA tramadol significantly reduced the consumption of tramadol at 6, 12, and 24 hours postoperatively, with no differences in the incidence of nausea and sedation (42). Diplopia was reported by two patients.

Magnesium sulfate

In 44 patients the addition of magnesium sulfate 30 mg/ml to PCA tramadol both significantly reduced the consumption of tramadol at 6, 12, and 24 hours postoperatively, with no differences in the incidence of nausea and sedation (42).

Morphine

In a double-blind, randomized, controlled study, the addition of a tramadol infusion to morphine for PCA in 69 patients undergoing elective abdominal surgery resulted in improved analgesic efficacy and reduced morphine requirements, with a relative lack of adverse effects (43).

Observational studies

The role of tramadol in the treatment of rheumatological pain has been reviewed (44). Tramadol causes fewer opioid adverse effects for a given level of analgesia compared with traditional opioids. Common adverse effects, such as nausea and dizziness, usually occur only at the beginning of therapy, abate with time, and are further minimized by up-titrating the dosage over several days (45).

When tramadol 1 mg/kg was given intravenously to 110 adults for postoperative shivering, few adverse effects were reported; two had transient hypotension and two complained of nausea without vomiting. Similarly, mild adverse effects were reported in 20% of patients in a trial of tramadol in cancer pain (SEDA-16, 86), and when it was used to relieve severe pain in sports injuries (SEDA-16, 86).

Organs and Systems

Cardiovascular

Pericarditis has been attributed to tramadol (46).

- An 88-year-old man took tramadol and 2 days later developed precordial chest pressure radiating to the scapula and increasing with inspiration and movement. His blood pressure was 75/45 mmHg and his heart rate 60/minute. There was a soft pericardial rub, mild cardiomegaly, diffuse ST segment elevation, and PR interval shortening, normal left ventricular systolic function, and no wall motion abnormalities or effusion on echocardiography.

The temporal relationship between the development of acute pericarditis and the resolution of symptoms on withdrawal of tramadol suggested a causal link.

Respiratory

Tramadol is said not to cause respiratory depression (SEDA-17, 84) (SEDA-18, 82), but it has been reported that equipotent doses of tramadol did produce respiratory depression, albeit less severe and for a shorter time than morphine (SEDA-17, 84) (47). This was confirmed in an extensive review of the literature (SEDA-21, 90).

The effect of oral tramadol on the ventilatory response to acute isocapnic hypoxia has been studied in 20 healthy volunteers. Tramadol had a small but significant depressive effect on the hypercapnic ventilatory response but no effect on the hypoxic ventilatory response (48). This is in contrast to morphine, which causes 50–60% suppression of the hypoxic ventilatory response.

Nervous system

Tramadol-associated seizures have been studied retrospectively in 9218 adult tramadol users and 37 232 non-users (49). Seizures occurred in under 1% of all tramadol users, but the risk of seizure was increased two- to six-fold among users adjusted for selected co-morbidities and polydrug prescription. The risk of seizure was higher in those aged 25–54 years, those who had more than four tramadol prescriptions, and those who had a history of alcohol abuse, stroke, or head injury.

In a nested case-control study of 11 383 patients, there were 21 cases of idiopathic seizures, only three of whom had been exposed to tramadol alone, the other having taken other analgesics (opioids or others) (50). The findings did not suggest an increased risk of seizures among patients taking tramadol alone.

Seizures followed by opioid withdrawal symptoms have been reported in a patient taking tramadol (51).

- A 29-year-old woman took tramadol 50 mg 6-hourly for pain associated with the carpal tunnel syndrome. She slowly increased the dose of tramadol and obtained it from several physicians and different hospitals, so that after 3 years she was taking 30 tramadol 50 mg tablets daily. She had two generalized seizures and stopped taking tramadol; 1 day later she developed severe opioid withdrawal symptoms, including diarrhea, headache, insomnia, and blurred vision. She was detoxified with tapering doses of tramadol and discharged after 6 days.

Psychological, psychiatric

Hallucinations have been attributed to tramadol, both visual (52) and auditory (53).

- A 66-year-old tetraparetic man developed hallucinations while taking tramadol, paroxetine, and dosulepin for chronic pain (52).
- A 74-year-old man with lung cancer took tramadol 200 mg/day for chest pain (53). Soon afterwards (time not specified) he had vivid auditory hallucinations in the form of "two voices singing accompanied by an accordion and a banjo." They resolved 48 hours after withdrawal.

Two elderly patients taking long-term tramadol for chronic back pain experienced fluctuating confusional states over 2 years, alleviated when tramadol was withdrawn (54).

Gastrointestinal

In one study the incidence of nausea was high (30–35%) when tramadol was used for postoperative pain (SEDA-20, 81).

Tramadol 2.0 mg/kg was associated with nausea and vomiting in six children undergoing tonsillectomy but not very different from that experienced by those who were given either saline (n = 8) or ketoprofen (n = 7), suggesting other causes (55). This dosage of tramadol did not provide sufficient analgesia control

Intravenous tramadol (1.25 mg/kg), codeine (1 mg/kg), morphine (0.125 mg/kg), and saline have been compared for their effect on gastric emptying (using the paracetamol absorption test) in 10 healthy subjects in a randomized, double-blind study (56). Tramadol had a measurable but statistically insignificant inhibitory effect on gastric emptying, whereas morphine and codeine significantly delayed gastric emptying. The implication of this is that the risk of regurgitation is less with tramadol than with the other opioids investigated and that tramadol is less likely to alter the pharmacokinetics of other drugs administered simultaneously.

There has been a randomized controlled study of the effects of tramadol on the pH of the gastric contents during anesthesia in 30 patients (57). They were given tramadol 100 micrograms (n=10), famotidine 20 micrograms (n=10), or saline (n=10) injected into the deltoid muscle. Both drugs significantly caused increased gastric pH.

In mild to moderate postoperative pain, rectal tramadol has been compared with standard treatment with co-codamol (paracetamol plus codeine) suppositories in 40 patients who were given either tramadol 100 mg suppositories 6-hourly or 1000/20 mg of co-codamol 6-hourly (58). Nausea and vomiting were significantly more frequent with tramadol (84%) than with co-codamol (31%).

The effect of tramadol on postoperative nausea and vomiting after ENT surgery has been studied in a prospective, randomized, double-blind comparison with nalbuphine, pethidine, or saline in 281 patients (59). The three opioids caused a similar incidence of postoperative nausea and vomiting (40, 52, and 37% respectively) and more than placebo (32%).

In a randomized, double-blind placebo-controlled study of 76 women undergoing abdominal hysterectomy, tramadol 100 mg was a more effective analgesic than ketorolac 30 mg given every 6 hours intravenously (60). However, of those given tramadol 38% had vomiting compared with only 8% of those who were given ketorolac.

Urinary tract

The Netherlands Pharmacovigilance Foundation (LAREB), has reported five cases of transient difficulty in urinating, which spontaneously resolved on withdrawal of tramadol and was suspected to be induced by tramadol; none needed catheterization (61). In all five cases tramadol had been prescribed for back pain in relatively healthy individuals in a dose range of 50–150 mg.

Skin

Dermatological adverse effects of tramadol are rare, the majority being itching and rash. Tramadol-induced subcutaneous nodules have been described (62).

- A 46-year-old woman with infiltrative ductal carcinoma of the breast with bone metastases was given tramadol for bone pain. She developed skin nodules 1 day later; they disappeared when tramadol was withdrawn but there was residual pigmentation.
- A 47-year-old man taking tramadol 100 mg for low back pain developed a maculopapular rash with secondary erythroderma, which resolved after withdrawal of tramadol (63).

Immunologic

Tramadol has been associated with angioedema, a rare but potentially life threatening adverse effect (64).

- A 52-year-old woman developed swelling of the tongue, peripheral sensory loss, difficulty in standing, and swelling below both eyes after taking tramadol 50 mg bd. Her symptoms resolved on withdrawal.
- A 36-year-old woman developed swelling of the tongue, difficulty swallowing, intense pruritus, sweating, hallucinations, vertigo, and, loss of sensory perception over the mouth and cheeks after taking tramadol.
- An 83-year-old woman with a history of heart failure, paroxysmal atrial fibrillation, chronic obstructive airways disease, and angina, was given tramadol 50 mg tds and 5 days later developed swelling of the throat due to edema of the oral mucous membrane, uvula, tongue, and supraglottis. Tramadol was withdrawn and she was treated with cortisone, antihistamines, and adrenaline by inhalation.
- A 79-year-old man with a history of myocardial infarctions, anemia, heart failure, and angina, was given tramadol for back pain. After 17 days he developed respiratory distress and a swollen tongue. He was treated with cortisone and adrenaline, and tramadol and ramipril were withdrawn.
- A 61-year-old woman was given tramadol 50 mg/day for sciatic pain and 2 hours later developed respiratory distress and difficulty opening her mouth. Anti-allergy treatment was given and tramadol was withdrawn.
- A 55-year-old man with a history of hypertension and chronic bronchitis was given tramadol 50–100 mg 2–3 times daily and 5 days later developed swelling of the tongue and edema of the oral cavity. Betamethasone and adrenaline were given and tramadol and enalapril were withdrawn.

Four of these patients were taking concomitant ACE inhibitors, which can also cause angioedema (SEDA-29, 207). Whether an interaction of tramadol and ACE inhibitors increases the risk of angioedema is not known.

Long-Term Effects

Drug abuse

Tramadol abuse was monitored in the USA during the 3 years (1995–1998) after the drug was marketed there, through the systematic collection and evaluation of reports of suspected abuse in high-risk populations from a network of drug abuse specialists and reports sent through the FDA's Med Watch system (65). The overall conclusion was that experimentation with tramadol during the first 18 months of its introduction peaked at two cases per 100 000 patients exposed. This figure subsequently fell to less than one case per 100 000 patients in the second 18 months of the study period. Of cases of abuse 97% occurred among individuals with a history of substance abuse.

In Munich 20 cases of tramadol-related dependence syndrome have been recorded (66). In 17 cases tramadol had been used for chronic non-malignant pain, including headache (n=4), back pain (n = 7), and generalized non-specific pain (n = 6). The other three patients had a history of polydrug abuse.

Susceptibility Factors

Genetic

In 300 patients recovering from abdominal surgery recruited into a prospective study, the CYP2D6 poor metabolizer genotype had a negative impact on the response to tramadol analgesia postoperatively (67).

The CYP2D6*10 allele commonly found in Chinese is associated with reduced metabolic activity. This affects the dose of tramadol needed to achieve adequate analgesia. In homozygotes for the CYP2D6*10 allele (n = 17) more tramadol was needed than in heterozygotes (n = 26) and those who did not have the allele at all (n = 20) (68).

Multiple sclerosis

A woman with multiple sclerosis had a generalized seizure during a febrile urinary tract infection while taking baclofen 45 mg/day and tramadol 100 mg/day (69). The authors suggested that the multiple sclerosis had increased her susceptibility to a tramadol-induced seizure.

Drug Administration

Drug formulations

The incidence of adverse effects is reduced with the use of an oral, modified-release formulation of tramadol in the treatment of chronic pain (70), starting at the lowest dose, increasing gradually according to the patient's response during chronic oral administration (71,72), and using a loading dose immediately after the start of surgery.

The results of postmarketing surveillance of modified-released tramadol in Germany have been published (73). Modified-release tramadol (mean daily dose 236 mg usually divided into two doses) was used in 3153 patients, of whom most had severe or very severe pain. During the 6-week trial, 316 adverse effects were reported by a total of 206 patients (6.5%). Adverse effects were, in decreasing order of frequency, nausea (3.4%), dizziness (1.5%), vomiting (1.1%), constipation (0.5%), tiredness (0.5%), sweating (0.4%), dry mouth (0.3%), and pruritus (0.3%). Confusion, hypotension, sleep disturbances, abdominal pain, stomach upset, gastrointestinal hemorrhage, and cerebral hemorrhage were all among the less frequently reported adverse events, and 28% of events were classified as severe. Age did not affect the frequency of events, but women reported a higher frequency of adverse events than men (7.3 versus 5.7%).

The use of modified-release tramadol in chronic malignant pain has been examined in an open, prospective study in 146 patients with moderate to severe cancer pain; 90 patients completed the 6-week trial (74). Dropouts were due to opioid adverse effects (20%), inadequate pain relief (9%), or both (2.5%). There was at least one adverse effect in 86%. Overall, 433 adverse effect events were reported but some reduced in frequency over the 6 weeks. Modified-release tramadol (400 mg/day) provided fast and efficient pain relief in almost 60% of patients both during initial dosing and long-term treatment.

Drug dosage regimens

In a randomized, controlled, double-blind, multicenter, parallel, pharmaceutical company-sponsored study a once-daily formulation of tramadol was compared with a twice-daily formulation in 431 patients with osteoarthritis of the knee (75). The two formulations in daily doses of 100-400 micrograms provided similar analgesia. Of the 70 patients (16%) who withdrew from the study, 41 did so because of adverse events. About 80% of the study population reported at least one adverse event, all of them considered mild to moderate. The twice-daily formulation was associated with more dizziness, vertigo, vomiting, and headache, and the once-daily formulation was associated with more somnolence.

A double-blind, randomized, controlled study has been performed in 60 patients undergoing knee arthroplasty in order to identify the appropriate initial dose of tramadol PCA to minimize the incidence of opioid-related adverse effects (76). The patients received tramadol 1.25, 2.5, 3.75, or 5 mg/kg. The results suggested that a 2.5 mg/kg intraoperative loading dose of tramadol is optimal, since it provided the right balance of effective analgesia and minimal adverse effects.

In a double-blind, randomized, crossover trial in 134 patients with moderate osteoarthritic pain tramadol 150 or 200 mg/day and normal-release tramadol capsules 50 mg 8 hourly had similar therapeutic efficacy, adherence to therapy, and tolerability (77). Nausea, constipation, itching, drowsiness, dizziness, and headache were recorded by over 10% of the patients in each of the three groups. However, at least 8% of the patients in each group recorded similar adverse events at entry into the study. On the basis of these results and patients' opinions, once-daily tramadol 150 mg was the preferred treatment.

Drug administration route

Pethidine 100 mg produced better analgesia and significantly fewer adverse effects than intramuscular tramadol 100 mg in 49 full-term parturients in active labor in a randomized study (78).

Drug overdose

Fatal overdoses of tramadol has been reported.

- A 67-year-old man with painful rib fractures was given tramadol 100 mg qds and 8 days later developed acute liver failure as a result of fulminant hepatic necrosis (79). He had a cardiorespiratory arrest and died soon after admission. It transpired that he had taken 168 tablets of tramadol, each of 50 mg. Post-mortem toxicology confirmed a blood tramadol concentration of 3.7 micrograms/ml, 12 times higher than the usual target range (0.1-0.3 micrograms/ml).

- A 26-year-old male nurse died of tramadol intoxication (80). The peripheral blood concentration of tramadol was 9.6 micrograms/ml (target concentration 0.1–0.3 micrograms/ml). There was no objective evidence at postmortem of any pre-existing disease or use/overuse of ethanol or other drugs that could have contributed to or caused death.

Drug–Drug Interactions

NSAIDs

In a multicenter, randomized, double-blind, placebo-controlled study in 227 patients, tramadol 37.5 micrograms + paracetamol 325 mg combination tablets was safely added to NSAID therapy in patients with osteoarthritis and increased the analgesic effect (81).

Ondansetron

Tramadol dosage requirements for patient-controlled analgesia increased when ondansetron was given as a prophylactic antiemetic in 40 patients undergoing lumbar laminectomy in an open, controlled study (82). During the first 4 hours postoperatively tramadol consumption increased by about 30% in those given ondansetron and remained 22–25% higher thereafter. A single dose of ondansetron 4 mg given during induction did not reduce the 24-hour incidence of nausea or vomiting.

In a randomized, controlled study of postoperative PCA using tramadol with or without ondansetron in 59 patients undergoing ear, nose, and throat surgery, ondansetron reduced the overall analgesic effect of tramadol, increased doses of tramadol being needed in the first 12 hours after surgery. This increase in tramadol requirements in those given ondansetron resulted in a significantly higher vomiting scores at 4 and 8 hours postoperatively and an overall increase in the number of episodes of vomiting, despite the use of ondansetron (83).

Oral anticoagulants

Tramadol may increase the anticoagulant effect of phenprocoumon or warfarin (SEDA-22, 103).

Seven patients in whom an interaction of tramadol with warfarin, with an increased International Normalized Ratio (INR), was confirmed carried a defective CYP2D6 allele (population prevalence 42%) (84). Tramadol is unlikely to displace warfarin because it is not extensively protein bound. Inhibition of serotonin uptake in platelets by tramadol may increase the tendency to bleeding, but would not increase the INR. A metabolic interaction is another possible explanation.

Quinidine

Inhibition of the hepatic metabolism of tramadol to morphine by quinidine may reduce its opioid effects (SEDA-21, 90).

Selective serotonin re-uptake inhibitors (SSRIs)

Serotonin syndrome has been attributed to the co-administration of tramadol with venlafaxine, mirtazapine (85), sertraline (86), and citalopram (87).

Fluoxetine

Serotonin syndrome and mania occurred in a 72-year-old woman taking fluoxetine 20 mg/day and tramadol 150 mg/day 18 days after she started to take the combination (88). Inhibition of CYP2D6 may have played a part (89).

Sertraline

The serotonin syndrome has been reported after concurrent use of tramadol and sertraline (SEDA-22, 103).

- Serotonin syndrome occurred in an 88-year-old woman who took sertraline 50–100 mg/day and tramadol 200–400 mg/day for 10 days; the symptoms subsided 15 days after withdrawal of tramadol (90).

Venlafaxine

The death of a 36-year-old patient with a history of alcohol dependence who was taking tramadol, venlafaxine, trazodone, and quetiapine has highlighted the increased risk of seizures with concomitant use of tramadol and selective serotonin re-uptake inhibitors (91).

References

1. Budd K, Langford R. Tramadol revisited. Br J Anaesth 1999;82(4):493–5.
2. Reig E. Tramadol in musculoskeletal pain—a survey. Clin Rheumatol 2002;21(Suppl 1):S9–S12.
3. Silverfield JC, Kamin M, Wu SC, Rosenthal NCAPSS-105 Study Group. Tramadol/acetaminophen combination tablets for the treatment of osteoarthritis flare pain: a multicenter, outpatient, randomized, double-blind, placebo-controlled, parallel-group, add-on study. Clin Ther 2002;24(2):282–97.
4. Günes Y, Gunduz M, Unlugenc H, Ozalevli M, Ozcengiz D. Comparison of caudal vs intravenous tramadol administered either preoperatively or postoperatively for pain relief in boys. Ped Anesth 2004;14:324–8.
5. Schug SA. Combination analgesia in 2005. A rational approach: focus on paracetamol–tramadol. Clin Rheumatol 2006;25(Suppl 7):S16–21.
6. Pendleton J, Costa J, Wludyka P, Carvin DM, Rosser CJ. Combination of oral Tramadol, acetaminophen and 1% lidocaine induced periprostatic nerve block for pain control during transrectal ultrasound guided biopsy of the prostate: a prospective, randomized, controlled trial. J Urol 2006;176(4):1372–5.
7. Senel AC, Akyol A, Dohman D, Solak M. Caudal bupivacaine-tramadol combination for postoperative analgesia in pediatric herniorrhaphy. Acta Anaesthesiol Scand 2001;45(6):786–9.
8. Eren GA, Cinar SO, Oba S, Zoylan G. Pediyatrik alt batin cerrahisinde postoperatif analjezi amacli kaudal tramadol kullanimi. Turk Anesteziyol Reanim 2001;29:39–43.
9. Mullican WS, Lacy JRTRAMAP-ANAG-006 Study Group. Tramadol/acetaminophen combination tablets and codeine/acetaminophen combination capsules for the management

of chronic pain: a comparative trial. Clin Ther 2001;23(9):1429–45.

10. Jeffrey HM, Charlton P, Mellor DJ, Moss E, Vucevic M. Analgesia after intracranial surgery: a double-blind, prospective comparison of codeine and tramadol. Br J Anaesth 1999;83(2):245–9.

11. Resim S, Gumusalan Y, Ekerbicer HC, Sahin MA, Sahinkanat T. Effectiveness of electro-acupuncture compared to sedo-analgesics in relieving pain during shockwave lithotripsy. Urol Res 2005;33(4):285–90.

12. Hirsh I, Vaissler A, Chernin J, Segol O, Pizov R. Fentanyl or tramadol, with midazolam, for outpatient colonoscopy: analgesia, sedation, and safety. Dig Dis Sci 2006;51:1946–51.

13. Gunduz M, Ozalevli M, Ozbek H, Ozcengiz D. Comparison of caudal ketamine with lidocaine or tramadol administration for postoperative analgesia of hypospadias surgery in children. Paediatr Anesth 2006;16(2):158–63.

14. Khosravi MB, Khezri S, Azemati S. Tramadol for pain relief in children undergoing herniotomy: a comparison with ilioinguinal and iliohypogastric blocks. Paediatr Anesth 2006;16(1):54–8.

15. Wilder-Smith CH, Hill L, Spargo K, Kalla A. Treatment of severe pain from osteoarthritis with slow-release tramadol or dihydrocodeine in combination with NSAID's. A randomised study comparing analgesia, antinociception and gastrointestinal effects. Pain 2001;91(1–2):23–31.

16. Fleischmann RM, Caldwell JR, Roth SH, Tesser JRP, Olson W, Kamin M. Tramadol for the treatment of joint pain associated with osteoarthritis: a randomised double-blind, placebo-controlled trial. Curr Ther Res 2001;62:113–28.

17. Pavelka K, Peliskova Z, Stehlikova H, Ratcliffe S, Repas C. Intraindividual differences in pain relief and functional improvement in osteoarthritis with diclofenac or tramadol. Clin Drug Invest 1998;16:421–9.

18. Engindeniz Z, Demircan C, Karli N, Armagan E, Bulut M, Aydin T, Zarifoglu M. Intramuscular tramadol vs. diclofenac sodium for the treatment of acute migraine attacks in emergency department: a prospective, randomised, double-blind study. J Headache Pain 2005;6(3):143–8.

19. Putland AJ, McCluskey A. The analgesic efficacy of tramadol versus ketorolac in day-case laparoscopic sterilisation. Anaesthesia 1999;54(4):382–5.

20. Ekman EF, Ruoff G, Kuehl K, Ralph L, Hormbrey P, Fiechtner J, Berger MF. The COX-2 specific inhibitor valdecoxib versus tramadol in acute ankle sprain: a multicenter randomized, controlled trial. Am J Sports Med 2006;34(6):945–55.

21. Joshi GP, Duffy L, Chehade J, Wesevich J, Gajraj N, Johnson ER. Effects of prophylactic nalmefene on the incidence of morphine-related side effects in patients receiving intravenous patient-controlled analgesia. Anesthesiology 1999;90(4):1007–11.

22. Turturro MA, Paris PM, Larkin GL. Tramadol versus hydrocodone–acetaminophen in acute musculoskeletal pain: a randomized, double-blind clinical trial. Ann Emerg Med 1998;32(2):139–43.

23. Coetzee JF, van Loggerenberg H. Tramadol or morphine administered during operation: a study of immediate postoperative effects after abdominal hysterectomy. Br J Anaesth 1998;81(5):737–41.

24. Wiebalck A, Tryba M, Hoell T, Strumpf M, Kulka P, Zenz M. Efficacy and safety of tramadol and morphine in patients with extremely severe postoperative pain. Acute Pain 2000;3:112–8.

25. Hopkins D, Shipton EA, Potgieter D, Van derMerwe CA, Boon J, De Wet C, Murphy J. Comparison of tramadol and morphine via subcutaneous PCA following major orthopaedic surgery. Can J Anaesth 1998;45(5 Pt 1):435–42.

26. Vergnion M, Degesves S, Garcet L, Magotteaux V. Tramadol, an alternative to morphine for treating posttraumatic pain in the prehospital situation. Anesth Analg 2001;92(6):1543–6.

27. Rawal N, Allvin R, Amilon A, Ohlsson T, Hallen J. Postoperative analgesia at home after ambulatory hand surgery: a controlled comparison of tramadol, metamizol, and paracetamol. Anesth Analg 2001;92(2):347–51.

28. Dejonckheere M, Desjeux L, Deneu S, Ewalenko P. Intravenous tramadol compared to propacetamol for postoperative analgesia following thyroidectomy. Acta Anaesthesiol Belg 2001;52(1):29–33.

29. Harati Y, Gooch C, Swenson M, Edelman SV, Greene D, Raskin P, Donofrio P, Cornblath D, Olson WH, Kamin M. Maintenance of the long-term effectiveness of tramadol in treatment of the pain of diabetic neuropathy. J Diabetes Complications 2000;14(2):65–70.

30. Russell IJ, Kamin M, Bennett RM, Schnitzer TJ, Green JA, Katz WA. Efficacy of tramadol in treatment of pain in fibromyalgia. J Clin Rheumatol 2000;6:250–7.

31. Viitanen H, Annila P. Analgesic efficacy of tramadol 2 mg kg^{-1} for paediatric day-case adenoidectomy Br J Anaesth 2001;86(4):572–5.

32. Ozcengiz D, Gunduz M, Ozbek H, Isik G. Comparison of caudal morphine and tramadol for postoperative pain control in children undergoing inguinal herniorrhaphy. Paediatr Anaesth 2001;11(4):459–64.

33. Mathews S, Al Mulla A, Varghese PK, Radim K, Mumtaz S. Postanaesthetic shivering—a new look at tramadol. Anaesthesia 2002;57(4):394–8.

34. Kaya M, Karakus D, Sariyildiz O, Ozalp G, Kodiogullari N. Genel anestezi sonrasi titreme tedavisinde tramadolum etkinligi. Turk Anesteziyol Reanim Cem Mecmuasi 2002;30:90–3.

35. Safarinejad MR, Hosseini SY. Safety and efficacy of tramadol in the treatment of idiopathic detrusor overactivity: a double-blind, placebo controlled, randomized study. Br J Clin Pharmacol 2006;61(4):456–63.

36. Safarinejad MR, Hosseini SY. Safety and efficacy of tramadol in the treatment of premature ejaculation: a double-blind, placebo-controlled, fixed dose, randomized study. Br J Clin Pharmacol. 2006;61(4):456–63.

37. Pang W, Huang S, Tung CC, Huang MH. Patient-controlled analgesia with tramadol versus tramadol plus lysine acetyl salicylate. Anesth Analg 2000;91(5):1226–9.

38. Tuncer S, Barikaner H, Yosunkaya A, Taulan A. Influence of dexamethasone on nausea and vomiting during patient-controlled analgesia with tramadol. Clin Drug Invest 2002;22:547–52.

39. Bloch MB, Dyer RA, Heijke SA, James MF. Tramadol infusion for postthoracotomy pain relief: a placebo-controlled comparison with epidural morphine. Anesth Analg 2002;94(3):523–8.

40. Ng KF, Tsui SL, Yang JC, Ho ET. Comparison of tramadol and tramadol/droperidol mixture for patient-controlled analgesia. Can J Anaesth 1997;44(8):810–5.

41. Zimmermann AR, Kibblewhite D, Sleigh J. Comparison of morphine/droperidol and tramadol/droperidol mixture for patient controlled analgesia (PCA) after cardiac surgery: a prospective, randomised, double-blind study. J Acute Pain 2002;4:65–9.

42. Unlugenc H, Gunduz M, Ozalevli M, Akman H. A comparative study on the analgesic effect of tramadol, tramadol plus magnesium, and tramadol plus ketamine for

postoperative pain management after major abdominal surgery. Acta Anaesthesiol Scand 2002;46(8):1025–30.

43. Webb AR, Leong S, Myles PS, Burn SJ. The addition of a tramadol infusion to morphine patient-controlled analgesia after abdominal surgery: a double-blinded, placebo-controlled randomized trial. Anesth Analg 2002;95(6):1713–8.

44. Desmeules JA. The tramadol option. Eur J Pain 2000;4(Suppl A):15–21.

45. Schnitzer TJ, Gray WL, Paster RZ, Kamin M. Efficacy of tramadol in treatment of chronic low back pain. J Rheumatol 2000;27(3):772–8.

46. Krantz MJ, Garcia JA, Mehler PS. Tramadol-associated pericarditis. Int J Cardiol 2005;99(3):497–8.

47. Duthie DJ. Remifentanil and tramadol. Br J Anaesth 1998;81(1):51–7.

48. Warren PM, Taylor JH, Nicholson KE, Wraith PK, Drummond GB. Influence of tramadol on the ventilatory response to hypoxia in humans. Br J Anaesth 2000;85(2):211–6.

49. Gardner JS, Blough D, Drinkard CR, Shatin D, Anderson G, Graham D, Alderfer R. Tramadol and seizures: a surveillance study in a managed care population. Pharmacotherapy 2000;20(12):1423–31.

50. Gasse C, Derby L, Vasilakis-Scaramozza C, Jick H. Incidence of first-time idiopathic seizures in users of tramadol. Pharmacotherapy 2000;20(6):629–34.

51. Yates WR, Nguyen MH, Warnock JK. Tramadol dependence with no history of substance abuse. Am J Psychiatry 2001;158(6):964.

52. Devulder J, De Laat M, Dumoulin K, Renson A, Rolly G. Nightmares and hallucinations after long-term intake of tramadol combined with antidepressants. Acta Clin Belg 1996;51(3):184–6.

53. Keeley PW, Foster G, Whitelaw L. Hear my song: auditory hallucinations with tramadol hydrochloride. BMJ 2000;321(7276):1608.

54. Künig G, Dätwyler S, Eschen A, Schreiter Gasser U. Unrecognized long-lasting tramadol-induced delirium in two elderly patients: a case report. Pharmacopsychiatry 2006;39(5):194–9.

55. Antila H, Manner T, Kuurila K, Salantera S, Kujala R, Aantaa R. Ketoprofen and tramadol for analgesia during early recovery after tonsillectomy in children. Paediatr Anesth 2006;16(5):548–53.

56. Crighton IM, Martin PH, Hobbs GJ, Cobby TF, Fletcher AJ, Stewart PD. A comparison of the effects of intravenous tramadol, codeine, and morphine on gastric emptying in human volunteers. Anesth Analg 1998;87(2):445–9.

57. Minami K, Ogata J, Hiroshita T, Shiraishi M, Okamoto T, Sata T, Shigematsu A. Intramuscular tramadol increases gastric pH during anesthesia. Can J Anaesth 2004;51:545–8.

58. Pluim MA, Wegener JT, Rupreht J, Vulto AG. Tramadol suppositories are less suitable for post-operative pain relief than rectal acetaminophen/codeine. Eur J Anaesthesiol 1999;16(7):473–8.

59. van den Berg AA, Halliday E, Lule EK, Baloch MS. The effects of tramadol on postoperative nausea, vomiting and headache after ENT surgery. A placebo-controlled comparison with equipotent doses of nalbuphine and pethidine. Acta Anaesthesiol Scand 1999;43(1):28–33.

60. Olle Fortuny G, Opisso Julia L, Oferil Riera F, Sanchez Pallares M, Calatayud Montesa R, Cabre Roca I. Ketorolaco frente a tramadol: estudio comparativo de la eficaciá analgesica en el dolor postoperatorio de histerectomias abdominal. [Ketorolac versus tramadol: comparative study of analgesic efficacy in the postoperative pain in abdominal hysterectomy.] Rev Esp Anestesiol Reanim 2000;47(4):162–7.

61. Meyboom RH, Brodie-Meijer CC, Diemont WL, van Puijenbroek EP. Bladder dysfunction during the use of tramadol. Pharmacoepidemiol Drug Saf 1999;8(Suppl 1):S63–4.

62. Senol Coskun H, Ozbalci D, Sahin M. An unusual side effect of tramadol: subcutaneous nodules. J Eur Acad Dermatol Venereol 2006;20(8):1008–9.

63. Ghislain PD, Wiart T, Bouhassoun N, Legout L, Alcaraz I, Caron J, Modiano P. Toxidermie au tramadol. [Toxic dermatitis caused by tramadol.] Ann Dermatol Venereol 1999;126(1):38–40.

64. Hallberg P, Brenning G. Angioedema induced by tramadol—a potentially life threatening condition. Eur J Clin Pharmacol 2005;60(12):901–3.

65. Cicero TJ, Adams EH, Geller A, Inciardi JA, Munoz A, Schnoll SH, Senay EC, Woody GE. A postmarketing surveillance program to monitor Ultram (tramadol hydrochloride) abuse in the United States. Drug Alcohol Depend 1999;57(1):7–22.

66. Soyka M, Backmund M, Hasemann S. Tramadol use and dependence in chronic non-cancer pain patients. Pharmacopsychiatry 2004;37:189–91.

67. Loughrey MB, Loughrey CM, Johnston S, O'Rourke D. Fatal hepatic failure following accidental tramadol overdose. Forensic Sci Int 2003;134:232–3.

68. Wang G, Zhang H, He F, Fang X. Effect of the CYP2D6*10 C188T polymorphism on postoperative tramadol analgesia in a Chinese population. Eur J Clin Pharmacol 2006;62(11):927–31.

69. Solaro C. Incidence of seizures in patients with multiple sclerosis treated with intrathecal baclofen. Neurology 2006;66(5):784.

70. Raber M, Hofmann S, Junge K, Momberger H, Kuhn D. Analgesic efficacy and tolerability of tramadol 100 mg sustained-release capsules in patients with moderate to severe chronic low back pain Clin Drug Invest 1999;17:415–23.

71. Ruoff GE. Slowing the initial titration rate of tramadol improves tolerability. Pharmacotherapy 1999;19(1):88–93.

72. Petrone D, Kamin M, Olson W. Slowing the titration rate of tramadol HCl reduces the incidence of discontinuation due to nausea and/or vomiting: a double-blind randomized trial. J Clin Pharm Ther 1999;24(2):115–23.

73. Nossol S, Schwarzbold M, Stadler T. Treatment of pain with sustained-release tramadol 100, 150, 200 mg: results of a post-marketing surveillance study Int J Clin Pract 1998;52(2):115–21.

74. Petzke F, Radbruch L, Sabatowski R, Karthaus M, Mertens A. Slow-release tramadol for treatment of chronic malignant pain—an open multicenter trial. Support Care Cancer 2001;9(1):48–54.

75. Mongin G, Yakusevich V, Kőpe A, Shostak N, Pikhlak E, Popdan L, Simon J, Navarro C, Fortier L, Robertson S, Bochard S. Efficacy and safety assessment of a novel once-daily tablet formulation of tramadol. Clin Drug Invest 2004;24:548–58.

76. Paing W-W, Wu H-S, Tung C-C. Tramadol 2.5 mg.kg^{-1} appears to be the optimal intraoperative loading dose before patient-controlled analgesia Can J Anesth 2003;50:48–51.

77. Bodalia B, Mcdonald CJ, Smith KJ, O'Brien C, Cousins L. A comparison of the pharmacokinetics, clinical efficacy and tolerability of once-daily tramadol tablets with normal release tramadol capsules. J Pain Symptom Manage 2003;25:142–9.

78. Keskin HL, Keskin EA, Avsar AF, Tabuk M, Caglar GS. Pethidine versus tramadol for pain relief during labour. Int J Gynaecol Obstet 2003;82:11–16.

79. Stamer UM, Lehnen K, Höthker F, Bayerer B, Wolf S, Hoeft A, Stuber F. Impact of CYP2D6 genotype on post-operative tramadol analgesia. Pain 2003;105:231–8.

80. Musshoff F, Madea B. Fatality due to ingestion of tramadol alone. Forensic Sci Int 2001;116(2–3):197–9.

81. Emkey R, Rosenthal N, Wu S-C, Jordan D, Kamin M. Efficacy and safety of tramadol/acetaminophen tablets (Ultracet®) as add-on therapy for osteoarthritis pain in subjects receiving a Cox-2 nonsteroidal anti-inflammatory drug: a multi-centre, randomized, double blind, placebo controlled trial. J Rheumatol 2004;31:150–6.

82. De Witte JL, Schoenmaekers B, Sessler DI, Deloof T. The analgesic efficacy of tramadol is impaired by concurrent administration of ondansetron. Anesth Analg 2001;92(5):1319–21.

83. Arcioni R, della Rocca M, Romano S, Romano R, Pietropaoli P, Gasparetto A. Ondansetron inhibits the analgesic effects of tramadol: a possible 5-HT(3) spinal receptor involvement in acute pain in humans. Anesth Analg 2002;94(6):1553–7.

84. Hedenmalm K, Lindh JD, Sawe J, Rane A. Increased liability of tramadol–warfarin interaction in individuals with mutations in the cytochrome P450 206 gene. Eur J Clin Pharmacol 2004;60:369–72.

85. Houlihan DJ. Serotonin syndrome resulting from co-administration of tramadol, venlafaxine and mirtazapine. Ann Pharmacother 2004;38:411–3.

86. Mittino D, Mula M, Monaco F. Serotonin syndrome associated with tramadol-sertraline co-administration. Clin Neuropharmacol 2004;27:150–1.

87. Mahlberg R, Kunz D, Sasse J, Kirchheiner J. Serotonin syndrome with tramadol and citalopram. Am J Psychiatry 2004;1612:1129.

88. Gonzalez-Pinto A, Imaz H, De Heredia JL, Gutierrez M, Mico JA. Mania and tramadol–fluoxetine combination. Am J Psychiatry 2001;158(6):964–5.

89. Ingelman-Sundberg M. Genetic susceptibility to adverse effects of drugs and environmental toxicants. The role of the CYP family of enzymes. Mutat Res 2001;482(1–2):11–9.

90. Sauget D, Franco PS, Amaniou M, Mazere J, Dantoine T. Possible syndrome sérotoninergiques induit par l'association de tramadol à de la sertraline chez une femme agée. [Possible serotonergic syndrome caused by combination of tramadol and sertraline in an elderly woman.] Thérapie. 57(3):309–10.

91. Ripple MG, Pestaner JP, Levine BS, Smialek JE. Lethal combination of tramadol and multiple drugs affecting serotonin. Am J Forensic Med Pathol 2000;21(4):370–4.

SALICYLATES, PARACETAMOL, AND OTHER NON-OPIOID ANALGESICS

Acetylsalicylic acid

See also Benorilate, Diflunisal, Lysine acetylsalicylate, Salicylates, topical, Salsalate

General Information

Over a century after its introduction, acetylsalicylic acid (aspirin) is by far the most commonly used analgesic, sharing its leading position with the relative newcomer paracetamol (acetaminophen), and notwithstanding the fact that other widely used anti-inflammatory drugs, like ibuprofen and naproxen, have in recent years been introduced in over-the-counter versions. Both are also still being prescribed by physicians and are generally used for mild to moderate pain, fever associated with common everyday illnesses, and disorders ranging from head colds and influenza to toothache and headache. Their greatest use is by consumers who obtain them directly at the pharmacy, and in many countries outside pharmacies as well. Perhaps this wide availability and advertising via mass media lead to a lack of appreciation by the lay public that these are medicines with associated adverse effects. Both have at any rate been subject to misuse and excessive use, leading to such problems as chronic salicylate intoxication with aspirin, and severe hepatic damage after overdose with paracetamol. Both aspirin and paracetamol have featured in accidental overdosage (particularly in children) as well as intentional overdosage.

In an investigation of Canadian donors who had not admitted to drug intake, 6–7% of the blood samples taken were found to have detectable concentrations of acetylsalicylic acid and paracetamol (1). Such drugs would be potentially capable of causing untoward reactions in the recipients.

To offer some protection against misuse of analgesics, many countries have insisted on the use of packs containing total quantities less than the minimum toxic dose (albeit usually the one obtained for healthy young volunteers and thus disregarding the majority of the population), and supplied in child-resistant packaging. Most important, however, is the need to provide education for the lay public to respect such medicines in general for the good they can do, but more especially for the harm that can arise but which can be avoided. There is a definite role for the prescribing physician, as informing the patient seems to prevent adverse events (2).

The sale of paracetamol or aspirin in dosage forms in which they are combined with other active ingredients offers considerable risk to the consumer, since the product as sold may not be clearly identified as containing either of these two analgesics. Brand names sometimes obscure the actual composition of older formulations that contain one or both of these analgesics in combination with, for example, a pyrazolone derivative and/or a potentially addictive substance. For instance, in Germany, with the EC harmonization of the Drug Law of 1990, the manufacturers of drugs already marketed before 1978 had the opportunity of exchanging even the active principles without being obliged to undergo a new approval procedure or to abandon their brand name. Combination formulations are still being promoted and sold, and not exclusively in developing countries. Consequently, the patient who is so anxious to allay all his symptoms that he takes several medications concurrently may without knowing it take several doses of aspirin or paracetamol at the same time, perhaps sufficient to cause toxicity. It is essential that product labels clearly state their active ingredients by approved name together with the quantity per dosage form (3).

The antipyretic analgesics, with the non-steroidal anti-inflammatory drugs (NSAIDs), share a common mechanism of action, namely the inhibition of prostaglandin synthesis from arachidonic acid and their release. More precisely their mode of action is thought to result from inhibition of both the constitutive and the inducible iso-enzymes (COX-1 and COX-2) of the cyclo-oxygenase pathway (4). However, aspirin and paracetamol are distinguishable from most of the NSAIDs by their ability to inhibit prostaglandin synthesis in the nervous system, and thus the hypothalamic center for body temperature regulation, rather than acting mainly in the periphery.

Endogenous pyrogens (and exogenous pyrogens that have their effects through the endogenous group) induce the hypothalamic vascular endothelium to produce prostaglandins, which activate the thermoregulatory neurons by increasing AMP concentrations. The capacity of the antipyretic analgesics to inhibit hypothalamic prostaglandin synthesis appears to be the basis of their antipyretic action. Neither aspirin nor paracetamol affects the synthesis or release of endogenous pyrogens and neither will lower body temperature if it is normal.

While aspirin significantly inhibits peripheral prostaglandin and thromboxane synthesis, paracetamol is less potent as a synthetase inhibitor than the NSAIDs, except in the brain, and paracetamol has only a weak anti-inflammatory action. It is simple to ascribe the analgesic activity of aspirin to its capacity to inhibit prostaglandin synthesis, with a consequent reduction in inflammatory edema and vasodilatation, since aspirin is most effective in the pain associated with inflammation or injury. However, such a peripheral effect cannot account for the analgesic activity of paracetamol, which is less well understood.

As a prostaglandin synthesis inhibitor, aspirin, like other NSAIDs, is associated with irritation of and damage to the gastrointestinal mucosa. In low doses it can also increase bleeding by inhibiting platelet aggregation; in high doses, prolongation of the prothrombin time will contribute to the bleeding tendency. Intensive treatment can also produce unwanted nervous system effects (salicylism).

Depending on the criteria used, the incidence of aspirin hypersensitivity is variously estimated as being as low as 1% or as high as 50%, the highest frequency being found in asthmatics. The condition is characterized by bronchospasm (asthma), urticaria, angioedema, and vasomotor rhinitis, each occurring alone or in combination, often leading to severe and even life-threatening reactions. There is no clear evidence of an association with tumors, apart from the possible peripheral contribution of aspirin to the development of urinary tract neoplasms in patients with analgesic nephropathy. Indeed, some authors have suggested a role for salicylates in reducing the incidence of colorectal tumors and breast tumors.

The following are absolute contraindications to the use of aspirin:

- children under 16;
- people with hypersensitivity to salicylates, NSAIDs, or tartrazine;
- people with peptic ulceration;
- people with known coagulopathies, including those induced as part of medical therapy.

The following are relative contraindications to the use of long-term analgesic doses of aspirin:

- gout, since normal analgesic doses impede the excretion of uric acid (high doses have a uricosuric effect); an additional problem in gout is that salicylates reduce the uricosuric effects of sulfinpyrazone and probenecid;
- variant angina; a daily dose of 4 g has been found to provoke attacks both at night-time and during the day (5,6), perhaps owing to direct triggering of coronary arterial spasm; blockade of the synthesis of PGI_z, which normally protects against vasoconstriction, could be involved;
- diabetes mellitus, in which aspirin can in theory interfere with the actions of insulin and glucagon sufficiently to derange control;
- some days before elective surgery (even in coronary artery bypass grafting) or delivery, especially if extradural anesthesia is used (7), although recent data seem reassuring (8); aspirin increases bleeding at dental extraction or perioperatively;
- in elderly people, who may develop gastrointestinal bleeding;
- anorectal inflammation (suppositories);
- pre-existing gastrointestinal disease, liver disease, hypoalbuminemia, hypovolemia, in the third trimester of pregnancy, perioperatively, or in patients with threatening abortion.

Assessing the benefit-to-harm balance of low-dose aspirin in preventing strokes and heart attacks

Although there is clear evidence of benefit of acetylsalicylic acid (aspirin) in secondary prevention of strokes and heart attacks, the question of whether aspirin should also be prescribed for primary prevention in asymptomatic people is still debatable. Trials in primary prevention have given contrasting results (9,10), and aspirin can cause major harms (for example severe gastrointestinal bleeding and hemorrhagic stroke).

Furthermore, despite evidence of the efficacy of aspirin in secondary prevention, its use in patients at high risk of strokes and heart attacks remains suboptimal (11). A possible explanation for this underuse may be concern about the relative benefit in relation to the potential risk for serious hemorrhagic events. Accurate evaluation of the benefits and harms of aspirin is therefore warranted.

Two meta-analyses have provided some information. The first examined the benefit and harms of aspirin in subjects without known cardiovascular or cerebrovascular disease (primary prevention) (12). The authors selected articles published between 1966 and 2000—five large controlled studies of primary prevention that lasted at least 1 year and nine studies of the effects of aspirin on gastrointestinal bleeding and hemorrhagic stroke. The five randomized, placebo-controlled trials included more than 50 000 patients and the meta-analysis showed that aspirin significantly reduced the risk of the combined outcome (confirmed non-fatal myocardial infarction or death from coronary heart disease) (OR = 0.72; 95% CI = 0.60, 0.87). However, aspirin increased the risk of major gastrointestinal bleeding (OR = 1.7; CI = 1.4, 2.1) significantly, while the small increase found for hemorrhagic stroke (OR = 1.4; CI = 0.9, 2.0) was not statistically significant. All-cause mortality was not significantly affected (OR = 0.93; CI = 0.84; 1.02). Most important was the finding that the net effect of aspirin improved with increasing risk of coronary heart disease. The meta-analysis showed that for 1000 patients with a 5% risk of coronary heart disease events over 5 years, aspirin would prevent 6–20 myocardial infarctions but would cause also 0–2 hemorrhagic strokes and 2–4 major gastrointestinal bleeds. For patients at lower risk (1% over 5 years), aspirin would prevent 1–4 myocardial infarctions but would still cause 0–2 hemorrhagic strokes and 2-4 major gastrointestinal bleeds.

Therefore when deciding to use aspirin in primary prophylaxis, one should take account of the relative utility of the different outcomes that are prevented or caused by aspirin.

The other meta-analysis (13) compared the benefits of aspirin in secondary prevention with the risk of gastrointestinal bleeding. An earlier analysis of this problem included patients at various levels of risk and doses of aspirin that would currently be regarded as too high (14), and may therefore have either under-represented the benefit or exaggerated the risk. In another analysis there was no difference in the risk of gastrointestinal bleeding across the whole range of doses used (15).

The meta-analysis reviewed all randomized, placebo-controlled, secondary prevention trials of at least 3-months duration published from 1970 to 2000. The dosage of aspirin was 50–325 mg/day. Six studies contributed 6300 patients to the analysis (3127 on aspirin and 3173 on placebo). Aspirin reduced all-cause mortality by 18%, the number of strokes by 20%, myocardial infarctions by 30%, and other vascular events by 30%. On the other hand, patients who took aspirin were 2.5 times more likely than those who took placebo to have gastrointestinal tract bleeds. The number of patients needed to be treated (NNT) to prevent one death from any cause was 67 and the NNT to cause one gastrointestinal bleeding event was 100. In other words 1.5 lives can be saved for every gastrointestinal bleed attributed to aspirin. Although the risk of gastrointestinal bleeding was increased by aspirin, the hemorrhagic events were manageable and led to no deaths. On the basis of these data we can conclude that the benefits–harm balance for low-dose aspirin in the secondary prevention of cardiovascular and cerebrovascular events is highly favorable. The same conclusions have been drawn from the systematic overview published by the Antithrombotic Trialists Collaboration Group, which analysed data from 287 studies involving 135 000 patients (16).

As far as primary prevention of cardiovascular events is concerned, it appears that aspirin can reduce heart attacks and strokes but increases gastrointestinal and intracranial bleeding. The decision to use aspirin in primary prevention should therefore take into account the fact that the net effect of aspirin improves with increasing risk of coronary heart disease as well as the values that patients attach to the main favorable and unfavorable outcomes.

Organs and Systems

Cardiovascular

Apart from rare reports of variant angina pectoris and vasculitis theoretically related to thromboxane, aspirin is not associated with adverse effects on the cardiovascular system (17,18), except an increase in circulating plasma volume after large doses.

The effects of aspirin on blood pressure have been investigated in 100 untreated patients with mild hypertension who took aspirin on awakening or before bedtime (19). There was no change in blood pressure after dietary recommendations alone or when aspirin was given on awakening. However, there was a highly significant reduction in blood pressure in those who took aspirin before bedtime (reductions of 6 and 4 mmHg in systolic and diastolic blood pressures respectively). As aspirin is given once a day for its cardioprotective effect, giving it in the evening could be of greater benefit if it also results in a reduction in blood pressure.

Respiratory

The effect of aspirin on bronchial musculature is discussed in the section on Immunologic in this monograph.

Salicylates can cause pulmonary edema, particularly in the elderly, especially if they are or have been heavy smokers (20).

Chronic salicylate toxicity can cause pulmonary injury, leading to respiratory distress. Lung biopsy may show diffuse alveolar damage and fibrosis (21).

Nervous system

Salicylism is a reaction to very high circulating concentrations of salicylate, characterized by tinnitus, dizziness, confusion, and headache.

Encephalopathy secondary to hyperammonemia has been reported in those rare cases of liver failure that are associated with high doses of aspirin, and this also forms a major feature of Reye's syndrome (see the section on Liver in this monograph).

One case-control study showed no increased risk of intracerebral hemorrhage in patients using aspirin or other NSAIDs in low dosages as prophylaxis against thrombosis (22). However, intracerebral hemorrhage has been reported with aspirin, even in low doses, and in the SALT study (23) and the Physicians Health Study of 1989

(24) hemorrhagic stroke and associated deaths occurred with aspirin.

In 208 subjects with intracerebral hemorrhage the 3-month mortality was 33% (25). The independent risk factors for death were regular aspirin use at the onset of intracerebral hemorrhage (RR = 2.5; 95% CI = 1.3, 4.6), warfarin use at the onset of intracerebral hemorrhage (RR = 3.2; 95% CI = 1.6, 6.1), and an intracerebral hemorrhage score over 2 on admission (RR = 14; 95% CI = 6.0, 31). Regular aspirin use (median dose 250 mg/day) preceding the onset of intracerebral hemorrhage was significantly associated with hematoma enlargement during the first week after intracerebral hemorrhage.

Sensory systems

Eyes
Well-documented acute myopia and increased ocular pressure attributed to aspirin has been described (26).

Ears
With the high concentrations achieved in attempted suicide, tinnitus and hearing loss, leading to deafness, develop within about 5 hours, usually with regression within 48 hours, but permanent damage can occur. Disturbed balance, often with vertigo, can develop, as well as nausea, usually with maintenance of consciousness, even without treatment. It has been postulated that in this state depolarization of the cochlear hair cells occurs, similar to the changes induced by pressure. Tinnitus is also a symptom of salicylism.

Aspirin has been reported to cause damage to the semicircular canals.

- A 61-year-old man with a monoclonal gammopathy developed severe persistent bilateral vestibular dysfunction after taking a high dose of aspirin (5-6 g/day for 3 days) (27). His symptoms (unsteadiness, a broad-based gait, blurred vision, and apparent visual motion when he moved his head and when he walked) persisted for 9 months. Investigations showed a bilateral dynamic deficit of his horizontal semicircular canal.

Metabolism

Aspirin lowers plasma glucose concentrations in C-peptide-positive diabetic subjects and in normoglycemic persons (28). This is of no clinical significance.

Fluid balance

NSAIDs can cause fluid retention, but this has rarely been reported with aspirin.

- Severe fluid retention, possibly due to impaired renal tubular secretion, has been reported in a 29-year-old woman taking aspirin (1.5 g/day for several days) for persistent headache (29). During rechallenge with aspirin (0.5 g tds for 3 days) a dynamic renal scintigram showed a substantial fall in tubular filtration. Withdrawal was followed by complete uneventful recovery.

Pulmonary edema is a feature of salicylate intoxication, but this patient was taking a therapeutic dosage.

Hematologic

Thrombocytopenia, agranulocytosis, neutropenia, aplastic anemia, and even pancytopenia have been reported in association with aspirin. The prospect for recovery from the latter is poor, mortality approaching 50%.

Hemolytic anemia can occur in patients with glucose-6-phosphate dehydrogenase deficiency or erythrocyte glutathione peroxidase deficiency (SED-9, 128) (30–32). Whether these reports have anything more than anecdotal value (SEDA-17, 97) is not known.

Simple iron deficiency caused by occult blood loss occurs with a frequency of 1%, and upper gastrointestinal bleeding resulting from regular aspirin ingestion is the reason for hospitalization in about 15 patients per 100 000 aspirin users per year. Aspirin causes bleeding of sufficient severity to lead to iron deficiency anemia in 10–15% of patients taking it continuously for chronic arthritis. Some individuals are particularly at risk because of pregnancy, age, inadequate diet, menorrhagia, gastrectomy, or malabsorption syndromes.

Macrocytic anemia associated with folate deficiency has been described in patients with rheumatoid arthritis (33) and also in patients who abuse analgesic mixtures containing aspirin (33).

Effects on coagulation

Aspirin in high doses for several days can reduce prothrombin concentrations and prolong the prothrombin time. This will contribute to bleeding problems initiated by other factors, including aspirin's local irritant effects on epithelial cells. It is therefore very risky to use aspirin in patients with bleeding disorders. The effect will contribute to increased blood loss at parturition, spontaneous abortion, or menorrhagia, and may be linked to persistent ocular hemorrhage, particularly in older people, with or without associated surgical intervention (34,35).

By virtue of its effects on both cyclo-oxygenase isoenzymes, aspirin inhibits platelet thromboxane A_2 formation. This effect in the platelet is irreversible and will persist for the lifetime of the platelet (that is up to 10 days), since the platelet cannot synthesize new cyclo-oxygenase. It is of clinical significance that the dose of aspirin necessary to inhibit platelet thromboxane A_2 (around 40 mg/day) is much lower than that needed to inactivate the subendothelial prostacyclin (PGI_2). Hence, platelet aggregation is inhibited, with some associated dilatation of coronary and cerebral arterioles, at doses that do not interfere with prostacyclin inhibition. It is important, in considering the dosage of aspirin for prophylaxis (see below), to appreciate that prostacyclin is a general inhibitor of platelet aggregation, while aspirin, as a cyclo-oxygenase inhibitor, affects aggregation from a limited number of stimuli, for example ADP, adrenaline, thromboxane A_2. It is also worth recalling that the vascular endothelium can synthesize new cyclo-oxygenase, so that any effect on prostacyclin synthesis is of limited duration only (SEDA-12, 74) (36).

Several long-term studies have been carried out since the 1980s to determine the prophylactic usefulness of these effects on clotting. It is now clear that aspirin in dosages of around 300 mg/day can be used successfully for secondary prophylaxis in patients with coronary artery disease, in order to reduce the incidence of severe myocardial infarction, and in patients with cerebrovascular disease to reduce the incidence of transient ischemic attacks and strokes. There is some suggestion that higher doses of aspirin may be required in women. A major drawback has been the high incidence of gastrointestinal adverse effects and particularly bleeding in aspirin-treated groups (5,6,10,37). In view of the age group involved, bleeding can have serious implications. In an attempt to avoid this high proportion of ill-effects and yet retain the benefits of prophylactic antithrombotic treatment, a few trials have been conducted using aspirin in a dose of 162 mg (ISIS-2) (38) and 75 mg (RISC) (39) in symptomatic coronary heart disease, with good evidence of efficacy. Two studies have been reported in patients with cerebrovascular events, namely the Dutch TIA trial with aspirin 30 versus 283 mg (22) and the SALT study with aspirin 75 mg (23). The former did not show any difference in efficacy between the 30 and 283 mg dose groups, but there was no placebo control. The latter study showed a significant reduction in thrombotic stroke. However, intracerebral hemorrhage has been reported with aspirin, even in low doses, and in this as well as in the Physicians Health Study of 1989 (24), hemorrhagic stroke and associated deaths occurred with aspirin. On the other hand, the incidence of serious gastrointestinal events was much lower than previously described.

In 711 patients, of whom 320 were taking aspirin at the time of surgical resection for cutaneous head and neck lesions, the incidence of significant postoperative hemorrhage was 1.6% (5 cases) versus none in the control group; the use of aspirin was the only susceptibility factor for significant postoperative hemorrhage (40).

However, in other studies there was no effect of aspirin on blood loss in patients with hip fractures (41), after coronary artery bypass surgery (42), or after tooth extraction (43).

As nearly all of the risks seem to be dose-related (SEDA-21, 96), there is a good prospect that an even lower daily dose of aspirin may offer advantages in antithrombotic prophylaxis without an increased risk of bleeding, but the results of further such studies are still awaited (9).

Relatively few patients developed a prolonged bleeding time while taking aspirin or other NSAIDs and only few had significant intraoperative blood loss. There is variation in the response of patients for unknown reasons and so the recommendation that NSAIDs should be withdrawn before elective surgery awaits confirmation (SEDA-19, 96).

Gastrointestinal

Gastric ulceration and hemorrhage

```
DoTS classification
Dose-relation: collateral effect
Time-course: intermediate
Susceptibility factors: age (over 65); sex (women);
disease (peptic ulceration)
```

The gastrointestinal adverse effects of aspirin and the other NSAIDs are the most common. While some argue against a causative relation between aspirin ingestion and chronic gastric ulceration, the current consensus favors such a relation, while admitting that other factors, such as *Helicobacter pylori*, are likely to play a part. Patients aged over 65 years and women are more at risk, as are those who take aspirin over prolonged periods in a daily dose of about 2 g or more.

However, there is no ambiguity about the association of aspirin with gastritis, gastric erosions, or extensions of existing peptic ulcers, all of which are demonstrable by endoscopy. Even after one or two doses, superficial erosions have been described in over 50% of healthy subjects. This association is now almost universally accepted as the standard basis for comparative testing of NSAIDs and other drugs (22,44–46). Whether it is of benefit to use other drugs concomitantly to prevent the effect of gastric acid on the mucosa, and thus reduce the risk of gastric ulceration, is discussed further in this monograph.

Dyspepsia, nausea, and vomiting occur in 2–6% of patients after aspirin ingestion. Patients with rheumatoid arthritis seem to be more sensitive, and the frequency of aspirin-induced dyspepsia in this group is 10–30% (SEDA-9, 129). However, these symptoms are generally poor predictors of the incidence of mucosal damage (SEDA-18, 90).

The bleeding that occurs is usually triggered by erosions and aggravated by the antithrombotic action of aspirin. While it is reported to occur in up to 100% of regular aspirin takers, bleeding tends to be asymptomatic in young adults, unless it is associated with peptic ulceration, but it is readily detectable by endoscopy and the presence of occult blood in the feces. Hematemesis and melena are less often seen, the odds ratio being 1.5–2.0 in an overview of 21 low-dose aspirin prevention studies (47). A degree of resultant iron deficiency anemia is common. Such events are more commonly seen in older people in whom there is a significant proportion of serious bleeding and even deaths. Major gastrointestinal bleeding has an incidence of 15 per 100 000 so-called heavy aspirin users. However, the interpretation of "heavy" and of quantities of aspirin actually taken is to a large extent subjective and very dependent on the questionable accuracy of patient reporting. The risk appears to be greater in women, smokers, and patients concurrently taking other NSAIDs, and is possibly affected by other factors not yet established (48). Gastrointestinal perforation can occur without prodromes. Aspirin increases the risk of major upper gastrointestinal bleeding and perforation two- to three-fold in a dose-related manner, but deaths are rare.

Incidence

Of the estimated annual 65 000 upper gastrointestinal emergency admissions in the UK, nearly 20% (including deaths in 3.4%) are attributable to the use of prostaglandin synthesis inhibitors (49). As might be expected with an inhibitor of prostaglandin synthesis, the cytoprotective effects of prostaglandin E and prostacyclin (PGI_2) are reduced by aspirin, as is the inhibitory action on gastric acid secretion. This effect may be both direct, as is the case with aspirin released in the stomach (or the lower rectum in the case of aspirin suppositories), and indirect following absorption and distribution via the systemic circulation; attempts to reduce the problems by coating and buffering can therefore have only limited success. The indirect type of effect is shown by the fact that these adverse gastric effects can also be exerted by parenteral lysine acetylsalicylate (SEDA-10, 72). The local effects depend in part on the tablet particle size, solubility, and rate of gastric absorption, while the most important variable appears to be gastric pH. On the other hand, within-day changes in the pharmacokinetics of the analgesic compounds may be involved in the prevalence of gastrointestinal adverse effects.

The estimates of gastrointestinal complication rates from aspirin are generally derived from clinical trials (SEDA-21, 100). However, the applicability of the results of such trials to the general population may be debatable, as protocols for these studies often are designed precisely to avoid enrollment of patients who are at risk of complications. Indeed differences in benefit-to-harm balance have been found in trials using the same dose of aspirin (50,51). For this reason, a population-based historical cohort study on frequency of major complications of aspirin used for secondary stroke prevention may be of interest (52). The study identified 588 patients who had a first ischemic stroke, transient ischemic attack, or amaurosis fugax during the study period. Of these, 339 patients had taken aspirin for an average of 1.7 years. The mean age of patients who had taken aspirin was 74 years. Complications occurred within 30 days of initiation of treatment in one patient, between 30 days and 6 months in 10 patients, between 6 months and 1 year in seven patients, and between 1 year and 2 years in two patients. Estimated standardized morbidity ratio of gastrointestinal hemorrhage (determined on the basis of 10 observed events and 0.661 expected events, during 576 person-years of observation) was 15 (95% CI = 7, 28). The estimated standardized morbidity ratio of intracerebral hemorrhage (determined on the basis of only one event and 0.59 expected events) was 1.7 (CI = 0.04, 9.4). One patient had a fatal gastrointestinal hemorrhage. Unfortunately these complication rates must be considered estimates, because aspirin therapy was not consistently recorded. However, the rates of complications were similar to those observed in some randomized clinical trials. On the basis of these data and of those of a meta-analysis of 16 trials involving more than 95 000 patients (52), the overall benefits of aspirin, measured in terms of preventing myocardial infarction and ischemic stroke, clearly outweigh the risks.

Dose-relatedness

The question of whether the risk of gastrointestinal hemorrhage with long-term aspirin is related to dose within the usual therapeutic dosage range (SEDA-12, 100) (15,53) merits attention. In a meta-analysis of the incidence of gastrointestinal hemorrhage associated with long-term aspirin and the effect of dose in 24 randomized, controlled clinical trials including almost 66 000 patients exposed for an average duration of 28 months to a wide range of different doses of aspirin (50–1500 mg/day), gastrointestinal hemorrhage occurred in 2.47% of patients taking aspirin compared with 1.42% taking placebo (OR = 1.68; 95% CI = 1.51, 1.88). In patients taking low doses of aspirin (50–162.5 mg/day; $n = 49\ 927$), gastrointestinal hemorrhage occurred in 2.3% compared with 1.45% taking placebo (OR = 1.56; 95% CI = 1.40, 1.81). The pooled OR for gastrointestinal hemorrhage with low-dose aspirin was 1.59 (95% CI = 1.4, 1.81). A meta-regression to test for a linear relation between the daily dose of aspirin and the risk of gastrointestinal hemorrhage gave a pooled OR of 1.015 (95% CI = 0.998, 1.047) per 100 mg dose reduction. The reduction in the incidence of gastrointestinal hemorrhage was estimated to be 1.5% per 100 mg dose reduction, but this was not significant.

In other studies the incidence of upper gastrointestinal haemorrhage has been reported to be similar in patients taking either 75 mg or 325 mg of aspirin per day (54,55).

These data are in apparent contrast with others previously reported (SEDA-21, 100) (14), which showed that gastrointestinal hemorrhage was related to dose in the usual dosage range. Many reasons may explain these contrasting results, the most important being differences in the definition of the hemorrhagic events, in study design, in the population studied, and in the presence of accessory risk factors (56–58).

The recent trends toward the use of lower doses of aspirin have been driven by the belief that these offer a better safety profile while retaining equivalent therapeutic efficacy. Despite the large number of patients enrolled in randomized clinical trials and included in meta-analyses, there is no firm evidence that dose reduction significantly lowers the risk of gastrointestinal bleeding. Patients and doctors therefore need to consider the trade-off between the benefits and harms of long-term treatment with aspirin. Meanwhile, it seems wise to use the lowest dose of proven efficacy.

A systematic review of 17 epidemiological studies conducted between 1990 and 2001 has provided further data on this topic (59). The effect of aspirin dosage was investigated in five studies. There was a greater risk of gastrointestinal complications with aspirin in dosages over 300 mg/day than in dosages of 300 mg/day or less. However, users of low-dose aspirin still had a two-fold increased risk of such complications compared with non-users, with no clear evidence of a dose-response relation at dosages under 300 mg/day, confirming previous findings (15). The study also addressed the question of whether the aspirin formulation affects gastrotoxicity. The pooled relative risks of gastrointestinal complications in four studies were 2.4 (95%; CI = 1.9, 2.9) for enteric-coated aspirin, 5.3 (3.0, 9.2) for buffered formulations, and 2.6 (2.3, 2.9) for plain aspirin, compared with non-use. These data confirm those from previous studies (SEDA-21, 100) (15), which negate any protective effect of the most frequently used aspirin formulations. Furthermore, there were higher relative risks, compared with non-use, for gastrointestinal complications in patients who used aspirin regularly (RR = 3.2; CI = 2.6, 5.9) than in patients who used it occasionally (2.1; 1.7,

2.6), and during the first month of use (4.4; 3.2, 6.1) compared with subsequent months (2.6; 2.1, 3.1).

Comparative studies

A comparative study of gastrointestinal blood loss after aspirin 972 mg qds for 4 days versus different doses of piroxicam (20 mg od, 5 mg qds, and 10 mg qds) showed that piroxicam did not increase fecal blood loss, whereas aspirin did. Gastroscopic evidence of irritation was also greater with aspirin (60).

In a randomized trial comparing ticlopidine (500 mg/day) with aspirin (1300 mg/day) for the prevention of stroke in high-risk patients, the incidence of bleeding was similar in both groups, although more patients treated with aspirin developed peptic ulceration or gastrointestinal hemorrhage (61).

Susceptibility factors

A study of the Susceptibility factors for gastrointestinal perforation, a much less frequent event than bleeding, has confirmed that aspirin and other NSAIDs increase the risk of both upper and lower gastrointestinal perforation (OR 6.7, CI 3.1–14.5 for NSAIDs) (62). Gastrointestinal perforation has been associated with other factors, such as coffee consumption, a history of peptic ulcer, and smoking. The combination of NSAIDs, smoking, and alcohol increased the risk of gastrointestinal perforation (OR 10.7, CI 3.8–30) (SEDA-21, 97).

The risks of adverse gastrointestinal effects of aspirin have been studied in relation to susceptibility factors using two major databases the General Practice Research Database in the UK and the Base de Datos para la Investigación Farmacoepidemiológica en Atención Primaria in Spain (63). The rates of upper gastrointestinal adverse effects varied depending on age, sex, the use of NSAIDs, and the presence of upper gastrointestinal pain or peptic ulceration. The highest rate was in men aged 80 years and over with complicated ulcers taking NSAIDs (300/1000 person years); the lowest rate was in women not taking NSAIDs and with no other susceptibility factors (0.8/1000 person-years).

Associated effects

Aspirin can also play a role in esophageal bleeding, ulceration, or benign stricture, and it should be considered as a possible cause in patients, particularly the elderly, who present with any of these features. There have also been reports of rectal stricture in the elderly, associated with the use of aspirin suppositories. Effects on both these strictures emphasize the significance of a direct local action of aspirin as well as a systemic action and underlines the relevance of the involvement of oxygen-derived free radicals in the pathogenesis of mucosal lesions in the gastrointestinal tract (64–66).

A gastrocolic fistula developed in a 47-year-old woman taking aspirin and prednisone for rheumatoid arthritis (67). Other similar case reports have been published (68,69).

Long-term effects

The effects on the stomach of continued exposure to aspirin remain controversial. While in short-term use, gastric mucosal erosions may often be recurrent but transient and comparatively trivial lesions, with longer administration there seems to be an increased risk of progression to ulceration.

Prophylaxis

Enteric-coated aspirin has been associated with gastroduodenal ulcer formation; the enteric coating has been shown to be toxic to the bowel and it is postulated that it is also toxic to the stomach (70).

Intravenous administration, or the use of enteric-coated formulations or modified-release products all appear to reduce the risk both of bleeding and more particularly of erosions/ulceration. However, because of the indirect effect noted above, such formulations do not eliminate the risk, although they may reduce the incidence of gastric or duodenal ulcer, as may buffered aspirin (71,72).

Considerable attention in recent years has been directed toward the efficacy of using synthetic forms of PGE_2, histamine H_2 receptor antagonists, proton pump inhibitors, or antacids, either to heal peptic ulcers associated with use of prostaglandin inhibitors or more significantly to act prophylactically to protect against ulceration or bleeding associated with aspirin or the NSAIDs. With the exception of PGE_2, there is no convincing evidence to justify their prophylactic use, as they do not reduce the risk of significant gastrointestinal events. In contrast, their soothing effect on gastrointestinal symptoms may ultimately result in more severe complications (73). Since all these agents carry their own potential risks, it is more than questionable whether administration to a patient with normal gastrointestinal mucosa is justified. Generally, use of prostaglandin inhibitors should be limited to the shortest possible duration, thereby minimizing, but not eliminating, the risk of gastrointestinal damage. Only high-risk patients should be eligible for prophylactic drug therapy. Well-known risk factors for the development of mucosal lesions of the gastrointestinal tract are age (over 75 years), a history of peptic ulcer, or gastrointestinal bleeding, and concomitant cardiac disease.

Liver

Aspirin can cause dose-related focal hepatic necrosis that is usually asymptomatic or anicteric. Much of the evidence for hepatotoxicity of aspirin and the salicylates has been shown in children (74,75), usually in patients with connective tissue disorders, taking relatively high long-term dosages for Still's disease, rheumatoid arthritis, or occasionally systemic lupus erythematosus. Rises in serum transaminases seem to be the most common feature (in up to 50% of patients) and are usually reversible on withdrawal, but they occasionally lead to fatal hepatic necrosis. Severe and even fatal metabolic encephalopathy can also occur, as in Reye's syndrome (see the section on Reye's syndrome in this monograph). One can easily overload the young patient's individual metabolic capacity. The co-existence of hypoalbuminemia may be a particular risk factor; in patients with hypoalbuminemia of 35 g/l or less, close monitoring of the aspartate transaminase is advisable, especially if the concentration of total serum salicylate is 1.1 mmol/l or higher (76). Plasma salicylate concentrations in serious cases have usually been in excess of 1.4 mmol/l and liver function tests return rapidly to normal when the drug is withdrawn. Finally, a very small number of cases of chronic active hepatitis have been attributed to aspirin (77).

Reye's syndrome

First defined as a distinct syndrome in 1963, Reye's syndrome came to be regarded some years later as an adverse effect of aspirin. In fact, the position is more complex, and the syndrome still cannot be assigned a specific cause. There is general agreement that the disorder presents a few days after the prodrome of a viral illness. Well over a dozen different viruses have so far been implicated, including influenza A and B, adenovirus, *Varicella*, and reovirus. Various other factors have also been incriminated, including aflatoxins, certain pesticides, and such antioxidants as butylated hydroxytoluene. Only in the case of aspirin have some epidemiological studies been conducted, and these appeared to show a close correlation with cases of Reye's syndrome. It was these studies that led to regulatory action against the promotion of salicylate use in children. However, doubt has been thrown on the clarity of the link, and it now seems increasingly likely that while there is some association with aspirin, the etiology is in fact multifactorial, including some genetic predisposition. Studies in Japan did not support the US findings, while studies in Thailand and Canada invoked other factors.

Two characteristic phenomena are present in Reye's syndrome.

1. Damage to mitochondrial structures, with pleomorphism, disorganization of matrix, proliferation of smooth endoplasmic reticulum, and an increase in peroxisomes; mitochondrial enzyme activity is severely reduced, but cytoplasmic enzymes are unaffected. The changes first appear in single cells, but may spread to all hepatocytes. Recovery may be complete by 5–7 days. While these changes are most evident in liver cells, similar effects have been seen in cerebral neurons and skeletal muscle. There appears to be a block in beta-oxidation of fatty acids (inhibition of oxidation of NAB-linked substrates). In vitro aspirin selectively inhibits mitochondrial oxidation of medium- and long-chain fatty acids.
2. An acute catabolic state with hypoglycemia, hyperammonemia, raised activities of serum aspartate transaminase and creatine phosphokinase, and increased urinary nitrogen and serum long chain dicarboxylic acid.

Despite our lack of understanding of the syndrome, the decision taken in many countries to advise against the use of salicylates in children under 12 made an impact, in terms of a falling incidence of Reye's syndrome (SEDA-16, 96; SEDA-17, 97).

Over the last 25 years, in the USA, the incidence of Reye's syndrome has fallen significantly—from the time that the advice was introduced up to 1999 there were 25 reported cases, but 15 were in adolescents aged 12–17 years, and 8% of cases occurred in patients aged 15 years or over (78). In the UK, in view of these findings, the Commission on Safety of Medicines (CSM) amended its original statement and advised that aspirin should be avoided in febrile illnesses or viral infections in patients aged under 16 years. However, the appropriateness of this decision has been challenged (79). This is because the incidence of Reye's syndrome is already low and is falling; furthermore, restricting the use of aspirin leaves paracetamol and ibuprofen as the only available therapeutic alternatives, and their safety is not absolutely guaranteed and might be even worse than that of aspirin.

Pancreas

There are conflicting findings in the literature regarding the possibility that long-term use of aspirin is associated with an increased risk of pancreatic cancer (80). New data from a recent study have suggested that extended periods of regular aspirin use appear to be associated with a statistically significant increased risk of pancreatic cancer among women (81). However, the results of this study were inconsistent and require confirmation.

Urinary tract

Aspirin is associated with a small but significant risk of hospitalization for acute renal insufficiency (SEDA-19, 95).

When aspirin is used by patients on sodium restriction or with congestive heart failure, there tends to be a reduction in the glomerular filtration rate, with preservation of normal renal plasma flow. Some renal tubular epithelial shedding can also occur.

Severe systemic disease involving the heart, liver, or kidneys seems to predispose the patient to the effects of aspirin and other NSAIDs on renal function (82).

In 106 elderly in-patients aspirin 100 mg/day for 2 weeks reduced creatinine clearance and uric acid clearance significantly in 70% and 62% of the patients respectively, with mean reductions of 19% and 17% (83). After withdrawal of aspirin renal function improved, but 67% of the patients were left with some impairment in creatinine clearance. Those who reacted adversely to aspirin had significantly better pre-study renal function, and lower hemoglobin and serum albumin concentrations.

Chronic renal disease

Renal papillary necrosis has been reported after long-term intake or abuse of aspirin and other NSAIDs (SEDA-11, 85; SEDA-12, 79). The relation between long-term heavy exposure to analgesics and the risk of chronic renal disease has been the object of intensive toxicological and epidemiological research for many years (SEDA-24, 120) (84). Most of the earlier reports suggested that phenacetin-containing analgesics probably cause renal papillary necrosis and interstitial nephritis. In contrast, there was no convincing epidemiological evidence that non-phenacetin-containing analgesics (including paracetamol, aspirin, mixtures of the two, and NSAIDs) cause chronic renal disease. Moreover, findings from epidemiological studies should be interpreted with caution, because of a number of inherent limitations and potential biases in study design (85). Two methodologically sound studies have provided information on this topic.

The first was the largest cohort study conducted thus far to assess the risk of renal dysfunction associated with analgesic use (86). Details of analgesic use were obtained from 11 032 men without previous renal dysfunction participating in the Physicians' Health Study (PHS), which lasted 14 years. The main outcome measure was a raised creatinine concentration defined as 1.5 mg/dl (133 µmol/l) or higher and a reduced creatinine clearance of 55 ml/minute or less. In all, 460 men (4.2%) had a raised creatinine concentration and 1258 (11%) had a reduced creatinine clearance. Mean creatinine concentrations and creatinine clearances were similar among men who did not use analgesics and those who did. This was true for all categories of analgesics (paracetamol and paracetamol-containing mixtures, aspirin and aspirin-containing mixtures, and other NSAIDs) and for higher-risk groups, such as those aged 60 years or over or those with hypertension or diabetes.

These data are convincing, as the large size of the PHS cohort should make it possible to examine and detect even modest associations between analgesic use and a risk of renal disease. Furthermore, this study included more individuals who reported extensive use of analgesics than any prior case-control study. However, the study had some limitations, the most important being the fact that the cohort was composed of relatively healthy men, most of whom were white. These results cannot therefore be generalized to the entire population. However, the study clearly showed that there is not a strong association between chronic analgesic use and chronic renal dysfunction among a large cohort of men without a history of renal impairment.

The second study was a Swedish nationwide, population-based, case-control study of early-stage chronic renal insufficiency in men whose serum creatinine concentration exceeded 3.4 mg/dl (300 µmol/l) or women whose serum creatinine exceeded 2.8 mg/dl (250 µmol/l) (87). In all, 918 patients with newly diagnosed renal insufficiency and 980 controls were interviewed and completed questionnaires about their lifetime consumption of analgesics. Compared with controls, more patients with chronic renal insufficiency were regular users of aspirin (37 versus 19%) or paracetamol (25 versus 12%). Among subjects who did not use aspirin regularly, the regular use of paracetamol was associated with a risk of chronic renal insufficiency that was 2.5 times as high as that for non-users of paracetamol. The risk increased with increasing cumulative lifetime dose. Patients who took 500 g or more over a year (1.4 g/day) during periods of regular use had an increased odds ratio for chronic renal insufficiency (OR = 5.3; 95% CI = 1.8, 15). Among subjects who did not use paracetamol regularly, the regular use of aspirin was associated with a risk of chronic renal insufficiency that was 2.5 times as high as that for non-users of aspirin. The risk increased significantly with an increasing cumulative lifetime dose of aspirin. Among the patients with an average intake of 500 g or more of aspirin per year during periods of regular use, the risk of chronic renal insufficiency was increased about three-fold (OR = 3.3; CI = 1.4, 8.0). Among patients who used paracetamol in addition to aspirin, the risk of chronic renal insufficiency was increased about two-fold when regular aspirin users served as the reference group (OR = 2.2; CI = 1.4, 3.5) and non-significantly when regular paracetamol users were used as controls (OR = 1.6; CI = 0.9, 2.7). There was no relation between the use of other analgesics (propoxyphene, NSAIDs, codeine, and pyrazolones) and the risk of chronic renal insufficiency. Thus, the regular use of paracetamol, or aspirin, or both was associated dose-dependently with an increased risk of chronic renal insufficiency. The OR among regular users exceeded 1.0 for all types of chronic renal insufficiency, albeit not always significantly. These results are consistent with exacerbating effects of paracetamol and aspirin on chronic renal insufficiency, regardless of accompanying disease.

How can we explain the contrasting results of these two studies? A possible explanation lies in the different populations studied. In the PHS study, relatively healthy individuals were enrolled while in the Swedish study all the patients had pre-existing severe renal or systemic disease, suggesting that such disease has an important role in causing analgesic-associated chronic renal insufficiency. People without pre-existing disease who use analgesics may have only a small risk of end-stage renal disease.

In a case-control study in 583 patients with end-stage renal disease and 1190 controls long-term use of any analgesic was associated with an overall non-significant odds ratio of 1.22 (CI = 0.89, 1.66) (88). For specific groups of drugs the risks were:

- aspirin 1.56 (1.05, 2.30);
- paracetamol 0.80 (0.39, 1.63);
- pyrazolones 1.03 (0.60, 1.76);
- other NSAIDs 0.94 (0.57, 1.56).

There was thus a small increased risk of end-stage renal disease associated with aspirin, which was related to the cumulative dose and duration of use; it was particularly high among the subset of patients with vascular nephropathy as underlying disease.

These results suggest that long-term use of non-aspirin analgesics and NSAIDs is not associated with an increased risk of end-stage renal disease but that long-term use of aspirin is associated with a small increase in the risk of end-stage renal disease.

Skin

Hypersensitivity reactions, such as urticaria and angioedema, are relatively common in subjects with aspirin hypersensitivity. Purpura, hemorrhagic vasculitis, erythema multiforme, Stevens–Johnson syndrome, and Lyell's

syndrome have also been reported, but much less often. Fixed drug eruptions, probably hypersensitive in origin, are periodically described. In some patients they do not recur on rechallenge, that is the sensitivity disappears (89).

Musculoskeletal

There is evidence that salicylates together with at least some NSAIDs suppress proteoglycan biosynthesis independently of effects on prostaglandin synthesis (90). Thus, prolonged use of these agents can accentuate deterioration of articular cartilage in weight-bearing arthritic joints. If this is proved, the problem will be of greatest relevance to elderly people with osteoarthritis, a condition in which this use of prostaglandin inhibitors is questionable.

Immunologic

Aspirin hypersensitivity

Aspirin-exacerbated respiratory disease has been reviewed (91,92,93). It consists of chronic hyperplastic eosinophilic sinusitis, nasal polyps, asthma, and aspirin hypersensitivity; respiratory complaints can be precipitated by other factors, such as exercise and inhalation of irritants. The term "aspirin triad disease" has been used since 1980 to describe the combination of asthma, nasal polyps, and aspirin intolerance (94). The main mechanisms appear to be related to reduced production of prostaglandin E_2, due to deficient COX-2 regulation, increased expression of leukotriene-C_4 synthase, and reduced production of metabolites (lipoxins) (95).

Of adult asthmatics 2–20% have aspirin hypersensitivity (9).

Oral challenge in asthmatic patients is an effective but potentially dangerous method for establishing the presence of aspirin hypersensitivity (74).

The term "aspirin allergy" is better avoided, in the absence of identification of a definite antigen–antibody reaction.

Prevalence
Aspirin hypersensitivity is relatively common in adults (about 20%). Estimates of the prevalence of aspirin-induced asthma vary from 3.3 to 44% in different reports (SEDA-5, 169), although it is often only demonstrable by challenge tests with spirometry, and only 4% have problems in practice. Patients with existing asthma and nasal polyps or chronic urticaria have a greater frequency of hypersensitivity (96), and women appear to be more susceptible than men, perhaps particularly during the childbearing period of life (97). Acute intolerance to aspirin can develop even in patients who have taken the drug for some years without problems.

In large questionnaire surveys the prevalence was 1.2% but the incidence of aspirin sensitivity was much higher in patients whose physicians made a diagnosis of asthma (8.8%) (98). In a survey of 12 971 adults in Poland, 4.3% of asthmatic subjects said that aspirin precipitated attacks of asthma (99). In 516 asthmatic patients and 1298 randomly selected individuals in Australia, the prevalence was 11% in subjects with asthma and 2.5% in the general population (100). In a meta-analysis of 15 studies in which oral aspirin challenge was used to detect aspirin hypersensitivity in patients with asthma, the prevalence was 21% (CI = 14, 29%) and in five studies in children it was 5% (CI = 0, 14%) (101).

There is considerable cross-reactivity with other NSAIDs and the now widely banned food colorant tartrazine (102). Cross-sensitization between aspirin and tartrazine is common; for example, in one series 24% of aspirin-sensitive patients also reacted to tartrazine (SEDA-9, 76).

Mechanism

The current theory of the mechanism relates to the inhibition of cyclo-oxygenases (103) and a greater degree of interference with PGE_2 synthesis, allowing the bronchoconstrictor PGF_2 to predominate in susceptible individuals.

Circulating and tissue concentrations of proinflammatory cytokines synthesized by epithelial cells, including IL-2, IL-3, IL-4, IL-5, IL-13, GM-CSF, and eotaxin, and numbers of activated TH_2 lymphocytes are increased in patients with aspirin-exacerbated respiratory disease (104,105,106). As a result, eosinophils and degranulated mast cells are found in nasal biopsies, although their pathophysiological role is not understood. There is also increased secretion of leukotrienes (107,108,109,110) and prostaglandin PGD_2 (111). The number of cysteinyl leukotriene receptors is also upregulated in nasal inflammatory cells (112). In contrast, there is reduced production of anti-inflammatory lipoxins (113) and of PGE_2 (114).

PGE_2 inhibition in macrophages may also unleash bronchial cytotoxic lymphocytes, generated by chronic viral infection, leading to destruction of virus-infected cells in the respiratory tract (115). When urticaria occurs, it may result from increased release of leukotrienes LTC_4, D_4, and E_4, which also induces bronchoconstriction, with a shunt of arachidonic acid toward lipoxygenation in aspirin-sensitive asthmatics (SEDA-18, 93). Aspirin-induced asthma patients show hyper-reactivity to inhaled metacholine and sulpyrine.

In 26 patients with nasal polyps (11 aspirin-sensitive and 15 aspirin-tolerant) and four controls without a history of nasal polyps or rhinosinusitis, cyclo-oxygenase activity was significantly higher in the nasal columnar epithelium and submucosal glands in those with polyps, irrespective of aspirin sensitivity; lipoxygenase activity was increased in the submucosal glands in the aspirin-sensitive subjects only (116)

In a study of the immunohistochemical expression of 5-lipoxygenase and cyclo-oxygenase pathway proteins in nasal polyps from 12 patients with asthma and aspirin intolerance and 13 with asthma and aspirin tolerance, cells that were immunopositive for LTC_4 synthase were four times more numerous in those with aspirin intolerance and cells that expressed 5-lipoxygenase were three times more numerous (117). LTC_4 synthase-positive cell counts correlated with mucosal eosinophils. There were no differences in 5-lipoxygenase activating protein (FLAP), COX-1, or COX-2.

In 34 healthy subjects aged 19–57 years, 39 subjects with mild persistent atopic asthma aged 18–66 years, 24 subjects with aspirin-induced asthma with rhinitis, aged 18–56 years, and 10 subjects with aspirin-induced asthma and nasal polyps aged 22–49 years, those with polyps had the highest concentrations of urinary LTE_4: asthma + polyps 432 pg/mg; asthma + rhinitis 331 pg/mg; atopic asthma 129 pg/mg; controls 67 pg/mg (118). Basal LTE_4 concentrations were inversely related to basal FEV_1.

The expression of the G-protein-coupled E-prostanoid receptors EP_1, EP_2, EP_3, and EP_4 has been studied in nasal biopsies from patients with aspirin-sensitive (n = 12) and non-aspirin-sensitive (n = 10) polypoid rhinosinusitis and in healthy controls (n = 9) (119). Global mucosal expression of EP_1 and EP_2 receptors, but not EP_3 or EP_4 receptors, was significantly increased in both groups with rhinosinusitis, which was principally attributable to increased expression on tubulin(+) epithelial cells and mucin 5 goblet cells subtypes A and B. In contrast, the percentages of neutrophils, mast cells, eosinophils, and T cells expressing EP_2 receptors, but not EP_1, EP_3, or EP_4 receptors, were significantly reduced in the aspirin-sensitive compared with non-aspirin-sensitive patients. The authors concluded that PGE_2 might be involved in the increased inflammatory infiltrate and production of cysteinyl leukotrienes that characterize aspirin-sensitive disease and in mediating epithelial repair in rhinitis and asthma.

IgE antibodies specific for staphylococcal superantigens have been implicated in the pathology of several allergic diseases, such as rhinosinusitis, nasal polyps, asthma, and aspirin sensitivity. In 80 patients with asthma and aspirin intolerance, 62 with asthma and aspirin tolerance, and 52 healthy controls, the prevalence of staphylococcal enterotoxin B-specific IgE and toxic shock syndrome toxin-1-specific IgE was significantly higher in the patients with asthma than in the controls, but there was no significant difference between the aspirin-tolerant and the aspirin-intolerant patients (120).

Expression of vascular cell adhesion molecule 1 (VCAM-1) and intercellular adhesion molecule I (ICAM-1) and their ligands, the integrins lymphocyte function-associated antigen 1 and very late activation antigen 4 (VLA-4) has been studied in nasal polyps from 21 patients with aspirin hypersensitivity and 23 aspirin-tolerant individuals (121). ICAM-1, VCAM-1, and VLA-4 were significantly increased in the patients with aspirin hypersensitivity, but the expression of lymphocyte function-associated antigen 1 did not differ. There was a correlation between the immunoexpression of VCAM-1 and its ligand VLA-4. The authors concluded that up-regulation of the adhesion molecules ICAM-1 and VCAM-1 and the integrin VLA-4 may play an important role in the development of chronic eosinophilic inflammation in nasal polyps in aspirin-hypersensitive patients.

Plasma concentrations of complement C3a and C4a were higher in 30 patients with aspirin-induced asthma than in 24 patients without (122). After an aspirin challenge, C3 fell in both groups, but the C3a concentration increased only in those with aspirin-induced asthma. C3a and C4a concentrations and the ratios C3a/C3 and C4a/C4 correlated with changes in FEV_1 after aspirin challenge.

Two studies have examined possible biochemical pathways in aspirin-induced asthma. In a study of the generation of 15-hydroxyeicosatetraenoic acid (15-HETE) and other eicosanoids by peripheral blood leukocytes from aspirin-sensitive and aspirin-tolerant asthmatics incubation with aspirin 2, 20, or 200 µmol/l resulted in a dose-dependent increase in 15-HETE generation (mean change +85%, +189%, and +284% at each aspirin concentration respectively) only in aspirin-sensitive patients (123). In a study of the cyclo-oxygenase pathways in airway fibroblasts from patients with aspirin-tolerant asthma (n=9), and patients with aspirin-intolerant asthma (n=7), patients with asthma had a low capacity for PGE_2 production after stimulation (124). In non-asthmatic patients mean PGE_2 production was 32 ng/ml (35 times basal production), in the patients with aspirin-tolerant asthma it was 16 ng/ml (16 times basal), and in the patients with aspirin-intolerant asthma it was only 5.3 ng/ml (4 times basal). These studies show biochemical differences in the effects of aspirin in patents with aspirin-induced asthma. That this is mediated by inhibition of cyclo-oxygenase type 1 is suggested by a study in 33 subjects with a typical history of aspirin-induced asthma, who tolerated the cyclo-oxygenase-2 selective celecoxib; there were no changes in lung function or in urinary excretion of leukotriene E4 (125).

Features

The features of aspirin hypersensitivity include bronchospasm, acute and usually generalized urticaria, angioedema, severe rhinitis, and shock. These reactions can occur alone or in various combinations, developing within minutes or a few hours of aspirin ingestion, and lasting until elimination is complete. They can be life-threatening. The bronchospastic type of reaction predominates in adults, only the urticarial type being found in children. The frequency of recurrent urticaria is significantly greater in adults (3.8 versus 0.3%).

The reactions usually occur within 30–60 minutes after a full therapeutic dose of aspirin, but can occur up to 3 hours later, particularly when the dose is low (30–100 mg). The average age of onset is around 30 years, and women outnumber men about 3–5 times (126,127).

People with asthma may be particularly sensitive to acetylsalicylic acid, which may be given alone or as a constituent of a combination medicine. The association between aspirin sensitivity, nasal polyps, and rhinitis in asthma is well known.

There is cross-reactivity with non-selective non-steroidal anti-inflammatory drugs (NSAIDs), but not generally with highly selective COX-2 inhibitors, including celecoxib (128,129,130), etoricoxib (131), parecoxib (132), rofecoxib (133,134,135,136), and valdecoxib (137). However, reactions to celecoxib (138,139,140,141), etoricoxib (142,143,144), and rofecoxib (145) have been reported. High doses of paracetamol can also cause reactions (146).

The natural history of asthma after endoscopic sinus surgery in patients with aspirin triad disease has been studied in a retrospective review of 65 patients, of whom 31 reported asthma symptoms preoperatively (147). Of those, 29 had long-term postoperative improvement and 21 reported further improvement of their asthma beyond the first postoperative year. Attacks of asthma were overall fewer and peak flow rates improved from an average of 60% of the predicted value preoperatively to 86% at the time of follow-up. The numbers of hospital visits and admissions for exacerbations of asthma were reduced.

Henoch–Schönlein purpura has been reported (148).

Life-threatening respiratory distress, facial edema, and lethargy occurred in a woman with a history of severe asthma and aspirin hypersensitivity (SEDA-22, 118).

Aspirin-sensitive subjects may have attacks induced by other NSAIDs (149).

Fish oil can also cause exacerbation of asthma in aspirin-sensitive patients (150).

Genetic factors

An increased prevalence of a genetic polymorphism in the LTC_4S promoter region has been identified in Polish patients with aspirin-induced asthma (151), although no polymorphisms in the flanking region of the LTC_4S gene were discovered (152,153). Two single nucleotide polymorphisms in the LTC_4S promoter region, –1702G>A and –444A>C, were not associated with aspirin hypersensitivity in a study in 110 Korean patients with aspirin-induced asthma, 125 aspirin-tolerant patients with asthma, and 125 controls (154)

Single nucleotide polymorphisms in the promoter region of the gene encoding an E-prostanoid receptor, EP_2, were significantly associated with aspirin-exacerbated respiratory disease (155). Reduced transcription of the EP_2 receptor for PGE_2 might prevent such patients from inhibiting 5-lipoxygenase and 5-lipoxygenase-activating protein activity

The HLA DPB1*0301 polymorphism is over-represented in aspirin-hypersensitive subjects with asthma (156).

ADAM33 (A Disintegrin And Metalloprotease 33) is an asthma susceptibility gene, and multiple single nucleotide polymorphisms in ADAM33 have been reported to be associated with asthma and bronchial hyper-responsiveness in Caucasians. Ten such polymorphisms (ST+4, ST+7, T1, T2, T+1, V-3, V-2, V-1, V4, V5) have been genotyped in a study of 102 Japanese patients with asthma and aspirin intolerance, 282 with asthma and aspirin tolerance, and 120 controls (157). Haplotypes at three sites, ST+7, V-1, and V5, were significantly different in the intolerant subjects compared with the tolerant subjects and the controls. The authors concluded that sequence variations in ADAM33 may correlate with susceptibility to aspirin intolerance in the Japanese population.

Polymorphisms of the MS4A2 gene (FcεR1β –109T > C and FcεR1β E237G) were determined in 164 Korean patients with aspirin-induced asthma, 144 with asthma and aspirin tolerance, and 264 healthy controls (158). The genotype frequencies of the FcεR1β –109T > C and

E237G polymorphisms were not significantly associated with the pathogenesis of aspirin-induced asthma. However, the FcεR1β −109T > C polymorphism was significantly associated with the presence of specific IgE to staphylococcal enterotoxin B; the number of subjects carrying both homozygous TT genotype of FcεR1β −109T > C and specific IgE to staphylococcal enterotoxin B was significantly higher in those with aspirin-induced asthma. The authors concluded that the FcεR1β −109T > C polymorphism may increase the expression of MS4A2 in mast cells, leading to enhanced release of inflammatory mediators, contributing to increased susceptibility to aspirin intolerance.

Diagnosis

Challenge with aspirin, oral, nasal, inhalational, or intravenous, is the only reliable method of diagnosis. Lysine aspirin can also be used (159). Antihistamines, short-acting beta-adrenoceptor agonists, and anticholinergic drugs should be withdrawn 24 hours before the challenge, since antihistamines can block reactions to aspirin and beta-adrenoceptor agonists and anticholinergic drugs can give false-positive reactions. Nasal challenge using a dilute solution of ketorolac 8 mg/ml in increasing doses every 30 minutes has also been used (160), as has oral ketoprofen (161).

In vitro tests may be helpful, including a leukotriene release test and a basophil activation test; these tests, alone or in combination, are positive in 70–75% of cases, with a specificity of over 85% (162,163).

Functional eicosanoid typing has been proposed as a method of diagnosing susceptibility to pseudoallergic reactions to aspirin (164). In one patient there were different patterns of eicosanoid secretion in response to aspirin and celecoxib (165).

- A 30-year-old woman with sinusitis and hypersensitivity reactions to naproxen and ibuprofen was challenged on separate occasions with aspirin and celecoxib. Oral challenge with celecoxib 400 mg caused flushing, dyspnea, a 21% fall in FEV_1, and urticaria. Urinary excretion of LTE_4 and PGE_2-M was unchanged (3132 pg/mg creatinine and 7.4 ng/mg creatinine respectively), and 9α11βPGF$_2$, rose from 1.3 to 2.6 pg/mg creatinine at 2 hours. Oral challenge with a cumulative dose of aspirin of 188 mg caused flushing, nasal blockage, throat irritation, dyspnea, and a 27% fall in FEV_1. Followed 20 minutes later by hypotension. Urinary eicosanoid concentrations all rose and peaked at the height of clinical symptoms after 2–4 hours: LTE_4 rose from 3448 to 14 310 pg/mg creatinine, 9α11βPGF$_2$ from 1.9 to 2.7 pg/mg creatinine, PGE_2-M from 15 to 56 ng/mg creatinine, and 11-dehydro-TXB$_2$ from 2.0 to 4.6 ng/mg creatinine.

The authors suggested that the changes in 9α11βPGF$_2$ (a urinary metabolite of PGD$_2$) after both challenges, without changes in the cysteinyl leukotrienes after celecoxib, implicated mast cell degranulation in the etiology of the sensitivity reactions in this patient.

Prophylaxis and treatment

Asthma induced by aspirin is often severe and resistant to treatment. Avoidance of aspirin and substances to which there is cross-sensitivity is the only satisfactory solution.

If a reaction occurs, topical corticosteroids, leukotriene receptor antagonists (such as montelukast and zafirlukast), and 5-lipoxygenase inhibitors are standard treatments; combined treatment may be necessary in those with severe disease. Antibacterial and antifungal drugs are also often required when infection has been demonstrated. In a study of the medical records of 676 patients who had undergone oral aspirin challenges followed by aspirin desensitization, leukotriene modifying drugs protected the lower airways from severe reactions, even in those who were already taking systemic corticosteroids (166).

Aspirin desensitization is sometimes helpful. Various methods have been described, including administration orally (167,168,169,170), nasally (171,172), and bronchially (173).

In 172 patients oral desensitization produced significant reductions in episodes of infectious sinusitis, olfactory scores, the need for hospital visits, and the need for systemic and nasal corticosteroids; however, there were no changes in the doses of the inhaled corticosteroids or leukotriene receptor antagonists (174). Most of the 16 patients who did not respond to aspirin desensitization had concomitant IgE-mediated rhinitis and asthma, with reactions to dust mites (n = 14), animals (n = 13), and molds (n = 7). Other cases of failed desensitization have been described (175) and repeated treatments may be needed to maintain any effect (176,177).

Patients with aspirin-exacerbated respiratory disease who are the best candidates for desensitization have been described (178):

1. Those with no concomitant respiratory diseases but who have moderate or severe asthma, intractable nasal congestion, or both, which have failed to respond to drug treatment.
2. Those with concomitant respiratory diseases that have not responded to drug treatment.
3. Those with multiple nasal polyps.
4. Those who require systemic corticosteroids for control of their symptoms.
5. Those who require aspirin for other diseases.

A suggested protocol for aspirin desensitization is given in Table 1. After desensitization, give aspirin 650 mg bd for 1 month and then reduce to 325 mg bd if the symptoms do not return. If the patient is taking systemic corticosteroids daily or every other day, reduce and withdraw the corticosteroids before reducing the dosage of aspirin. After reducing the dose, if symptoms return, increase the dosage of aspirin.

Successful rapid desensitization has been described in performed in four pregnant women with antiphospholipid syndrome and aspirin sensitivity, using increasing doses of aspirin (0.1–125 mg) over 24 hours (179).

Desensitization was attempted in 16 patients with acute coronary artery disease and a history of aspirin hypersensitivity (of whom three had a history of angioedema) in a protocol that lasted a few hours (180). None received pretreatment with antihistamines or glucocorticoids, and

Table 1 A suggested protocol for out-patient aspirin desensitization

Before desensitization
At 1–7 days before, determine airway stability.
1. Measure FEV$_1$—must be over 60% of predicted value and 1.5 liters absolute.
2. Measure FEV$_1$ every hour for 3 hours—must be less than 10% variability.
3. Start or continue montelukast 10 mg/day.
4. Start or continue an inhaled corticosteroid and/or a long-acting bronchodilator.
5. Start systemic corticosteroids for a low FEV$_1$ or any bronchial instability.
6. Discontinue antihistamines 48 hours before the challenge.

Oral aspirin challenge
1. Day 1: insert an intravenous line (keep in throughout the period of challenge).
2. Examples of doses of aspirin that can be used are 20 or 40 mg (first dose), followed by 60, 80, 100, 162.5, 325, and 650 mg, increasing the dose every 3 hours; doses at the lower end of this range can be modified according to the type of formulation available.
3. Measure FEV$_1$ and assess clinically every hour or when symptoms occur.
4. A reaction will probably occur at doses between 20 and 100 mg; this is called the provoking dose.
5. Treat reactions as described below until the patient is completely stable.
6. Start again with the provoking dose and increase the dose every 3 hours (on day 1 if there is time, otherwise on day 2).
7. If nasal, gastrointestinal, or cutaneous reactions occur on day 1, pretreat with H$_1$ and H$_2$ receptor antagonists for the rest of the challenge sequence.
8. The chance of a reaction to a repeated threshold dose is small; if it occurs, repeat that dose until reactions stop and then proceed to the next dose.
9. If a reaction occurs, continue as in 5.

Treatment of aspirin-induced reactions
1. Ocular: topical antihistamine.
2. Nasal: antihistamine (oral) or diphenhydramine 50 mg intravenously; topical decongestant.
3. Laryngeal: nebulized adrenaline 2.5 mg/2 ml, five inhalations and pause.
4. Bronchial: five inhalations of a β-adrenoceptor agonist every 5 minutes until comfortable.
5. Gastrointestinal cramping: intravenous ranitidine, 50 mg.
6. Urticaria/angioedema: intravenous diphenhydramine 50 mg.
7. Hypotension: adrenaline 0.3 ml of a 1:1000 solution intramuscularly.

beta-blockers were withheld. The first seven received eight oral doses of aspirin, starting at 1 mg and doubling each 30 minutes; the next nine patients underwent a shorter version using five doses (5, 10, 20, 40, and 75 mg). The patients were monitored in the coronary care unit; blood pressure, pulse, and peak expiratory flow were measured every 30 minutes, and cutaneous, naso-ocular, and pulmonary reactions were monitored closely until 3 hours after the procedure. Immediate tolerance was obtained in 14 patients, all of whom continued treatment uneventfully. One patient developed angioedema 3 hours after the procedure, which resolved immediately with a glucocorticoid and adrenaline. The patient was rechallenged successfully 2 days later and continued to take aspirin. Another patient, who had had a severe recent attack of asthma, developed nasal swelling and shortness of breath 1 hour after the last dose; although the symptoms resolved rapidly with inhaled salbutamol, rechallenge was not attempted. In 11 patients who then underwent coronary stenting aspirin + clopidogrel was given for 9–12 months; four were treated with aspirin alone. There were no major adverse cardiac events or new revascularization during a median follow-up of 14 months (range 1–35).

Long-Term Effects

Drug resistance
Aspirin resistance can be defined in two ways—clinical resistance (failure to respond to aspirin) and in vitro resistance (a reduced effect of aspirin on platelet function in vitro). These two are not necessarily related to each other. Resistance has been attributed to two mechanisms: the capability of platelets to produce thromboxane A$_2$, even at very low concentrations, despite aspirin treatment, because of pharmacokinetic or pharmacodynamic problems; and platelet activation independently of TxA$_2$ formation, possibly linked to polymorphisms in platelet receptors or pro-aggregating molecule. The production by other circulating cells of thromboxane or its precursors, bypassing COX-1, may also play a role.

Thromboxane biosynthesis and platelet aggregation have been studied in 50 patients taking aspirin 81 mg/day and 38 controls and have been related to clinical outcomes (181). Platelet COX-1 activity only accounted for 6–20% of the individual aggregatory responses. A common factor (other than platelet COX-1) explained 48% of the variation in platelet aggregation induced by collagen, adenosine diphosphate (ADP), and collagen-related peptide. In a prospective study of 136 patients taking aspirin, independent susceptibility factors for cardiovascular events were being in the upper quartile of light transmission or having large aggregate formation induced by collagen (i.e. having poor aggregation). The authors concluded that aspirin resistance, expressed as unsuppressed platelet COX-1 activity, is rare in out-patients and that other factors that affect collagen-induced platelet aggregation may affect outcomes in patients taking aspirin.

The contribution of poor systemic availability to apparent clinical resistance to aspirin has been studied in 71 healthy volunteers who took modified-release dipyridamole 200 mg bd plus different formulations of aspirin: three different enteric-coated formulations, dispersible aspirin, and a standard-release formulation, each containing 75 mg (182). Dispersible aspirin had a significantly larger effect on serum TXB_2 concentrations than all the other formulations, and there was treatment failure (less than 95% inhibition of serum TXB_2 formation) in 14 subjects, none of whom was taking dispersible aspirin. The authors concluded that poor systemic availability of aspirin from some formulations could result in inadequate platelet inhibition.

The role of aspirin resistance in the risk of major adverse coronary events has been studied prospectively after percutaneous coronary intervention in 146 patients with acute myocardial infarction (183). Aspirin resistance was characterized in vitro using the collagen–adrenaline closure time. After 1 year there were major adverse coronary events in 44 patients (30%). A significantly higher percentage of patients with major adverse coronary events had aspirin resistance (39% versus 23%); the difference persisted after adjustment for age, sex, cardiovascular risk factors, systolic left ventricular function, number of stenosed coronary arteries, and previous myocardial infarction, percutaneous coronary intervention, or coronary artery bypass grafting. The hazard ratio for aspirin resistance as a significant and independent risk factor for major adverse coronary events was 2.9 (95% CI = 1.1, 9.2).

Aspirin resistance has been described in a patient with a myocardial infarction in whom two stents occluded 2 days after insertion, despite standard antiplatelet drug therapy (184). Plasma thromboxane B_2 concentrations were raised and there was no thrombophilia.

A procedure for evaluating aspirin resistance in vitro using platelets from a single blood sample has been described (185) and is summarized in Figure 1.

Tumorigenicity

Studies on the tumor-inducing effects of heavy use of analgesics, especially those that contain phenacetin, have given contrasting results (SEDA-21, 100) (186,187). There has been a case-control study of the role of habitual intake of aspirin on the occurrence of urothelial cancer and renal cell carcinoma (188). In previous studies there was a consistent association between phenacetin and renal cell carcinoma, but inconclusive results with respect to non-phenacetin analgesics. In 1024 patients with renal cell carcinoma and an equal number of matched controls, regular use of analgesics was a significant risk factor for renal cell carcinoma (OR = 1.6; CI = 1.4, 1.9). The risk was significantly increased by aspirin, NSAIDs, paracetamol, and phenacetin, and within each class of analgesic the risk increased with increasing exposure. Individuals in the highest exposure categories had about a 2.5-fold increase in risk relative to non-users or irregular users of analgesics. However, exclusive users of aspirin who took aspirin 325 mg/day or less for cardiovascular problems were not at an increased risk of renal cell carcinoma (OR = 0.9; CI = 0.6, 1.4).

Second-Generation Effects

Pregnancy

The association between aspirin and miscarriage has been investigated in a prospective case-control study using data from the Collaborative Perinatal Project in 54 000 pregnant women at 12 sites in the USA from 1959 to 1965 (189). Women who had miscarriages (n = 542) were matched by clinic and time in pregnancy when they came under observation with 2587 women who had live births. During pregnancy 29% of cases and 34% of controls used aspirin, which was not associated with an increased risk of miscarriage (adjusted OR = 0.64–0.92;

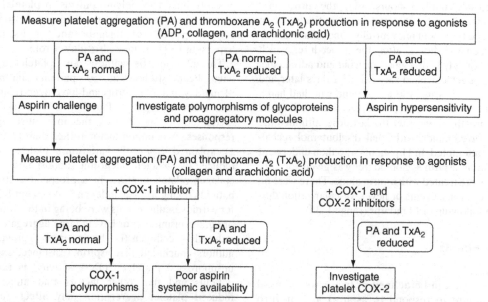

Figure 1 A procedure for evaluating aspirin resistance in vitro using platelets from a single blood sample

95% CI = 0.48, 1.38) for individual lunar months and combinations of lunar months.

Teratogenicity

It is perhaps surprising that aspirin, which is teratogenic in rodents, and which by virtue of its capacity to inhibit prostaglandin synthesis would be expected to affect the development of the renal and cardiovascular systems, has shown no evidence of teratogenesis in humans, despite very widespread use in pregnant women. Perhaps increased production of prostaglandins during pregnancy overrides the effects of aspirin in the usual dosages, and the intervention of placental metabolism protects the human fetus from exposure to aspirin. Whatever the explanation, there are very few reports in which aspirin can be implicated as a human teratogen and a few studies (190,191) have provided positive reassurance.

Fetotoxicity

Because aspirin is an antithrombotic agent and can promote bleeding, it should be avoided in the third trimester of pregnancy and at parturition (192). At parturition there is a second reason for avoiding aspirin, since its prostaglandin-inhibiting capacity could mean that it will delay parturition and induce early closure of the ductus arteriosus in the near-term fetus, as other NSAIDs do (193). However, its use in low doses in pregnancy may prevent retardation of fetal growth (194).

Susceptibility Factors

Genetic

Genetic polymorphisms in patients with aspirin-induced chronic urticaria have been reviewed (195,196).

HLA
The role of HLA class I phenotypes and the HLA-DRB1* genotype in patients with chronic idiopathic urticaria associated with aspirin and NSAIDs has been studied in 69 patients and 200 healthy subjects (197). There were more subjects with HLA-B44 and HLA-Cw5 antigens among patients with chronic idiopathic urticaria than among the controls; conversely, there were more subjects with HLA-A11, HLA-B13, HLACw4, and HLA-Cw7 among the controls. HLA-Cw4 and HLA-Cw7 were associated with a lower risk of chronic idiopathic urticaria and the HLA-B44 phenotype with a higher risk. There was no association with the HLA-DRB1* genotype.

An association between HLA DRB1*1302 and HLA DQB1*0609 alleles and aspirin-induced urticaria has been demonstrated (198). Patients with these alleles developed urticaria at an earlier age.

Leukotriene C₄ synthase (LCT₄S)
In patients with chronic urticaria, the frequency of those carrying the C allele of LTC$_4$S –444A>C was significantly higher among those with aspirin sensitivity than among those who did not react to aspirin; aspirin-induced urticaria aggregated in families with the LTC$_4$S –444C allele (199); the frequency of the –444C allele was significantly higher in patients who were sensitive to aspirin than in those who were not sensitive. However, there was no association between the LTC$_4$S –444A>C polymorphism and the phenotype of non-steroidal anti-inflammatory drug-induced isolated periorbital angioedema in Spain (200) or Korea (201).

Polymorphisms of the LTC$_4$S gene (AA, AC, CC) and the glutathione S-transferase M1 and P1 genes (GSTM1 and GSTP1) have been studied in 74 patients with chronic idiopathic urticaria and a history of aspirin hypersensitivity, two of whom had a family history of aspirin intolerance (202). In both families, the variant genotypes of LTC$_4$S (AC or CC) were present in the parents, but only one of them had urticaria. In one family both parents were healthy but the three children had urticaria, and in two of them it was associated with a variant LTC$_4$S genotype. In the other family, urticaria after aspirin ingestion was present only in those with a variant LTC$_4$S genotype. In the patients of both families with positive aspirin challenge tests, there was deletion of the GSTM1 gene.

In a study of nine single-nucleotide polymorphisms of four leukotriene-related genes, 5-lipoxygenase (ALOX5 –1708G>A, 270G>A, and 1728G>A), 5-lipoxygenase-activating protein (ALOX5AP 218A>G), cyclo-oxygenase 2 (PTGS2 –162C>G, 10T>G, and 228G>A), LTC$_4$S (–444A>C), and CYSLTR1 (–634C>T), there were significant differences in the frequencies of polymorphisms of ALOX5 (–1708G>A) and CYSLTR1 (–634C>T) between patients with aspirin-induced urticaria or angioedema and controls (200).

In another study there were no significant differences in single-nucleotide polymorphisms of the genes that encode high-affinity IgE receptor Iβ (FcεRIβ), histamine N-methyltransferase (HNMT), histamine receptors type 1 (H$_1$), histamine receptors type 2 (H$_2$), or their haplotypes between patients with aspirin-induced urticaria, patients with other drug allergies, and healthy controls (203). However, there was a significant association between two promoter polymorphisms of the FcεRIβ receptor (–344C>T and –95 T>C) and aspirin-induced chronic urticaria. The rare –344C>T polymorphism was significantly more common in the patients with chronic idiopathic urticaria than in controls and was significantly associated with total serum IgE concentrations and a higher rate of atopy (204).

Age

In view of the association with Reye's syndrome, aspirin should be avoided in children aged under 16.

Drug Administration

Drug formulations

Although the use of enteric-coated aspirin can reduce its direct adverse effect on the stomach (SEDA-10, 72), it could in principle transfer these to some extent to the intestine; modified-release NSAIDs have sometimes caused intestinal perforation.

Enteric coating reduces the rate of absorption of aspirin. In cases of severe overdosage this can cause difficulties in diagnosis and treatment, since early plasma salicylate measurements are unreliable, maximum blood concentrations sometimes not being reached until 60 or 70 hours after overdose (205,206). Another complication of the use of enteric-coated aspirin is the risk of gastric outlet obstruction and the resulting accumulation of tablets because of subclinical pyloric stenosis.

Drug overdose

Acute poisoning

Acute salicylate poisoning is a major clinical hazard (207), although it is associated with low major morbidity and mortality, in contrast to chronic intoxication (SEDA-17, 98). It can cause alkalemia or acidemia, alkaluria or aciduria, hyperglycemia or hypoglycemia, and water and electrolyte imbalances. However, the usual picture is one of hypokalemia with metabolic acidosis and respiratory alkalosis. Effects on hearing have been referred to in the section on Sensory systems in this monograph. Nausea, vomiting, tinnitus, hyperpnea, hyperpyrexia, confusion, disorientation, dizziness, coma, and/or convulsions are common. They are expressions of the nervous system effects of the salicylates. Gastrointestinal hemorrhage is frequent.

Serum salicylate concentrations above 3.6 mmol/l are likely to be toxic, and concentrations of 5.4 mmol/l can easily prove fatal.

After ingestion, drug absorption can be prevented by induction of emesis, gastric lavage, and the administration of active charcoal; drug excretion is enhanced by administering intravenous alkalinizing solutions, hemoperfusion, and hemodialysis (208). Forced diuresis is dangerous and unnecessary.

Fluid and electrolyte management is the mainstay of therapy. The immediate aim must be to correct acidosis, hyperpyrexia, hypokalemia, and dehydration. In severe cases vitamin K_1 should be given to counteract hypoprothrombinemia.

Aspirin overdose in children can be particularly serious.

- A 5-year-old girl died after taking an aspirin overdose. Autopsy showed a pattern of necrosis resembling acute toxic myocarditis (209).

Salicylate poisoning, including poisoning by excessive application of topical agents, ingestion of salicylate-containing ointments, use of keratolytic agents or agents containing methylsalicylate (for example oil of wintergreen), has been reviewed (210). Liquid formulations are highly concentrated and lipid soluble and can therefore cause severe, rapid salicylate poisoning.

- A 34-year-old woman took a large amount of aspirin for ear pain and developed a metabolic acidosis with a serum salicylate concentration of 668 mg/l (4.84 mmol/l; toxic range above 200 mg/l, 1.45 mmol/l) (211). Autopsy showed venous congestion of the brain, cardiac dilatation, and pulmonary edema. Brain histology

showed myelin disintegration and caspase-3 activation in glial cells, but sparse grey matter changes.

The authors suggested that acute white matter damage underlies cerebral dysfunction in salicylate intoxication.

Chronic poisoning

Chronic salicylate intoxication is commonly associated with chronic daily headaches, lethargy, confusion, or coma. Since headache is a feature, it can easily be misdiagnosed if the physician is not aware that aspirin has been over-used. Depression of mental status is usually present at the time of diagnosis, when the serum salicylate concentration is at a peak. The explanation of depression, manifested by irritability, lethargy, and unresponsiveness, occurring 1–3 days after the start of therapy for aspirin intoxication, lies in a persistently high concentration of salicylate in the central nervous system, while the serum salicylate concentration falls to non-toxic values. The delayed unresponsiveness associated with salicylate intoxication appears to be closely associated with the development of cerebral edema of uncertain cause. The encephalopathy that ensues appears to be directly related to increased intracranial pressure, a known effect of prostaglandin synthesis inhibitors; it responds to mannitol (212).

Drug–Drug Interactions

ACE inhibitors

Many large, prospective, randomized studies have shown that aspirin and ACE inhibitors reduce the risk of death and major adverse cardiovascular events in patients who have left ventricular dysfunction with or without congestive heart failure. Thus, both drugs are often taken concomitantly.

Shortly after the first demonstration of the favorable effects of ACE inhibitors (213) a controversy arose about whether there is a risk of a negative interaction between ACE inhibitors and COX inhibitors, in particular aspirin.

It is important to understand the theoretic basis for this potential interaction. ACE not only converts angiotensin I to angiotensin II, but it is also responsible for the degradations of kinins; thus, ACE inhibitors can increase bradykinin concentrations. Bradykinin, a potent vasodilator, activates endothelial β_2-kinin receptors, which promote the formation of vasodilatory prostaglandins through the action of phospholipase A_2 and cyclooxygenase (COX). ACE inhibitors reduce arterial blood pressure by reducing angiotensin II production and increasing the vasodilators bradykinin, PGI_2, and PGE_3. Some investigators have suggested that aspirin (and other NSAIDs) blunt the blood pressure lowering effects of ACE inhibitors by inhibiting the production of vasodilatory prostaglandins. Others have suggested that aspirin causes reduced synthesis of renal PGE_2, which might augment unwanted ACE inhibitor-induced impairment of renal function, resulting in increased retention of sodium and water. Consequently, it has been postulated that the beneficial effects of ACE inhibitors might be reduced in patients taking concomitant aspirin.

All of the studies of the clinical relevance of this possible interaction were post-hoc analyses or retrospective cohort studies of large trials of ACE inhibitors, and these studies have given different results. Some of them have shown possible interactions (213,214), while others have given conflicting results (215,216) or have not supported the hypothesis that aspirin has a negative effect on survival in patients taking ACE inhibitors (217,218,219,220).

More recently a systematic review and two retrospective studies have provided more information on this topic.

The systematic review assessed the effects of ACE inhibitors in patients with or without aspirin use at baseline (221). Individual patient data were collected on 22 060 patients from six long-term, randomized, placebo-controlled studies of ACE inhibitors (222,223,224,225,226,227) each of which included more than 1000 patients. The results from all of the trials, except SOLVD, did not suggest any significant differences between the proportional reductions in risk with ACE inhibitors in the presence or absence of aspirin for the major clinical outcomes (death; myocardial infarction and reinfarction; stroke; hospital admission for congestive heart failure; revascularization; and a combination of major vascular events) or in the risk of any of its individual components, except myocardial infarction. Overall ACE inhibitors significantly reduced the risk of the major clinical outcomes by 22% with clear reductions in risk among those taking aspirin at baseline (OR 0.80; 99% CI=0.73, 0.88) and those who were not (OR 0.71; 99% CI=0.62, 0.81).

Considering the totality of evidence on all major vascular outcomes in these studies, there is only weak evidence of any reduction in the benefit of ACE inhibitor therapy when added to aspirin. On the other hand, there is strong evidence of clinically important benefits with respect to these major clinical outcomes with ACE inhibitors, irrespective of whether aspirin is used concomitantly.

The authors of this meta-analysis concluded that at least some of the differences in the effects of ACE inhibitors on outcomes in SOLVD (228) among patients taking aspirin, compared with those who were not, might have suggested differences in the effects of ACE inhibitors in different types of patients rather than an interaction between ACE inhibitor and aspirin.

Evidence that aspirin does not interact with ACE inhibitors has come from two retrospective studies.

The first was a retrospective analysis of 755 stable patients with left ventricular systolic dysfunction and congestive heart failure, 92% of whom were taking ACE inhibitors (229). Compared with previous retrospective trials this study had some specific favorable features. It was a single-center study with the same kind of management used for all patients (including diagnostic procedures), all the patients had congestive heart failure related to left ventricular systolic dysfunction, and treatment (including aspirin and its dosage) was precisely recorded at entry. The mean dose of aspirin at entry was

183 mg/day and 74% of the patients took under 200 mg/day. Using a Cox regression model there were no interactions among aspirin, ACE inhibitors, and survival in the overall population or in subgroups of patient with ischemic or non-ischemic cardiomyopathies. Therefore, small doses of aspirin did not affect survival in patients with stable congestive heart failure taking ACE inhibitors.

The importance of the dose of aspirin was confirmed in the second study, a retrospective analysis of 344 patients taking ACE inhibitors admitted to hospital for congestive heart failure, in whom information was available about aspirin therapy during a follow-up period of 37 months (230). Cox proportional hazards regression analysis showed that the combination of high dose aspirin (325 mg/day and over) with an ACE inhibitor was independently associated with the risk of death, but that the combination with low-dose aspirin (under 160 mg/day) was not.

The results of these two studies must be interpreted with caution. Not only do they have the limitations common to cohort studies, including their retrospective nature and lack of randomization, but they were also small and biased by potential confounders related to patient characteristics.

However, taken together, the evidence for a significant interaction between low-dose aspirin and ACE inhibitors in patient with congestive heart failure is probably negligible and all patients should receive low-dose aspirin together with full-dose ACE inhibition if both are needed.

Alcohol

Although ethanol itself has no effect on bleeding time, it enhances the effect of aspirin when given simultaneously or up to at least 36 hours after aspirin ingestion (231). Ethanol also promotes gastric bleeding.

The FDA has announced its intention to require alcohol warnings on all over-the-counter pain medications that contain acetylsalicylic acid, salicylates, paracetamol, ibuprofen, ketoprofen, or naproxen. The proposed warnings are aimed at alerting consumers to the specific risks incurred from heavy alcohol consumption and its interaction with analgesics. For products that contain paracetamol, the warning indicates the risks of liver damage in those who drink more than three alcoholic beverages a day. For formulations that contain salicylates or the mentioned NSAIDs, three or more alcoholic beverages will increase the risk of stomach bleeding (232).

Anticoagulants

The effects on coagulation are additive if aspirin is used concurrently with anticoagulants. There are also other interaction mechanisms: the effect of the coumarins is temporarily increased by protein binding displacement, and if aspirin causes gastric hemorrhages, the latter may well be more severe when anticoagulants are being given.

In the SPORTIF III and IV randomized trials of anticoagulation with warfarin (INR 2–3) or fixed-dose ximelagatran, 14% of the patients took aspirin, the addition of which did not reduce strokes or episodes of systemic embolism (233). However, major bleeding occurred significantly more often with aspirin plus warfarin (3.9% per year) than with warfarin alone (2.3% per year), aspirin + ximelagatran (2.0% per year), or ximelagatran alone (1.9% per year). The authors concluded that the harms associated with the addition of aspirin to anticoagulation in patients with atrial fibrillation outweigh the benefits.

In 107 consecutive patients who underwent coronary stenting and were given aspirin + clopidogrel + warfarin and 107 who were given aspirin + clopidogrel, the former had significantly more major bleeding (6.6 versus 0%) and minor bleeding (15 versus 3.8%) than the latter (234).

Aspirin should therefore generally be avoided in patients adequately treated with anticoagulants. The most relevant information on hemorrhagic complications occurring during prophylaxis with antiplatelet drugs, whether used singly or in combination, has been provided by well-controlled prospective trials with aspirin (17), aspirin combined with dipyridamole (235), or aspirin compared with oral anticoagulants (236).

Antihypertensive drugs

An increase in mean supine blood pressure has been reported with aspirin (SEDA-19, 92). Aspirin may therefore interfere with antihypertensive pharmacotherapy, warranting caution, especially in the elderly.

Captopril

Aspirin is thought to reduce the antihypertensive effect of captopril (237).

Carbonic anhydrase inhibitors

In two children, aspirin potentiated the slight metabolic acidosis induced by carbonic anhydrase inhibitors (SEDA-9, 79) (238).

Clopidogrel

The combination of aspirin with clopidogrel can increase the risk of bleeding (239).

- A 76-year-old man with a history of myocardial infarction and unstable angina developed spontaneous hemarthrosis in his knee 2 weeks after starting to take clopidogrel 75 mg/day and aspirin 100 mg/day. He suddenly developed pain in the right knee while resting in bed. There was massive swelling, tenderness, and an intra-articular effusion; an X-ray showed osteoarthritis. Hemorrhagic fluid was aspirated. His coagulation status was normal. Treatment was withdrawn and recovery was uneventful.

In the CAPRIE study clopidogrel was superior to aspirin in patients with previous manifestations of atherothrombotic disease, and its benefit was amplified in some high-risk subgroups of patients (240). To assess whether the addition of aspirin to clopidogrel could have a greater benefit than clopidogrel alone in preventing vascular events with a potentially higher bleeding risk, patients who had recently had an ischemic stroke or a transient ischemic attack and were taking clopidogrel

75 mg/day, were randomized to receive additional aspirin 75 mg/day (n=3797) or placebo (n=3802) for 18 months (241). The primary end-point was a composite of ischemic stroke, myocardial infarction, vascular death, or rehospitalization for acute ischemia. Aspirin was associated with a small non-significant reduction in the risk of the primary end-point (relative risk reduction of 6.4%; CI= –4.6, 16); absolute risk reduction 1.1%; (CI= –0.6, 2.7). However, the incidence of life-threatening bleeding was higher with aspirin than placebo: 96 (2.6%) versus 49 (1.3%). The absolute increase in risk was 1.3% (CI= –0.6, 1.9) as was the incidence of major bleeding. These possibly increased risks might therefore offset any beneficial effect of adding aspirin to clopidogrel treatment in these patients.

Case reports documenting an increased risk of bleeding with the concomitant use of clopidogrel with aspirin in perioperative setting have been published (242).

Fish oils

In eight healthy men who took a total of 485 mg of aspirin over 3 days before beginning 2 weeks of fish oil supplementation (4.5 g of n-3 fatty acids/day), aspirin alone prolonged the bleeding time by 34% and fish oil alone prolonged it by only 9%; however, aspirin + fish oil prolonged the bleeding time by 78% (259). Although fish oil alone did not significantly raise aggregation thresholds for collagen, arachidonic acid, or platelet activating factor, it did reduce the extent of aggregation with collagen. When challenged by single or dual agonists, the combination of fish oil and aspirin did not make platelets less sensitive than aspirin alone.

However, in 18 healthy men randomly allocated to N-3 polyunsaturated fatty acids 10 g/day or placebo for 14 days, the addition of a single intravenous dose of acetylsalicylic acid 100 mg did not alter the small effect of polyunsaturated fatty acids on platelet aggregation (260).

In four subjects given a single oral dose of aspirin 37.5 mg before and after a natural stable fish oil daily for 1 week, serum thromboxane A_2 fell by 40% after aspirin alone, but by 62% after fish oil + aspirin, and leukotriene B_4 rose by 19% after aspirin and fell by 69% after fish oil + aspirin; serum prostacyclin fell equally in both cases (261).

In healthy subjects who took either fish oil or olive oil (control) daily for 3 weeks before exposure to aspirin or no aspirin, fish oil had no significant effect on mucosal prostaglandin E_2 or $F_{2\alpha}$ content or on the damaging effect of aspirin on the stomach, despite the fact that fish oil reduced serum triglyceride concentrations significantly (262).

Glucocorticoids

The effects of aspirin on gastrointestinal mucosa will lead to additive effects if it is used concurrently with other drugs that have an irritant effect on the stomach, notably other NSAIDs or glucocorticoids (243,244).

Heparin

Risk factors for heparin-induced bleeding include concomitant use of aspirin (245).

Intrauterine contraceptive devices

The supposed mechanisms of action of intrauterine contraceptive devices (IUCDs) include a local inflammatory response and increased local production of prostaglandins that prevent sperm from fertilizing ova (246,247). As aspirin has both anti-inflammatory and antiprostaglandin properties, the contraceptive effectiveness of an IUCD can be reduced by the drug, although the effect on periodic bleeding may prevail.

Methotrexate

Aspirin displaces methotrexate from its binding sites and also inhibits its renal tubular elimination, so that the dosage of concurrently used methotrexate should be reduced (except once-a-week low-dose treatment in rheumatoid arthritis) (248).

Nitrates

Aspirin in low dosages (under 300 mg/day) is widely used in cardiovascular prophylaxis, but its use is accompanied by an increased risk of gastrointestinal bleeding (SEDA-21, 100). Of particular interest therefore are data from a retrospective case-control study showing that nitrate therapy may reduce the risk of aspirin-induced gastrointestinal bleeding (249). As nitrates are often used in the same population of patients, such data merit further confirmation from larger prospective studies.

NSAIDs

The effects of aspirin on gastrointestinal mucosa will lead to additive effects if it is used concurrently with other drugs that have an irritant effect on the stomach, notably other NSAIDs or glucocorticoids (243,244). Salicylates can be displaced from binding sites by some NSAIDs such as naproxen, or in turn displace others such as piroxicam.

Pemetrexed

In a randomized, crossover study in patients with cancer with a creatinine clearance below 60 ml/minute, oral aspirin 325 mg every 6 hours, starting 2 days before intravenous administration of pemetrexed 500 mg/m^2 and continuing until 1 hour before the infusion, had no effect on the pharmacokinetics of pemetrexed (250).

Sodium valproate

Aspirin displaces sodium valproate from protein binding sites (251) and reduces its hepatic metabolism (252).

When aspirin displaces other drugs from protein-binding sites on serum albumin, it increases the unbound fraction, producing a toxic unbound concentration. This can affect the actions of drugs that are highly protein bound and have low volumes of distribution, such as warfarin and phenytoin. However, the clearance of these low-clearance drugs increases in response to the increase in the unbound fraction, the total concentration falls, and the unbound concentration once again becomes nontoxic. Thus, the effects of such interactions are generally transient. If the physician then increases the dose in order to increase the total concentration, toxicity can occur, since the unbound concentration will then be increased to toxic values. This has been reported in a patient taking aspirin and valproate (253).

- A 76-year-old man with bipolar I disorder was given divalproex sodium 750 mg/day and the total serum valproate concentration was 14 ng/ml. Aspirin 325 mg/day was added, and during a subsequent admission to hospital his total serum valproate concentration was 19 ng/ml. A psychiatrist suggested titrating the dose of divalproex to produce a total serum trough concentration of 50–70 ng/ml, and the dose was gradually titrated from 750 to 2500 mg/day. After 2 weeks he started to have increasing difficulty in transferring from bed to a wheelchair, and 3 weeks later he became dizzy and had a painful fall. His difficulties with transfers steadily increased. His trough total valproate concentration was 64 ng/ml and the trough unbound concentration was 25 ng/ml. Throughout this time he had hypoalbuminemia below 30 g/l. The dose of divalproex was reduced to 1250 mg/day.

Displacement of valproate by aspirin and hypoalbuminemia probably both contributed to the high unbound concentration of valproate in this case. Aspirin may also have inhibited the metabolism of valproate, contributing to an increase in total valproate concentration.

Streptokinase

Major hemorrhagic complications, including cerebral hemorrhage, can occur with aspirin (SEDA-23, 116) and the same is also true for thrombolytic therapy of acute ischemic stroke (254). A post hoc analysis of the Multicenter Acute Stroke Trial in Italy showed a negative interaction of aspirin and streptokinase in acute ischemic stroke (255). In 156 patients who received streptokinase plus aspirin and 157 patients treated with streptokinase alone, the combined regimen significantly increased early case fatality at days 3–10 (53 versus 30; OR = 2.5; CI = 1.2, 3.6). The excess in deaths was solely due to treatment and was not explained by the main prognostic predictors. Deaths in the combination group were mainly cerebral (42 versus 24; OR = 2.0; CI = 1.3, 3.7) and associated with hemorrhagic transformation (22 versus 11; OR = 2.2; CI = 1.0, 5.0). The data suggest that aspirin should be avoided when thrombolytic agents are used for acute ischemic stroke.

Uricosuric drugs

In low dosages (up to 2 g/day), aspirin reduces urate excretion and blocks the effects of probenecid and other uricosuric agents (256). However, in 11 patients with gout, aspirin 325 mg/day had no effect on the uricosuric action of probenecid (257). In higher dosages (over 5 g/day), salicylates increase urate excretion and inhibit the effects of spironolactone, but it is not clear that these phenomena are of importance.

Food–Drug Interactions

Food allergens

Aspirin seems to potentiate the effects of food allergens, but this is uncertain (SEDA-10, 72).

Interference with Diagnostic Tests

Thyroid function tests

Through competitive binding to thyroid-binding globulin, salicylates in high concentrations can displace thyroxine and triiodothyronine, thus interfering with the results of diagnostic thyroid function tests (258).

References

1. MacIntyre A, Gray JD, Gorelick M, Renton K. Salicylate and acetaminophen in donated blood. CMAJ 1986;135(3):215–6.
2. Wynne HA, Long A. Patient awareness of the adverse effects of non-steroidal anti-inflammatory drugs (NSAIDs). Br J Clin Pharmacol 1996;42(2):253–6.
3. National Drugs Advisory Board. Availability of aspirin and paracetamol. Annual Report 1987;24.
4. Mitchell JA, Akarasereenont P, Thiemermann C, Flower RJ, Vane JR. Selectivity of nonsteroidal antiinflammatory drugs as inhibitors of constitutive and inducible cyclooxygenase. Proc Natl Acad Sci USA 1993; 90(24):11693–7.
5. Antiplatelet Trialists' Collaboration. Secondary prevention of vascular disease by prolonged antiplatelet treatment. BMJ (Clin Res Ed) 1988;296(6618):320–31.
6. Hennekens CH, Buring JE, Sandercock P, Collins R, Peto R. Aspirin and other antiplatelet agents in the secondary and primary prevention of cardiovascular disease. Circulation 1989;80(4):749–56.
7. Macdonald R. Aspirin and extradural blocks. Br J Anaesth 1991;66(1):1–3.
8. de Swiet M, Redman CW. Aspirin, extradural anaesthesia and the MRC Collaborative Low-dose Aspirin Study in Pregnancy (CLASP). Br J Anaesth 1992;69(1):109–10.
9. Steering Committee of the Physicians' Health Study Research Group. Final report on the aspirin component of the ongoing Physicians' Health Study. N Engl J Med 1989;321(3):129–35.
10. Peto R, Gray R, Collins R, Wheatley K, Hennekens C, Jamrozik K, Warlow C, Hafner B, Thompson E, Norton S, et al. Randomised trial of prophylactic daily aspirin in British male doctors. BMJ (Clin Res Ed) 1988;296(6618): 313–6.
11. Stafford RS. Aspirin use is low among United States outpatients with coronary artery disease. Circulation 2000; 101(10):1097–101.
12. Hayden M, Pignone M, Phillips C, Mulrow C. Aspirin for the primary prevention of cardiovascular events: a summary of the evidence for the U.S. Preventive Services Task Force Ann Intern Med 2002;136(2):161–72.
13. Weisman SM, Graham DY. Evaluation of the benefits and risks of low-dose aspirin in the secondary prevention of cardiovascular and cerebrovascular events. Arch Intern Med 2002;162(19):2197–202.
14. Roderick PJ, Wilkes HC, Meade TW. The gastrointestinal toxicity of aspirin: an overview of randomised controlled trials. Br J Clin Pharmacol 1993;35(3):219–26.
15. Derry S, Loke YK. Risk of gastrointestinal haemorrhage with long term use of aspirin: meta-analysis. BMJ 2000;321(7270):1183–7.
16. Antithrombotic Trialists' Collaboration. Collaborative meta-analysis of randomised trials of antiplatelet therapy for prevention of death, myocardial infarction, and stroke in high risk patients. BMJ 2002;324(7329):71–86.
17. Aspirin Myocardial Infarction Study Research Group. A randomized, controlled trial of aspirin in persons recovered from myocardial infarction. JAMA 1980;243(7):661–9.
18. Habbab MA, Szwed SA, Haft JI. Is coronary arterial spasm part of the aspirin-induced asthma syndrome? Chest 1986;90(1):141–3.
19. Hermida RC, Ayala DE, Calvo C, Lopez JE, Fernandez JR, Mojon A, Dominguez MJ, Covelo M. Administration time-dependent effects of aspirin on blood pressure in untreated hypertensive patients. Hypertension 2003;41:1259–67.
20. Heffner JE, Sahn SA. Salicylate-induced pulmonary edema. Clinical features and prognosis. Ann Intern Med 1981;95(4):405–9.
21. Grabe DW, Manley HJ, Kim JS, McGoldrick MD, Bailie GR. Respiratory distress caused by salicylism confirmed by lung biopsy. Clin Drug Invest 1999;17:79–81.
22. The Dutch TIA Trial Study Group. A comparison of two doses of aspirin (30 mg vs. 283 mg a day) in patients after a transient ischemic attack or minor ischemic stroke N Engl J Med 1991;325(18):1261–6.
23. The SALT Collaborative Group. Swedish Aspirin Low-Dose Trial (SALT) of 75 mg aspirin as secondary prophylaxis after cerebrovascular ischaemic events Lancet 1991;338(8779):1345–9.
24. Steering Committee of the Physicians' Health Study Research Group. Final report on the aspirin component of the ongoing Physicians' Health Study. N Engl J Med 1989;321(3):129–35.
25. Saloheimo P, Ahonen M, Juvela S, Pyhtinen J, Savolainen ER, Hillbom M. Regular aspirin-use preceding the onset of primary intracerebral hemorrhage is an independent predictor for death. Stroke 2006;37(1):129–33.
26. Rohr WD. Transitorische Myopisierung und Drucksteigerung als Medikamentennebenwirkung. [Transitory myopia and increased ocular pressure as side effects of drugs.] Fortschr Ophthalmol 1984;81(2):199–200.
27. Strupp M, Jahn K, Brandt T. Another adverse effect of aspirin: bilateral vestibulopathy. J Neurol Neurosurg Psychiatry 2003;74:691.
28. Prince RL, Larkins RG, Alford FP. The effect of acetylsalicylic acid on plasma glucose and the response of glucose regulatory hormones to intravenous glucose and arginine in insulin treated diabetics and normal subjects. Metabolism 1981;30(3):293–8.
29. Manfredini R, Ricci L, Giganti M, La Cecilia O, Kuwornu Afi H, Chierici F, Gallerani M. An uncommon case of fluid retention simulating a congestive heart failure after aspirin consumption. Am J Med Sci 2000;320(1):72–4.
30. Necheles TF, Steinberg MH, Cameron D. Erythrocyte glutathione-peroxidase deficiency. Br J Haematol 1970;19(5):605–12.
31. Meloni T, Forteleoni G, Ogana A, Franca V. Aspirin-induced acute haemolytic anaemia in glucose-6-phosphate dehydrogenase-deficient children with systemic arthritis. Acta Haematol 1989;81(4):208–9.
32. Levy M, Heyman A. Hematological adverse effects of analgesic anti-inflammatory drugs. Hematol Rev 1990;4:177.
33. Williams JO, Mengel CE, Sullivan LW, Haq AS. Megaloblastic anemia associated with chronic ingestion of an analgesic. N Engl J Med 1969;280(6):312–3.
34. Kingham JD, Chen MC, Levy MH. Macular hemorrhage in the aging eye: the effects of anticoagulants. N Engl J Med 1988;318(17):1126–7.
35. Werblin TP, Peiffer RL. Persistent hemorrhage after extracapsular surgery associated with excessive aspirin ingestion. Am J Ophthalmol 1987;104(4):426.

36. Hanley SP, Bevan J, Cockbill SR, Heptinstall S. Differential inhibition by low-dose aspirin of human venous prostacyclin synthesis and platelet thromboxane synthesis. Lancet 1981;1(8227):969–71.

37. The Canadian Cooperative Study Group. A randomized trial of aspirin and sulfinpyrazone in threatened stroke. N Engl J Med 1978;299(2):53–9.

38. ISIS-2 (Second International Study of Infarct Survival) Collaborative Group. Randomised trial of intravenous streptokinase, oral aspirin, both, or neither among 17,187 cases of suspected acute myocardial infarction: ISIS-2. Lancet 1988;2(8607):349–60.

39. The RISC Group. Risk of myocardial infarction and death during treatment with low dose aspirin and intravenous heparin in men with unstable coronary artery disease. Lancet 1990;336(8719):827–30.

40. Dhiwakar M, Khan NA, McClymont LG. Surgical resection of cutaneous head and neck lesions: does aspirin use increase hemorrhagic risk? Arch Otolaryngol Head Neck Surg 2006;132(11):1237–41.

41. Kennedy MT, Roche S, Fleming SM, Lenehan B, Curtin W. The association between aspirin and blood loss in hip fracture patients. Acta Orthop Belg 2006;72(1):29–33.

42. Sirvinskas E, Veikutiene A, Grybauskas P, Cimbolaityte J, Mongirdiene A, Veikutis V, Raliene L. Influence of aspirin or heparin on platelet function and postoperative blood loss after coronary artery bypass surgery. Perfusion 2006;21(1):61–6.

43. Hemelik M, Wahl G, Kessler B. Zahnextraktionen unter Medikation mit Acetylsalicylsäure (ASS). [Tooth extraction under medication with acetylsalicylic acid.] Mund Kiefer Gesichtschir 2006 Jan;10(1):3–6.

44. Blower AL, Brooks A, Fenn GC, Hill A, Pearce MY, Morant S, Bardhan KD. Emergency admissions for upper gastrointestinal disease and their relation to NSAID use. Aliment Pharmacol Ther 1997;11(2):283–91.

45. Piper DW, McIntosh JH, Ariotti DE, Fenton BH, MacLennan R. Analgesic ingestion and chronic peptic ulcer. Gastroenterology 1981;80(3):427–32.

46. Petroski D. Endoscopic comparison of various aspirin preparations-gastric mucosal adaptability to aspirin restudied. Curr Ther Res 1989;45:945.

47. Szabo S. Pathogenesis of gastric mucosal injury. S Afr Med J 1988;74(Suppl):35.

48. Faulkner G, Prichard P, Somerville K, Langman MJ. Aspirin and bleeding peptic ulcers in the elderly. BMJ 1988;297(6659):1311–3.

49. Freeland GR, Northington RS, Hedrich DA, Walker BR. Hepatic safety of two analgesics used over the counter: ibuprofen and aspirin. Clin Pharmacol Ther 1988;43(5):473–9.

50. Hansson L, Zanchetti A, Carruthers SG, Dahlof B, Elmfeldt D, Julius S, Menard J, Rahn KH, Wedel H, Westerling SHOT Study Group. Effects of intensive blood-pressure lowering and low-dose aspirin in patients with hypertension: principal results of the Hypertension Optimal Treatment (HOT) randomised trial. Lancet 1998;351(9118):1755–62.

51. Meade TW, Brennan PJ, Wilkes HC, Zuhrie SR. Thrombosis prevention trial: randomised trial of low-intensity oral anticoagulation with warfarin and low-dose aspirin in the primary prevention of ischaemic heart disease in men at increased risk. The Medical Research Council's General Practice Research Framework. Lancet 1998;351(9098):233–41.

52. Petty GW, Brown RD Jr, Whisnant JP, Sicks JD, O'Fallon WM, Wiebers DO. Frequency of major complications of aspirin, warfarin, and intravenous heparin for secondary stroke prevention. A population-based study. Ann Intern Med 1999;130(1):14–22.

53. Sorensen HT, Mellemkjaer L, Blot WJ, Nielsen GL, Steffensen FH, McLaughlin JK, Olsen JH. Risk of upper gastrointestinal bleeding associated with use of low-dose aspirin. Am J Gastroenterol 2000;95(9):2218–24.

54. Fisher M, Knappertz V. Comments in response to "Analysis of risk of bleeding complications after different doses of aspirin in 192,036 patients enrolled in 31 randomised controlled trials". Am J Cardiol 2005;96(10):1467.

55. Laine L, McQuaid K. Bleeding complications related to aspirin dose. Am J Cardiol 2005;96(7):1035–6.

56. Tramèr MR, Moore RA, Reynolds DJ, McQuay HJ. Quantitative estimation of rare adverse events which follow a biological progression: a new model applied to chronic NSAID use. Pain 2000;85(1–2):169–82.

57. Weil J, Langman MJ, Wainwright P, Lawson DH, Rawlins M, Logan RF, Brown TP, Vessey MP, Murphy M, Colin-Jones DG. Peptic ulcer bleeding: accessory risk factors and interactions with non-steroidal anti-inflammatory drugs. Gut 2000;46(1):27–31.

58. Tramèr MR. Aspirin, like all other drugs, is a poison. BMJ 2000;321(7270):1170–1.

59. Garcia Rodriguez LA, Hernandez-Diaz S, de Abajo FJ. Association between aspirin and upper gastrointestinal complications: systematic review of epidemiologic studies. Br J Clin Pharmacol 2001;52(5):563–71.

60. Bianchine JR, Procter RR, Thomas FB. Piroxicam, aspirin, and gastrointestinal blood loss. Clin Pharmacol Ther 1982;32(2):247–52.

61. Hass WK, Easton JD, Adams HP Jr, Pryse-Phillips W, Molony BA, Anderson S, Kamm BTiclopidine Aspirin Stroke Study Group. A randomized trial comparing ticlopidine hydrochloride with aspirin for the prevention of stroke in high-risk patients. N Engl J Med 1989;321(8):501–7.

62. Lanas A, Serrano P, Bajador E, Esteva F, Benito R, Sainz R. Evidence of aspirin use in both upper and lower gastrointestinal perforation. Gastroenterology 1997;112(3):683–9.

63. Hernández-Díaz S, García Rodríguez LA. Cardioprotective aspirin users and their excess risk of upper gastrointestinal complications. BMC Med 2006;4:22.

64. Bonavina L, DeMeester TR, McChesney L, Schwizer W, Albertucci M, Bailey RT. Drug-induced esophageal strictures. Ann Surg 1987;206(2):173–83.

65. Schreiber JB, Covington JA. Aspirin-induced esophageal hemorrhage. JAMA 1988;259(11):1647–8.

66. Barrier CH, Hirschowitz BI. Controversies in the detection and management of nonsteroidal antiinflammatory drug-induced side effects of the upper gastrointestinal tract. Arthritis Rheum 1989;32(7):926–32.

67. Suazo-Barahona J, Gallegos J, Carmona-Sanchez R, Martinez R, Robles-Diaz G. Nonsteroidal anti-inflammatory drugs and gastrocolic fistula. J Clin Gastroenterol 1998;26(4):343–5.

68. Gutnik SH, Willmott D, Ziebarth J. Gastrocolic fistula-secondary to aspirin abuse. S D J Med 1993;46(10):358–60.

69. Levine MS, Kelly MR, Laufer I, Rubesin SE, Herlinger H. Gastrocolic fistulas: the increasing role of aspirin. Radiology 1993;187(2):359–61.

70. Graham D, Chan F. Endoscopic ulcers with low-dose aspirin and reality testing. Gastroenterology 2005;128(3):807.

71. Mielants H, Verbruggen G, Schelstraete K, Veys EM. Salicylate-induced gastrointestinal bleeding: comparison

between soluble buffered, enteric-coated, and intravenous administration. J Rheumatol 1979;6(2):210–8.

72. Malfertheiner P, Stanescu A, Rogatti W, Ditschuneit H. Effects of microencapsulated vs. enteric-coated acetylsalicylic acid on gastric and duodenal mucosa: an endoscopic study. J Clin Gastroenterol 1988;10(3):269–72.

73. Singh G, Ramey DR, Morfeld D, Shi H, Hatoum HT, Fries JF. Gastrointestinal tract complications of nonsteroidal anti-inflammatory drug treatment in rheumatoid arthritis. A prospective observational cohort study. Arch Intern Med 1996;156(14):1530–6.

74. Ward MR. Reye's syndrome: an update. Nurse Pract 1997;22(12):45–649–50, 52–3.

75. Food and Drug Administration, HHS. Labeling for oral and rectal over-the-couter drug products containing aspirin and nonaspirin salicylates; Reye's Syndrome warning. Final rule. Fed Regist 2003;68(74):18861–9.

76. Zimmerman HJ. Effects of aspirin and acetaminophen on the liver. Arch Intern Med 1981;141(3 Spec No):333–42.

77. Gitlin N. Salicylate hepatotoxicity: the potential role of hypoalbuminemia. J Clin Gastroenterol 1980;2(3):281–5.

78. Belay ED, Bresee JS, Holman RC, Khan AS, Shahriari A, Schonberger LB. Reye's syndrome in the United States from 1981 through 1997. N Engl J Med 1999; 340(18): 1377–82.

79. Langford NJ. Aspirin and Reye's syndrome: is the response appropriate? J Clin Pharm Ther 2002;27(3):157–60.

80. Baron JA. What now for aspirin and cancer prevention? J Natl Cancer Inst 2004;96:22–8.

81. Schernhammer ES, Kang JH, Chan AT, Michaud DS, Skinner HG, Giovannucci E, Colditz GA, Fuchs CS. A prospective study of aspirin use and the risk of pancreatic cancer in women. J Natl Cancer Inst 2004;96:22–8.

82. Plotz PH, Kimberly RP. Acute effects of aspirin and acetaminophen on renal function. Arch Intern Med 1981; 141(3 Spec No):343–8.

83. Segal R, Lubart E, Leibovitz A, Iaina A, Caspi D. Renal effects of low dose aspirin in elderly patients. Isr Med Assoc J 2006;8(10):679–82.

84. Delzell E, Shapiro S. A review of epidemiologic studies of nonnarcotic analgesics and chronic renal disease. Medicine (Baltimore) 1998;77(2):102–21.

85. McLaughlin JK, Lipworth L, Chow WH, Blot WJ. Analgesic use and chronic renal failure: a critical review of the epidemiologic literature. Kidney Int 1998;54(3):679–86.

86. Rexrode KM, Buring JE, Glynn RJ, Stampfer MJ, Youngman LD, Gaziano JM. Analgesic use and renal function in men. JAMA 2001;286(3):315–21.

87. Fored CM, Ejerblad E, Lindblad P, Fryzek JP, Dickman PW, Signorello LB, Lipworth L, Elinder CG, Blot WJ, McLaughlin JK, Zack MM, Nyren O. Acetaminophen, aspirin, and chronic renal failure. N Engl J Med 2001;345(25):1801–8.

88. Ibáñez L, Morlans M, Vidal X, Martínez MJ, Laporte J-R. Case-control study of regular analgesic and nonsteroidal anti-inflammatory use and end-stage renal disease. Kidney Int 2005;67:2393–8.

89. Kanwar AJ, Belhaj MS, Bharija SC, Mohammed M. Drugs causing fixed eruptions. J Dermatol 1984;11(4):383–5.

90. Brandt KD, Palmoski MJ. Effects of salicylates and other nonsteroidal anti-inflammatory drugs on articular cartilage. Am J Med 1984;77(1A):65–9.

91. Pfaar O, Klimek L. Eicosanoids, aspirin-intolerance and the upper airways—current standards and recent improvements of the desensitization therapy. J Physiol Pharmacol 2006;57 Suppl 12:5–13.

92. Stevenson DD, Szczeklik A. Clinical and pathologic perspectives on aspirin sensitivity and asthma. J Allergy Clin Immunol 2006;118(4):773–86.

93. Szczeklik A, Sanak M. The broken balance in aspirin hypersensitivity. Eur J Pharmacol 2006;533(1-3):145–55.

94. Jackowski L, Nowakowski T, Sokal K, Sadłecki W. Zespok ASA-triad u 21-letniej kobiety w 24 tygodniu ciazy. [ASA-triad syndrome in a 21-year-old woman in the 24th week of pregnancy.] Wiad Lek 1980;33(1):53–5.

95. Picado C. Mechanisms of aspirin sensitivity. Curr Allergy Asthma Rep 2006;6(3):198–202.

96. Oates JA, FitzGerald GA, Branch RA, Jackson EK, Knapp HR, Roberts LJ 2nd. Clinical implications of prostaglandin and thromboxane A2 formation (1). N Engl J Med 1988;319(11):689–98.

97. Settipane RA, Constantine HP, Settipane GA. Aspirin intolerance and recurrent urticaria in normal adults and children. Epidemiology and review. Allergy 1980;35(2):149–54.

98. Hedman J, Kaprio J, Poussa T, Nieminen MM. Prevalence of asthma, aspirin intolerance, nasal polyps and chronic obstructive pulmonary disease in a population-based study. Int J Epidemiol 1999;28(4):717–22.

99. Kasper L, Sladek K, Duplaga M, Bochenek G, Liebhart J, Gladysz U, Malolepszy J, Szczeklik A. Prevalence of asthma with aspirin hypersensitivity in the adult population of Poland. Allergy 2003;58(10):1064–6.

100. Vally H, Taylor M, Thompson PJ. The prevalence of aspirin intolerant asthma in Australian asthmatic patients. Thorax 2002;57(7):569–74.

101. Jenkins C, Costello J, Hodge L. Systematic review of prevalence of aspirin-induced asthma and its implications for clinical practice. BMJ 2004;328(7437):434–7.

102. Farr RS, Spector SL, Wangaard CH. Evaluation of aspirin and tartrazine idiosyncrasy. J Allergy Clin Immunol 1979;64(6 pt 2):667–8.

103. Szczeklik A. The cyclooxygenase theory of aspirin-induced asthma. Eur Respir J 1990;3(5):588–93.

104. Bachert C, Wagenmann M, Hauser U, Rudack C. IL-5 synthesis is upregulated in human nasal polyp tissue. J Allergy Clin Immunol 1997;99(6 Pt 1):837–42.

105. Bachert C, Wagenmann M, Rudack C, Höpken K, Hillebrandt M, Wang D, van Cauwenberge P. The role of cytokines in infectious sinusitis and nasal polyposis. Allergy 1998;53(1):2–13.

106. Hamilos DL, Leung DY, Wood R, Cunningham L, Bean DK, Yasruel Z, Schotman E, Hamid Q. Evidence for distinct cytokine expression in allergic versus nonallergic chronic sinusitis. J Allergy Clin Immunol 1995;96(4):537-44.

107. Sladek K, Dworski R, Soja J, Sheller JR, Nizankowska E, Oates JA, Szczeklik A. Eicosanoids in bronchoalveolar lavage fluid of aspirin-intolerant patients with asthma after aspirin challenge. Am J Respir Crit Care Med 1994;149(4 Pt 1):940–6.

108. Szczeklik A, Sladek K, Dworski R, Nizankowska E, Soja J, Oates J. Bronchial aspirin challenge causes specific eicosanoid response in aspirinsensitive asthmatics. Am J Respir Crit Care Med 1996;154 (6 Pt 1):1608–14.

109. Christie PE, Tagari P, Ford-Hutchinson AW, Charlesson S, Chee P, Arm JP, Lee TH. Urinary leukotriene E4 concentrations increase after aspirin challenge in aspirin-sensitive asthmatic subjects. Am Rev Respir Dis 1991;143(5 Pt 1):1025–9.

110. Smith CM, Hawksworth RJ, Thien FC, Christie PE, Lee TH. Urinary leukotriene E4 in bronchial asthma. Eur Respir J 1992;5(6):693–9.

111. Bochenek G, Nagraba K, Nizankowska E, Szczeklik A. A controlled study of 9α11β-PGF2 (a PGD2 metabolite) in plasma and urine of patients with bronchial asthma and healthy controls after aspirin challenges. J Allergy Clin Immunol 2003;111(4):743–9.

112. Sousa A, Parikh A, Scadding G, Corrigan CJ, Lee TH. Leukotriene-receptor expression on nasal mucosal inflammatory cells in aspirin-sensitive rhinosinusitis. N Engl J Med 2002;347(19):1524–6.

113. Sanak M, Levy BD, Clish CB, Chiang N, Gronert K, Mastalerz L, et al. Aspirin-tolerant asthmatics generate more lipoxins than aspirin- intolerant asthmatics. Eur Respir J 2000;16(1):44–9.

114. Schäfer D, Schmid M, Göde UC, Baenkler HW. Dynamics of eicosanoids in peripheral blood cells during bronchial provocation in aspirin-intolerant asthmatics. Eur Respir J 1999;13(3):638–46.

115. Szczeklik A. Aspirin-induced asthma: pathogenesis and clinical presentation. Allergy Proc 1992;13(4):163–73.

116. Owens JM, Shroyer KR, Kingdom TT. Expression of cyclooxygenase and lipoxygenase enzymes in nasal polyps of aspirin-sensitive and aspirin-tolerant patients. Arch Otolaryngol Head Neck Surg 2006;132(6):579–87.

117. Adamjee J, Suh YJ, Park HS, Choi JH, Penrose JF, Lam BK, Austen KF, Cazaly AM, Wilson SJ, Sampson AP. Expression of 5-lipoxygenase and cyclooxygenase pathway enzymes in nasal polyps of patients with aspirin-intolerant asthma. J Pathol 2006;209(3):392–9.

118. Micheletto C, Visconti M, Tognella S, Facchini FM, Dal Negro RW. Aspirin induced asthma (AIA) with nasal polyps has the highest basal LTE4 excretion: a study vs AIA without polyps, mild topic asthma, and normal controls. Eur Ann Allergy Clin Immunol 2006;38(1):20–3.

119. Ying S, Meng Q, Scadding G, Parikh A, Corrigan CJ, Lee TH. Aspirin-sensitive rhinosinusitis is associated with reduced E-prostanoid 2 receptor expression on nasal mucosal inflammatory cells. J Allergy Clin Immunol 2006;117(2):312–8.

120. Lee JY, Kim HM, Ye YM, Bahn JW, Suh CH, Nahm D, Lee HR, Park HS. Role of staphylococcal superantigen-specific IgE antibodies in aspirin-intolerant asthma. Allergy Asthma Proc 2006;27(5):341–6.

121. Kupczyk M, Kupryś I, Danilewicz M, Bocheńska-Marciniak M, Murlewska A, Górski P, Kuna P. Adhesion molecules and their ligands in nasal polyps of aspirin-hypersensitive patients. Ann Allergy Asthma Immunol 2006;96(1):105–11.

122. Lee SH, Rhim T, Choi YS, Min JW, Kim SH, Cho SY, Paik YK, Park CS. Complement C3a and C4a increased in plasma of patients with aspirin-induced asthma. Am J Respir Crit Care Med 2006;173(4):370–8.

123. Kowalski ML, Ptasinska A, Bienkiewicz B, Pawliczak R, DuBuske L, Differential effects of aspirin and misoprostol on 15-hydroxyeicosatetraenoic acid generation by leukocytes from aspirin-sensitive asthmatic patients. J Allergy Clin Immunol 2003;112:505–12.

124. Pierzchalska M, Szabo Z, Sanak M, Soja J, Szczeklik A. Deficient prostaglandin E2 production by bronchial fibroblasts of asthmatic patients, with special reference to aspirin-induced asthma. J Allergy Clin Immunol 2003;111:1041–8.

125. Gyllfors P, Bochenek G, Overholt J, Drupka D, Kumlin M, Sheller J, Nizankowska E, Isakson PC, Mejza F, Lefkowith JB, Dahlen SE, Szczeklik A, Murray JJ, Dahlen B. Biochemical and clinical evidence that aspirin-intolerant asthmatic subjects tolerate the cyclooxygenase 2-selective analgetic drug celecoxib. J Allergy Clin Immunol 2003;111:1116–21.

126. Berges-Gimeno M, Simon RA, Stevenson DD. The natural history and clinical characteristics of aspirin exacerbated respiratory disease. Ann Allergy Asthma Immunol 2002;89(5):474–8.

127. Szczeklik A, Nizankowska E, Duplaga M. Natural history of aspirin-induced asthma. AIANE Investigators. European Network on Aspirin-Induced Asthma. Eur Respir J 2000;16(3):432–6.

128. Yoshida S, Ishizaki Y, Onuma K, Shoji T, Nakagawa H, Amayasu H. Selective cyclo-oxygenase 2 inhibitor in patients with aspirin-induced asthma. J Allergy Clin Immunol 2000;106(6):1201–2.

129. Woessner KM, Simon RA, Stevenson DD. The safety of celecoxib in aspirin exacerbated respiratory disease. Arthritis Rheum 2002;46(8):2201–6.

130. Gyllfors P, Bochenek G, Overholt J, Drupka D, Kumlin M, Sheller J, Nizankowska E, Isakson PC, Mejza F, Lefkowith JB, Dahlén SE, Szczeklik A, Murray JJ, Dahlén B. Biochemical and clinical evidence that aspirin-intolerant asthmatic subjects tolerate the cyclooxygenase 2-selective analgetic drug celecoxib. J Allergy Clin Immunol 2003;111(5):1116–21.

131. El Miedany Y, Youssef S, Ahmed I, El Gaafary M. Safety of etoricoxib, a specific cyclooxygenase-2 inhibitor, in asthmatic patients with aspirin-exacerbated respiratory disease. Ann Allergy Asthma Immunol 2006;97(1):105–9.

132. Viola M, Quaratino D, Volpetti S, Gaeta F, Romano A. Parecoxib tolerability in patients with hypersensitivity to nonsteroidal anti-inflammatory drugs. J Allergy Clin Immunol 2006;117(5):1189–90.

133. Stevenson DD, Simon RA. Lack of cross-reactivity between rofecoxib and aspirin in aspirin sensitive asthmatic patients. J Allergy Clin Immunol 2001;108(1):47–51.

134. Martin-Garcia C, Hinojosa M, Berges P. Safety of a cyclooxygenase-2 inhibitor in patients with aspirin-sensitive asthma. Chest 2002;121(6):1812–7.

135. Szczeklik A, Nizankowska E, Bochenek G, Nagraba K, Mejza F, Swierczynska M. Safety of a specific COX-2 inhibitor in aspirin-induced asthma. Clin Exp Allergy 2001;31(2):219–25.

136. Micheletto C, Tognella S, Guerriero M, Dal Negro R. Nasal and bronchial tolerability of rofecoxib in patients with aspirin induced asthma. Eur Ann Allergy Clin Immunol 2006;38(1):10–14.

137. Woessner K. Cross-reacting drugs and chemicals. Clin Rev Allergy Immunol 2003;24(2):149–58.

138. Mastalerz L, Sanak M, Gawlewicz A, Gielicz A, Faber J, Szczeklik A. Different eicosanoid profile of the hypersensitivity reactions triggered by aspirin and celecoxib in a patient with sinusitis and asthma. J Allergy Clin Immunol 2006;118(4):957–8.

139. Baldassarre S, Schandene L, Choufani G, Michils A. Asthma attacks induced by low doses of celecoxib, aspirin, and acetaminophen. J Allergy Clin Immunol 2006;117(1):215–7.

140. Roll A, Wüthrich B, Schmid-Grendelmeier P, Hofbauer G, Ballmer-Weber BK. Tolerance to celecoxib in patients with a history of adverse reactions to nonsteroidal anti-inflammatory drugs. Swiss Med Wkly 2006;136(43-44):684–90.

141. Wyplosz B, Vautier S, Lillo-Le Louët A, Capron L. Tolerance of diclofenac after hypersensitivity to celecoxib and to nabumetone. Br J Clin Pharmacol 2006;61(4):474.

142. Rodríguez SC, Olguín AM, Miralles CP, Viladrich PF. Characteristics of meningitis caused by ibuprofen: report of 2 cases with recurrent episodes and review of the literature. Medicine (Baltimore) 2006;85(4):214–20.

143. Passero M. Cyclo-oxygenase-2 inhibitors in aspirin-sensitive asthma. Chest 2003;123(6):2155–6.

144. Bavbek S, Celik G, Ozer F, Mungan D, Misirligil Z. Safety of selective COX-2 inhibitors in aspirin/NSAID intolerant patients: comparison of nimesulide, meloxicam and rofecoxib. J Asthma 2004;41(1):67–75.

145. Morias-Almeida Marinho S, Rosa S, Rosado-Pinto JE. Multiple drug intolerance, including etoricoxib. Allergy 2006;61(1):144–5.

146. Settipane RA, Stevenson DD. Cross sensitivity with acetaminophen in aspirin-sensitive subjects with asthma. J Allergy Clin Immunol 1989;84(1):26–33.

147. Loehrl TA, Ferre RM, Toohill RJ, Smith TL. Long-term asthma outcomes after endoscopic sinus surgery in aspirin triad patients. Am J Otolaryngol 2006;27(3):154–60.

148. Sola Alberich R, Jammoul A, Masana L. Henoch-Schonlein purpura associated with acetylsalicylic acid. Ann Intern Med 1997;126(8):665.

149. Martelli NA. Bronchial and intravenous provocation tests with indomethacin in aspirin-sensitive asthmatics. Am Rev Respir Dis 1979;120(5):1073–9.

150. Ritter JM, Taylor GW. Fish oil in asthma. Thorax 1988;43(2):81–3.

151. Sanak M, Simon HU, Szczeklik A. Leukotriene C4 synthase promotor polymorphism and risk of aspirin-induced asthma. Lancet 1997;350(9091):1599–600.

152. Van Sambeek R, Stevenson DD, Baldasaro M, Lam BK, Zhao J, Yoshida S, et al. 5' flanking region polymorphism of the gene encoding leukotriene C4 synthase does not correlate with the aspirin-intolerant asthma phenotype in the United States. J Allergy Clin Immunol 2000;106(1 Pt 1):72–6.

153. Sanak M, Szczeklik A. Leukotriene C4 synthase polymorphism and aspirin-induced asthma. J Allergy Clin Immunol 2001;107(3):561–2.

154. Choi JH, Kim SH, Bae JS, Yu HL, Suh CH, Nahm DH, Park HS. Lack of an association between a newly identified promoter polymorphism (−1702G>A) of the leukotriene C4 synthase gene and aspirin-intolerant asthma in a Korean population. Tohoku J Exp Med 2006;208(1):49–56.

155. Jinnai N, Sakagami T, Sekigawa T, Kakihara M, Nakajima T, Yoshida K, Goto S, Hasegawa T, Koshino T, Hasegawa Y, Inoue H, Suzuki N, Sano Y, Inoue I. Polymorphisms in the prostaglandin E2 receptor subtype 2 gene confer susceptibility to aspirin-intolerant asthma: a candidate gene approach. Hum Mol Genet 2004;13(24):3203–17.

156. Choi JH, Lee KW, Oh HB, Lee KJ, Suh YJ, Park CS, Park HS. HLA association in aspirin intolerant asthma: DPB1*0301 as a strong marker in a Korean population. J Allergy Clin Immunol 2004;113(3):562–4.

157. Sakagami T, Jinnai N, Nakajima T, Sekigawa T, Hasegawa T, Suzuki E, Inoue I, Gejyo F. ADAM33 polymorphisms are associated with aspirin-intolerant asthma in the Japanese population. J Hum Genet 2007;52(1):66–72.

158. Kim SH, Bae JS, Holloway JW, Lee JT, Suh CH, Nahm DH, Park HS. A polymorphism of MS4A2 (−109T > C) encoding the beta-chain of the high-affinity immunoglobulin E receptor (FcεR1β) is associated with a susceptibility to aspirin-intolerant asthma. Clin Exp Allergy 2006;36(7):877–83.

159. Modrzyński M, Mazurek H, Zawisza E. Ocena przydatności testu donosowej prowokacji z aspiryna lizynowa w diagnostyce przewlekłych eozynofilowych nieżytów nosa. [Nasal provocation test with lysine aspirin in diagnosis of nonallergic rhinitis with eosinophilia.] Otolaryngol Pol 2006;60(1):25–31.

160. White A, Bigby T, Stevenson D. Intranasal ketorolac challenge for the diagnosis of aspirin-exacerbated respiratory disease. Ann Allergy Asthma Immunol 2006;97(2):190–5.

161. Asero R. Use of ketoprofen oral challenges to detect cross-reactors among patients with a history of aspirin-induced urticaria. Ann Allergy Asthma Immunol 2006;97(2):187–9.

162. de Weck AL, Gamboa PM, Esparza R, Sanz ML. Hypersensitivity to aspirin and other nonsteroidal anti-inflammatory drugs (NSAIDs). Curr Pharm Des 2006;12(26):3347–58.

163. Kleine-Tebbe J, Erdmann S, Knol EF, MacGlashan DW Jr, Poulsen LK, Gibbs BF. Diagnostic tests based on human basophils: potentials, pitfalls and perspectives. Int Arch Allergy Immunol 2006;141(1):79–90.

164. Velten FW, Bayerl C, Baenkler HW, Schaefer D. Functional eicosanoid test and typing (FET) in acetylsalicylic acid intolerant patients with urticaria. J Physiol Pharmacol 2006;57 Suppl 12:35–46.

165. Mastalerz L, Sanak M, Gawlewicz A, Gielicz A, Faber J, Szczeklik A. Different eicosanoid profile of the hypersensitivity reactions triggered by aspirin and celecoxib in a patient with sinusitis, asthma, and urticaria. J Allergy Clin Immunol 2006;118(4):957–8.

166. White A, Ludington E, Mehra P, Stevenson DD, Simon RA. Effect of leukotriene modifier drugs on the safety of oral aspirin challenges. Ann Allergy Asthma Immunol 2006;97(5):688–93.

167. Stevenson DD, Simon RA, Mathison DA. Aspirin-sensitive asthma: tolerance to aspirin after positive oral aspirin challenges. J Allergy Clin Immunol 1980;66(1):82–8.

168. Stevenson DD, Pleskow WW, Simon RA, Mathison DA, Lumry WR, Schatz M, Zeiger RS. Aspirin-sensitive rhinosinusitis asthma: a double blind cross over study of treatment with aspirin. J Allergy Clin Immunol 1984;73(4):500–7.

169. Sweet J, Stevenson DD, Simon RA, Mathison DA. Long-term effects of aspirin desensitization—treatment for aspirin-sensitive rhinosinusitis–asthma. J Allergy Clin Immunol 1990;85(1 Pt 1):59–65.

170. Stevenson DD, Hankammer MA, Mathison DA, Christiansen SC, Simon RA. Aspirin desensitization treatment of aspirin-sensitive patients with rhinosinusitis-asthma: long-term outcomes. J Allergy Clin Immunol 1996;98(4):751–8.

171. Parikh AA, Scadding GK. Intranasal lysine-aspirin in aspirin-sensitive nasal polyposis: a controlled trial. Laryngoscope 2005;115(8):1385–390.

172. Patriarca G, Schiavino D, Nucera E, Papa G, Schinco G, Fais G. Prevention of relapse in nasal polyposis. Lancet 1991;337(8755):148.

173. Schmitz-Schumann M, Schaub E, Virchow C. Inhalative Provokation mit Lysin-Azetylsalizylsaure bei Analgetika-Asthme-Syndrom. [Inhalation provocation test with lysine-acetylsalicylic acid in patients with analgesic-induced asthma.] Prax Klin Pneumol 1982;36(1):17–21.

174. Berges-Gimeno MP, Simon RA, Stevenson DD. Long-term treatment with aspirin desensitization in asthmatic patients with aspirin-exacerbated respiratory disease. J Allergy Clin Immunol 2003;111(1):180–6.

175. White AA, Hope AP, Stevenson DD. Failure to maintain an aspirin-desensitized state in a patient with aspirin-exacerbated respiratory disease. Ann Allergy Asthma Immunol 2006;97(4):446–8.

176. Anonymous. Aspirin sensitivity in asthmatics. BMJ 1980;281(6246):958–9.

177. Pleskow WW, Stevenson DD, Mathison DA, Simon RA, Schatz M, Zeiger RS. Aspirin desensitization in aspirin-sensitive asthmatic patients: clinical manifestations and characterization of the refractory period. J Allergy Clin Immunol 1982;69(1 Pt 1):11–9.

178. Stevenson DD, Simon RA. Selection of patients for aspirin desensitization treatment. J Allergy Clin Immunol 2006;118(4):801–4.

179. Alijotas-Reig J, San Miguel-Moncín M, Cisteró-Bahíma A. Aspirin desensitization in the treatment of antiphospholipid syndrome during pregnancy in ASA-sensitive patients. Am J Reprod Immunol 2006;55(1):45–50.

180. Silberman S, Neukirch-Stoop C, Steg PG. Rapid desensitization procedure for patients with aspirin hypersensitivity undergoing coronary stenting. Am J Cardiol 2005;95(4):509–10.

181. Ohmori T, Yatomi Y, Nonaka T, Kobayashi Y, Madoiwa S, Mimuro J, Ozaki Y, Sakata Y. Aspirin resistance detected with aggregometry cannot be explained by cyclooxygenase activity: involvement of other signaling pathway(s) in cardiovascular events of aspirin-treated patients. J Thromb Haemost 2006;4(6):1271–8.

182. Cox D, Maree AO, Dooley M, Conroy R, Byrne MF, Fitzgerald DJ. Effect of enteric coating on antiplatelet activity of low-dose aspirin in healthy volunteers. Stroke 2006;37(8):2153–8.

183. Marcucci R, Paniccia R, Antonucci E, Gori AM, Fedi S, Giglioli C, Valente S, Prisco D, Abbate R, Gensini GF. Usefulness of aspirin resistance after percutaneous coronary intervention for acute myocardial infarction in predicting one-year major adverse coronary events. Am J Cardiol 2006;98(9):1156–9.

184. Ruef J, Kranzhöfer R. Coronary stent thrombosis related to aspirin resistance: what are the underlying mechanisms? J Interv Cardiol 2006;19(6):507–9.

185. Pulcinelli FM, Riondino S. More on aspirin resistance: position paper of the Working Group on Aspirin Resistance. Proposal for a laboratory test guiding algorithm. J Thromb Haemost 2006;4(2):485–7.

186. Dubach UC, Rosner B, Pfister E. Epidemiologic study of abuse of analgesics containing phenacetin. Renal morbidity and mortality (1968-1979). N Engl J Med 1983;308(7):357–62.

187. Dubach UC, Rosner B, Sturmer T. An epidemiologic study of abuse of analgesic drugs. Effects of phenacetin and salicylate on mortality and cardiovascular morbidity (1968 to 1987). N Engl J Med 1991;324(3):155–60.

188. Gago-Dominguez M, Yuan JM, Castelao JE, Ross RK, Yu MC. Regular use of analgesics is a risk factor for renal cell carcinoma. Br J Cancer 1999;81(3):542–8.

189. Keim SA, Klebanoff MA. Aspirin use and miscarriage risk. Epidemiology 2006;17(4):435–9.

190. Slone D, Siskind V, Heinonen OP, Monson RR, Kaufman DW, Shapiro S. Aspirin and congenital malformations. Lancet 1976;1(7974):1373–5.

191. Werler MM, Mitchell AA, Shapiro S. The relation of aspirin use during the first trimester of pregnancy to congenital cardiac defects. N Engl J Med 1989;321(24):1639–42.

192. Rumack CM, Guggenheim MA, Rumack BH, Peterson RG, Johnson ML, Braithwaite WR. Neonatal intracranial hemorrhage and maternal use of aspirin. Obstet Gynecol 1981;58(Suppl 5):S52–6.

193. Shapiro S, Siskind V, Monson RR, Heinonen OP, Kaufman DW, Slone D. Perinatal mortality and birthweight in relation to aspirin taken during pregnancy. Lancet 1976;1(7974):1375–6.

194. Uzan S, Beaufils M, Breart G, Bazin B, Capitant C, Paris J. Prevention of fetal growth retardation with low-dose aspirin: findings of the EPREDA trial. Lancet 1991; 337(8755):1427–31.

195. Kim SH, Ye YM, Lee SK, Park HS. Genetic mechanism of aspirin-induced urticaria/angioedema. Curr Opin Allergy Clin Immunol 2006;6(4):266–70.

196. Kim SH, Park HS. Genetic markers for differentiating aspirin-hypersensitivity. Yonsei Med J 2006;47(1):15–21.

197. Pacor ML, Di Lorenzo G, Mansueto P, Martinelli N, Esposito-Pellitteri M, Pradella P, Uxa L, Di Fede G, Rini G, Corrocher R. Relationship between human leucocyte antigen class I and class II and chronic idiopathic urticaria associated with aspirin and/or NSAIDs hypersensitivity. Mediators Inflamm 2006;2006(5):6248.

198. Kim SH, Choi JH, Lee KW, Kim SH, Shin ES, Oh HB, Suh CH, Nahm DH, Park HS. The human leucocyte antigen-DRB1*1302-DQB1*0609-DPB1*0201 haplotype may be a strong genetic marker for aspirin-induced urticaria. Clin Exp Allergy 2005;35(3):339–44.

199. Mastalerz L, Setkowicz M, Sanak M, Rybarczyk H, Szczeklik A. Familial aggregation of aspirin-induced urticaria and leukotriene C synthase allelic variant. Br J Dermatol 2006;154(2):256–60.

200. Torres-Galván MJ, Ortega N, Sánchez-García F, Blanco C, Carrillo T, Quiralte J. LTC4-synthase A-444C polymorphism: lack of association with NSAID-induced isolated periorbital angioedema in a Spanish population. Ann Allergy Asthma Immunol 2001;87(6):506–10.

201. Kim SH, Choi JH, Holloway JW, Suh CH, Nahm DH, Ha EH, Park CS, Park HS. Leukotriene-related gene polymorphisms in patients with ASA-induced urticaria and ASA-intolerant asthma: differing contributions of ALOX5 polymorphism in Korean population. J Korean Med Sci 2005;20(6):926–31.

202. Mastalerz L, Setkowicz M, Sanak M, Rybarczyk H, Szczeklik A. Familial aggregation of aspirin-induced urticaria and leukotriene C synthase allelic variant. Br J Dermatol 2006;154(2):256–60.

203. Choi JH, Kim SH, Suh CH, Nahm DH, Park HS. Polymorphisms of high-affinity IgE receptor and histamine-related genes in patients with ASA-induced urticaria/angioedema. J Korean Med Sci 2005;20(3):367–72.

204. Bae JS, Kim SH, Ye YM, Yoon HJ, Suh CH, Nahm DH, Park HS. Significant association of FcεRIα promoter polymorphisms with aspirin-intolerant chronic urticaria. J Allergy Clin Immunol 2007;119(2):449–56.

205. Anonymous. Poisoning with enteric-coated aspirin. Lancet 1981;2(8238):130.

206. Pierce RP, Gazewood J, Blake RL Jr. Salicylate poisoning from enteric-coated aspirin. Delayed absorption may complicate management. Postgrad Med 1991;89(5):61–4.

207. Temple AR. Acute and chronic effects of aspirin toxicity and their treatment. Arch Intern Med 1981;141(3 Spec No):364–9.

208. Meredith TJ, Vale JA. Non-narcotic analgesics. Problems of overdosage. Drugs 1986;32(Suppl 4):177–205.

209. Pena-Alonso YR, Montoya-Cabrera MA, Bustos-Cordoba E, Marroquin-Yanez L, Olivar-Lopez V. Aspirin intoxication in a child associated with myocardial necrosis: is a drug-related lesion? Pediatr Dev Pathol 2003;6:342–7.

210. Reingardiene D, Lazauskas R. Apsinuodijimas salicilatais. [Acute salicylate poisoning.] Medicina (Kaunas) 2006;42(1):79–83.

211. Rauschka H, Aboul-Enein F, Bauer J, Nobis H, Lassmann H, Schmidbauer M. Acute cerebral white matter damage in lethal salicylate intoxication. Neurotoxicology 2007;28(1):33–7.

212. Dove DJ, Jones T. Delayed coma associated with salicylate intoxication. J Pediatr 1982;100(3):493–6.

213. Al-Khadra AS, Salem DN, Rand WM, Udelson JE, Smith

JJ, Konstam MA. Antiplatelet agents and survival: a cohort analysis from the Studies on Ventricular Dysfunction (SOLVD) trial. J Am Coll Cardiol 1998;31:419–25.

214. Nguyen KN, Aursnes I, Kjekshus J. Interaction between enalapril and aspirin on mortality after acute myocardial infarction: subgroup analysis of the Cooperative New Scandinavian Enalapril Survival Study II (CONSENSUS II). Am J Cardiol 1997;79:115–19.

215. Baur LH, Schipperheyn JJ, Van den Laarse A, Souverijin JH, Frolich M, De Groot Voogd PJ, Vroom TF, Cats VM, Keirse MJ, Bruschke AVG. Combining salicylate and enalapril in patients with coronary artery disease and heart failure. Br Heart J 1995;73:227–36.

216. Van Wijngaarden J, Smit AJ, De Graeff PA, Van Glist WH, Van der Broek SA, Van Veldhuisen DJ, Lie KI, Wesseling H. Effects of acetylsalicylic acid on peripheral hemodynamics in patients chronic heart failure treated with angiotensin-converting enzyme inhibitors. J Cardiovasc Pharmacol 1994;23:240–5.

217. Oosterga M, Anthonio RL, de Kam PJ, Kingma JH, Crijns HJ, Van Gilst WH. Effects of aspirin on angiotensin-converting enzyme inhibition and left ventricular dilatation one year after acute myocardial infarction. Am J Cardiol 1998;81:1178–81.

218. Leor J, Reicher-Reiss H, Goldbourt U, Boyko V, Gottlieb S, Battler A, Behar S. Aspirin and mortality in patients treated with angiotensin-converting enzyme inhibitors: a cohort study of 11,575 patients with coronary artery disease. J Am Coll Cardiol 2000;35:817–9.

219. Latini R, Tognoni G, Maggioni AP, Baigent C, Braunwald E, Chen ZM, Collins R, Flather M, Franzosi MG, Kjekashus J, Kober L, Liu LS, Peto R, Pfeffer M, Pizzetti F, Santoro E, Sleight P, Swedberg K, Tavazzi L, Wang W, Yusuf S. Clinical effects of early angiotensin-converting enzyme inhibitor treatment for acute myocardial infarction are similar in the presence and absence of aspirin: systematic overview of individual data from 96,712 randomized patients. Angiotensin-converting Enzyme Inhibitor Myocardial Infarct Collaborative Group. J Am Coll Cardiol 2000;35:1801–7.

220. Nawarskas JJ, Spinler SA. Does aspirin interfere with the therapeutic efficacy of angiotensin-converting enzyme inhibitors in hypertension or congestive heart failure. Pharmacotherapy 1998;18:1041–52.

221. Teo KK, Yusuf S, Pfeffer M, Torp-Pedersen C, Kober L, Hall A, Pogue J, Latini R, Collins R. ACE Inhibitors Collaborative Group. Effects of long-term treatment with angiotensin-converting-enzyme inhibitors in the presence or absence of aspirin: a systematic review. Lancet 2002;360:1037–43.

222. The SOLVD investigators. Effect of enalapril on survival in patients with reduced left ventricular ejection fractions and congestive heart failure. N Engl J Med 1991;325:293-30.

223. The SOLVD investigators. Effects of enalapril on mortality and the development of heart failure in asymptomatic patients with reduced left ventricular ejection fractions. N Engl J Med 1991;327:685–91.

224. Pfeffer MA, Braunwald E, Moye LA, Basta L, Brown EJ Jr, Cuddy TE, Davis BR, Geltman EM, Goldman S, Flaker GC, Klein M, Lamas GA, Packer M, Rouleau J, Rouleau JL, Rutherford J, Wertheimer JH, Hawkins CM. Effect of captopril on mortality and morbidity in patients with left ventricular dysfunction after myocardial infarction. Results of the survival and ventricular enlargement trial. The SAVE Investigators. N Engl J Med 1992;327:669–77.

225. The Acute Infarction Ramipril Efficacy (AIRE) Study Investigators. Effect of ramipril on mortality and morbidity of survivors of acute myocardial infarction with clinical evidence of heart failure. Lancet 1993;342:821–8.

226. Kober L, Torp-Pederson C, Carlsen JE, Bagger H, Eliasen P, Lyngborg K, Videbaek J, Cole DS, Aucler L, Pauly NC. A clinical trial of the angiotensin-converting-enzyme inhibitor trandolapril in patients with left ventricular dysfunction after myocardial infarction. Trandolapril Cardiac Evaluation (TRACE) Study Group. N Engl J Med 1995;333:1670–6.

227. The Heart Outcomes Prevention Evaluation Investigators. Effect of an angiotensin converting enzyme inhibitors ramipril, on cardiovascular events in high risk patients. N Engl J Med 2000;324:145–53.

228. Langman M, Kong SX, Zhang Q, Kahler KH, Finch E. Safety and patient tolerance of standard and slow-release formulation. NSAIDs. Pharmacoepidemiol Drug Saf 2003;12:61–6.

229. Aumègeat V, Lamblin N, De Groote P, Mc Fadden EP, Millaire A, Bauters C, Lablanche JM. Aspirin does not adversely affect survival in patients with stable congestive heart failure treated with angiotensin-converting enzyme inhibitors. Chest 2003;124:1250–8.

230. Guazzi M, Brambilla R, Reina G, Tuminello G, Guazzi MD. Aspirin-angiotensin-converting enzyme inhibitor coadministration and mortality in patients with heart failure a dose-related adverse effect of aspirin. Arch Intern Med 2003;163:1574–9.

231. Deykin D, Janson P, McMahon L. Ethanol potentiation of aspirin-induced prolongation of the bleeding time. N Engl J Med 1982;306(14):852–4.

232. Anonymous. Alcohol warning on over-the-counter pain medications. WHO Drug Inf 1998;12:16.

233. Flaker GC, Gruber M, Connolly SJ, Goldman S, Chaparro S, Vahanian A, Halinen MO, Horrow J, Halperin JL; SPORTIF Investigators. Risks and benefits of combining aspirin with anticoagulant therapy in patients with atrial fibrillation: an exploratory analysis of stroke prevention using an oral thrombin inhibitor in atrial fibrillation (SPORTIF) trials. Am Heart J 2006;152(5):967–73.

234. Khurram Z, Chou E, Minutello R, Bergman G, Parikh M, Naidu S, Wong SC, Hong MK. Combination therapy with aspirin, clopidogrel and warfarin following coronary stenting is associated with a significant risk of bleeding. J Invasive Cardiol 2006;18(4):162–4.

235. Diener HC, Cunha L, Forbes C, Sivenius J, Smets P, Lowenthal AEuropean Stroke Prevention Study. 2. Dipyridamole and acetylsalicylic acid in the secondary prevention of stroke. J Neurol Sci 1996;143(1-2):1–13.

236. Enquete de prevention secondaire de l'infarctus du Myocarde' Research Group. A controlled comparison of aspirin and oral anticoagulants in prevention of death after myocardial infarction. N Engl J Med 1982;307(12):701–8.

237. Moore TJ, Crantz FR, Hollenberg NK, Koletsky RJ, Leboff MS, Swartz SL, Levine L, Podolsky S, Dluhy RG, Williams GH. Contribution of prostaglandins to the antihypertensive action of captopril in essential hypertension. Hypertension 1981;3(2):168–73.

238. Cowan RA, Hartnell GG, Lowdell CP, Baird IM, Leak AM. Metabolic acidosis induced by carbonic anhydrase inhibitors and salicylates in patients with normal renal function. BMJ (Clin Res Ed) 1984;289(6441):347–8.

239. Gille J, Bernotat J, Bohm S, Behrens P, Lohr JF. Spontaneous hemarthrosis of the knee associated with clopidogrel and aspirin treatment. Z Rheumatol 2003;62:80–1.

240. CAPRIE Steering Committee. A randomised, blinded, trial of clopidogrel versus aspirin in patients at risk of ischaemic events (CAPRIE). Lancet 1996;348(9038):1329–39.

241. Diener HC, Bogousslavsky J, Brass LM, Cimminiello C, Csiba L, Kaste M, Leys D, Matias-Guiu J, Rupprecht HJ; Match investigators. Aspirin and clopidogrel compared with clopidogrel alone after recent ischaemic stroke or transient ischaemic attack in high-risk patients (MATCH): randomised, double-blind, placebo-controlled trial. Lancet 2004;364:331–7.

242. Moore M, Power M. Perioperative hemorrhage and combined clopidogrel and aspirin therapy. Anesthesiology 2004;101:792–4.

243. Brooks PM, Day RO. Nonsteroidal antiinflammatory drugs—differences and similarities. N Engl J Med 1991;324(24):1716–25.

244. McInnes GT, Brodie MJ. Drug interactions that matter. A critical reappraisal. Drugs 1988;36(1):83–110.

245. Levine MN, Raskob G, Landefeld S, Kearon C. Hemorrhagic complications of anticoagulant treatment. Chest 1998;114(Suppl 5):S511–23.

246. World Health Organization (WHO). Mechanism of action, safety and efficacy of intrauterine devices. In: Technical Report Series 753. Geneva: WHO, 1987:91.

247. Croxatto HB, Ortiz ME, Valdez E. IUD mechanisms of action. In: Bardin CW, Mishell DR, editors. Proceedings from the 4th International Conference on IUDs. Boston: Butterworth-Heinemann, 1994:44.

248. Offerhaus L. Drug interactions at excretory mechanisms. Pharmacol Ther 1981;15(1):69–78.

249. Lanas A, Bajador E, Serrano P, Arroyo M, Fuentes J, Santolaria S. Effects of nitrate and prophylactic aspirin on upper gastrointestinal bleeding: a retrospective case-control study. J Int Med Res 1998;26(3):120–8.

250. Sweeney CJ, Takimoto CH, Latz JE, Baker SD, Murry DJ, Krull JH, Fife K, Battiato L, Cleverly A, Chaudhary AK, Chaudhuri T, Sandler A, Mita AC, Rowinsky EK. Two drug interaction studies evaluating the pharmacokinetics and toxicity of pemetrexed when coadministered with aspirin or ibuprofen in patients with advanced cancer. Clin Cancer Res 2006;12(2):536–42.

251. Orr JM, Abbott FS, Farrell K, Ferguson S, Sheppard I, Godolphin W. Interaction between valproic acid and aspirin in epileptic children: serum protein binding and metabolic effects. Clin Pharmacol Ther 1982;31(5):642–9.

252. Abbott FS, Kassam J, Orr JM, Farrell K. The effect of aspirin on valporic acid metabolism. Clin Pharmacol Ther 1986;40(1):94–100.

253. Sandson NB, Marcucci C, Bourke DL, Smith-Lamacchia R. An interaction between aspirin and valproate: the relevance of plasma protein displacement drug–drug interactions. Am J Psychiatry 2006;163(11):1891–6.

254. Multicentre Acute Stroke Trial—Italy (MAST-I) Group. Randomised controlled trial of streptokinase, aspirin, and combination of both in treatment of acute ischaemic stroke. Lancet 1995;346(8989):1509–14.

255. Ciccone A, Motto C, Aritzu E, Piana A, Candelise L. Negative interaction of aspirin and streptokinase in acute ischemic stroke: further analysis of the Multicenter Acute Stroke Trial—Italy. Cerebrovasc Dis 2000;10(1):61–4.

256. Akyol SM, Thompson M, Kerr DN. Renal function after prolonged consumption of aspirin. BMJ (Clin Res Ed) 1982;284(6316):631–2.

257. Harris M, Bryant LR, Danaher P, Alloway J. Effect of low dose daily aspirin on serum urate levels and urinary excretion in patients receiving probenecid for gouty arthritis. J Rheumatol 2000;27(12):2873–6.

258. Samuels MH, Pillote K, Ashex D, Nelson JC. Variable effects of nonsteroidal antiinflammatory agents on thyroid test results. J Clin Endocrinol Metab 2003;88(12):5710–6.

259. Harris WS, Silveira S, Dujovne CA. The combined effects of N-3 fatty acids and aspirin on hemostatic parameters in man. Thromb Res 1990;57(4):517–26.

260. Svaneborg N, Kristensen SD, Hansen LM, Bullow I, Husted SE, Schmidt EB. The acute and short-time effect of supplementation with the combination of N-3 fatty acids and acetylsalicylic acid on platelet function and plasma lipids. Thromb Res 2002;105(4):311–6.

261. Engstrom K, Wallin R, Saldeen T. Effect of low-dose aspirin in combination with stable fish oil on whole blood production of eicosanoids. Prostaglandins Leukot Essent Fatty Acids 2001;64(6):291–7.

262. Faust TW, Redfern JS, Podolsky I, Lee E, Grundy SM, Feldman M. Effects of aspirin on gastric mucosal prostaglandin E2 and F2 alpha content and on gastric mucosal injury in humans receiving fish oil or olive oil. Gastroenterology 1990;98(3):586–91.

Ademetionine

General Information

Ademetionine (S-adenosylmethionine) has anti-inflammatory and analgesic effects in animals. Convincing evidence of these effects in man is still lacking. In trials in osteoarthritis, as presented at a symposium organized by the manufacturers (and thus open to selection bias), ademetionine was well tolerated (1). In a large, uncontrolled, short-term Phase IV trial, adverse effects (moderate or severe) were reported by 21% of the patients, with withdrawal in 5.2%. Adverse effects were mainly gastrointestinal (nausea, stomachache, heartburn, diarrhea), CNS symptoms (headache, dizziness, sleep disturbances, fatigue), and skin rashes.

Reference

1. di Padova C. S-adenosylmethionine in the treatment of osteoarthritis. Review of the clinical studies. Am J Med 1987;83(5A):60–5.

Aminophenazone (amidopyrine)

General Information

Aminophenazone (amidopyrine) is the most toxic and most dangerous anti-inflammatory analgesic. Blood dyscrasias have been documented beyond any doubt, perhaps due to a hypersensitivity mechanism. The Committee on the Safety of Drugs of the Japanese Pharmaceutical Affairs Bureau has ordered its withdrawal because of its serious adverse effects (SEDA-12, 82) and it has been withdrawn in most developed countries. However, aminophenazone is still used in some developing countries (1).

Organs and Systems

Hematologic

Aminophenazone causes severe bone marrow depression, usually with a fulminant course and a high mortality (SED-9, 146) (2,3). Specific antibodies and leukoagglutinins are sometimes found (4). Agranulocytosis is caused by arrest of maturation at the metamyelocyte stage (5).

Fatal thrombocytopenia has been reported in a breast-feeding infant after the administration of aminophenazone suppositories (6).

Gastrointestinal

Gastrotoxicity with aminophenazone is less common than with other analgesic/anti-inflammatory drugs, probably because of its weaker anti-inflammatory effect.

Liver

Aminophenazone is not hepatotoxic, but liver damage can occur in the course of a general hypersensitivity reaction (7).

Urinary tract

Albuminuria, hematuria, and acute renal insufficiency have been observed, and aminophenazone causes direct renal damage even at therapeutic doses. It can also contribute to analgesic nephropathy (SED-8, 211) (8,9).

Skin

Toxic epidermal necrolysis, exfoliative dermatitis, and Stevens–Johnson syndrome have been described (SED-8, 210) (10–13).

Immunologic

A range of allergic skin reactions, acute anaphylactic shock, acute bronchospasm (in predisposed patients), and cross-sensitivity to aspirin have been reported (14).

Long-Term Effects

Tumorigenicity

Aminophenazone and its derivatives may be metabolized to carcinogenic nitrosamines. The clinical importance of this is not clear (SEDA-2, 389) (15).

Drug Administration

Drug overdose

In overdose, aminophenazone mainly affects the central nervous system, causing coma and convulsions, and the liver (16). Fatal intoxication has occurred in infants (17).

References

1. Epstein P, Yudkin JS. Agranulocytosis in Mozambique due to amidopyrine, a drug withdrawn in the west. Lancet 1980;2(8188):254–5.
2. Pisciotta AV. Drug-induced leukopenia and aplastic anemia. Clin Pharmacol Ther 1971;12(1):13–43.
3. Pisciotta V. Drug-induced agranulocytosis. Drugs 1978;15(2):132–43.
4. Barrett AJ, Weller E, Rozengurt N, Longhurst P, Humble JG. Amidopyrine agranulocytosis:drug inhibition of granulocyte colonies in the presence of patient's serum. BMJ 1976;2(6040):850–1.
5. Goudemand J, Plouvier J, Bauters F, Goudemand M. Les agranulocytoses aigues induites parle pyramidon ou les phenothiazines. A propos de 31 observations. [Acute agranulocytosis induced by pyramidon or phenothiazines. Apropos of 31 cases.] Sem Hop 1976;52(25–28):1513–20.
6. Ionescu D, Lunganoiu N. Sindrom hemoragipar trombocitopenic letal dupa aminofenazona la sugar. [A fatal thrombocytopenic hemorrhagiparous syndrome following aminophenazone in an infant.] Pediatrie (Bucur) 1991;40(1–2):169–72.
7. Scholz H, Meyer W. Akute Agranulozytose und intrahepatische Cholestase nach Aminophenazon bei einem 12 jahrigen Madchen. [Aminophenazone induced agranulocytosis and intrahepatic cholestasis in a 12-year-old girl.] Dtsch Gesundheitsw 1972;27(5):205–9.
8. Eknoyan G, Matson JL. Acute renal failure caused by aminopyrine. JAMA 1964;90:34–5.
9. Baumgartner H, Scheitlin W, von Rechenberg HK. [Bilateral renal cortical necrosis following pyrazolone treatment.]Dtsch Med Wochenschr 1967;2(23):1075–7.
10. Zombai E, Grof PA. Lyellbetegseg allergias jellegerol. Borgyogy Venerol Sz 1971;7:119.
11. Huriez C, Bergoend H, Bertez M. Vingt-trois cas de toxidermies bulleuses graves avec epidermolyse: part predominante d'anti-infectieux retard et de plurimedications. [23 cases of severe bullous toxicoderma with epidermolysis: predominant role of delayed-action anti-infectious agents and of plurimedications.] Bull Acad Natl Med 1972;156(1):12–8.
12. Kauppinen K. Lyellin syndrooma. [Lyell's syndrome.] Duodecim 1971;7(5):355–61.
13. Schmidt JG, Lischka G. Zur ophthalmologischen Symptomatologie, Therapie und Prognose des Fuchs- und Lyell-syndroms. [Ophthalmological symptomatology, therapy and prognosis of Fuch's and Lyell's syndromes.] Klin Monatsbl Augenheilkd 1970;157(3):342–57.
14. Bartoli E, Faedda in Masala R, Chiandussi L. Letter: Drug-induced asthma. Lancet 1976;1(7973):1357.
15. World Health Organisation. Aminophenazone a possible cancer hazard? WHO Drug Info 1977;9Jul-Sep.
16. Cervini C. Ipirazolonici: gli effetti indesiderati. [Pyrazolones: undesired effects.] Clin Ter 1972;60(4):305–18.
17. Tronzano L. Avvelenamento acuto mortale da iperdosaggio di piramidone in un lattante. [Fatal acute poisoning caused by an overdose of pyramidon in an infant.] Minerva Medicoleg 1968;88(1):71–6.

Benorilate

See also Acetylsalicylic acid

General Information

Benorilate is an acetylsalicylic ester of paracetamol. It is slowly absorbed unchanged from the gastrointestinal tract but is rapidly hydrolysed to its components, aspirin and paracetamol. Thereafter its effects and kinetics are those of the two moieties. However, the delay in its metabolism reduces the incidence of direct gastric irritation, delays its onset of action, and prolongs its duration of action (1,2).

Drug Administration

Drug overdose

In cases of suspected benorilate overdosage, both salicylate and paracetamol should be assayed.

References

1. Reizenstein P, Doberl A. Relevance of gastrointestinal symptoms and blood loss after long term treatment with a salicylate-paracetamol ester. A new anti-inflammatory agent (benorylate). Rheum and Rehab Suppl 1973;75:.
2. Wright V. A review of benorylate – a new antirheumatic drug. Scand J Rheumatol Suppl 1975;(13):5–8.

Benzydamine

General Information

Benzydamine is 1-benzyl-3-(3-dimethylaminopropoxy)-*H*-indazole, used for medical purposes as the hydrochloride. It has analgesic, anti-inflammatory, antipyretic, and local anesthetic effects. In the past it has been especially used in the symptomatic treatment of edematous postoperative or traumatic swelling, non-specific inflammation of the upper respiratory tract, and inflammation of connective tissues and joints. Nowadays, Tantum verde is the only such formulation listed in Germany; it is used for the treatment of oral and pharyngeal inflammation from any cause, for example radiotherapy-induced mucositis, stomatitis, Vincent's angina, necrotic oropharyngeal neoplasms, after surgical operations on the mouth and pharynx, after intubation, and after endoscopic laryngeal surgery. It can be administered as a spray, a gargle solution, a rinsing solution, or lozenges.

Organs and Systems

Skin

Skin reactions, including photosensitivity and contact dermatitis (when used topically), have been reported (1–7).

- A 67-year-old woman with pharyngitis gargled with Tantum verde, and after 3 weeks, during a holiday, developed an erythematous rash on sun-exposed skin, worsening within the next few days (8). She had not used a sunscreen. There were mainly well-demarcated areas of eczema on the face, neck, neckline, forearms, and lower legs. After oral and topical corticosteroids, the skin lesions improved within a few days.

There have been two other case reports of photoallergic dermatitis after local pharyngeal treatment with formulations containing benzydamine (6). This presumably occurs because of oral or intestinal absorption.

References

1. Turner M, Laitt R. Benzydamine oral rinse and rash. BMJ (Clin Res Ed) 1988;296(6628):1071.
2. Bruynzeel DP. Contact allergy to benzydamine. Contact Dermatitis 1986;14(5):313–4.
3. Anonymous. Difflam—a topical NSAID. Drug Ther Bull 1986;24(5):19–20.
4. Goncalo S, Souso L, Greitas JD. Dermatitis de fotosensibilizacion por benzidamine. Dermatitis Contacto 1982;3:21.
5. Vincenzi C, Cameli N, Tardio M, Piraccini BM. Contact and photocontact dermatitis due to benzydamine hydrochloride. Contact Dermatitis 1990;23(2):125–6.
6. Fernandez de Corres L. Photodermatitis from benzydamine. Contact Dermatitis 1980;6(4):285.
7. Frosch PJ, Weickel R. Photokontaktallergie durch Benzydamin (Tantum). [Photocontact allergy caused by benzydamine (Tantum).] Hautarzt 1989;40(12):771–3.
8. Henschel R, Agathos M, Breit R. Photocontact dermatitis after gargling with a solution containing benzydamine. Contact Dermatitis 2002;47(1):53.

Cinchophen

General Information

Cinchophen is a uricosuric drug that was formerly used in the treatment of gout (1). In 1991 the Spanish authorities withdrew cinchophen. It had been known for some time that it can cause severe hepatitis (SEDA-17, 114).

Reference

1. Cutrin Prieto C, Nieto Pol E, Batalla Eiras A, Casal Iglesias L, Perez Becerra E, Lorenzo Zuniga V. Hepatitis toxica por cincofeno: descripcion de tres enfermos. [Toxic hepatitis from cinchophen: report of 3 cases.] Med-Clin-(Barc) 1991;97(3):104–6.

Cloximate

General Information

Cloximate is approved in only a few countries, so experience with its use is limited. The usual adverse effects of NSAIDs (headache, insomnia, drowsiness, anorexia, gastrointestinal symptoms, a transient increase in blood urea, leukopenia, thrombocytopenia, and rashes) have been reported (1).

Reference

1. Kolarz G, Lieni KS, Richel H, Scherak O. Doppelblindstudie zwischen Indometacin und Cloximat, einem neuen nichtsteroidalen Anti-rheumatikum. Therapiewoche 1979;29:5898.

Diacerein

General Information

Diacerein (diacetylrhein), an anthraquinone derivative, is said to be effective in the treatment of osteoarthritis. Its active metabolite is rhein, about which there are very few clinical data. Diacerein does not affect arachidonic acid metabolism and might be better tolerated than other NSAIDs with regards to renal and gastric toxicity. Epigastric or abdominal pain and diarrhea are the most frequent adverse effects. Diarrhea occurred in 37% of patients with osteoarthritis taking diacerein (1). Acute hepatitis has been described (SEDA-22, 119), as have skin reactions.

Reference

1. Nguyen M, Dougados M, Berdah L, Amor B. Diacerhein in the treatment of osteoarthritis of the hip. Arthritis Rheum 1994;37(4):529–36.

Diflunisal

General Information

Diflunisal is a fluorinated salicylic acid derivative, which is absorbed unchanged from the gastrointestinal tract, reaching peak concentrations after about 2 hours, and is metabolized by glucuronidation (1). Its adverse effects and other characteristics are those of aspirin, although gastrointestinal haemorrhage may be less common (2).

References

1. Davies RO. Review of the animal and clinical pharmacology of diflunisal. Pharmacotherapy 1983;3(2 pt 2):9S–22S.

2. Turner RA, Shackleford RW, Whipple JP. Comparison of diflunisal and aspirin in long-term treatment of patients with rheumatoid arthritis. Clin Ther 1986;9(Suppl C):37–46.

Diftalone

General Information

Because of hepatotoxicity and carcinogenicity (hepatoma) detected in preclinical studies, and hemotoxicity and gastrointestinal adverse effects in man, diftalone has been withdrawn by its manufacturer (1).

Reference

1. Anonymous. Dow Lepetit drops diftalone. Scrip 1977; October 15;22.

Emorfazone

General Information

Emorfazone is a pyridazinone NSAID that was developed in Japan. Sleepiness, dry mouth, rash, and various gastrointestinal disturbances are its most important adverse effects (1).

Reference

1. Anonymous. Emorfazone. Drugs Today 1985;21:63.

Flosulide

General Information

Flosulide is a COX-2 inhibitor.

Organs and Systems

Gastrointestinal

Flosulide caused less damage to the mucosa and was better tolerated than naproxen in a 2-week endoscopic study, but the clinical relevance of endoscopic studies of this sort is debatable (SEDA-14, 79).

Urinary tract

Clinical development of flosulide, a COX-2 selective inhibitor, has been discontinued because of nephrotoxicity (1). Measurement of renal prostaglandin synthesis did not predict the nephrotoxicity of flosulide in single-dose and short-term studies (2).

References

1. Kaplan-Machlis B, Klostermeyer BS. The cyclooxygenase-2 inhibitors: safety and effectiveness. Ann Pharmacother 1999;33(9):979–88.
2. Brunel P, Hornych A, Guyene TT, Sioufi A, Turri M, Menard J. Renal and endocrine effects of flosulide, after single and repeated administration to healthy volunteers. Eur J Clin Pharmacol 1995;49(3):193–201.

Flupirtine

General Information

Flupirtine is a non-opiate, centrally acting analgesic, with muscle relaxant properties. It causes predominantly nervous system adverse effects (visual, disorientation, confusion, tremor). About 26% of patients develop minor adverse reactions (1).

Reference

1. Galasko CS, Courtenay PM, Jane M, Stamp TC. Trial of oral flupirtine maleate in the treatment of pain after orthopaedic surgery. Curr Med Res Opin 1985;9(9):594–601.

Isoxepac

General Information

Evidence about the properties of the NSAID isoxepac is minimal; only increases in gastrointestinal blood loss over pretreatment levels have been described (1).

Reference

1. Mitchell H, Barraclough D, Muirden KD. Blood-loss studies for new non-steroidal anti-inflammatory drugs. Med J Aust 1982;1(8):328.

IX 207-887

General Information

IX 207-887 (10-methoxy-4H-benzo-(4,5)-cyclohepta-(1,2–6)-thiophene-4-ylidene acetic acid) is a slow-acting drug for use in rheumatoid arthritis. Its mechanism of action involves inhibition of the release of interleukin-1.

Adverse effects have occurred in 22% of cases, most commonly skin reactions, but also hepatitis and gastrointestinal disorders (1).

Reference

1. Dougados M, Combe B, Beveridge I, Bourdeix I, Lallemand A, Amor B, Sany J. IX 207–887 in rheumatoid arthritis. A double-blind placebo-controlled study. Arthritis Rheum 1992;35(9):999–1006.

Lysine acetylsalicylate

General Information

Lysine acetylsalicylate is a soluble form of salicylate developed for intravenous administration in acute pain. Its mode of action and scope of adverse effects are similar to those of aspirin (1), although it has a faster onset of action (2) and causes less gastrointestinal bleeding (3).

References

1. Majluf-Cruz A, Chavez-Ochoa AR, Majluf-Cruz K, Coria-Ramirez E, Pineda Del Aguila I, Trevino-Perez S, Matias-Aguilar L, Lopez-Armenta JC, Corona de la Pena N. Effect of combined administration of clopidogrel and lysine acetyl-salicylate versus clopidogrel and aspirin on platelet aggregation and activated GPIIb/IIIa expression in healthy volunteers. Platelets 2006;17(2):105–7.
2. Gurfinkel EP, Altman R, Scazziota A, Heguilen R, Mautner B. Fast Platelet suppression by lysine acetylsalicylate in chronic stable coronary patients. Potential clinical impact over regular aspirin for coronary syndromes. Clin Cardiol 2000;23(9):697–700.
3. Bretagne JF, Fevillu A, Gosselin M, Gastard J. Aspirine et toxicite gastroduodenale. Etude endoscopique en double insu des effects d'un placébo, de l'aspirine et de l'acétylsalicylate de lysine chez le sujet sain. [Aspirin and gastroduodenal toxicity. A double-blind endoscopic study of the effects of placebo, aspirin and lysine acetylsalicylate in healthy subjects.] Gastroenterol Clin Biol 1984;8(1):28–32.

Metamizole DIPYRONE

General Information

Metamizole and phenyldimethylaminophenazone are the main derivatives of aminophenazone (amidopyrine) and are expected to provoke the same adverse reactions as aminophenazone itself.

Metamizole is still widely prescribed and openly sold as a headache remedy in some developing countries, but has been withdrawn from the market in many parts of the world. Curiously, in some Western countries it still enjoys a reputation as an injectable product that relieves renal colic. In other places it is entirely unknown and apparently not missed. Although it was German in origin, in 1987 the German authorities decided to subject all metamizole products to prescription-only regulations, a clear message to the regulatory authorities in other countries where it is sold without prescription (SEDA-12, 82). According to the Japanese authorities, suppositories and injectable formulations should be used only as a last resort, and warnings should be included in the package insert (SEDA-12, 83).

Metamizole was the single most commonly used agent causing adverse reactions (mainly hypersensitivity reactions, anaphylactic shock, and two deaths) in India, based on reports to an adverse drug reactions monitoring center by general practitioners (SEDA-16, 108).

The balance of benefit and harm for metamizole is controversial. It is used most commonly to treat postoperative pain, colic pain, cancer pain and migraine, and in many countries, for example Russia, Spain, Brazil, and in many parts of South-America and Africa, it is the most popular non opioid first line analgesic. In others (for example the USA and the UK) it has been banned because of its association with blood dyscrasias such as agranulocytosis. It is often also associated with severe anaphylactic reactions, especially when it is infused intravenously for analgesia (1).

Systematic reviews

In a systematic review of 15 studies, of which eight involved placebo and seven an active control (oral dexketoprofen 12.5 mg or 25 mg, oral ketorolac 10 mg, intramuscular pethidine 100 mg, intramuscular ketorolac 30 mg, intravenous tramadol 100 mg, or rectal suprofen 300 mg) (2). Adverse effects were too poorly reported for it to be possible to carry out a formal analysis. The commonest adverse effects were somnolence, gastric discomfort, and nausea. There were no reports of agranulocytosis, reflecting the general poor reporting of adverse effects in these trials.

Organs and Systems

Cardiovascular

In one case, intravenous injection of metamizole caused arterial hypotension (3).

Fluid balance

Fluid and salt retention have been observed in small children given metamizole (4).

Hematologic

The absolute risk of blood dyscrasias associated with the use of metamizole, particularly agranulocytosis (5,6), is unacceptably high.

In the International Agranulocytosis and Aplastic Anemia study (7), an epidemiological study organized by the manufacturers (Hoechst) of metamizole, the overall annual community agranulocytosis incidence was 4.4 per million (6.2 including hospital cases), with a fatality rate of 10% and an annual mortality rate of 0.4 per million. Analgesics significantly associated with agranulocytosis were metamizole, indometacin, oxyphenbutazone, and phenylbutazone. The International Agranulocytosis Study has been both criticized (8) and strongly defended (9).

An analysis of all reports of blood disorders attributed to NSAIDs that were submitted to the Finnish National Board of Health during 1973–85 showed that metamizole was suspected of causing 14· cases of agranulocytosis (three fatal), other pyrazolones four cases, indometacin two cases, and ibuprofen one case (10).

In a study of all spontaneous reports of serious blood dyscrasias associated with metamizole and an analysis of prescription data the incidence was estimated to be at least one in 1439 prescriptions (95% CI = 850, 4684), of which 92% occurred during the first 2 months of treatment (11). These results stimulated comments and criticisms (12,13), but despite criticisms about the small number of cases identified in the study, this result confirms earlier ones (13).

In a case-control study in patients identified from a large database designed for the surveillance of blood dyscrasias, during 78.73 million person-years follow-up there were 396 confirmed cases of agranulocytosis, 177 of which were analysed, with 586 matched controls (14). In the week before agranulocytosis developed, 30 cases (17%) and 9 controls (1.5%) had been exposed to metamizole (adjusted RR = 26; CI = 8.4, 79). Among exposed patients there was a trend towards an increased risk of agranulocytosis, with increased duration of exposure. However, the risk disappeared 10 days after the last dose of metamizole.

Hemolysis has also been reported with metamizole (15). It is possibly due to cell membrane absorption of drug-antibody immune complexes.

Urinary tract

Nephrotoxicity from metamizole is rare (SEDA-17, 108).

Skin

An active amide group on metamizole has been shown to cause pemphigus vulgaris (16,17).

Second-Generation Effects

Pregnancy

Adverse effects of metamizole have been described in pregnancy.

- A 21-year-old woman developed acute renal insufficiency during her 30th week of pregnancy (18). She had been taking metamizole 1.5-3 g/day for 10 days for back pain. Laboratory investigations showed renal insufficiency, generalized edema and a skin rash. Ultrasound showed oligohydramios. Metamizole was withdrawn and her rash disappeared, amniotic fluid production rose, and her laboratory values normalized. Delivery was uneventful.

Oligohydramnios has been attributed to metamizole (19).

- A 26 year old woman in the 35th week of her first pregnancy took metamizole 6 g/day for 3 days and papaverine hydrochloride to relieve urinary symptoms. Ultrasonography showed oligohydramnios with an amniotic fluid index of 40 mm (reference range 50–240 mm) and a restricted ductus arteriosus. Metamizole was replaced by paracetamol. Serial fetal ultrasonography showed an improvement in the width of the ductus arteriosus and in amniotic fluid volume 2 days after metamizole withdrawal, and gradual return to normal within 1 week. A normal healthy baby was born vaginally at 40 weeks.

Drug Administration

Drug overdose

In a retrospective review of 243 patients who had taken an overdose of metamizole, median age 17 years (range 4 months to 83 years), median amount 5 g (250 mg to 45 g), and median time to consultation 2 hours (5 minutes to 48 hours), there were toxic effects in 39 (16%); 57% of these were gastrointestinal and all were mild (20). The time to consultation was longer in the symptomatic patients (4 versus 1.5 hours) and in children (8 versus 3.5 hours in adults). There were no cases of agranulocytosis. Suggested treatment includes gastrointestinal decontamination and supportive measures.

The pattern of episodes of overdose with metamizole reported to six Texas poison centers from 1998 to 2004 has been identified (21). Of 81 cases 52 were isolated and 29 non-isolated. Most of the episodes occurred at the patient′s own residence (72/76) and the patients were more likely to be women (54/81). Children under 6 years of age accounted for a higher proportion of isolated exposures (33% versus 10%), while a higher proportion of non-isolated exposures involved older children (28% versus 8%); 22% (11/51) of isolated cases were intentional, compared with 59% (17/29) of non-isolated cases. When the medical outcome was known, there was no adverse clinical effect in 76% (16/21) of isolated exposures and 42% (8/19) of non-isolated exposures. The specific adverse effects in isolated exposures were primarily neurological (n = 6), gastrointestinal (n = 4), and dermal (n = 3).

References

1. Eckle T, Ghanayim N, Trick M, Unertl K, Eltzsching HK. Intraoperative metamizol as cause for acute anaphylactic collapse. Eur J Anaesthesiol 2005;22:810–.
2. Edwards JE, Meseguer F, Faura CC, Moore RA, McQuay HJ. Single-dose dipyrone for acute postoperative pain. Cochrane Database Syst Rev 2001;(3):CD00322.
3. Zoppi M, Hoigne R, Keller MF, Streit F, Hess T. Blutdruckabfall unter Dipyron (Novaminsulfon-Natrium). [Reducing blood pressure with Dipyron (novaminsulfone sodium).] Schweiz Med Wochenschr 1983;113(47):1768–70.
4. Bajoghli M, Ajudani TS, Gharavi M. Generalized oedema of newborn associated with the administration of dipyrone. Eur J Pediatr 1977;126(4):271–4.
5. Heimpel H, Kewitz H. Agranulozytose und Schock nach Metamizol. Dtsch Arztebl 1982;79:48.
6. Garcia S, Canionero M, Lopes G. Dipyrone-induced granulocytopenia: a case for awareness. Pharmacotherapy 2006;26(3):440–.
7. The International Agranulocytosis and Aplastic Anemia Study. Risks of agranulocytosis and aplastic anemia. A first report of their relation to drug use with special reference to analgesics. JAMA 1986;256(13):1749–57.
8. Offerhaus L. Metamizol: een honderdjarige treurnis. [Metamizole: 100 years of grief.] Ned Tijdschr Geneeskd 1987;131(12):479–81.
9. Levy M, Shapiro S. Metamizol: een honderdjarige treurnis. [Metamizole: a 100-year-old grief.] Ned Tijdschr Geneeskd 1987;131(38):1680–3.
10. Palva ES, Eranko PO. Dipyrone and agranulocytosis in Finland. Paper presented at Conference of the International Union of Pharmacology, August, 198.
11. Hedenmalm K, Spigset O. Agranulocytosis and other blood dyscrasias associated with dipyrone (metamizole). Eur J Clin Pharmacol 2002;58(4):265–74.
12. Edwards JE, McQuay HJ. Dipyrone and agranulocytosis: what is the risk? Lancet 2002;360(9344):1438.
13. Schonhofer P, Offerhaus L, Herxheimer A. Renal tolerability of three commonly employed non-steroidal anti-inflammatory drugs in elderly patients with osteoarthritis. Lancet 2003;361:968.
14. Ibàñèz L, Vidal X, Ballarìn E, Laporte JR. Population-based drug-induced agranulocytosis. Arch Intern Med 2005;165:869–74.
15. Ribera A, Monasterio J, Acebedo G, Triginer J, Martin C. Dipyrone-induced immune haemolytic anaemia. Vox Sang 1981;41(1):32–5.
16. Brenner S, Bialy-Golan A, Crost N. Dipyrone in the induction of pemphigus. J Am Acad Dermatol 1997;36(3 Pt 1):488–90.
17. Wolf R, Brenner S. An active amide group in the molecule of drugs that induce pemphigus: a casual or causal relationship? Dermatology 1994;189(1):1–4.
18. Sanchez MD de la Nieta, Rivera F, De la Torre M, Alcazar R, Caparros G, Pac Alcaide M, Vozmediano C, Sanchez A. Acute renal failure and oligohydramnios induced by magnesium dipyrone (metamizol) in a pregnant woman. Nephrol Dial Transplant. 2003;18:1679–80.
19. Weintraub A, Mankuta D. Dipyrone-induced oligohydramnios and ductus arteriosus restriction. Isr Med Assoc J 2006;8(10):722–3.
20. Bentur Y, Cohen O. Dipyrone overdose. J Toxicol Clin Toxicol 2004;42(3):261–5.
21. Forrester MB. Pattern of dipyrone exposure in Texas, 1998 to 2004. J Med Toxicol 2006;2(3):101–7.

Nefopam

General Information

Nefopam, an orphenadrine derivative, is a centrally acting non-opioid analgesic.

Nefopam

with both supraspinal and spinal sites of action. It inhibits the reuptake of serotonin, dopamine, and noradrenaline and is neither an opiate nor a non-steroidal anti-inflammatory drug. It does not cause respiratory depression. The usual intravenous dose is 20 micrograms and the equianalgesic ratio with morphine is 3.5:1 95).

Various adverse effects have been reported, including nausea, vomiting, epigastric pain, dizziness, drowsiness and mental confusion, hypotension, tachycardia, skin rashes, xerostomia, and urinary retention(1,2); some of these may be related to its anticholinergic properties (SEDA-11, 100). Its unsatisfactory adverse effects profile was confirmed in two studies of pain control in cancer and rheumatoid arthritis (SEDA-15, 104)

In one study, five of 33 patients (15%) stopped treatment because of the severity of adverse effects attributed to nefopam (3).

In an open trial 120 patients undergoing elective hepatic resection were randomized to receive postoperative intravenous patient-controlled analgesia with morphine either alone or in combination with nefopam (20 mg 4-hourly) or propacetamol (2 g 6-hourly) (4). Nefopam plus morphine was the most effective treatment. Adverse effects, especially sedation, were comparable in the three groups, but there was significantly more nausea in the morphine group and more sweating in the nefopam group (requiring early drug withdrawal in three cases). Tachycardia was seen more often in the nefopam group but did not reach significance.

Organs and Systems

Urinary tract

There have been 53 cases of reversible urinary retention, hesitancy, a poor stream, or dribbling reported to the UK Committee on Safety of Medicines.

Long-Term Effects

Drug abuse

Three cases of nefopam abuse have been reported (5). The patients had the same pattern of a history of chronic pain, concomitant anxiolytic and antidepressant drug therapy, and abuse of nefopam due to its primarily psychostimulant-like symptoms. The recommended dose of nefopam is 20 mg intramuscularly every 6 hours, with a maximum recommended dose of 120 mg/day. Daily consumption in the three patients was 120–1840 mg/day.

Susceptibility Factors

The UK Committee on Safety of Medicines received 12 reports of confusion and 22 of hallucinations and recommended that nefopam be used with caution in the elderly, in patients with symptoms of urinary retention, or in conjunction with other drugs that have anticholinergic activity (6).

References

1. Bobeil H, Delage N, Nègre I, Mezoit J-X, Benhamou D. The median effective dose of nefopam and morphine administered intravenously for post-operative pain after minor

surgery: a prospective, randomized double-blinded isobolographic study of their analgesic action. Anesth Analg 2004;98:395–40.
2. Alfonsi P, Adam F, Passard A, Guignard B, Sessler DI, Chauvin M. Nefopam, a non-sedative benzoxazocine analgesic selectively reduces the shivering threshold in unanaesthetized subjects. Anaesthesiology 2004;100:37–43.
3. Minotti V, Patoia L, Roila F, Basurto C, Tonato M, Pasqualucci V, Maresca V, Del Favero A. Double-blind evaluation of analgesic efficacy of orally administered diclofenac, nefopam, and acetylsalicylic acid (ASA) plus codeine in chronic cancer pain. Pain 1989;36(2):177–83.
4. Mimoz O, Incagnoli P, Josse C, Gillon MC, Kuhlman L, Mirand A, Soilleux H, Fletcher D. Analgesic efficacy and safety of nefopam vs. propacetamol following hepatic resection. Anaesthesia 2001;56(6):520–5.
5. Villier C, Mallaret MP. Nefopam abuse. Ann Pharmacother 2002;36(10):1564–6.
6. D'Arcy PF. Drug reactions and interactions. Int Pharm J 1989;3:91.

Oxaceprol

General Information

Oxaceprol, a hydroxyproline derivative, has been used to treat osteoarthritis (1,2). Gastrointestinal reactions, nervous system reactions (headache, dizziness), and skin reactions have been reported (3), but oxaceprol is reportedly tolerated at least as well as diclofenac (1) or better (2).

References

1. Bauer HW, Klasser M, von Hanstein KL, Rolinger H, Schladitz G, Henke HD, Gimbel W, Steinbach K. Oxaceprol is as effective as diclofenac in the therapy of osteoarthritis of the knee and hip. Clin Rheumatol 1999;18(1):4–9.
2. Herrmann G, Steeger D, Klasser M, Wirbitzky J, Furst M, Venbrocks R, Rohde H, Jungmichel D, Hildebrandt HD, Parnham MJ, Gimbel W, Dirschedl H. Oxaceprol is a well-tolerated therapy for osteoarthritis with efficacy equivalent to diclofenac. Clin Rheumatol 2000;19(2):99–104.
3. Diehl K, Fallot-Burghardt W, Frie A. Die Therapie der Gonarthrose mit Oxaceprol. Therapiewoche 1985;35:51.

Paracetamol

General Information

A century after its introduction, acetylsalicylic acid (aspirin) is by far the most commonly used analgesic, sharing its leading position with the relative newcomer paracetamol (acetaminophen), and notwithstanding the fact that other widely used compounds, such as ibuprofen, have in recent years been introduced in over-the-counter versions. Both are also still being prescribed by physicians and are generally used for mild to moderate pain, fever associated with common everyday illnesses, and disorders ranging from head colds and influenza to toothache and headache. However, their greatest use is by consumers who obtain them directly from the pharmacy, and in many countries outside pharmacies as well.

Perhaps this wide availability and advertising via mass media leads to a lack of appreciation by the lay public that these are medicines with adverse effects. Both have at any rate been subject to misuse and excessive use, leading to such problems as chronic salicylate intoxication with aspirin and severe hepatic damage with paracetamol overdose. Both aspirin and paracetamol have also featured in accidental overdosage (particularly in children) as well as intentional overdosage.

In an investigation of Canadian donors who had not admitted to drug intake, 6–7% of the blood samples taken were found to have detectable concentrations of acetylsalicylic acid and paracetamol (1). Such drugs would be potentially capable of causing untoward reactions in the recipients.

To offer some protection against misuse of analgesics, many countries have insisted on the use of packs containing total quantities less than the minimum toxic dose (albeit usually the one obtained for healthy young volunteers and thus disregarding the majority of the population), and supplied in child-resistant packaging. Most important, however, is the need to provide education for the lay public to respect such medicines in general for the good they can do, but more especially for the harm that can arise, but can be avoided. There is a definite role for the prescribing physician, since informing the patient seems to prevent adverse events (2).

The sale of paracetamol or aspirin in dosage forms in which they are combined with other active ingredients offers considerable risk to the consumer, since the product as sold may not be clearly identified as containing either of these two analgesics. Brand names sometimes obscure the actual composition of older formulations that contain one or both of these analgesics in combination with, for example, a pyrazolone derivative and/or a potentially addictive substance. For instance, in Germany, with the EC harmonization of the Drug Law of 1990, the manufacturers of drugs already marketed before 1978 had the opportunity of exchanging even the active principles without being obliged to undergo a new approval procedure or to abandon their brand name. Combination formulations are still being promoted and sold, and not exclusively in developing countries. Consequently the patient who is so anxious to allay all his symptoms that he takes several medications concurrently may without knowing it take several doses of aspirin or paracetamol at the same time, perhaps sufficient to cause toxicity. It is essential that product labels clearly state their active ingredients by approved name, together with the quantity per dosage form (3).

The antipyretic analgesics share with the non-steroidal anti inflammatory drugs (NSAIDs) a common mechanism of action, namely the inhibition of prostaglandin synthesis from arachidonic acid and their release. More precisely their mode of action is thought to result from inhibition of both the constitutive and the inducible isoenzymes (COX-1 and COX-2) of the cyclo-oxygenase pathway (4). However, aspirin and paracetamol are distinguishable from most of the NSAIDs by their ability to inhibit prostaglandin synthesis in the nervous system, and thus the hypothalamic center for body temperature regulation, rather than acting mainly in the periphery.

Endogenous pyrogens (and exogenous pyrogens that have their effects through the endogenous group) induce the hypothalamic vascular endothelium to produce prostaglandins, which activate the thermoregulatory neurons by increasing AMP concentrations. The capacity of the antipyretic analgesics to inhibit hypothalamic prostaglandin synthesis appears to be the basis of their antipyretic action. Neither aspirin nor paracetamol affects the synthesis or release of endogenous pyrogens and neither will lower body temperature if it is normal.

While aspirin significantly inhibits peripheral prostaglandin and thromboxane synthesis, paracetamol is less potent as a synthetase inhibitor than the NSAIDs, except in the brain, and paracetamol has only a weak anti-inflammatory action. It is simple to ascribe the analgesic activity of aspirin to its capacity to inhibit prostaglandin synthesis, with a consequent reduction in inflammatory edema and vasodilatation, since aspirin is most effective in the pain associated with inflammation or injury. However, such a peripheral effect cannot account for the analgesic activity of paracetamol, which is less well understood.

The use of paracetamol as an antipyretic increased rapidly once phenacetin was no longer available and has received a boost more recently with wide acknowledgement of the role of aspirin as a causative agent in Reye's syndrome, resulting in the virtual disappearance of children's dosage forms of aspirin. While the incidence of adverse effects is reassuringly low, satisfaction must be tempered by appreciation of the relatively short duration of extensive clinical experience with paracetamol, its close relation to phenacetin, its low potency as an analgesic, and low public awareness of its potential adverse effects.

General adverse reactions

Although paracetamol is acceptably safe in usual dosages, there have been some reports that in patients with significant hepatic dysfunction or those taking substances that induce hepatic enzymes (for example ethanol, phenobarbital, isoniazid) even these doses may aggravate liver dysfunction, sometimes to the point of causing hepatic failure. The problem of overdosage is substantial. Allergic reactions, including urticaria, are seen occasionally. Anaphylactic shock has been reported.

Organs and Systems

Cardiovascular

Despite the high prevalence of the use of minor analgesics (aspirin and paracetamol) there is little information available on the association between the use of these analgesics and the risk of hypertension. A prospective cohort study in 80 020 women aged 31–50 years has provided some useful information (5). The women had participated in the Nurses' Health Study II and had no previous history of hypertension. The frequency of use of paracetamol, aspirin, and NSAIDs was collected by mailed questionnaires and cases of physician-diagnosed hypertension were identified by self-report. During 164 000 person-years of follow-up, 1650 incident cases of hypertension were identified. Overall, 73% of the cohort had used paracetamol at least 1–4 days/month, 51% had used aspirin, and 77% had used an NSAID. Compared with non-users of paracetamol the age-adjusted relative risk (RR) of hypertension was significantly increased even in women who had used paracetamol for only 1–4 days/month (RR = 1.22; CI = 1.07, 1.39). There seemed to be a dose–response relation, as the RR of hypertension compared with non-users was 2.00 (CI = 1.52, 2.62) in women who had taken paracetamol for 29 days/month or more. For women using aspirin or NSAIDs at a frequency of 1–4 days/month the RRs were 1.18 (CI = 1.02, 1.35) and 1.17 (CI = 1.02, 1.36) respectively. However, after adjusting for age and other potential risk factors, only paracetamol and NSAIDs, but not aspirin, remained significantly associated with a risk of hypertension. In summary, the data from this study support the view that paracetamol and NSAIDs are strongly associated with an increased risk of hypertension in women, the risk increasing with increasing frequency of use. Aspirin did not seem to be associated with an increased risk. This conclusion contrasts with the results of some short-term studies that have shown no effect of paracetamol on blood pressure (6,7).

This study suggests that paracetamol can raise arterial blood pressure in a dose-related fashion, interfere with the actions of antihypertensive drugs, and prompt the need for new antihypertensive therapy. However, these results must be interpreted with caution, as there were some limitations: the assessments of analgesic use and hypertension were made using a self-reported questionnaire; relative risk can be influenced by many potentially confounding variables; the results are relevant only for young women and cannot be extrapolated to the general population.

Respiratory

Paracetamol can aggravate bronchospasm in patients who are sensitive to aspirin and other analgesics (8). In severe poisoning, paracetamol depresses respiratory function centrally through metabolic acidosis and coma (9).

The prevalence of asthma has risen worldwide in recent years, but the reason for this increase is unclear. A number of hypotheses have been formulated, and among them attention has been paid to epidemiological and pathophysiological evidence underlying the hypothesis that paracetamol may be a risk factor for asthma (10).

The first study to suggest a link between asthma and paracetamol was one using data from the International Study of Asthma and Allergies in Childhood of the European Community Respiratory Health Survey (ECHRIS) (11). There was a positive correlation between

paracetamol sales and asthma symptoms. For each gram increase in per capita paracetamol sales in 1994–5 the prevalence of wheeze increased by 0.52% among 13- to 14-year-old subjects in this study. Similarly, wheezing rose by 0.26% per gram increase among young adults.

While ecological findings such as these are helpful for the description of group-level (in this case country-level) patterns of association, inferences about individuals cannot be made. However, an association between paracetamol and asthma at the individual level has been seen in a large case-control study

Of dietary antioxidants and asthma, has shown an association between the regular use of paracetamol and the incidence of asthma and rhinitis in adults (12). After controlling for potential confounding factors the OR for asthma in daily users, compared with never users, was 2.38 (CI = 1.22, 4.64). Not unexpectedly, there was also an association in users and non-users of aspirin, strongest when cases with more severe disease were compared with controls.

However, the study had limitations, such as selection bias, and did not take into account factors such as respiratory tract infections. Furthermore, the cross-sectional design of the study makes it unclear whether the use of paracetamol contributed to asthma or vice versa (13).

Further evidence came from the Nurses' Health Study, a prospective cohort study of 121 200 women (14). The objective was to examine the relation between paracetamol use and new-onset asthma. During 352 719 person-years of follow-up, 346 participants reported a new diagnosis of asthma. Increasing frequency of paracetamol use was positively associated with newly diagnosed asthma. The multivariate rate ratio for asthma for participants who took paracetamol for more than 14 days/month was 1.65 (CI = 1.11, 2.39) compared with non-users. The positive association were not affected by the use of aspirin. In a multivariate analysis aspirin was inversely related to newly diagnosed asthma. There was no association with NSAIDs. However, these results cannot be generalized, as the study was conducted in an older, female, and predominantly white population not representative of the general population.

A more recent study using data from the US-based Third National Health and Nutrition Examination Survey has provided further evidence that use of paracetamol is associated with asthma in a dose-related way (adjusted OR = 1.20; C.I.= 1.12, 1.28) (15). Increased use of paracetamol was also dose-dependently associated with COPD.

In a well conducted, double-blind, randomized study aimed at determining the safety of ibuprofen in children with febrile illnesses, there was a significant association between increased out-patient visits for asthma and use of paracetamol (16). However, the lack of a placebo group in this study made it unclear whether ibuprofen reduced the risk of asthma, paracetamol increased the risk, or a combination of the two.

Finally, there have been multiple case reports and case series of respiratory symptoms and acute reductions in respiratory function indexes after ingestion of paracetamol among both aspirin-sensitive and aspirin tolerant patients (10). Plausible mechanisms that explain the association of paracetamol with asthma include depletion of pulmonary glutathione and thereby a reduced capability of the host to mitigate oxidative stress produced by reactive oxygen species.

In 3000 children aged 6–7 years and 3000 teenagers aged 13–14 years the prevalence of ever wheezing in the younger children who had taken paracetamol in the first year of life was 11% (OR = 1.54; 95% CI = 1.00, 2.38) and the prevalence of ever wheezing in older children who had taken paracetamol at least once a month was 25% (OR = 1.7; 95% CI = 1.43, 2.04) (17). Taking more paracetamol during the previous 12 months led to a higher prevalence of dry cough at night and symptoms of rhinitis in the younger children and eczema and rhinitis symptoms in the teenagers.

In a cross-sectional questionnaire study in 3493 children aged 6–7 years old children were classified as cases if they had had wheezing, rhinitis, or eczema either at any time since their neonatal period or in the 12 months before the study (18). Paracetamol exposure was considered positive if it had occurred often during the first year of life (first analysis) or in the previous 12 months (second analysis). Paracetamol intake in the first year of life was significantly associated with an increased risk of wheezing (adjusted OR = 1.69; 95% CI = 1.23, 2.34) and rhinitis (adjusted OR = 1.37; 95% CI =1.20, 1.59) but not eczema (adjusted OR = 1.45; 95% CI = 0.91, 2.32). Frequent paracetamol intake in the previous year increased the risk of wheezing (OR = 3.3; 95% CI = 1.54, 7.18), rhinitis (OR = 1.61; 95% CI = 1.33, 1.95), or eczema (OR = 1.82; 95% CI = 1.24, 2.66).

Nervous system

In patients who suffer from recurrent headaches, for example migraine, cluster headache, or tension headache, temporary relief for the constant or intermittent pains is obtained from each analgesic dose, but wears off after a few hours with the arrival of a new episode. The patient gets accustomed to this pattern and may use excessive doses of analgesics. This in turn can cause, worsen, and perpetuate headaches, leading to what is called analgesic-induced or rebound headache. Like migraine, analgesic-induced headache is more likely to occur in women and is associated with depression.

It is postulated that the mechanism by which analgesic abuse transforms a primary headache into a rebound headache involves serotonin: both platelet serotonin concentrations and uptake were lower in patients with analgesic-induced headache compared with migraine sufferers and non-headache sufferers. At the same time, there was upregulation of serotonin receptors on the platelet membrane (19,20). Extrapolating these findings to the nervous system, it has been suggested that excessive analgesic use suppresses serotonin pathways, contributing to aggravation of headaches. Paracetamol and codeine were the major culprits of the analgesics investigated.

Analgesic-induced headache has also been described in children. One report (21) described 12 children, aged 6–16 years, who gave a history of headaches on at least 4 days a week, for 3 months to 10 years. Eleven of the children had been taking paracetamol, six in combination with codeine, and one was taking ibuprofen alone. They were taking at least one dose of an analgesic for each headache and eight were taking analgesics every day. The headaches presented with increasing frequency and were related to overuse of analgesics, a typical finding in analgesic-induced headache. The analgesics were withdrawn; in six children the headaches resolved completely, another five children experienced a reduced frequency of headaches, and one resumed analgesic abuse.

A second report (22) was of a retrospective study of patients seen in a pediatric headache clinic. During 8 months, 98 patients were seen for headache; 46 of them suffered from daily or near daily headache and 30 were consuming analgesics daily. Follow-up information was available in 25. The average number of doses of analgesics per week they consumed was 26. The most commonly used medications were paracetamol and ibuprofen. In addition, a minority were taking combinations that contained aspirin, codeine, caffeine, propoxyphene, or butalbital, or other NSAIDs. Abrupt withdrawal of all analgesics concomitant with the use of amitriptyline 10 mg/day (in 22 patients) prompted a significant reduction in the frequency and severity of headache.

The data from these studies are comparable to previous observations reported in adults (SEDA-21, 95) and suggest that daily use of analgesics can cause daily or near daily headaches in children and adolescents. However, additional controlled prospective studies are needed to address the true frequency of analgesics rebound headache among children and to evaluate possible treatments.

Metabolism

Hypoglycemia has been recorded with paracetamol, particularly in children (23).

Acid-base balance

Acidosis without liver damage, a rare presentation, has been reported in a case of paracetamol poisoning in a child (24).

- A previously healthy 27-month-old girl started vomiting and became somnolent without a history of drug exposure. She was intubated and given activated charcoal. The serum paracetamol concentration was 5.3 mmol/l (804 μg/ml) 2.5 hours after the onset of symptoms. The pH was 7.32, P_aCO_2 4.6 kPA, P_aO_2 46 kPa, and bicarbonate 17 mmol/l. The lactate was 4.6 mmol/l. The serum transaminases were not raised. A urine toxicology screen was negative, and the aspirin concentration was less than 20 mg/l. Four hours after the development of symptoms, she was given intravenous N-acetylcysteine, which was continued for 36 hours, until the paracetamol concentration was undetectable. Her liver function tests remained normal, the acidosis resolved, and her mental status returned to normal.

Hematologic

Agranulocytosis was recorded in a series in France (25), but does not appear to have been a significant clinical problem elsewhere.

Two patients developed immune thrombocytopenia attributed to metabolites of paracetamol (26).

- A 30-year-old man and a 66-year-old woman had taken paracetamol 1 g intermittently for headaches and other non-specific indications. Routine blood testing showed thrombocytopenia (50×10^9/l and 45×10^9/l respectively). They both stopped taking paracetamol, and their platelet counts rose to normal within 7–10 days. Their sera contained antibodies (IgG or IgA) that recognized normal platelets in the presence of the metabolite paracetamol sulfate.

This suggests that in patients with drug-induced immune thrombocytopenia, tests for metabolite-dependent antibodies can be helpful in identifying the responsible agent.

A hemolytic crisis has been recorded in a patient with glucose-6-phosphate dehydrogenase deficiency (27).

Gastrointestinal

The association between paracetamol and upper gastrointestinal complications has been investigated in a nested case-control study using the UK General Practice Research Database and a systematic review of 12 twelve studies (28). Paracetamol was associated with a small increased risk of upper gastrointestinal complications (RR = 1.3; 95% CI = 1.1, 1.5). The relative risk was 3.6 (95% CI = 2.6, 5.1) among paracetamol users of more than 2 g/day, whereas smaller doses did not increase the risk. Among the 12 studies identified in the systematic review, estimates were 0.2–2.0, with a summary estimate of 1.3 (95% CI = 1.2, 1.5). These findings suggest that paracetamol does not greatly increase the risk of upper gastrointestinal complications.

Liver

Paracetamol is directly hepatotoxic and can cause severe hepatic damage in dosages over 6–10 g (12–20 tablets).

Liver damage due to paracetamol is usually associated with suicidal overdosage. However, it has been suggested that the use of paracetamol in children with acute febrile illnesses can cause fulminant hepatic failure (29). In a case-control study 25 children with fulminant hepatic failure were compared with 33 age-matched controls. All of the former and none of the latter had taken supratherapeutic doses of paracetamol (mean 145 mg/kg/day). The mean paracetamol concentration was 1.78 mmol/l. There was no serological evidence of hepatitis A, hepatitis B, or dengue. Three children died.

In an analysis of alanine transaminase activity in seven controlled clinical trials involving the use of paracetamol alone 1950–4000 mg/day for 4 weeks up to 12 months, there were no reports of hepatotoxicity or hepatic failure in 1530 patients (30). While they were taking long-term paracetamol, 181 of 1039 patients (17%) had an alanine transaminase activity that exceeded the upper limit of the reference range, but none was more than three times the upper limit of the reference range in conjunction with a serum bilirubin over the upper limit of the reference range, and no patient had an alanine transaminase activity more than 10 times the upper limit of the reference range. All the changes were transient.

Biliary tract

Acute biliary pain with cholestasis is an occasional complication (31,32).

Pancreas

Pancreatitis has been reported, but only in overdose (33).

Urinary tract

Apart from renal tubular necrosis, which is usually associated with hepatic toxicity, but is occasionally seen without hepatic damage, there have been reports of a nephropathy similar to that seen with phenacetin, after prolonged use of paracetamol alone or in combination with other NSAIDs (34–39).

Analgesic nephropathy

> *DoTS classification (BMJ 2003;327:1222–5)*
> Dose-relation: collateral effect
> Time-course: delayed
> Susceptibility factors: age (over 65); sex (women)

In a series of papers that appeared from 1950 onwards (40), Spüler and Zollinger in Switzerland recognized analgesic nephropathy as a condition resulting from prolonged excessive consumption of analgesic mixtures, usually containing phenacetin. The disease is characterized by renal papillary necrosis and interstitial nephritis. The prevalence is variable, being especially high when the use of minor analgesics is intensive. The evidence linking the disorder primarily to phenacetin has been reviewed extensively (SED-8, 169) (SED-8, 178) (SED-9, 123) (SED-10, 135) (SEDA-9, 75).

Over the last 50 years there has been a steady evolution in our knowledge of drug-related renal pathology, including the role of prostaglandins in the kidneys and the concept of two cyclo-oxygenase isozymes. In the 1960s a distinct clinical entity was identified, separate from NSAID-induced renal toxicity, comprising interstitial nephritis and renal papillary necrosis. The condition, named analgesic nephropathy, was not uncommon and was serious. In a number of cases malignancies in the urinary tract also occurred.

The relation between long-term heavy exposure to analgesics and the risk of chronic renal disease has been the object of intensive toxicological and epidemiological research for many years (SEDA-24, 120) (41). Most of the earlier reports suggested that phenacetin-containing analgesics probably cause renal papillary necrosis and interstitial nephritis.

Nephropathy due to non-phenacetin-containing analgesics

There is no convincing epidemiological evidence that non-phenacetin-containing analgesics (including paracetamol, aspirin, mixtures of the two, and NSAIDs) cause chronic renal disease. Findings from epidemiological studies should be interpreted with caution, because of a number of inherent limitations and potential biases in study design (42). However, two methodologically sound studies have provided information on this topic.

The first was the largest cohort study conducted thus far to assess the risk of renal dysfunction associated with analgesic use (43). Details of analgesic use were obtained from 11 032 men without previous renal dysfunction participating in the Physicians' Health Study (PHS), which lasted 14 years. The main outcome measure was a raised creatinine concentration defined as 1.5 mg/dl (133 μmol/l) or higher and a reduced creatinine clearance of 55 ml/minute or less. In all, 460 men (4.2%) had a raised creatinine concentration and 1258 (11%) had a reduced creatinine clearance. Mean creatinine concentrations and creatinine clearances were similar among men who did not use analgesics and those who did. This was true for all categories of analgesics (paracetamol and paracetamol-containing mixtures, aspirin and aspirin-containing mixtures, and other NSAIDs) and for higher risk groups, such as those aged 60 years or over or those with hypertension or diabetes.

These data are convincing, because the large size of the PHS cohort should have made it possible to examine and detect even modest associations between analgesic use and a risk of renal disease. Furthermore, this study included more individuals who reported extensive use of analgesics than any prior case-control study. However, the study had some limitations, the most important being the fact that the cohort was composed of relatively healthy men, most of whom were white. These results cannot therefore be generalized to the entire population. However, the study clearly showed that there is not a strong association between chronic analgesic use and chronic renal dysfunction among a large cohort of men without a history of renal impairment.

The second study was a Swedish nationwide, population-based, case-control study of early-stage chronic renal insufficiency in men whose serum creatinine concentration exceeded 3.4 mg/dl (300 μmol/l) or women whose serum creatinine exceeded 250 μmol/l (2.8 mg/dl) (44). In all, 918 patients with newly diagnosed renal insufficiency and 980 controls were interviewed and completed questionnaires about their lifetime consumption of analgesics. Compared with controls, more patients with chronic renal insufficiency were regular users of aspirin (37 versus 19%) or paracetamol (25 versus 12%). Among subjects who did not use aspirin regularly, the regular use of paracetamol was associated with a risk of chronic renal insufficiency that was 2.5 times as high as that for non-users of paracetamol. The risk increased with increasing cumulative lifetime dose. Patients who took 500 g or more over a year (1.4 g/day) during periods of regular use had an increased odds ratio for chronic renal insufficiency (OR = 5.3; 95% CI = 1.8, 15). Among subjects who did not use paracetamol regularly, the regular use of aspirin was associated with a risk of chronic renal insufficiency that was 2.5 times as high as that for non-users of aspirin. The risk increased significantly with an increasing cumulative lifetime dose of aspirin. Among the patients with an average intake of 500 g or more of aspirin per year during periods of regular use, the risk of chronic renal insufficiency was increased about three-fold (OR = 3.3; CI = 1.4, 8.0). Among patients who used paracetamol in addition to aspirin, the risk of chronic renal insufficiency was increased about two-fold when regular aspirin users served as the reference group (OR = 2.2; CI = 1.4, 3.5) and non-significantly when regular paracetamol users were used as controls (OR = 1.6; CI = 0.9, 2.7). There was no relation between the use of other analgesics (propoxyphene, NSAIDs, codeine, and pyrazolones) and the risk of chronic renal insufficiency. Thus, the regular use of paracetamol, or aspirin, or both was associated dose-dependently with an increased risk of chronic renal insufficiency. The OR among regular users exceeded 1.0 for all types of chronic renal insufficiency, albeit not always significantly. These results are consistent with exacerbating effects of paracetamol and aspirin on chronic renal insufficiency, regardless of accompanying disease.

How can we explain the contrasting results of these two studies? A possible explanation lies in the different populations studied. In the PHS study, relatively healthy individuals were enrolled, while in the Swedish study all the patients had pre-existing severe renal or systemic disease, suggesting that such disease has an important role in causing analgesic-associated chronic renal insufficiency. People without pre-existing disease who use analgesics may have only a small risk of end-stage renal disease.

As up to 10% of about 42 000 dialysis patients have suffered from renal insufficiency due to analgesic nephropathy (in the postphenacetin era), German nephrologists have demanded the withdrawal from the market of medications that contain fixed combinations of analgesics (paracetamol, aspirin, or propyphenazone) plus caffeine, following the example of their American colleagues in the National Kidney Foundation (45).

Despite the fact that a careful evaluation of all epidemiological studies on non-narcotic analgesics showed no evidence that phenacetin-free combination drugs are more nephrotoxic than simple analgesics (41), the Belgian Public Health Authorities decided that combination analgesics are to become "prescription only" (46), as they have a "devastating" effect on the kidneys. However, contrasting opinions have been published (42,47).

The effect of the withdrawal of phenacetin in Germany in 1986 and its replacement with paracetamol in most analgesic mixtures resulted in a significant fall in the incidence of end-stage analgesic nephropathy from 30% in 1981–82 to 21% in 1991–92 and 12% in 1995–97 (48). However, whether this reduction can be taken as proof that only phenacetin and not paracetamol is nephrotoxic in compound analgesics is debatable (49). In fact, the German authors found that other factors, such as advanced age and an increasing prevalence of type II diabetes mellitus, affected the relative frequencies of primary renal disease in patients with end-stage renal disease to such a degree that the observed relative reduction in analgesic nephropathy may not have been related to a change from phenacetin to paracetamol. Thus, the relative reduction in the incidence of analgesic nephropathy cannot be used as an argument for the non-toxicity of compound analgesics that contain paracetamol.

Furthermore, despite withdrawal of phenacetin from the market, analgesic nephropathy has continued to occur. It has been estimated that analgesic-associated nephropathy still accounts for 20% of patients in the USA with interstitial nephritis. As recently as the mid-1990s, a German study showed that up to 10% of dialysis patients had suffered from renal insufficiency owing to analgesic nephropathy (SEDA-20, 89). There is evidence that paracetamol, which replaced phenacetin in analgesic combination formulations, is nephrotoxic as well (50,51). The withdrawal of combination analgesic products from over-the-counter sales in Sweden and Australia has markedly reduced analgesic nephropathy as a cause of end-stage renal disease in those countries (SEDA-21, 99). It is therefore not surprising that nephrologists on both sides of the Atlantic have suggested a ban on the advertising and over-the-counter sales of these medications.

Symptoms and signs

Clinical evidence suggestive of analgesic nephropathy includes nocturia, renal insufficiency with severe acidosis, persistent urinary tract infection with colic, hematuria, and hypertension (52,53). Nocturia resulting from failure to concentrate urine is usually the earliest functional defect, but like the other symptoms it is non-specific, rendering the diagnosis of analgesic nephropathy difficult. A CT scan showing bilateral small kidneys with bumpy contours, and papillary calcification is accepted to be of sufficient specificity (50,51).

Epidemiology

Analgesic nephropathy is mostly diagnosed between the ages of 30 and 70 years, with a peak in the fourth decade, and there is a familial predisposition (SEDA-6, 80).

The prevalence of analgesic nephropathy is particularly high when there is intensive use of analgesics. There is evidence from animal and clinical work to suggest that hypovolemia plays a part, and that the risk of nephropathy is greatest in women and the elderly. Because of the long latent period of over 10 years, the condition has continued to appear despite the withdrawal of phenacetin.

In Australia, where phenacetin was withdrawn from antipyretic analgesic formulations during 1962–75 (54), analgesic nephropathy continued to be a major problem for a considerable time thereafter, reflecting the long latent period before the disorder develops; 22% of patients newly admitted to the Australian Kidney Foundation's dialysis and transplant registry in 1980 had analgesic nephropathy. The consumption of phenacetin-containing analgesics increased the risk of renal papillary necrosis in Australian women some 17-fold compared with non-consumers, while analgesics not containing phenacetin did not increase the risk of kidney damage (55).

In Belgium, the distribution of analgesic nephropathy in patients with terminal renal insufficiency was well correlated with the sale of drugs containing either aspirin + phenacetin or paracetamol + caffeine (SEDA-7, 75), and it is estimated that Belgium, after Australia, had the second highest incidence of analgesic nephropathy in the world.

Statistics published in 1981 from the European Dialysis and Transplant Association on the causes of chronic renal insufficiency suggested that in Europe about 3.1% of cases up to that time had been drug-induced; the figures cited varied from 0.4% in Spain to 17.5% in Switzerland. Some of the best-documented reports were those from Switzerland, where per capita consumption of phenacetin reached a peak of some 10 g annually between 1955 and 1968 (56). Between 1962 and 1978 the proportion of phenacetin users coming to autopsy increased from 1.8 to 3.1%.

In the USA only a very small proportion of phenacetin patients (in one series 2.8%) have a history of analgesic abuse (57).

True geographic differences cannot be proven from such figures, since the variation from country to country is largely due to inconsistent classification and differences in the selection of patients for dialysis and transplantation (58).

By the early 1980s, most countries had severely restricted or entirely prohibited the sale of phenacetin. Subsequent data from several of these countries suggested that the number of new patients with analgesic nephropathy fell as a result of the prohibition of phenacetin in analgesic mixtures.

Cause

It soon became clear that the major causative agent in analgesic nephropathy was phenacetin, improperly used long-term and especially in combinations with other analgesics, and this identification led to its virtual disappearance in the mid-1970s, following regulatory action.

In recent years it has become obvious that many of the NSAIDs are associated with renal disorders arising de novo or by aggravation of existent renal dysfunction. Inhibition of prostaglandin synthesis intrarenally leads to reduced vasodilator activity of PGE_1, which normally contributes to the maintenance of renal functional balance and protection against the vasoconstrictor effects of noradrenaline and angiotensin-II and the action of antidiuretic hormone. Some experimental work suggests a tendency for phenacetin and its metabolite paracetamol to concentrate in the renal medulla, possibly accounting for the papillary lesions most often associated with them.

There is no evidence that short-term use of cyclo-oxygenase inhibitors has any major deleterious effect on renal function in healthy individuals.

Although some authors have stressed the possible role of aspirin as a causal factor (SED-8, 169), a study of the safety of long-term ingestion of large cumulative doses did not confirm this (59). The patients in question, with seropositive rheumatoid arthritis, had taken aspirin continuously for 10 or more years (mean total dose per patient 36 kg, range 16–82 kg). Their normal creatinine and BUN concentrations, with maximum recorded specific gravities of urine greater than 1019 in 93% of patients, suggested that long-term salicylate ingestion does not cause renal damage or that the magnitude and long-term clinical significance of such damage is not significant. The fact remains, however, that the overwhelming sale of phenacetin was in the form of fixed combinations with aspirin (and sometimes with caffeine, codeine, and other components), and the possibility of some additive effect cannot retrospectively be excluded.

As the debate developed, the safety of paracetamol and its combination with aspirin, which had only come to the fore on a large scale as phenacetin disappeared, also came to be questioned. The difficulty in assigning specific roles to the various analgesics is partly related to the use of drug combinations but largely because of the prolonged time over which the disorder develops.

Susceptibility factors

The association between analgesic abuse and renal papillary necrosis is well established, but the existence of other unrecognized factors is highly probable (SEDA-6, 80). The female/male ratio of analgesic abusers as a whole in the Australian community is 2:1, but the ratio in analgesic nephropathy is about 6.5:1. Swiss data also point to a higher incidence than expected in women and in elderly subjects (40). Climatic factors and fluid intake have also been incriminated, since dehydration can aggravate the risk. Reports of an association between HLA genotype and analgesic nephropathy might explain why only a few of the many individuals who take large quantities of analgesics develop renal insufficiency (60).

Pathology

The primary renal lesions in phenacetin abusers are those involving the capillaries (61,62). In some 80% of cases there is capillary sclerosis, with reduplication of laminar transformation of the intima, due to reduplication of the basement membrane in the capillaries just below the urothelium in the papillae, renal pelvis, and lower urinary tract. It is these changes that make it possible to diagnose analgesic abuse from surgical or postmortem specimens, even when the clinical history is unknown. A morphological study of 21 transitional cell carcinomas in an Australian histopathology department disclosed 16 cases with papillary changes of the analgesic type. Of these patients, only two were known to be analgesic abusers (SEDA-6, 82).

The renal cortical and medullary tubules are similarly affected, since overuse of analgesic-containing formulations can affect the metabolism of the basement membranes of capillaries and tubules and result in thickening of the walls. In skin biopsy specimens from patients with a history of excessive intake of analgesics, thickening of dermal capillaries suggested that the microangiopathy was not confined to the renal tract but also occurred in other organs (SEDA-6, 81).

Associated disorders

In the prospective Swiss Analgesic Study the risk of bacteriuria was about three times higher in those who abused analgesics heavily than in matched controls (63). The primary causes of mortality in this study were tumors and cardiovascular disease; only 7.5% died from primary renal disease due to pyelonephritis.

Renal papillary necrosis with retroperitoneal fibrosis secondary to analgesic abuse (involving aspirin, propoxyphene, and numerous other analgesics taken in large quantities for many years) has also incidentally been reported (SEDA-7, 94).

Patients with analgesic nephropathy have an increased risk of atherosclerosis. In a retrospective study their serum cholesterol and triglyceride concentrations were significantly higher than in a control group of similar age and with a similar degree of renal insufficiency due to other renal diseases (SEDA-6, 81). Some possible mechanisms of hyperlipidemia in analgesic nephropathy have been discussed, as this phenomenon is not sufficiently explained by end-stage renal insufficiency or by protein loss, as in the nephrotic syndrome (SEDA-7, 94).

Urinary tract tumors

Renal carcinoma has been associated with analgesic abuse an order of magnitude greater than in non-abusers (64–66), and the causal association has been recognized since 1965 (SEDA-6, 81) and repeatedly confirmed. In 1984 an authoritative consensus conference in the USA pointed to the evidence that very heavy and sustained use of some analgesic mixtures without phenacetin can also predispose to cancer of the urinary tract, particularly transitional cell carcinoma of the renal pelvis (67).

Of 422 inhabitants of Basel with malignant tumors of the lower urinary tract, 18.5% were users of phenacetin-containing analgesics, which means that carcinomas and sarcomas of the lower urinary tract were nearly 13 times as common in abusers as in non-abusers (66). Carcinoma of the renal pelvis was increased 77-fold, carcinoma of the ureter 89-fold, and carcinoma of the urinary bladder 7-fold. In Australia, in 274 urological patients who had abused phenacetin-containing products, renal symptoms appeared after an average latent period of 10 years; within the last decade of the period studied, 8% of this group (22 patients) had tumors of the urothelium.

In an Australian investigation of renal papillary carcinoma (SEDA-6, 81) the overall crude incidence rate was 1.6 per 100 000 population per year; 47% of the tumors were associated with analgesic abuse and analgesic nephropathy. The risk of renal papillary carcinoma among patients who regularly took analgesics was estimated to be 8 per 100 000 patients per year. Renal papillary carcinoma had a female-to-male ratio among analgesic abusers of 2.6:1, compared with 1:2 among those without analgesic-associated nephropathy. A similar epidemiological study from the USA (65) supported this association between analgesic nephropathy and tumors; 5.2% of patients with transitional carcinoma of the urinary tract diagnosed over 3 years had analgesic-associated nephropathy. The patients were predominantly younger women, who had renal pelvis tumors instead of bladder tumors and a higher mortality rate. In a historical prospective study of 146 patients with interstitial nephritis, 84 cases were associated with analgesics and in four patients transitional cell carcinoma developed. None of the 98 nephritic patients without analgesic-associated nephropathy developed transitional cell carcinoma. In 300 urological patients (75% women) in whom renal and extrarenal manifestations appeared after an average latency period of 20 years, 31 patients had a tumor of the urothelium.

Studies on the tumor-inducing effects of heavy use of analgesics, especially those that contain phenacetin, have given contrasting results (SEDA-21, 100; 68,69). Two case-control studies have been published on the role of habitual intake of analgesics on the occurrence of urothelial cancer and renal cell carcinoma.

In the first study, 647 cases of urothelial cancer (571 bladder, 25 ureter, and 51 renal pelvis) and an identical number of controls were enrolled (70). Exposure to compound analgesic (at least 1 kg of analgesic substances lifelong) showed a substance-specific association, with an increased risk ratio for renal pelvis cancer but not for cancers of the ureter or bladder. Among the different analgesics, anilide derivatives (intake over 1 kg) were associated with the highest risks of renal pelvis cancer, with respective odds ratios of 5.28 for phenacetin (CI = 0.34, 81) and 3.27 for paracetamol (CI = 0.25, 43); however, these odds ratios were not statistically significant. This lack of significance was due mainly to two factors, the high proportion of heavy analgesic use in controls and the low number of cases with renal pelvis cancer, which had the highest risk.

The second study (71) was aimed at clarifying the possible relation between analgesic use and renal cell carcinoma. In previous studies there was a consistent association between phenacetin and renal cell carcinoma, but inconclusive results with respect to non-phenacetin analgesics. In 1024 patients with renal cell carcinoma and an equal number of matched controls, regular use of analgesics was a significant risk factor for renal cell carcinoma (OR = 1.6; CI = 1.4, 1.9). The risk was significantly increased by all four major classes of analgesics (aspirin, NSAIDs, paracetamol, and phenacetin) and within each class of analgesic, the risk increased with increasing exposure. Individuals in the highest exposure categories had about a 2.5-fold increase in risk relative to non-users or irregular users of analgesics. However, exclusive users of aspirin who took aspirin 325 mg/day or less for cardiovascular problems were not at an increased risk of renal cell carcinoma (OR = 0.9; CI = 0.6, 1.4).

In contrast to these results, another large case-control study (72) in 1732 patients with renal cell carcinoma and 2039 controls showed no increase in the risk of renal cell carcinoma among regular users of phenacetin, paracetamol, and aspirin. There is no clear explanation of these disparate findings.

Conclusions

The history of analgesic nephropathy must not be dismissed as involving only a drug now obsolete. Phenacetin, alone or in combination with other analgesics, was unwisely taken chronically by a large section of the public, and unless such misuse of analgesics can be avoided, there is much reason to fear that the story will be repeated with other agents and combinations.

If analgesics are discontinued in the early phases of nephropathy, there is a reasonable possibility of a return to normal renal function. It is wise to ensure that the dosage of aspirin or paracetamol, or of any NSAID, is kept as low as possible, that renal function is regularly assessed, and that prolonged use is avoided, especially in patients over 65 years of age, who seem to be at particular risk of analgesic nephropathy and who may also have pre-existing renal dysfunction, including marginally compensated asymptomatic renal insufficiency (52).

There is no evidence that short-term use of single cyclo-oxygenase inhibitors has any major deleterious effect on renal function in healthy, non-hypovolemic individuals, but even short-term use of a compound of this class is never a guarantee that nephropathy will not occur.

Skin

Rashes, usually erythematous, occur occasionally (73–75).

Paracetamol can rarely cause fixed drug eruptions (76,77), including an unusual non-pigmented fixed drug eruption (78).

Henoch–Schönlein purpura has been attributed to paracetamol + codeine (co-codamol) (79).

- A 69-year-old man took Co-efferalgan (co-codamol) for 1 week and developed a fever, hematuria, acute renal failure, palpable purpura on the legs, feet, and arms, arthralgias, and abdominal discomfort. His serum creatinine and C-reactive protein were raised but there was no thrombocytopenia or hypocomplementemia. Co-codamol was withdrawn. The hematuria resolved in 2 days, the purpura disappeared in 10 days, renal function returned to normal after 2 weeks, and the abdominal pain and arthralgias improved during the following 2–3 weeks.

This appears to be the only case of Henoch–Schönlein purpura that has been attributed to co-codamol.

Immunologic

Acute hypersensitivity reactions due to paracetamol are rare (SEDA-22, 114), but can be life-threatening (80).

Long-Term Effects

Mutagenicity

Animal studies have indicated a carcinogenic effect when paracetamol has been administered for prolonged periods in relatively high dosages. However, no clinical data are so far available to corroborate this. The matter cannot be dismissed entirely for the time being, in view of a report (81) of the development of chromosomal aberrations after prolonged use.

Tumorigenicity

In a questionnaire study of the effects of paracetamol on the risk of acute leukemia in 169 adult with leukemia and 676 age- and sex-matched hospital controls with non-neoplastic conditions ever use of paracetamol was associated with a slightly increased risk of leukemia (adjusted OR = 1.53; 95% CI = 1.03, 2.26) (82). There was no difference between men and women.

Second-Generation Effects

Fetotoxicity

Paracetamol crosses the placenta readily. However, there has been no published evidence of a teratogenic effect in the offspring of mothers who have taken paracetamol during pregnancy. A case of fetal death after a maternal overdose of paracetamol (30 g) has been described (SEDA-10, 73), but in another similar case, in which 22.5 g was taken in the 36th week, the fetus survived (SEDA-9, 96). Preliminary data from a longitudinal study have shown no adverse effects of therapeutic doses of paracetamol on either pregnancy or infant development (83).

Susceptibility Factors

Hepatic disease

It is generally considered inadvisable to use paracetamol in patients with active liver disease or severe liver dysfunction, patients with cachexia, or chronic alcoholics. Stable mild chronic liver disease does not seem to be a contraindication (84).

In a retrospective review of all cases of exposure to paracetamol that occurred over 3 years in children under 18 years of age who were managed in a regional poison control center, there were 473 exposures; 76% were in those under 6 years, 3% in those aged 6–12 years, and 21% in those aged 13–17 years (85). Unintentional ingestion was the most common type of exposure in the first two age groups (100 and 94% respectively), but in the older children intentional ingestion was more common (91%); girls represented far more of these exposures than boys (87 versus 14%).

Drug Administration

Drug overdose

Paracetamol is one of the most commonly ingested medications in deliberate self-poisoning and accidental ingestion by children.

Fulminant hepatic failure occurs in 1–5% of cases of paracetamol overdosage 3–6 days after ingestion (86), with frequent deaths in people who take 20–25 g. There is only a narrow margin between the normal maximum 24-hour dosage and that which can cause liver damage and acute hepatic failure. Undoubtedly, some people are more susceptible than most to paracetamol toxicity, since although 6 g has been reported as toxic in some cases, most toxicity is seen with 12 g upwards (87,88). Nomograms have been developed to show the relation between plasma paracetamol concentrations over time and the risk of a serious outcome (SEDA-18, 94).

Epidemiology

Paracetamol is a widely-used, effective, and well-tolerated analgesic, but thanks also to its ready availability, it is the most commonly used substance in self-poisoning (SEDA-18, 94) (89) and a frequent cause of accidental overdose, especially in children (SEDA-22, 114), although children of 6 years and under are rarely subject to hepatotoxicity, even with accidental overdosage (90), possibly owing to age-dependent differences in paracetamol kinetics (91).

From prospective data (89,92), it has been estimated that around 58 000 people take paracetamol in overdose each year in England and Wales and that these episodes of poisoning prompted 3.3% of inquiries to US regional poisons centers (93), 10% of inquiries to the UK National Poisons Information Service (94), and up to 43% of all admissions to hospital with self-poisoning in the UK (95). Despite the availability of effective antidotes for patients who seek medical intervention early after an overdose, in the USA paracetamol alone accounted for 4.1% of deaths from poisoning reported to American poison centers in 1997 (93).

Paracetamol plus dextropropoxyphene, the combination known as co-proxamol, is available as a prescription-only analgesic in many countries. Self-poisoning can be lethal, as respiratory depression can occur from an excessive dose of dextropropoxyphene. In England and Wales, co-proxamol alone accounts for 5% of all suicides, and overdose is more likely to result in death than overdose with paracetamol alone or tricyclic antidepressants (96). Furthermore, although it is often prescribed, it is no more effective than paracetamol for short-term relief of pain. It should not be prescribed without good reason.

Nutrition

In patients who develop liver damage after moderate or even recommended doses of paracetamol, recent fasting or severe nutritional impairment have been described as possible susceptibility factors for hepatotoxicity (97).

Symptoms and signs

While damage to the liver is effected within hours of ingestion, major clinical manifestations are seldom seen until some 24–48 hours. However, they can be prevented by early treatment. Thus, early history taking, a high index of suspicion, and prompt and repeated assays of plasma paracetamol concentrations are essential in emergency management. Primary signs, when they do appear, are those of liver failure, for example abdominal pain and tenderness, followed by jaundice, raised serum transaminases, and reduced concentrations of coagulation factors, resulting in a prolonged prothrombin time. It may be up to a week before severe liver failure ensues. Consciousness is not usually lost early on, but resistant cerebral edema can intervene in a few days secondary to hepatic failure.

Acute renal tubular damage occurs in association with the liver damage, together with muscle necrosis and hyperkalemia. The muscle necrosis, as demonstrated at autopsy in fatal cases (98), can itself exacerbate the severe electrolyte derangement, particularly marked hyperkalemia, that occurs in liver failure. The measurement of serum concentrations of coagulation factors V (below 10%) and VIII (VIII/V ratio over 30) can have predictive value and can thus be helpful in selecting patients who require liver transplantation (SEDA-17, 99).

In 8 patients aged 16–32 years old who for suicidal purposes took paracetamol, average 17.8 g, there were changes in renal function compared with 21 healthy individuals (99). There were transient increases in the activities of N-acetyl-β-D-glucosaminidase, α-glutathione transferase, β-glucuronidase, γ-glutamyltransferase, and the efficiency of nephron resorption through β_2-microglobulin enzymes. However, there were no cases of acute renal failure.

- A 29-year-old woman with a psychiatric disorder took an overdose of paracetamol on nine separate occasions. On the last three occasions she developed a dose-dependent, late-onset, delayed hypersensitivity reaction, characterized by an erythematous rash over the entire body (100).

Risk factors
Alcohol

Alcohol abuse can predispose to paracetamol hepatotoxicity (101–108), even in moderate social drinkers who take therapeutic or modestly excessive doses (109), and there have been anecdotal reports of severe hepatotoxicity in chronic ethanol abusers after ingestion of 4 g/day (110). Alcoholics are more likely to exceed the recommended dosage of paracetamol and consequently may be at higher risk of hepatotoxicity than non-alcoholics (108,111).

The theory behind this effect involves induction by alcohol of CYP2E1, which metabolizes about 5% of a typical dose of paracetamol, producing the reactive hepatotoxic metabolite named N-acetylparabenzoquinone-imine (NAPQI), which is normally metabolized by glutathione (112). The rest of a therapeutic dose of paracetamol is conjugated to non-toxic forms of glucuronide and sulfate. Saturation of the detoxification pathway occurs with overdose of paracetamol (87), or sometimes in certain individuals who make long-term use of normal dosages (113), in patients with compromised hepatic function, with certain drug combinations, and in other conditions of glutathione deficiency. Ingestion of alcohol induces the activity of CYP2E1 and therefore predisposes the alcoholic patient to injury even at therapeutic doses of paracetamol (114).

Despite this theory, the evidence that therapeutic doses of paracetamol can produce liver injury in alcoholics is scanty (115,116). There has been only one study of the hepatotoxicity of paracetamol in therapeutic doses in alcoholic patients, a double-blind, randomized, placebo-controlled study in which 200 long-term alcoholic patients took placebo or paracetamol 1 g qds on two consecutive days (117). Paracetamol was not given until alcohol had been eliminated from the body. Liver injury, documented by increased serum transaminases, was not detected. Mean aspartate transaminase activity on day 4 was 38 U/l with paracetamol and 38 U/l with placebo. Only five patients who took placebo and four who took paracetamol had an increase in serum aspartate transaminase to greater than 120 U/l, and it did not exceed 200 U/l in any patient. Thus, repeated administration of the maximum recommended daily doses of paracetamol to alcoholic patients was not associated with liver damage. An older report also provided evidence that alcoholic patients are not at risk from therapeutic doses of paracetamol (84). The researchers concluded that the usual recommendations that alcoholic patients should use reduced doses of paracetamol or avoid it entirely are not based on firm evidence. However, the study had some limitations, as paracetamol was given for only 2 days in doses that did not exceed the maximum therapeutic daily dose. Moreover, the alcoholic patients enrolled in the study may not have been representative of those who would be at increased risk of paracetamol toxicity (118–120). It therefore seems wise to suggest that caution is still warranted with paracetamol in alcoholic patients.

Other drugs

Analgesic cocktails or the concurrent use of potentially hepatotoxic drugs increase the risk of paracetamol toxicity.

Drugs that induce liver microsomal enzymes, such as phenobarbital, phenytoin, carbamazepine, rifampicin, and isoniazid, can make paracetamol poisoning more severe (121,122). In patients taking such drugs the serum paracetamol concentration should be doubled before consulting the usual treatment nomogram.

Fasting

Potentiation of the toxic effects of paracetamol by fasting has been previously shown in animals. In 21 cases of paracetamol hepatotoxicity not due to intentional overdosage, fasting was significantly more common than recent alcohol use among patients who developed hepatotoxicity after a dosage of 4–10 g/day (SEDA-20, 96).

Prevention
Restricting supplies

The easy availability of paracetamol is reported to be the most common reason for its common use in overdose (123), and so reducing its availability might be an effective strategy. Therefore, in September 1998 legislation was introduced in the UK limiting the pack size of paracetamol to 20 units of 500 mg; at the same time nearly all formulations became available only in blister packs. The justification for this legislation was that analgesic self-poisoning is highly impulsive and is associated with both low suicidal intent and limited knowledge of the possible consequences; it was expected that the number of cases of paracetamol overdose might be reduced by limiting its availability.

The impact of this legislation on mortality from paracetamol overdose has been assessed in a prospective study of mortality from paracetamol overdose before and after the new legislation (124). The evaluation included the number of patients referred to liver units or listed for liver transplantation, the number of episodes of overdose and tablets taken, the plasma concentration of paracetamol, and sales of paracetamol to pharmacies. In the years after the legislation the number of tablets of paracetamol formulations per packet fell markedly, as did the number of deaths from self-poisoning with paracetamol, the number of liver transplants and admissions to liver units with hepatic damage after paracetamol poisoning, and the number of episodes of overdose in which a large number of tablets was taken. On the basis of these results it seems that the legislation was relatively successful. The results suggested that the main factor was the reduction in the number of tablets per pack available for impulsive self-poisoning. However, the study had some limitations. The period assessed may have been too short for a full assessment of the impact of the legislation (125), and the effect of legislation on self-poisoning with other drugs was not examined (126).

It may be that limiting access to one type of drug simply increases the incidence of overdose with other potentially more dangerous medicines. If that is so, unless the availability of other medications is also controlled, the removal of one readily available medication, such as paracetamol, could lead to an increase in the use of other compounds with similar or even greater toxicity (for example aspirin, ibuprofen).

In Australia, paracetamol-containing medications were recalled during two periods in 2000, presenting a unique opportunity for a retrospective observational study of the effect of reduced availability of paracetamol on the incidence of deliberate self-poisoning and accidental pediatric poisoning with paracetamol and other over-the-counter analgesics (127). During the recall periods there was a significant increase in ibuprofen deliberate self-poisoning (RR = 1.86; 95% CI = 1.41, 2.44), while there was no statistically significant change in paracetamol and aspirin deliberate self-poisoning. In children there was a significant increase in the proportion of ibuprofen accidental poisoning but no significant change for aspirin and paracetamol.

These results suggest that reduced paracetamol availability increased poisoning with alternative analgesics (in particular ibuprofen) but had little effect on the incidence of paracetamol poisoning. Restriction of paracetamol-containing medications should be critically reconsidered as an effective strategy for preventing deliberate and accidental poisoning.

Adding antidotes to oral formulations
Because restricting the packet size cannot completely resolve the problem of paracetamol overdose, alternative measures have been proposed (SEDA-22, 114). Because of the beneficial effect of acetylcysteine in paracetamol overdose, it has been suggested that toxicity caused by paracetamol overdoses, whether intentional or not, could be prevented by formulating paracetamol with added acetylcysteine. It has been estimated that including 200 mg acetylcysteine for every 500 mg of paracetamol would prevent toxicity (128,129). Methionine has previously been added to oral paracetamol formulations for the same reason. For example, Paradote contains paracetamol 500 mg and methionine 100 mg, and the combination is called co-methiamol. However, adding methionine to every paracetamol tablet prompted contrasting opinions (SEDA-22, 114) (130,131). Pameton (paracetamol 500 mg + methionine 250 mg) was voluntarily withdrawn in the UK because of safety concerns, before any evaluation of its impact on overdose had been carried out (130). Paradote remains available in the UK, but similar formulations are not currently available in the rest of Europe or the USA.

Treatment
Gastric lavage, especially in the first hour after ingestion, is recommended.

Glutathione donors
Since the mechanism of damage appears to be the exhaustion or depletion of sulfhydryl groups, as available in glutathione, treatment consists of early replacement of those groups by administration of an alternative source of glutathione, either oral methionine or, better, N-acetylcysteine, either orally or intravenously. To be most effective, a glutathione donor should be given within 8–12 hours of ingestion of the overdosage, but even up to 24 hours administration can improve the outcome (132). Acetylcysteine is usually given intravenously, but a 20-hour treatment protocol for acute paracetamol overdose using oral acetylcysteine has also been proposed (133) and was effective in preventing hepatic injury after an acute overdose of paracetamol when therapy was begun within 8 hours after ingestion.

To reduce the chance of liver damage and death in cases of paracetamol overdosage, guidelines have been produced in many countries (89,134,135) to identify patients at high risk who need to be treated soon with acetylcysteine.

In general, such guidelines recommend that the antidote should be given to all patients with a serum paracetamol concentration over 200 µg/ml (1.32 mmol/l) 4 hours after ingestion. A nomogram, in which this value is joined to an end-point of 25 µg/ml (0.16 mmol/l) at 16 hours, allows identification over this period of the patients who must receive the antidote. If acetylcysteine is not administered, it has been calculated that over 60% of patients with serum concentration of paracetamol above the described treatment line develop serious liver damage and of these about 5% will die (136). No deaths have been reported in any of the major treatment trials, however high the initial serum paracetamol concentrations, provided acetylcysteine was given within 10 hours of paracetamol ingestion. These data support the hypothesis that serious liver damage and death should be very uncommon if treatment guidelines are followed and if the patient presents for medical advice within the critical time of 10 hours from poisoning.

However, a report (136) has described fatal overdose of paracetamol in four patients who presented within 10 hours with serum paracetamol concentrations below the treatment line who, in accord with the established guidelines, were not treated with the antidote and developed fatal acute liver failure. The report generated considerable debate by advocating changing the treatment line for the use of antidotes in patients at standard risk from paracetamol poisoning from that currently recommended to a lower line passing through 150 µg/ml at 4 hours and 30 µg/ml at 12 hours.

A second "high-risk patient" line, at about half the concentration of the conventional treatment line, has already been adopted in some guidelines for patients considered at adjunctive risk of liver damage, such as those taking long-term enzyme-inducing drugs, abusing alcohol chronically, or with poor nutrition and cachexia.

However, an absolute cut-off point between a non-toxic and a toxic paracetamol overdose does not exist. Many factors should be taken into consideration in correctly interpreting the measured serum concentrations. First, the timing of the blood sample in relation to the overdose is often uncertain, and when using treatment nomogram clinicians should assume the longest interval between poisoning and blood sampling that is consistent with the history. Secondly, the current treatment nomogram is useless when paracetamol overdosage has occurred over several hours or more rather than as a single episode. Thirdly, apart from the already mentioned known risk factors, some individual differences in susceptibility to paracetamol are not well understood.

Therefore, owing to these uncertainties, it seems wise to suggest that in judging whether or not to use an antidote, clinicians should always err on the side of caution: "If there is doubt about the timing or the need of treatment, treat" (89).

Oral and intravenous N-acetylcysteine in the management of paracetamol overdose have been compared (137). The advantages and disadvantages are listed in Table 1. The authors concluded that acetylcysteine can be given orally to patients who present within 8–10 hours of paracetamol overdose and intravenously to those who present after 10 hours or have underlying conditions that prevent oral administration.

Other methods of treatment

The only alternatives to glutathione donors are charcoal hemoperfusion and hemodialysis, which can be effective up to 18 hours after dosage. However, the longer the time from ingestion to treatment, the less likely the condition is to be reversible and the more likely a fatal outcome.

The use of activated charcoal in addition to standard N-acetylcysteine therapy after paracetamol overdose has been assessed in a 1-year non-randomized, prospective, multicenter, observational case series of 145 patients, of whom 58 received N-acetylcysteine only and 87 received N-acetylcysteine + activated charcoal (138). Activated charcoal was associated with a reduced incidence of liver injury, as assessed by serum transaminases and prothrombin time.

Theoretically, inhibitors of cytochrome P450, like cimetidine, might be of value in the treatment of paracetamol overdosage, and preliminary animal data also suggest this (132).

Drug–Drug Interactions

Alcohol

The FDA has announced its intention to require alcohol warnings on all over-the-counter pain medications that contain acetylsalicylic acid, salicylates, paracetamol, ibuprofen, ketoprofen, or naproxen. The proposed warnings are aimed at alerting consumers to the specific risks incurred from heavy alcohol consumption and its interaction with analgesics. For products that contain paracetamol, the warning indicates the risks of liver damage in those who drink more than three alcoholic beverages a day. For formulations that contain salicylates or the mentioned NSAIDs three or more alcoholic beverages will increase the risk of stomach bleeding (139).

Argatroban

The thrombin inhibitor argatroban had no effect on the pharmacokinetics of five oral doses of paracetamol 1 g 6-hourly in 12 healthy volunteers; the argatroban was given as an intravenous infusion of 1.5 µg/kg/minute from hours 12 to 30 (140).

Table 1 The advantages and disadvantages of oral and intravenous N-acetylcysteine in the management of paracetamol ovedose

Formulation	Advantages	Disadvantages
Oral	Cheap	Putrid odor; taste very difficult to mask
	Easy to prepare and administer	Nausea and vomiting common
	Non-IgE-mediated anaphylactic (anaphylactoid) reactions rare	Delayed action, depending on rate of absorption (delayed by anticholinergic drugs)
		Reduces the binding of activated charcoal to paracetamol
		High concentrations in the liver during first-pass—potential for hepatotoxicity
Intravenous	Rapidly effective	Difficult to prepare and administer reliably—errors can occur
	Reliable access to the systemic circulation, not affected by vomiting	Adverse effects include non-IgE-mediated anaphylactic (anaphylactoid) reactions, asthma, and epilepsy; severe adverse effects are rare

Chlormezanone

The concomitant use of paracetamol may increase the chance of adverse effects, especially erythema and urticaria (154).

Hormonal contraceptives—oral

Paracetamol might have a similar effect to ascorbic acid, that is competition with ethinylestradiol for sulfation capacity in the gut. Paracetamol significantly reduced the AUC of ethinylestradiol sulfate but had no effect on plasma levonorgestrel concentrations

In six healthy women, a single dose of paracetamol 1 g significantly increased the AUC of ethinylestradiol by 22% and reduced the AUC of ethinylestradiol sulfate (155). Plasma concentrations of levonorgestrel were unaltered. This interaction could be of clinical significance in women taking oral contraceptives who take paracetamol regularly or suddenly stop taking it, but it is doubtful whether it has any practical repercussions.

The clearance of paracetamol was 22% greater in men than women, entirely because of increased glucuronidation, there being no sex-related differences in the sulfation or oxidative metabolism of paracetamol (156). Paracetamol clearance in women using oral contraceptive steroids was 49% greater than in the control women. Glucuronidation and oxidative metabolism were both induced in contraceptive users (by 78% and 36% respectively) but sulfation was not altered. Although sex-related differences in paracetamol metabolism are unlikely to be of clinical importance, induction of paracetamol metabolism by oral contraceptive steroids may have clinical and toxicological consequences.

Phenytoin

Paracetamol is metabolized in part by CYP2E1, and inducers of CYP2E1 predispose patients to paracetamol hepatotoxicity. However, a possible interaction leading to hepatotoxicity with phenytoin has been reported in a 55-year-old woman taking paracetamol 1300–6200 mg/day over 10 days (141). Phenytoin induces CYP2C and CYP3A4 but not CYP2E1. As CYP3A4 may participate in paracetamol metabolism the induction of this isoform may also be responsible for paracetamol-induced hepatotoxicity.

Drugs that induce hepatic drug-metabolizing enzymes increase the toxicity of paracetamol after overdose, and another case has been reported in which liver transplantation was necessary (142).

- A 22-year-old man taking steady-state phenytoin took 25 ibuprofen tablets 400 mg plus paracetamol 25 g. He was given oral N-acetylcysteine. The serum phenytoin concentration was 128 μmol/l (32 μg/ml) and the paracetamol concentration at 6 hours after the overdose was 0.87 μmol/l (131 μg/ml) which was judged to be below the treatment threshold of about 1.06 μmol/l (160 μg/ml). On day 3 he developed hepatic encephalopathy and acute renal failure requiring hemodialysis. His arterial pH was 7.19, alanine transaminase over 3500 U/l, total bilirubin 205 μmol/l, and prothrombin time over 50 sec (INR over 30). He underwent successful liver transplantation on day 4. The liver explant showed massive hepatic necrosis.

The usual criterion for acetylcysteine therapy when a patient is taking an enzyme-inducing drug is to double the serum paracetamol concentration before using the nomogram. There were many deficiencies in this report (143), and it is not clear whether this patient was given appropriate therapy.

Rifampicin

The addition of rifampicin in patients taking paracetamol can reportedly cause liver failure and encephalopathy (144).

- A 32-year-old woman, who had been taking paracetamol 2–4 g/day for several weeks, was given rifampicin 600 mg bd, and 2 days later developed agitation, confusion, and laboratory abnormalities indicative of severe liver injury. Both rifampicin and paracetamol were withdrawn and she was given acetylcysteine. Her liver dysfunction resolved.

The severe hepatotoxicity in this case was probably due to induction of CYP3A4 by rifampicin, but rifampicin-induced liver damage could not be excluded.

Warfarin

The anticoagulant effect of warfarin is potentiated by concomitant long-term paracetamol administration.

In an early, double-blind, placebo-controlled study of the interaction between coumarin anticoagulants and paracetamol, there was a statistically significant lengthening of the prothrombin time (145). The effect, although statistically significant, was very small and was considered to be clinically unimportant.

However, in a case-control study of the risk factors for excessive warfarin anticoagulation the investigators studied 289 patients prospectively, 93 with an International Normalized Ratio (INR) over 6.0 and 196 with an INR of 1.7–3.3 during warfarin therapy (146). Paracetamol intake was independently associated with a high INR and the effect was dose-related. At a dosage of about 2–4 g/week the adjusted odds ratio (OR) for having an INR over 6 was 3.5 (95% CI = 1.2, 10) compared with no intake of paracetamol. At an intake of 4–9 g/week the adjusted OR was 6.9 (95% CI = 2.2, 22), and at an intake over 10 g/week the OR was 10 (95% CI = 2.6, 38).

However, the results of this study must be interpreted with caution, for many reasons. First, despite these data and the widespread use of paracetamol as an analgesic in patients taking warfarin, only few reports from the literature have described serious hemorrhagic complications due to potentiation of anticoagulant effect of warfarin or acenocoumarol by paracetamol (147,148). Secondly, numerous factors in the Hylex study were independently associated with an increased likelihood of having an INR over 6.0 and it is therefore possible that overlap could have occurred between these factors and paracetamol intake. Thirdly, the biochemical mechanism by which paracetamol may interfere with warfarin is not well understood. The normal metabolism of warfarin, which occurs via hepatic cytochrome P450, is a complex mechanism that can be competitively and non-competitively inhibited by many drugs. The normal metabolism of paracetamol, particularly when large doses of paracetamol are ingested, also involves cytochrome P450. Thus, paracetamol can exhaust the capacity of cytochrome P450 and prevent the normal metabolism of warfarin. When the normal metabolism of warfarin is prevented by paracetamol, the amount of active, non-protein bound warfarin promptly increases and may double or triple in concentration in the blood. Some pharmacological data, however, makes this explanation uncertain. CYP2E1 and CYP1A2 partially metabolize paracetamol. CYP2E1 is not involved in warfarin metabolism, CYP1A2 partially metabolizes paracetamol and is responsible for metabolism of *R*-warfarin, the less potent anticoagulant of the two warfarin stereoisomers. While *R*-warfarin and paracetamol may compete for metabolism, it is unlikely that a drug that competes for or inhibits metabolism of the less potent *R*-warfarin would significantly increase the INR. Finally, despite sporadic case reports this potential interaction has been suggested to be clinically irrelevant on the basis of the extensive collective experience of many clinicians in managing patients who require anticoagulation (149,150).

Some pharmacokinetic studies have failed to show such an interaction (151). However, if this interaction happens in only a few individuals at risk, a formal pharmacokinetic study in a small number of subjects would probably fail to include enough of such individuals to detect an effect. A case-control study, on the other hand, would be the appropriate design for detecting this type of interaction.

Thus, the key message from this study is that in patients taking a stable warfarin regimen who begin to take repeated doses of paracetamol a possible interaction should be considered. The dose and duration of paracetamol therapy should be as low as possible and INR values should be monitored.

Zidovudine

Concomitant administration of paracetamol and zidovudine leads to inhibition of glucuronidation and to potentiation of the toxicity of each drug (152,153).

Interference with Diagnostic Tests

YSI glucose analyser

Paracetamol can cause false-positive reactions for glucose in serum and blood specimens examined using the YSI glucose analyser. The effect could be of considerable importance in patients admitted with suspected paracetamol overdosage.

References

1. MacIntyre A, Gray JD, Gorelick M, Renton K. Salicylate and acetaminophen in donated blood. CMAJ 1986;135(3):215–6.
2. Wynne HA, Long A. Patient awareness of the adverse effects of non-steroidal anti-inflammatory drugs (NSAIDs). Br J Clin Pharmacol 1996;42(2):253–6.
3. National Drugs Advisory Board. Availability of aspirin and paracetamol. Annual Report 1987;24.
4. Mitchell JA, Akarasereenont P, Thiemermann C, Flower RJ, Vane JR. Selectivity of nonsteroidal antiinflammatory drugs as inhibitors of constitutive and inducible cyclooxygenase. Proc Natl Acad Sci USA 1993;90(24):11693–7.
5. Curhan GC, Willett WC, Rosner B, Stampfer MJ. Frequency of analgesic use and risk of hypertension in younger women. Arch Intern Med 2002;162(19):2204–8.
6. Radack KL, Deck CC, Bloomfield SS. Ibuprofen interferes with the efficacy of antihypertensive drugs. A randomized, double-blind, placebo-controlled trial of ibuprofen compared with acetaminophen. Ann Intern Med 1987;107(5):628–35.
7. Chalmers JP, West MJ, Wing LM, Bune AJ, Graham JR. Effects of indomethacin, sulindac, naproxen, aspirin, and paracetamol in treated hypertensive patients. Clin Exp Hypertens A 1984;6(6):1077–93.
8. Schenck NL. Nasal polypectomy in the aspirin-sensitive asthmatic. Trans Am Acad Ophthalmol Otolaryngol 1973;77:30.
9. Roth B, Woo O, Blanc P. Early metabolic acidosis and coma after acetaminophen ingestion. Ann Emerg Med 1999;33(4):452–6.
10. Eneli I, Sadri K, Camargo C Jr, Barr RG. Acetaminophen and the risk of asthma: the epidemiologic and pathophysiologic evidence. Chest 2005;127:604–12.
11. Newson RB, Shaheen SO, Chinn S, Burney PG. Paracetamol sales and atopic disease in children and adults: an ecological analysis. Eur Respir J 2000;16:817–23.
12. Shaheen SO, Sterne JA, Songhurst CE, Burney PG. Frequent paracetamol use and asthma in adults. Thorax 2000;55(4):266–70.
13. Shaheen SO, Newson RB, Sherriff A, Henderson AJ, Heron JE, Burney PG, Golding J, ALSPAC Study Team. Paracetamol use in pregnancy and wheezing in early childhood. Thorax 2002;57:958–63.
14. Barr RG, Wentowsky CC, Curhan GC, Somers SC, Stampfer MJ, Schwarts J, Speizer FE, Camargo CA. Prospective study of acetaminophen use and newly diagnosed asthma among women. Am J Respir Crit Care Med 2004;169:836–41.
15. McKeever TM, Lewis SA, Smit HA, Burney P, Britton JR, Cassano PA. The association of acetaminophen, aspirin, and ibuprofen with respiratory disease and lung function. Am J Respir Crit Care Med 2005;171:966–71.
16. Lesko SM, Mitchell AA. The safety of acetaminophen and ibuprofen among children younger than two years old. Pediatrics 1999;104:39.
17. Karimi M, Mirzaei M, Ahmadieh MH. Acetaminophen use and the symptoms of asthma, allergic rhinitis and eczema in children. Iran J Allergy Asthma Immunol 2006;5(2):63–7.
18. Barragán-Meijueiro MM, Morfín-Maciel B, Nava-Ocampo AA. A Mexican population-based study on exposure to paracetamol and the risk of wheezing, rhinitis, and eczema in childhood. J Investig Allergol Clin Immunol 2006;16(4):247–52.
19. Srikiatkhachorn A, Anthony M. Serotonin receptor adaptation in patients with analgesic-induced headache. Cephalalgia 1996;16(6):419–22.
20. Srikiatkhachorn A, Anthony M. Platelet serotonin in patients with analgesic-induced headache. Cephalalgia 1996;16(6):423–6.
21. Symon DN. Twelve cases of analgesic headache. Arch Dis Child 1998;78(6):555–6.

22. Vasconcellos E, Pina-Garza JE, Millan EJ, Warner JS. Analgesic rebound headache in children and adolescents. J Child Neurol 1998;13(9):443–7.

23. Ruvalcaba RH, Limbeck GA, Kelley VC. Acetaminophen and hypoglycemia. Am J Dis Child 1966;112(6):558–60.

24. Mendoza CD, Heard K, Dart RC. Coma, metabolic acidosis and normal liver function in a child with a large serum acetaminophen level. Ann Emerg Med 2006;48(5):637.

25. Duhamel G, Najman A, Gorin NC, Stachowiak. Aspects actuels de l'agranulocytose (àpropos de 15 observations). [Current aspects of agranulocytosis (15 cases).] Ann Med Interne (Paris) 1977;128(3):303–6.

26. Bougie D, Aster R. Immune thrombocytopenia resulting from sensitivity to metabolites of naproxen and acetaminophen. Blood 2001;97(12):3846–50.

27. Heintz B, Bock TA, Kierdorf H, Maurin N. Haemolytic crisis after acetaminophen in glucose-(6)-phosphate dehydrogenase deficiency. Klin Wochenschr 1989;67(20):1068.

28. González-Pérez A, Rodríguez LA. Upper gastrointestinal complications among users of paracetamol. Basic Clin Pharmacol Toxicol 2006;98(3):297–303.

29. Ranganathan SS, Sathiadas MG, Sumanasena S, Fernandopulle M, Lamabadusuriya SP, Fernandopulle BM. Fulminant hepatic failure and paracetamol overuse with therapeutic intent in febrile children. Indian J Pediatr 2006;73(10):871–5.

30. Kuffner EK, Temple AR, Cooper KM, Baggish JS, Parenti DL. Retrospective analysis of transient elevations in alanine aminotransferase during long-term treatment with acetaminophen in osteoarthritis clinical trials. Curr Med Res Opin 2006;22(11):2137–48.

31. Waldum HL, Hamre T, Kleveland PM, Dybdahl JH, Petersen H. Can NSAIDs cause acute biliary pain with cholestasis? J Clin Gastroenterol 1992;14(4):328–30.

32. Wong V, Daly M, Boon A, Heatley V. Paracetamol and acute biliary pain with cholestasis. Lancet 1993;342(8875):869.

33. Gilmore IT, Tourvas E. Paracetamol-induced acute pancreatitis. BMJ 1977;1(6063):753–4.

34. Schwarz A, Kunzendorf U, Keller F, Offermann G. Progression of renal failure in analgesic-associated nephropathy. Nephron 1989;53(3):244–9.

35. McCredie M, Stewart JH. Does paracetamol cause urothelial cancer or renal papillary necrosis? Nephron 1988;49(4):296–300.

36. Walker RJ. Paracetamol, nonsteroidal antiinflammatory drugs and nephrotoxicity. NZ Med J 1991;104(911):182–3.

37. Pommer W, Bronder E, Greiser E, Helmert U, Jesdinsky HJ, Klimpel A, Borner K, Molzahn M. Regular analgesic intake and the risk of end-stage renal failure. Am J Nephrol 1989;9(5):403–12.

38. Sandler DP, Smith JC, Weinberg CR, Buckalew VM Jr, Dennis VW, Blythe WB, Burgess WP. Analgesic use and chronic renal disease. N Engl J Med 1989;320(19):1238–43.

39. Steenland NK, Thun MJ, Ferguson CW, Port FK. Occupational and other exposures associated with male end-stage renal disease: a case/control study. Am J Public Health 1990;80(2):153–7.

40. Spuhler O, Zollinger HU. Die chronische interstitielle Nephritis. [Chronic interstitial nephritis.] Helv Med Acta 1950;17(4–5):564–7.

41. Delzell E, Shapiro S. A review of epidemiologic studies of nonnarcotic analgesics and chronic renal disease. Medicine (Baltimore) 1998;77(2):102–21.

42. McLaughlin JK, Lipworth L, Chow WH, Blot WJ. Analgesic use and chronic renal failure: a critical review of the epidemiologic literature. Kidney Int 1998;54(3):679–86.

43. Rexrode KM, Buring JE, Glynn RJ, Stampfer MJ, Youngman LD, Gaziano JM. Analgesic use and renal function in men. JAMA 2001;286(3):315–21.

44. Fored CM, Ejerblad E, Lindblad P, Fryzek JP, Dickman PW, Signorello LB, Lipworth L, Elinder CG, Blot WJ, McLaughlin JK, Zack MM, Nyren O. Acetaminophen, aspirin, and chronic renal failure. N Engl J Med 2001;345(25):1801–8.

45. Tuffs A. German nephrologists demand painkiller ban. Lancet 1996;348:952.

46. Anonymous. Analgesics combos go Rx in Belgium. Scrip 1999;2424:4.

47. De Broe ME, Elseviers MM. Analgesic nephropathy. N Engl J Med 1998;338(7):446–52.

48. Schwarz A, Preuschof L, Zellner D. Incidence of analgesic nephropathy in Berlin since 1983. Nephrol Dial Transplant 1999;14(1):109–12.

49. Fox JM. Doubts about a particularly high nephrotoxicity of combination analgesics. Nephrol Dial Transplant 1999;14(12):2966–8.

50. Elseviers MM, Bosteels V, Cambier P, De Paepe M, Godon JP, Lins R, Lornoy W, Matthys E, Moeremans C, Roose R, et al. Diagnostic criteria of analgesic nephropathy in patients with end-stage renal failure: results of the Belgian study. Nephrol Dial Transplant 1992;7(6):479–86.

51. Elseviers MM, Waller I, Nenoy D, Levora J, Matousovic K, Tanquerel T, Pommer W, Schwarz A, Keller E, Thieler H, et al. Evaluation of diagnostic criteria for analgesic nephropathy in patients with end-stage renal failure: results of the ANNE study. Analgesic Nephropathy Network of Europe. Nephrol Dial Transplant 1995;10(6):808–14.

52. Prescott LF. Analgesic nephropathy: a reassessment of the role of phenacetin and other analgesics. Drugs 1982;23(1–2):75–149.

53. Cove-Smith JR, Knapp MS. Analgesic nephropathy: an important cause of chronic renal failure. Q J Med 1978;47(185):49–69.

54. Kincaid-Smith P. Analgesic nephropathy. BMJ (Clin Res Ed) 1981;282(6278):1790–1.

55. McCredie M, Stewart JH, Mahony JF. Is phenacetin responsible for analgesic nephropathy in New South Wales? Clin Nephrol 1982;17(3):134–40.

56. Murray RM. Analgesic nephropathy: removal of phenacetin from proprietary analgesics. BMJ 1972;4(833):131–2.

57. McAnally JF, Winchester JF, Schreiner GE. Analgesic nephropathy. An uncommon cause of end-stage renal disease. Arch Intern Med 1983;143(10):1897–9.

58. Schreiner GE, McAnally JF, Winchester JF. Clinical analgesic nephropathy. Arch Intern Med 1981;141(3 Spec No):349–57.

59. Emkey RD, Mills JA. Aspirin and analgesic nephropathy. JAMA 1982;247(1):55–7.

60. MacDonald IM, Dumble LJ, Doran T, et al. Increased frequency of HLA-B12 in analgesic nephropathy. Aust NZ J Med 1978;8:233.

61. Torhorst J. Nierenschädigung durch Analgetika: pathologische Anatomie und Morphogenese. Nephrol Klin Prax 1976;3:134.

62. Zollinger HU. 25 Jahre Phenacetinabusus. [25 years of phenacetin abuse.] Schweiz Med Wochenschr 1980;110(4):106–7.

63. Dubach UC. Die Bedeutung des Analgetikaabusus für chronische Harninfektionen. Therapiewoche 1981;31:7891.

64. Kung LG. Hypernephroides Karzinom und Karzinome der ableitenden Harnwege nach Phenacetinabusus. [Hypernephroid carcinoma and carcinoma of the urinary tract following phenacetin abuse.] Schweiz Med Wochenschr 1976;106(2):47–51.

65. Gonwa TA, Corbett WT, Schey HM, Buckalew VM Jr. Analgesic-associated nephropathy and transitional cell carcinoma of the urinary tract. Ann Intern Med 1980;93(2):249–52.

66. Mihatsch MJ, Manz T, Knusli C, Hofer HO, Rist M, Guetg R, Rutishauser G, Zollinger HU. [Phenacetin abuse III. Malignant urinary tract tumors in phenacetin abuse in Basle 1963–1977.]Schweiz Med Wochenschr 1980;110(7):255–64.

67. Consensus conference: Analgesic-associated kidney disease. JAMA 1984;251(23):3123–5.

68. Dubach UC, Rosner B, Pfister E. Epidemiologic study of abuse of analgesics containing phenacetin. Renal morbidity and mortality (1968–1979). N Engl J Med 1983;308(7):357–62.

69. Dubach UC, Rosner B, Sturmer T. An epidemiologic study of abuse of analgesic drugs. Effects of phenacetin and salicylate on mortality and cardiovascular morbidity (1968 to 1987). N Engl J Med 1991;324(3):155–60.

70. Pommer W, Bronder E, Klimpel A, Helmert U, Greiser E, Molzahn M. Urothelial cancer at different tumour sites: role of smoking and habitual intake of analgesics and laxatives. Results of the Berlin Urothelial Cancer Study. Nephrol Dial Transplant 1999;14(12):2892–7.

71. Gago-Dominguez M, Yuan JM, Castelao JE, Ross RK, Yu MC. Regular use of analgesics is a risk factor for renal cell carcinoma. Br J Cancer 1999;81(3):542–8.

72. McCredie M, Pommer W, McLaughlin JK, Stewart JH, Lindblad P, Mandel JS, Mellemgaard A, Schlehofer B, Niwa S. International renal-cell cancer study. II. Analgesics. Int J Cancer 1995;60(3):345–9.

73. Valsecchi R. Fixed drug eruption to paracetamol. Dermatologica 1989;179(1):51–2.

74. Thomas RH, Munro DD. Fixed drug eruption due to paracetamol. Br J Dermatol 1986;115(3):357–9.

75. Dussarat GV, Dalger J, Mafart B, Chagnon A. Purpura vasculaire au paracétamol: une observation. [Vascular purpura caused by paracetamol. A case.] Presse Méd 1988;17(31):1587.

76. Zemtsov A, Yanase DJ, Boyd AS, Shehata B. Fixed drug eruption to Tylenol: report of two cases and review of the literature. Cutis 1992;50(4):281–2.

77. Silva A, Proenca E, Carvalho C, Senra V, Rosario C. Fixed drug eruption induced by paracetamol. Pediatr Dermatol 2001;18(2):163–4.

78. Galindo PA, Borja J, Feo F, Gomez E, Encinas C, Garcia R. Nonpigmented fixed drug eruption caused by paracetamol. J Investig Allergol Clin Immunol 1999;9(6):399–400.

79. Santoro D, Stella M, Castellino S. Henoch–Schönlein purpura associated with acetaminophen and codeine. Clin Nephrol 2006;66(2):131–.

80. Ayonrinde OT, Saker BM. Anaphylactoid reactions to paracetamol. Postgrad Med J 2000;76(898):501–2.

81. Fyfe AI, Wright JM. Chronic acetaminophen ingestion associated with (1;7) (p11) translocation and immune deficiency syndrome. Am J Med 1990;88(4):443–4.

82. Weiss JR, Baker JA, Baer MR, Menezes RJ, Nowell S, Moysich KB. Opposing effects of aspirin and acetaminophen use on risk of adult acute leukemia. Leuk Res 2006;30(2):164–.

83. Anonymous. Paracetamol in pregnancy. Pharm J 1996;257:921.

84. Benson GD. Acetaminophen in chronic liver disease. Clin Pharmacol Ther 1983;33(1):95–101.

85. Angalakuditi MV, Coley KC, Krenzelok EP. Children's acetaminophen exposures reported to a regional poison control center. Am J Health Syst Pharm 2006;63(4):323–.

86. Brotodihardjo AE, Batey RG, Farrell GC, Byth K. Hepatotoxicity from paracetamol self-poisoning in western Sydney: a continuing challenge. Med J Aust 1992;157(6):382–5.

87. Meredith TJ, Prescott LF, Vale JA. Why do patients still die from paracetamol poisoning? BMJ (Clin Res Ed) 1986;293(6543):345–6.

88. Stricker BHC, Spoelstra P. Paracetamol (acetaminophen). In: Drug-Induced Hepatic Injury. Amsterdam: Elsevier, 1985:51–4.

89. Thomas SHL. Paracetamol (acetaminophen) poisoning. BMJ 1998;317:1609–10.

90. Penna A, Buchanan N. Paracetamol poisoning in children and hepatotoxicity. Br J Clin Pharmacol 1991;32(2):143–9.

91. Rumore MM, Blaiklock RG. Influence of age-dependent pharmacokinetics and metabolism on acetaminophen hepatotoxicity. J Pharm Sci 1992;81(3):203–7.

92. Thomas SH, Horner JE, Chew K, Connolly J, Dorani B, Bevan L, Bhattacharyya S, Bramble MG, Han KH, Rodgers A, Sen B, Tesfayohannes B, Wynne H, Bateman DN. Paracetamol poisoning in the north east of England: presentation, early management and outcome. Hum Exp Toxicol 1997;16(9):495–500.

93. Litovitz TL, Klein-Schwartz W, Dyer KS, Shannon M, Lee S, Powers M. 1997 Annual Report of the American Association of Poison Control Centers Toxic Exposure Surveillance System. Am J Emerg Med 1998;16(5):443–97.

94. Vale JA, Proudfoot AT. Paracetamol (acetaminophen) poisoning. Lancet 1995;346(8974):547–52.

95. Bialas MC, Reid PG, Beck P, Lazarus JH, Smith PM, Scorer RC, Routledge PA. Changing patterns of self-poisoning in a UK health district. QJM 1996;89(12):893–901.

96. Hawton K, Simkin S, Deeks J. Co-proxamol and suicide: a study of national mortality statistics and local non-fatal self poisonings. BMJ 2003;326(7397):1006–8.

97. Kurtovic J, Riordan SM. Paracetamol-induced hepatotoxicity at recommended dosage. J Intern Med 2003;253:240–.

98. Ojeda VJ, Shilkin KB, Wright EA, Williams R. Massive hepatic necrosis and focal necrotising myopathy. Lancet 1982;1(8264):172–3.

99. Marchewka Z, Przewłocki M, Lepka M, Długosz A, Kochman K. Wybrane wskazniki biochemiczne w moczu w ocenie nefrotoksycznosci paracetamolu. [Selected biochemical parameters of urine in the evaluation of paracetamol nephrotoxicity.] Przegl Lek 2006;63(12):1299–30.

100. Huitema AD, Soesan M, Meenhorst PL, Koks CH, Beijnen JH. A dose-dependent delayed hypersensitivity reaction to acetaminophen after repeated acetaminophen intoxications. Hum Exp Toxicol 1998;17(7):406–8.

101. Emby DJ, Fraser BN. Hepatotoxicity of paracetamol enhanced by ingestion of alcohol: report of two cases. S Afr Med J 1977;51(7):208–9.

102. Barker JD Jr, de Carle DJ, Anuras S. Chronic excessive acetaminophen use and liver damage. Ann Intern Med 1977;87(3):299–301.

103. Goldfinger R, Ahmed KS, Pitchumoni CS, Weseley SA. Concomitant alcohol and drug abuse enhancing acetaminophen toxicity. Report of a case. Am J Gastroenterol 1978;70(4):385–8.

104. McClain CJ, Kromhout JP, Peterson FJ, Holtzman JL. Potentiation of acetaminophen hepatotoxicity by alcohol. JAMA 1980;244(3):251–3.

105. Licht H, Seeff LB, Zimmerman HJ. Apparent potentiation of acetaminophen hepatotoxicity by alcohol. Ann Intern Med 1980;92(4):511.

106. Johnson MW, Friedman PA, Mitch WE. Alcoholism, nonprescription drug and hepatotoxicity. The risk from

unknown acetaminophen ingestion. Am J Gastroenterol 1981;76(6):530–3.

107. Leist MH, Gluskin LE, Payne JA. Enhanced toxicity of acetaminophen in alcoholics: report of three cases. J Clin Gastroenterol 1985;7(1):55–9.

108. Seeff LB, Cuccherini BA, Zimmerman HJ, Adler E, Benjamin SB. Acetaminophen hepatotoxicity in alcoholics. A therapeutic misadventure. Ann Intern Med 1986;104(3):399–404.

109. Draganov P, Durrence H, Cox C, Reuben A. Alcohol–acetaminophen syndrome. Even moderate social drinkers are at risk. Postgrad Med 2000;107(1):189–95.

110. Zimmerman HJ, Maddrey WC. Acetaminophen (paracetamol) hepatotoxicity with regular intake of alcohol: analysis of instances of therapeutic misadventure. Hepatology 1995;22(3):767–73.

111. Seeff L, Zimmerman H. Acetaminophen hepatotoxicity in alcoholics. Ann Intern Med 1986;105(4):624–5.

112. Hinson JA, Pohl LR, Monks TJ, Gillette JR. Acetaminophen-induced hepatotoxicity. Life Sci 1981;29(2):107–16.

113. Itoh S, Matsuo S, Shiomi M, Ichinoe A. Cirrhosis following 12 years of treatment with acetaminophen. Hepato-Gastroenterology 1983;30:58.

114. Thummel KE, Slattery JT, Ro H, Chien JY, Nelson SD, Lown KE, Watkins PB. Ethanol and production of the hepatotoxic metabolite of acetaminophen in healthy adults. Clin Pharmacol Ther 2000;67(6):591–9.

115. Dart RC, Kuffner EK, Rumack BH. Treatment of pain or fever with paracetamol (acetaminophen) in the alcoholic patient: a systematic review. Am J Ther 2000;7(2):123–34.

116. Dart RC. The use and effect of analgesics in patients who regularly drink alcohol. Am J Manag Care 2001;7(Suppl 19):S597–601.

117. Kuffner EK, Dart RC, Bogdan GM, Hill RE, Casper E, Darton L. Effect of maximal daily doses of acetaminophen on the liver of alcoholic patients: a randomized, double-blind, placebo-controlled trial. Arch Intern Med 2001;161(18):2247–52.

118. Holtzman JL. The effect of alcohol on acetaminophen hepatotoxicity. Arch Intern Med 2002;162(10):1193.

119. Soll AH, Sees KL. Is acetaminophen really safe in alcoholic patients? Arch Intern Med 2002;162(10):1194.

120. Oviedo J, Wolfe MM. Alcohol, acetaminophen, and toxic effects on the liver. Arch Intern Med 2002;162(10):1194–5.

121. Marsepoils T, Mahassani B, Roudiak N, et al. Potentialisation de la toxicité hépatique et rénal du paracétamol par le phénobarbital. Jeur 1989;2:118.

122. Dossing M, Sonne J. Drug-induced hepatic disorders. Incidence, management and avoidance. Drug Saf 1993;9(6):441–9.

123. Hawton K, Ware C, Mistry H, Hewitt J, Kingsbury S, Roberts D, Weitzel H. Why patients choose paracetamol for self poisoning and their knowledge of its dangers. BMJ 1995;310(6973):164.

124. Hawton K, Townsend E, Deeks J, Appleby L, Gunnell D, Bennewith O, Cooper J. Effects of legislation restricting pack sizes of paracetamol and salicylate on self poisoning in the United Kingdom: before and after study. BMJ 2001;322(7296):1203–7.

125. Dargan P, Jones A. Effects of legislation restricting pack sizes of paracetamol on self poisoning. It's too early to tell yet. BMJ 2001;323(7313):633.

126. Isbister G, Balit C. Effects of legislation restricting pack sizes of paracetamol on self poisoning. Authors did not look at effects on all deliberate and accidental self poisoning. BMJ 2001;323(7313):633–4.

127. Balit CR, Isbister GK, Peat J, Dawson AH, Whyte IM. Paracetamol recall: a natural experiment influencing analgesic poisoning. Med J Aust 2002;176(4):162–5.

128. Andrus JP, Herzenberg LA, Herzenberg LA, DeRosa SC. Effects of legislation restricting pack sizes of paracetamol on self poisoning. Paracetamol should be packaged with its antidote. BMJ 2001;323(7313):634.

129. Law R. Severity of overdose after restriction of paracetamol availability. Why hasn't strategy for minimising paracetamol poisoning been enacted? BMJ 2001;322(7285):554.

130. Jones AL, Hayes PC, Proudfoot AT, Vale JA, Prescott LF. Should methionine be added to every paracetamol tablet? (No: the risks are not well enough known). BMJ 1997;315(7103):301–3.

131. Krenzelok EP. Should methionine be added to every paracetamol tablet? (Yes: but perhaps only in developing countries). BMJ 1997;315(7103):303–4.

132. Lewis RK, Paloucek FP. Assessment and treatment of acetaminophen overdose. Clin Pharm 1991;10(10):765–74.

133. Yip L, Dart RC. A 20-hour treatment for acute acetaminophen overdose. N Engl J Med 2003;348(24):2471–2.

134. UK National Poisons Information Service. National guidelines: management of acute paracetamol poisoningParacetamol Information Centre in collaboration with the British Association for Accident and Emergency Medicine;. 1995.

135. Bialas MC, Evans RJ, Hutchings AD, Alldridge G, Routledge PA. The impact of nationally distributed guidelines on the management of paracetamol poisoning in accident and emergency departments. National Poison Information Service. J Accid Emerg Med 1998;15(1):13–17.

136. Bridger S, Henderson K, Glucksman E, Ellis AJ, Henry JA, Williams R. Deaths from low dose paracetamol poisoning. BMJ 1998;316(7146):1724–5.

137. Kanter MZ. Comparison of oral and i.v. acetylcysteine in the treatment of acetaminophen poisoning. Am J Health Syst Pharm 2006;63(19):1821–.

138. Spiller HA, Winter ML, Klein-Schwartz W, Bangh SA. Efficacy of activated charcoal administered more than four hours after acetaminophen overdose. J Emerg Med 2006;30(1):1–.

139. Anonymous. Alcohol warning on over-the-counter pain medications. WHO Drug Inf 1998;12:16.

140. Inglis AM, Sheth SB, Hursting MJ, Tenero DM, Graham AM, DiCicco RA. Investigation of the interaction between argatroban and acetaminophen, lidocaine, or digoxin. Am J Health Syst Pharm 2002;59(13):1258–66.

141. Brackett CC, Bloch JD. Phenytoin as a possible cause of acetaminophen hepatotoxicity: case report and review of the literature. Pharmacotherapy 2000;20(2):229–33.

142. Suchin SM, Wolf DC, Lee Y, Ramaswamy G, Sheiner PA, Facciuto M, Marvin MR, Kim-Schluger L, Lebovics E. Potentiation of acetaminophen hepatotoxicity by phenytoin, leading to liver transplantation. Dig Dis Sci 2005;50(10):1836–.

143. Cook MD, Williams SR, Clark RF. Phenytoin-potentiated hepatotoxicity following acetaminophen overdose? A closer look. Dig Dis Sci 2007;52(1):208–.

144. Stephenson I, Qualie M, Wiselka MJ. Hepatic failure and encephalopathy attributed to an interaction between acetaminophen and rifampicin. Am J Gastroenterol 2001;96(4):1310–1.

145. Boeijinga JK, Boerstra EE, Ris P, et al. De invloed van paracetamol op antistollingsbehandeling met coumarine-derivaten. Pharm Weekbl 1983;118:209.

146. Hylek EM, Heiman H, Skates SJ, Sheehan MA, Singer DE. Acetaminophen and other risk factors for excessive warfarin anticoagulation. JAMA 1998;279(9):657–62.

147. Bell WR. Acetaminophen and warfarin: undesirable synergy. JAMA 1998;279(9):702–3.

148. Bagheri H, Bernhard NB, Montastruc JL. Potentiation of the acenocoumarol anticoagulant effect by acetaminophen. Ann Pharmacother 1999;33(4):506.

149. Riser J, Gilroy C, Hudson P, McCay L, Willis TA. Acetaminophen and risk factors for excess anticoagulation with warfarin. JAMA 1998;280(8):696.

150. Amato MG, Bussey H, Farnett L, Lyons R. Acetaminophen and risk factors for excess anticoagulation with warfarin. JAMA 1998;280(8):695–6.

151. Kwan D, Bartle WR, Walker SE. The effects of acetaminophen on pharmacokinetics and pharmacodynamics of warfarin. J Clin Pharmacol 1999;39(1):68–75.

152. Shriner K, Goetz MB. Severe hepatotoxicity in a patient receiving both acetaminophen and zidovudine. Am J Med 1992;93(1):94–6.

153. Ameer B. Acetaminophen hepatotoxicity augmented by zidovudine. Am J Med 1993;95(3):342.

154. Verbov J. Fixed drug eruption due to a drug combination but not to its constituents. Dermatologica 1985;171(1):60–1.

155. Rogers SM, Back DJ, Stevenson PJ, Grimmer SF, Orme ML. Paracetamol interaction with oral contraceptive steroids: increased plasma concentrations of ethinyloestradiol. Br J Clin Pharmacol 1987;23(6):721–5.

156. Miners JO, Attwood J, Birkett DJ. Influence of sex and oral contraceptive steroids on paracetamol metabolism. Br J Clin Pharmacol 1983;16(5):503–9.

Phenazone (antipyrine)

General Information

Phenazone, commonly known as antipyrine, is still used therapeutically in some countries, although it is now used mainly as a marker of hepatic enzyme drug metabolizing activity. It is an old compound with little recent investigation, usually taken in combination with other analgesics, and an exact analysis of its adverse effects is impossible. Phenazone seems to have a low toxicity index, in correspondence with its weak anti-inflammatory effect. Allergic reactions are very rare (SEDA-6, 92; SEDA-14, 92; SEDA-16, 108), but subjects undergoing the phenazone test should be informed of the potential risk.

Dichloralphenazone is a complex of phenazone (antipyrine) and chloral hydrate, which dissociates in aqueous solution. It has been used as a hypnotic but is obsolete. Its adverse effects are those of its components (1,2).

Organs and Systems

Hematologic

Hemolysis can occur in patients with glucose-6-phosphate dehydrogenase deficiency. An immediate reaction after a single test dose, in the form of latent leukopenia, has also been reported (3), with previous sensitization to pyrazolone derivatives as the most probable explanation. Agranulocytosis has been observed in six women after the use of a phenazone-containing cream (SEDA-18, 101).

Gastrointestinal

Only chronic abuse of phenazone, probably together with other more aggressive antipyretics, can cause gastric symptoms (4).

Urinary tract

Phenazone nephrotoxicity is well-established, but information is limited. Experimental papillary necrosis can easily be provoked; analgesic nephropathy is probably a real danger with antipyrine, especially when it is combined with a stronger inhibitor of prostaglandin synthesis. The effect is probably toxic, since inhibition of prostaglandins is not a marked characteristic of phenazone. Two reports have suggested a causal link between phenazone and renal carcinoma, as is well-known for phenacetin (5,6), but this has not been confirmed.

Skin

Urticarial rashes and erythema are the most common adverse effects of phenazone, followed by maculopapular eruptions, erythema multiforme, erythema nodosum, or even angioedema (7).

Erythema multiforme has been rarely reported with phenazone.

- In a 70-year-old man erythema multiforme occurred in association with a reticular exanthema after the use of phenazone in combination with epirizole (8).

References

1. Limb DG. Anaphylaxis after dichloralphenazone treatment. BMJ 1977;2(6100):1480.

2. Perl S. Anaphylaxis after dichloralphenazone treatment. BMJ 1977;2(6096):1187–8.

3. Kadar D, Kalow W. Acute and latent leukopenic reaction to antipyrine. Clin Pharmacol Ther 1980;28(6):820–2.

4. Drtil J, Sandz Z. Veranderungen der Magenschleimhaut nach Gebrauch einiger Antiasthmatika und Analgetika Antipyretika. [Changes in the gastric mucosa following the use of various antiasthmatics and analgesics-antipyretics.] Z Gesamte Inn Med 1968;23(8):236–40.

5. Johansson S, Angervall L, Bengtsson U, Wahlqvist L. Uroepithelial tumors of the renal pelvis associated with abuse of phenacetin-containing analgesics. Cancer 1974;33(3):743–53.

6. Shabert P, Nagel R, Leistenschneider W. Zur Frage der Koinzidenz von Tumoren der oberen Harnwege mit chronischer Einnahme analgetischer Substanzen. In: Haschek H, editor. Internationales Symposium uber Probleme des Phenacetin Abusus. Vienna: Facta Publication, Verlag H, Egerman, 1973:257.

7. Zurcher K, Krebs A. Nebenwirkungen interner Arzneimittel auf die Haut unter besonderer Berudcksichtigung neuerer Medikamente. [Cutaneous side effects of systemic drugs with special reference to recently introduced medicaments. I.] Dermatologica 1970;141(2):119–29.

8. Chen W, Hsieh FS. Dimorphic exanthema manifested as reticular maculopapular exanthema and erythema multiforme major associated with pyrazolon derivative. Eur J Dermatol 2002;12:488–9.

5. Mulvaney WP, Beck CW, Brown RR. Urinary phenazopyridine stones. A complication of therapy. JAMA 1972;221(13):1511–2.
6. Amit G, Halkin A. Lemon-yellow nails and long-term phenazopyridine use. Ann Intern Med 1997;127(12):1137.

Phenazopyridine

General Information

Phenazopyridine, an azo dye, is used as a urinary tract analgesic. However, because of toxicity, the standard use of phenazopyridine as part of a fixed-dose combination no longer seems justified.

Organs and Systems

Nervous system

Aseptic meningitis was diagnosed in a patient who had three distinct episodes of fever and confusion after taking phenazopyridine (SEDA-13, 84).

Hematologic

Hematological adverse effects of phenazopyridine include methemoglobinemia and hemolytic anemia, particularly after overdosage (1,2).

Liver

Liver toxicity has been reported with phenazopyridine (3).

Urinary tract

Because of nephrotoxicity (oliguria, cylindruria, and reduced creatinine clearance, with crystal deposits in renal tubules and interstitial tissue) (4) phenazopyridine should not be used in patients with suspected renal disease and insufficiency, or in patients with glucose-6-phosphate dehydrogenase deficiency. Bladder stones have also been described (5).

Skin

Yellow discoloration of the nails has been attributed to long-term therapy with phenazopyridine (6).

References

1. Jeffery WH, Zelicoff AP, Hardy WR. Acquired methemoglobinemia and hemolytic anemia after usual doses of phenazopyridine. Drug Intell Clin Pharm 1982;16(2):157–9.
2. Green ED, Zimmerman RC, Ghurabi WH, Colohan DP. Phenazopyridine hydrochloride toxicity: a cause of drug-induced methemoglobinemia. JACEP 1979;8(10):426–31.
3. Goldfinger SE, Marx S. Hypersensitivity hepatitis due to phenazopyridine hydrochloride. N Engl J Med 1972;286(20):1090–1.
4. Alano FA Jr, Webster GD Jr. Acute renal failure and pigmentation due to phenazopyridine (Pyridium). Ann Intern Med 1970;72(1):89–91.

Propyphenazone

General Information

Propyphenazone is a pyrazolone derivative that has been incorporated into many over-the-counter analgesic combinations in many countries. There is no evidence that it has a lower incidence of adverse effects than phenazone (antipyrine), as was originally supposed, since neither compound has been widely studied alone.

In a systematic review of comparisons of Saridon (propyphenazone 150 mg + paracetamol 250 mg + caffeine 50 mg), paracetamol 500 mg + aspirin 500 mg + ibuprofen 200 mg, and placebo in 500 healthy adults, of whom 329 (66%) had moderate and 171 (34%) severe acute dentoalveolar pain, more of the patients who received Saridon reported "pain gone/partly gone" and fewer reported "pain unchanged or worse" at 30 and 60 minutes (1). There were adverse events in 20 patients (4.0%), with no significant differences between the groups. The most common adverse events were gastrointestinal disorders, followed by nervous system, skin, subcutaneous tissue, respiratory, cardiac, and general disorders.

Organs and Systems

Liver

Hepatitis has been attributed to Saridon, which contains propyphenazone, phenacetin, and apronalide.

- A 30-year-old women developed hepatitis with hepatic granulomata after taking long-term Saridon for headaches (2). The drug was withdrawn and within 10 weeks her liver enzymes had returned to normal.

Immunologic

Severe type I hypersensitivity reactions have been reported (SEDA-16, 108). Serious generalized urticaria with angioedema has occurred (3). Rechallenge with oral propyphenazone caused a severe anaphylactic reaction in a patient with a negative skin test. Although the report stressed the importance of oral challenge, it also drew attention to its risks (SEDA-12, 83).

In 44 of 53 patients, all of whom developed symptoms suggestive of IgE-mediated anaphylaxis within 30 minutes of taking propyphenazone, skin tests showed typical wheal and flare reactions and significant amounts of propyphenazone-specific serum IgE was detected in 31 (4). In seven of nine patients with negative skin tests, propyphenazone-specific IgE was detected.

Drug Administration

Drug overdose

In overdose, propyphenazone, like other pyrazolones, mainly affects the central nervous system, causing coma and convulsions, and the liver; dysrhythmias and cardiogenic shock can occur; hemoperfusion has been recommended for patients with severe pyrazolone intoxication (5).

References

1. Kiersch TA, Minic MR. The onset of action and the analgesic efficacy of Saridon (a propyphenazone/paracetamol/caffeine combination) in comparison with paracetamol, ibuprofen, aspirin and placebo (pooled statistical analysis). Curr Med Res Opin 2002;18(1):18–25.
2. Abe M, Kumagi T, Nakanishi S, Yamagami T, Michitaka K, Abe K, Okura I, Yam H, Horiike N, Onji M. Drug-induced hepatitis with hepatic granuloma due to Saridon. J Gastroenterol 2002;37:1068–72.
3. Kienlein-Kletschka B, Baurle G. Epicutane sofort Reaktion. Aktuelle Derm 1981;7:88.
4. Himly M, Jahn-Schmid B, Pittertschatscher K, Bohle B, Grubmayr K, Ferreira F, Ebner H, Ebner C. IgE-mediated immediate-type hypersensitivity to the pyrazolone drug propyphenazone. J Allergy Clin Immunol 2003;111(4):882–8.
5. Okonek S, Reinecke HJ. Acute toxicity of pyrazolones. JAMA 1983;75(5A):94–8.

Rimazolium

General Information

Rimazolium is a non-narcotic analgesic that strongly potentiates the analgesic and antagonizes the respiratory depressant effect of morphine alkaloids in animals and prevents the development of tolerance to morphine in animals and humans (1). Although rimazolium is not a new drug, experience with it is very limited.

Organs and Systems

Nervous system

Vertigo, drowsiness, and nausea have been attributed to rimazolium (SED-10, 172) (SEDA-7, 117) (2).

References

1. Furst S, Gyires K, Knoll J. Analgesic profile of rimazolium as compared to different classes of pain killers. Arzneimittelforschung 1998;38(4):552–7.
2. Anonymous. Rimazolio metilsulfato. [Rimazolium methyl-sulfate.] Drugs of Today 1981;17:567.

Salicylates, topical

General Information

Salicylic acid is widely used in dermatology because of its keratolytic properties. Methylsalicylate (the main constituent of oil of wintergreen) is a topical analgesic that is also a constituent of Red Flower Oil and White Flower Oil formulations, popular herbal analgesics used topically in Southeast Asia (1). Some users take small amounts of the oil orally to enhance its analgesic effects. It has been responsible for rare cases of allergic skin reactions.

Salicylism

Many reports have described "salicylism," intoxication due to percutaneous absorption of salicylates, such as methyl salicylate (2). The first symptoms of salicylism are pallor, fatigue and drowsiness, and altered respiration, which becomes more frequent and at the same time deeper, and which can be heard from a distance. Other early signs of intoxication with salicylic acid are nausea, vomiting, changes in the ability to hear, and mental confusion. Several deaths have been recorded, mainly in children.

Other signs and symptoms of salicylism (3–5) include:

fatigue, changes in hearing ability, nuchal rigidity, fever, profuse sweating, and pallor (6);
frequent deep respiration, Cheyne-Stokes respiration, dyspnea, hyperpnea;
drowsiness, mental confusion, stupor, hallucinations, headache, dizziness, tinnitus, slurred speech, agitation, disorientation, lethargy, delusions, aggression, retrograde amnesia, depression, coma, somnolence;
hypoglycemia (SEDA-16, 158) and metabolic acidosis (6);
nausea, vomiting, thirst, anorexia, diarrhea.

Accidental ingestion of methylsalicylate in young children has resulted in severe salicylate poisoning, in one case with laryngeal edema (7). A suicide attempt by deliberate ingestion of about 100 ml resulted in severe salicylate poisoning (8).

References

1. Chan TY. Ingestion of medicated oils by adults: the risk of severe salicylate poisoning is related to the packaging of these products. Hum Exp Toxicol 2002;21(4):171–4.
2. Morra P, Bartle WR, Walker SE, Lee SN, Bowles SK, Reeves RA. Serum concentrations of salicylic acid following topically applied salicylate derivatives. Ann Pharmacother 1996;30(9):935–40.
3. Chiaretti A, Schembri Wismayer D, Tortorolo L, Piastra M, Polidori G. Salicylate intoxication using a skin ointment. Acta Paediatr 1997;86(3):330–1.
4. Brubacher JR, Hoffman RS. Salicylism from topical salicylates: review of the literature. J Toxicol Clin Toxicol 1996;34(4):431–6.
5. Treguer H, Le Bihan G, Coloignier M, Le Roux P, Bernard JP. Intoxication salicylée par application locale de vaseline salicylée à 20% chez un psoriasique. [Salicylate poisoning by local application of 20% salicylic acid petrolatum to a psoriatic patient.] Nouv Presse Med 1980;9(3):192–3.

6. Smith WO, Lyons D. Metabolic acidosis associated with percutaneous absorption of salicylic acid. J Okla State Med Assoc 1980;73(1):7–8.
7. Botma M, Colquhoun-Flannery W, Leighton S. Laryngeal oedema caused by accidental ingestion of Oil of Wintergreen. Int J Pediatr Otorhinolaryngol 2001; 58(3):229–32.
8. Chan TH, Wong KC, Chan JC. Severe salicylate poisoning associated with the intake of Chinese medicinal oil ("red flower oil"). Aust N Z J Med 1995;25(1):57.

Salsalate

General Information

Salsalate is a compound that contains two salicylate molecules joined by a diazo bond, which is hydrolysed after absorption, yielding two molecules of salicylate.

Organs and Systems

Mouth

Salicylates can cause ulceration in the mouth from local contact (1).

- A 77-year-old man developed three ulcerated lesions on his tongue because he had difficulty in swallowing salsalate tablets. He was taught how to swallow tablets and instructed to take them with water to avoid prolonged contact of salsalate with the tongue. Three weeks later, his lesions had healed and no new ones had appeared (2).

Gastrointestinal

There is some evidence that salsalate causes less gastric toxicity than aspirin, but salsalate can produce dyspepsia and occult bleeding when used therapeutically in effective doses. In an open study in 66 patients taking salsalate 3 g/day for 6 weeks, three patients were withdrawn because of gastrointestinal upsets; the most common adverse effect was dyspepsia (3).

References

1. Sapir S, Bimstein E. Cholinsalicylate gel induced oral lesion: report of case. J Clin Pediatr Dent 2000;24(2):103–6.
2. Ruscin JM, D'Astroth JD. Lingual lesions secondary to prolonged contact with salsalate tablets. Ann Pharmacother 1998;32(11):1248.
3. Regalado RG. The use of salsalate for control of long-term musculo-skeletal pain: an open, non-comparative assessment. Curr Med Res Opin 1978;5(6):454–60.

NON-STEROIDAL ANTI-INFLAMMATORY DRUGS (NSAIDs)

NSAIDs

General Information

Non-steroidal anti-inflammatory drugs (NSAIDs) form a heterogeneous group of organic acids (Table 1) that have analgesic, antipyretic, anti-inflammatory, and platelet inhibitory actions.

More than 100 NSAIDs are marketed or at an advanced stage of development worldwide. Their use is constantly expanding and the search for more efficacious and better-tolerated compounds is still being pursued, and has received renewed impulse with studies on selective inhibitors of cyclo-oxygenase type 2 (COX-2), nitric oxide-releasing NSAIDs, peroxidase inhibitors, enantiomers of already known NSAIDs, NSAIDs associated with zwitterionic phospholipids, and cytokine-modulating antirheumatic drugs.

Predominantly used in the management of rheumatological conditions, NSAIDs are drugs of choice in the treatment of inflammatory arthropathies. However, their use has also been extended to many non-rheumatological problems (for example dysmenorrhea, pain of different origin, neoplastic fever, migraine, thromboembolic disease, and patent ductus arteriosus; they are also used for tocolysis and in some neoplastic diseases) (1). Several clinical, epidemiological, and animal studies have suggested that NSAIDs can reduce the occurrence or progression of colorectal cancer, polyps, and perhaps other gastrointestinal tumors (2–4). Reports and epidemiological studies have shown that NSAIDs can protect against the risk of Alzheimer's disease (5,6). NSAIDs are used locally in the eye to prevent and treat postoperative cystoid macular edema, to control postoperative ocular inflammation and pain, for example after radial keratotomy or photorefractive keratectomy, and for non-surgically induced inflammatory disorders, such as allergic conjunctivitis.

The range and incidence of these conditions clearly justifies extensive use of suitable drugs, and explains the pharmaceutical industry's interest in exploiting the potential revenues of such a large market.

The effort to find new compounds is medically justified by the unsatisfactory benefit-to-harm balance of the NSAIDs that are currently available.

The adverse reactions profiles of many NSAIDs have proved to be unacceptable. Over the last 20 years, 18 NSAIDs have been withdrawn from the market or their clinical studies have been terminated because of unexpected toxicity (7). Selection of an NSAID can be difficult, since reliable information about their relative efficacy and adverse reactions is usually meager.

Although the physicochemical features, pharmacokinetics, and pharmacodynamics of individual NSAIDs differ, it is not known to what extent these differences are significant in the benefit-to-harm balance in the individual patient (8). Certainly they influence the adverse reactions and the general pattern of action of a particular subgroup of NSAIDs or a specific

compound within a class, but this still provides no reliable prediction of what the individual patient will experience.

The acidic nature and lipid solubility of these compounds are important. The lipid solubility of an NSAID determines its penetration into the central nervous system and hence the incidence of nervous system-related adverse effects and perhaps adverse skin reactions (9,10). The weak acid nature affects tissue distribution, which explains why NSAIDs have actions at certain sites (for example synovial tissue of inflamed joints) and also contribute to triggering particular adverse reactions at others (for example the stomach and renal medulla) (11).

Pharmacokinetic aspects can play a critical role in the onset of certain adverse effects in some patients (12). NSAIDs are almost entirely absorbed from the gastrointestinal tract (13). The rate and the site of absorption from the gastrointestinal tract can be important; formulations designed to spare the stomach from NSAID toxicity can instead damage the intestinal wall, which seems to have been the case with Osmosin (SEDA-8, 103). There have been a few studies of the chronopharmacology of NSAIDs (SEDA-20, 90). NSAID absorption is probably better in the morning, but there are more adverse effects than when the drug is taken in the evening.

NSAIDs bind avidly to plasma proteins. High protein binding can theoretically predispose patients to drug interactions, which occur most frequently with certain NSAIDs (for example the butazones) in patients who are concomitantly taking drugs such as hypoglycemic agents or oral anticoagulants. The unbound fraction responsible for the pharmacological action of NSAIDs varies with the plasma albumin concentrations, which can be influenced by active rheumatoid arthritis, genetic factors, sex, age, pregnancy, other drugs, and diseases, particularly when the kidney and liver are involved. A correlation between anti-inflammatory action and dose or plasma concentration has been documented for only a few NSAIDs, and there is no direct evidence that an increase in unbound drug concentration is associated with greater toxicity. However, there is convincing evidence that the dose contributes to certain adverse effects (for example gastrointestinal and renal). A record-linkage study has shown an association between NSAID dosage and upper gastrointestinal bleeding (14).

NSAIDs can be roughly divided into those with short and long half-lives. Although the difference in clinical effects between these two categories is poorly understood, half-lives have served as a rough guide for NSAID dosage regimens, compounds with long half-lives being administered only once a day. These NSAIDs also have a greater potential to cause adverse effects, at least in some patients. As the half-lives of this type of NSAID vary widely in different patients, drug accumulation can occur in some individuals. When using an NSAID with a long half-life, loading doses can be given to achieve high drug concentrations quickly, but can be associated with increased adverse effects, particularly gastrointestinal intolerance.

NSAIDs are mainly cleared by the liver, and their clearances would be expected to fall with age (13). Their metabolites are generally inactive and excreted in the urine, which as a rule contains very little unchanged drug. Conversely, several NSAIDs that are themselves inactive can be used as prodrugs, since they have active metabolites; some of these compounds, such as sulindac, undergo enterohepatic recycling. Claims that these pro-drugs are less toxic than other compounds are not sup-ported by any firm evidence. Some NSAIDs, including carprofen, fenoprofen, indometacin, ketoprofen, and naproxen are metabolized to acylglucuronides; the meta-bolites are retained and hydrolysed to re-form the parent compound. This is probably one of the mechanisms of toxicity in patients with renal insufficiency.

Pharmacodynamic mechanisms can also be crucial. The main mechanism of action is inhibition of cyclo-oxygenase (COX) activity and consequently of prosta-glandin synthesis (15–17). Two forms of COX have been identified: COX-1, which is constitutively expressed in many cells and tissues, and COX-2, which is selectively induced by proinflammatory cytokines at the site of inflammation. The discovery of a second COX enzyme has led to the hypothesis that the toxicity associated with the clinically useful NSAIDs is caused by inhibition of COX-1, whereas the anti-inflammatory properties are caused by the inhibition of COX-2 (18). A selective COX-2 inhibitor may therefore have better anti-inflam-matory activity with greater safety than existing NSAIDs. The in vitro potency of NSAIDs as inhibitors of prostaglandin synthesis, which tends to match their anti-inflammatory potency in vivo, varies from one anti-inflammatory agent to the next (19,20). Other mechan-isms that are poorly understood may be implicated in determining both a drug's activity and its adverse effects.

These data provide a basis for the practical use of NSAIDs. There can be no doubt that some NSAIDs are more toxic than others, notably those that have the greatest inhibitory effect on cyclo-oxygenase. NSAIDs that inhibit both cyclo-oxygenase and lipoxygenase are particularly toxic. The fact that some NSAIDs are more toxic to single organs than others seems to depend on the physicochemical and metabolic characteristics of single drugs or groups of similar drugs. Despite numerous stu-dies, reliable comparisons of the adverse effects of the different drugs are scanty. However, some data have been produced from the data bank centers of the Arthritis Rheumatism and Aging Medical Information System (ARAMIS) and have been reviewed (SEDA-17, 102). If selective COX-2 inhibitors are confirmed to have less gastrointestinal toxicity than the old NSAIDs, we should have new drugs with fewer risks. However, doubts are emerging about whether COX-1 inhibition makes a contribution to the anti-inflammatory activity of NSAIDs and whether COX-2 activity is implicated in mucosal healing and protective processes (SEDA-22, 109).

The categories of patients who are at higher risk of adverse reactions when treated with NSAIDs are well known and can largely be deduced from what has been said above. They include the elderly (especially women), pregnant women (and their fetuses), neonates, patients with liver, kidney, or cardiac disorders, and those with hypertension, multiple myeloma, peptic disorders, or active rheumatoid arthritis. Greater awareness of these risk factors among medical practitioners, limiting the use of NSAIDs to cases in which there is a precise indication, informing patients, developing systems for monitoring unwanted adverse effects, and carrying out adequate well-designed experimental studies would do much to ensure better use of these drugs. Many of the adverse effects of NSAIDs are, with negligible differences, com-mon to all of them.

Table 1 NSAIDs by structural class

Arylalkanoic acid derivatives	Anthranilic acid derivatives
Aceclofenac	Antrafenine
Alclofenac	Etofenamate
Benoxaprofen	Floctafenine
Bromfenac	Flufenamic acid
Bucloxic acid	Glafenine
Bufexamac	Meclofenamate
Butibufen	Mefenamic acid
Carprofen	Niflumic acid
Clobuzarit	Talinflumate
Dexibuprofen	Tolfenamic acid
Dexindoprofen	**Butazone derivatives**
Diclofenac	Dexketoprofen
Diphenpyramidex	Azapropazone
Etodolac	Bumadizone
Felbinac	Feprazone
Fenbufen	Ketophenylbutazone
Fenclofenac	Monophenylbutazone
Fenoprofen	Oxyphenbutazone
Fentiazac	Phenylbutazone
Flunoxaprofen	Pipebuzone
Flurbiprofen	Pyrazine-butazone
Ibuprofen	Suxibuzone
Ibuproxam	Trimethazone
Indoprofen	**Coxibs (COX-2 inhibitors)**
Ketoprofen	Celecoxib
Ketorolac	Etoricoxib
Lonazolac	Lumaricoxib
Loxoprofen	Parecoxib
Nabumetone	Rofecoxib
Naproxen	Valdecoxib
Oxaprozin	**Indoleacetic acid derivatives**
Pirproxen	Acemetacin
Pranoprofen	Cinmetacin
Romazarit	Clometacin
Tiaprofenic acid	Glucametacin
Tolmetin	Indometacin
Tropesin	Oxametacin
Suprofen	Proglumetacin
Zomepirac	Sulindac
	Zidometacin

Organs and Systems

Cardiovascular

The effects that NSAIDs have on the cardioprotective effects of aspirin are dicusssed in the section on drug-drug interactions below.

Hypertension

NSAIDs can cause or aggravate hypertension and interact negatively with the effects of antihypertensive drugs, including diuretics, although contrasting data from experimental and clinical studies have been published (21).

The mechanisms by which NSAIDs affect cardiovascular function are complex and controversial. They may include reduced blood flow, a reduction in the filtered load of sodium, an increase in tubular reabsorption of sodium, and a reduction in the synthesis of PGE-1, which may be associated with raised blood viscosity and increased peripheral vascular resistance. This is perhaps the primary mechanism, which is due to increased renal synthesis of endothelin-1.

Meta-analyses

In a meta-analysis of the hypertensive effects of NSAIDs or aspirin (1.5 g/day or greater) in short-term intervention studies; 54 studies and 123 NSAID treatment arms were included (22). Of the 1324 participating subjects, 92% were hypertensive; they had a mean age of 46 years and none was over 65 years. The major outcome studied was the change in mean arterial pressure. The effects of NSAIDs on blood pressure were found solely in hypertensive subjects; among these, the increase in mean arterial pressure, after adjusting for possible confounders (for example dietary salt intake) was different among different NSAIDs. The increase in mean arterial pressure was 3.59 mmHg for indometacin (57 treatment arms), 3.74 mmHg for naproxen (4 arms), and 0.45 mmHg for piroxicam (4 arms). However, mean arterial pressure fell by 2.59 mmHg with placebo (10 arms), by 0.83 mmHg with ibuprofen (6 arms), 1.76 mmHg with aspirin (4 arms), and 0.16 mmHg with sulindac (23 arms).

Overall, only the effects of indometacin on mean arterial pressure were statistically significantly different from those found with placebo, showing that in this population the effects of NSAIDs on blood pressure were modest and varied considerably among different drugs. However, one must take into account the important limitations of the analysis: the patients were mostly young, the studies included in the meta-analysis were small and short-term, and information on possible confounders was incomplete. The significance of the results of this study is therefore doubtful.

Another meta-analysis provided more complete and useful results (23). Its primary aim was to produce an estimate of the overall effect of NSAIDs on blood pressure, and its secondary aims were to evaluate the mechanisms by which NSAIDs alter blood pressure and to determine susceptibility factors. Moreover, as NSAIDs have been associated with raised blood pressure in normotensive individuals and in both treated and untreated hypertensive subjects, the authors tried to discover different effects in these subgroups. Finally, they studied whether different NSAIDs alter blood pressure to the same degree.

In all, 50 randomized placebo-controlled trials and 16 randomized comparisons of two or more NSAIDs met the selection criteria. These studies included 771 young volunteers or patients aged 47 years or younger. The studies were small (the mean sample size per trial was 16); many different NSAIDs and antihypertensive drugs were used, but indometacin was used in more than half of all the trials; the duration of therapy with NSAIDs or antihypertensive drugs was 1 week or longer, but in most studies it was less than 3 months. NSAIDs raised supine mean blood pressure by 5.0 mmHg (95% CI = 1.2, 8.7), but had no significant effect on variables measured to assess possible mechanisms (such as body weight, daily urinary sodium output, creatinine clearance, or urinary prostaglandin excretion). Overall, the data suggested that NSAIDs do not appear to increase blood pressure primarily by increasing salt and water retention, because weight and urinary sodium were not altered by NSAIDs and inhibition of blood pressure control was not more marked in patients taking diuretics compared with other antihypertensive drugs. In addition NSAIDs did not significantly alter plasma renin activity or 24-hour urinary excretion of prostaglandin E_2 and 6-ketoprostaglandin $F_{1\alpha}$. Other factors may therefore contribute to the increase in blood pressure caused by NSAIDs. In particular, a potential effect of NSAIDs on peripheral vascular resistance should be considered (24,25). There is good evidence to suggest an important role for prostaglandins in the modulation of two major determinants of blood pressure, vasoconstriction of arteriolar smooth muscle and control of extracellular volume.

NSAIDs inhibited the effects of all antihypertensive drug categories. However, in patients taking beta-blockers and vasodilators, NSAIDs produced a greater increase in supine mean blood pressure than in patients taking diuretics, but only the pooled inhibitory effect of NSAIDs on the effects of beta-blockers achieved statistical significance. When the data were analysed by type of NSAID the meta-analysis showed that all NSAIDs increased supine blood pressure, and that piroxicam, indometacin, and ibuprofen produced the most marked increases. However, only piroxicam had a statistically significant effect with respect to placebo. Aspirin, sulindac, and flurbiprofen caused the smallest increases in blood pressure.

In conclusion this meta-analysis has provided more clear evidence that, as a group, NSAIDs significantly increase arterial pressure and can antagonize the blood pressure-lowering effect of some antihypertensive drugs, by mechanisms that are still unclear. Although the hypertensive effect of NSAIDs was more marked in hypertensive subjects taking antihypertensive drugs than in normotensive subjects not taking antihypertensive drugs, the difference was not statistically significant and its clinical relevance is unclear. It is worth noting that the effects of NSAIDs on blood pressure were similar in patients taking antihypertensive drugs for months or only a few days.

This study also had two main limitations: first, most of the trials were small, which precluded definitive conclusions about the effects of individual NSAIDs or individual antihypertensive drug classes; secondly, in most studies, therapy was short term and the patients were relatively young, making generalization of the results difficult, as

NSAIDs are most often prescribed long term and for elderly people.

The effects of NSAIDs on blood pressure have been studied in a systematic review of two meta-analyses, 11 randomized controlled trials, four prospective studies, two retrospective observational trials, and one case-control study (26). The results were highly variable, but a few general conclusions can be drawn. In normotensive adults NSAIDs caused a small but non-significant average increase in mean arterial pressure of 1–2 mmHg. In hypertensive adults there was a small but statistically significant increase in mean arterial pressure of about 3–5 mmHg; before and after adjustment for salt intake, naproxen, indometacin, and piroxicam were associated with an increase in mean arterial pressure, whereas ibuprofen and placebo were associated with a reduction. When non-steroidal anti-inflammatory drugs were used in combination with different antihypertensive drugs, beta-blockers + NSAIDs produced a statistically significant increase in mean arterial pressure of about 6 mmHg; enalapril + NSAIDS increased blood pressure by a similar amount; no other combinations changed the blood pressure.

Prospective studies

A case-control study of the effects of NSAID therapy on arterial pressure has been performed in subjects aged 65 years and over, drawn from a large database (the State of New England Medicaid Program) to determine whether NSAIDs affect blood pressure (27). The investigators calculated the odds ratio (OR) for the initiation of antihypertensive therapy in patients taking NSAIDs relative to non-users after adjusting for possible confounding factors. The 9411 patients had started taking antihypertensive drugs between 1981 and 1990, and a similar number of controls were randomly selected. The date of the first prescription for an antihypertensive drug was defined as the index date. Of those who took antihypertensive drugs, 41% had taken an NSAID during the year before the index date, compared with 26% of the control subjects. This risk increased with the recency of NSAID therapy, and was greatest among recent users (those with a supply of NSAIDs ending more than 60 days before the index date) (OR = 2.10; 95% CI = 1.95, 2.26). For former users (those with a supply of NSAIDs ending more than 60 days before the index date) the adjusted OR compared with non-users was 1.66 (CI = 1.54, 1.80). There was a dose-response relation, with adjusted ORs of 1.55 (CI = 1.38, 1.74), 1.64 (CI = 1.44, 1.87), and 1.82 (CI = 1.62, 2.05) for low, medium, and high daily doses of NSAIDs respectively. The unadjusted ORs for ibuprofen, piroxicam, meclofenamate, and indometacin, were separately calculable, and for each of these drugs the OR increased with increasing dose. The relation between cumulative duration of NSAID use and the initiation of antihypertensive therapy was also examined in recent users. The risk was greatest in those who had used an NSAID for 30–90 days and was less for those who had used an NSAID for less than 30 days or for more than 90 days.

The results of this study suggest that the effects of NSAIDs on blood pressure in older patients taking NSAIDs may be clinically important. Given that 15% of the control group were recent users of NSAIDs, and assuming that the adjusted OR of 1.66 represents a causal association of these drugs with the initiation of antihypertensive therapy, the proportion of cases attributable to the use of these drugs in this sample of elderly population was nearly one in ten.

Despite the high prevalence of the use of minor analgesics (aspirin and paracetamol) there is little information available on the association between the use of these analgesics and the risk of hypertension. A prospective cohort study in 80 020 women aged 31–50 years has provided some useful information (28). The women had participated in the Nurses' Health Study II and had no previous history of hypertension. The frequency of use of paracetamol, aspirin, and NSAIDs was collected by mailed questionnaires and cases of physician-diagnosed hypertension were identified by self-report. During 164 000 person-years of follow-up, 1650 incident cases of hypertension were identified. Overall 73% of the cohort had used paracetamol at least 1–4 days/month, 51% had used aspirin, and 77% had used an NSAID. Compared with non-users of paracetamol the age-adjusted relative risk (RR) of hypertension was significantly increased even in women who had used paracetamol for only 1–4 days/month (RR = 1.22; CI = 1.07, 1.39). There seemed to be a dose-response relation, as the RR of hypertension compared with non-users was 2.00 (CI = 1.52, 2.62) in women who had taken paracetamol for 29 days/month or more. For women using aspirin or NSAIDs at a frequency of 1–4 days/month the RRs were 1.18 (CI = 1.02, 1.35) and 1.17 (CI = 1.02, 1.36) respectively. However, after adjusting for age and other potential risk factors, only paracetamol and NSAIDs, but not aspirin, remained significantly associated with a risk of hypertension. In summary, the data from this study support the view that paracetamol and NSAIDs are strongly associated with an increased risk of hypertension in women, the risk increasing with increasing frequency of use. Aspirin did not seem to be associated with an increased risk. This conclusion contrasts with the results of some short-term studies that have shown no effect of paracetamol on blood pressure (29,30).

However, the results from this study must be interpreted with caution, as there were some limitations: the assessments of analgesic use and hypertension were made using a self-reported questionnaire; relative risk can be influenced by many potentially confounding variables; the results are relevant only for young women and cannot be extrapolated to the general population.

The impact of NSAIDs on blood pressure in elderly people has been evaluated in three epidemiological studies, with similar findings (SEDA-19, 92). The use of NSAIDs was significantly associated with hypertension or the use of antihypertensive drugs. Reliable data are available for hypertension in the elderly. Recent users of NSAIDs have a 1.7-fold increase in the risk of initiating antihypertensive therapy compared with non-users, and the use of NSAIDs significantly predicts the presence of hypertension (OR = 1.4; 95% CI = 1.1, 1.7) (21).

Anecdotal reports

The Australian Adverse Drug Reaction Advisory Committee received six reports of severe hypertension in women after post-partum administration of indometacin, ibuprofen, or diclofenac (31). Four of the women had a history of pre-eclampsia and the other two had no prior history of hypertension. One of the women with pre-eclampsia died of a hypertensive crisis and intracranial hemorrhage. Only two were taking antihypertensive drugs at the time of the adverse event. The committee suggested that the severe hypertension in these cases may have been caused by the underlying condition, but it is plausible that the administration of an NSAID made a significant contribution. While waiting for more data on this potential risk, careful monitoring of the blood pressure in women with a history of pre-eclampsia or hypertension who are given an NSAID in the post-partum period is wise.

Conclusions

The overall results of these studies have provided convincing evidence that NSAIDs and paracetamol can raise arterial blood pressure in a dose-related fashion, interfere with the actions of antihypertensive drugs, and prompt the need for new antihypertensive therapy.

Even if the increase in mean blood pressure is probably modest (less than 5.0 mmHg) the clinical relevance of such an increase can be large, especially in elderly people. In fact, an overview of randomized clinical trials of antihypertensive treatment has shown that a 5–6 mmHg increase in diastolic blood pressure over a few years can be associated with a 67% increase in the incidence of strokes and a 15% increase in coronary heart disease (32). These effects are apparent in both normotensive and hypertensive patients.

Whether these results apply with certainty to patients taking NSAIDs is not known, because these studies included patients not taking NSAIDs, but it is wise to consider this probability. The type and dose of NSAID may be important, but more studies are needed to document this. Hypertensive and elderly patients seem to be particularly at risk. In patients taking long-term NSAIDs, or even paracetamol, periodic monitoring of blood pressure appears to be warranted.

Congestive heart failure

Much less is known about the risk of congestive heart failure with NSAIDs. The rate of hospitalization for congestive heart failure in more than 10 000 patients over 55 years of age during exposure to both diuretics and NSAIDs was compared with the rate in those exposed to diuretics alone (33). At mean follow up of 4.7 years, there was an increased risk of hospitalization when diuretics and NSAIDs were used concomitantly (RR = 1.8; 95% CI = 1.4, 2.4).

In 600 elderly patients with documented congestive cardiac failure there was a possible or probable link

between NSAIDs and heart failure in 27 cases (34). In some, the mechanism was apparently a reduction in the effect of furosemide. In others the NSAID may have caused an imbalance in circulatory homeostasis. Pre-existing renal impairment was not observed in any of the 27 cases. This study suggests that in elderly people congestive heart failure may be a complication of NSAIDs.

In a matched case-control study the relation between the recent use of NSAIDs and hospitalization with congestive heart failure in elderly patients has been analysed (35). Cases (n = 365) were patients admitted to hospital with a primary diagnosis of congestive heart failure; controls (n = 658) were patients without congestive heart failure. Structured interviews were used to obtain information on several possible risk factors, such as a history of heart disease and the type and dosage of NSAIDs used. The use of NSAIDs (other than low-dose aspirin) in the previous week was associated with a doubling of the chance of a hospital admission with congestive heart failure (adjusted OR = 2.5, CI = 1.2, 3.3). The risk was even higher in patients with a history of heart disease, in whom the use of NSAIDs was associated with an increased risk of a first admission with congestive heart failure (OR = 11; CI = 0.7, 45), but not in those without a history of heart disease (OR = 1.6; CI = 0.7, 3.7). In contrast to the results of a previous study (33), the risk of admission to hospital with congestive heart failure was positively related to the dose of NSAID consumed in the previous week and was higher with long half-life NSAIDs than with short half-life NSAIDs. The authors estimated that, assuming that these relations were causal, NSAIDs might be responsible for about 19% of hospital admissions with congestive heart failure. If confirmed, this burden of illness resulting from NSAID-related congestive heart failure may rival that resulting from damage to the gastrointestinal tract and would represent an under-recognized public health problem. In any case, this study reinforces the timely suggestion that NSAIDs should be used with great caution in patients with a history of cardiovascular disease. This recommendation must also include the use of the selective COX-2 inhibitors, until more information is available.

Major cardiovascular events

The effects of NSAIDs and paracetamol on the risk of major cardiovascular events (non-fatal myocardial infarction, fatal coronary heart disease, non-fatal and fatal stroke) have been studied prospectively in 70 971 women, aged 44–69 years, free of known cardiovascular disease or cancer, who provided medication data biennially for 12 years, during which there were 2041 major cardiovascular events (36). Women who reported occasional use of NSAIDs or paracetamol (1–21 days/month) did not have a significant increase in the risk of cardiovascular events. However, after adjustment for cardiovascular risk factors, women who frequently used NSAIDs (on at least 22 days/month) had a relative risk for a cardiovascular event of 1.44 (95% CI = 1.27, 1.65) compared with non-users, and those who frequently consumed paracetamol had a relative risk of 1.35 (95% CI = 1.14, 1.59). The increased risk associated with frequent NSAID use was most marked among current smokers (RR = 1.82; 95% CI = 1.38, 2.42) and was absent among never smokers. Risk was also related to dose. The authors concluded that NSAIDs and paracetamol, if taken in high enough dosages, are associated with a significantly increased risk of major cardiovascular events.

In an analysis of data from the Taiwanese Bureau of National Health Insurance database of 16 326 patients aged 18 years or over who had taken etodolac (n = 2014), nabumetone (n = 2262), ibuprofen (n = 5239), naproxen (n = 3049), or celecoxib (n = 3762) for at least 180 days, there were higher prevalences of acute myocardial infarction (4.76 versus 0.99%), angina (4.11 versus 0.43%), strokes (7.74 versus 1.51%), and transient ischemic attacks (4.03 versus 0.52%) in long-term users with a history of cardiovascular disease than in those without (37). There were no differences between the non-selective NSAIDs and celecoxib. A history of cardiovascular disease increased the risks, with hazard ratios of 2.29 (1.22, 4.32), 6.19 (3.56, 10.78), 3.56 (2.80, 4.52), and 6.60 (3.72, 11.73) for the four complications respectively. Pre-existing hypertension, dyslipidemia, diabetes mellitus, congestive heart failure, and chronic renal disease also significantly affected the risks.

In a prespecified pooled analysis of data from three trials in which patients with osteoarthritis or rheumatoid arthritis were randomly assigned to etoricoxib 60 or 90 mg/day or diclofenac 150 mg/day for an average of 18 months (SD 11.8), there were equal numbers of thrombotic cardiovascular events with etoricoxib (n = 320) and diclofenac(n = 323), giving event rates of 1.24 and 1.30 per 100 patient-years and a hazard ratio of 0.95 (95% CI = 0.81, 1.11) for etoricoxib compared with diclofenac (38). Rates of upper gastrointestinal events (perforation, bleeding, obstruction, ulcer) were lower with etoricoxib (0.67 versus 0.97 per 100 patient-years; HR = 0.69; 95% CI = 0.57, 0.83), but the rates of complicated upper gastrointestinal events were similar (0.30 versus 0.32).

The time-course of the effects of NSAIDs in increasing the risk of cardiovascular events has been assessed in a cohort study in 74 838 users of non-selective NSAIDs or coxibs and 23 532 comparable users of other drugs (39). There was a significant increase in the event rate for rofecoxib (RR = 1.15; 95% CI = 1.06, 1.25) and a significant reduction in the rate for naproxen (RR = 0.75; 95% CI = 0.62, 0.92). No other coxib or NSAID had an effect. The increased rate associated with rofecoxib was seen in the first 60 days of use and persisted thereafter.

In a meta-analysis of studies in 7462 patients exposed to (a) celecoxib 200–800 mg/day for 1268 patient-years compared with 4057 patients treated with placebo for 585 patient-years and (b) 19 773 patients treated with celecoxib 200–800 mg/day for 5651 patient-years compared with 13 990 patients treated with non-selective NSAIDs (diclofenac, ibuprofen, naproxen, ketoprofen, and loxoprofen) for 4386 patient-years, the incidence rates of the combined cardiovascular events were not significantly different between patients treated with celecoxib and placebo or between those treated with celecoxib and non-selective NSAIDs (40). The dose of celecoxib, the use of aspirin, or the presence of cardiovascular risk factors did not alter these results. The authors concluded that there was no evidence of an increased cardiovascular risk with celecoxib relative to placebo and a comparable rate of cardiovascular events with celecoxib compared with non-selective NSAIDs.

Intracerebral hemorrhage

The use of acetylsalicylic acid has been associated with an increased risk of intracerebral hemorrhage (41,42), but the effect of non-aspirin NSAIDs on the risk of intracerebral hemorrhage is unclear. This issue is particularly important, as NSAIDs are widely used and therefore even small risks of adverse effects, especially serious ones, may have considerable clinical and public health implications. Furthermore, most NSAIDs are prescribed for people over 65 years, often with other susceptibility factors (for example hypertension) for intracerebral hemorrhage or subarachnoid hemorrhage.

Two recent studies have helped to clarify this issue.

The first (43) study was a population-based case-control study aimed at estimating the risk of intracerebral hemorrhage, subarachnoid hemorrhage, and ischemic stroke in users of NSAIDs versus non-users. The diagnosis was validated if the patient had clinical evidence of stroke, according to the World Health Organization definition, and appropriate neuroimaging or autopsy. The investigators compared the use of NSAIDs in 659 patients with intracerebral hemorrhage, 208 with subarachnoid hemorrhage, and 40 000 random controls using a nested case-control design. Compared with non-user, NSAID users did not have an increased risk of intracerebral hemorrhage or subarachnoid hemorrhage or a reduced risk of ischemic stroke. The adjusted odds ratio of stroke in current NSAIDs users compared with never users was 1.2 (95% CI=0.9, 1.6) for intracerebral hemorrhage and 1.2 (0.7, 2.1) for subarachnoid hemorrhage. This study had several strengths: potential cases were identified from a long-standing population-based registry, neurologists who assessed the records were blinded to drug exposure information, drug exposure was assessed through a prescription database and was therefore not susceptible to recall bias, and the analysis was adjusted for many potential confounding medical conditions.

The second study was a population-based case-control study of the risk of being hospitalized for intracerebral hemorrhage among users of non-aspirin NSAIDs (44). There were 912 cases and 9059 sex-matched and age-matched controls. The use of non-aspirin NSAIDs was not associated with a significant increase in the risk of hospital admission for intracerebral hemorrhage. There was no overall association between prescription of NSAIDs in the preceding 30, 60, or 90 days and the risk of intracerebral hemorrhage. The odds ratios ranged from 0.92 (95% CI=0.70, 1.21) to 1.19 (0.81, 1.58). This absence of association was present in all subgroups analysed, including those with higher baseline risks of intracerebral hemorrhage, such as the elderly and patients with hypertension.

The validity of these studies of the association between the use of NSAIDs and intracerebral hemorrhage depends on accurate identification of cases, including methods used to diagnose intracerebral hemorrhage and assessment of exposure to NSAIDs. Despite the potential limitations of case-control studies, the evidence provided by these two studies suggests that non-aspirin NSAIDs are unlikely to be a major contributor to the risk of intracerebral hemorrhage (45).

Respiratory

As 2–20% of adult asthmatics have aspirin hypersensitivity (46), they must be considered at risk from NSAIDs. The mechanism is related to a deficiency in bronchodilator prostaglandins; prostaglandin inhibition may make arachidonic acid produce more leukotrienes with bronchoconstrictor activity. Oral challenge in asthmatic patients is an effective but potentially dangerous method for establishing the presence of aspirin hypersensitivity (47). Occasionally, bronchospasm may be part of an anaphylactoid reaction to NSAIDs; zomepirac was withdrawn for this reason. Intriguingly bee-keepers may be at increased risk for severe reactions from bee stings if they are taking NSAIDs, and it has been suggested that NSAIDs should be prescribed with particular caution for them (48).

Nervous system

NSAIDs cause headaches and confusion in a relatively small number of patients. Headache and dizziness are common with indometacin, and it has been suggested that its chemical similarity to serotonin, which can cause severe headaches, may be responsible (49). Headache due to long-term use of ibuprofen has been reported in children (50,51).

The Australian Drug Reaction Advisory Committee has reported paresthesia as a class effect of NSAIDs, although it is rare and reversible (52).

Studies on the link between falls in elderly people and NSAIDs have yielded conflicting and inconsistent data (53,54), and an increased risk of falls with NSAIDs is difficult to explain.

Some rarer adverse effects, such as aseptic meningitis, have been reported with ibuprofen, sulindac, and tolmetin (49) in patients with systemic lupus erythematosus. A case-control study showed no increased risk of intracerebral hemorrhage in patients using aspirin or other NSAIDs in low dosages as prophylaxis against thrombosis (55).

Sensory systems

Eye disorders, such as blurred vision, ocular discomfort, irritation, and more severe problems, such as optic or retrobulbar neuritis and papilledema, have been described (SEDA-19, 96).

Psychological, psychiatric

Behavioral changes have been reported with indometacin (56).

- A 92-year-old man with a history of senile dementia of the Alzheimer type, glaucoma, and constipation took indometacin 25 mg for pseudogout. After six doses he became very agitated and confused and was physically and verbally aggressive. Indometacin was withdrawn and he recovered over 10 days with the help of haloperidol 0.5 mg/day (57).

NSAIDs should probably be included as one of the many groups of drugs that can cause confusion in the elderly.

Cognitive function in elderly out-patients was assessed in a large retrospective study by a questionnaire; there were no significant differences in the total scores of users and non-users of NSAIDs (SEDA-17, 106). Another study showed that performance in sensorimotor coordination and short-term memory tests can improve in healthy elderly volunteers who take indometacin (58). NSAIDs have also been associated with a reduced risk of Alzheimer's disease (59).

Electrolyte balance

NSAIDs can interfere with fluid and electrolyte homeostasis, thereby causing edema, hyponatremia, hyperkalemia, and blunting of the natriuretic effects of diuretics (60,61).

Hematologic

NSAIDs have been reported to cause potentially severe hematological disorders: thrombocytopenia, agranulocytosis, aplastic anemia, and hemolytic anemia (62). Thrombocytopenia is generally mild and reversible and has a low case-fatality rate, but deaths from bleeding have been reported, particularly with indometacin, oxyphenbutazone, and phenylbutazone (62).

Pyrazolone derivatives and butazones are most frequently blamed for causing agranulocytosis and aplastic anemia (SEDA-9, 85) (SEDA-11, 89). Unfortunately, no reasonably accurate estimate of the overall incidence of either disease or of the risk associated with the use of any particular NSAID is available. The results of the International Agranulocytosis and Aplastic Anemia study (63) have been reviewed in detail (SEDA-11, 89) (SED-11, 171). This epidemiological study was organized by the manufacturer (Hoechst) of the widely incriminated drug dipyrone. The overall annual community agranulocytosis incidence was 4.4 per million (6.2 including hospital cases), with a fatality rate of 10% and an annual mortality rate of 0.4 per million. Analgesics significantly associated with agranulocytosis were dipyrone, indometacin, and two butazones (oxyphenbutazone and phenylbutazone). Other pyrazolones, such as amidopyrine (which is an acknowledged cause of agranulocytosis), or other NSAIDs could not be evaluated because of the small number of cases.

A population-based, case-control study in patients hospitalized with neutropenia has confirmed both the association between NSAIDs and neutropenia and the differences between different classes of NSAID (64). The data on aplastic anemia are also of interest, since this was the first study to provide excess risk estimates of this adverse effect in NSAID users. The overall annual incidence was 2.2 per million, with a 2-year fatality rate of 40%. A significantly increased risk for aplastic anemia was associated with any exposure to three drugs: indometacin (multivariate rate ratio 13), butazones (8.7), and, unexpectedly, diclofenac (8.8). Whatever the interpretations by different manufacturers, the study confirmed that dipyrone can cause agranulocytosis and that indometacin can cause aplastic anemia (65). The high relative risk of diclofenac for aplastic anemia is unexpected and requires confirmation.

Hemolytic anemia has occasionally been associated with NSAIDs; many reports involved mefenamic acid, ibuprofen and sulindac (66). No evidence has been found that any NSAID, except aspirin, constitutes a particular risk for subjects with glucose-6-phosphate dehydrogenase deficiency.

A prospective study on bleeding complications in 23 patients undergoing dermatological surgery has shown that NSAIDs and aspirin need not be withdrawn routinely preoperatively, unless the bleeding time is prolonged (67). Relatively few patients developed a prolonged bleeding time while taking aspirin or other NSAIDs and only few had significant intraoperative blood loss. There is variation in the response of patients for unknown reasons and so the recommendation that NSAIDs should be withdrawn before elective surgery awaits confirmation (SEDA-19, 96).

Gastrointestinal

Dyspepsia

Dyspepsia is common in patients taking NSAIDs and is the most common reason for discontinuation of therapy or for beginning symptomatic "gastroprotective" therapy. NSAIDs differ in their capability to cause dyspepsia, but despite the high prevalence, understanding of the relation between NSAID use and dyspepsia is scanty.

Meta-analysis of randomized studies
The risk of upper gastrointestinal damage by NSAIDs has been estimated in five meta-analyses (68,69,70,71,72), but these reviews mainly focused on estimating the risk of severe ulcer complications (hemorrhage, perforation) rather than the dyspeptic syndrome caused by NSAIDs. In only one of them (68) was dyspepsia addressed, and it had two important limitations: first, the definition of dyspepsia was not specified and secondly, information was not provided about the effect of different NSAIDs or dosages, which can be important factors associated with dyspepsia.

Interesting and more accurate information on this topic has come from a recent meta-analysis (73). The authors identified studies in which defined upper gastrointestinal outcomes were reported in patients who had used oral NSAIDs for more than 4 days. Unpublished data from the Food and Drug Administration (FDA) were also obtained from new drug application reviews for the most common NSAIDs used in the USA.

The authors identified 55 randomized comparisons of NSAIDs with placebo; 86 randomized comparisons of NSAIDs versus NSAIDs; 23 large exposure trials; and 37 previously unpublished placebo-controlled trials (data from the FDA).

Of the 55 NSAID versus placebo trials and the 37 FDA reviews, 48 studies (37 published and 11 from the FDA) reported data on dyspepsia, encompassing nearly 12 000 patients. The overall percentage of patients with dyspepsia in the NSAID treated group was 4.8% (95% CI=3.8, 5.8) and the percentage in the placebo group was 2.3% (95 CI=1.6, 3.1), with a significant risk ratio of 1.4 (95% CI=1.1, 1.8). Meta-regression identified an increased risk of dyspepsia among users of specific NSAIDs (indometacin, meclofenamate, and piroxicam) (OR=2.8), and for high dosages of other NSAIDs (OR=3.1), but not for other NSAIDs in low dosage (OR=1.1).

The risk of dyspepsia varied according to the type of patient. The overall percentage of patients with NSAID-associated dyspepsia increased from 4.8% (12 000 patients in 48 studies) in the NSAID versus placebo studies to 7.1% (11 299 patients in 66 studies) in the NSAID versus NSAID comparisons, and to 11% (80 000 patients in 8 studies) in the large exposure studies. The percentage of patients who reported dyspepsia in the NSAID-treated arm of the NSAID versus placebo randomized trials may be lower in the general population because these studies tend to enrol healthier patients, who are least likely to have complications. The duration of NSAID use was not significantly associated with an increased percentage of patients reporting dyspepsia or with an increased risk of NSAID-associated dyspepsia, but only two studies lasted longer than 12 weeks. Thus, the risk of dyspepsia in patients taking long-term NSAIDs may be different from that reported in this meta-analysis. COX_2-selective NSAIDs were not considered.

In conclusion this meta-analysis suggests that the combination of a high dosage of any NSAID along with any dosage of indometacin, meclofenamate, or piroxicam increases the risk of dyspepsia by about three-fold. Other NSAIDs at lower dosages were not associated with an increased risk of dyspepsia.

Are modified-release formulations of NSAIDs any better? Despite claims of better gastroduodenal tolerability and improved adherence, evidence that modified-release NSAIDs should be preferred to standard formulations is at best scanty (SEDA-9, 83).

Standard and modified-release formulations of NSAIDs have been compared in a study from a practice database of 36 908 patients over 4 months who had an initial prescription for a standard NSAID formulation, most commonly ibuprofen (58%), and 4195 patients who received a prescription for a modified-release NSAID, most commonly diclofenac (73%) (74I). The measures that were used to document better tolerability were: prescriptions of gastroprotective drugs, the need for gastrointestinal investigations, switching from the modified-release formulation to a standard formulation. Patients who took modified-release formulations were more likely to receive concomitant gastroprotective agents, were more likely to need gastrointestinal investigations, and more commonly switched from modified-release to standard formulations than vice versa. Thus, it appears that modified-release NSAID formulations are no better tolerated than standard formulations. However, these conclusions must be interpreted with caution, as the possibility of confounding by indication could not be excluded.

Peptic ulceration

Prostaglandins have a protective effect on the gastrointestinal mucosa. All NSAIDs that non-selectively inhibit prostaglandin synthesis cause gastrointestinal mucosal damage. Direct NSAID-mediated acid damage has been identified as a mechanism of gastrointestinal toxicity (75). Several in vitro and animal studies have provided evidence of early vascular changes and have highlighted the role of leukocyte adhesion to the endothelium in NSAID-induced gastropathy. The pathogenesis of NSAID-associated gastrointestinal damage has been reviewed (SEDA-17, 104).

Clinical presentation

Features of upper gastrointestinal toxicity during NSAID therapy range from relatively mild symptoms (such as heartburn, dyspepsia, and stomach discomfort) to more severe and potentially life-threatening states (for example gastrointestinal erosion or ulceration, bleeding, or perforation). Although dyspepsia is one of the major factors that limit the use of NSAIDs in patients with rheumatic diseases, it does not necessarily predict mucosal damage. There is no close correlation between objective gastroscopy findings and subjective intolerance of medications, or between acute or chronic damage and complications. Epigastric pain was the most common symptom in patients admitted to hospital with hematemesis and/or melena, whether treated or not with NSAIDs in the 14 days before admission (SEDA-17, 103).

"NSAID gastropathy" is the term proposed by Roth and Bennett to describe upper gastrointestinal lesions associated with NSAID therapy. It has its own specific features (primarily antral and prepyloric localization, especially in elderly women), which differentiate it from classic peptic ulcer disease (76). Damage to the upper gastrointestinal tract can also involve the duodenum and, albeit infrequently, the esophagus.

Frequency

Gastrointestinal damage by NSAIDs is a major health problem. Estimates of the absolute risk vary from about two cases of serious upper gastrointestinal adverse effects per 10 000 person-months (77) to a seven-fold increase in the risk of hospitalization in patients with rheumatoid arthritis (78). Estimates of hospitalization for ulcer complications and the excess of gastrointestinal deaths in the UK have shown that 20–30% of all cases of ulcer complications in subjects aged over 60 which result in hospitalization are directly attributable to the use of NSAIDs, and that some 10% culminate in death (79). For the UK, this means that at least 2000 cases of bleeding are caused every year with about 200 deaths (80), in association with about 11 million prescriptions. The relative risk reported in different studies has generally been in the range of 3:1 to 5:1 (81).

In 2747 patients with rheumatoid arthritis, those taking NSAIDs were five times more likely (hazard ratio of 5.2) to be hospitalized for an upper gastrointestinal event (82). The risk of hospitalization for a gastrointestinal event was 15.8 per 1000 person-years in individuals taking NSAIDs, compared with 3.2 per 1000 person-years for controls. Such figures mean that on average one to two out of every 100 patients taking NSAIDs for 1 year are hospitalized for a gastrointestinal event (most commonly an ulcer).

The conclusion of a meta-analysis of 16 studies was that NSAID users have an approximately three-fold greater relative risk of developing serious adverse gastrointestinal events than non-users (83). This has been confirmed by a review (84).

Several authors have suggested that the upper gastrointestinal toxicity shortly after exposure does not persist (SEDA-22, 108), either because there is adaptation to NSAID-induced mucosal damage or because in these studies susceptible patients were selected. However, a population-based, cohort study has provided evidence that upper gastrointestinal toxicity is constant during exposure to NSAIDs and continues for some time after treatment stops (85).

Susceptibility factors

Case-control and surveillance studies have confirmed that the susceptibility factors for peptic ulcer disease are age, a history of ulcers and/or gastric bleeding, combination with corticosteroids, combination with other NSAIDs, and possibly smoking (SEDA-14, 84). The combination of NSAIDs, smoking, and alcohol increased the risk of gastrointestinal perforation nearly 11 times (OR = 10.7; CI = 3.8, 30) (SEDA-21, 97). Data on patients with rheumatoid arthritis taking NSAIDs show that the predisposition to gastrointestinal events is related to the severity of the disease (82). Other potential risk factors are sex (female), the musculoskeletal diseases for which NSAIDs are used, the NSAID taken, and dosage. The presence of gastric mucosal erosions at endoscopy was associated with an increased risk of a gastric ulcer, irrespective of prophylactic treatment (misoprostol versus sucralfate) in chronic NSAID users with osteoarthritis evaluated in a large randomized controlled trial (86). This was confirmed in other studies (SEDA-20, 86) (87,88), suggesting that the presence or absence of erosions is a better predictor of the risk of ulceration than the number of erosions.

The role of Helicobacter pylori

Helicobacter pylori and non-steroidal anti-inflammatory drugs (NSAIDs) account for nearly all gastroduodenal ulcers and serious ulcer complications, but the interaction between infection with *H. pylori* and the use of NSAIDs in the pathogenesis of NSAID-induced gastropathy is controversial. In fact, studies that have examined these two susceptibility factors have yielded conflicting results about whether *H. pylori* infection increases the risk of toxicity in NSAID users, has no effect, or may even be protective (89–91).

Since we reviewed this topic 10 years ago (SEDA-16, 103) (SEDA-17, 105) a large amount of information has accumulated and merits further attention.

The pathophysiological mechanisms Among possible common pathophysiological mechanisms of importance are those that compromise the effectiveness of the gastro-duodenal mucus–bicarbonate barrier, those that cause recruitment and activation of neutrophils, and those that can interfere with the process of mucosal adaptation (89). Both NSAIDs and aspirin can reduce the effectiveness of mucosal defences, by inhibiting gastroduodenal prosta-glandin synthesis and by reducing mucosal blood flow (92). On the other hand *H. pylori* infection can damage the mucus–bicarbonate barrier, by increasing gastric acid secretion and reducing the viscosity of gastric mucus (93). Contrasting data have been reported on the effect of *H. pylori* on mucosal blood flow (94,95) and on mucosal prostaglandin production. However, although *H. pylori* increases mucosal prostaglandin synthesis, the combina-tion of *H. pylori* with NSAIDs or aspirin causes a marked fall in mucosal prostaglandin synthesis, showing that the stimulatory effect of prostaglandin production by *H. pylori* is insignificant in the presence of NSAIDs or aspirin (95,96).

Gastric ulceration induced by NSAIDs is a neutrophil-dependent process (97) and the association of *H. pylori* infection with neutrophil infiltration has also been well documented. Gastric injury by NSAIDs is minimal in neutropenic animals, and the cumulative incidence of peptic ulcers in long-term NSAID users is increased in the presence of neutrophil infiltration in the mucosa of patients who are *H. pylori*-positive, suggesting a possible link between NSAIDs and *H. pylori* in the pathogenesis of peptic ulcers (98,99).

The ability of the gastroduodenal mucosa to adapt to repeated exposure to NSAIDs and aspirin is well docu-mented, and some reports have shown the possible invol-vement of *H. pylori* in this process (95,100). In one endoscopic study in volunteers, mucosal adaptation to naproxen after 4 weeks of treatment occurred in 53% of *H. pylori*-positive subjects and in 81% in *H. pylori*-nega-tive subjects (101). Similar results were found in another study in volunteers who took aspirin for 2 weeks; mucosal adaptation to the injury caused by aspirin was clearly impaired in the presence of *H. pylori* and was restored after *H. pylori* eradication (102).

In summary, NSAIDs and *H. pylori* can cause adverse effects on gastroduodenal mucosal protective mechan-isms in different ways, and so the interaction between these two susceptibility factors might allow damage to occur more readily when NSAIDs are taken in the presence of *H. pylori* infection. However, despite this experimental evidence, the interaction between *H. pylori* infection and use of NSAIDs in the pathogenesis of peptic ulcers and their complications is still unclear from clinical studies.

Clinical studies Most of the early studies of the inter-action between *H. pylori* infection and the use of NSAIDs were based on observational studies in long-term NSAID users and gave conflicting results (98,103–110). In some studies there were significantly more ulcers in NSAID users who were *H. pylori*-positive then in users who were not infected (98,103,104). However, these findings were not confirmed by other investigators (105–108), and they probably reflect a com-plex relation between *H. pylori* infection and NSAID-associated gastropathy, as well as heterogeneity of methods across studies. For example, differences in population studied (for example the type of NSAID exposure, the age of the patient) and even in the defini-tion of ulcer at endoscopy make direct comparison of results difficult. Most of the few published prospective trials did not show that *H. pylori* is a susceptibility factor for NSAID-induced gastroduodenal damage (96,111–113), and two long-term longitudinal studies (88,114) gave conflicting results, although the data have mostly been derived from studies in small numbers of young healthy volunteers at very low risk of gastropathy, and the results must therefore be treated with great caution. Thus, despite numerous studies we do not have convin-cing evidence for or against a link between *H. pylori* and NSAIDs in the development of peptic ulcers.

A meta-analysis has helped to clarify this issue (115). The aim was to assess the presence and magnitude of any possible interaction in peptic ulcer disease between these two susceptibility factors, with particular attention to bleeding peptic ulcer disease, the sites of ulceration, and the effect of *H. pylori* eradication. In all, 61 relevant studies were identified, 36 of which were excluded for various reasons. Thus, 25 studies were left for analysis, of which 16 observational studies (eight cross-sectional studies, seven case-control studies, and one cohort study) provided data on the prevalence of peptic ulcer disease in 1633 NSAID users, with data on *H. pylori* status for 1625 patients. The pooled frequency of peptic ulcer disease in NSAID users was 42% in those who were *H. pylori*-positive and 25% in those who were *H. pylori*-negative (OR = 2.12; 95% CI = 1.68, 2.67).

The frequencies of uncomplicated peptic ulcer disease in NSAID users and non-users were compared in eight case-control studies; however, the NSAID users and con-trols were not matched by age in three studies and so, because *H. pylori* infection is age-dependent, the preva-lence of infection was analysed in only five studies. Overall, *H. pylori* infection was diagnosed in 47% of the NSAID users and 46% of the controls, but peptic ulcer disease was significantly more common in the NSAID users (36% versus 8.3%; OR = 5.14; CI = 1.35, 20). Compared with patients who were *H. pylori*-negative and were not taking NSAIDs, the risk of ulcer in *H.*

pylori-infected NSAID users was very high (OR = 61; CI = 10, 373). *H. pylori* infection increased the risk of peptic ulcer disease in NSAID users 3.53 times in addition to the risk associated with NSAID use (OR = 19). Similarly, in the presence of a risk of peptic ulcer disease associated with *H. pylori* infection (OR = 18) the use of NSAIDs increased the risk of peptic ulcer disease 3.55 times. *H. pylori* infection and NSAID use, respectively, increased the risk of ulcer bleeding 1.79 times and 4.85 times; the risk of ulcer bleeding increased to 6.13 when both factors were present.

From these data we can conclude that both *H. pylori* infection and NSAID use independently and significantly increase the risk of peptic ulcer and ulcer bleeding and that there is synergism in the development of peptic ulcer and ulcer bleeding between *H. pylori* infection and NSAID use.

The meta-analysis also showed that one-third of patients taking long-term NSAIDs have gastric or duodenal ulcers, irrespective of *H. pylori* status and study design. However, peptic ulcer disease was significantly more common in *H. pylori*-infected NSAID users than in non-infected users, suggesting a possible interaction between NSAID use and *H. pylori* infection for the development of peptic ulcers.

Moreover, the meta-analysis clarified another uncertainty: whether in NSAID takers *H. pylori* infection is as important a risk factor for gastric ulcer as it is for duodenal ulcer. A pooled analysis of four studies (94,116–118) showed that *H. pylori* infection is less closely associated with gastric ulcer than with duodenal ulcer in both NSAID users and non-users, and that while NSAID use has a major role in the development of gastric ulcer, duodenal ulcer is more closely related to *H. pylori* infection.

Further convincing evidence for the existence of a possible interaction between *H. pylori* and NSAIDs in the pathogenesis of ulcer has been obtained by investigating the effects of *H. pylori* eradication on the occurrence of NSAID-related ulcers and their complications (for example bleeding), although some divergent findings have been reported from these studies (119,120).

In a prospective, randomized trial of the effect of eradication of *H. pylori* before the start of NSAID therapy on the subsequent risk of ulcer occurrence, patients who required new NSAID treatment and who had *H. pylori* infection but no pre-existing ulcers on baseline endoscopy were recruited (119). Of these patients, 100 were randomly allocated to naproxen for 8 weeks, either alone or preceded by a 1-week course of *H. pylori* eradication. Endoscopy was repeated after 8 weeks or if naproxen was withdrawn early because of adverse effects. The primary end-point of the study was the cumulative rate of gastric and duodenal endoscopic ulcers. At 8 weeks *H. pylori* was eradicated in 40 patients (89%) who took eradication therapy and in none of those who had no pretreatment. Twelve (26%) of those who had no eradication therapy developed ulcers compared with three (7%) who had eradication therapy, two of whom had failure of eradication. Thus, only one patient with successful eradication developed ulcers with naproxen. These data suggest that NSAID-induced

ulceration can be reduced by eradication of *H. pylori* before naproxen administration and suggest that *H. pylori* infection is a susceptibility factor for NSAID-induced ulcer disease. Some therefore believe that determination of *H. pylori* infection and eradication in infected patients should be recommended before starting NSAID therapy.

However, the data from this study contrasted with those from another randomized, controlled trial, the HELP study, in which the effect of *H. pylori* eradication was investigated in a different population of 285 patients who had used long-term NSAID therapy, those with current or previous peptic ulcers, or dyspepsia, or both (120). The patients were randomly assigned to omeprazole plus 1 week of eradication therapy (n = 142) or to omeprazole plus placebo for 1 week (n = 143). They took omeprazole until their ulcer healed or dyspepsia resolved, after which they continued taking the NSAID, with follow-up assessment of ulcer and dyspepsia at 1, 3, and 6 months. The estimated probabilities of being ulcer-free at 6 months were similar in the two groups: 0.56% (95% CI = 0.47, 0.65) with eradication treatment and 0.53 (0.44, 0.62) with control treatment. Moreover, fewer gastric ulcers healed in those who had taken eradication therapy than in the controls (7% versus 100% at 8 weeks). These data suggest that *H. pylori* eradication therapy not only did not reduce the rate of development of peptic ulcer or dyspepsia at 6 months, but actually led to impaired healing of gastric ulcers. On the basis of these results *H. pylori* eradication seems not to be justified.

These conflicting results can probably be explained by important differences in the characteristics of the patients and the study methods. The inclusion criteria in the two studies were mutually exclusive: patients with long-term NSAID use and a history of ulceration were excluded in the first study and included in the second. Furthermore, there were differences in the definition of endoscopic ulcers, the eradication regimen, the definition of *H. pylori* infection, and the length of follow-up.

Data from a later eradication study helped to clarify these uncertainties. The aim of the study was to determine whether among NSAID-naive patients positive for *H. pylori* who have dyspepsia or a history of ulcer and who are about to start long-term NSAID treatment, eradication of *H. pylori* infection reduces the risk of ulcers (121). Bismuth was replaced by omeprazole in the eradication regimen, the observation period was increased to 6 months, and the frequencies of both complicated and symptomless ulcers were assessed. Patients were randomly assigned to omeprazole triple therapy (eradication group, n = 51) or omeprazole with placebo antibiotics (control group, n = 51) for 1 week. All took diclofenac 100 mg/day for 6 months. The 6-month probability of having ulcers was 12% (95% CI = 3.1, 21) in the eradication group and 34% (21, 48) in the placebo group. The 6-month probability of complicated ulcers was 4.2% (1.3, 9.7) in the eradication group and 27% (15, 40) in the placebo group. These statistically significant differences suggested that screening and treatment for *H. pylori* infection significantly reduces the risk of ulceration and bleeding in patients who take long-term NSAIDs.

However, these conclusions may not be valid for patients who take low-dose aspirin for prevention of cardiovascular events, as there are data that suggest that *H. pylori* increases (122), has no effect (123,124), or even reduces (125) the risk of bleeding among users of low-dose aspirin as well as other NSAIDs. This question has been addressed in 400 patients with a history of upper gastrointestinal bleeding who were infected with *H. pylori* and who were taking low-dose aspirin ($n = 250$) or other NSAIDs ($n = 150$) (126). Their ulcers were healed with omeprazole 20 mg/day for 8 weeks. Those who had been taking aspirin were given aspirin 80 mg/day, and those who had been taking other NSAIDs were given naproxen 500 mg bd for 6 months. The patients in each group were then randomly assigned separately to receive omeprazole 20 mg/day for 6 months or 1 week of eradication therapy followed by placebo for 6 months.

Among patients taking aspirin the probability of recurrent bleeding during the 6 months was 1.9% for patients who had taken eradication therapy and 0.9% for patients who had taken omeprazole, a non-statistically significant difference of 1% (95% CI = −1.9, 3.9). Among users of naproxen the probability of recurrent bleeding was significantly greater among patients who had taken eradication therapy (19%) than among those who had taken omeprazole (4.4%). Unfortunately, the absolute reduction in the risk of recurrent bleeding attributable to eradication of *H. pylori* could not be determined, because a placebo group was not included.

This study has therefore shown that in patients infected with *H. pylori* who take low-dose aspirin, eradication of *H. pylori* is as effective as prophylactic therapy with omeprazole in preventing recurrent upper gastrointestinal bleeding. Therefore, patients taking aspirin for cardiovascular prophylaxis could be tested for *H. pylori* infection and treated for it if infection is confirmed. In contrast, omeprazole is superior to eradication of *H. pylori* for the secondary prevention of upper gastrointestinal bleeding in *H. pylori*-infected users of naproxen and presumably other non-aspirin NSAIDs.

More information comes from a randomized study of omeprazole or eradication therapy in patients with a history of upper gastrointestinal bleeding who were infected with *Helicobacter pylori* and who were taking low-dose aspirin or other NSAIDs (127). Among patients with *Helicobacter pylori* infection and a history of upper gastrointestinal bleeding who were taking low-dose aspirin, eradication was equivalent to treatment with omeprazole in preventing recurrent bleeding. However, omeprazole was superior to eradication in preventing recurrent bleeding in patients who were taking other NSAIDs, such as naproxen, and by implication other non-aspirin NSAIDs.

In light of the increasing use of aspirin for cardiovascular prophylaxis, these findings suggest that patients who are at risk of bleeding from ulcers should be tested for *Helicobacter pylori* infection and treated if necessary.

The role of gastric acid suppression with a proton pump inhibitor (lansoprazole) in preventing the recurrence of ulcer complications after eradication of *Helicobacter pylori* in patients taking long-term low-dose aspirin has been further better defined in another randomized study,

in which patients with healed ulcers in whom *Helicobacter pylori* had been eradicated were randomized for 12 months to aspirin 100 mg + either lansoprazole 30 mg or placebo (128). Those who took lansoprazole were significantly less likely to have recurrent ulcer complications while taking low-dose aspirin, compared with those in whom only eradication was used.

Conclusions   Whether the eradication of *H. pylori* can reduce the risk of ulcers appears to vary according to the characteristics of the patient. For people who have never taken a non-aspirin NSAID, eradication of *H. pylori* before NSAID treatment is begun reduces the risk of ulcers (119). However, for long-term users of non-aspirin NSAIDs, eradication of *H. pylori* has not been shown to prevent gastroduodenal injury. Moreover, eradication alone is not sufficient to prevent recurrent bleeding in susceptible long-term users.

The divergent outcomes in patients taking aspirin or other NSAIDs suggest that *H. pylori* may have a more important role in ulcer bleeding associated with low-dose aspirin than in bleeding associated with other NSAIDs. A possible explanation is that infection with *H. pylori* impairs gastric adaptation to aspirin (95); eradication restores this capability and increases the mucosal resistance to aspirin.

There are several conclusions from these results.

First, eradication of *H. pylori* is a useful strategy in preventing upper gastrointestinal damage caused by NSAIDs or aspirin in some patients.

Secondly, there are doubts about the correct interpretation and generalizability of the results of some relevant studies on the efficacy of omeprazole and misoprostol in the prevention of gastroduodenal ulcer in chronic NSAID users. In fact in these studies, OMNIUM (129), ASTRONAUT (130), and MUCOSA (131), the patients' *H. pylori* status was not considered and may have modified their outcomes (ulcer recurrence and ulcer healing). Some evidence supporting this hypothesis comes from a reanalysis of the data, taking into account the presence or absence of *H. pylori* (132). The superiority of omeprazole over ranitidine or misoprostol claimed in OMNIUM and ASTRONAUT in preventing NSAID-induced ulcers was markedly affected by *H. pylori* status. In a dosage of 40 mg/day, omeprazole was not superior to the full dose of misoprostol in healing unequivocal NSAID-induced gastric ulcers in chronic NSAID users, but it was superior in those whose NSAID use was complicated by *H. pylori* infection. Duodenal ulcers were markedly over-represented as a cause of ulcer recurrence in the *H. pylori*-infected patients and most of the effect of omeprazole occurred in this population. Therefore, the therapeutic advantages of using omeprazole to prevent recurrent ulcers or their complications in chronic NSAID users may be different in those with and without *H. pylori* infection.

We have no data on the possible interaction between *H. pylori* status and the ability of COX-2-selective inhibitors to cause gastrointestinal toxicity. However, one would expect that when patients use COX-2 inhibitors

H. pylori infection would remain a source of continuing ulcer risk, requiring eradication. Although there are no trials, this approach is supported by data from the VIGOR study, in which the residual risk of ulcers in patients taking rofecoxib was approximately doubled in *H. pylori*-infected compared with non-infected patients (133).

Comparative studies of different NSAIDs

Although some reports suggest that some NSAIDs are more gastrotoxic than others, data on individual drugs have been at best fragmentary (SEDA-14, 85). Two well-conducted studies have provided convincing data for clarifying whether some compounds are more likely to cause serious adverse gastrointestinal events (134,135) than others. Ibuprofen was associated with the lowest risk of gastrointestinal toxicity; diclofenac, naproxen, and possibly indometacin were intermediate, while piroxicam and in particular azapropazone had much higher risks. The differences appeared to be due to the fairly low dosage of ibuprofen; there were also dose–response relations for naproxen and indometacin. These results have practical implications. When NSAID treatment is needed the least toxic compound should be selected, on the basis of the data provided by these studies and, because of the substantial increase in risk from low-dose to high-dose NSAID therapy, it is wise to start treatment with low dosages.

The search for less toxic drugs or formulations has been discouraging. Several new formulations may be less gastrotoxic than standard formulations in short-term studies, but their long-term merit has not yet been proven. Equally, prodrugs have not protected users against gastric complications (14). Parenteral and rectal administration of NSAIDs does not spare the stomach.

Prevention

NSAID-induced gastrointestinal damage is an important cause of hospital admissions and deaths world wide. It has been responsible every year for about 7000 deaths in the USA and 1000 in the elderly population in the UK (136,137). Other estimates suggest that the number of cases of bleeding ulcers attributable to NSAIDs in the UK is about 2400. It is therefore not surprising that guidelines have been produced to assist clinicians in choosing the most appropriate preventive strategies in patients with varying degrees of gastrointestinal risk (138,139). Clinical trials have also been carried out to explore possible preventive strategies. Several theoretical options are available in clinical practice, but the best preventive choice depends on a careful consideration of several factors, such as: the intrinsic gastrotoxic potential of the NSAID used; the treatment regimen adopted, with particular attention to dose and duration of therapy; the characteristics of the individual subject, i.e. the identification of high-risk patients; and the availability and appropriate use of the most efficacious pharmacological prophylactic regimen.

1. Choosing the least toxic NSAID in the first step on the way to choosing the best prophylaxis

Table 1. Odds ratios (and 95% CI) for gastrointestinal adverse effects of NSAIDs

	Odds ratio for gastrointestinal bleeding and perforation (95% CI)	Odds ratio for acute gastrointestinal bleeding (95% CI)
Ibuprofen	2.9 (1.8, 5.0)	2.0 (1.4, 2.8)
Naproxen	3.1 (1.7, 5.9)	9.1 (5.5, 15)
Diclofenac	3.9 (2.3, 6.5)	4.2 (2.6, 6.8)
Indometacin	6.3 (3.3, 12)	11.3 (6.3, 20)
Ketoprofen	5.4 (2.6, 11)	23.7 (7.6, 74)
Piroxicam	18 (8.2, 40)	14 (7.1, 26)
Azapropazone	23 (6.9, 80)	32 (10.3, 97)
Overall	4.7 (3.8, 5.7)	4.5 (3.6, 5.6)
Low dose	2.6 (1.8, 3.8)	2.5 (1.7, 3.8)
Intermediate dose	–	4.5 (3.3, 6.0)
High dose	7.0 (5.2, 9.6)	8.6 (5.8, 13)

There is a consistent body of evidence that traditional NSAIDs are not all the same with respect to gastrointestinal toxicity (SEDA-18, 99; Table 1) (140,141), and the clinical and epidemiological relevance of this fact should not be ignored (137,142,143). In fact, if one takes in account epidemiological data on the frequency of bleeding ulcers and deaths attributable to NSAIDs as well as the relative risks associated with different NSAIDs, substitution of ibuprofen (which has the least gastrointestinal toxicity at a dose of 2.4 g/day) for all other NSAIDs would reduce the number of such events in the UK from 2431 to 695 annually. Substituting ibuprofen (or another "safe" NSAID) at a lower dose of 1200 g/day would be likely to reduce events nearly to zero. Similarly, substitution of ibuprofen 1.2 g/day, or another relatively safe NSAID, would be likely to reduce events nearly to zero. These estimates should be interpreted with caution, as the overall incidence of bleeding ulcers may be inaccurate, and reduced efficacy at a lower dose, albeit accompanied by better tolerability, may affect the benefit to harm balance.

Similar data are obtained for patients taking low-dose aspirin. The total number of excess cases attributable to aspirin in the UK is 753 annually. If prophylactic aspirin was prescribed solely at a dose of 75 mg/day, the safest efficacious dose for cardiovascular prophylaxis, the number of cases would fall to 445 annually, and the number of related deaths from 87 to 51.

On the basis of these data it is likely that an appropriate clinical strategy could prevent many episodes of peptic ulcer bleeding by selecting the least toxic NSAIDs at the lowest effective doses and using them only in patients who do not respond to simple analgesics.

2. Identification of patients at high risk of complicated ulcers

Epidemiological data show that about 50% of patients who regularly take NSAIDs have gastric erosions and 15–30% have endoscopic ulcers. However, the clinical relevance of these manifestations varies greatly, and the incidence of clinically significant gastrointestinal events caused by NSAIDs is much lower. In fact, upper gastrointestinal events may occur in 3.0–4.5% of patients taking NSAIDs, and serious complicated events (upper gastrointestinal bleeding and perforation) develop in about 1.5% (142,143).

There have been several studies of the factors that increase the risk of serious gastrointestinal complications and of methods to reduce the risk. Advanced age (over 65 years) has been consistently found to be a primary risk factor for gastrointestinal toxicity; the risk increases linearly with age and remains constant over an extended period of observation. Other risk factors that have been identified in multiple studies are higher doses of NSAIDs, including the use of two or more NSAIDs; a history of ulceration or gastrointestinal bleeding; concomitant use of some drugs, such as glucocorticoids and anticoagulants, and consumption of alcohol. Concomitant disease should also be considered (144). Not all of these possible risk factors have the same quality of evidence, as many of them have been based on univariate analyses and have not considered the interactions among multiple factors and co-existing conditions.

However, these risk factors should be carefully considered when choosing to start a NSAID.

3. Eradication of Helicobacter pylori

See above.

4. COX-2 selective inhibitors in preventing upper gastro-intestinal bleeding

There is a consistent body of evidence that concurrent therapy with non-selective NSAIDs and a proton pump inhibitor can reduce the risk of ulceration or ulcer complications (145,146,147), and this approach is therefore recommended for prophylaxis in patients at high risk for ulcer complications. COX-2 selective inhibitors (coxibs) were developed with the goal of delivering effective pain relief without causing the serious gastrointestinal adverse effects (mainly complicated ulcers) linked to the non-selective NSAIDs (SEDA-25, 126). Unfortunately the claims of better gastrointestinal safety of coxibs relative to traditional NSAIDs were open to criticism (SEDA-29, 116). Most of the data on gastric safety profile of coxibs came from a study (CLASS) that failed to demonstrate a significant reduction in ulcer complications in patients taking celecoxib compared with patients taking non-selective NSAIDs. However, the coxibs were widely adopted, both in clinical practice and official guidelines (139). Moreover, more recent data have linked coxibs with serious cardiovascular, renal, and cutaneous adverse reactions, prompting regulatory authorities to withdraw some compounds from the market.

There have been two studies of the efficacy of selective COX-2 inhibitors with respect to co-therapy with proton pump inhibitors and NSAIDs.

The aim of the first study was to assess whether celecoxib is similar to diclofenac plus omeprazole in reducing the risk of recurrent ulcer bleeding in high-risk patients. Patients who used NSAIDs for arthritis and who developed ulcer bleeding were randomly assigned to either celecoxib 200 mg bd or diclofenac 75 mg bd + omeprazole 20 mg/day for 6 months (148). The therapeutic and point was recurrent ulcer bleeding. The probability of recurrent bleeding during 6 months was 4.9% (CI = 3.1,

6.7) in patients taking celecoxib and 6.4% (4.3, 8.4) in those taking diclofenac + omeprazole, a non-significant difference. In the second trial eligible patients were randomly assigned to celecoxib 200 mg/day or naproxen 250 mg tds + lansoprazole 30 mg/day (149). The primary therapeutic end point was recurrent ulcer complications. During a median follow-up of 24 weeks 3.7% (CI = 0, 7.3%) of those who took celecoxib compared with 6.3% (1.6, 16%) of those who took lansoprazole developed recurrent ulcer complications. Celecoxib was therefore as effective as lansoprazole co-therapy in preventing recurrences of ulcer complications in subjects with a history of NSAID related complicated peptic ulcers.

The results of these studies should be interpreted with caution, for two reasons.

Firstly, in both studies a significant proportion (4–6%) of patients still had recurrent ulcer complications over the period of follow-up, showing that neither prophylactic regimen was completely protective in high-risk patients. In view of these data an important question is whether the addition of a proton pump inhibitor to celecoxib (or other COX-2 inhibitors) will further reduce upper gastrointestinal events. The problem awaits the results of further studies.

Secondly, there was an unexpectedly high rate of renal adverse effects, including acute renal insufficiency, in both studies. Careful monitoring of patients taking proton pump inhibitors + NSAIDs or celecoxib is wise.

S. Ulcer-preventing drugs

The limited data available indicate that H_2 receptor antagonists do not prevent NSAID-induced gastric ulceration. Two studies on ranitidine, reporting that it reduces the incidence of duodenal ulcers, conflict with others that did not find that it offers protection against gastroduodenal mucosal lesions (SEDA-14, 86). Only high-dose famotidine significantly reduced the cumulative incidence of both gastric and duodenal ulcers in patients taking long-term NSAIDs (87). Other trials gave contrasting results (150,151). A large prospective observational cohort study showed that patients taking antacids and H_2 receptor antagonists in combination with NSAIDs did not have a lower risk of significant gastrointestinal events, and asymptomatic patients who started taking these anti-ulcer drugs prophylactically had a higher risk of a serious gastrointestinal complication than those who did not (OR = 2.69; 95% CI = 1.36, 5.81) (152). The risk might have been increased because these drugs suppress gastrointestinal symptoms and so encourage the use of higher doses of NSAIDs for longer periods, which finally results in more severe gastrointestinal complications.

Co-administration of misoprostol and NSAIDs significantly reduced the frequency of NSAID-induced gastric ulcer in patients with osteoarthritis (153) and misoprostol reduced serious upper gastrointestinal complications (perforation, gastric outlet obstruction, and perhaps bleeding) by 40% compared with placebo in older patients with rheumatoid arthritis treated with NSAIDs (131,154).

Two studies on the proton pump inhibitor omeprazole (155,156) have provided evidence of effective prophylaxis in patients at low and high risks of developing NSAID-associated ulcers, erosions, or dyspeptic symptoms. Two other trials have shown that in patients with ulcers or multiple erosions in the stomach or duodenum who require continuous NSAID treatment, omeprazole gives greater benefit than ranitidine but not misoprostol (129,130). However, misoprostol may be less effective in healing duodenal ulcers and it is not as well tolerated as omeprazole. A daily dose of omeprazole over 20 mg does not confer any clinical advantage. As far as maintenance therapy is concerned, in patients taking NSAIDs, omeprazole 20 mg od prevents gastroduodenal damage more effectively than ranitidine or misoprostol.

Taking into account the limitations of these studies (SEDA-22, 110), these results should not lead to uncritical prescription of proton pump inhibitors for primary prophylaxis in patients taking NSAIDs. Prophylactic therapy may be justified only in high-risk patients, such as the elderly, patients with a history of peptic ulcer, gastrointestinal bleeding, or concomitant cardiovascular disease, or patients who are concurrently taking warfarin or high-dosage glucocorticoids. Whether patients who start taking NSAIDs should routinely have prophylaxis with antiulcer drugs is not at all clear. The costs of therapy are obviously high (appropriate pharmacoeconomic evaluations on the prophylactic use of omeprazole are lacking), the adverse effects of prophylactic drugs must be taken into consideration, and it would seem logical to limit it to high-risk cases (see below).

Conclusions

What are the practical implications of these data? To reduce the substantial risk of ulcer-related bleeding and perforation associated with all NSAIDs we must take into account all possible strategies that might prevent complications in as many patients as possible. Too many patients continue to take NSAIDs when simple analgesics, such as paracetamol, would provide the same benefit with less toxicity and cost. Moreover, when an NSAID is needed, the least toxic compound should be selected on the basis of available data. Finally, because of the substantial increase in risk from low-dose to high-dose NSAID therapy, it is wise, whenever possible, to start treatment with low dosages.

Individual risk factors must lead clinicians to choose the best prophylaxis. However, the gastrointestinal advantage of a combination of a traditional NSAID with a proton pump inhibitor should not be interpreted without careful consideration of competing risks from the cardiovascular perspective. For NSAIDS with competing cardiovascular and gastrointestinal risks, the trade off between reducing gastrointestinal adverse events must be weighed against concerns about cardiovascular adverse effects.

These simple guidelines, if followed, would provide a realistic strategy for preventing many complications related to the use of NSAID.

Patient education

The relevance of patient information to the prevention of adverse effects of NSAIDs has been well illustrated in a study of 50 consecutive patients who were admitted to hospital with acute gastrointestinal bleeding and who had taken NSAIDs 3 days before admission, compared with 100 matched control patients who had not bled (157). Despite the limitations of the study (158), it looks as if ignorance of adverse effects can lead to inappropriate compliance and failure to recognize warning symptoms. In fact, if the patients who bled had reduced their intake of NSAIDs in response to epigastric pain to the same extent as the apparently better informed control patients, some episodes of acute gastrointestinal bleeding might have been avoided. Consequently we should consider patient education as one of the main strategies for preventing NSAID-related toxicity.

Esophageal damage

Esophageal damage by NSAIDs, usually considered a rare adverse reaction, has been underestimated, perhaps because the symptoms of esophagitis can be misinterpreted as being of gastric origin. The clinical pattern is characterized by inflammatory changes (erosive and/or ulcerative esophagitis), ulceration with or without bleeding, and/or perforation and strictures. Data suggest that the frequency of erosive/ulcerative esophagitis in patients taking NSAIDs is not as low as was previously thought (SEDA-15, 100). Erosive or ulcerative esophagitis was present in 12 of 60 arthritic patients taking long-term NSAIDs (159). There were esophageal symptoms in 83% of the patients with esophagitis.

Long-term NSAID users have fewer esophageal histological abnormalities than controls (160). However, more epidemiological and experimental prospective studies are needed to define the role of NSAIDs in causing esophageal injury. Data on esophageal function suggest that naproxen does not cause reflux and has no significant effect on motility in healthy subjects (161).

Small bowel damage

The capacity of NSAIDs to cause intestinal damage has been demonstrated in a case-control study (162) as well as by experience with a special formulation of indometacin (Osmosin) (SEDA-15, 93). Severe intestinal damage perforation and bleeding is a very rare complication of therapy with conventionally formulated NSAIDs. The expected incidences of lower bowel perforations and bleeding are about ten and seven per 100 000 patients, respectively (162). Uncomplicated intestinal mucosal lesions are more frequent, particularly when NSAIDs are given in the long term (163). Small intestine enteropathy is characterized by inflammation and/or malfunction, with an increase in intestinal permeability. Most patients are asymptomatic, although a few taking long-term treatment have symptoms that mimic the features of Crohn's disease. As NSAIDs can exacerbate Crohn's disease (SEDA-10, 76), the differential diagnosis is difficult in symptomatic patients.

Adverse effects on the small intestine may be more frequent than previously thought and range from asymptomatic enteropathy to severe complications, such as ulceration, bleeding, perforation, and stricture (164). A prospective autopsy study in 713 patients provided an estimate of the prevalence of such lesions (165). Non-specific ulcers in the small intestine were more frequent in the NSAID group than in the control group (8.6 versus 0.6%) and the percentage was slightly higher in long-term users. Most lesions were subclinical, but perforation leading to peritonitis and death was documented in three patients taking long-term NSAIDs. The pathogenesis of NSAID-induced enteropathy is still unknown (SEDA-17, 106).

Whether the "diaphragm disease" (166–168) that is found in a few patients is a distinct NSAID-related disease or only a variant form of congenital intestinal diaphragm remains to be clarified.

Large bowel damage

"Diaphragm disease" has been reported in the ascending colon; these lesions are identical to those in the small bowel and are found only in patients who have taken modified-release NSAIDs for more than a year, because they are probably delivered unabsorbed to the large intestine (SEDA-20, 88) (169).

The causal connection between NSAIDs and large bowel inflammation needs to be confirmed by appropriate epidemiological studies. Many publications have associated NSAID and colonic inflammation (SEDA-10, 77) (SEDA-15, 95), but the differential diagnosis between colonic inflammation arising de novo and exacerbation of underlying inflammatory bowel disease can be difficult, and the role of NSAIDs in aggravating ulcerative colitis or Crohn's disease or other inflammatory bowel disease is controversial (SEDA-10, 76) (SEDA-15, 95). A case-control study showed no association between appendicectomy for acute appendicitis and the use of NSAIDs (SEDA-22, 111).

The evidence that NSAIDs can cause exacerbation of inflammatory bowel disease is at best scanty (SEDA-10, 76; SEDA-15, 92; SEDA-17, 102). In the few studies in which drugs as a cause of relapse of chronic inflammatory bowel disease have been investigated, NSAIDs have not been shown to be major contributors.

However, well-documented published series of patients with quiescent inflammatory bowel disease whose colitis became active shortly after they were given NSAIDs make the causal relation probable, at least in some patients (170–173). Because the pathogenesis of inflammatory bowel disease is unknown, it is difficult to say whether episodes of colitis are exacerbations of the underlying disease or unrelated events caused by NSAIDs in predisposed patients.

Consecutive new patients with colitis (n=105) were questioned about their recent use of NSAIDs and salicylates and compared with two groups of 105 age- and sex-matched controls taken from hospital in-patients and community cases attending the Accident and Emergency Department (174). Of the patients with colitis, 78 (74%) had taken NSAIDs or salicylates before or during the development of their disease. By comparison, significantly fewer of the community controls (20%; OR=9.1; CI=4.5, 22) and hospital in-patients (30%; OR=6.2; CI=3.2, 14) were using NSAIDs or salicylates. The

authors concluded that in new patients with colitis there is a significantly high frequency of antecedent exposure to NSAIDs or salicylates, supporting the concept that these agents may be important in the pathogenesis of colitis.

Two other studies of the possible association between NSAIDs and the onset or exacerbation of inflammatory bowel disease have given contrasting results. In the first study (175) the authors interviewed 60 patients (mean age 42 years) with either Crohn's disease or ulcerative colitis who required admission to hospital owing to symptoms of their disease, and 62 matched controls (mean age 46 years) with irritable bowel syndrome who did not require hospitalization. Patients were asked about their use of NSAIDs and the relation in time and duration to the exacerbation or onset of the inflammatory bowel disease. There was an association with the use of NSAIDs in 31% of the patients with inflammatory bowel disease, but in only 2% of those with irritable bowel syndrome. Compared with patients with irritable bowel syndrome the odds ratio (OR) for an exacerbation or new onset of symptoms of inflammatory bowel disease after recent use of NSAIDs (defined as use within 1 month of symptom exacerbation or onset of disease) was 20 (95% CI = 2.6, 160).

In contrast, the second study (176) showed that the use of NSAIDs was not associated with a higher incidence of active inflammatory bowel disease. The authors retrospectively examined the records of 192 outpatients with inflammatory bowel disease: 112 with Crohn's disease (mean age 53 years) and 80 with ulcerative colitis (mean age 61 years). The use of NSAIDs was more common in patients with inactive inflammatory bowel disease than in those with active disease. Of 40 patients with active Crohn's disease, three were using NSAIDs compared with 14 of 72 with inactive disease. Of 58 patients with active ulcerative colitis, eight were using NSAIDs compared with five of 21 patients with ulcerative colitis in remission.

These contrasting results may have been due to different patient populations studied (inpatients versus outpatients) or to other limitations: in the case-control study, the number of patients enrolled was small and the confidence intervals of the odds ratio were very large; in the observational study, the analysis was retrospective and the possibility that some patients had used over-the-counter NSAIDs could not be excluded.

The adverse effects of NSAIDs on the lower gastrointestinal tract have been studied in a systematic review of 18 randomized studies, 14 case-control studies, eight cohort studies, and seven before-and-after studies (177). Nonselective NSAIDs had significantly more adverse effects than no NSAIDs in 20 of 22 studies of lower gastrointestinal integrity, five of seven visualization studies, seven of 11 bleeding studies (OR = 1.9–18 in case-control studies), two of two perforation studies (OR = 2.5–8.1), and five of seven diverticular disease studies (OR = 1.5–11). Coxibs had significantly less effect than non-selective NSAIDs in three of four integrity studies, one endoscopic study (RR for mucosal breaks = 0.3), and two randomized studies (RR for lower gastrointestinal clinical events = 0.5; RR for hematochezia = 0.4).

Despite the clinical importance of the problem, we lack a firm answer to the question of whether patients with inflammatory bowel disease should refrain from using NSAIDs.

When administered long-term, the fenamates cause watery diarrhea in more patients than other NSAIDs. Although colonic ulceration has been reported after oral ingestion of several NSAIDs (SEDA-7, 105; SEDA-10, 77; SEDA-15, 95), the evidence is not entirely convincing. On the other hand, there is firm reason to conclude that there is a direct causal relation between rectally administered NSAID and rectal ulceration, which seems to occur more frequently when doses are high or treatment is prolonged.

Liver

Serious liver reactions to NSAIDs are rare and unpredictable (SEDA-17, 107) (178), suggesting that most reactions are due to hypersensitivity. However, the FDA has recognized liver reactions as a class effect of NSAIDs. Severe injury and even deaths have been reported (179).

Because of hepatotoxicity, particularly problematic in the elderly, benoxaprofen was withdrawn from the market in 1982, and ibufenac is not on sale for the same reason. Serious hepatocellular reactions have been well-documented with phenylbutazone and the death rate is high (180). Hepatotoxicity has been reported with all of the structural classes of NSAIDs.

Hepatic reactions are more often reported with the pyrazolone, indole, and propionic acid groups of compounds than with the fenamate and oxicam classes (62). Some national monitoring centers have published their experience on liver toxicity with NSAIDs, and the Swedish and Australian agencies have both drawn attention to an apparently higher frequency of liver reactions with sulindac and diclofenac (181,182). Reactions to sulindac are characterized by cholestasis. Diclofenac is associated with more acute hepatocellular derangement and is recognized as a rare cause of acute hepatocellular damage (183).

Cirrhosis with esophageal or cardiac varices

Aspirin can increase the risk of variceal bleeding in patients with cirrhosis. In fact, according to a case-control study (184), patients with cirrhosis and esophageal or cardiac varices who take NSAIDs are three times more likely to have a first episode of variceal bleeding compared with similar patients who are not taking NSAIDs.

In 125 patients with cirrhosis who were admitted to hospital with a first episode of bleeding related to esophageal or cardiac varices, compared with 75 patients with cirrhosis, but no previous or current history of variceal bleeding, who were admitted to the same hospitals, a questionnaire showed that more patients with a first episode of bleeding had used aspirin, either alone or in combination with other NSAIDs compared with controls (OR = 4.9). This increased risk of bleeding was seen only in patients with grade 2 or grade 3 varices.

The results of this small hospital-based study should be interpreted with caution, but as variceal bleeding is a life-threatening event and in cirrhosis other factors (thrombocytopenia and coagulation defects) can also predispose to bleeding, the possible benefit of therapy with aspirin or other NSAIDs should be carefully weighed against the risks of major gastrointestinal bleeding.

Pancreas

Case reports have suggested that the use of newer COX-2 selective inhibitors can cause acute pancreatitis. This has been assessed in a case-control study in 3083 patients with acute pancreatitis and 30 830 controls (185). For current use the relative risk estimate for celecoxib was 1.4 (95% CI = 0.8, 2.3) and for rofecoxib 1.3 (95% CI = 0.7, 2.3). The overall relative risk for other non-steroidal anti-inflammatory drugs was 2.7 (95% CI = 2.4, 3.0) with substantial variation in risk between individual drugs. The highest relative risk was for diclofenac (OR = 5.0; 95% CI = 4.2, 5.9) and the lowest for naproxen (OR = 1.1; 95% CI = 0.7, 1.7).

Urinary tract

Many of the NSAIDs are associated with renal disorders arising de novo or by aggravation of existent renal dysfunction. Inhibition of PGE-1 synthesis intrarenally leads to a reduction in the vasodilator activity of this prostaglandin, which normally contributes to maintenance of renal functional balance and protection against the vasoconstrictor effects of noradrenaline and angiotensin-II and the action of antidiuretic hormone.

NSAIDs can produce a spectrum of renal diseases: functional renal insufficiency, nephrotic syndrome with or without interstitial nephritis, renal papillary necrosis and chronic interstitial nephritis, acute tubular necrosis, vasculitis, glomerulonephritis, and obstructive nephropathy.

Incidence

Two studies have suggested that the overall incidence of clinical nephrotoxicity with NSAIDs is small (186,187). However, some patients (see below) are at increased risk of particular effects (SEDA-11, 82), and patients with sickle cell anemia can probably be added to the list (SEDA-15, 97).

Although some compound-related variations do occur, every nephrotoxic effect seems to have been reported with every NSAID at some time and no NSAID is free of nephrotoxic potential. This applies to sulindac as to other NSAIDs, although its renal function-sparing effect is disputed (SEDA-15, 99) (188,189). One study suggested that renal effects were more likely to occur with ibuprofen than with piroxicam or sulindac (190), but it was criticized for flawed experimental design (191). There is other evidence that sulindac is relatively safer: short-term sulindac 400 mg/day had no effect on glomerular filtration rate, renal plasma flow, or renal prostaglandin excretion in ten patients with arthritis and impaired renal function, while naproxen 750 mg/day reduced all three (192). Such short-term evidence clearly does not eliminate the problems of long-term use, which constitute the real challenge.

A study of the risk of chronic renal disease associated with the regular use of NSAIDs showed that it was twice as high in men over 65 years and tended to be even higher in patients with heart disease or other disorders that might compromise renal circulation (193). The results of a second investigation, a case control study of 340 patients with end-stage renal disease on a hemodialysis maintenance program and 678 hospitalized controls, confirmed the trend (SEDA-16, 105), but more reliable epidemiological data are needed to show that regular consumption of NSAIDs increases the risk of chronic renal disease. NSAID-associate analgesic nephropathy has been reviewed (SEDA-18, 100).

The actual risk of NSAID-associated acute renal dysfunction also continues to be the subject of controversy. There is adequate evidence that underlying renal insufficiency, congestive heart failure, or hepatic cirrhosis are conditions that carry a high risk of NSAID-related renal functional impairment. It is still not known whether old age is a risk factor, whether the risk of renal impairment varies with different NSAIDs, or whether renal function continues to deteriorate, stabilize, or even improve in affected patients with continued use of NSAIDs. Three cases of renal insufficiency caused by topical NSAIDs have been described (SEDA-18, 100).

Types of complication

Of all the potentially serious adverse effects of NSAIDs, functional renal insufficiency, which is probably the most common, results from the hemodynamic changes secondary to inhibition of prostaglandin synthesis. Renal insufficiency and interference with fluid and electrolyte homeostasis occur in disease states in which prostaglandins are significant determinants of renal function, such as those characterized by hypovolemic states due to salt depletion or hypoalbuminemia and those in which there is pre-existing renal impairment due to age, atherosclerosis, hypertensive renal disease, or other intrinsic renal disease. Although the functional renal insufficiency is usually mild and reversible within a few days of withdrawing NSAIDs, it can also be severe and irreversible, so early recognition is essential. All NSAIDs can cause this complication.

A case-control study on recent use of NSAIDs and functional renal impairment at the time of hospitalization showed that there was a weak association between the use of NSAIDs and renal dysfunction. Patients at higher risk had a history of renal disease or of gout and hyperuricemia. While NSAID dosages were only weakly related to renal impairment, there was a statistically significant difference between compounds with half-lives under or over 4 hours: the OR increased from 1.2 (95% CI = 0.6, 2.4) to 4.8 (CI = 1.5, 16) for compounds with half-lives over 12 hours (194). Therefore, long half-life drugs should be avoided in subjects at risk of renal impairment.

A case-control study provided convincing epidemiological evidence that the use of NSAIDs was associated with the risk of hospitalization for acute renal insufficiency (relative risk about 2.0) (SEDA-19, 95; 195).

Acute interstitial nephritis, which is distinct from the methicillin-like form, is the most important type of organic renal damage caused by NSAIDs. Distinguished by a nephrotic syndrome, often with renal insufficiency, the histological picture is an acute interstitial nephritis combined plus a glomerular lesion with fusion of the epithelial foot process. Patients had usually been taking NSAIDs over a long period of time. Acute interstitial nephritis has been reported relatively often in patients taking fenoprofen.

The acute flank pain syndrome associated with reversible renal insufficiency is very rare. It has usually been reported with suprofen (SEDA-12, 89), but flurbiprofen and ibuprofen have also been implicated (SEDA-18, 100).

Membranous nephropathy is rare and causes the nephrotic syndrome, usually with minimal-change glomerulopathy, with or without interstitial nephritis (SEDA-11, 85). A retrospective study provided more data on the frequency and clinical characteristics of membranous nephropathy associated with NSAIDs (196). It confirmed that it is rare (13 of 125 patients diagnosed during the last 20 years met the strict criteria for NSAID-associated membranous nephropathy), and the nephrotic syndrome is reversible after prompt withdrawal. The pathogenesis is unknown but seems to be immune-mediated, given the characteristic deposition of IgG and C3.

Renal papillary necrosis has been reported after long-term intake or abuse of aspirin and other NSAIDs (SEDA-11, 85; SEDA-12, 79).

The risk of acute renal insufficiency when NSAIDs are used in combination with ACE inhibitors is discussed below under drug-drug interactions

Prostaglandins play an important role in genitourinary function, as they provoke contraction of the detrusor muscle. Relaxation of the detrusor muscle by inhibition of prostaglandin synthesis by NSAIDs could therefore result in acute urinary retention. In a population-based case-control study of 536 men each matched with up to 10 controls (n = 5348 in all) from a source population of 72 114, the risk of acute urinary retention in current users of NSAIDs was twice that in non-users (CI = 1.23, 3.31) (197). The highest risk (adjusted OR = 3.3; CI = 1.2, 9.2) was in those who had recently started using NSAIDs and in those using high doses.

Chronic renal disease

The relation between long-term heavy exposure to analgesics and the risk of chronic renal disease has been the object of intensive toxicological and epidemiological research for many years (SEDA-24, 120) (198). Most of the earlier reports suggested that phenacetin-containing analgesics probably cause renal papillary necrosis and interstitial nephritis. In contrast, there is no convincing epidemiological evidence that non-phenacetin-containing analgesics (including paracetamol, aspirin, mixtures of the two, and NSAIDs) cause chronic renal disease. Moreover, findings from epidemiological studies should be interpreted with caution, because of a number of inherent limitations and potential biases in study design (199). Two methodologically sound studies have provided information on this topic.

The first was the largest cohort study conducted thus far to assess the risk of renal dysfunction associated with analgesic use (200). Details of analgesic use were obtained from 11 032 men without previous renal dysfunction participating in the Physicians' Health Study (PHS), which lasted 14 years. The main outcome measure was a raised creatinine concentration defined as 1.5 mg/dl (133 µmol/l) or higher, and a reduced creatinine clearance of 55 ml/minute or less. In all, 460 men (4.2%) had a raised creatinine concentration and 1258 (11%) had a reduced creatinine clearance. Mean creatinine concentrations and creatinine clearances were similar among men who did not use analgesics and those who did. This was true for all categories of analgesics (paracetamol and paracetamol-containing mixtures, aspirin and aspirin-containing mixtures, and other NSAIDs) and for higher risk groups, such as those aged 60 years or over or those with hypertension or diabetes.

These data are convincing, as the large size of the PHS cohort should make it possible to examine and detect even modest associations between analgesic use and a risk of renal disease. Furthermore, this study included more individuals who reported extensive use of analgesics than any prior case-control study. However, the study had some limitations, the most important being the fact that the cohort was composed of relatively healthy men, most of whom were white. These results cannot therefore be generalized to the entire population. However, the study clearly showed that there is not a strong association between chronic analgesic use and chronic renal dysfunction among a large cohort of men without a history of renal impairment.

The second study was a Swedish nationwide, population-based, case-control study of early-stage chronic renal insufficiency in men whose serum creatinine concentration exceeded 3.4 mg/dl (300 µmol/l) or women whose serum creatinine exceeded 2.8 mg/dl (250 µmol/l) (201). In all, 918 patients with newly diagnosed renal insufficiency and 980 controls were interviewed and completed questionnaires about their lifetime consumption of analgesics. Compared with controls, more patients with chronic renal insufficiency were regular users of aspirin (37% versus 19%) or paracetamol (25% versus 12%). Among subjects who did not use aspirin regularly, the regular use of paracetamol was associated with a risk of chronic renal insufficiency that was 2.5 times as high as that for non-users of paracetamol. The risk increased with increasing cumulative lifetime dose. Patients who took 500 g or more over a year (1.4 g/day) during periods of regular use had an increased odds ratio for chronic renal insufficiency (OR = 5.3; 95% CI = 1.8, 15). Among subjects who did not use paracetamol regularly, the regular use of aspirin was associated with a risk of chronic renal insufficiency that was 2.5 times as high as that for non-users of aspirin. The risk increased significantly with an increasing cumulative lifetime dose of aspirin. Among the patients with an average intake of 500 g or more of aspirin per year during periods of regular use, the risk of chronic renal insufficiency was increased about three-fold (OR = 3.3; CI = 1.4, 8.0). Among patients who used paracetamol in addition to aspirin, the risk of chronic renal

insufficiency was increased about two-fold when regular aspirin users served as the reference group, (OR = 2.2; CI = 1.4, 3.5) and non-significantly when regular paracetamol users were used as controls (OR = 1.6; CI = 0.9, 2.7). There was no relation between the use of other analgesics (propoxyphene, NSAIDs, codeine, and pyrazolones) and the risk of chronic renal insufficiency. Thus, the regular use of paracetamol, or aspirin, or both was associated dose-dependently with an increased risk of chronic renal insufficiency. The OR among regular users exceeded 1.0 for all types of chronic renal insufficiency, albeit not always significantly. These results are consistent with exacerbating effects of paracetamol and aspirin on chronic renal insufficiency, regardless of accompanying disease.

How can we explain the contrasting results of these two studies? A possible explanation lies in the different populations studied. In PHS, relatively healthy individuals were enrolled while in the Swedish study all the patients had pre-existing severe renal or systemic disease, suggesting that such disease has an important role in causing analgesic-associated chronic renal insufficiency. People without pre-existing disease who use analgesics may have only a small risk of end-stage renal disease.

Prevention

While misoprostol has been shown to limit NSAID-induced gastric damage, three studies failed to show that misoprostol prevents NSAID-induced impairment of renal function. However, another showed that it prevents ciclosporin-induced renal damage in renal transplant patients (202). Further studies are therefore required to assess the protective effect of misoprostol on renal function (SEDA-16, 106).

Skin

Skin reactions are often reported with NSAIDs, but the true incidences with individual NSAIDs are unknown. There are very few specific epidemiological studies, and most information comes from single case reports and data from national spontaneous reporting systems. A major study on nearly 20 000 patients showed that 0.3% of 9118 patients taking analgesics and NSAIDs developed skin reactions that could be attributed to these drugs (203).

Although usually mild, skin reactions very often require withdrawal of treatment. At times they can be severe, and isoxicam was withdrawn from the market because of the high frequency of severe adverse skin reactions (SEDA-10, 88).

There are various types of NSAID-induced rashes. The main morphological patterns are urticarial, maculopapular, vesicular, and exfoliative. Skin reactions to NSAIDs are probably of phototoxic origin and can be associated with systemic hypersensitivity or other allergic reactions. More rarely, NSAIDs can exacerbate pre-existing skin disease (for example psoriasis, acne). Phototoxic reactions were very common with benoxaprofen (30–50% of patients treated in the UK), and were one reason why it did not receive licensing approval in Australia or the

Benelux countries. Other NSAIDs, such as azapropazone, piroxicam, and fenbufen, have been reported to cause higher than average rates of photosensitivity (204). NSAIDs were among the causal agents of phototoxic reactions most commonly reported to the Australian Adverse Drug Reactions Advisory Committee (205,206).

Widespread use of naproxen, sulindac, diclofenac, and diflunisal probably explains why they were the most frequently implicated, rather than because they have a greater tendency to cause these adverse effects. NSAIDs differ in their ability to cause adverse skin reactions in terms of both frequency and severity: pyrazolones, butazones, and oxicams are most often blamed, and among the arylalkanoic acid derivatives fenbufen and carprofen are most often incriminated.

The types of skin adverse effect also vary with different compounds. The most serious life-threatening reactions, such as erythema multiforme and its variants (Stevens–Johnson syndrome, toxic epidermal necrolysis, exfoliative erythroderma) are uncommon and occur mainly with the butazone derivatives and to a lesser extent with piroxicam, sulindac, and possibly fenbufen. In large series reported in France, Germany, and the USA, NSAIDs are most often implicated: 12 (44%) of the most commonly implicated 29 drugs (207).

Although all NSAIDs can cause urticaria, particularly in aspirin-sensitive patients, it is more common with pyrazolone derivatives. Photosensitivity is principally a problem with azapropazone, carprofen, tiaprofenic acid, and piroxicam (SEDA-9, 84).

The reasons for these different effects of different NSAIDs are poorly understood. The only physicochemical characteristic that seems to be important in determining a particular propensity for adverse skin reactions is lipophilicity (10), which probably affects NSAID distribution to the skin. The longer half-lives of lipophilic compounds may concomitantly facilitate the persistence of skin reactions. Although there are no clear relations between the other pharmacological and kinetic characteristics of NSAIDs and effects on the skin, less lipophilic drugs with short half-lives might be preferable.

There are no clearly identifiable predisposing factors for most adverse skin reactions. Urticaria and photosensitivity are exceptions. Many NSAIDs can cause urticaria (sometimes associated with angioedema) in aspirin-sensitive patients. Probably not immunological in origin, the reaction may be related to prostaglandin inhibition in a patient whose cutaneous mastocytes are more susceptible to the stabilizing effect of prostaglandins. Skin testing in patients with a history of urticarial and/or anaphylactic reactions to analgesics is of little value in identifying patients at risk and can be dangerous (208,209). Skin pigmentation and environmental factors that influence the radiant exposure dose are clearly very important in determining the risk of a phototoxic reaction.

Since the extreme rarity of life-threatening reactions, such as erythema multiforme and toxic epidermal necrolysis, suggests individual susceptibility, efforts have been made to identify subjects at risk. In 25 cases of erythema multiforme and toxic epidermal necrolysis there was a slight, non-significant increase in the frequency of the HLA-B12 and DR4 phenotypes, suggesting that genetic factors are involved (210). Genetic predisposition also seems to be confirmed by the finding of a fixed drug eruption in four members of a single family taking feprazone (SEDA-17, 108). From a practical point of view, if a mild reaction occurs it is wise to withdraw treatment, even if the reaction disappears spontaneously in some patients despite continuing treatment. Withdrawal of treatment and prompt referral to hospital is imperative if the reaction is severe and/or tends to progress.

Careful clinical monitoring is probably necessary for all patients with underlying skin diseases (for example acne, psoriasis), as some NSAIDs can exacerbate them (211,212). NSAIDs should not be used for apparently benign inflammatory cutaneous lesions, unless the possibility of infection has been ruled out.

Lichenoid photoeruptions have been reported not infrequently in HIV-positive people, often in association with photosensitizing drugs, especially NSAIDs (213). Facial scars have been described in adults and children treated with NSAIDs, usually in connection with sun exposure (214).

Contact sensitivity to topical NSAIDs

Topical NSAIDs can cause allergic, photoallergic, and phototoxic contact dermatitis. There have been two systematic studies of photosensitivity to these compounds and their cross-reactivity (215,216). Eleven patients with confirmed photocontact dermatitis were photopatch tested with seven topical NSAIDs. Ketoprofen was the commonest cause. In five cases there was cross-sensitivity with fenofibrate, which was explained by a common benzoylketone or benzophenone molecule, and in one patient there was cross-sensitivity to tiaprofenic acid, an arylpropionic acid derivate that is not available in topical form in Europe. There was also one case of photocontact dermatitis from diclofenac, which was discovered by 1% dilution in alcohol, while 5% in petrolatum was negative in the same patient (215). In contrast to these findings, all 12 patients tested in another study reacted to both ketoprofen and tiaprofenic acid, mainly after UVA irradiation, but were negative to other arylpropionic acids (216). Furthermore, there were positive reactions to both ketoprofen and fenofibrate in eight of the 12 patients. The authors concluded that photoallergy to ketoprofen and fenofibrate is due to the molecular benzophenone structure and confirmed cross-reactivity with other benzophenones, used as sunscreens. Cross-reactivity between ketoprofen and tiaprofenic acid was supposed to be due to the benzophenone moiety of ketoprofen, or to the very similar thiophene-phenylketone part of tiaprofenic acid, but not to their arylpropionic function.

The topical use of NSAIDs, such as bufexamac, can provoke contact allergic reactions (217–219) and a case has been reported with bendazac (220).

- A 28-year-old man had been using a bendazac-containing ointment for his atopic dermatitis for 6 months, together with topical corticosteroids. Patch testing showed positive reactions to bendazac in petrolatum on days 2, 3, and 7 and a positive reaction to alclometasone dipropionate.

Contact allergy to topical indometacin has rarely been reported (221).

- A 14-year-old boy had contact allergy to indometacin gel used for a sprained ankle (222). He had previously taken NSAIDs orally, but not topically. Patch tests with the indometacin gel and pure indometacin 1% in petrolatum were positive.

Photocontact allergy to NSAIDs is not uncommon, but the incidence may differ from NSAID to NSAID. A case of photoallergy from local piketoprofen has been reported (223), as have two cases of prolonged photosensitivity after contact photoallergy from ketoprofen, persisting for more than a year after withdrawal (224,225).

Contact pemphigus has been attributed to ketoprofen.

- A 65-year-old Caucasian woman developed a localized skin eruption within hours of using ketoprofen gel on her knees to relieve arthralgia (226). The lesions were pruritic, well-demarcated, and erythematous, and later became studded with vesicles and small bullae. Histology and immunopathology suggested autoimmune pemphigus.

Photosensitivity to topical NSAIDs

The arylpropionic acid derivatives often cause allergic and photoallergic contact dermatitis, and photoallergic dermatitis to ketoprofen, with cross-photosensitivity to benzophenone and tiaprofenic acid, has been reported (227). Photopatch tests to these substances were positive but patch tests were negative.

A case of photoallergic contact dermatitis from aceclofenac has been reported (228). Photopatch tests were positive with aceclofenac 10% in petrolatum, but not with either aceclofenac 1% or 5% in petrolatum or with a series of NSAIDs and other analgesics (benzydamine hydrochloride 3 and 5%, bufexamac 5%, diclofenac 1, 5, and 10%, fepradinol 1%, ibuprofen 5%, indometacin 1, 5, and 10%, ketoprofen 1%, naproxen 5%, paracetamol 1, 5, and 10%, phenylbutazone 1%, piroxicam 1%, salicylic acid 1 and 5%, and thiosalicylic acid 0.1%, all in petrolatum).

Photocontact dermatitis has been reported after topical application of dexketoprofen (Enangel), with positive photopatch tests to dexketoprofen 1% and piketoprofen 2% (229).

Local pharyngeal treatment with benzydamine hydrochloride 0.15% (Tantum verde) by a 67-year-old man resulted in systemic photocontact dermatitis in the third week of treatment (230). Photopatch tests with Tantum verde as is and in 10% aqueous solution were positive: D1+, D2+, D3++.

Photosensitization potentials and cross-reactivities of ketoprofen, suprofen, tiaprofenic acid, and benzophenone have been studied in guinea pigs (231). Ketoprofen and benzophenone were the strongest photosensitizers. Cross-reactivity was most frequent after sensitization with ketoprofen. Benzophenone photosensitization did not induce cross-reactivity. The benzoyl radical was identified as the key structure for both photosensitization and cross-reactivity among the NSAIDs.

Pseudoporphyria

Pseudoporphyria is a photodistributed bullous disorder with clinical and histological features similar to those of porphyria cutanea tarda, but without accompanying abnormalities of porphyrin metabolism. Drugs, in particular NSAIDs and sulfur-containing diuretics, often cause pseudoporphyria (232). Pseudoporphyria associated with naproxen (15 mg/kg/day) has been reported in a child (233).

Musculoskeletal

Suspected but unproven harmful effects of NSAIDs on joints, cartilage, and bone have been reviewed (SEDA-11, 87). Inhibition of glycosaminoglycan synthesis in joint cartilage, inhibition of necrotic bone repair by reduced synthesis of vasodilator prostaglandins, which have been shown both in vitro and in animals, and deprivation of protective painful stimuli are possible mechanisms. As these data derive from experimental models, they cannot be extrapolated with certainty to the effects of NSAIDs on the pathophysiological characteristics of the human osteoarthritic joint. Evidence for harmful effects of NSAIDs on the human hip joint comes from single case reports and a small series of clinical observations, two retrospective studies, and two prospective investigations. The first prospective study showed that hip osteoarthritis progressed more rapidly in patients taking indometacin, a potent inhibitor of prostaglandin synthesis, than in those taking azapropazone, a weak inhibitor (234). This suggests that one should be cautious with long-term use of the more potent cyclo-oxygenase inhibitors in patients whose joints are severely compromised by osteoarthritis. The second study showed that the risk of progression of knee osteoarthritis increased in patients treated with indometacin for 1 year (235). Other studies have reported that some NSAIDs have a protective effect on cartilage (236). A study on a small group of patients treated with piroxicam for osteoarthritis of the knee supported the hypothesis that deprivation of painful stimuli lets the patient put more load on the joint, increasing the risk of more rapid progression of the disease (237).

The suggestion that NSAIDs should not be used as analgesics after orthopedic surgery because they might inhibit fracture healing (238) elicited strong disagreement (239,240). The belief that NSAIDs could cause more harm then benefit in patients undergoing orthopedic surgery in based on some experimental data in animals. In diverse rodent models NSAIDs inhibited bone healing, but other animal studies have shown no effect (239,241,242). In humans, published evidence is almost non-existent (239). In the absence of well-designed trials showing important effects on bone healing, NSAIDs should continue to be used as effective analgesics after orthopedic surgery.

Reproductive system

There have been several case reports that non-selective NSAIDs (diclofenac, naproxen, piroxicam) can cause infertility, attributed to "luteinized unruptured ovarian follicles" syndrome (243–245). Women who are trying to become pregnant should avoid taking any NSAIDs if possible, and those who need one for a chronic rheumatic disorder should be aware of possible infertility; in such cases further investigation is not required, as withdrawal of the drug restores fertility.

Immunologic

There is considerable difficulty and controversy in identifying and classifying allergic reactions to NSAIDs, for many reasons (246). First, the difficulty in making a definite diagnosis in patients who have these reactions without provocative challenge with the suspected drug and other NSAIDs. Secondly, reactions are characterized by a large spectrum of target organ responses to NSAIDs, and the same drug may cause different types of reactions in different organs in the same or different individuals. Thirdly, a patient can have a similar reaction to a structurally different NSAID. Finally, reports of these reactions include different, often imprecise, terms, making interpretation difficult.

Anaphylactic or anaphylactoid reactions to NSAIDs are probably relatively rare. Even today, the only data available are from 1981, when the FDA's Division of Drug Experience was notified of 131 cases attributable to various NSAIDs (247). Tolmetin was the most frequently implicated compound. However, the figures are distorted, because some of these drugs are much more widely used than others. A retrospective cohort study using 1980–84 Medicaid billing data from three states in the USA, designed to assess the relative risk of hypersensitivity reactions from different NSAIDs, failed to confirm that tolmetin is associated with a higher risk of hypersensitivity reactions than other NSAIDs (248). However, two drugs (glafenine and zomepirac) have been withdrawn from the market because of their propensity to cause severe hypersensitivity reactions.

The clinical picture of hypersensitivity reactions varies from vasomotor rhinitis, urticaria, and angioedema to serious bronchoconstriction and in some cases anaphylactic shock.

Two pathogenic mechanisms have been proposed: an allergic immunological hypersensitivity reaction and a pseudoallergic reaction characterized by mast-cell degranulation by complement components, histamine liberation by drugs, and interference with endogenous eicosanoid biosynthesis (249). The first mechanism appears to be responsible for anaphylactic shock and/or urticaria after amidopyrine or noramidopyrine, and the second for bronchoconstriction after aspirin, noramidopyrine, or aminophenazone and other pyrazole drugs. It is important to distinguish the two mechanism, since the first type of intolerance is fairly structure-specific and can be avoided by switching from a drug to which the patient has proved sensitive to an NSAID with a distinct structure, whereas pseudoallergic aspirin-sensitive

patients must avoid all drugs that inhibit fatty acid cyclo-oxygenase.

There have been reports of exaggerated responses (angioedema and malaise) to bee stings in patients taking NSAIDs (SEDA-11, 88). More recently a report of resensitization to bee stings associated with diclofenac has been received by the Centre for Adverse Reactions Monitoring in New Zealand. The patient, who had been successfully desensitized to bee venom many years before, developed life-threatening anaphylaxis after a bee sting while taking diclofenac (250).

Autacoids

The risks of angioedema among users of the newer cyclo-oxygenase, COX-2 selective inhibitors celecoxib and rofecoxib and other non-aspirin NSAIDs have been studied in a case-control study of 377 patients and 10 matched population controls per case (n = 3747) selected from the Civil Registration System (251). After adjustment for confounding, the relative risk for current use of the COX-2 selective inhibitors was 0.96 (95% CI = 0.46, 2.03), whereas the risk for other NSAIDs was 1.77 (95% CI = 1.23, 2.58).

Infection risk

NSAIDs can mask signs of infection, such as fever and pain, which can delay appropriate treatment. Furthermore they can impair the host defence mechanism against infection and can modulate the acute inflammatory response in such a way as to alter the course of infection, predisposing the patient to bacteremia, shock, and multiorgan failure (252,253). Until appropriate studies have defined the relation between NSAIDs and severe soft tissue infections, it is better to avoid using them, if possible, until the cause of the fever is known.

There have been sporadic case reports of a possible association between NSAIDs and necrotizing fasciitis due to Group A *Streptococcus pyogenes* (SEDA-12, 79) (254,255). It has been suggested that NSAIDs may increase the risk of the infection, impede its timely recognition and management, and/or accelerate the course of infection, and these questions have been examined in a systematic review of case reports, retrospective studies, and prospective studies (256). To be included in the analysis documentation of invasive streptococcal infection and necrotizing fasciitis was required. To assess the relation between NSAID use and the development of necrotizing fasciitis, cases were analysed for the presence of risk factors for necrotizing fasciitis (co-morbidity), a putative portal of entry for Streptococcus pyogenes, the timing of NSAID use, the concomitant use of immunosuppressive agents, and the development of complications.

Of eight patients with necrotizing fasciitis identified in the published case reports, only one had used an NSAID on a long-term basis (an elderly man with alcoholism and osteoarthritis), three had used 3 NSAIDs before the onset of symptoms suggestive of necrotizing fasciitis, and four had no identifiable susceptibility factors.

There were 12 retrospective studies of necrotizing fasciitis including data on the use of NSAIDs. Of these, 10 were case series, often including duplicate publications, and two were case-control studies. There were detailed data on 31 patients. Of these 15 had no identifiable susceptibility factor, and in 22 NSAIDs had been started after the onset of symptoms.

In the first case-control study of NSAID use in childhood *Varicella* infection there were only three cases of necrotizing fasciitis and there was no significant association between NSAIDs and fasciitis. In the second case-control study of 16 children with necrotizing fasciitis, always in the setting of primary *Varicella* infection, the cases were more likely than controls to have taken ibuprofen before hospitalization, suggesting an association between the use of ibuprofen and necrotizing fasciitis.

There were five prospective studies of the association between NSAIDs and necrotizing fasciitis, and three were conducted by the same group in Canada. These studies included a larger number of patients who had been exposed to NSAIDs, and there was no association between their use and necrotizing fasciitis.

Thus, establishing an adverse effect of NSAIDs on the course of necrotizing fasciitis associated with Streptococcus pyogenes is difficult on the basis of the available data. However, some conclusions can be reached. First, published data show no evidence of necrotizing fasciitis in young healthy persons taking long-term NSAIDs and no evidence that NSAIDs adversely affect the severity of necrotizing fasciitis once it is established. Secondly, it is likely that some sign and symptoms (swelling, erythema, fever, and pain), which characterize the initial presentation of necrotizing fasciitis, may be attenuated by NSAIDs, thus delaying diagnosis and treatment. Thirdly, it is possible that NSAIDs could reduce host immunity by many different mechanisms (257); however, the evidence in humans that they adversely affect the outcome of infection is still lacking.

Long-Term Effects

Tumorigenicity

Studies on the tumor-inducing effects of heavy use of analgesics, especially those that contain phenacetin, have given contrasting results (SEDA-21, 100) (258,259). There has been a case-control study of the role of habitual intake of NSAIDs on the occurrence of urothelial cancer and renal cell carcinoma (260). In previous studies there was a consistent association between phenacetin and renal cell carcinoma, but inconclusive results with respect to non-phenacetin analgesics. In 1024 patients with renal cell carcinoma and an equal number of matched controls, regular use of analgesics was a significant risk factor for renal cell carcinoma (OR = 1.6; CI = 1.4, 1.9). The risk was significantly increased by aspirin, NSAIDs, paracetamol, and phenacetin, and within each class of analgesic the risk increased with increasing exposure. Individuals in the highest exposure categories had about a 2.5-fold increase in risk relative to non-users or irregular users of analgesics.

NSAIDs and aspirin are associated with a reduced risk of colon cancer. In rheumatoid arthritis the risk of colon cancer is reduced, but the risk of non-Hodgkin's lymphoma is increased. The association between the use of NSAIDs and aspirin, a history of arthritis, and the risk of non-Hodgkin's lymphoma has been evaluated in a prospective cohort of 27 290 postmenopausal women (261). During 7 years of follow-up, 131 cases of non-Hodgkin's lymphoma were identified. Compared with women who did not use either aspirin or non-aspirin NSAIDs, there was an increased risk of non-Hodgkin's lymphoma in women who used aspirin exclusively (RR=1.71; 95% CI=0.94, 3.13), non-aspirin NSAIDs exclusively (RR=2.39; 95% CI=1.18, 4.83), or both types of drugs (RR=1.97; 95% CI=1.06, 3.68). A diagnosis of rheumatoid arthritis (RR=1.75; 95% CI=1.09, 2.79), but not osteoarthritis (RR=1.06; 95% CI=0.67, 1.68), was associated with an increased risk of non-Hodgkin's lymphoma, but the positive association between the use of aspirin and other NSAIDs and non-Hodgkin's lymphoma was independent of a history of rheumatoid arthritis.

Second-Generation Effects

Pregnancy

NSAIDs are among the commonest drugs prescribed for pregnant woman (262). However, the risk of adverse birth outcomes in women who take NSAIDs other than aspirin during pregnancy is largely unknown.

In a comparison, too small to allow firm conclusions, pregnancies in 88 patients with rheumatic diseases in which NSAIDs had or had not been used, there were no differences in pregnancy outcome, duration of labor, complications at delivery, neonatal health, and the health or development of offspring at follow-up (263).

However, there is no doubt that NSAIDs can alter fetal physiology in the last trimester of pregnancy and prolong gestation and labor (SEDA-5, 101; SEDA-6, 93; SEDA-7, 108; SEDA-8, 102; SEDA-9, 88; SEDA-11, 88; SEDA-12, 84; SEDA-15, 99; SEDA-21, 96; SEDA-22, 112).

There has been a study in a Danish county (population about 490 000), including data on all women who between 1991 and 1998 had a live birth or a stillbirth after the 28th week of gestation, or who had a miscarriage (including missed abortions) (264). The researchers performed a case-control study using data from the Danish birth registry, the county hospital discharge registry, and the county's prescriptions database. The risk of miscarriage was examined. The study involved 4268 women who had had their first miscarriage, 63 of whom had filled a prescription for an NSAID in the 12 weeks before being discharged from hospital after the miscarriage, and 29 750 primiparous controls who had live births. There was a significant association with miscarriage both when the prescription for the NSAID was filled during the week before the miscarriage (OR = 7.0; CI = 2.8, 17) and when it was filled at 7–9 weeks before the miscarriage (OR = 2.6; CI = 1.8, 4.0).

The validity of these findings has been challenged on the grounds of possible bias and other methodological problems (265,266). However, according to a statement issued by the UK Royal College of Obstetricians and

Gynaecologists (RCOG) NSAIDs should be avoided by women who know that they are pregnant. According to the RCOG, although the study did not establish a causative link between NSAID use and miscarriage, pregnant women should avoid NSAIDs and in the meantime prefer to use effective alternative drugs, such as paracetamol (267).

Teratogenicity

Many NSAIDs have provoked teratogenic effects in animals, but there is no evidence from epidemiological studies that NSAIDs are embryotoxic in humans. The lack of clinical and epidemiological studies makes any firm recommendations about the use of NSAIDs during the first 6 months of pregnancy impossible. However, the possibility of unrecognized dysmorphogenic effects of NSAIDs needs to be considered before prescribing, so it is wise to use compounds with short elimination half-lives and to give them at the longest possible dosage intervals. When NSAIDs are used for dysmenorrhea, administration should be delayed until menstruation has started, so as to avoid ingestion during an unrecognized pregnancy; in any case, there is no need to give them earlier.

There has been a study in a Danish county (population about 490 000), including data on all women who between 1991 and 1998 had a live birth or a stillbirth after the 28th week of gestation, or who had a miscarriage (including missed abortions) (264). The researchers performed a cohort study using data from the Danish birth registry, the county hospital discharge registry, and the county's prescriptions database. The risk of an adverse birth outcome (congenital abnormality, low birth weight, and preterm birth) was examined. The study included 1462 women who gave birth after 28 weeks and who had filled a prescription for an NSAID, a total of 1742 prescriptions. The control group consisted of 17 259 pregnant women who did not take any drugs during pregnancy. There was no significant association between the uptake of prescriptions for NSAIDs during pregnancy and the risks of congenital abnormalities, low birth weight, or preterm births.

The teratogenic risk of non-steroidal anti-inflammatory drugs has been investigated using a population-based pregnancy registry in 36 387 mothers of live singleton infants who took an NSAID or other medications during pregnancy (268). For each infant with any congenital anomaly diagnosed in the first year of life, up to 10 controls, infants with no congenital anomalies, were selected. There were 93 births with congenital anomalies in 1056 women (8.8%) who filled prescriptions for NSAIDs in the first trimester of pregnancy, compared with 2478 in 35 331 (7%) who did not. The adjusted OR for any congenital anomalies for the former was 2.21 (95% CI = 1.72, 2.85) and for anomalies related to cardiac septal closure 3.34 (95% CI = 1.87, 5.98). There were no significant associations with anomalies in other major organ systems.

Fetotoxicity

Several studies have shown that the use of indometacin as a tocolytic agent is associated with severe adverse effects in the fetus (for example fetal ductal constriction, oligohydramnios), which limit this indication (SEDA-16, 108) (269).

Lactation

Although the newer NSAIDs are all secreted into milk, the amounts are probably too small to affect the breast-fed infant. However, serious adverse effects in breast-fed children have been described with pyrazolones and indometacin (SEDA-10, 78). The choice of NSAID, if it is indispensable, should therefore be directed to compounds that have short half-lives. In order to reduce the quantity of drug reaching the child, the mother should take the drug at the time of breast feeding or immediately afterwards, so that the next feed occurs after a time equivalent to the half-life of the drug.

Susceptibility Factors

Genetic factors

Anaphylactic reactions induced by NSAIDs are associated with HLA-DRB1 genes encoding HLA-DR11 molecules, according to the results of a study in 21 patients who suffered from anaphylactic reactions to NSAIDs and 47 patients who had exclusively skin reactions to these drugs (270). A control group of 167 patients was studied. Patients and controls were challenged, single-blind, with aspirin, salsalate, paracetamol, piroxicam, or diclofenac. There were 88 episodes of skin reactions to NSAIDs and 26 episodes of anaphylaxis. The frequency of HLA-DR11 alleles was 59% in the anaphylaxis group compared with 16% in the control group. Neither HLA-DR nor HLA-DQ alleles was associated with NSAID-induced skin reactions.

Drug Administration

Drug administration route

Topical NSAIDs

Despite official approval and wide use as either over-the-counter or prescription drugs, there is skepticism that topical NSAIDs have any action other than as rubefacients (271). There has been a systematic review of the efficacy and safety of these drugs in 86 randomized controlled clinical trials in more than 10 000 patients with acute or chronic pain (272). Topical NSAIDs were significantly more effective than placebo for pain relief. Local tolerability was good: local skin reactions were rare (3.6%) and systemic effects even rarer (less than 0.5%). Local or systemic unwanted effects of sufficient severity to cause withdrawal from the study were also rare (0.5%) and no more common than with placebo.

In two case-control studies, topical NSAIDs were not significantly associated with upper gastrointestinal bleeding or perforation, after adjustment for the confounding effect of concomitant use of oral NSAIDs (273), nor with hospitalization for acute renal insufficiency (195), although renal adverse effects have been described, albeit rarely, with these topical formulations (SEDA-18, 100).

Drug–Drug Interactions

General interactions with NSAIDs

General interactions with NSAIDs are summarized in Table 2 (pharmacokinetic interactions) and Table 3 (pharmacodynamic interactions).

Widespread use of NSAIDs, particularly in the elderly, who often take other drugs at the same time, leads to a high risk of clinically significant drug interactions, both pharmacokinetic and pharmacodynamic. The inhibitory effects of azapropazone, oxyphenbutazone, and phenylbutazone on the metabolism of other drugs, such as oral anticoagulants, oral hypoglycemic drugs, and phenytoin, is an example of a pharmacokinetic mechanism. Other NSAIDs inhibit the renal excretion of lithium (although toxicity is less likely with aspirin, ibuprofen, and sulindac) and methotrexate. Pharmacodynamic mechanisms are exemplified by the interactions between indometacin and other NSAIDs (except perhaps sulindac) and with antihypertensive agents (including beta-blockers, diuretics, and ACE inhibitors). Interactions of NSAIDs with other drugs (274) are summarized in Tables 2 and 3.

To explore the frequency of continuous use of over-the-counter drugs and the potential for harmful interactions between OTC drugs and prescribed drugs, a population-based interview survey was conducted in 10 477 subjects (275). Daily use of over-the-counter drugs was reported by 7% of the subjects and 4% of those who used over-the-counter drugs had taken combinations with potential for clinically significant interactions. Interactions were most common for NSAIDs such as ketoprofen (15% of ketoprofen users), ibuprofen (10%), and aspirin (6%). Unfortunately, this study did not provide information on whether the potential interactions led to actual clinical problems.

In a population-based study in Finland of co-prescription of NSAIDs and other drugs that may potentiate their gastrointestinal toxicity, combining NSAIDs with corticosteroids, anticoagulants, or selective serotonin reuptake inhibitors (SSRIs) increased the risk of upper gastrointestinal haemorrhage by 15, 15, and 13 times respectively (276).

ACE inhibitors

Whenever renal blood flow is compromised the kidneys respond by releasing prostaglandins and angiotensin II. Angiotensin II has a vasoconstrictor effect on the renal efferent arterioles and prostaglandins have a vasodilator effect on the afferent arterioles; thus, both preserve glomerular filtration rate. Under conditions of renal hypoperfusion or renal impairment, the administration of a combination of NSAIDs with ACE inhibitors will interfere with these physiological compensatory mechanisms, and so cause acute impairment of renal function through a

fall in glomerular filtration by combined renal blood flow changes: NSAIDs inhibit dilatation by renal prostaglandins and the vasoconstrictor effect on the efferent arterioles is inhibited by ACE inhibitors.

It is not surprising, therefore, that various combinations of ACE inhibitors, diuretics, NSAIDs (including COX_2 selective inhibitors) and angiotensin receptor antagonists have been implicated in a significant number of reports of drug-induced renal insufficiency. More specifically, the combined use of ACE inhibitors, diuretics, and NSAIDs has been implicated most often (277) in single cases or small series of cases of nephrotoxicity (278,279,280,281), in spontaneous reports to pharmacovigilance agencies, or in epidemiological studies.

In 2002, 28 of the 129 reports to the Australian Drug Reaction Advisory Committee (ADRAC) of acute renal insufficiency implicated one of the above-mentioned combinations (282). Most of the events reported to ADRAC related to elderly patients and appeared to be precipitated by mild stress (for example diarrhea, dehydration) in a patient taking the triple combination or by the addition of a third drug, usually an NSAID, to the stable use of the other two. If promptly recognized and the offending drug is withdrawn, the renal dysfunction can be reversible, but the fatality rate for ADRAC cases of renal insufficiency with the "triple whammy" was as high as 10%.

More recently, a case-control study has shown an increased risk of hospitalization for renal insufficiency in patients taking ACE inhibitors who started using NSAIDs (283). The study included 144 users of ACE inhibitors aged over 40 years, who were admitted to hospital with renal insufficiency during treatment and 1189 controls without any hospital admission for renal problems during ACE inhibitor therapy. Of the 144 cases, 22% had taken an NSAID in the 90 days before hospital admission (adjusted OR=2.2; 95% CI=1.1, 4.5). The increased risk was most pronounced in patients aged over 70 years and in those who had received a larger number of prescriptions for an ACE inhibitor.

Convincing evidence is now available that there is an increased risk of acute renal insufficiency in patients taking ACE-inhibitors with or without a diuretic who start using NSAIDs (including COX_2 selective agents). The risk of this interaction seems to be underestimated and the syndrome under-recognized. NSAIDs should be avoided in these patients, especially if they are elderly and have predisposing factors to renal insufficiency.

Alcohol

The FDA has announced its intention to require alcohol warnings on all over-the-counter pain medications that contain acetylsalicylic acid, salicylates, paracetamol, ibuprofen, ketoprofen, or naproxen. The proposed warnings are aimed at alerting consumers to the specific risks incurred from heavy alcohol consumption and its interaction with analgesics. For products that contain paracetamol, the warning indicates the risks of liver damage in those who drink more than three alcoholic beverages a day. For formulations that contain salicylates or the mentioned NSAIDs three or more alcoholic beverages will increase the risk of stomach bleeding (284).

Antihypertensive drugs

All NSAIDs interfere with hypertension control in patients taking diuretics, beta-blockers, or vasodilators, although contrasting data have been published on the effects of these drugs on blood pressure (285). Moreover, they interact diversely with different antihypertensive drugs, antagonizing the effect of beta-blockers and ACE inhibitors more than calcium channel blockers, diuretics, and centrally acting alpha-adrenoceptor agonists (286,287). In one study there was no significant change in blood pressure in patients taking calcium channel blockers (verapamil or nifedipine) with NSAIDs (288). Among ACE inhibitors, perindopril reduces blood pressure in patients taking NSAIDs (289).

Aspirin

Ibuprofen antagonizes the cardioprotective effects of aspirin in patients with cardiovascular disease. (SEDA-26, 115; SEDA-27, 111). In one study, 7107 patients who were discharged after a first admission for cardiovascular disease, who were taking low-dose aspirin (less than 325 mg/day), and who survived for at least 1 month, were studied (290). Compared with those who used aspirin alone, patients taking aspirin plus ibuprofen had increased risks of all-cause mortality (hazard ratio = 1.93; 95% CI = 1.30, 2.87) and cardiovascular mortality (1.73; 1.05, 2.84). The theoretical basis for this interaction came from experimental data (291), which suggest that ibuprofen may limit the cardioprotective effect of aspirin by competitively inhibiting the binding of aspirin to platelets.

If this interaction were demonstrated with all NSAIDs its clinical relevance could be enormous, because NSAIDs are among the most frequently used drugs. This question has been examined in two studies.

The first study was a subgroup analysis of the results of a randomized, double-blind, placebo-controlled study of aspirin (325 mg on alternate days) in 22 071 individuals participating in the Physicians Health Study (292). During a mean follow-up period of 5 years, there were 378 myocardial infarctions among the study participants, 139 of which occurred in those taking aspirin and 239 in those taking placebo (RR = 0.56; 95% CI = 0.45, 0.70). While intermittent NSAID use was not associated with an increased risk of myocardial infarction in either the aspirin or placebo groups, the use of NSAIDs on more than 60 days/year in those taking aspirin was significantly associated with an increased risk of myocardial infarction. Compared with no NSAID use, the relative risks of myocardial infarction among participants randomized to receive aspirin were 1.21 (95% CI = 0.78, 1.87) for NSAID use on 1–59 days/year and 2.86 (95% CI = 1.25, 6.25) for NSAID use on more than 60 days/year. In contrast, among hose who took placebo, NSAID use did not significantly alter the risk of myocardial infarction. Thus, this post-hoc subgroup analysis from a large randomized trial showed a more than twofold increase in the risk of a first myocardial infarction among participants taking aspirin who also take NSAIDs for more than 60 days/year.

The second study gave contrasting results (293). Compared with aspirin alone, the concomitant use of aspirin and ibuprofen did not increased the risk of death in elderly patients after myocardial infarction. The authors conducted a retrospective cohort study of 234 769 Medicare patients aged over 65 years, discharged from hospital after a myocardial infarction between 1994 and 1996, of whom 70 316 were taking aspirin at discharge; 66 739 took aspirin alone, 844 took aspirin + ibuprofen, and 2733 took aspirin + other NSAIDs. A total of 11 546 patients (17.5%) who took aspirin alone, 118 (14%) who took aspirin + ibuprofen, and 432 (16%) who took aspirin + other NSAIDs died within 1 year of discharge. Patients who took aspirin +ibuprofen had a comparable risk of death to those who took aspirin alone (hazard ratio = 0.84; 95% CI = 0.7, 1.01) or aspirin + another NSAID (0.96; 0.86.1.06). Thus, in this study in elderly patients discharged after myocardial infarction aspirin and ibuprofen did not adversely interact.

These studies have been criticized for many different reasons: study design poor; population studied not representative of the general population; bias in data collection; use of concomitant medications not addressed; only a small number of events measured (294,295,296,297); the results must be interpreted with caution. Although an interaction of ibuprofen with aspirin is potentially clinically important, the current evidence is not sufficient to make definitive recommendations for or against the sue of concomitant ibuprofen in patients who may need prophylactic aspirin. The place of aspirin in primary and secondary prevention of coronary artery disease is well established (298), while the evidence supporting the hypothesis that regular use of NSAIDs may negate the cardioprotective benefit of aspirin is not. While waiting for further research to clarify this, aspirin avoidance in patients taking long-term NSAIDs, and vice versa, is probably not justified.

Ciclosporin

An interaction resulting in additive deterioration of renal function has been documented in patients taking ciclosporin together with different NSAIDs (SEDA-17, 107). The mechanism is still uncertain, but may involve prostaglandin production, and the known effects of NSAIDs on cyclo-oxygenase suggest an additive effect in the kidney. The concomitant use of NSAIDs and ciclosporin requires caution. Sulindac, which may be less toxic to the kidneys, can increase whole blood ciclosporin concentrations by inhibiting hepatic cytochrome P450 (SEDA-17, 107). Inhibition by ciclosporin of diclofenac first-pass metabolism has been hypothesized (SEDA-21, 104).

Table 2 Pharmacokinetic drug interactions with NSAIDs

Drug(s) affected by NSAIDs	NSAID(s) implicated	Effect(s)	Management
Oral anticoagulants	Phenylbutazone	Inhibition of metabolism of S-warfarin, increasing anticoagulant effect	Avoid NSAIDs if possible; careful monitoring when unavoidable (note also pharmacodynamic interactions)
	Oxyphenbutazone Azapropazone		
Lithium	Probably all NSAIDs (?except sulindac, aspirin)	Inhibition of renal excretion of lithium, increasing lithium serum concentrations and increasing risk of toxicity	Use sulindac or aspirin if an NSAID is unavoidable; careful monitoring of serum lithium concentration and appropriate dosage reduction
Oral hypoglycemic drugs	Phenylbutazone	Inhibition of metabolism of sulfonylureas, prolonging half-lives and increasing the risk of hypoglycemia	Avoid these NSAIDs if possible; if not, monitor blood glucose closely
	Oxyphenbutazone Azapropazone		
Phenytoin	Phenylbutazone	Inhibition of metabolism of phenytoin, increasing plasma concentration and risk of toxicity	Avoid these NSAIDs if possible; if not, intensive plasma concentration monitoring
	Oxyphenbutazone Other NSAIDs	Displacement of phenytoin from plasma albumin, reducing total concentration for the same unbound (active) concentration	Careful interpretation of serum total phenytoin concentration; measurement of unbound concentration can be helpful, if available
Methotrexate	Probably all NSAIDs	Reduced clearance of methotrexate (mechanism unclear), increasing plasma concentration and risk of severe toxicity	Simultaneous dosing is contraindicated; use of NSAIDs between cycles of chemotherapy is probably safe
Sodium valproate	Aspirin	Inhibition of valproate metabolism, increasing plasma concentration	Avoid aspirin; monitor plasma concentration if other NSAIDs are used
Digoxin	All NSAIDs	Potential reduction in renal function (particularly in the very young and very old), reducing digoxin clearance and increasing plasma concentrations and the risk of toxicity; no interaction if renal function is normal	Avoid NSAIDs if possible; if not, frequent checks of serum digoxin concentration and serum creatinine
Aminoglycosides	All NSAIDs	Reduction in renal function in susceptible individuals, reducing aminoglycoside clearance and increasing plasma concentrations	Careful plasma concentration monitoring and dosage adjustment
Antacids	Indometacin (?other NSAIDs)	Variable effects of different formulations: aluminium-containing antacids reduce the rate and extent of absorption of indometacin; sodium bicarbonate increases the rate and extent of absorption of indometacin	No action required, unless a marked reduction in absorption results in a poor response to the NSAID, in which case dosages may need to be increased or the antacid withdrawn
Probenecid	Probably all NSAIDs	Reduction in the metabolism and renal clearance of NSAIDs and their acylglucuronide metabolites, which are hydrolysed back to the parent drug	Can be used therapeutically to increase the response to a given dose of an NSAID
Barbiturates	Phenylbutazone (?other NSAIDs)	Increased metabolic clearance of NSAIDs	May require higher dosages of phenylbutazone
Caffeine	Aspirin	Increased rate of absorption of aspirin	No action required
Colestyramine	Naproxen and probably other NSAIDs	The anion exchange resin binds NSAIDs in gut, reducing the rate (?and extent) of absorption	Separate dosing times by 4 hours; may need higher than expected dosages of NSAIDs
Metoclopramide	Aspirin	Increased rate and extent of absorption of aspirin in patients with migraine	Can be used therapeutically

Table 3 Pharmacodynamic drug interactions with NSAIDs

Drug affected by NSAIDs	NSAID(s) implicated	Effect(s)	Management
Antihypertensive drugs	Indometacin	Reduction in hypotensive effect, probably related to impaired prostaglandin synthesis (causing salt and water retention) and vascular prostaglandin synthesis (causing vasoconstriction)	Avoid all NSAIDs in treated hypertensive patients if possible; if not, use sulindac preferentially; may need additional antihypertensive therapy
Diuretics	Indometacin	Reduction in natriuretic and diuretic effects; can exacerbate congestive cardiac failure	Avoid NSAIDs in patients with cardiac failure; use sulindac; monitor clinical signs of fluid retention
Anticoagulants	All NSAIDs	Gastrointestinal tract mucosal damage; inhibition of platelet aggregation; increased risk of gastrointestinal bleeding in patients taking anticoagulants	Avoid all NSAIDs if possible
Hypoglycemic drugs	Salicylates (high dosages)	Potentiation of hypoglycemic effects (mechanism unknown)	Monitor blood glucose concentration
Combinations with increased risk of toxicity Management	NSAID(s)	implicated	Effect(s)
All diuretics	All NSAIDs	Combination associated with increased risk of hemodynamic renal insufficiency	Avoid combination if possible
Triamterene	Indometacin	Potentiation of nephrotoxicity, including subjects with normal renal function	Combination contraindicated
Potassium-sparing diuretics	All NSAIDs	Potassium retention and hyperkalemia	Avoid combination; monitor plasma potassium concentration

Methotrexate

Interactions of NSAIDs with methotrexate have been reviewed (SEDA-20, 89). Severe toxicity has been attributed to different dosages of methotrexate in concomitant use with several NSAIDs. The mechanisms are unclear. Both methotrexate and the NSAIDs are secreted by the organic acid secretory pathway in the kidney and both are highly bound to plasma albumin. In a study on the pharmacokinetics of methotrexate in patients with rheumatoid arthritis there was no significant interaction between a single low dose of methotrexate and piroxicam (299). A second study in patients with rheumatoid arthritis showed no significant differences in the pharmacokinetics of methotrexate 7.5 mg/week with or without NSAIDs. At higher dosages (10–25 mg/week) the renal clearance of methotrexate was reduced by both salicylate and non-salicylate NSAIDs (300). These data confirm that simultaneous dosing of methotrexate (over 7.5 mg/week) and NSAIDs must be avoided, since methotrexate toxicity can be severe. Differences between NSAIDs in interactions with methotrexate require other studies (301).

Misoprostol

Two reports of adverse neurological effects (dizziness, unsteadiness in walking, and ataxic symptoms) in patients treated with misoprostol and NSAIDs require confirmation (SEDA-16, 108).

Selective serotonin reuptake inhibitors (SSRIs)

The interaction between SSRIs and NSAIDs has been reviewed in the light of four retrospective studies of gastrointestinal adverse outcomes (302). The risk ratio for an upper gastrointestinal bleed from this drug combination (compared with not receiving either agent) was 3.3–16, and the risk ratio for gastrointestinal adverse effects was 12. In two studies the risk for an upper gastrointestinal bleed from the drug combination exceeded the additive risk of the agents alone. The risk ratio for an upper gastrointestinal bleed from an SSRI–aspirin interaction was 1.9–7.2. The number needed to harm (NNT_H) in terms of an upper gastrointestinal bleed from an SSRI–NSAID combination was 62–75 patient-years, and the NNT_H for gastrointestinal adverse effects was 2 patient-years.

Warfarin

Despite the clinical and epidemiological importance of the problem, there is little information on the comparative safety of coxibs and NSAIDs in patients taking warfarin. A nested case-control study has provided some information about the risk of upper gastrointestinal hemorrhage in patients taking warfarin and a non-selective NSAID or a COX-2 inhibitor (303). The patients had had an upper gastrointestinal hemorrhage while taking warfarin. After adjusting for potential confounders, patients taking warfarin were more likely to have been taking celecoxib (OR = 1.7; CI = 1.2, 3.6), rofecoxib (OR = 2.4; CI = 1.7, 3.6), or a non-selective NSAID (OR = 1.9; CI = 1.4, 3.7) relative to controls. These findings suggest that the risk of upper gastrointestinal hemorrhage is equally increased in warfarin users taking either a coxib or a traditional NSAID. If there is co-prescription, careful monitoring of the INR is mandatory and gastric protection wise.

References

1. Evens RP. Nonrheumatologic uses of NSAIDS. Drug Intell Clin Pharm 1984;18(1):52–5.
2. Peleg II, Maibach HT, Brown SH, Wilcox CM. Aspirin and nonsteroidal anti-inflammatory drug use and the risk of subsequent colorectal cancer. Arch Intern Med 1994;154(4):394–9.
3. Waterhouse DM, Brenner D. Aspirin, NSAIDs, and risk reduction of colorectal cancer. The problem is translation. Arch Intern Med 1994;154(4):366–8.
4. Muscat JE, Stellman SD, Wynder EL. Nonsteroidal anti-inflammatory drugs and colorectal cancer. Cancer 1994;74(7):1847–54.
5. Andersen K, Launer LJ, Ott A, Hoes AW, Breteler MM, Hofman A. Do nonsteroidal anti-inflammatory drugs decrease the risk for Alzheimer's disease? The Rotterdam Study. Neurology 1995;45(8):1441–5.
6. Rich JB, Rasmusson DX, Folstein MF, Carson KA, Kawas C, Brandt J. Nonsteroidal anti-inflammatory drugs in Alzheimer's disease. Neurology 1995;45(1):51–5.
7. Rainsford KD. Introduction and historical aspects of the side-effects of anti-inflammatory analgesic drugs. In: Rainsford KD, Velo GP, editors. Side-effects of Anti-inflammatory Drugs. Part I: Clinical and Epidemiological Aspects. Lancaster: MTP Press, 1987:3.
8. Furst DE. The basis for variability of response to anti-rheumatic drugs. Baillière's Clin Rheumatol 1988;2(2):395–424.
9. Brooks PM, Day RO. Nonsteroidal antiinflammatory drugs—differences and similarities. N Engl J Med 1991;324(24):1716–25.
10. Fenner H. Hautreaktionen durch nicht-steroidale Antirheumatica. Dtsch Apoth Ztg 1985;125:2654.
11. Brune K, Graft P. Non-steroid anti-inflammatory drugs: influence of extra-cellular pH on biodistribution and pharmacological effects. Biochem Pharmacol 1978;27(4): 525–30.
12. Day RO, Graham GG, Williams KM, Champion GD, de Jager J. Clinical pharmacology of non-steroidal anti-inflammatory drugs. Pharmacol Ther 1987;33(2–3): 383–433.
13. Day RO, Graham GG, Williams KM. Pharmacokinetics of non-steroidal anti-inflammatory drugs. Baillière's Clin Rheumatol 1988;2(2):363–93.
14. Carson JL, Strom BL, Morse ML, West SL, Soper KA, Stolley PD, Jones JK. The relative gastrointestinal toxicity of the nonsteroidal anti-inflammatory drugs. Arch Intern Med 1987;147(6):1054–9.
15. Shea TY. Anti-inflammatory drugs. In: Vane JR, Ferreira SH, editors. Handbook Exp Pharmacol 50 1979:305–42 11.
16. Moncada S, Vane JR. Mode of action of aspirin-like drugs. Adv Intern Med 1979;24:1–22.
17. Abramson SB, Weissmann G. The mechanisms of action of nonsteroidal antiinflammatory drugs. Arthritis Rheum 1989;32(1):1–9.
18. Vane J. Towards a better aspirin. Nature 1994;367(6460): 215–6.
19. Higgs GA, Moncada S, Vane JR. The mode of action of anti-inflammatory drugs which prevent peroxidation of arachidonic acid. Clin Rheum Dis 1980;6:675.
20. Kitchen EA, Dawson W, Rainsford KD, Cawston T. Inflammation and possible modes of action of anti-inflammatory drugs. In: Rainsford KD, editor. Anti-inflammatory and Antirheumatic Drugs 1. Boca Raton, FL: CRC Press, 1985:21.
21. Johnson AG. NSAIDs and blood pressure. Clinical importance for older patients. Drugs Aging 1998;12(1):17–27.
22. Pope JE, Anderson JJ, Felson DT. A meta-analysis of the effects of nonsteroidal anti-inflammatory drugs on blood pressure. Arch Intern Med 1993;153(4):477–84.
23. Johnson AG, Nguyen TV, Day RO. Do nonsteroidal anti-inflammatory drugs affect blood pressure? A meta-analysis. Ann Intern Med 1994;121(4):289–300.
24. Nowak J, Wennmalm A. Influence of indomethacin and of prostaglandin E1 on total and regional blood flow in man. Acta Physiol Scand 1978;102(4):484–91.
25. Johnson AG, Nguyen TV, Owe-Young R, Williamson DJ, Day RO. Potential mechanisms by which nonsteroidal anti-inflammatory drugs elevate blood pressure: the role of endothelin-1. J Hum Hypertens 1996;10(4):257–61.
26. Wilson SL, Poulter NR. The effect of non-steroidal anti-inflammatory drugs and other commonly used non-narcotic analgesics on blood pressure level in adults. J Hypertens 2006;24(8):1457:1457–69.
27. Gurwitz JH, Avorn J, Bohn RL, Glynn RJ, Monane M, Mogun H. Initiation of antihypertensive treatment during nonsteroidal anti-inflammatory drug therapy. JAMA 1994;272(10):781–6.
28. Curhan GC, Willett WC, Rosner B, Stampfer MJ. Frequency of analgesic use and risk of hypertension in younger women. Arch Intern Med 2002;162(19):2204–8.
29. Radack KL, Deck CC, Bloomfield SS. Ibuprofen interferes with the efficacy of antihypertensive drugs. A randomized, double-blind, placebo-controlled trial of ibuprofen compared with acetaminophen. Ann Intern Med 1987;107(5):628–35.
30. Chalmers JP, West MJ, Wing LM, Bune AJ, Graham JR. Effects of indomethacin, sulindac, naproxen, aspirin, and paracetamol in treated hypertensive patients. Clin Exp Hypertens A 1984;6(6):1077–93.
31. Australian Adverse Drug Reactions Advisory Committee. Post-partum NSAIDs may cause hypertension. Aust Adv Drug React Bull 2003;22:23–4.
32. Collins R, Peto R, MacMahon S, Hebert P, Fiebach NH, Eberlein KA, Godwin J, Qizilbash N, Taylor JO, Hennekens CH. Blood pressure, stroke, and coronary heart disease. Part 2. Short-term reductions in blood pressure: overview of randomised drug trials in their epidemiological context. Lancet 1990;335(8693):827–38.
33. Heerdink ER, Leufkens HG, Herings RM, Ottervanger JP, Stricker BH, Bakker A. NSAIDs associated with increased risk of congestive heart failure in elderly patients taking diuretics. Arch Intern Med 1998;158(10):1108–12.
34. Van den Ouweland FA, Gribnau FW, Meyboom RH. Congestive heart failure due to nonsteroidal anti-inflammatory drugs in the elderly. Age Ageing 1988;17(1):8–16.
35. Page J, Henry D. Consumption of NSAIDs and the development of congestive heart failure in elderly patients: an underrecognized public health problem. Arch Intern Med 2000;160(6):777–84.

36. Chan AT, Manson JE, Albert CM, Chae CU, Rexrode KM, Curhan GC, Rimm EB, Willett WC, Fuchs CS. Nonsteroidal antiinflammatory drugs, acetaminophen, and the risk of cardiovascular events. Circulation 2006;113(12):1578–87.

37. Huang WF, Hsiao FY, Wen YW, Tsai YW. Cardiovascular events associated with the use of four nonselective NSAIDs (etodolac, nabumetone, ibuprofen, or naproxen) versus a cyclooxygenase-2 inhibitor (celecoxib): a population-based analysis in Taiwanese adults. Clin Ther 2006;28(11):1827–36.

38. Cannon CP, Curtis SP, FitzGerald GA, Krum H, Kaur A, Bolognese JA, Reicin AS, Bombardier C, Weinblatt ME, van der Heijde D, Erdmann E, Laine L; MEDAL Steering Committee. Cardiovascular outcomes with etoricoxib and diclofenac in patients with osteoarthritis and rheumatoid arthritis in the Multinational Etoricoxib and Diclofenac Arthritis Long-term (MEDAL) programme: a randomised comparison. Lancet 2006;368(9549):1771–81.

39. Solomon DH, Avorn J, Stürmer T, Glynn RJ, Mogun H, Schneeweiss S. Cardiovascular outcomes in new users of coxibs and nonsteroidal antiinflammatory drugs: high-risk subgroups and time course of risk. Arthritis Rheum 2006;54(5):1378–89.

40. White WB, West CR, Borer JS, Gorelick PB, Lavange L, Pan SX, Weiner E, Verburg KM. Risk of cardiovascular events in patients receiving celecoxib: a meta-analysis of randomized clinical trials. Am J Cardiol 2007;99(1):91–8.

41. Saloheima P, Juvela S, Hillbom M. Use of aspirin, epistaxis, and untreated hypertension as risk factors for primary intracerebral hemorrhage in middle-aged and elderly people. Stroke 2001;32:399–404.

42. Thrift AG, McNeil JJ, Forbes A, Donnan G. Risk of primary intracerebral haemorrhage associated with aspirin and non-steroidal anti-inflammatory drugs: case-control study. BMJ 1999;318:759–64.

43. Bak S, Andersen M, Tsiropoulos I, Garcia Rodriguez LA, Hallas J, Christensen K, Gaist D. Risk of stroke associated with nonsteroidal anti-inflammatory drugs. A nested case–control study. Stroke 2003;34:379–86.

44. Johnsen SP, Oedersen L, Friis S, Blot WJ, McLaughlin JK, Olsen JH, Sorensen HT. Nonaspirin nonsteroidal anti-inflammatory drugs and risk of hospitalisation for intracerebral hemorrhage: a population-based case control study. Stroke 2003;34:387–91.

45. Qureshi AI. Nonsteroidal anti-inflammatory drugs and risk of intracerebral hemorrhage. Stroke 2003;34:385–6.

46. O'Brien WM, Bagby GF. Rare adverse reactions to nonsteroidal antiinflammatory drugs. J Rheumatol 1985;12(1):13–20.

47. Simon RA. Oral challenges to detect aspirin and sulfite sensitivity in asthma. Allerg Immunol (Paris) 1994; 26(6):216–8.

48. Bernard AA, Kersley JB. Sensitivity to insect stings in patients taking anti-inflammatory drugs. BMJ (Clin Res Ed) 1986;292(6517):378–9.

49. O'Brien WM, Bagby GF. Rare adverse reactions to nonsteroidal antiinflammatory drugs. J Rheumatol 1985; 12(4):785–90.

50. Symon DN. Twelve cases of analgesic headache. Arch Dis Child 1998;78(6):555–6.

51. Vasconcellos E, Pina-Garza JE, Millan EJ, Warner JS. Analgesic rebound headache in children and adolescents. J Child Neurol 1998;13(9):443–7.

52. Anonymous. Paraesthesia with NSAIDs. Aust Adv Drug React Bull 1997;167 May.

53. Myers AH, Baker SP, Van Natta ML, Abbey H, Robinson EG. Risk factors associated with falls and injuries among elderly institutionalized persons. Am J Epidemiol 1991;133(11):1179–90.

54. Yip YB, Cumming RG. The association between medications and falls in Australian nursing-home residents. Med J Aust 1994;160(1):14–8.

55. Thrift AG, McNeil JJ, Forbes A, Donnan GA. Risk of primary intracerebral haemorrhage associated with aspirin and non-steroidal anti-inflammatory drugs: case-control study. BMJ 1999;318(7186):759–64.

56. Carney MW. Paranoid psychosis with indomethacin. BMJ 1977;2(6093):994–5.

57. Mallet L, Kuyumjian J. Indomethacin-induced behavioral changes in an elderly patient with dementia. Ann Pharmacother 1998;32(2):201–3.

58. Bruce-Jones PN, Crome P, Kalra L. Indomethacin and cognitive function in healthy elderly volunteers. Br J Clin Pharmacol 1994;38(1):45–51.

59. Stewart WF, Kawas C, Corrada M, Metter EJ. Risk of Alzheimer's disease and duration of NSAID use. Neurology 1997;48(3):626–32.

60. Murray MD, Brater DC. Renal toxicity of the nonsteroidal anti-inflammatory drugs. Annu Rev Pharmacol Toxicol 1993;33:435–65.

61. Harris K. The role of prostaglandins in the control of renal function. Br J Anaesth 1992;69(3):233–5.

62. O'Brien WM, Bagby GF. Rare adverse reactions to nonsteroidal antiinflammatory drugs. J Rheumatol 1985;12(2):347–53.

63. The International Agranulocytosis and Aplastic Anemia Study. Risks of agranulocytosis and aplastic anemia. A first report of their relation to drug use with special reference to analgesics. JAMA 1986;256(13):1749–57.

64. Strom BL, Carson JL, Schinnar R, Snyder ES, Shaw M, Lundin FE Jr. Nonsteroidal anti-inflammatory drugs and neutropenia. Arch Intern Med 1993;153(18):2119–24.

65. DeGruchy GC. Drug-Induced Blood Disorders. Melbourne: Blackwell Scientific Publications;. 1979.

66. Sanford-Driscoll M, Knodel LC. Induction of hemolytic anemia by nonsteroidal antiinflammatory drugs. Drug Intell Clin Pharm 1986;20(12):925–34.

67. Lawrence C, Sakuntabhai A, Tiling-Grosse S. Effect of aspirin and nonsteroidal antiinflammatory drug therapy on bleeding complications in dermatologic surgical patients. J Am Acad Dermatol 1994;31(6):988–92.

68. Chalmers TC, Berrier J, Hewitt P, Berli J, Reitmen D, Nagalingaun R, Sacks H. Meta-analysis of randomized controlled trials as a method of estimate rare complications of non-steroidal anti-inflammatory drug therapy. Aliment Pharmacol Ther 1988;Suppl 1:9–26.

69. Gabriel SE, Jaakkimainen L, Bombardier C. Risk for serious gastrointestinal complications related to use of nonsteroidal anti-inflammatory drugs. A meta-analysis. Ann Intern Med 1991;115:787–96.

70. Garcia RL. Nonsteroidal antiinflammatory drugs, ulcers and risk: collaborative meta-analysis. Semin Arthritis Rheum 1997;26:16–20.

71. Henry D, Lim LL, Garcia Rodriguez LA, Perez Gutthann S, Carson JL, Griffin M, Savage R, Logan R, Moride Y, Hawkey C, Hill S, Fries JT. Variability in risk of gastrointestinal complications with individual non steroidal anti-inflammatory drugs: results of a collaborative meta-analysis. BMJ 1996;312:1563–6.

72. Stalnikowicz R, Rachmilewitz D. NSAID-induced gastroduodenal damage: is prevention needed? A review and metaanalysis. J Clin Gastroenterol 1993;17:238–43.

73. Ofman JJ, Maclean CH, Straus WL, Morton SC, Berger ML, Roth EA, Shekelle P. Meta-analysis of dyspepsia and nonsteroidal anti-inflammatory drugs. Arthritis Rheum 2003;49:508–18.

74. Langman M, Kong SX, Zhang Q, Kahler KH, Finch E. Safety and patient tolerance of standard and slow-release formulation. NSAIDs. Pharmacoepidemiol Drug Saf 2003;12:61–6.

75. Schoen RT, Vender RJ. Mechanisms of nonsteroidal anti-inflammatory drug-induced gastric damage. Am J Med 1989;86(4):449–58.

76. Roth SH, Bennett RE. Nonsteroidal anti-inflammatory drug gastropathy. Recognition and response. Arch Intern Med 1987;147(12):2093–100.

77. Langman MJ. Epidemiologic evidence on the association between peptic ulceration and antiinflammatory drug use. Gastroenterology 1989;96(2 Pt 2 Suppl):640–6.

78. Fries JF, Miller SR, Spitz PW, Williams CA, Hubert HB, Bloch DA. Toward an epidemiology of gastropathy associated with nonsteroidal antiinflammatory drug use. Gastroenterology 1989;96(2 Pt 2 Suppl):647–55.

79. Henry DA, Johnston A, Dobson A, Duggan J. Fatal peptic ulcer complications and the use of non-steroidal anti-inflammatory drugs, aspirin, and corticosteroids. BMJ (Clin Res Ed) 1987;295(6608):1227–9.

80. Somerville K, Faulkner G, Langman M. Non-steroidal anti-inflammatory drugs and bleeding peptic ulcer. Lancet 1986;1(8479):462–4.

81. Pincus T, Griffin M. Gastrointestinal disease associated with nonsteroidal anti-inflammatory drugs: new insights from observational studies and functional status questionnaires. Am J Med 1991;91(3):209–12.

82. Fries JF, Williams CA, Bloch DA, Michel BA. Nonsteroidal anti-inflammatory drug-associated gastropathy: incidence and risk factor models. Am J Med 1991;91(3):213–22.

83. Gabriel SE, Jaakkimainen L, Bombardier C. Risk for serious gastrointestinal complications related to use of non-steroidal anti-inflammatory drugs. A meta-analysis. Ann Intern Med 1991;115(10):787–96.

84. Willett LR, Carson JL, Strom BL. Epidemiology of gastrointestinal damage associated with nonsteroidal anti-inflammatory drugs. Drug Saf 1994;10(2):170–81.

85. MacDonald TM, Morant SV, Robinson GC, Shield MJ, McGilchrist MM, Murray FE, McDevitt DG. Association of upper gastrointestinal toxicity of non-steroidal anti-inflammatory drugs with continued exposure: cohort study. BMJ 1997;315(7119):1333–7.

86. Agrawal NM, Roth S, Graham DY, White RH, Germain B, Brown JA, Stromatt SC. Misoprostol compared with sucralfate in the prevention of nonsteroidal anti-inflammatory drug-induced gastric ulcer. A randomized, controlled trial. Ann Intern Med 1991;115(3):195–200.

87. Taha AS, Hudson N, Hawkey CJ, Swannell AJ, Trye PN, Cottrell J, Mann SG, Simon TJ, Sturrock RD, Russell RI. Famotidine for the prevention of gastric and duodenal ulcers caused by nonsteroidal antiinflammatory drugs. N Engl J Med 1996;334(22):1435–9.

88. Taha AS, Sturrock RD, Russell RI. Mucosal erosions in longterm non-steroidal anti-inflammatory drug users: predisposition to ulceration and relation to *Helicobacter pylori*. Gut 1995;36(3):334–6.

89. Sung J, Russell RI, Nyeomans, Chan FK, Chen S, Fock K, Goh KL, Kullavanijaya P, Kimura K, Lau C, Louw J, Sollano J, Triadiafalopulos G, Xiao S, Brooks P. Non-steroidal anti-inflammatory drug toxicity in the upper gastrointestinal tract. J Gastroenterol Hepatol 2000;15(Suppl):G58–68.

90. Marshall B. NSAIDs and *Helicobacter pylori*: therapeutic options. Lancet 1998;352(9133):1001–3.

91. Pounder RE. *Helicobacter pylori* and NSAIDs—the end of the debate? Lancet 2002;359(9300):3–4.

92. Hirose H, Takeuchi K, Okabe S. Effect of indomethacin on gastric mucosal blood flow around acetic acid-induced gastric ulcers in rats. Gastroenterology 1991;100(5 Pt 1):1259–65.

93. Sarosiek J, Slomiany A, Slomiany BL. Evidence for weakening of gastric mucus integrity by *Campylobacter pylori*. Scand J Gastroenterol 1988;23(5):585–90.

94. Taha AS, Angerson W, Nakshabendi I, Beekman H, Morran C, Sturrock RD, Russell RI. Gastric and duodenal mucosal blood flow in patients receiving non-steroidal anti-inflammatory drugs—influence of age, smoking, ulceration and *Helicobacter pylori*. Aliment Pharmacol Ther 1993;7(1):41–5.

95. Konturek JW, Dembinski A, Stoll R, Domschke W, Konturek SJ. Mucosal adaptation to aspirin induced gastric damage in humans. Studies on blood flow, gastric mucosal growth, and neutrophil activation. Gut 1994;35(9):1197–204.

96. Laine L, Cominelli F, Sloane R, Casini-Raggi V, Marin-Sorensen M, Weinstein WM. Interaction of NSAIDs and *Helicobacter pylori* on gastrointestinal injury and prostaglandin production: a controlled double-blind trial. Aliment Pharmacol Ther 1995;9(2):127–35.

97. Wallace JL, Keenan CM, Granger DN. Gastric ulceration induced by nonsteroidal anti-inflammatory drugs is a neutrophil-dependent process. Am J Physiol 1990;259(3 Pt 1):G462–7.

98. Taha AS, Nakshabendi I, Lee FD, Sturrock RD, Russell RI. Chemical gastritis and *Helicobacter pylori* related gastritis in patients receiving non-steroidal anti-inflammatory drugs: comparison and correlation with peptic ulceration. J Clin Pathol 1992;45(2):135–9.

99. Taha AS, Dahill S, Morran C, Hudson N, Hawkey CJ, Lee FD, Sturrock RD, Russell RI. Neutrophils, *Helicobacter pylori*, and nonsteroidal anti-inflammatory drug ulcers. Gastroenterology 1999;116(2):254–8.

100. Konturek JW, Konturek SJ, Stachura J, Domschke W. *Helicobacter pylori*-positive peptic ulcer patients do not adapt to aspirin. Aliment Pharmacol Ther 1998;12(9):857–64.

101. Lipscomb GR, Campbell F, Rees WD. The influence of age, gender, *Helicobacter pylori* and smoking on gastric mucosal adaptation to non-steroidal anti-inflammatory drugs. Aliment Pharmacol Ther 1997;11(5):907–12.

102. Konturek JW, Dembinski A, Konturek SJ, Stachura J, Domschke W. Infection of *Helicobacter pylori* in gastric adaptation to continued administration of aspirin in humans. Gastroenterology 1998;114(2):245–55.

103. Martin DF, Montgomery E, Dobek AS, Patrissi GA, Peura DA. *Campylobacter pylori*, NSAIDS, and smoking: risk factors for peptic ulcer disease. Am J Gastroenterol 1989;84(10):1268–72.

104. Li EK, Sung JJ, Suen R, Ling TK, Leung VK, Hui E, Cheng AF, Chung S, Woo J. *Helicobacter pylori* infection increases the risk of peptic ulcers in chronic users of non-steroidal anti-inflammatory drugs. Scand J Rheumatol 1996;25(1):42–6.

105. Heresbach D, Raoul JL, Bretagne JF, Minet J, Donnio PY, Ramee MP, Siproudhis L, Gosselin M. *Helicobacter pylori*: a risk and severity factor of non-steroidal anti-inflammatory drug induced gastropathy. Gut 1992;33(12):1608–11.

106. Loeb DS, Talley NJ, Ahlquist DA, Carpenter HA, Zinsmeister AR. Long-term nonsteroidal anti-inflammatory drug use and gastroduodenal injury: the role of *Helicobacter pylori*. Gastroenterology 1992;102(6):1899–905.

107. Graham DY, Lidsky MD, Cox AM, Evans DJ Jr, Evans DG, Alpert L, Klein PD, Sessoms SL, Michaletz PA, Saeed ZA. Long-term nonsteroidal

antiinflammatory drug use and *Helicobacter pylori* infection. Gastroenterology 1991;100(6):1653–7.

108. Shallcross TM, Rathbone BJ, Wyatt JI, Heatley RV. *Helicobacter pylori* associated chronic gastritis and peptic ulceration in patients taking non-steroidal anti-inflammatory drugs. Aliment Pharmacol Ther 1990;4(5):515–22.

109. Upadhyay R, Howatson A, McKinlay A, Danesh BJ, Sturrock RD, Russell RI. *Campylobacter pylori* associated gastritis in patients with rheumatoid arthritis taking non-steroidal anti-inflammatory drugs. Br J Rheumatol 1988;27(2):113–6.

110. Publig W, Wustinger C, Zandl C. Non-steroidal anti-inflammatory drugs (NSAID) cause gastrointestinal ulcers mainly in *Helicobacter pylori* carriers. Wien Klin Wochenschr 1994;106(9):276–9.

111. Lanza FL, Evans DG, Graham DY. Effect of *Helicobacter pylori* infection on the severity of gastroduodenal mucosal injury after the acute administration of naproxen or aspirin to normal volunteers. Am J Gastroenterol 1991;86(6):735–7.

112. Thillainayagam AV, Tabaqchali S, Warrington SJ, Farthing MJ. Interrelationships between *Helicobacter pylori* infection, nonsteroidal antiinflammatory drugs and gastroduodenal disease. A prospective study in healthy volunteers. Dig Dis Sci 1994;39(5):1085–9.

113. Goggin PM, Collins DA, Jazrawi RP, Jackson PA, Corbishley CM, Bourke BE, Northfield TC. Prevalence of *Helicobacter pylori* infection and its effect on symptoms and non-steroidal anti-inflammatory drug induced gastrointestinal damage in patients with rheumatoid arthritis. Gut 1993;34(12):1677–80.

114. Kim JG, Graham DYThe Misoprostol Study Group. *Helicobacter pylori* infection and development of gastric or duodenal ulcer in arthritic patients receiving chronic NSAID therapy. Am J Gastroenterol 1994;89(2): 203–7.

115. Huang JQ, Sridhar S, Hunt RH. Role of *Helicobacter pylori* infection and non-steroidal anti-inflammatory drugs in peptic-ulcer disease: a meta-analysis. Lancet 2002;359(9300):14–22.

116. Voutilainen M, Sokka T, Juhola M, Farkkila M, Hannonen P. Nonsteroidal anti-inflammatory drug-associated upper gastrointestinal lesions in rheumatoid arthritis patients. Relationships to gastric histology, *Helicobacter pylori* infection, and other risk factors for peptic ulcer. Scand J Gastroenterol 1998;33(8):811–6.

117. Santucci L, Fiorucci S, Patoia L, Di Matteo FM, Brunori PM, Morelli A. Severe gastric mucosal damage induced by NSAIDs in healthy subjects is associated with *Helicobacter pylori* infection and high levels of serum pepsinogens. Dig Dis Sci 1995;40(9):2074–80.

118. Caselli M, Pazzi P, LaCorte R, Aleotti A, Trevisani L, Stabellini G. *Campylobacter*-like organisms, nonsteroidal anti-inflammatory drugs and gastric lesions in patients with rheumatoid arthritis. Digestion 1989;44(2):101–4.

119. Chan FK, Sung JJ, Chung SC, To KF, Yung MY, Leung VK, Lee YT, Chan CS, Li EK, Woo J. Randomised trial of eradication of *Helicobacter pylori* before non-steroidal anti-inflammatory drug therapy to prevent peptic ulcers. Lancet 1997;350(9083):975–9.

120. Hawkey CJ, Tulassay Z, Szczepanski L, van Rensburg CJ, Filipowicz-Sosnowska A, Lanas A, Wason CM, Peacock RA, Gillon KR. Randomised controlled trial of *Helicobacter pylori* eradication in patients on non-steroidal anti-inflammatory drugs: HELP NSAIDs study. Helicobacter Eradication for Lesion Prevention. Lancet 1998;352(9133):1016–21.

121. Chan FK, To KF, Wu JC, Yung MY, Leung WK, Kwok T, Hui Y, Chan HL, Chan CS, Hui E, Woo J, Sung JJ. Eradication of *Helicobacter pylori* and risk of peptic ulcers in patients starting long-term treatment with non-steroidal anti-inflammatory drugs: a randomised trial. Lancet 2002;359(9300):9–13.

122. Aalykke C, Lauritsen JM, Hallas J, Reinholdt S, Krogfelt K, Lauritsen K. *Helicobacter pylori* and risk of ulcer bleeding among users of nonsteroidal anti-inflammatory drugs: a case-control study. Gastroenterology 1999;116(6):1305–9.

123. Labenz J, Peitz U, Kohl H, Kaiser J, Malfertheiner P, Hackelsberger A, Borsch G. *Helicobacter pylori* increases the risk of peptic ulcer bleeding: a case-control study. Ital J Gastroenterol Hepatol 1999;31(2):110–5.

124. Cullen DJ, Hawkey GM, Greenwood DC, Humphreys H, Shepherd V, Logan RF, Hawkey CJ. Peptic ulcer bleeding in the elderly: relative roles of *Helicobacter pylori* and non-steroidal anti-inflammatory drugs. Gut 1997; 41(4):459–62.

125. Santolaria S, Lanas A, Benito R, Perez-Aisa M, Montoro M, Sainz R. *Helicobacter pylori* infection is a protective factor for bleeding gastric ulcers but not for bleeding duodenal ulcers in NSAID users. Aliment Pharmacol Ther 1999;13(11):1511–8.

126. Chan FK, Chung SC, Suen BY, Lee YT, Leung WK, Leung VK, Wu JC, Lau JY, Hui Y, Lai MS, Chan HL, Sung JJ. Preventing recurrent upper gastrointestinal bleeding in patients with *Helicobacter pylori* infection who are taking low-dose aspirin or naproxen. N Engl J Med 2001;344(13):967–73.

127. Chan FK, Chung SC, Suen BY, Lee YT, Leung WK, Leung VK, Wu JC, Lau JY, Hui Y, Lai MS, Chan HL, Sung JJ. Preventing recurrent upper gastrointestinal bleeding in patients with *Helicobacter pylori* infection who are taking low-dose aspirin or naproxen. N Engl J Med 2001;344:967–73.

128. Lai KC, Lam SK, Chu KM, Wong BC, Hui WM, HUWH, Lau GK, Wong WM, Yuen MF, Chan AO, Lai CL, Wong J. Lansoprazole for the prevention of recurrences of ulcer complications from long-term low-dose aspirin use. N Engl J Med 2002;346:2033–8.

129. Hawkey CJ, Karrasch JA, Szczepanski L, Walker DG, Barkun A, Swannell AJ, Yeomans ND. Omeprazole compared with misoprostol for ulcers associated with nonsteroidal antiinflammatory drugs. Omeprazole versus Misoprostol for NSAID-induced Ulcer Management (OMNIUM) Study Group. N Engl J Med 1998;338(11):727–34.

130. Yeomans ND, Tulassay Z, Juhasz L, Racz I, Howard JM, van Rensburg CJ, Swannell AJ, Hawkey CJ. A comparison of omeprazole with ranitidine for ulcers associated with nonsteroidal antiinflammatory drugs. Acid Suppression Trial: Ranitidine versus Omeprazole for NSAID-associated Ulcer Treatment (ASTRONAUT) Study Group. N Engl J Med 1998;338(11):719–26.

131. Silverstein FE, Graham DY, Senior JR, Davies HW, Struthers BJ, Bittman RM, Geis GS. Misoprostol reduces serious gastrointestinal complications in patients with rheumatoid arthritis receiving nonsteroidal anti-inflammatory drugs. A randomized, double-blind, placebo-controlled trial. Ann Intern Med 1995;123(4):241–9.

132. Graham DY. Critical effect of *Helicobacter pylori* infection on the effectiveness of omeprazole for prevention of gastric or duodenal ulcers among chronic NSAID users. Helicobacter 2002;7(1):1–8.

133. Hawkey CJ, Langman MJ. Non-steroidal anti-inflammatory drugs: overall risks and management. Complementary roles for COX-2 inhibitors and proton pump inhibitors. Gut 2003;52(4):600–8.

134. Garcia Rodriguez LA, Jick H. Risk of upper gastrointestinal bleeding and perforation associated with individual non-steroidal anti-inflammatory drugs. Lancet 1994;343(8900):769–72.

135. Langman MJ, Weil J, Wainwright P, Lawson DH, Rawlins MD, Logan RF, Murphy M, Vessey MP, Colin-Jones DG. Risks of bleeding peptic ulcer associated with individual non-steroidal anti-inflammatory drugs. Lancet 1994;343(8905):1075–8.

136. Roth SH, Fries JF, Abadi IA, Hubscer O, Mintz G, Samara AM. Prophylaxis of nonsteroidal anti-inflammatory drug gastropathy: a clinical opinion. J Rheumatol 1991;18:956–8.

137. Langman MJ. Ulcer complications associated with anti-inflammatory drug use. What is the extent of the disease burden? Pharmacoepidemiol Drug Saf 2001;10:13–19.

138. Dubois RW, Melmed GY, Henning JM, Bernal M. Risk of upper gastrointestinal injury and events in patients treated with cyclooxygenase (COX)-1/COX-2 nonsteroidal anti-inflammatory drugs (NSAIDs), COX-2 selective NSAIDs, and gastroprotective co-therapy: an appraisal of the literature 2004;10:178–89.

139. Schnitzer TJ. Update on guidelines for the treatment of chronic musculoskeletal pain. Clin Rheumatol 2006;25:S22–9.

140. Langman MJ, Weil J, Wainwright P, Lawson DH, Rawlins MD, Logan RF, Murphy M, Vessey MP, Colin-Jones DG. Risks of bleeding peptic ulcer associated with individual non-steroidal anti-inflammatory drugs. Lancet 1994;343:1075–8.

141. Garcia Rodriguez LA, Ruigòmez A. Secondary prevention of upper gastrointestinal bleeding associated with maintenance acid-suppressing treatment in patients with peptic ulcer bleed. Epidemiology 1999;10:228–32.

142. Laine L. Approaches to nonsteroidal anti-inflammatory drug use in the high-risk patient. Gastroenterology 2001;120:594–606.

143. Langman M. Population impact of strategies designed to reduce peptic ulcer risks associated with NSAID use. Int J Clin Pract Suppl 2003;135:38–42.

144. Wolfe MM, Lichtenstein DR, Singh G. Gastrointestinal toxicity of nonsteroidal anti-inflammatory drugs. N Engl J Med 1999;340:1888–99.

145. Graham DY, Agrawal NM, Campbell DR, Haber MM, Collis C, Lukasik NL, Huang B, NSAID-Associated Gastric Ulcer Prevention Study Group. Ulcer prevention in long-term users of nonsteroidal anti-inflammatory drugs: results of a double-blind, randomized, multicenter, active-and placebo-controlled study of misoprostol vs lansoprazole. Arch Intern Med 2002;162:169–75.

146. Silverstein FE, Graham Dy, Senior JR, Davies HW, Struthers BJ, Bittman RM, Geis GS. Misoprostol reduces serious gastrointestinal complications in patients with rheumatoid arthritis receiving nonsteroidal anti-inflammatory drugs. A randomized, double-blind, placebo-controlled trial. Ann Intern Med 1995;123:241–9.

147. Garcia Rodriguez LA, Ruigomez A. Secondary prevention of upper gastrointestinal bleeding associated with maintenance acid-suppressing treatment in patients with peptic ulcer bleed. Epidemiology 1999;10:*228–32*.

148. Chan FK, Hung LC, Suen BY, Wu JC, Lee KC, Leung VK, Hui AJ, To KF, Leung WK, Wong VW, Chung SC, Sung JJ. Celecoxib versus diclofenac and omeprazole in reducing the risk of recurrent ulcer bleeding in patients with arthritis. N Engl J Med 2002;347:2104–10.

149. Lai KC, Chu KM, Hui WM, Wong BC, Hu WH, Wong WM, Chan AO, Wong J, Lam SK. Celecoxib compared with lansoprazole and naproxen to prevent gastrointestinal ulcer complications. Am J Med 2005;118:1271–8.

150. Koch M, Capurso L, Dezi A, Ferrario F, Scarpignato C. Prevention of NSAID-induced gastroduodenal mucosal injury: meta-analysis of clinical trials with misoprostol and H2-receptor antagonists. Dig Dis 1995;13(Suppl 1):62–74.

151. Simon TJ, Berger ML, Hoover ME, Stauffer LA, Berline RG. A dose ranging study of famotidine in prevention of gastroduodenal lesions associated with non-steroidal anti-inflammatory drugs (NSAIDs): results of a US multicenter trial. Am J Gastroenterol 1994;89:1644.

152. Singh G, Ramey DR, Morfeld D, Shi H, Hatoum HT, Fries JF. Gastrointestinal tract complications of nonsteroidal anti-inflammatory drug treatment in rheumatoid arthritis. A prospective observational cohort study. Arch Intern Med 1996;156(14):1530–6.

153. Graham DY, Agrawal NM, Roth SH. Prevention of NSAID-induced gastric ulcer with misoprostol: multicentre, double-blind, placebo-controlled trial. Lancet 1988;2(8623):1277–80.

154. Levine JS. Misoprostol and nonsteroidal anti-inflammatory drugs: a tale of effects, outcomes, and costs. Ann Intern Med 1995;123(4):309–10.

155. Ekstrom P, Carling L, Wetterhus S, Wingren PE, Anker-Hansen O, Lundegardh G, Thorhallsson E, Unge P. Prevention of peptic ulcer and dyspeptic symptoms with omeprazole in patients receiving continuous non-steroidal anti-inflammatory drug therapy. A Nordic multicentre study. Scand J Gastroenterol 1996;31(8):753–8.

156. Cullen D, Bardhan KD, Eisner M, Kogut DG, Peacock RA, Thomson JM, Hawkey CJ. Primary gastroduodenal prophylaxis with omeprazole for non-steroidal anti-inflammatory drug users. Aliment Pharmacol Ther 1998;12(2):135–40.

157. Wynne HA, Long A. Patient awareness of the adverse effects of non-steroidal anti-inflammatory drugs (NSAIDs). Br J Clin Pharmacol 1996;42(2):253–6.

158. Herxheimer A. Many NSAID users who bleed don't know when to stop. BMJ 1998;316(7130):492.

159. Semble EL, Wu WC, Castell DO. Nonsteroidal antiinflammatory drugs and esophageal injury. Semin Arthritis Rheum 1989;19(2):99–109.

160. Taha AS, Dahill S, Nakshabendi I, Lee FD, Sturrock RD, Russell RI. Oesophageal histology in long term users of non-steroidal anti-inflammatory drugs. J Clin Pathol 1994;47(8):705–8.

161. Scheiman JM, Patel PM, Henson EK, Nostrant TT. Effect of naproxen on gastroesophageal reflux and esophageal function: a randomized, double-blind, placebo-controlled study. Am J Gastroenterol 1995;90(5):754–7.

162. Langman MJ, Morgan L, Worrall A. Use of anti-inflammatory drugs by patients admitted with small or large bowel perforations and haemorrhage. BMJ (Clin Res Ed) 1985;290(6465):347–9.

163. Bjarnason I, Macpherson A. The changing gastrointestinal side effect profile of non-steroidal anti-inflammatory drugs. A new approach for the prevention of a new problem. Scand J Gastroenterol Suppl 1989;163:56–64.

164. Bjarnason I, Hayllar J, MacPherson AJ, Russell AS. Side effects of nonsteroidal anti-inflammatory drugs on the small and large intestine in humans. Gastroenterology 1993;104(6):1832–47.

165. Allison MC, Howatson AG, Torrance CJ, Lee FD, Russell RI. Gastrointestinal damage associated with the use of nonsteroidal antiinflammatory drugs. N Engl J Med 1992;327(11):749–54.

166. Lang J, Price AB, Levi AJ, Burke M, Gumpel JM, Bjarnason I. Diaphragm disease: pathology of disease of the small intestine induced by non-steroidal anti-inflammatory drugs. J Clin Pathol 1988;41(5):516–26.

167. Kwo PY, Tremaine WJ. Nonsteroidal anti-inflammatory drug-induced enteropathy: case discussion and review of the literature. Mayo Clin Proc 1995;70(1):55–61.

168. Speed CA, Bramble MG, Corbett WA, Haslock I. Nonsteroidal anti-inflammatory induced diaphragm disease of the small intestine: complexities of diagnosis and management. Br J Rheumatol 1994;33(8):778–80.

169. Gargot D, Chaussade S, d'Alteroche L, Desbazeille F, Grandjouan S, Louvel A, Douvin J, Causse X, Festin D, Chapuis Y, et al. Nonsteroidal anti-inflammatory drug-induced colonic strictures: two cases and literature review. Am J Gastroenterol 1995;90(11):2035–8.

170. Giardiello FM, Hansen FC 3rd, Lazenby AJ, Hellman DB, Milligan FD, Bayless TM, Yardley JH. Collagenous colitis in setting of nonsteroidal antiinflammatory drugs and antibiotics. Dig Dis Sci 1990;35(2):257–60.

171. Rampton DS, McNeil NI, Sarner M. Analgesic ingestion and other factors preceding relapse in ulcerative colitis. Gut 1983;24(3):187–9.

172. Rampton DS, Sladen GE. Relapse of ulcerative proctocolitis during treatment with non-steroidal anti-inflammatory drugs. Postgrad Med J 1981;57(667):297–9.

173. Kaufmann HJ, Taubin HL. Nonsteroidal anti-inflammatory drugs activate quiescent inflammatory bowel disease. Ann Intern Med 1987;107(4):513–6.

174. Gleeson MH, Davis AJ. Non-steroidal anti-inflammatory drugs, aspirin and newly diagnosed colitis: a case-control study. Aliment Pharmacol Ther 2003;17:817–25.

175. Felder JB, Korelitz BI, Rajapakse R, Schwarz S, Horatagis AP, Gleim G. Effects of nonsteroidal antiinflammatory drugs on inflammatory bowel disease: a case-control study. Am J Gastroenterol 2000;95(8):1949–54.

176. Bonner GF, Walczak M, Kitchen L, Bayona M. Tolerance of nonsteroidal antiinflammatory drugs in patients with inflammatory bowel disease. Am J Gastroenterol 2000;95(8):1946–8.

177. Laine L, Smith R, Min K, Chen C, Dubois RW. Systematic review: the lower gastrointestinal adverse effects of non-steroidal anti-inflammatory drugs. Aliment Pharmacol Ther 2006;24(5):751–67.

178. Garcia Rodriguez LA, Williams R, Derby LE, Dean AD, Jick H. Acute liver injury associated with nonsteroidal anti-inflammatory drugs and the role of risk factors. Arch Intern Med 1994;154(3):311–6.

179. Fry SW, Seeff LB. Hepatotoxicity of analgesics and anti-inflammatory agents. Gastroenterol Clin North Am 1995;24(4):875–905.

180. Benjamin SB, Ishak KG, Zimmerman HJ, Grushka A. Phenylbutazone liver injury: a clinical-pathologic survey of 23 cases and review of the literature. Hepatology 1981;1(3):255–63.

181. ADRAC. Diclofenac sodium and hepatic injury. Aust Adv Drug React Bull 1986;June.

182. Wilholm BE, Myrhed M, Ekman E. Trends and patterns in adverse drug reactions to non-steroidal anti-inflammatory drugs reported in Sweden. In: Rainsford KD, Velo GP, editors. Side-effects of Anti-inflammatory Drugs, Part I. Clinical and Epidemiological Aspects. Lancaster: MTP Press, 1987:55.

183. Brooks PM. Side-effects of non-steroidal anti-inflammatory drugs. Med J Aust 1988;148(5):248–51.

184. De Ledinghen V, Heresbach D, Fourdan O, Bernard P, Liebaert-Bories MP, Nousbaum JB, Gourlaouen A, Becker MC, Ribard D, Ingrand P, Silvain C, Beauchant M. Anti-inflammatory drugs and variceal bleeding: a case-control study. Gut 1999;44(2):270–3.

185. Sørensen HT, Jacobsen J, Nørgaard M, Pedersen L, Johnsen SP, Baron JA. Newer cyclo-oxygenase-2 selective inhibitors, other non-steroidal anti-inflammatory drugs and the risk of acute pancreatitis. Aliment Pharmacol Ther 2006;24(1):111–6.

186. Richards IM, Fraser SM, Capell HA, Fox JG, Boulton-Jones JM. A survey of renal function in outpatients with rheumatoid arthritis. Clin Rheumatol 1988;7(2):267–71.

187. Allred J, Wong W, Kafetz K. Elderly people taking nonsteroidal anti-inflammatory drugs are unlikely to have excess renal impairment. Postgrad Med J 1989;65(768):735–7.

188. Dunn MJ, Simonson M, Davidson EW, Scharschmidt LA, Sedor JR. Nonsteroidal anti-inflammatory drugs and renal function. J Clin Pharmacol 1988;28(6):524–9.

189. Stillman MT, Schlesinger PA. Nonsteroidal anti-inflammatory drug nephrotoxicity. Should we be concerned? Arch Intern Med 1990;150(2):268–70.

190. Whelton A, Stout RL, Spilman PS, Klassen DK. Renal effects of ibuprofen, piroxicam, and sulindac in patients with asymptomatic renal failure. A prospective, randomized, crossover comparison. Ann Intern Med 1990;112(8):568–76.

191. Murray MD, Brater DC. Adverse effects of nonsteroidal anti-inflammatory drugs on renal function. Ann Intern Med 1990;112(8):559–60.

192. Eriksson LO, Sturfelt G, Thysell H, Wollheim FA. Effects of sulindac and naproxen on prostaglandin excretion in patients with impaired renal function and rheumatoid arthritis. Am J Med 1990;89(3):313–21.

193. Sandler DP, Burr FR, Weinberg CR. Nonsteroidal anti-inflammatory drugs and the risk for chronic renal disease. Ann Intern Med 1991;115(3):165–72.

194. Henry D, Page J, Whyte I, Nanra R, Hall C. Consumption of non-steroidal anti-inflammatory drugs and the development of functional renal impairment in elderly subjects. Results of a case-control study. Br J Clin Pharmacol 1997;44(1):85–90.

195. Evans JM, McGregor E, McMahon AD, McGilchrist MM, Jones MC, White G, McDevitt DG, MacDonald TM. Non-steroidal anti-inflammatory drugs and hospitalization for acute renal failure. QJM 1995;88(8):551–7.

196. Radford MG Jr, Holley KE, Grande JP, Larson TS, Wagoner RD, Donadio JV, McCarthy JT. Reversible membranous nephropathy associated with the use of nonsteroidal anti-inflammatory drugs. JAMA 1996;276(6):466–9.

197. Verhamme KM, Dieleman JP, Van Wijk MA, van der Lei J, Bosch JL, Stricker BH, Sturkenboom MC. Nonsteroidal anti-inflammatory drugs and increased risk of acute urinary retention. Arch Intern Med 2005;165:1547–51.

198. Delzell E, Shapiro S. A review of epidemiologic studies of nonnarcotic analgesics and chronic renal disease. Medicine (Baltimore) 1998;77(2):102–21.

199. McLaughlin JK, Lipworth L, Chow WH, Blot WJ. Analgesic use and chronic renal failure: a critical review of the epidemiologic literature. Kidney Int 1998;54(3):679–86.

200. Rexrode KM, Buring JE, Glynn RJ, Stampfer MJ, Youngman LD, Gaziano JM. Analgesic use and renal function in men. JAMA 2001;286(3):315–21.

201. Fored CM, Ejerblad E, Lindblad P, Fryzek JP, Dickman PW, Signorello LB, Lipworth L, Elinder CG, Blot WJ, McLaughlin JK, Zack MM, Nyren O. Acetaminophen, aspirin, and chronic renal failure. N Engl J Med 2001;345(25):1801–8.

202. Moran M, Mozes MF, Maddux MS, Veremis S, Bartkus C, Ketel B, Pollak R, Wallemark C, Jonasson O. Prevention of acute graft rejection by the prostaglandin E1 analogue misoprostol in renal-transplant recipients treated with cyclosporine and prednisone. N Engl J Med 1990;322(17):1183–8.

203. Kaiser U, Sollberger J, Hoigné R, Wymann R, Fritschy D, Maibach R. Haut-Nebenwirkungen unter richt-Steroidalen Analgetika-Entzundungshemmexn und sogenannten leichten Analgetika. Mitteilung aus dem komprehensiven Spital Drug Monitorin Bern (CHDMB). [Skin side effects of non-steroidal anti-inflammatory analgesics and so-called minor analgesics. Report from the Berne Comprehensive Hospital Monitor.] Schweiz Med Wochenschr 1987;117(49):1966–70.

204. Fowler PD. Aspirin, paracetamol and non-steroidal anti-inflammatory drugs. A comparative review of side effects. Med Toxicol Adverse Drug Exp 1987;2(5):338–66.

205. ADRAC. Photosensitivity reactions: a sunburnt country. Aust Adv Drug React Bull 1983;March.

206. ADRAC. A sunburnt country revisited. Aust Adv Drug React Bull 1987;February.

207. Roujeau JC, Stern RS. Severe adverse cutaneous reactions to drugs. N Engl J Med 1994;331(19):1272–85.

208. Paul E, Hellwich M. Die Wertigkeit des intracutanen Hauttestes bei Analgetika-Unverträglichkeit im Vergleich zur oralen Provokation. [Value of the intracutaneous skin test in analgesic intolerance in comparison with oral provocation.] Z Hautkr 1987;62(9):705–14.

209. Maucher OM, Fuchs A. Kontakturtikaria im Epikutantest bei Pyrazolonallergie. [Contact urticaria caused by skin test in pyrazolone allergy.] Hautarzt 1983;34(8):383–6.

210. Roujeau JC, Bracq C, Huyn NT, Chaussalet E, Raffin C, Duedari N. HLA phenotypes and bullous cutaneous reactions to drugs. Tissue Antigens 1986;28(4):251–4.

211. Powles AV, Griffiths CE, Seifert MH, Fry L. Exacerbation of psoriasis by indomethacin. Br J Dermatol 1987;117(6):799–800.

212. Sendagorta E, Allegue F, Rocamora A, Ledo A. Generalized pustular psoriasis precipitated by diclofenac and indomethacin. Dermatologica 1987;175(6):300–1.

213. Berger TG, Dhar A. Lichenoid photoeruptions in human immunodeficiency virus infection. Arch Dermatol 1994;130(5):609–13.

214. Wallace CA, Farrow D, Sherry DD. Increased risk of facial scars in children taking nonsteroidal antiinflammatory drugs. J Pediatr 1994;125(5 Pt 1):819–22.

215. Adamski H, Benkalfate L, Delaval Y, Ollivier I, le Jean S, Toubel G, le Hir-Garreau I, Chevrant-Breton J. Photodermatitis from non-steroidal anti-inflammatory drugs. Contact Dermatitis 1998;38(3):171–4.

216. Le Coz CJ, Bottlaender A, Scrivener JN, Santinelli F, Cribier BJ, Heid E, Grosshans EM. Photocontact dermatitis from ketoprofen and tiaprofenic acid: cross-reactivity study in 12 consecutive patients. Contact Dermatitis 1998;38(5):245–52.

217. Kranke B, Szolar-Platzer C, Komericki P, Derhaschnig J, Aberer W. Epidemiological significance of bufexamac as a frequent and relevant contact sensitizer. Contact Dermatitis 1997;36(4):212–5.

218. Ophaswongse S, Maibach H. Topical nonsteroidal antiinflammatory drugs: allergic and photoallergic contact dermatitis and phototoxicity. Contact Dermatitis 1993;29(2):57–64.

219. Gniazdowska B, Rueff F, Przybilla B. Delayed contact hypersensitivity to non-steroidal anti-inflammatory drugs. Contact Dermatitis 1999;40(2):63–5.

220. Iwakiri K, Hata M, Miura Y, Numano K, Yuge M, Sasaki E. Allergic contact dermatitis due to bendazac and alclometasone dipropionate. Contact Dermatitis 1999;41(4):218–39.

221. Beller U, Kaufmann R. Contact dermatitis to indomethacin. Contact Dermatitis 1987;17(2):121.

222. Pulido Z, Gonzalez E, Alfaya T, Alvarez JA, Cena M, de la Hoz B. Allergic contact dermatitis from indomethacin. Contact Dermatitis 1999;41(2):112.

223. Bujan JJ, Morante JM, Guemes MG, Del Pozo Losada J, Capdevila EF. Photoallergic contact dermatitis from piketoprofen. Contact Dermatitis 2000;43(5):315.

224. Albes B, Marguery MC, Schwarze HP, Journe F, Loche F, Bazex J. Prolonged photosensitivity following contact photoallergy to ketoprofen. Dermatology 2000;201(2):171–4.

225. Offidani A, Cellini A, Amerio P, Simonetti O, Bossi G. A case of persistent light reaction phenomenon to ketoprofen? Eur J Dermatol 2000;10(2):153–4.

226. Kanitakis J, Souillet AL, Faure M, Claudy A. Ketoprofen-induced pemphigus-like dermatosis: localized contact pemphigus? Acta Derm Venereol 2001;81(4):304–5.

227. Kawada A, Aragane Y, Asai M, Tezuka T. Simultaneous photocontact sensitivity to ketoprofen and oxybenzone. Contact Dermatitis 2001;44(6):370.

228. Goday Bujan JJ, Garcia Alvarez-Eire GM, Martinez W, del Pozo J, Fonseca E. Photoallergic contact dermatitis from aceclofenac. Contact Dermatitis 2001;45(3):170.

229. Valenzuela N, Puig L, Barnadas MA, Alomar A. Photocontact dermatitis due to dexketoprofen. Contact Dermatitis 2002;47(4):237.

230. Henschel R, Agathos M, Breit R. Photocontact dermatitis after gargling with a solution containing benzydamine. Contact Dermatitis 2002;47(1):53.

231. Sugiura M, Hayakawa R, Xie Z, Sugiura K, Hiramoto K, Shamoto M. Experimental study on phototoxicity and the photosensitization potential of ketoprofen, suprofen, tiaprofenic acid and benzophenone and the photocross-reactivity in guinea pigs. Photodermatol Photoimmunol Photomed 2002;18(2):82–9.

232. Green JJ, Manders SM. Pseudoporphyria. J Am Acad Dermatol 2001;44(1):100–8.

233. Maerker JM, Harm A, Foeldvari I, Hoger PH. Naproxeninduzierte pseudoporphyrie. [Naproxen-induced pseudoporphyria.] Hautarzt 2001;52(11):1026–9.

234. Rashad S, Revell P, Hemingway A, Low F, Rainsford K, Walker F. Effect of non-steroidal anti-inflammatory drugs on the course of osteoarthritis. Lancet 1989;2(8662):519–22.

235. Huskisson EC, Berry H, Gishen P, Jubb RW, Whitehead J. Effects of antiinflammatory drugs on the progression of osteoarthritis of the knee. LINK Study Group. Longitudinal Investigation of Nonsteroidal Antiinflammatory Drugs in Knee Osteoarthritis. J Rheumatol 1995;22(10):1941–6.

236. al Arfag A, Davis P. Osteoarthritis 1991. Current drug treatment regimens. Drugs 1991;41(2):193–201.

237. Schnitzer TJ, Popovich JM, Andersson GB, Andriacchi TP. Effect of piroxicam on gait in patients with osteoarthritis of the knee. Arthritis Rheum 1993;36(9):1207–13.

238. Varghese D, Kodakat S, Patel H. Non-steroidal anti-inflammatories should not be used after orthopaedic surgery. BMJ 1998;316(7141):1390–1.

239. Stone PG, Richards E. NSAIDs need not usually be withheld after orthopaedic surgery. BMJ 1998;317(7165):1079.

240. Godden D. Effects of NSAIDs on bone healing have been widely reported in maxillofacial journals. BMJ 1999;318(7191):1141.

241. Dimar JR 2nd, Ante WA, Zhang YP, Glassman SD. The effects of nonsteroidal anti-inflammatory drugs on posterior spinal fusions in the rat. Spine 1996;21(16):1870–6.

242. Altman RD, Latta LL, Keer R, Renfree K, Hornicek FJ, Banovac K. Effect of nonsteroidal antiinflammatory drugs on fracture healing: a laboratory study in rats. J Orthop Trauma 1995;9(5):392–400.

243. Smith G, Roberts R, Hall C, Nuki G. Reversible ovulatory failure associated with the development of luteinized unruptured follicles in women with inflammatory arthritis taking non-steroidal anti-inflammatory drugs. Br J Rheumatol 1996;35(5):458–62.

244. Akil M, Amos RS, Stewart P. Infertility may sometimes be associated with NSAID consumption. Br J Rheumatol 1996;35(1):76–8.

245. Mendonca LL, Khamashta MA, Nelson-Piercy C, Hunt BJ, Hughes GR. Non-steroidal anti-inflammatory drugs as a possible cause for reversible infertility. Rheumatology (Oxford) 2000;39(8):880–2.

246. Stevenson DD, Sanchez-Borges M, Szczeklik A. Classification of allergic and pseudoallergic reactions to drugs that inhibit cyclooxygenase enzymes. Ann Allergy Asthma Immunol 2001;87(3):177–80.

247. Eaton RA. A comparison of anaphylactoid reactions associated with non-steroidal anti-inflammatory drugs. ADR Highlights 1981;8116:.

248. Strom BL, Carson JL, Schinnar R, Sim E, Morse ML. The effect of indication on the risk of hypersensitivity reactions associated with tolmetin sodium vs other nonsteroidal anti-inflammatory drugs. J Rheumatol 1988;15(4):695–9.

249. Czerniawska-Mysik G, Szczeklik A. Idiosyncrasy to pyrazolone drugs. Allergy 1981;36(6):381–4.

250. Anonymous. Sensitisation to bee and wasp stings with NSAIDs/ACE inhibition. Reactions 1999;3:747.

251. Downing A, Jacobsen J, Sorensen HT, McLaughlin JK, Johnsen SP. Risk of hospitalization for angio-oedema among users of newer COX-2 selective inhibitors and other nonsteroidal anti-inflammatory drugs. Br J Clin Pharmacol 2006;62(4):496–501.

252. Stevens DL. Could nonsteroidal antiinflammatory drugs (NSAIDs) enhance the progression of bacterial infections to toxic shock syndrome? Clin Infect Dis 1995;21(4):977–80.

253. Barnham M, Anderson AW. Non-steroidal anti-inflammatory drugs (NSAIDs). A predisposing factor for streptococcal bacteraemia? Adv Exp Med Biol 1997;418:145–7.

254. Rivey MP, Allington DR, Henry Dunham AL. Necrotising fasciitis in an elderly patient: case report. Pharm Technol 1998;14:58–62.

255. Kahn LH, Styrt BA. Necrotizing soft tissue infections reported with nonsteroidal antiinflammatory drugs. Ann Pharmacother 1997;31(9):1034–9.

256. Aronoff DM, Bloch KC. Assessing the relationship between the use of nonsteroidal anti-inflammatory drugs and necrotizing fasciitis caused by group A streptococcus. Medicine 2003;82:225–35.

257. Aronoff DM, Neilson EG. Antipyretics: mechanisms of action and clinical use in fever suppress. Am J Med 2001;111:304–15.

258. Dubach UC, Rosner B, Pfister E. Epidemiologic study of abuse of analgesics containing phenacetin. Renal morbidity and mortality (1968–1979). N Engl J Med 1983;308(7):357–62.

259. Dubach UC, Rosner B, Sturmer T. An epidemiologic study of abuse of analgesic drugs. Effects of phenacetin and salicylate on mortality and cardiovascular morbidity (1968 to 1987). N Engl J Med 1991;324(3):155–60.

260. Gago-Dominguez M, Yuan JM, Castelao JE, Ross RK, Yu MC. Regular use of analgesics is a risk factor for renal cell carcinoma. Br J Cancer 1999;81(3):542–8.

261. Cerhan JR, Anderson KE, Janney CA, Vachon CM, Witzig TE, Habermann TM. Association of aspirin and other non-steroidal anti-inflammatory drug use with incidence of non-Hodgkin lymphoma. Int J Cancer 2003;106:784–8.

262. Bonati M, Bortolus R, Marchetti F, Romero M, Tognoni G. Drug use in pregnancy: an overview of epidemiological (drug utilization) studies. Eur J Clin Pharmacol 1990;38(4):325–8.

263. Ostensen M, Ostensen H. Safety of nonsteroidal antiinflammatory drugs in pregnant patients with rheumatic disease. J Rheumatol 1996;23(6):1045–9.

264. Nielsen GL, Sorensen HT, Larsen H, Pedersen L. Risk of adverse birth outcome and miscarriage in pregnant users of non-steroidal anti-inflammatory drugs: population based observational study and case-control study. BMJ 2001;322(7281):266–70.

265. Chan LY, Yuen PM, Kristensen P. Risk of miscarriage in pregnant users of NSAIDs. BMJ 2001;322(7298):1365–6.

266. Kristensen P. Risk of miscarriage in pregnant users of NSAIDs. Miscarriages also occur in women intending to have induced abortions. BMJ 2001;322(7298):1366.

267. Anonymous. Pregnant woman should avoid NSAIDs, says RCOG. Pharm J 2001;266:178.

268. Ofori B, Oraichi D, Blais L, Rey E, Bérard A. Risk of congenital anomalies in pregnant users of non-steroidal anti-inflammatory drugs: a nested case-control study. Birth Defects Res B Dev Reprod Toxicol 2006;77(4):268–79.

269. Keirse MJNC. Indomethacin tocolysis in preterm labour. In: Cochrane Library. CDROM and online versions. Cochrane Collection. Issue 22, Review number 04383. Oxford: Update Software,1995:283.

270. Quiralte J, Sanchez-Garcia F, Torres MJ, Blanco C, Castillo R, Ortega N, de Castro FR, Perez-Aciego P, Carrillo T. Association of HLA-DR11 with the anaphylactoid reaction caused by nonsteroidal anti-inflammatory drugs. J Allergy Clin Immunol 1999;103(4):685–9.

271. Eccles M, Freemantle N, Mason J. North of England evidence based guideline development project: summary guideline for non-steroidal anti-inflammatory drugs versus basic analgesia in treating the pain of degenerative arthritis. The North of England Non-Steroidal Anti-Inflammatory Drug Guideline Development Group. BMJ 1998;317(7157):526–30.

272. Moore RA, Tramer MR, Carroll D, Wiffen PJ, McQuay HJ. Quantitative systematic review of topically applied non-steroidal anti-inflammatory drugs. BMJ 1998;316(7128):333–8.

273. Evans JM, McMahon AD, McGilchrist MM, White G, Murray FE, McDevitt DG, MacDonald TM. Topical non-steroidal anti-inflammatory drugs and admission to hospital for upper gastrointestinal bleeding and perforation: a record linkage case-control study. BMJ 1995;311(6996):22–6.

274. Tonkin AL, Wing LM. Interactions of non-steroidal anti-inflammatory drugs. Baillière's Clin Rheumatol 1988;2(2):455–83.

275. Sihvo S, Klaukka T, Martikainen J, Hemminki E. Frequency of daily over-the-counter drug use and potential clinically significant over-the-counter-prescription drug interactions in the Finnish adult population. Eur J Clin Pharmacol 2000;56(6–7):495–9.

276. Helin-Salmivaara A, Huupponen R, Virtanen A, Lammela J, Klaukka T. Frequent prescribing of drugs with potential gastrointestinal toxicity among continuous users of non-steroidal anti-inflammatory drugs. Eur J Clin Pharmacol 2005;61:425–31.

277. Thomas MC. Diuretics, ACE inhibitors and NSAIDs—the triple whammy. Med J Aust 2000;172:184–5.

278. Seelig CB, Maloley PA, Campbell JR. Nephrotoxicity associated with concomitant ACE inhibitor and NSAID therapy. South Med J 1990;83:1144–8.

279. Sturrock NS, Struthers AD. Non-steroidal anti-inflammatory drugs and angiotensin converting enzyme inhibitors: a commonly prescribed combination with variable effects on renal function. Br J Clin Pharmacol 1993;35:343–8.

280. Badid C, Chambrier C, Aouifi A, Boucaud C, Bouletreau P. Anti-inflammatoire non steroidien et inhibiteur de l'enzyme de conversion: association dangereuse en periode postoperatoire. Ann Fr Anesth Réanim 1997;161:55–7.

281. Adhiyaman V, Asghar M, Oke A, Whithe AD, Shah IU. Nephrotoxicity in the elderly due to co-prescription of angiotensin converting enzyme inhibitors and nonsteroidal anti-inflammatory drugs. J R Soc Med 2001;94:512–4.

282. Anonymous. ACE inhibitor, diuretic and NSAID: a dangerous combination. Aust Adv Drug React Bull 2003;22:14–15.

283. Bouvy ML, Heerdink ER, Hoes AW, Lefkens HG. Effects of NSAIDs on the incidence of hospitalisation for renal dysfunction in users of ACE inhibitors. Drug Saf 2003;26:983–9.

284. Anonymous. Alcohol warning on over-the-counter pain medications. WHO Drug Inf 1998;12:16.

285. Radack K, Deck C. Do nonsteroidal anti-inflammatory drugs interfere with blood pressure control in hypertensive patients? J Gen Intern Med 1987;2(2):108–12.

286. Mene P, Pugliese F, Patrono C. The effects of nonsteroidal anti-inflammatory drugs on human hypertensive vascular disease. Semin Nephrol 1995;15(3):244–52.

287. Klassen DK, Jane LH, Young DY, Peterson CA. Assessment of blood pressure during naproxen therapy in hypertensive patients treated with nicardipine. Am J Hypertens 1995;8(2):146–53.

288. Houston MC, Weir M, Gray J, Ginsberg D, Szeto C, Kaihlenen PM, Sugimoto D, Runde M, Lefkowitz M. The effects of nonsteroidal anti-inflammatory drugs on blood pressures of patients with hypertension controlled by verapamil. Arch Intern Med 1995;155(10):1049–54.

289. Overlack A, Adamczak M, Bachmann W, Bonner G, Bretzel RG, Derichs R, Krone W, Lederle RM, Reimann HJ, Zschiedrich H, et al. ACE-inhibition with perindopril in essential hypertensive patients with concomitant diseases. The Perindopril Therapeutic Safety Collaborative Research Group. Am J Med 1994; 97(2):126–34.

290. MacDonald TM, Wie L. Effect of ibuprofen on cardioprotective effect of aspirin. Lancet 2003;361:573–4.

291. Catella-Lawson F, Reilly MP, Kapoor SC, Cucchiara AJ, DeMarco S, Tournier B, Fitzgerald SN, GA. Cyclooxygenase inhibitors and the antiplatelet effects of aspirin. New Engl J Med 2001;345:1809–17.

292. Kurth T, Glynn RJ, Walker AM, Chan KA, Buring JE, Hennekens CH, Gaziano JM. Inhibition of clinical benefit of aspirin on first myocardial infarction by nonsteroidal antiinflammatory drugs. Circulation 2003;108:1191–5.

293. Curtis JP, Wang Y, Portnay EL, Masoudi FA, Havranek EP, Krumholz HM. Aspirin, Ibuprofen, and mortality after myocardial infarction: retrospective cohort study. BMJ 2003;327:1322–3.

294. Kimmel SE, Strom BL. Giving aspirin and ibuprofen after myocardial infarction Clinical consequences are still unknown. BMJ 2003;327:1298–9.

295. Singh SM, Alter DA. Do NSAIDs inhibit the cardioprotective effects of ASA? Can Med Assoc J 2004;170:1094.

296. Gottemberg JE, Sordet C, Sibilia J. Inhibition of clinical benefits of aspirin on first myocardial infarction nonsteroidal antiinflammatory drugs. Circulation 2004;109:157.

297. Eliasziw M, Hill MD. Throw away the aspirin and take nonsteroidal anti-inflammatory drugs for the primary prevention of myocardial infarction. Circulation 2004;109:65–6.

298. Eldelman RS, Hebert PR, Weisman SM, Hennekens CH. An update on aspirin in the primary prevention of cardiovascular disease. Arch Intern Med 2003;163:2006–10.

299. Combe B, Edno L, Lafforgue P, Bologna C, Bernard JC, Acquaviva P, Sany J, Bressolle F. Total and free methotrexate pharmacokinetics, with and without piroxicam, in rheumatoid arthritis patients. Br J Rheumatol 1995;34(5):421–8.

300. Kremer JM, Hamilton RA. The effects of nonsteroidal antiinflammatory drugs on methotrexate (MTX) pharmacokinetics: impairment of renal clearance of MTX at weekly maintenance doses but not at 7.5 mg J Rheumatol 1995;22(11):2072–7.

301. Tracy TS, Worster T, Bradley JD, Greene PK, Brater DC. Methotrexate disposition following concomitant administration of ketoprofen, piroxicam and flurbiprofen in patients with rheumatoid arthritis. Br J Clin Pharmacol 1994;37(5):453–6.

302. Mort JR, Aparasu RR, Baer RK. Interaction between selective serotonin reuptake inhibitors and nonsteroidal antiinflammatory drugs: review of the literature. Pharmacotherapy 2006;26(9):1307–13.

303. Battistella M, Mamdami MM, Juurlink DN, Rabeneck L, Laupacis A. Risk of upper gastrointestinal hemorrhage in warfarin users treated with nonselective NSAIDs or COX-2 inhibitors. Arch Intern Med 2005;24:158-60.

COX-2 inhibitors

See also Individual names

General Information

The cyclo-oxygenase (COX) that is responsible for prostaglandin synthesis exists in two isoforms, COX-1 and COX-2, which differ in their structure, regulation, expression, and function. COX-1 is expressed normally in a constant amount in almost all body tissues and produces prostaglandins important for the maintenance of normal homeostasis. In particular, among other important functions, they help to protect the gastrointestinal mucosa against ulceration and regulate renal function and platelet activity. COX-1 appears to be largely unaffected by inflammatory stimuli. In contrast, the COX-2 isoform is constitutively expressed only in the brain, in bone (associated with osteoblast activity), in the female reproductive tract (associated with both the ovulatory cycle and implantation of fertilized ova), and in the kidney, where it may play an important role in regulating renal function. In many other cells COX-2 is expressed at very low levels or is undetectable, but it is readily induced by inflammatory cytokines, mitogens, and endotoxins. Therefore, prostaglandins generated by COX-2 mediate pain and inflammation in many tissues and probably also have a role in renal, brain, and reproductive physiology, and in tissue repair (1–4).

Traditional NSAIDs inhibit both COX-1 and COX-2, providing benefit at sites of inflammation, but at the cost of potential adverse effects related to COX-1 inhibition, particularly in areas such as the gastrointestinal mucosa, platelets, and the kidney. The development of a drug that inhibits only COX-2 would offer the promise of relieving pain and inflammation without some, if not all, of these adverse effects. However, the concept that selective inhibition of COX-2 is only a positive event and inhibition of COX-1 a bad one may be simplistic, as it is flawed by many experimental data that have also implicated COX-2 as an integral component in the maintenance of physiological homeostasis (3). In particular, COX-2 may reduce inflammation by generating anti-inflammatory prostanoids (5); COX-2, like COX-1, may be present in normal gastric mucosa (6,7) and can play a physiological role there in defense mechanisms (8,9), and there is evidence that prostaglandins derived from COX-2 may be important in the healing of gastric ulcers (9–12). Furthermore, COX-2 inhibition alone may be insufficient to resolve inflammation and pain (13), suggesting that COX-1 inhibition may play a role in reducing inflammation as well (14). Although the relevance of these experimental observations to the possible beneficial role of COX-2 activity is uncertain, they cannot be simply dismissed.

Nearly all of the traditional NSAIDs are predominantly COX-1-selective. In fact, only two of them, meloxicam and nimesulide (1,2), have been shown to have some COX-2 selectivity in humans. Two other NSAIDs, etodolac and nabumetone, may be COX-2 preferential inhibitors, but the evidence is less convincing than for meloxicam or nimesulide. Unfortunately, despite their wide use, clinical and epidemiological evidence that supports the claim of better tolerability of these preferential inhibitors with respect to other NSAIDs, is scanty and even controversial (1,4). Furthermore, for both meloxicam and nimesulide there are data consistent with reduced COX-2 selectivity at high doses, those usually used in clinical practice. These considerations have prompted research for more selective COX-2 inhibitors, and three compounds, celecoxib, parecoxib, and rofecoxib, have become available. These compounds are much more selective than previous preferential inhibitors and they have no effect on COX-1 (COX-1 sparing drugs) over the whole range of doses used and concentrations achieved in clinical use. In particular, they have been shown in humans to spare gastric COX-1 to a much greater extent than traditional NSAIDs.

Is there convincing evidence that COX-2-selective NSAIDs offer a distinct therapeutic advantage over non-selective ones? To prove the usefulness of these compounds, clinical studies should show:

- whether the COX-2 selective inhibitors are as effective as older NSAIDs in the relief of pain and/or inflammation;
- whether in the effective dosage range there is evidence of less damage to the mucosa of the upper gastrointestinal tract than with conventional NSAIDs;
- whether there are any effects on platelet in effective doses;
- whether unexpected adverse drug reactions compromise the safety of these compounds.

As far as the last of these criteria is concerned, the finding that rofecoxib increases the risk of cardiovascular disease (heart attacks and strokes) during long-term therapy has led to a reappraisal of the role of the COX-2 inhibitors. Furthermore, both rofecoxib and valdecoxib have been withdrawn by their manufacturers, the former because of its adverse cardiovascular effects and the latter because of an increased risk of cardiovascular events after coronary artery bypass surgery and reports of potentially fatal skin reactions.

Clinical studies

Both celecoxib and rofecoxib have been evaluated in large randomized trials lasting from weeks to 1 year, for the relief of the signs and symptoms of osteoarthritis or rheumatoid arthritis in adults (1,15–21). In all of these studies both compounds have been shown to be more effective than placebo and at least as effective as traditional NSAIDs (that is ibuprofen, diclofenac, nabumetone, naproxen). However, there is less information about their efficacy as analgesics. A few randomized, double-blind trials have shown that both compounds are more effective than placebo; rofecoxib was as effective as non-selective NSAIDs (ibuprofen, naproxen) in relieving the pain of osteoarthritis or after dental surgery, but celecoxib was less effective (22–26). Rofecoxib was also analgesic in patients with primary dysmenorrhea (27). However, there are no published data on the usefulness of COX-2-selective NSAIDs in other types of acute pain, such as that related to acute gout, migraine, cancer, or biliary or ureteric colic.

General adverse effects

Although the scientific literature has been flooded by articles and reviews on the use of selective COX-2 inhibitors (coxibs), the safe prescribing and use of these compounds is controversial (28–31).

COX-2 selectivity may be a double-edged sword. Because the cardiovascular risk outweighs the gastrointestinal risk in adults with rheumatoid arthritis or osteoarthritis, the harm would outweigh the benefits in most clinical settings. This means that the total number of serious adverse events would be increased by COX-2-selective NSAIDs compared with non-selective NSAIDs. COX-2 selectivity, which is an appealing theoretical concept, might be a clinical failure (30).

Much information on celecoxib and rofecoxib has come from two large pivotal randomized clinical trials, the Celecoxib Long-term Arthritis Safety Study (CLASS) and Vioxx Gastrointestinal Outcomes Research (VIGOR) studies, in which the efficacy and safety of the two coxibs and various non-selective NSAIDs were compared (32,33).

Summary

The COX-2-selective inhibitors are as efficacious as traditional NSAIDs in treating inflammation and pain due to osteoarticular diseases. However, there are questions to be addressed before COX-2-selective inhibitors can be considered to be definitely safer than traditional NSAIDs (4). Among these questions the most important relate to the possibility that COX-2 inhibitors may cause complicated ulceration in some subgroup of patients and may retard ulcer healing in others. Therefore, whether the COX-2 inhibitors in place of non-selective NSAIDs will prove to be cost-effective by reducing ulcer-related morbidity remains to be demonstrated. Moreover, it is likely that such drugs can cause the same renal problems as traditional NSAIDs do. Finally, the effect of COX-2 inhibitors on the incidence of vascular disease will need strict scrutiny, since vascular disease is a commoner cause of death than ulcer perforation or bleeding and since some of them clearly increase the long-term risk of heart attacks and strokes. Only their continuing use and post-marketing surveillance studies will demonstrate their strengths and weaknesses with respect to non-selective NSAIDs.

Criticisms of outcome studies that support the safety of COX-2 inhibitors continue to appear. A number of flaws in both the design and analysis of these studies have been identified in a recent review (34), casting doubts on the available evidence of the safety profile of coxibs.

Organs and Systems

Cardiovascular

Major cardiovascular events
Selective inhibitors of the cyclo-oxygenase type 2 isoenzyme (COX-2) were developed with the expectation that their use would be accompanied by a reduction in the severe gastrointestinal and renal adverse effects associated with conventional non-steroidal anti-inflammatory drugs (NSAIDs), adverse effects that were thought to be largely a result of inhibition of the COX-1 isoenzyme (35). However, evidence has since accumulated that COX-2 selective inhibitors (coxibs) not only cause gastro-intestinal and renal toxicity but can also contribute to an increased risk of adverse cardiovascular events. The possible explanation of this phenomenon came from pharmacological studies that identified COX-2 inhibition as a plausible, albeit not the only, pharmacological mechanism for induction of thrombotic events. In fact, suppression of COX-2 dependent formation of PGI2 by coxibs, without significant concomitant inhibition of thromboxane A2 biosynthesis, can predispose patients to acute thromboembolic events. The pharmacological evidence that supports the mechanism for prothrombotic effects of coxibs has been reviewed (SEDA-26, 116; SEDA-27, 102; SEDA-28, 128) (36,37,38). Figure 1 shows the physiological effects of COX-2 inhibition and the potential clinical implications (39).

There is also evidence from experimental and clinical studies that COX-2 may be atherogenic and thrombogenic and that selective COX-2 inhibitors may actually reduce, rather than cause, atherothrombotic vascular events (40). Some evidence supporting this hypothesis comes from laboratory and clinical studies. A recent randomized trial suggested that simvastatin reduces inflammation and suppresses the expression of cycloxigenase-2 and prostaglandin E synthase in plaque macrophages, and this effect may in turn contribute to plaque stabilization by inhibition of metalloproteinase-induced plaque rupture (41). Inhibition of COX-2 by celecoxib compared with placebo improved endothelium-dependent vasodilatation and reduced oxidative stress in men with severe coronary artery disease (42).

Rofecoxib
Information about comes from the two large studies, CLASS and VIGOR, from a pooled cardiovascular safety analysis using individual patient data derived from all rofecoxib phase IIb to V trials conducted by the manufacturer that lasted at least 2 weeks, and from the adverse events reporting system in the USA (43). As a result of these and other studies the COX-2 inhibitors, rofecoxib and valdecoxib, have been voluntarily withdrawn from the market by their manufacturers, and other COX-2 inhibitors are under scrutiny.

In VIGOR, rofecoxib 50 mg/day was associated with a higher rate of non-fatal myocardial infarction (0.4%) than the non-selective COX-2 inhibitor naproxen 500 mg bd (0.1%) (RR = 0.2; CI = 0.1, 0.7) (33). In CLASS there was no difference in the rates of myocardial infarction in patients taking celecoxib (0.5%) and those taking ibuprofen or diclofenac (0.4%). However, the protocols of the two studies differed substantially with respect to the use of aspirin. In VIGOR, the patients were not allowed to take aspirin or any other antiplatelet drug, while in CLASS one-fifth of the patients took aspirin. A re-analysis of CLASS for cardiovascular thromboembolic events, including myocardial infarction, stroke, cardiovascular deaths, and peripheral events, showed no significant increase with celecoxib versus NSAIDs (44).

The results of VIGOR might be explained by a significant prothrombotic effect of rofecoxib and/or an antithrombotic effect of naproxen, which may have a significant antiplatelet effect. To clarify this, the annualized myocardial infarction rates in both VIGOR and CLASS were compared with those found in placebo-treated patients with similar cardiac risk factors enrolled in three meta-analyses of four aspirin primary prevention trials (43,45). The analysis showed 0.24 and 0.30% increases over placebo in cardiovascular events for rofecoxib and celecoxib respectively, suggesting a prothrombotic potential of both COX-2 inhibitors. However, these results have been heavily criticized (46–52), because of many potential pitfalls in the comparisons of patient populations in different trials. The results from a recently reported pooled analysis of individual patient data combined across rofecoxib phase IIb to phase V trials seem to be more reliable (53). Cardiovascular events were assessed across 23 studies. Comparisons were made between patients taking rofecoxib and those taking placebo, naproxen, or other non-selective NSAIDs (diclofenac, ibuprofen, and nabumetone). The major outcome measure was the combined end-point used by the Anti-platelet Trialist Collaboration, which includes cardiovascular death, hemorrhagic death, death of unknown cause, non-fatal myocardial infarction, and non-fatal stroke. More than 28 000 patients, representing more than 14 000 patient-years at risk, were analysed. The relative risk for an end-point was 0.84 (95% CI = 0.51, 1.38) when comparing rofecoxib with placebo; 0.79 (95% CI = 0.40, 1.55) when comparing rofecoxib with non-selective NSAIDs; and 1.69 (95% CI = 1.07, 2.69) when comparing rofecoxib with naproxen. These data provide no evidence for an excess of cardiovascular events for rofecoxib relative to either placebo or the non-selective NSAIDs that were studied. Instead, the difference between rofecoxib and naproxen showed that naproxen was associated with a reduced risk of cardiovascular events.

The cardiovascular results in VIGOR may have occurred simply by chance, given the low number of events, or because naproxen may have a cardioprotective effect similar to that of aspirin, or because rofecoxib 50 mg/day could have prothrombotic effects, especially in the absence of concomitant COX-1 inhibition in patients at increased risk of cardiovascular thromboembolic events. Because there was no untreated group in VIGOR, we do not know whether this finding suggests a protective effect of naproxen or a harmful effect of rofecoxib. All three explanations are plausible, and they are not mutually exclusive.

It has been suggested that the increase in thrombotic cardiovascular events in rofecoxib-treated patients probably represents the antiplatelet effect of naproxen (43,54,55). Naproxen has a long pharmacodynamic half-life and inhibits platelet aggregation by 88% for up to 8 hours (56).

In VIGOR (30,33), the incidence of confirmed thrombotic cardiovascular events was 0.6% higher with rofecoxib than with naproxen (RR = 2.4; 95% CI = 3.9, 4.0).

Some data may help to answer the important question of whether the relative difference in the incidence of myocardial infarction in VIGOR was due to a harmful effect of rofecoxib or a beneficial effect of naproxen. Although contrasting data have been published (57), the hypothesis that naproxen has a cardioprotective effect has gained wider support (58). Only one of the four most recently published studies negated a potential cardioprotective effect of naproxen.

However, an analysis of FDA data suggested an increase in serious cardiac events with celecoxib (30). The incidence of serious cardiac adverse events (myocardial infarction, combined anginal events, and atrial dysrhythmias) was 0.6% higher with celecoxib than with other NSAIDs (RR = 1.55; CI = 1.04, 2.30). The reasons for these inconsistencies are not clear.

In an 11-year observational study in new users of non-selective, non-aspirin NSAIDs ($n = 181\ 441$) and an equal number of non-users there was no evidence of a protective effect of naproxen (59). During 532 634 person-years of follow-up there were 6382 cases of serious coronary heart disease (11.9 per 1000 person-years). Multivariate-adjusted rate ratios for current and former use of non-

aspirin NSAIDs were 1.05 (95% CI = 0.97, 1.14) and 1.02 (0.97, 1.08) respectively. Rate ratios for ibuprofen, naproxen, and other NSAIDs were 1.15 (1.02, 1.28), 0.95 (0.82, 1.09), and 1.03 (0.92, 1.16) respectively. There was no protection in long-term users with uninterrupted use; the rate ratio among current users with more than 60 days of continuous use was 1.05 (0.91, 1.21). When naproxen was directly compared with ibuprofen, the rate ratio in current users was 0.83 (0.69, 0.98). This study therefore seems to have shown no cardioprotective effect of naproxen. However, the study had a number of important limitations, including: lack of information about some important confounders (smoking, obesity), possible exposure misclassification, and lack of information about over-the-counter use of aspirin.

Opposite evidence has emerged from three case-control studies from the USA, Canada, and the UK, which showed that the rates of myocardial infarction in patients taking naproxen were lower than in patients not taking any NSAIDs (60,61) and those taking other NSAIDs (62).

In the first study, 4425 patients hospitalized with acute myocardial infarction who used NSAIDs were compared with 17 700 controls in a large health-care database in the USA (51). Multivariate models were constructed to control for potential confounders. A quarter of the cases and controls had also filled a prescription for an NSAID in the 6 months before the study. Overall, the NSAID users had the same risk of acute myocardial infarction as non-users, but naproxen users had a significantly lower risk of acute myocardial infarction compared with those who were not taking NSAIDs (adjusted OR = 0.84; 95% CI = 0.72, 0.98). The cardioprotective effect of naproxen was very modest compared with aspirin (a 44% reduction in the risk of acute myocardial infarction in the Physician Health Study (63)).

The second study was a case-control study sponsored by Merck & Co (the manufacturers of celecoxib), in which the risk of acute thromboembolic cardiovascular events among 16 937 patients aged 40–75 years with rheumatoid arthritis using naproxen was examined using the British General Practice Research Database (61). Each patient with a first thromboembolic event ($n = 809$: 435 myocardial infarctions, 347 strokes, 27 sudden deaths) was matched with four controls. The results suggested that patients with rheumatoid arthritis who currently use naproxen have a significantly lower risk of thromboembolic events relative to those who have not used naproxen in the past year (RR = 0.61; 0.39, 0.94). However, the risk was not lower with previous use of naproxen, suggesting that any effect of naproxen is likely to be short-lived. Moreover, the significantly lower risk of myocardial infarction with current naproxen was not found when myocardial infractions were analysed separately (RR = 0.57; 0.3, 1.06). There was no protective effect for thromboembolic events with current use of non-naproxen NSAIDs.

The third study was also sponsored by Merck & Co and was designed to examine the association between the use of naproxen and other non-selective NSAIDs and hospitalization for acute myocardial infarction (62). In a database of 14 163 patients aged 65 years or older who were hospitalized for acute myocardial infarction and an equal number of age-matched controls, concurrent exposure to naproxen had a protective effect against myocardial infarction compared with the other non-selective non-aspirin NSAIDs (RR = 0.79; CI = 0.63, 0.99). This effect was present only with concurrent naproxen exposure and was stronger in long-term users. However, this study also had several limitations: some important risk factors, such as smoking and obesity, could not be assessed, patients who died of myocardial infarction before reaching the hospital were not included, and there was uncertainty about concurrent use of over-the-counter drugs, especially aspirin.

Unexpectedly, in September 2004, Merck Sharp & Dohme announced the voluntary worldwide withdrawal of rofecoxib. This followed the release of data from a long-term, randomized, placebo-controlled trial, the Adenomatous Polyp Prevention on Vioxx the APPROVe trial, which showed that the use of rofecoxib was associated with an increased risk of thrombotic events (64,65). The study was designed to evaluate the hypothesis that treatment with rofecoxib for 3 years would reduce the risk of recurrent adenomatous polyps among patients with a history of colorectal adenomas. A total of 2586 patients underwent randomization (1287 were assigned to rofecoxib 25 mg/day and 1299 to placebo). All investigator-reported serious adverse events that represented potential thrombotic cardiovascular events were adjudicated in a blinded fashion by an independent committee, and all the safety data were monitored by an external safety monitoring committee. The mean duration of treatment was 2.4 years with rofecoxib and 2.6 years with placebo. In the rofecoxib group 46 patients had confirmed thrombotic events during 3059 patient-years of follow-up (1.50 events per 100 patient years) compared with 26 patients who took placebo during 3327 patient-years of follow up (0.78 events per 100 patient years). The relative risk was 1.92 (95% CI=1.19, 3.11). However, the increased relative risk became apparent only after 18 months of treatment; during the first 18 months the events rates were similar in the two groups. The difference between the two groups was mainly due to an increased number of myocardial infarctions and strokes in those taking rofecoxib.

Those who took rofecoxib also had higher risks of non-adjudicated cardiovascular events (hypertension and edema-related events) compared with those who took placebo. The Kaplan–Meier curves for the cumulative incidence of congestive heart failure, pulmonary edema, and cardiac failure showed an early separation of the two groups, at about 5 months.

Further data consistent with the results of APPROVe were found in a standard and cumulative random effects meta-analysis (66). This study aimed at establishing whether robust evidence on the adverse cardiovascular effects of rofecoxib had been available before September 2004, the date on which rofecoxib was withdrawn. The meta-analysis identified 18 randomized controlled trials, including 25 273 patients with chronic musculoskeletal disorders, in which rofecoxib was compared with other NSAIDs or placebo, and 11

observational studies on naproxen and cardiovascular risk. Myocardial infarction was the primary end-point. By the end of 2000 (52 myocardial infarctions, 20 742 patients) the relative risk in randomized controlled trials was 2.30 (95% CI=1.22, 4.33), and 1 year later (64 events, 21 432 patients) it was 2.24 (1.24, 4.02). There was no evidence that the relative risk differed depending on the control group (placebo, a non-naproxen NSAID, or naproxen) or the duration of the trial. In observational studies, the cardioprotective effect of naproxen was small (combined estimate 0.86; CI=0.75, 0.99) and could not have explained the findings of VIGOR. These findings suggest that evidence of the adverse cardiovascular effects was available before September 2004 and that rofecoxib should have been withdrawn several years earlier. The reasons why the manufacturers and regulatory authorities did not continuously monitor and summarize the accumulating evidence need to be clarified (64).

Besides the VIGOR and APPROVe studies, a number of other clinical and epidemiological studies have signalled an increased risk of harmful cardiovascular effects with rofecoxib. Among them three epidemiological studies merit attention.

The first study (67) was a retrospective cohort study of individuals on the expanded Tennessee Medicaid programme, in which the occurrence of serious coronary heart disease was assessed both in non-users (n=202 916) and users of rofecoxib (n=24 132) and other NSAIDs (n=15 728). The patients were aged 50–84 years, lived in the community, and had no life-threatening non-cardiovascular illnesses. The incidence of acute myocardial infarction or cardiac death in new users of rofecoxib at doses above 25 mg/day was almost twice that in non-users (24 versus 13 events per 1000 patient years; RR=1.93; 95% CI=1.00, 3.43). In contrast, there was no evidence of an increased risk of coronary heart disease among users of rofecoxib at doses of 25 mg/day or less or among users of other NSAIDs.

The second study was a matched case-control study of the relation between coxibs, non-selective NSAIDs, and hospitalization for acute myocardial infarction in a large population of patients aged 65 years or over (68). The study database contained information on more than 50 000 patients and included 10 895 cases of acute myocardial infarction. Current use of rofecoxib was associated with an increased relative risk of acute myocardial infarction compared with celecoxib (OR=1.24; CI=1.05, 1.46) and with no NSAIDs (OR=1.14; CI=1.00, 1.31). A dosage of rofecoxib of over 25 mg/day was associated with a higher risk than 25 mg/day or less. The risk was increased in the first 90 days but not thereafter.

The timing of cardiovascular risks associated with the use of COX-2 inhibitors is unclear. The APPROVe trial reported a two-fold increase in cardiovascular toxicity after 18 months of use, while in the VIGOR study a similar increase in risk was reported after only 9 months of treatment. However, the risk curves in the VIGOR study started to diverge after the first month of therapy (69). In the APC trial celecoxib was associated with a dose-dependent increase in risk after 3 years of use, but the combination of intravenous parecoxib plus oral valdecoxib resulted in an increased risk after only 10 days of exposure. A more recent study has provided new insights into the timing of the cardiovascular risks associated with the use of rofecoxib and celecoxib (70). The study, which was a time-matched, nested, case-control study, showed that among elderly users of rofecoxib and celecoxib the cardiovascular risks associated with the use of rofecoxib were more acute than has previously been recognized. The risk was highest in the first 6-13 days (median 9 days) after starting treatment and did not increase with further treatment. Indeed, the risk of myocardial infarction appeared to reduce over time despite continued exposure, presumably owing to attrition of susceptible individuals, i.e. the healthy survivor effect that is seen in an adverse effect of intermediate time course (71).

Further evidence that rofecoxib increases the risk of serious coronary heart disease comes from a third case-control study commissioned by the US Food and Drug Administration (72). Cases of serious coronary heart disease (acute myocardial infarction and sudden cardiac death) in a cohort of NSAID-treated patients were risk-matched with four controls. Current exposure to coxibs (rofecoxib and celecoxib) and standard NSAIDs was compared with remote exposure to any NSAID, and rofecoxib was compared with celecoxib. During 2 302 029 person-years of follow up, there were 8143 cases of serious coronary heart disease, of which 2210 were fatal. Multivariate adjusted odds ratios for rofecoxib versus celecoxib were: 1.59 (all doses; CI=1.10, 2.32); 1.47 (rofecoxib 25 mg/day or less; CI=0.99, 2.17); and 3.58 (rofecoxib over 25 mg/day; CI=1.00, 4.30). For naproxen versus remote NSAIDs the adjusted OR was 1.14 (1.00, 1.30). The interpretation of these results was that rofecoxib increases the risk of acute myocardial infarction and sudden death compared with celecoxib and that naproxen does not protect against serious coronary heart disease. This study also provided data relevant to some other controversies about the cardiovascular safety of coxibs. In particular there was a substantially higher risk with high-dose rofecoxib, in accordance with the results of other studies (67,68). Moreover the mean duration of use before the occurrence of an event was identical with high doses and standard doses of rofecoxib (about 110 days), consistent with the idea that the risk of cardiovascular toxicity begins early in treatment. That is in accord with the analysis by the FDA of data from VIGOR, which showed that the survival curve for acute myocardial infarction with high-dose rofecoxib began to diverge from the naproxen curve after 1 month. There was no evidence that the relative risk differed depending on the control group (placebo, a non-naproxen NSAID, or naproxen) or the duration of treatment. This suggests that patients are at risk of myocardial infarction even if rofecoxib is taken for a few months only. Therefore, the reassuring statement by Merck that there is no excess risk in the first 18 months is not supported by this meta-analysis.

In contrast to these findings, two earlier meta-analyses from Merck laboratories showed no evidence for an excess of cardiovascular thrombotic events for rofecoxib relative to either placebo or non-naproxen NSAIDs

(ibuprofen, nabumetone, diclofenac) or an increased risk in trials in which rofecoxib and naproxen were compared (53,73).

In conclusion these data provide further convincing evidence that naproxen does not have a cardioprotective effect, in accordance with the results of some studies (74,75) although not others (60,61,62). Indeed, the current data show even a possibility of a small increased risk of coronary heart disease.

The demonstration of a lack of protective effect of naproxen is important, because it is often used as a comparator in clinical trials of new coxibs. Thus, a result that shows that a new drug has an increased risk of cardiovascular disease relative to naproxen should alert prescribers to potential cardiotoxic effects.

There are two further crucial questions:

- Is the apparent treatment-associated increase in severe cardiovascular events unique to rofecoxib or does it apply to other COX-2 selective drugs, suggesting a COX-2 class effect, and even to NSAIDs in general?
- Does it apply to all patients or only to a subset, such as those with known susceptibility factors for vascular disease?

Two recently published reports help in answering these questions. The first is a meta-analysis of randomized controlled trials of selective COX-2 inhibitors versus placebo or traditional NSAIDs or both (76). Eligible studies were randomized trials that lasted at least 4 weeks, with information on serious vascular events (defined as myocardial infarction, stroke, and vascular death). Data were available from 138 randomized trials involving a total of 143 373 participants. NSAIDs were subdivided into naproxen and others. In placebo comparisons, allocation to a COX-2 selective inhibitor was associated with a 42% relative increase in the incidence of serious vascular events: 1.2% per year versus 0.9% per year (RR=1.42; 95% CI=1.13, 1.78) with no significant heterogeneity among the different coxibs. This increase was chiefly attributable to an increased risk of myocardial infarction (0.6% per year versus 0.3% per year; RR=1.86; 95% CI=1.93, 2.59), with little apparent difference in other vascular outcomes. Among trials of at least 1 year duration (mean 2.7 years) the rate ratio for vascular events was 1.45 (CI=1.12, 1.89). There were too few vascular events to allow an assessment of the dose-response relation in placebo-controlled trials of all coxibs, with the exception of celecoxib, for which there was a significant trend towards an increased incidence of serious vascular events with higher daily doses. The size of the risk of vascular events in placebo-controlled trials that allowed concomitant use of aspirin was similar among aspirin users and non-users.

Comparisons of selective COX-2 inhibitors versus traditional NSAIDs showed a similar incidence of serious vascular events (1.0% per year versus 0.9% per year; RR=1.16; CI=0.97, 138). However, there was marked heterogeneity across the rate ratios for vascular events in trials that compared a coxib with naproxen and trials that compared a selective COX-2 inhibitor with a non-naproxen NSAID. Overall, compared with naproxen, allocation to a selective COX-2 inhibitor was associated with a highly significant increase in the incidence of a serious vascular event (RR=1.57; CI=1.21, 2.03) and a two-fold increased risk of a myocardial infarction (RR=2.04; CI=1.41, 2.96), but no difference in the incidences of stroke or vascular death. In contrast the comparison of COX-2 selective inhibitors with non-naproxen NSAIDs showed non-significant differences in the incidences of vascular events, myocardial infarctions, and vascular deaths, but selective COX-2 inhibitors were associated with a significantly lower incidence of stroke than any non-naproxen NSAIDs (RR=0.62; CI=0.41, 0.95).

The time-course of the effects of NSAIDs in increasing the risk of cardiovascular events has been assessed in a cohort study in 74 838 users of non-selective NSAIDs or coxibs and 23 532 comparable users of other drugs (77). There was a significant increase in the event rate for rofecoxib (RR = 1.15; 95% CI = 1.06, 1.25) and a significant reduction in the rate for naproxen (RR = 0.75; 95% CI = 0.62, 0.92). No other coxib or NSAID had an effect. The increased rate associated with rofecoxib was seen in the first 60 days of use and persisted thereafter.

When the rate ratio of serious vascular events with traditional NSAIDs was compared with that of placebo, high-dose ibuprofen and high-dose diclofenac were both associated with an increased risk of cardiovascular events (ibuprofen RR=1.51; CI=0.96, 2.37; diclofenac RR=1.63; CI=1.12, 237), while naproxen was not.

Thus, it appears that allocation to a selective COX-2 inhibitor is associated with about three extra vascular events per 1000 patients per year. Most of this excess is attributable to myocardial infarction.

The other study that has contributed to better evaluation of the data on cardiovascular risk due to inhibition of cyclo-oxygenase is a systematic review of the available controlled pharmacoepidemiological studies (78). There were 23 eligible studies that reported on cardiovascular events (predominantly myocardial infarction) with COX-2 inhibitors, NSAIDs, or both, with non-use/remote use of the drug as the reference exposure for calculation of the relative risk. The studies were 17 case-control studies involving 86 193 cases with cardiovascular events and about 52 800 controls and six cohort studies involving 75 520 users of selective COX-2 inhibitors, 375 619 users of non-selective NSAIDs, and 594 720 unexposed participants. The results confirmed that there is an increased risk of cardiovascular events with rofecoxib. The summary relative risk with doses in excess of 25 mg/day was 2.19 (CI=1.64, 2.91) compared with 1.33 (CI=1.00, 1.79) with 25 mg/day or less. The risk was increased during the first month of treatment. In contrast to the evidence from the meta-analysis of randomized trials, this study showed no increase in risk with celecoxib 200 mg/day. However, one must remember that the randomized clinical trials only showed an increased risk with doses of celecoxib of 400 mg/day and above. The study also provided more data on the cardiovascular toxicity of traditional NSAIDs. Naproxen was not associated with a reduction in risk, as was suggested in previous comparisons with rofecoxib.

Of more concern is evidence, from both randomized and non-randomized trials, that diclofenac increases the risk of cardiovascular events (RR=1.63; CI=1.12, 2.37). Less convincing is the evidence of potential cardiovascular risk with other NSAIDs, such as ibuprofen, meloxicam, and indometacin.

Celecoxib

In December 2004 the results of the Adenoma Prevention with Celecoxib trial (the APC trial) were presented. This was a randomized, double-blind, multicenter study of the effects of two doses of celecoxib (200 mg or 400 mg bd) or placebo in the prevention of colorectal adenomas (79). All potentially serious cardiovascular events among 2035 patients with a history of colorectal neoplasia were identified, with a follow up of 2.8–3.1 years. Celecoxib was associated with a dose-related increase in the composite end-point of death from cardiovascular causes, myocardial infarction, stroke, or heart failure. The composite end-point was reached in seven of 679 patients in the placebo group (1%) compared with 16 of 685 patients who took celecoxib 200 mg bd (2.3%; hazard ratio=2.3; CI=0.9, 5.5) and 23 of 671 patients who took celecoxib 400 mg bd (3.4%; hazard ratio=3.4; CI=1.4, 7.8). The annualized incidence of death due to cardiovascular causes per 1000 patient years was 3.4 events in the placebo group; there were 7.5 events in patients who took celecoxib 200 mg bd and 11.4 in those who took 400 mg bd. The hazard ratio associated with celecoxib was not significantly affected by any baseline characteristics, including use of aspirin. Moreover, the results were also consistent among the individual components of the composite end-point. Based on these statistically significant findings, the sponsor of the study, the USA National Cancer Institute suspended the study.

However, to underscore the uncertainty of the available data on cardiovascular risk, we should consider the results of another large long-term trial with celecoxib 400 mg/day, designed to investigate the role of NSAIDs in preventing Alzheimer's disease, the Alzheimer Disease Anti-inflammatory Prevention Trial (ADAPT), in which celecoxib was compared with naproxen (440 mg/day). The unpublished results of the study showed that celecoxib did not increase cardiovascular risk, while naproxen was associated with an increased risk (80). The results from the APC and ADAPT studies are disturbing, because they are inconsistent with the results of most previous studies. The following data summarize the currently available information on the cardiovascular safety of celecoxib.

In two retrospective re-analyses of randomized controlled trial data for celecoxib (81,82) the cardiovascular events in patients enrolled in the CLASS study (83) were examined, as were those reported across the entire controlled arthritis clinical trial database for celecoxib. The results of the reanalysis of CLASS showed no evidence of an increase in investigator-reported serious cardiovascular adverse events in patients taking celecoxib. In the analysis of the celecoxib comparative trials database the incidence of cardiovascular events was not significantly different between celecoxib and placebo or between celecoxib and naproxen, regardless of aspirin use. Thus, these comparative analyses failed to show an increased risk of thrombotic events associated with celecoxib compared with conventional NSAIDs, naproxen specifically, or placebo.

In a meta-analysis of studies in 7462 patients exposed to (a) celecoxib 200–800 mg/day for 1268 patient-years compared with 4057 patients treated with placebo for 585 patient-years and (b) 19 773 patients treated with celecoxib 200–800 mg/day for 5651 patient-years compared with 13 990 patients treated with non-selective NSAIDs (diclofenac, ibuprofen, naproxen, ketoprofen, and loxoprofen) for 4386 patient-years, the incidence rates of the combined cardiovascular events were not significantly different between patients treated with celecoxib and placebo or between those treated with celecoxib and non-selective NSAIDs (84). The dose of celecoxib, the use of aspirin, or the presence of cardiovascular risk factors did not alter these results. The authors concluded that there was no evidence of an increased cardiovascular risk with celecoxib relative to placebo and a comparable rate of cardiovascular events with celecoxib compared with non-selective NSAIDs.

Most information on the potential cardiovascular toxicity of celecoxib has come from a number of observational studies (67,68,82,821,188,85,86). Most of them were population-based case-control studies in which the relative risk of acute myocardial infarction was assessed in patients who took celecoxib, rofecoxib, conventional NSAIDs, or no NSAIDs at all. None of these studies identified a significantly increased risk of severe cardiovascular events with celecoxib. However, the results of these observational studies must be interpreted with caution. In fact, although findings from observational studies are more generalizable, as they are larger and include less carefully selected patients than randomized controlled trials, they suffer from potential bias and confounding, which could have contributed to the failure to confirm the hypothesis of a consistent difference in severe cardiovascular risk between all the coxibs and other NSAIDs. Whether this safety concern represents a class effect requires additional information from other randomized controlled trials, not yet available (87).

The risk of cardiovascular events with celecoxib has been studied in a systematic review and meta-analysis of randomized double-blind trials of at least 6 weeks' duration with data on serious thromboembolic events [88]. Four placebo-controlled trials in 4422 patients were analysed. The odds ratio for myocardial infarction with celecoxib was 2.26 (95% CI = 1.0, 5.1). There was no significant increase in risk with celecoxib for composite cardiovascular events, cardiovascular deaths, or stroke. A secondary meta-analysis of six studies with placebo, diclofenac, ibuprofen, and paracetamol as comparators in 12 780 patients showed similar findings: there was a significantly increased risk of myocardial infarction with celecoxib (OR = 1.88; 95% CI = 1.15, 3.08) but not other outcome measures.

Etoricoxib

Data on the efficacy and safety of this highly selective COX-2 inhibitor are still limited. A combined analysis of all randomized, double-blind trials of long-term treatment showed a significantly lower incidence of peptic ulcer bleeding with etoricoxib (n=9226) than with conventional NSAIDs (n=2215), but there was no information about potential cardiovascular toxicity (89).

There has been a systematic review and meta-analysis of double-blind, randomized, placebo-controlled trials of etoricoxib of at least 6 weeks duration (five studies with a total of 2919 patients); the main outcome measure was cardiovascular thromboembolic events (90). There were seven cardiovascular thromboembolic events in 1441 patients (0.5%) taking etoricoxib, and one event in 906 patients (0.1%) taking placebo. The pooled fixed-effects estimate of the absolute risk difference was 0.5% (CI=0.1, 1.0). The odds ratio for the risk of cardiovascular events was 1.49 (0.42, 5.31). These limited data provide weak evidence of an increased cardiovascular risk with etoricoxib.

In a prespecified pooled analysis of data from three trials in which patients with osteoarthritis or rheumatoid arthritis were randomly assigned to etoricoxib 60 or 90 mg/day or diclofenac 150 mg/day for an average of 18 months (SD 11.8), there were equal numbers of thrombotic cardiovascular events with etoricoxib (n = 320) and diclofenac(n = 323), giving event rates of 1.24 and 1.30 per 100 patient-years and a hazard ratio of 0.95 (95% CI = 0.81, 1.11) for etoricoxib compared with diclofenac (91). Rates of upper gastrointestinal events (perforation, bleeding, obstruction, ulcer) were lower with etoricoxib (0.67 versus 0.97 per 100 patient-years; HR = 0.69; 95% CI = 0.57, 0.83), but the rates of complicated upper gastrointestinal events were similar (0.30 versus 0.32).

Lumiracoxib

Lumiracoxib is a novel COX-2 selective inhibitor, a phenylacetic acid derivative with a short half-life and a higher selectivity than any other coxib. Clinical data on its efficacy and safety are still limited.

The cardiovascular safety of lumiracoxib has been assessed in the Therapeutic Arthritis and Gastrointestinal Event Trial (TARGET) in 18 325 patients aged 50 years or older with osteoarthritis, who were randomized to lumiracoxib (400 mg/day; n=9156), ibuprofen (800 mg tds; n=4415), or naproxen (500 mg bd; n=4754) for 52 weeks in two substudies of identical design (lumiracoxib versus ibuprofen and lumiracoxib versus naproxen) (92). Randomization was stratified for low-dose aspirin and age. The primary cardiovascular end points were the ATC end-points of non-fatal and silent myocardial infarction, stroke, or cardiovascular death. At 1 year of follow up, the incidence of the primary end-point was low and did not differ between treatment groups: lumiracoxib 59 events (0.65%), NSAIDs 50 events (0.55%; hazard ratio 1.14; CI=0.28, 1.66). The incidence of myocardial infarction in the overall population in the individual substudies was 0.38% with lumiracoxib (18 events) versus 0.21% with naproxen (10 events), and 0.11% with lumiracoxib (5 events) versus 0.16% (7 events) with ibuprofen. In both substudies the rates of myocardial infarction did not differ significantly between lumiracoxib and NSAIDs, irrespective of aspirin use.

These TARGET trial data suggest that lumiracoxib does not have the potential to precipitate adverse cardiovascular events more often than NSAIDs. However, these results must be interpreted with caution (93) for several reasons:

- patients with known and significant pre-existing coronary artery disease were excluded, which explains the overall low frequency of cardiovascular events and introduced bias into the generalizability of the TARGET results;
- the statistical power was inadequate to detect significant differences in the rates of myocardial infarction, again raising concern about an excess, albeit not a statistically significant one, of myocardial infarctions with lumiracoxib compared with naproxen: 18 events (0.38%) versus 10 events (0.21%); hazard ratio 1.77 (0.82, 3.84).
- lumiracoxib significantly reduced the frequency of upper gastrointestinal ulcer complications (NNT to prevent one ulcer complication 139) but only in patients not taking low-dose aspirin (94), confirming the results of other coxib trials (CLASS).
- the data raised a concern about possible hepatotoxicity of lumiracoxib; the proportion of patients with transaminase activities more than three times the upper limit of the reference range differed significantly between lumiracoxib (2.57%, n=230) and NSAIDs (0.63%, n=56; hazard ratio 3.97; CI=2.96, 5.32).

Valdecoxib and parecoxib

Further support of the hypothesis that the increase in cardiovascular risk is a COX-2 class effect has come from an analysis of clinical trials of valdecoxib and its pro-drug parecoxib.

The cardiovascular safety of valdecoxib was initially assessed in a study that pooled results from 10 clinical trials that included nearly 8000 patients with osteoarthritis and rheumatoid arthritis and compared the incidence of cardiovascular events in patients taking valdecoxib (10–80 mg/day) with those of controls taking diclofenac, ibuprofen, naproxen, or placebo (87). The incidences of cardiovascular thrombotic events (cardiac, cerebrovascular, and peripheral vascular or arterial thrombotic) were similar with valdecoxib, the conventional NSAIDs, and placebo. Short-term and intermediate-term treatment with valdecoxib in therapeutic doses (10 or 20 mg/day) and supratherapeutic doses (40–80 mg/day) was not associated with an increased incidence of thrombotic events. In contrast, recent studies have raise serious doubts about the safety of valdecoxib in patients who are at high risk of thrombotic complications, such those undergoing coronary artery bypass surgery.

The cardiovascular toxicity of valdecoxib and its prodrug parecoxib has been studied in two randomized placebo-controlled trial and one meta-analysis. The first study involved 462 patients and evaluated the safety and efficacy of intravenous parecoxib (parecoxib 40 mg intravenously every 12 hours for 3 days postoperatively), followed by oral valdecoxib (40 mg every 12 hours for a total of 14 days) (95). In the second study, which involved more than 1600 patients, a similar schedule of administration was used, but the dosage and duration of treatment were reduced (20 mg bd for 10 days) (96). In both studies there were clusters of cardiovascular adverse events, including myocardial infarction, stroke, deep vein thrombosis, and pulmonary embolism, which were more frequent in those who were given parecoxib than in the controls, although the difference was not statistically significant. However, when the coronary and cerebrovascular events were combined in a meta-analysis parecoxib/valdecoxib was associated with a three-fold risk of cardiovascular events compared with placebo: 31/1399 events versus 5/699 (RR=3.08; CI=1.20, 7.87) (97).

Following this important information a new warning contraindicating the use of parecoxib/valdecoxib in patients undergoing coronary artery bypass grafting was added to the label by many drug control agencies. Meanwhile the FDA received reports of 87 cases of severe skin reactions associated with valdecoxib, including Stevens–Johnson syndrome and toxic epidermal necrolysis, with four deaths; 20 of the 87 cases involved patients with a known allergy to sulfa-containing drugs, of which valdecoxib is one; thus, patients allergic to sulfa drugs may be at greater risk of severe skin reactions with valdecoxib. These data have raised concerns not only about the cardiovascular safety of valdecoxib in the general population but also about its overall benefit to harm profile. The drug manufacturers and regulatory agencies in the USA and Europe agreed to suspend valdecoxib in April 2005 (98).

Conclusions

At present at least three important questions about the adverse cardiovascular effects of COX-2 selective inhibitors remain unanswered.

First, the mechanism whereby COX-2 inhibitors facilitate ischemic cardiovascular events is unclear. The major unanswered question is whether unopposed COX-2 inhibition or other drug-specific mechanisms cause the increased cardiovascular risk. It is worth noting that in addition to ischemic cardiovascular disease, COX-2 inhibitors are associated with other adverse cardiovascular effects, such as heart failure (99,100), hypertension (101,102), and edema (103).

Secondly, it is still unknown whether the cardiovascular risk is or is not a class effect. Since at least three separate drugs in the class (rofecoxib, valdecoxib, and celecoxib) have now been associated with increased cardiovascular morbidity, the burden of proof has been shifted to those who deny a class effect. We must remember that absence of evidence is not evidence of absence (36).

Thirdly, there is uncertainty about what physicians should do if they decide to prescribe an NSAID. In light of the current uncertainty about whether cardiotoxicity is a class effect, coxibs, in particular at high dosages and for long-term use, should not be prescribed, particularly in populations at high risk, such as elderly patients and those with established cardiovascular disease. This recommendation is fully justified in light of the possible consequences of the current heavy unjustified promotion of these compounds to both patients and prescribers. A recent epidemiological study in Ontario, Canada showed that the use of NSAIDs in patients aged 66 years or older increased by 41% after the introduction of coxibs (104). This rise was entirely attributable to the use of coxibs and was accompanied by a 10% increase in hospitalization for upper gastrointestinal bleeding.

The continued commercial availability of coxibs is therefore troubling, and probably unjustified, in the light of their marginal efficacy, heightened risk, and higher costs compared with traditional NSAIDs.

The coxib debate will not go away until these safety and efficacy questions have been answered (92).

Hypertension

The shift in hemostatic balance toward a prothrombotic state might not be the only mechanism by which COX-2 inhibitors could increase the risk of cardiovascular adverse effects. In fact, non-selective NSAIDs can raise blood pressure and antagonize the hypotensive effect of antihypertensive medications to an extent that may increase hypertension-related morbidity (105,106). The problem is clinically relevant, as arthritis and hypertension are common co-morbid conditions in elderly people, requiring concurrent therapy.

Information on the effect of COX-2-selective inhibitors on arterial blood pressure is scanty. In VIGOR, more patients developed hypertension with rofecoxib than naproxen. For rofecoxib, the mean increase in blood pressure was 4.6/1.7 mmHg compared with a 1.0/0.1 mmHg increase with naproxen (43). Previous work has shown that a 2 mmHg reduction in diastolic blood pressure can result in about a 40% reduction in the rate of stroke and a 25% reduction in the rate of myocardial infarction (107). The effect of celecoxib on blood pressure was evaluated in a post hoc analysis using the safety database generated during the celecoxib clinical development program in more than 13 000 subjects (108). The incidence of hypertension after celecoxib was greater than that after placebo but similar to that after non-selective NSAIDs. Hypertension and exacerbation of pre-existing hypertension occurred, respectively, in 0.8 and 0.6% of patients. Furthermore, there was no evidence of interactions between celecoxib and other antihypertensive drugs.

The safety profiles of celecoxib (200 mg/day) and rofecoxib (25 mg/day) have recently been compared in a 6-week, randomized, parallel-group, double-blind trial in 810 patients with osteoarthritis aged 65 years or over taking antihypertensive drugs (109). The primary endpoints were edema and changes in systolic and diastolic blood pressures, measured at baseline and after 1, 2, and 6 weeks. Systolic blood pressure rose significantly in 17% of rofecoxib-treated patients ($n = 399$) compared with 11% of celecoxib-treated patients ($n = 411$), a statistically significant difference, at any time in the study. Diastolic blood pressure rose in 2.3% of rofecoxib-treated patients

compared with 1.5% of celecoxib-treated patients, a non-significant difference. At week 6, the change from baseline in mean systolic blood pressure was +2.6 mmHg for rofecoxib compared with –0.5 mmHg for celecoxib, a highly significant difference. Nearly twice as many rofecoxib-treated than celecoxib-treated patients had edema. Despite some limitations, this study provides some evidence that COX-2-selective inhibitors may differ in their ability to alter arterial blood pressure.

Cardiac dysrhythmias

There have been reports of celecoxib-associated torsade de pointes in three patients who had never had any complaints before celecoxib administration; the dysrhythmia did not recur after the drug was withdrawn (110). However, all three patients had cardiac abnormalities that might have predisposed them to the development of torsade de pointes, and the follow-up period was too short to evaluate possible spontaneous recurrence. The hypothesis that celecoxib is dysrhythmogenic requires confirmation.

Respiratory

Most people tolerate aspirin well, but not patients with asthma, of whom there is a subgroup in whom aspirin precipitates asthmatic attacks (111,112). This is a distinct clinical syndrome, called aspirin-induced asthma, which affects about 10% of adults with asthma (113). Aspirin-induced asthma is usually accompanied by naso-ocular symptoms and can be triggered not only by aspirin, but by several NSAIDs, a fact that makes immunological cross-reactivity most unlikely. The propensity of an NSAID to precipitate an attack of asthma is probably related to inhibition of COX. There is evidence that potent inhibitors of COX-1 (such as ibuprofen, indometacin, and naproxen) are more likely to precipitate bronchoconstriction than NSAIDs that inhibit COX-2 preferentially (such as meloxicam and nimesulide) (114,115). A widely accepted hypothesis is that in patients with asthma and aspirin intolerance, NSAID-induced COX inhibition results in increased products from the 5-lipoxygenase pathway, the leukotrienes, which are both potent bronchoconstrictors and also inducers of mucous hypersecretion and airway edema. The leukotrienes implicated in aspirin intolerance are cysteinyl leukotrienes (111,113), but leukotriene release is probably not the only pathogenic mechanism.

The hypothesis that in aspirin-induced asthma the attacks are triggered by inhibition of COX-1 and not COX-2 has been tested in three small studies, two of which were double-blind and placebo-controlled (116–118). In the first study (116) 12 patients with aspirin-induced asthma were challenged with increasing doses of rofecoxib (1.25–25 mg/day for 5 days); no patients had any adverse symptoms, and biochemical markers that reflect intolerance to aspirin in asthma (urinary leukotriene E4 and 9α-11β-PGF-2) were unchanged.

In the second study, 60 aspirin-sensitive asthmatics were challenged with oral rofecoxib (12.5 and 25 mg/day for 2 days) (117). There were no signs or symptoms of asthma in any patient and no reductions in FEV_1.

In the third study, 27 patients with stable chronic asthma in whom inhalation of lysine aspirin caused a 20% fall in FEV_1 were challenged with increasing doses of oral celecoxib (from 10 to 200 mg/day); they do not develop bronchoconstriction or other extrapulmonary reactions (118).

So, is the safety of COX-2 inhibitors in patients with aspirin-induced asthma sufficiently well documented? Avoidance of NSAIDs is crucial in patients with asthma who have aspirin sensitivity, and hitherto two alternative analgesic options have been available: paracetamol and non-acetylated salicylates. Paracetamol is a generally safe substitute; however, it is a weak COX inhibitor and, albeit very rarely, patients who are sensitive to aspirin have an adverse reaction to high-dose paracetamol (119). Choline magnesium salicylate and salicylic acid are also weak COX inhibitors and should therefore be used with care in these patients. The results of the above-mentioned studies suggest that rofecoxib and celecoxib can be taken safely by patients with aspirin-induced asthma. However, this conclusion must be treated with caution, as only a few patients were studied and this does not exclude COX-2 inhibitors from participating in other types of reactions, including immune recognition after prior treatment.

Nervous system

Aseptic meningitis is a rare complication of NSAID therapy. Five serious cases of aseptic meningitis associated with rofecoxib have been reported (120).

- A 55-year-old woman who had taken rofecoxib for 1 month reported numbness and tingling on the left side of the tongue and left hand (121). The association between paresthesia and rofecoxib was supported by the time-course of the reaction and resolution after withdrawal.

Because this patient was using other medications (paroxetine, zolpidem, and sumatriptan), which can have a similar effect, this report requires confirmation.

Sensory systems

There is evidence that celecoxib and rofecoxib can be associated with visual impairment (122), and visual disturbances associated with standard or COX-2 selective NSAIDs may be more frequent than previously thought and may be under-recognized. There have been two cases of more severe visual disturbances, one of temporary blindness related to celecoxib, and one that suggested a visual field defect related to rofecoxib. There have also been another five less specific reports of blurred or abnormal vision. One patient who had blurred vision while taking celecoxib had similar symptoms many years before while taking indometacin. Four of seven patients had an onset time of visual impairment of 1 week or less. One patient regularly had problems for a few hours after each dose. All the patients recovered rapidly (within one or two days of withdrawal), which suggests the absence of vascular embolism or thrombosis. A likely mechanism for the visual impairment is inhibition of the synthesis of prostaglandins and other related compounds that control retinal blood flow. As these adverse reactions have also been reported with conventional NSAIDs, it is likely that inhibition of either COX-1 or COX-2 alters the cyclo-oxygenase pathway and in turn alters regulation of retinal blood flow, with potential changes in vision.

Psychiatric

Psychiatric effects have been previously reported with celecoxib (SEDA-26, 123), and may represent a class effect of the COX-2 inhibitors, according to the Australian Adverse Reactions Advisory Committee (ADRAC), which has received 142 reports of acute neuropsychiatric reactions attributed to celecoxib and 49 to rofecoxib (123). The most common reactions associated with celecoxib were: confusion (n=23) somnolence (n=22), and insomnia (n=21), while those associated with rofecoxib were confusion (n=18) and hallucinations (n=11). In many cases the onset of the reaction occurred within 24 hours of the first dose of the drug.

Hematologic

Platelets have only the COX-1 isoform for generating thromboxane to precipitate platelet aggregation. Therefore, selective COX-2 inhibitors have no effect on platelet aggregation or bleeding time (3,124). On the other hand, COX-2 plays a role in the production of endothelial PGI2. In vitro studies have shown that COX-2 expression is up-regulated in endothelial cells by laminar shear stress (125). Furthermore, selective COX-2 inhibitors reduce systemic PGI-2 production in healthy volunteers (126). The clinical implications of these observations are unknown. In theory, COX-2 selective NSAIDs might increase the risk of thromboembolic cardiovascular events because of preferential inhibition of endothelial prostacyclin synthesis without corresponding inhibition of platelet thromboxane synthesis, but no reliable data are available on the occurrence of cardiovascular events in patients treated with COX-2 selective or non-selective NSAIDs.

Gastrointestinal

Gastric damage

Evidence that the COX-2 selective agents cause less damage to the gastrointestinal mucosa than traditional NSAIDs is still limited. Gastrointestinal tolerability has been evaluated by measuring the frequency and severity of gastrointestinal adverse effects during randomized comparative efficacy trials, by performing microbleeding or endoscopic studies, and by evaluating the incidence of severe ulcer complications. Evidence from efficacy trials suggests an incidence of unwanted gastrointestinal effects (dyspepsia, epigastric abdominal pain, nausea, or diarrhea) similar to that caused by the traditional NSAIDs (1,15–17,20,127). The withdrawal rate from clinical trials because of unwanted effects (gastrointestinal or as a whole) was also similar, the only exception being one study in which fewer patients with rheumatoid arthritis stopped taking celecoxib than stopped taking diclofenac

(16). However, the clinical importance of the frequency and severity of symptoms is uncertain. In fact, it is well known that symptoms do not necessarily predict the presence of mucosal damage, and it is still unclear if patients who have dyspeptic symptoms associated with NSAIDs are at greater or lesser risk of serious gastrointestinal complications (SEDA-15, 92) (SEDA-17, 103), the crucial question in evaluating these drugs.

In endoscopic comparisons of the new compounds with placebo or older NSAIDs, in both healthy volunteers and patients with rheumatoid arthritis or osteoarthritis, endoscopically observed lesions (erosions, ulcers) in the stomach and duodenum were undoubtedly fewer with the two COX-2-selective compounds than with non-selective NSAIDs (16,127–130) and were similar to those found with placebo (1).

However, the clinical significance of endoscopically detected erosions and ulcers is debatable (SEDA-14, 131) (SEDA-20, 97), as there is much controversy about whether endoscopic ulcers are surrogates for clinical outcomes such as perforation, obstruction, and gastrointestinal bleeding (130). Thus, although endoscopic studies are an important step in the evaluation of COX-2-selective inhibitors, large-scale, prospective, randomized outcome studies are necessary before we can definitively determine if these drugs will indeed represent significantly safer alternatives to the older NSAIDs. Unfortunately, these prospective comparative complication trials are difficult to perform, as the absolute rate of serious gastrointestinal complications (perforation, obstruction, and bleeding) is low (about 2% per year) (130) and so a large number of patients must be studied.

Suggestions for improved gastrointestinal safety of COX-2-selective inhibitors have come from two studies, which addressed the problem of sample size by pooling published and unpublished randomized, double-blind trials of varying design and duration, comparing celecoxib, rofecoxib, non-selective NSAIDs (diclofenac, ibuprofen, nabumetone), and placebo in patients with osteoarthritis and/or rheumatoid arthritis.

In the first study the results of eight studies were pooled (131). The sample size of 5435 patients was large enough to detect even small differences in rates of complicated ulcers (perforation, symptomatic ulcers, and bleeding ulcers). Over 12 months complicated ulcers occurred at a rate of 1.33 per 100 patient-years with rofecoxib and 2.60 per 100 patient-years with non-selective NSAIDs. The analysis of confirmed upper gastrointestinal perforations, symptomatic ulcers, and upper gastrointestinal bleeding showed a relative risk (RR) with rofecoxib versus NSAIDs of 0.51 (95% CI = 0.26, 1.00). The difference between rofecoxib and the usual NSAIDs in the incidence of perforation, symptomatic ulcers, and bleeding ulcers became statistically significant as early as 6 weeks and remained so up to 12 months. However, this study has some limitations: first, it was not a prospective analysis or a properly conducted meta-analysis; secondly, there were only enough patient-years of exposure to compare rofecoxib with pooled traditional NSAIDs rather than individual drugs; thirdly, the confidence intervals were wide and compatible with no difference between the two

treatment groups; fourthly, the time to exposure with any selective drug or placebo was too short to give a good prediction of actual complication rates with typical use.

In the second analysis, data from 14 studies of the efficacy of celecoxib in osteoarthritis or rheumatoid arthritis in 11 007 patients were pooled (132,133). Gastrointestinal complications (bleeding, obstruction, or perforation) occurred in 0.2% of the patients per year of exposure to celecoxib and in 1.7% per year of exposure to traditional NSAIDs. The absolute risk reduction was 1.5% (CI = 0.4, 2.6). This study, too, had some limitations. In fact, ulcer complication was not the specified end-point of the studies that were pooled, and about 15% of celecoxib-treated patients took a dose below that indicated for arthritis.

Assuming that a COX-2-selective inhibitor will prevent complicated ulcers in 50% of patients, it has been calculated that the NNT for avoiding one complicated ulcer each year in low-risk patients with rheumatoid arthritis (that is with a 0.4% risk of ulcer complications) is 500. On the other hand, in patients at higher risk (that is a 5% risk for ulcer complications) the NNT is 40 (134). It is therefore of paramount importance that studies currently under way confirm the same benefit from COX-2-selective agents in patients with a high risk of ulcer complications (that is aged 75 years or older, with a prior history of ulcer and gastrointestinal tract bleeding, taking low-dose aspirin for cardiovascular disease).

Two large trials have addressed the efficacy of COX-2 selective inhibitors and the associated risk of gastrointestinal complications: the CLASS and the VIGOR trial (32,33).

The CLASS consisted of two separate studies, in which celecoxib was compared with ibuprofen and diclofenac; the results obtained from the two traditional NSAIDs were pooled for analysis. Overall, 3987 patients with osteoarthritis and rheumatoid arthritis took celecoxib (400 mg bd), 1985 patients took ibuprofen (800 mg tds), and 1996 took diclofenac (75 mg bd). The study lasted 13 months, but only the data from 6 months of follow-up were published initially.

There was no statistically significant difference between the two groups in the incidence of the primary end-point of complicated ulcers (upper gastrointestinal bleeding, ulcer perforation, gastric outlet obstruction); the annualized incidence of complicated ulcers in patients taking celecoxib was 0.76% (11 events per 1441 patient-years) versus an incidence of 1.45% (20 events per 1384 patient-years) in patients taking the non-selective NSAIDs, a non-significant difference. However, for the composite end-point of upper gastrointestinal ulcer complications plus symptomatic gastroduodenal ulcers, celecoxib was significantly better tolerated than traditional NSAIDs; the annualized incidence was 2.08% (30 events per 1441 patient-years) with celecoxib versus 3.54% (49 events per 1384 patient-years) for patients taking traditional NSAIDs, significantly different.

The lack of difference in the rate of ulcer complications between the two treatments appeared to be a function of the higher-than-expected rate of complicated ulcers in those taking celecoxib compared with previous studies

(133). Further analysis showed that this increase in complications was likely to be attributable to concurrent low-dose aspirin; the annualized incidence of upper gastrointestinal tract ulcer complications and of symptomatic gastroduodenal ulcers in patients not taking low-dose aspirin was significantly lower with celecoxib than with non-selective NSAIDs (0.44% or 5 events per 1143 patient-years versus 1.27% or 14 events per 1101 patient-years respectively). In patients taking aspirin, the annualized incidence of upper gastrointestinal complications and symptomatic ulcers were not significantly different (4.7% or 14 events per 298 patient-years in patients taking celecoxib versus 6.0% or 17 events per 283 patient-years in those taking traditional NSAIDs).

Moreover, the overall incidence of gastrointestinal symptoms in patients taking celecoxib was only slightly lower than that of patients taking the traditional NSAIDs, as was the rate of withdrawal due to gastrointestinal intolerance in both users and non-users of low-dose aspirin.

This subgroup analysis shows what might be called "competing co-morbidity"; that is, in the subgoup of patients taking aspirin as prophylaxis against ischemic heart disease, the gastrointestinal safety advantage of celecoxib over traditional NSAIDs was almost totally wiped out by the use of aspirin (135).

Despite that, the authors of CLASS concluded by stating that celecoxib caused fewer symptomatic ulcers and ulcer complications than ibuprofen or diclofenac at 6 months.

However, these conclusions were not only contradicted by the published data (32), but were also called into question by subsequent information on the trial available to the FDA (136,137). As was first described on the FDA website, the published account of CLASS differed from the original protocol in many respects (in primary outcomes, statistical analysis, and trial duration). In particular, the published article represented selective reporting of the combined analysis of only the first 6 months of two separate protocols of longer duration: the first a 12-month comparison of celecoxib with diclofenac and the other a 16-month comparison of celecoxib with ibuprofen. The unpublished data show that by week 65 celecoxib was associated with a similar number of ulcer complications as diclofenac and ibuprofen and that the relative risks of both complicated ulcers and all serious gastrointestinal adverse events were higher at 12–16 months than they were at 6 months, suggesting an increased risk of serious adverse events with celecoxib long-term therapy.

Serious criticism was therefore aimed at the authors on the grounds of design, data analysis, and misleading presentation of the results. They were charged with having published and circulated overoptimistic short-term pooled data from different protocols, and of omitting disappointing long-term data. They replied to these criticisms, but their explanations were not considered to be convincing (138–140). Furthermore, Pharmacia, the manufacturers of celecoxib, continue to present inappropriately pooled short-term results from different protocols performed in different continents with different comparator drugs for the SUCCESS 1 trial, the successor to CLASS (138–140).

In the VIGOR study, 8076 patients with rheumatoid arthritis were randomly assigned to receive rofecoxib 50 mg/day or naproxen 500 mg bd. The primary end-point was a confirmed clinical upper gastrointestinal event (gastroduodenal perforation or obstruction, upper gastrointestinal bleeding, and symptomatic gastroduodenal ulcer).

Overall, confirmed upper gastrointestinal events occurred in 177 patients, 56 with rofecoxib ($n = 4047$), and 121 in those taking naproxen ($n = 4029$). In 53 of these patients (16 taking rofecoxib and 37 taking naproxen) the event was complicated. That means that during a median follow-up of 9.0 months, there were 2.1 confirmed gastrointestinal events per 100 patient-years with rofecoxib compared with 4.5 per 100 patient-years with naproxen (RR = 0.5; 95% CI = 0.2, 0.8). The respective rates of complicated ulcers (perforation, obstruction, and bleeding) were 0.6 per 100 patient-years and 1.4 per 100 patient-years (RR = 0.4; 95% CI = 0.2, 0.8).

It is also worth noting that the most common adverse events that led to withdrawal of treatment, excluding the primary gastrointestinal end-points, were dyspepsia, abdominal pain, epigastric discomfort, nausea, and heartburn and that significantly fewer patients discontinued treatment as a result of any one of these five upper gastrointestinal symptoms in the rofecoxib group (3.5%) than in the naproxen group (4.9%).

Problems have also occurred in interpreting the results of VIGOR (33). There were significantly fewer upper gastrointestinal adverse events with rofecoxib compared with naproxen, but an unexpected substantial excess of serious cardiovascular events, making the overall safety of rofecoxib uncertain. When the complete data from VIGOR were presented and all serious adverse events were included (not just gastrointestinal events) the patients who took naproxen had fewer overall serious events: 9.3% of the patients who took rofecoxib had a serious adverse event, compared with 7.8% of those who took naproxen (RR = 0.81; 95% CI = 0.62, 0.97).

The reasons for the discrepancy between celecoxib and rofecoxib in the frequency of upper gastrointestinal complications are not clear, but some hypotheses have been proposed. First, aspirin was used concomitantly with celecoxib (20% of patients) in CLASS but not in VIGOR, increasing the risk of gastrointestinal damage. Secondly, diclofenac (which has greater COX-2 selectivity than naproxen) was used as a comparator in CLASS. Thirdly, the dosages of celecoxib were too high and at the doses studied in CLASS celecoxib might not have had true selectivity for COX-2. Finally, the selectivity of celecoxib for COX-2 is probably lower than that of rofecoxib. Therefore, given major differences in study design and data analysis between the two trials, a valid comparison of the two coxibs is not possible from these data alone; a head-to-head comparison in a large outcome study is needed (141).

Two recently published articles have helped to clarify this point: a systematic review of randomized clinical trials on the upper gastrointestinal safety of celecoxib (142) and a population-based retrospective cohort comparison of the rate of upper gastrointestinal hemorrhages in over 40 000 NSAID-naïve elderly users of non-selective NSAIDs, celecoxib, or rofecoxib with the rate in 100 000 patients who had not been exposed to NSAIDs (143).

In the systematic review, all published and unpublished randomized clinical trials that compared at least 12 weeks of celecoxib treatment with placebo or a traditional NSAID (diclofenac, ibuprofen, naproxen) were analysed. Nine of 17 trials fulfilled the inclusion criteria (a total of 15 187 patients). Withdrawals because of drug-related gastrointestinal adverse effects, ulcers detected at endoscopy, and complicated ulcers were used as measures of gastrointestinal tolerability. Compared with those taking non-selective NSAIDs, the patients who took celecoxib had a lower rate of withdrawals because of adverse gastrointestinal effects at 12 weeks (3.2 versus 6.2%), but there was no significant difference between celecoxib and NSAIDs in the incidence of withdrawals for all adverse events. The incidence of ulcers detected at routine endoscopy at 12 weeks was also lower in patients who took celecoxib compared with those who took non-selective NSAIDs (6.2 versus 23%). In four trials that provided information on the incidence of ulcers detected by endoscopy according to whether or not patients were taking concomitant aspirin up to 325 mg/day, the benefit provided by celecoxib was greater in patients not taking aspirin. The incidences of ulcers were as follows:

- celecoxib alone 6.2%;
- celecoxib + aspirin 12%;
- non-selective NSAID alone 25%;
- non-selective NSAID + aspirin 26%.

However, these results must be treated with great caution, as the total number of patients who took prophylactic aspirin was small (150 taking celecoxib and 140 taking non-selective NSAIDs) and the largest number of patients came from a single trial (CLASS).

The same warning applies to evaluation of the incidence of complicated ulcers (bleeds, perforation, and obstructions). The incidence of these serious events with celecoxib was 2.7% (11 events) versus 5% (20 events) in patients taking diclofenac or ibuprofen, a non-significant difference.

This meta-analysis has provided further evidence that celecoxib has better upper gastrointestinal tolerability that some traditional NSAIDs when withdrawal from trials due to drug-related adverse effects or ulceration detected during routine endoscopy are used as measures of tolerability. However, not all ulcers detected by endoscopy progress to a serious event, and many probably heal spontaneously; the clinical relevance of this measure is therefore controversial. On the other hand, there is a consensus that ulcer complications, the prime cause of concern with NSAIDs, should be the primary end-point of outcome studies aimed at evaluating the gastrointestinal toxicity of NSAIDs. Unfortunately, this consensus is counterbalanced by the problems of doing such studies, as they need to be very large to achieve even marginal power and there are also problems in evaluating the clinical outcomes (141).

Another study that deserves attention was an observational study of upper gastrointestinal hemorrhage in over 40 000 elderly patients taking COX-2-selective drugs (celecoxib, rofecoxib) or non-selective NSAIDs with and without misoprostol, compared with 100 000 non-NSAID users (143). Of about 1.3 million potential subjects aged 65 years and over, 364 686 (28%) were given an NSAID during the study period (about 1 year). From the total elderly population, the authors identified 5391 users of non-selective NSAIDs, 5087 users of diclofenac plus misoprostol, 14 583 users of rofecoxib, 18 908 users of celecoxib, and 100 000 controls. Most of the users of non-selective NSAIDs were taking naproxen (32%), ibuprofen (23%), or diclofenac (20%). During over 55 000 person-years of follow-up, there were 187 hospitalizations for upper gastrointestinal hemorrhage. Relative to the non-users, there was a significantly greater risk of upper gastrointestinal hemorrhage in the patients who took non-selective NSAIDs (adjusted risk ratio 4.0; 95% CI = 2.3, 6.9), diclofenac plus misoprostol (3.0; 1.7, 5.6), or rofecoxib (1.9; 1.3, 2.6), but not celecoxib (1.0; 0.7, 1.6). There were also significant differences in the risks of upper gastrointestinal hemorrhage. Relative to celecoxib users, there was a higher risk of hospitalization for upper gastrointestinal hemorrhage, not only among users of non-selective NSAIDs and diclofenac plus misoprostol but also among users of rofecoxib.

This study has provided further evidence that the risk of upper gastrointestinal hemorrhage with COX-2 inhibitors is significantly lower than with conventional NSAIDs, whether or not they are taken with misoprostol. The apparently greater risk of gastrointestinal hemorrhage with rofecoxib than with celecoxib needs confirmation, as the study had some limitations, of which the most important were the low absolute number of events in the study group and the retrospective design.

What are the implications of these data on the use of the coxibs? Overall they suggest that COX-2 selective inhibitors are less likely to cause upper gastrointestinal damage than some traditional NSAIDs. This advantage is measured by a lower number of events that represent a composite end-point of gastrointestinal toxicity, such as endoscopically detected symptomatic ulcers and serious ulcer complications (perforation, obstruction, bleeding). However, this may not be true in all patients, especially in those who simultaneously take aspirin. This question is of major clinical importance, as many patients with osteoarthritis or rheumatoid arthritis use low-dose aspirin for cardiovascular prophylaxis. We do not know whether gastrointestinal safety is preserved with the use of such combinations, nor whether a proton pump inhibitor should be added in this situation. Furthermore, the data on which of the coxibs has better gastrointestinal tolerability are inconclusive. Large outcome studies will be necessary to solve these questions.

A final consideration is worthwhile. To focus attention only on gastrointestinal events may provide an incomplete picture of the benefit/harm profile of the COX-2 inhibitors. Meta-analysis of mortality and morbidity outcomes from CLASS and VIGOR has suggested that total mortality was higher with coxibs than with non-selective

NSAIDs, although the difference was not statistically significant (30). Moreover, if one takes into account the incidence of serious adverse events (including death, admission to hospital, and any life-threatening event or events leading to serious disability) as a combined measure of harm, the incidence was significantly higher with COX-2 selective compounds than with other NSAIDs, and complicated gastrointestinal ulcers accounted for only a small proportion of total serious adverse events. Non-gastrointestinal serious adverse events call for more attention.

Two other aspects of gastrointestinal toxicity have yet to be studied. First, the use of COX-2 inhibitors in patients with inflammatory bowel disease, in whom it is likely that COX-2 activity is upregulated (144) and in whom traditional NSAIDs may exacerbate the disease. Experimental colitis has been induced both in COX-2-deficient mice and in rats treated with COX-2-selective inhibitors (145). However, in healthy volunteers, rofecoxib did not alter intestinal permeability, in contrast to indometacin, which increased it (146). Studies in patients with inflammatory bowel disease are necessary before considering COX-2 selective inhibitors to be safe in these patients (147).

Secondly, a possible beneficial role of COX-2 on the stomach should also be taken into account. In mice, COX-2 is expressed at the borders of gastric ulcers and has been implicated as a critical factor in promoting repair (11). Whether these experimental data have any clinical relevance is unknown, but this issue raises the possibility that individuals with pre-existing peptic ulcers who take COX-2 selective drugs may be at risk of delayed ulcer healing and potential complications. This issue may be of particular concern in patients with ulcers due to *Helicobacter pylori* infection.

In conclusion, clinical trials have shown that COX-2-selective NSAIDs seem to be less toxic to the gastrointestinal mucosa than traditional ones. However, life-threatening ulcer complications have been reported in patients taking both celecoxib (133,148,149) and rofecoxib (131). The FDA and other regulatory authorities require that drug information sheets for celecoxib and rofecoxib carry gastrointestinal ulcer warnings similar to those for older NSAIDs.

Large bowel damage

Little is known about the effects of COX-2 inhibitors on the colon, although animal evidence suggests that they can worsen or precipitate acute colitis. Features similar to those seen in cases of ischemic colitis have been reported in a patient taking rofecoxib (150).

- A 52-year-old woman with a colostomy for a tumor of the sigmoid colon developed low back pain that radiated to the legs. A bone scan showed no evidence of tumor. She was given rofecoxib 25 mg/day and 4 days later noticed bloody diarrhea from the colostomy. At colonoscopy a large portion of the transverse colon was seen to be hemorrhagic, with nodularity, a superficial exudate, and mucosal edema, with a well-demarcated transition to normal areas. Despite extensive

investigations, no plausible cause of the bloody diarrhea and colitis were found, except the possible involvement of rofecoxib. She stopped taking it and was given intravenous fluids. After 4 days the colostomy stopped oozing blood; colonoscopy showed no evidence of hemorrhage and the mucosa was regenerative. Bleeding did not recur.

Liver

The hepatotoxicity of celecoxib and rofecoxib compared with non-selective NSAIDs (other than bromfenac, nimesulide, and sulindac) has been studied using the US Food and Drug Administration Freedom of Information (FDA/FOI) database and the Uppsala Monitoring Centre (UMC) database (151). There were 158 539 and 185 253 reports relating to NSAIDs in the FDA/FOI and UMC databases respectively; 25% and 16% involved other hepatotoxic drugs. The proportions of reports of hepatic disorders for all COX-2 selective inhibitors and non-selective NSAIDs were 3.0% in the FDA/FOI database and 2.7% in the UMC database. Nimesulide (17% and 14%), bromfenac (12% and 21%), diclofenac (8.1% and 4.7%), and sulindac (6.1 % and 9.9%) were associated with higher rates of hepatic disorders than other NSAIDs. Crude and adjusted reported odds ratios for the prevalences of overall hepatic disorders and hepatic failure with celecoxib and rofecoxib versus the other NSAIDs were all less than 1.0 in both databases. Thus, bromfenac, nimesulide, sulindac, and diclofenac had higher proportions of reports of hepatic disorders compared with other NSAIDs. The analysis did not raise concerns about celecoxib or rofecoxib compared with NSAIDs.

Pancreas

Two case reports have suggested a potential association between the sulfonamide group in celecoxib and the development of acute pancreatitis (152,153). The cause of acute pancreatitis in patients taking celecoxib is speculative, but sulfonamides are known to cause pancreatitis, and one of these patients reported an allergy to sulfa medication. Thus, the reaction might have been allergic in nature.

Urinary tract

Kidneys

Renal dysfunction after therapy with COX-2 inhibitors is not unexpected. COX-2 is expressed in the normal human kidney, especially in endothelial and smooth muscle cells of the vasculature and glomerular epithelial cells. Angiotensin II and endothelin induce and upregulate COX-2 and prostaglandin synthesis. Furthermore, it seems reasonable to hypothesize that intrarenal dependence on COX-2-synthesized prostaglandins increases in heart failure, liver failure, volume depletion, and chronic renal disease (154). It is thought that in healthy kidneys COX-2 plays an important role in the balance of water and electrolytes, and its activity is upregulated in patients with reduced left ventricular filling pressure, to help maximize renal blood flow.

As experience with COX-2-selective inhibitors accumulates, it appears that the pattern of nephrotoxicity is similar to that of traditional NSAIDs (155,156). Non-selective NSAIDs can cause hemodynamically mediated acute renal insufficiency in predisposed patients and can cause sodium and water retention, causing peripheral edema and hypertension. Efficacy trials have shown a similar incidence of pedal edema, renal adverse effects, and hypertension with COX-2 selective and non-selective NSAIDs (18,127).

- A 43-year-old woman with rheumatoid arthritis developed dizziness having taken celecoxib 200 mg/day for 2 weeks. At the start of treatment she had normal renal function (157). Her serum creatinine was 670 µmol/l (7.4 mg/dl) and blood urea nitrogen 30 mmol/l (90 mg/dl). Creatinine clearance was 16 ml/minute. Urinalysis was normal and casts were not present. Urinary chemical analysis showed a sodium concentration of 18 mmol/l, a fractional excretion of sodium of 0.3, and a renal failure index of 0.493, consistent with prerenal acute renal insufficiency. Celecoxib was withdrawn. Although her renal function then improved, her serum creatinine was still abnormal (4.7 mg/dl) 1 month later.

In a randomized comparison of celecoxib and diclofenac plus omeprazole, renal adverse events, including hypertension, peripheral edema, and renal insufficiency, were common and similar in the two groups (158). They occurred in the 24% of the patients who took celecoxib and in 31% of those who took diclofenac plus omeprazole. Among patients with renal impairment at baseline, 51% of those who took celecoxib and 41% of those who took diclofenac plus omeprazole had renal adverse events. Careful monitoring of renal function in patients taking COX-2 inhibitors or traditional NSAIDs is mandatory, especially in high-risk subjects (for example those with pre-existing renal disease, diabetes, or heart failure).

Two studies in healthy volunteers have shown that the effects of COX-2 inhibitors on renal function are similar to those of traditional non-selective NSAIDs (159,160). The first was a short-term crossover study on renal function in healthy elderly subjects treated with rofecoxib and naproxen. Although there was a greater fall in glomerular filtration rate with naproxen, reductions in the urinary excretion of sodium, prostaglandin E-2, and 6-keto-prostaglandin F-1α were similar with the two compounds (159). In the second study in elderly people taking a low-salt diet, rofecoxib and indometacin significantly lowered the glomerular filtration to a similar extent (160).

However, these data are limited and must be interpreted with caution, since NSAIDs have significant toxic effects on the kidney only in patients at risk (that is those with volume depletion, heart failure, cirrhosis, intrinsic renal disease, and hypercalcemia), in whom the secretion of vasodilator prostaglandins is increased in an attempt to counteract the effect of increased renal vasoconstrictors, such as angiotensin II.

The incidence of adverse effects related to renal function in CLASS and VIGOR was low and similar (0.9% with celecoxib and 1.2% with rofecoxib). The incidence of increased creatinine and urea nitrogen concentrations was slightly lower in patients taking celecoxib than in those taking ibuprofen or diclofenac. Similar results have been documented in two other clinical trials. The first compared celecoxib with diclofenac in long-term management of rheumatoid arthritis in 430 patients (16). There were only small increases in serum creatinine concentration (from 93 µmol/l at baseline to 96 µmol/l at the final visit) and serum urea concentration (from 6.0 to 6.4 mmol/l). There was a similar increase in patients taking diclofenac. The second trial, in 1149 patients, compared celecoxib with naproxen; serum creatinine concentrations were not affected by either celecoxib or naproxen (127). However, data from these clinical trials must be interpreted with caution, as patients at major risk of renal adverse events were likely to be excluded.

In contrast, published case reports and case series have provided more insight into the potential nephrotoxicity associated with COX-2-selective inhibitors. Taken together, these case reports suggest that COX-2 inhibitors, like non-selective NSAIDs, produce similar and consistent renal adverse effects in patients with one or more risk factors that induce prostaglandin-dependent renal function (that is patients with renal and cardiovascular disease and taking a number of culprit medications, such as diuretics and ACE inhibitors). Acute renal insufficiency, disturbances in volume status (edema, heart failure), metabolic acidosis, hyperkalemia, and hyponatremia have been commonly described. The duration of treatment with COX-2 inhibitors before the development of clinically recognized renal impairment ranged from a few days to 3–4 weeks. Withdrawal of COX-2 inhibitors and supportive therapy most often resulted in resolution of renal dysfunction, but in some patients hemodialysis was required (155,161–165).

The renal safety of rofecoxib and celecoxib has been studied using the database of spontaneous reports of adverse drug reactions in the WHO Monitoring Center in Uppsala (166). Disproportionality in the association between COX-2 selective inhibitors and renal-related adverse drug reactions was evaluated using a Bayesian confidence propagation neural network method, in which a statistical parameter (the information component: IC) was calculated for each drug-reaction combination. In this method an IC value significantly greater than 0 implies that the association of a drug-reaction pair is stronger than background; the higher the IC value, the more the combination stands out from the background. As with non-selective NSAIDs, both COX-2 selective inhibitors were associated with renal-related adverse drug reactions. IC values were significantly different for the following comparisons: water retention, abnormal renal function, renal insufficiency, cardiac failure, and hypertension. However, the adverse renal impact of rofecoxib was significantly greater than that of celecoxib. Renal-related events for rofecoxib were two- to four-fold higher than for celecoxib and the severity of these reported adverse reactions was also more serious. Studies based on spontaneous reports have many limitations and their results must therefore be confirmed by additional epidemiological studies that can provide more accurate information on incidence rates and risk factors.

Rare reports of acute reversible renal impairment have been recorded in patients with predisposing factors (162).

Whether selective COX-2 inhibitors can cause the other types of renal toxicity that are associated with non-selective NSAIDs (that is acute interstitial nephritis, nephrotic syndrome with or without renal insufficiency) is not known.

Bladder

The use of NSAIDs to treat and prevent bladder spasms has been documented in clinical trials (167) and their role in relaxing bladder smooth muscle has experimental support (168). Three elderly patients who used rofecoxib or celecoxib developed acute but reversible urinary retention (169). Each had co-morbidities likely to cause bladder dysfunction, and the administration of a COX-2 inhibitor may have caused further relaxation of the detrusor muscle, resulting in urinary retention.

Skin

There have been reports of maculopapular rash (170) and severe erythema multiforme (toxic epidermal necrolysis) (171) with celecoxib. Three patients developed erythema multiforme while taking rofecoxib (172). All were well documented, and oral rechallenge with rofecoxib, positive in two of them, confirmed the role of rofecoxib in the pathogenesis of this adverse reaction.

- Swelling and wrinkling of the palms soon after exposure to water occurred in an 18-year-old-woman taking rofecoxib for mixed connective tissue disease (173). The swelling followed exposure for 1 to a few minutes to water at any temperature. The swelling developed rapidly and was accompanied by symptoms of mild pain and discomfort. Over the following 2 hours, the palms would return to normal. Because of the temporal correlation with the use of rofecoxib, it was withdrawn, and 3 weeks later her symptoms had almost completely resolved.

The authors speculated that this phenomenon might have been due to increased salt content of the skin caused by the rofecoxib, resulting in increased water-binding capacity of keratin.

Musculoskeletal

An in vitro experiment on cartilage explants from patients with osteoarthritis showed upregulation of COX-2 activity, which may be linked to cartilage repair (174). If this is true, long-term use of COX-2 inhibitor NSAIDs could have harmful effect on joints. Preliminary data suggest that these drugs are efficacious in osteoarthritis, at least in the short term.

There have been few human studies of the effects of NSAIDs on fracture healing. The results of a recent retrospective study suggested that NSAID therapy delays fracture healing (175). Overall 20 of 29 NSAID users in a comparable patient population had non-union of femoral fractures compared with 12 of 70 patients who did not took any NSAIDs. In an experimental study this NSAID-induced delay in fracture healing was attributable to inhibition of COX-2, since absent COX-2 gene function prevented normal fracture healing in animals (176).

Although it is difficult to extrapolate from animal studies to humans the available data suggest caution in the long term use of NSAIDs, including COX-2 selective inhibitors, after bone fractures or certain orthopedic procedures until prospective human clinical studies show otherwise.

Reproductive system

Many reproductive processes (ovulation, fertilization, implantation, decidualization, and parturition) depend on prostaglandin ligand–receptor interactions. It is therefore not surprising that selective COX-2 inhibition has a negative local effect on ovulation, resulting in delayed follicular rupture and infertility, without affecting peripheral hormonal cyclicity (177,178).

There have been several case reports that non-selective NSAIDs (diclofenac, naproxen, piroxicam) can cause infertility, attributed to "luteinized unruptured ovarian follicles" syndrome (179–181). Now the syndrome has been documented in a double-blind, randomized, placebo-controlled study, in which women were assessed over two menstrual cycles while taking rofecoxib (178). Women who are trying to become pregnant should avoid taking any NSAIDs if possible, and those who need one for a chronic rheumatic disorder should be aware of possible infertility; in such cases further investigation is not required, as withdrawal of the drug restores fertility.

Immunologic

There is considerable difficulty and controversy in identifying and classifying allergic reactions to NSAIDs, for many reasons (182). First, the difficulty in making a definite diagnosis in patients who have these reactions without provocative challenge with the suspected drug and other NSAIDs. Secondly, reactions are characterized by a large spectrum of target organ responses to NSAIDs, and the same drug can cause different types of reactions in different organs in the same or different individuals. Thirdly, a patient can have a similar reaction to a structurally different NSAID. Finally, reports of these reactions include different, often imprecise, terms, making interpretation difficult. It is worth evaluating the safety of new coxibs in patients who cannot tolerate non-selective NSAIDs.

Anaphylaxis due to celecoxib has been described (SEDA 26, 121). Life-threatening anaphylaxis, with urticaria, angioedema, and bronchospasm, has also been described 30 minutes after a dose of celecoxib for arthritis of the hip (183).

Allergic vasculitis has been reported in association with various NSAIDs, and has been attributed to celecoxib (184,185), including one case with a fatal outcome (186).

Whether allergic reactions to celecoxib occur more often in patients who report a previous reaction to sulfonamides, and should therefore be contraindicated in such patients, is still unknown (187).

Angioedema has been attributed to rofecoxib (SEDA-26, 121).

- A 60-year-old man developed angioedema after taking two doses of rofecoxib 12.5 mg 18 and 12 hours before (188). Despite intensive treatment he developed pulmonary hemorrhagic edema and died a day later. He had fibrotic lung disease, which may have predisposed him to the lethal event.

The tolerability of rofecoxib in patients with cutaneous allergic and pseudoallergic adverse reactions to non-selective NSAIDs has been confirmed in a study in 139 patients with NSAID-induced adverse reactions: 60 with urticaria alone (43%), 34 with angioedema (25%), 34 with angioedema plus urticaria (2.9%), and 2 with Stevens–Johnson syndrome (1.4%) (189). They all underwent a single-blind, placebo-controlled oral challenge with increasing doses of rofecoxib, and 138 of them tolerated it without adverse reactions. Only one had mild urticaria on the arms. Rofecoxib may be a useful alternative in patients with NSAID hypersensitivity.

Anaphylaxis

Among the anaphylactic reactions to NSAIDs that result in different types of reaction (urticaria, angioedema, asthma, or hypotension), there have been very few reports of anaphylactic shock. However, anaphylaxis has been described in patients taking celecoxib (190,191) or rofecoxib (192). Rofecoxib caused anaphylaxis in a patient who had had a similar reaction to diclofenac, suggesting that COX-2 inhibitors may be not safe in all individuals who have adverse reactions to non-selective COX inhibitors. It also suggests that different mechanisms may be involved in patients with asthma and in those with anaphylactoid reactions to NSAIDs.

Sulfonamide-like allergic adverse reactions

Concerns that COX-2 inhibitors may be associated with an increased risk of allergic reactions in patients with a history of sulfonamide hypersensitivity arise from the molecular structures of these compounds (SEDA-24, 119) (193).

A sulfur component is necessary for the receptor binding of both celecoxib and rofecoxib, but their structures differ and they have different potentials for causing allergic reactions. Consequently, celecoxib is thought to be contraindicated in patients with a history of allergy to sulfonamides. The available data on the immunological tolerability profile of celecoxib and rofecoxib are scanty but merit attention.

Sulfonamide-like adverse drug reactions seem to occur more frequently with celecoxib than with rofecoxib, according to a report from Sweden (194). The investigators identified a profile of 19 typical sulfonamide-like adverse reactions from published papers and the WHO Adverse Drug Reactions database from 1968 to 2000, and compared this profile with reported adverse drug reactions associated with celecoxib and rofecoxib. The WHO database contained 11 514 reports about celecoxib describing 21 292 suspected adverse drug reactions and 10 200 reports about rofecoxib describing 18 585 suspected drug reactions. The relative reporting rate of sulfonamide-like adverse drug reactions was almost twice as high for celecoxib as for rofecoxib (RR = 1.8; 95% CI = 1.6, 1.9) for all reports and for reports that listed a COX-2 inhibitor as the only suspected drug. The reporting rate for 15 of the 19 sulfonamide-like adverse drug reactions was higher for celecoxib than for rofecoxib, with significant differences for rash (RR = 2.3; CI = 2.0, 2.6), urticaria (RR = 2.0; CI = 1.6, 24), Stevens–Johnson syndrome (RR = 3.6; CI = 1.4, 12), and photosensitivity (RR = 2.4; CI = 1.5, 4.0). Fatal adverse drug reactions fitting the typical sulfonamide profile also occurred more often with celecoxib than with rofecoxib (1.8; CI = 0.9, 4.0).

Even though serious sulfonamide reactions are rare, their clinical impact warrants close monitoring as more data become available, and physicians should be aware of possible sulfonamide allergy when prescribing COX-2 inhibitors, in particular celecoxib.

There have been single case reports of sulfonamide-like allergic reactions in patients taking celecoxib; in two cases sulfonamide allergy was ignored and was discovered only after an adverse reaction to celecoxib (195) or rofecoxib (196) had occurred.

Urticaria and angioedema

Of 110 patients with a history of urticaria and angioedema triggered by one or more non-selective NSAIDs, who were submitted to 184 single-blind, placebo-controlled oral challenges with the suspected NSAID, patients with a positive challenge underwent further oral challenge with various COX-2 inhibitors (celecoxib and rofecoxib, and also nimesulide and meloxicam, which are relatively selective COX-2 inhibitors) (197). The maximal challenge doses were celecoxib 200 mg, rofecoxib 25 mg, meloxicam 15 mg, and nimesulide 100 mg. Reactions (expressed as a percentage of tested patients with a positive test) varied among the COX-2 inhibitors: 33% (10/30) for celecoxib, 21% (16/75) for nimesulide, 17% (8/46) for meloxicam, and 3% (1/33) for rofecoxib. This suggests that the degree of cross-reactivity of COX-2 inhibitors was related to the degree of in vitro COX-1 inhibition, since meloxicam, nimesulide, and celecoxib inhibit COX-1 to a similar extent (198). The results also suggested that the most selective COX-2 inhibitor (rofecoxib) might be relatively safe in a patient with NSAID-induced urticaria/angioedema.

In another study, 34 patients with a history of urticaria and/or angioedema after ingestion of at least two chemically unrelated non-selective NSAIDs, 22 of whom also had chronic urticaria, all underwent a single-blind, placebo-controlled oral tolerance test with rofecoxib (12 and 25 mg 1 hour apart) (199). Rofecoxib caused urticaria and/or angioedema in 6/34 patients (18%), with no difference between patients with or without a history of chronic urticaria.

There was even better tolerability of rofecoxib in another study in 33 patients with documented urticaria/angioedema after ingestion of two different NSAIDs (200). The patients underwent provocative tests with increasing doses of rofecoxib (from 6.25 to 25 mg); at the end of the challenge all tolerated rofecoxib 25 mg.

Other single case reports have supported the evidence of better tolerability of COX-2-selective inhibitors (in particular rofecoxib) in patients with a history of urticaria/angioedema (64,201). However, contrasting data have shown cross-reactivity of celecoxib with other NSAIDs and between celecoxib and rofecoxib (202).

Why are COX-2-selective drugs better tolerated? The mechanisms underlying intolerance to chemically unrelated NSAIDs are unknown, but it has been hypothesized that intolerant patients may have exaggerated sensitivity to the effects of leukotrienes, which are more active than histamine in inducing wheal and flare reactions. Blockade of both COX-1 and COX-2 by non-selective NSAIDs increases the production of leukotrienes by the lipoxygenase pathway, whereas COX-2-selective agents do not increase the production of LTB_4 or cysteinyl LTS. However, this may not be the only pathogenic mechanism, as some drugs probably trigger histamine release from mast cells and basophils non-specifically, and others may trigger immunological cross-reactivity. Overall, the above-mentioned studies and clinical experience suggest that urticaria and angioedema can occur with COX-2 inhibitors, albeit with a lower frequency than with non-selective NSAIDs.

Second-Generation Effects

Fetotoxicity

A single case report supports the hypothesis that a COX-2-selective NSAID might have the efficacy of indometacin as a tocolytic agent without its adverse effects in the fetus (203).

Susceptibility Factors

Children

Despite the abundance of studies on coxibs in adults, there is a dearth of published data on their use in children (204). One study showed that ibuprofen was better than rofecoxib but equally well tolerated in patients undergoing tonsillectomy when added to paracetamol (205). Children had faster drug clearance of celecoxib and a shorter half-life than adults in a single-dose pharmacokinetic study (206).

While the coxibs appear, at least in the short term, safe and effective in adults, more investigations are needed before widespread use in children can be recommended.

Drug–Drug Interactions

Lithium

A possible interaction of rofecoxib with lithium has been reported (207).

- A 73-year-old man with manic-depressive illness, who had taken lithium for 40 years, underwent coronary bypass surgery and was given long-term warfarin. He developed signs of lithium intoxication (confusion, irritability, tremor, and gait disturbance) after having taken rofecoxib 12.5 mg/day for 9 days for arthritis.

Rofecoxib had been chosen in order to avoid a possible drug interaction with warfarin. Lithium and rofecoxib were withdrawn and the signs resolved within 1 week. His serum lithium concentration was 1.5 mmol/l and his serum creatinine 1430 µmol/l.

Both lithium and rofecoxib have been associated with nephrotoxicity, and it is likely that lithium intoxication was caused by concomitant administration of rofecoxib, causing a reversible reduction in renal function.

In one study, there was a mean increase of only 17% in healthy volunteers taking celecoxib 200 mg bd (210). When celecoxib was co-administered with lithium, celecoxib concentrations were higher for the first 6 hours after the dose but the AUC was not altered significantly (211). In another review it was mentioned that clinically significant interactions with lithium (increased lithium concentrations) had been identified, but no detail was presented (212). Both celecoxib and naproxen reduced the renal clearance of lithium (used as a measure of proximal tubular sodium reabsorption) (213).

There have been several reports of raised serum lithium concentrations and neurotoxic symptoms when COX-2 inhibitors (celecoxib and rofecoxib) were added to an otherwise stable lithium regimen (214,215,216). In 10 patients taking lithium who took rofecoxib 50 mg/day for 5 days serum lithium concentrations increased in 9 and reached 1.26, 1.47, and 1.63 mmol/l in three (details not provided) (217).

- A 44-year-old woman taking nimesulide and ciprofloxacin developed lithium intoxication (serum concentration 3.23 mmol/l) complicated by renal insufficiency; the interaction was attributed to nimesulide (218).

All in all, the COX-2 inhibitors appear to be similar to non-selective NSAIDs with regard to the likelihood of increasing lithium concentrations.

Propofol

A single perioperative dose of parecoxib did not alter the disposition or the clinical effects of a bolus of propofol (208).

Sex hormones

Rofecoxib did not cause any clinically important changes in ethinylestradiol and norethindrone pharmacokinetics in 18 subjects (209).

Warfarin

The Australian Adverse Drug Reactions Advisory Committee (ADRAC) and the New Zealand Pharmacovigilance Centre have received and published case reports of raised International Normalized Ratios (INR) and hemorrhage when celecoxib and rofecoxib were given to patients stabilized on warfarin. Small increases in INR have also been reported with valdecoxib (219,220,221,222). This possible interaction could be mediated by several mechanisms. Firstly, many NSAIDs are substrates for CYP2C9 and may interfere with the oxidative metabolism of S-warfarin, thereby increasing the hypoprothrombinemic response. Secondly, the non-selective NSAIDs may significantly inhibit COX-1 generated thromboxane A_2, impairing platelet aggregation, impairing hemostasis if bleeding occurs. Thirdly, NSAIDs can cause gastric damage and further increase the risk of gastrointestinal bleeding in patients taking warfarin. Differences in the risk of gastrointestinal toxicity may be relevant when evaluating the risk of the interaction in an individual.

Despite the clinical and epidemiological importance of the problem, there is little information on the comparative safety of coxibs and NSAIDs in patients taking warfarin. A nested case-control study has provided some information about the risk of upper gastrointestinal hemorrhage in patients taking warfarin and a non-selective NSAID or a COX-2 inhibitor (223). The patients had had an upper gastrointestinal hemorrhage while taking warfarin. After adjusting for potential confounders, patients taking warfarin were more likely to have been taking celecoxib (OR = 1.7; CI = 1.2, 3.6), rofecoxib (OR = 2.4; CI = 1.7, 3.6), or a non-selective NSAID (OR = 1.9; CI = 1.4, 3.7) relative to controls. These findings suggest that the risk of upper gastrointestinal hemorrhage is equally increased in warfarin users taking either a coxib or a traditional NSAID. If there is co-prescription, careful monitoring of the INR is mandatory and gastric protection wise.

References

1. Feldman M, McMahon AT. Do cyclooxygenase-2 inhibitors provide benefits similar to those of traditional non-steroidal anti-inflammatory drugs, with less gastrointestinal toxicity? Ann Intern Med 2000;132(2):134–43.
2. Hawkey CJ. COX-2 inhibitors. Lancet 1999;353(9149): 307–14.
3. Crofford LJ, Lipsky PE, Brooks P, Abramson SB, Simon LS, van de Putte LB. Basic biology and clinical application of specific cyclooxygenase-2 inhibitors. Arthritis Rheum 2000;43(1):4–13.
4. Brooks P, Emery P, Evans JF, Fenner H, Hawkey CJ, Patrono C, Smolen J, Breedveld F, Day R, Dougados M, Ehrich EW, Gijon-Banos J, Kvien TK, Van Rijswijk MH, Warner T, Zeidler H. Interpreting the clinical significance of the differential inhibition of cyclooxygenase-1 and cyclooxygenase-2. Rheumatology (Oxford) 1999;38(8): 779–88.
5. Gilroy DW, Colville-Nash PR, Willis D, Chivers J, Paul-Clark MJ, Willoughby DA. Inducible cyclooxygenase may have anti-inflammatory properties. Nat Med 1999;5(6):698–701.
6. Zimmermann KC, Sarbia M, Schror K, Weber AA. Constitutive cyclooxygenase-2 expression in healthy human and rabbit gastric mucosa. Mol Pharmacol 1998;54(3):536–40.
7. Iseki S. Immunocytochemical localization of cyclooxygenase-1 and cyclooxygenase-2 in the rat stomach. Histochem J 1995;27(4):323–8.
8. Robert A, Nezamis JE, Lancaster C, Davis JP, Field SO, Hanchar AJ. Mild irritants prevent gastric necrosis through "adaptive cytoprotection" mediated by prostaglandins. Am J Physiol 1983;245(1):G113–21.
9. Gretzer B, Ehrlich K, Maricic N, Lambrecht N, Respondek M, Peskar BM. Selective cyclo-oxygenase-2 inhibitors and their influence on the protective effect of a mild irritant in the rat stomach. Br J Pharmacol 1998;123(5):927–35.
10. Schmassmann A. Mechanisms of ulcer healing and effects of nonsteroidal anti-inflammatory drugs. Am J Med 1998;104(3A):S43–51.
11. Mizuno H, Sakamoto C, Matsuda K, Wada K, Uchida T, Noguchi H, Akamatsu T, Kasuga M. Induction of cyclooxygenase 2 in gastric mucosal lesions and its inhibition by the specific antagonist delays healing in mice. Gastroenterology 1997;112(2):387–97.
12. Takahashi S, Shigeta J, Inoue H, Tanabe T, Okabe S. Localization of cyclooxygenase-2 and regulation of its mRNA expression in gastric ulcers in rats. Am J Physiol 1998;275(5 Pt 1):G1137–45.
13. Seibert K, Zhang Y, Leahy K, Hauser S, Masferrer J, Perkins W, Lee L, Isakson P. Pharmacological and biochemical demonstration of the role of cyclooxygenase 2 in inflammation and pain. Proc Natl Acad Sci USA 1994;91(25):12013–7.
14. Wallace JL, Bak A, McKnight W, Asfaha S, Sharkey KA, MacNaughton WK. Cyclooxygenase 1 contributes to inflammatory responses in rats and mice: implications for gastrointestinal toxicity. Gastroenterology 1998;115(1):101–9.
15. Bensen WG, Fiechtner JJ, McMillen JI, Zhao WW, Yu SS, Woods EM, Hubbard RC, Isakson PC, Verburg KM, Geis GS. Treatment of osteoarthritis with celecoxib, a cyclooxygenase-2 inhibitor: a randomized controlled trial. Mayo Clin Proc 1999;74(11):1095–105.
16. Emery P, Zeidler H, Kvien TK, Guslandi M, Naudin R, Stead H, Verburg KM, Isakson PC, Hubbard RC, Geis GS. Celecoxib versus diclofenac in long-term management of rheumatoid arthritis: randomised double-blind comparison. Lancet 1999;354(9196):2106–11.
17. Zhao SZ, McMillen JI, Markenson JA, Dedhiya SD, Zhao WW, Osterhaus JT, Yu SS. Evaluation of the functional status aspects of health-related quality of life of patients with osteoarthritis treated with celecoxib. Pharmacotherapy 1999;19(11):1269–78.
18. Schnitzer TJ, Truitt K, Fleischmann R, Dalgin P, Block J, Zeng Q, Bolognese J, Seidenberg B, Ehrich EW. The safety profile, tolerability, and effective dose range of rofecoxib in the treatment of rheumatoid arthritis. Phase II Rofecoxib Rheumatoid Arthritis Study Group. Clin Ther 1999;21(10):1688–702.
19. Ehrich EW, Schnitzer TJ, McIlwain H, Levy R, Wolfe F, Weisman M, Zeng Q, Morrison B, Bolognese J, Seidenberg B, Gertz BJRofecoxib Osteoarthritis Pilot Study Group. Effect of specific COX-2 inhibition in osteoarthritis of the knee: a 6 week double blind, placebo controlled pilot study of rofecoxib. J Rheumatol 1999;26(11):2438–47.
20. Day R, Morrison B, Luza A, Castaneda O, Strusberg A, Nahir M, Helgetveit KB, Kress B, Daniels B, Bolognese J, Krupa D, Seidenberg B, Ehrich ERofecoxib/Ibuprofen Comparator Study Group. A randomized trial of the efficacy and tolerability of the COX-2 inhibitor rofecoxib vs ibuprofen in patients with osteoarthritis. Arch Intern Med 2000;160(12):1781–7.
21. Cannon GW, Caldwell JR, Holt P, McLean B, Seidenberg B, Bolognese J, Ehrich E, Mukhopadhyay S, Daniels BRofecoxib Phase III Protocol 035 Study Group. Rofecoxib, a specific inhibitor of cyclooxygenase 2, with

clinical efficacy comparable with that of diclofenac sodium: results of a one-year, randomized, clinical trial in patients with osteoarthritis of the knee and hip. Arthritis Rheum 2000;43(5):978–87.

22. Anonymous. Celecoxib for arthritis. Med Lett Drugs Ther 1999;41(1045):11–2.

23. Anonymous. Rofecoxib for osteoarthritis and pain. Med Lett Drugs Ther 1999;41(1056):59–61.

24. Morrison BW, Christensen S, Yuan W, Brown J, Amlani S, Seidenberg B. Analgesic efficacy of the cyclooxygenase-2-specific inhibitor rofecoxib in post-dental surgery pain: a randomized, controlled trial. Clin Ther 1999;21(6):943–53.

25. Malmstrom K, Daniels S, Kotey P, Seidenberg BC, Desjardins PJ. Comparison of rofecoxib and celecoxib, two cyclooxygenase-2 inhibitors, in postoperative dental pain: a randomized, placebo- and active-comparator-controlled clinical trial. Clin Ther 1999;21(10):1653–63.

26. Ehrich EW, Dallob A, De Lepeleire I, Van Hecken A, Riendeau D, Yuan W, Porras A, Wittreich J, Seibold JR, De Schepper P, Mehlisch DR, Gertz BJ. Characterization of rofecoxib as a cyclooxygenase-2 isoform inhibitor and demonstration of analgesia in the dental pain model. Clin Pharmacol Ther 1999;65(3):336–47.

27. Morrison BW, Daniels SE, Kotey P, Cantu N, Seidenberg B. Rofecoxib, a specific cyclooxygenase-2 inhibitor, in primary dysmenorrhea: a randomized controlled trial. Obstet Gynecol 1999;94(4):504–8.

28. Juni P, Rutjes AW, Dieppe PA. Are selective COX 2 inhibitors superior to traditional non steroidal anti-inflammatory drugs? BMJ 2002;324(7349):1287–8.

29. Jones R. Efficacy and safety of COX 2 inhibitors. BMJ 2002;325(7365):607–8.

30. Wright JM. The double-edged sword of COX-2 selective NSAIDs. CMAJ 2002;167(10):1131–7.

31. McCormack JP, Rangno R. Digging for data from the COX-2 trials. CMAJ 2002;166(13):1649–50.

32. Silverstein FE, Faich G, Goldstein JL, Simon LS, Pincus T, Whelton A, Makuch R, Eisen G, Agrawal NM, Stenson WF, Burr AM, Zhao WW, Kent JD, Lefkowith JB, Verburg KM, Geis GS. Gastrointestinal toxicity with celecoxib vs nonsteroidal anti-inflammatory drugs for osteoarthritis and rheumatoid arthritis: the CLASS study: a randomized controlled trial. Celecoxib Long-term Arthritis Safety Study. JAMA 2000;284(10):1247–55.

33. Bombardier C, Laine L, Reicin A, Shapiro D, Burgos-Vargas R, Davis B, Day R, Ferraz MB, Hawkey CJ, Hochberg MC, Kvien TK, Schnitzer TJVIGOR Study Group. Comparison of upper gastrointestinal toxicity of rofecoxib and naproxen in patients with rheumatoid arthritis. N Engl J Med 2000;343(21):1520–8.

34. Cerezo JG, Hristov RL, Caracas Sansuàn AJ, Vàzques Rodriguez JJ. Outcome trials of COX-2 selective inhibitors: global safety evaluation does not promise benefits. Eur J Pharmacol 2003;59:169–75.

35. Aronson JK. The NSAID roller coaster: more about rofecoxib. Br J Clin Pharmacol 2006;62:257–9.

36. Fitzgerald GA. Coxibs and cardiovascular disease. N Engl J Med 2004;351:1709–11.

37. Linton MRF, Fazio S. Cyclooxygenase-2 and inflammation in atherosclerosis. Curr Opin Pharmacol 2004;4:116–23.

38. Clark DW, Layton D, Shakir SA. Do some inhibitors of COX-2 increase the risk of thromboembolic events? Linking pharmacology with pharmacoepidemiology. Drug Saf 2004;27:427:427–56.

39. Armstrong PW. Balancing the cyclooxygenase portfolio. CMAJ 2006;174:1581–2.

40. Hankey GJ, Eikelboom JW. Cyclooxygenase-2 inhibitors: are they really atherothrombotic, and if not why not? Stroke 2003;34:2736–40.

41. Cipollone F, Fazia M, Iezzi A, Zucchelli M, Pini B, De Cesare D, Ucchino S, Spigon··· F, Bajocchi G, Bei R, Muraro R, Artese L, Piattelli A, Chiarelli F, Cuccurullo F, Mezzetti A. Suppression of the functionally coupled cyclooxygenase-2/prostglandin E synthase as a basis of simvastatin-dependent plaque stabilization in humans. Circulation 2003;107:1479–85.

42. Chenevard R, Hurlimann D, Bechir M, Enseleit F, Spiker L, Hermann M, Riesen Gay S, Gay RE, Neidhart M, Michel B, Luscher TF, Noll G, Ruschitzka F. Selective COX-2 inhibition improves endothelial function in coronary artery disease. Circulation 2003;107:405–9.

43. Mukherjee D, Nissen SE, Topol EJ. Risk of cardiovascular events associated with selective COX-2 inhibitors. JAMA 2001;286(8):954–9.

44. White WB, Faich G, Whelton A, Maurath C, Ridge NJ, Verburg KM, Geis GS, Lefkowith JB. Comparison of thromboembolic events in patients treated with celecoxib, a cyclooxygenase-2 specific inhibitor, versus ibuprofen or diclofenac. Am J Cardiol 2002;89(4):425–30.

45. Sanmuganathan PS, Ghahramani P, Jackson PR, Wallis EJ, Ramsay LE. Aspirin for primary prevention of coronary heart disease: safety and absolute benefit related to coronary risk derived from meta-analysis of randomised trials. Heart 2001;85(3):265–71.

46. Fleming M. Cardiovascular events and COX-2 inhibitors. JAMA 2001;286(22):2808.

47. Burnakis TG. Cardiovascular events and COX-2 inhibitors. JAMA 2001;286(22):2808.

48. Konstam MA, Demopoulos LA. Cardiovascular events and COX-2 inhibitors. JAMA 2001;286(22):2809.

49. Grant KD. Cardiovascular events and COX-2 inhibitors. JAMA 2001;286(22):2809.

50. Haldey EJ, Pappagallo M. Cardiovascular events and COX-2 inhibitors. JAMA 2001;286(22):2809–10.

51. McGeer PL, McGeer EG, Yasojima K. Cardiovascular events and COX-2 inhibitors. JAMA 2001;286(22):2810.

52. White WB, Whelton A. Cardiovascular events and COX-2 inhibitors. JAMA 2001;286(22):2811–2.

53. Konstam MA, Weir MR, Reicin A, Shapiro D, Sperling RS, Barr E, Gertz BJ. Cardiovascular thrombotic events in controlled, clinical trials of rofecoxib. Circulation 2001;104(19):2280–8.

54. FitzGerald GA, Cheng Y, Austin S. COX-2 inhibitors and the cardiovascular system. Clin Exp Rheumatol 2001;19(6 Suppl 25):S31–6.

55. Wooltorton E. What's all the fuss? Safety concerns about COX-2 inhibitors rofecoxib (Vioxx) and celecoxib (Celebrex). CMAJ 2002;166(13):1692–3.

56. Van Hecken A, Schwartz JI, Depre M, De Lepeleire I, Dallob A, Tanaka W, Wynants K, Buntinx A, Arnout J, Wong PH, Ebel DL, Gertz BJ, De Schepper PJ. Comparative inhibitory activity of rofecoxib, meloxicam, diclofenac, ibuprofen, and naproxen on COX-2 versus COX-1 in healthy volunteers. J Clin Pharmacol 2000;40(10):1109–20.

57. Cleland JG. No reduction in cardiovascular risk with NSAIDs-including aspirin? Lancet 2002;359(9301):92–3.

58. Dalen JE. Selective COX-2 Inhibitors, NSAIDs, aspirin, and myocardial infarction. Arch Intern Med 2002;162(10):1091–2.

59. Ray WA, Stein CM, Hall K, Daugherty JR, Griffin MR. Non-steroidal anti-inflammatory drugs and risk of serious

coronary heart disease: an observational cohort study. Lancet 2002;359(9301):118–23.

60. Solomon DH, Glynn RJ, Levin R, Avorn J. Nonsteroidal anti-inflammatory drug use and acute myocardial infarction. Arch Intern Med 2002;162(10):1099–104.

61. Watson DJ, Rhodes T, Cai B, Guess HA. Lower risk of thromboembolic cardiovascular events with naproxen among patients with rheumatoid arthritis. Arch Intern Med 2002;162(10):1105–10.

62. Rahme E, Pilote L, LeLorier J. Association between naproxen use and protection against acute myocardial infarction. Arch Intern Med 2002;162(10):1111–5.

63. Steering Committee of the Physicians' Health Study Research Group. Final report on the aspirin component of the ongoing Physicians' Health Study. N Engl J Med 1989;321(3):129–35.

64. Topol EJ. Failing the public health—rofecoxib, Merck, and the FDA. N Engl J Med 2004;351:1707–9.

65. Bresalier RS, Sandler RS, Quan H, Bolognese JA, Oxenius B, Horgan K, Lines C, Riddell R, Morton D, Lanas A, Konstam MA, Baron JA, Adenomatous Polyp Prevention on Vioxx (APPROVe) Trial Investigators. Cardiovascular events associated with rofecoxib in a colorectal adenoma chemoprevention trial. N Engl J Med 2005;352:1092–102.

66. Jüni P, Nartey L, Reinchenbach S, Sterchi R, Dieppe PA, Egger M. Risk of cardiovascular events and rofecoxib: cumulative meta-analysis. Lancet 2004;364:2021–29.

67. Ray WA, Stein CM, Daugherty JR, Hall K, Arbogast PG, Griffin MR. COX-2 selective non-steroidal anti-inflammatory drugs and risk of serious coronary heart disease. Lancet 2002;360:1071–3.

68. Solomon DH, Schneeweiss S, Glynn RJ, Kiyota Y, Levin R, Mogun H, Avorn J. Relationship between selective cyclooxygenase-2 inhibitors and acute myocardial infarction in older adults. Circulation 2004;109:2068–73.

69. Nissen SE. Adverse cardiovascular effects of rofecoxib. N Engl J Med 2006;355:203–4.

70. Lévesque LE, Brophy JM, Zhang B. Time variations in the risk of myocardial infarction among elderly users of COX-2 inhibitors. CMAJ 2006;174:1563–9.

71. Aronson JK, Ferner RE. Joining the DoTS. New approach to classifying adverse drug reactions. BMJ 2003;327:1222–5.

72. Graham DJ, Campen D, Hui R, Spence M, Cheetham C, Levy G, Shoor S, Ray WA. Risk of acute myocardial infarction and sudden cardiac death in patients treated with cyclo-oxygenase 2 selective and non-selective non-steroidal anti-inflammatory drugs: nested Solomon 21068case-control study. Lancet 2005;365:475–81.

73. Reicin AS, Shapiro D, Sperling RS, Barr E, Yu Q. Comparison of cardiovascular thrombotic events in patients with osteoarthritis treated with rofecoxib versus nonselective nonsteroidal anti-inflammatory drugs (ibuprofen, diclofenac, and nabumetone). Am J Cardiol 2002;89:971–2.

74. Mamdani M, Rochon P, Juurlink DN, Anderson GM, Kopp A, Naglie G, Austin PC, Laupacies A. Effect of selective cyclooxygenase 2 inhibitors and naproxen on short-term risk of acute myocardial infarction in the elderly. Arch Intern Med 2003;163:481–6.

75. Ray WA, Stein CM, Hall K, Daugherty JR, Griffin MR. Non-steroidal anti-inflammatory drugs and risk of serious coronary heart disease: an observational cohort study. Lancet 2002;359:118–23.

76. Kearney P, Baigent C, Godwin J, Halls H, Emberson JR, Patrono C. Do selective cyclo-oxygenease-2 inhibitors and traditional non-steroidal anti-inflammatory drugs increase the risk of atherothrombosis? Meta-analysis of randomised trials. BMJ 2006;332:1302–8.

77. Solomon DH, Avorn J, Stürmer T, Glynn RJ, Mogun H, Schneeweiss S. Cardiovascular outcomes in new users of coxibs and nonsteroidal antiinflammatory drugs: high-risk subgroups and time course of risk. Arthritis Rheum 2006;54(5):1378–89.

78. McGettigan P, Henry D. Cardiovascular risk and inhibition of cyclooxygenase: a systematic review of the observational studies of selective and nonselective inhibitors of cyclooxygenase 2. JAMA 2006;296:1633–44.

79. Solomon SD, McMurray JJV, Pfeffer MA, Wittes J, Fowler R, Finn P, Anderson WF, Zauber A, Hawk W, Bertagnolli M; Adenoma Prevention with Celecoxib (APC) Study Investigators. Cardiovascular risk associated with celecoxib in a clinical trial for colorectal adenoma prevention. N Engl J Med 2005;352:1071–80.

80. Brophy JM. Cardiovascular risk associated with celecoxib. N Engl J Med 2005;352:2648–50.

81. White WB, Faich G, Whelton A, Maurath C, Ridge NJ, Verburg KM, Geis GS, Lefkowith JB. Comparison of thromboembolic events in patients treated with celecoxib, a cyclooxygenase-2 specific inhibitor, versus ibuprofen or diclofenac. Am J Cardiol 2002;89:425–30.

82. White WB, Faich G, Borer JS, Makuch RW. Cardiovascular thrombotic events in arthritis trials of the cyclooxygenase-2 inhibitor celecoxib. Am J Cardiol 2003;92:411–8.

83. Silverstein FE, Faich G, Goldstein JL, Simon LS, Pincus T, Whelton A, Makuch R, Eisen G, Agrawal NM, Stenson WF, Burr AM, Zhao WW, Kent JD, Lefkowith JB, Verburg KM, Geis GS. Gastrointestinal toxicity with celecoxib vs nonsteroidal anti-inflammatory drugs for osteoarthritis and rheumatoid arthritis: the CLASS study: a randomized controlled trial. Celecoxib Long-term Arthritis Safety Study. JAMA 2000;284:1247–55.

84. White WB, West CR, Borer JS, Gorelick PB, Lavange L, Pan SX, Weiner E, Verburg KM. Risk of cardiovascular events in patients receiving celecoxib: a meta-analysis of randomized clinical trials. Am J Cardiol 2007;99(1):91–8.

85. Kimmel SE, Berlin JA, Reilly M, Jaskowiak J, Kishel L, Chittams J, Strom BL. Patients exposed to rofecoxib and celecoxib have different odds of nonfatal myocardial infarction. Ann Intern Med 2005;142:157–64.

86. Shaya FT, Blume SW, Blanchette CM, Weir MR, Mullins CD. Selective cyclooxygenase-2 inhibition and cardiovascular effects: an observational study of a Medicaid population. Arch Intern Med 2005;165:181–6.

87. White WB, Strand V, Roberts R, Whelton A. Effects of the cycloxygenase-2 specific inhibitor valdecoxib versus nonsteroidal antiinflammatory agents and placebo on cardiovascular thrombotic events in patients with arthritis. Am J Ther 2004;11:244–50.

88. Caldwell B, Aldington S, Weatherall M, Shirtcliffe P, Beasley R. Risk of cardiovascular events and celecoxib: a systematic review and meta-analysis. J R Soc Med 2006;99(3):132–40.

89. Ramey DR, Watson DJ, Yu C, Bolognese JA, Curtis SP, Reicin AS. The incidence of upper gastrointestinal adverse events in clinical trials of etoricoxib vs. non-selective NSAIDs: an updated combined analysis. Curr Med Res Opin 2005;21:715–22.

90. Aldington S, Shirtcliffe P, Weatherall M, Beasley R. Systematic review and meta-analysis of the risk of major cardiovascular events with etoricoxib therapy. N Z Med J 2005;118:U1684.

91. Cannon CP, Curtis SP, FitzGerald GA, Krum H, Kaur A, Bolognese JA, Reicin AS, Bombardier C, Weinblatt ME, van der Heijde D, Erdmann E, Laine L; MEDAL Steering Committee. Cardiovascular outcomes with etoricoxib and diclofenac in patients with osteoarthritis and rheumatoid arthritis in the Multinational Etoricoxib and Diclofenac Arthritis Long-term (MEDAL) programme: a randomised comparison. Lancet 2006;368(9549):1771–81.

92. Farkouh ME, KirshnerH, Harrington RA, Ruland S, Verheugt FWA, Schnitzer TJ, Burmster GR, Mysler E, Hochberg MC, Doherty M, Ehrsam E, Gitton X, Krammer G, Mellein B, Gimona A, Matchaba P, Hawkey CJ, Chesebro J, on behalf of the TARGET Study Group. Comparison of lumiracoxib with naproxen and ibuprofen in the therapeutic arthritis research and gastrointestinal event trial (TARGET), cardiovascular outcomes: randomised controlled trial. Lancet 2004;364:675–84.

93. Topol EJ, Falk GW. A coxib a day won't keep the doctor away. Lancet 2004;364:639–40.

94. Schnitzer T, Burmester GR, Mysler E, Hochberg MC, Doherty M, Ehrsam E, Gitton X, Krammer G, Mellein B, Matchaba P, Gimona A, Hawkey CJ, on behalf of the TARGET Study Group. Comparison of lumiracoxib with naproxen and ibuprofen in the therapeutic arthritis research and gastrointestinal event trial (TARGET), reduction in ulcer complications: randomised controlled trial. Lancet 2004;364:665–74.

95. Ott E, Nussmeier NA, Duke PC, Feneck RO, Alston RP, Snabes MC, Hubbard RC, Hsu PH, Saidman LJ, Mangano DT. Efficacy and safety of the cyclooxygenase 2 inhibitors parecoxib and valdecoxib in patients undergoing coronary artery bypass surgery. J Thorac Cardiovasc Surg 2003;125:1481–92.

96. Nussmeier NA, Whelton AA, Brown MT, Langford RM, Hoeft A, Parlow JL, Boyce SW, Verburg KM. Complications of the COX-2 inhibitors parecoxib and valdecoxib after cardiac surgery. N Engl J Med 2005;352:1081–91.

97. Furberg CD, Psaty BM, FitzGerald GA. Parecoxib, valdecoxib, and cardiovascular risk. Circulation 2005;111:249.

98. Ray WA, Griffin MR, Stein CM. Cardiovascular toxicity of valdecoxib. N Engl J Med 2004;361:2767.

99. Mandani M, Juurlink DN, Lee DS, Rochon PA, Kopp A, Naglie G, Austin PC, Laipacis A, Stukel TA. Cyclo-oxygenase-2 inhibitors versus non-selective non-steroidal anti-inflammatory drugs and congestive heart failure outcomes in elderly patients: a population-based cohort study. Lancet 2004;363:1751–6.

100. Hudson M, Richard H, Pilote L. Differences in outcomes of patients with congestive heart failure prescribed celecoxib, rofecoxib, or non-steroidal anti-inflammatory drugs: population based study. BMJ 2005;330:1370.

101. Solomon DH, Scheneewciss S, Levin R, Avorn J. Relationship between COX-2 specific inhibitors and hypertension. Hypertension 2004;44:140–5.

102. Aw TJ, Haas SJ, Liew D, Krum H. Meta-analysis of cyclooxygenase-2 inhibitors and their effects on blood pressure. Arch Intern Med 2005;165:490–6.

103. Wolfe F, Zhao S, Pettitt D. Blood pressure destabilization and edema among 8538 users of celecoxib, rofecoxib, and nonselective nonsteroidal anti-inflammatory drugs (NSAID) and nonusers of NSAID receiving ordinary clinical care. J Rheumatol 2004;31:1035–7.

104. Mamdani M, Juurlink DN, Kopp A, Naglie G, Austin PC, Laupacis A. Gastrointestinal bleeding after the introduction of COX 2 inhibitors: ecological study. BMJ 2004;328:1415–6.

105. Johnson AG, Nguyen TV, Day RO. Do nonsteroidal anti-inflammatory drugs affect blood pressure? A meta-analysis. Ann Intern Med 1994;121(4):289–300.

106. Whelton A. Renal and related cardiovascular effects of conventional and COX-2-specific NSAIDs and non-NSAID analgesics. Am J Ther 2000;7(2):63–74.

107. Collins R, Peto R, MacMahon S, Hebert P, Fiebach NH, Eberlein KA, Godwin J, Qizilbash N, Taylor JO, Hennekens CH. Blood pressure, stroke, and coronary heart disease. Part 2. Short-term reductions in blood pressure: overview of randomised drug trials in their epidemiological context. Lancet 1990;335(8693):827–38.

108. Whelton A, Maurath CJ, Verburg KM, Geis GS. Renal safety and tolerability of celecoxib, a novel cyclooxygenase-2 inhibitor. Am J Ther 2000;7(3):159–75.

109. Whelton A, Fort JG, Puma JA, Normandin D, Bello AE, Verburg KMSUCCESS VI Study Group. Cyclooxygenase-2-specific inhibitors and cardiorenal function: a randomized, controlled trial of celecoxib and rofecoxib in older hypertensive osteoarthritis patients. Am J Ther 2001;8(2):85–95.

110. Pathak A, Boveda S, Defaye P, Mansourati J, Mallaret M, Thebault L, Galinier M, Blanc JJ, Montastruc JL. Celecoxib-associated torsade de pointes. Ann Pharmacother 2002;36(7–8):1290–1.

111. Levy S, Volans G. The use of analgesics in patients with asthma. Drug Saf 2001;24(11):829–41.

112. Szczeklik A, Nizankowska E, Duplaga M. Natural history of aspirin-induced asthma. AIANE Investigators. European Network on Aspirin-Induced Asthma. Eur Respir J 2000;16(3):432–6.

113. Szczeklik A, Stevenson DD. Aspirin-induced asthma: advances in pathogenesis and management. J Allergy Clin Immunol 1999;104(1):5–13.

114. Kosnik M, Music E, Matjaz F, Suskovic S. Relative safety of meloxicam in NSAID-intolerant patients. Allergy 1998;53(12):1231–3.

115. Bianco S, Robuschi M, Petrigni G, Scuri M, Pieroni MG, Refini RM, Vaghi A, Sestini PS. Efficacy and tolerability of nimesulide in asthmatic patients intolerant to aspirin. Drugs 1993;46(Suppl 1):115–20.

116. Szczeklik A, Nizankowska E, Bochenek G, Nagraba K, Mejza F, Swierczynska M. Safety of a specific COX-2 inhibitor in aspirin-induced asthma. Clin Exp Allergy 2001;31(2):219–25.

117. Stevenson DD, Simon RA. Lack of cross-reactivity between rofecoxib and aspirin in aspirin-sensitive patients with asthma. J Allergy Clin Immunol 2001;108(1):47–51.

118. Dahlen B, Szczeklik A, Murray JJCelecoxib in Aspirin-Intolerant Asthma Study Group. Celecoxib in patients with asthma and aspirin intolerance. N Engl J Med 2001;344(2):142.

119. Settipane RA, Stevenson DD. Cross sensitivity with acetaminophen in aspirin-sensitive subjects with asthma. J Allergy Clin Immunol 1989;84(1):26–33.

120. Bonnel RA, Villalba ML, Karwoski CB, Beitz J. Aseptic meningitis associated with rofecoxib. Arch Intern Med 2002;162(6):713–5.

121. Daugherty KK, Gora-Harper ML. Idiopathic paresthesia reaction associated with rofecoxib. Ann Pharmacother 2002;36(2):264–6.

122. Coulter DM, Clark DW, Savage RL. Celecoxib, rofecoxib, and acute temporary visual impairment. BMJ 2003;327:1214–5.

123. ADRAC. Acute neuropsychiatric events with celecoxib and rofecoxib. Aust Adv Drug React Bull 2003;22:3.

124. Simon LS, Lanza FL, Lipsky PE, Hubbard RC, Talwalker S, Schwartz BD, Isakson PC, Geis GS. Preliminary study of the safety and efficacy of SC-58635, a novel cyclooxygenase 2 inhibitor: efficacy and safety in two placebo-controlled trials in osteoarthritis and rheumatoid arthritis, and studies of gastrointestinal and platelet effects. Arthritis Rheum 1998;41(9):1591–602.

125. Topper JN, Cai J, Falb D, Gimbrone MA Jr. Identification of vascular endothelial genes differentially responsive to fluid mechanical stimuli: cyclooxygenase-2, manganese superoxide dismutase, and endothelial cell nitric oxide synthase are selectively up-regulated by steady laminar shear stress. Proc Natl Acad Sci USA 1996;93(19):10417–22.

126. McAdam BF, Catella-Lawson F, Mardini IA, Kapoor S, Lawson JA, Fitzgerald GA. Systemic biosynthesis of prostacyclin by cyclooxygenase (COX)-2: the human pharmacology of a selective inhibitor of COX-2. Proc Natl Acad Sci USA 1999;96(1):272–7.

127. Simon LS, Weaver AL, Graham DY, Kivitz AJ, Lipsky PE, Hubbard RC, Isakson PC, Verburg KM, Yu SS, Zhao WW, Geis GS. Anti-inflammatory and upper gastrointestinal effects of celecoxib in rheumatoid arthritis: a randomized controlled trial. JAMA 1999;282(20):1921–8.

128. Lanza FL, Rack MF, Simon TJ, Quan H, Bolognese JA, Hoover ME, Wilson FR, Harper SE. Specific inhibition of cyclooxygenase-2 with MK-0966 is associated with less gastroduodenal damage than either aspirin or ibuprofen. Aliment Pharmacol Ther 1999;13(6):761–7.

129. Laine L, Harper S, Simon T, Bath R, Johanson J, Schwartz H, Stern S, Quan H, Bolognese JRofecoxib Osteoarthritis Endoscopy Study Group. A randomized trial comparing the effect of rofecoxib, a cyclooxygenase 2-specific inhibitor, with that of ibuprofen on the gastroduodenal mucosa of patients with osteoarthritis. Gastroenterology 1999;117(4):776–83.

130. Wolfe MM, Lichtenstein DR, Singh G. Gastrointestinal toxicity of nonsteroidal antiinflammatory drugs. N Engl J Med 1999;340(24):1888–99.

131. Langman MJ, Jensen DM, Watson DJ, Harper SE, Zhao PL, Quan H, Bolognese JA, Simon TJ. Adverse upper gastrointestinal effects of rofecoxib compared with NSAIDs. JAMA 1999;282(20):1929–33.

132. Goldstein JL, Agrawal NM, Silverstein F, Kaiser J, Burr AM, Verburg KM, et al. Celecoxib is associated with a significantly lower incidence of clinically significant upper gastrointestinal (UGI) events in osteoarthritis (OA) and rheumatoid arthritis (RA) patients as compared to NSAIDs. Gastroenterology 1999;116:A174.

133. Goldstein JL, Silverstein FE, Agrawal NM, Hubbard RC, Kaiser J, Maurath CJ, Verburg KM, Geis GS. Reduced risk of upper gastrointestinal ulcer complications with celecoxib, a novel COX-2 inhibitor. Am J Gastroenterol 2000;95(7):1681–90.

134. Peterson WL, Cryer B. COX-1-sparing NSAIDs—is the enthusiasm justified? JAMA 1999;282(20):1961–3.

135. Boers M. NSAIDS and selective COX-2 inhibitors: competition between gastroprotection and cardioprotection. Lancet 2001;357(9264):1222–3.

136. Hrachovec JB, Mora M. Reporting of 6-month vs 12-month data in a clinical trial of celecoxib. JAMA 2001;286(19):2398.

137. Wright JM, Perry TL, Bassett KL, Chambers GK. Reporting of 6-month vs 12-month data in a clinical trial of celecoxib. JAMA 2001;286(19):2398–400.

138. Geis GS. CLASS clarification: reaffirms the medical importance of the analyses and results. BMJ USA 2002;2:522–3.

139. Juni P, Rutjes AWS, Dieppe P. Pharmacia addresses June 1 editorial regarding CLASS study: authors' response. BMJ 2002;324:1287–8.

140. Budenholzer BR, Geis GS, Mamdani M, Juurlink DN, Anderson GM, Stover RR, Juni P, Rutjes AW, Dieppe PA. Are selective COX 2 inhibitors superior to traditional NSAIDs? BMJ 2002;325:161.

141. Hawkey CJ. Outcomes studies of drug induced ulcer complications: do we need them and how should they be done? BMJ 2000;321(7256):291–3.

142. Deeks JJ, Smith LA, Bradley MD. Efficacy, tolerability, and upper gastrointestinal safety of celecoxib for treatment of osteoarthritis and rheumatoid arthritis: systematic review of randomised controlled trials. BMJ 2002;325(7365):619.

143. Mamdani M, Rochon PA, Juurlink DN, Kopp A, Anderson GM, Naglie G, Austin PC, Laupacis A. Observational study of upper gastrointestinal haemorrhage in elderly patients given selective cyclo-oxygenase-2 inhibitors or conventional non-steroidal anti-inflammatory drugs. BMJ 2002;325(7365):624.

144. Hendel J, Nielsen OH. Expression of cyclooxygenase-2 mRNA in active inflammatory bowel disease. Am J Gastroenterol 1997;92(7):1170–3.

145. Reuter BK, Asfaha S, Buret A, Sharkey KA, Wallace JL. Exacerbation of inflammation-associated colonic injury in rat through inhibition of cyclooxygenase-2. J Clin Invest 1996;98(9):2076–85.

146. Sigthorsson G, Crane R, Simon T, Hoover M, Quan H, Bolognese J, Bjarnason I. COX-2 inhibition with rofecoxib does not increase intestinal permeability in healthy subjects: a double blind crossover study comparing rofecoxib with placebo and indomethacin. Gut 2000;47(4):527–32.

147. Bjarnason I, Thjodleifsson B. Gastrointestinal toxicity of non-steroidal anti-inflammatory drugs: the effect of nimesulide compared with naproxen on the human gastrointestinal tract. Rheumatology (Oxford) 1999;38(Suppl 1):24–32.

148. Reuben SS, Steinberg R. Gastric perforation associated with the use of celecoxib. Anesthesiology 1999;91(5):1548–9.

149. Mohammed S, Croom DW 2nd. Gastropathy due to celecoxib, a cyclooxygenase-2 inhibitor. N Engl J Med 1999;340(25):2005–6.

150. Freitas J, Farricha V, Nascimento I, Borralho P, Parames A. Rofecoxib: a possible cause of acute colitis. J Clin Gastroenterol 2002;34(4):451–3.

151. Sanchez-Matienzo D, Arana A, Castellsague J, Perez-Gutthann S. Hepatic disorders in patients treated with COX-2 selective inhibitors or nonselective NSAIDs: a case/noncase analysis of spontaneous reports. Clin Ther 2006;28(8):1123–32.

152. Godino J, Butani RC, Wong PWK, Murphy FT. Acute drug-induced pancreatitis associated with celecoxib. J Clin Rheumatol 1999;5:305–7.

153. Carrillo-Jimenez R, Nurnberger M. Celecoxib-induced acute pancreatitis and hepatitis: a case report. Arch Intern Med 2000;160(4):553–4.

154. Dunn MJ. Are COX-2 selective inhibitors nephrotoxic? Am J Kidney Dis 2000;35(5):976–7.

155. Perazella MA, Tray K. Selective cyclooxygenase-2 inhibitors: a pattern of nephrotoxicity similar to traditional nonsteroidal anti-inflammatory drugs. Am J Med 2001;111(1):64–7.

156. Noroian G, Clive D. Cyclo-oxygenase-2 inhibitors and the kidney: a case for caution. Drug Saf 2002;25(3):165–72.

157. Alkhuja S, Menkel RA, Alwarshetty M, Ibrahimbacha AM. Celecoxib-induced nonoliguric acute renal failure. Ann Pharmacother 2002;36(1):52–4.

158. Chan FK, Hung LC, Suen BY, Wu JC, Lee KC, Leung VK, Hui AJ, To KF, Leung WK, Wong VW, Chung SC, Sung JJ. Celecoxib versus diclofenac and omeprazole in reducing the risk of recurrent ulcer bleeding in patients with arthritis. N Engl J Med 2002;347(26):2104–10.

159. Whelton A, Schulman G, Wallemark C, Drower EJ, Isakson PC, Verburg KM, Geis GS. Effects of celecoxib and naproxen on renal function in the elderly. Arch Intern Med 2000;160(10):1465–70.

160. Swan SK, Rudy DW, Lasseter KC, Ryan CF, Buechel KL, Lambrecht LJ, Pinto MB, Dilzer SC, Obrda O, Sundblad KJ, Gumbs CP, Ebel DL, Quan H, Larson PJ, Schwartz JI, Musliner TA, Gertz BJ, Brater DC, Yao SL. Effect of cyclooxygenase-2 inhibition on renal function in elderly persons receiving a low-salt diet. A randomized, controlled trial. Ann Intern Med 2000;133(1):1–9.

161. Boyd IW, Mathew TH, Thomas MC. COX-2 inhibitors and renal failure: the triple whammy revisited. Med J Aust 2000;173(5):274.

162. Perazella MA, Eras J. Are selective COX-2 inhibitors nephrotoxic? Am J Kidney Dis 2000;35(5):937–40.

163. Pfister AK, Crisalli RJ, Carter WH. Cyclooxygenase-2 inhibition and renal function. Ann Intern Med 2001;134(11):1077.

164. Graham MG. Acute renal failure related to high-dose celecoxib. Ann Intern Med 2001;135(1):69–70.

165. Wolf G, Porth J, Stahl RA. Acute renal failure associated with rofecoxib. Ann Intern Med 2000;133(5):394.

166. Zhao SZ, Reynolds MW, Lejkowith J, Whelton A, Arellano FM. A comparison of renal-related adverse drug reactions between rofecoxib and celecoxib, based on the World Health Organization/Uppsala Monitoring Centre safety database. Clin Ther 2001;23(9):1478–91.

167. Park JM, Houck CS, Sethna NF, Sullivan LJ, Atala A, Borer JG, Cilento BG, Diamond DA, Peters CA, Retik AB, Bauer SB. Ketorolac suppresses postoperative bladder spasms after pediatric ureteral reimplantation. Anesth Analg 2000;91(1):11–5.

168. Park JM, Schnermann JB, Briggs JP. Cyclooxygenase-2. A key regulator of bladder prostaglandin formation Adv Exp Med Biol 1999;462:171–81.

169. Gruenenfelder J, McGuire EJ, Faerber GJ. Acute urinary retention associated with the use of cyclooxygenase-2 inhibitors. J Urol 2002;168(3):1106.

170. Verbeiren S, Morant C, Charlanne H, Ajebbar K, Caron J, Modiano P. Toxidermie au célécoxib (Cerebrex®) avec test epicutané positif. [Celecoxib induced toxiderma with positive patch-test.] Ann Dermatol Venereol 2002;129(2):203–5.

171. Berger P, Dwyer D, Corallo CE. Toxic epidermal necrolysis after celecoxib therapy. Pharmacotherapy 2002;22(9):1193–5.

172. Sarkar R, Kaur C, Kanwar AJ. Erythema multiforme due to rofecoxib. Dermatology 2002;204(4):304–5.

173. Carder KR, Weston WL. Rofecoxib-induced instant aquagenic wrinkling of the palms. Pediatr Dermatol 2002;19(4):353–5.

174. Amin AR, Attur M, Patel RN, Thakker GD, Marshall PJ, Rediske J, Stuchin SA, Patel IR, Abramson SB. Superinduction of cyclooxygenase-2 activity in human osteoarthritis-affected cartilage. Influence of nitric oxide. J Clin Invest 1997;99(6):1231–7.

175. Giannoudis PV, MacDonald DA, Matthews SJ, Smith RM, Furlong AJ, De Boer P. Nonunion of the femoral diaphysis. The influence of reaming and nonsteroidal anti-antiinflammatory drugs. J Bone Joint Surg Br 2000;82:655–8.

176. Simon AM, Manigrasso MB, O'Connor JP. Cyclo-oxygenase 2 function is essential for bone fracture healing. J Bone Miner Res 2002;17:963–76.

177. Norman RJ. Reproductive consequences of COX-2 inhibition. Lancet 2001;358(9290):1287–8.

178. Pall M, Friden BE, Brannstrom M. Induction of delayed follicular rupture in the human by the selective COX-2 inhibitor rofecoxib: a randomized double-blind study. Hum Reprod 2001;16(7):1323–8.

179. Smith G, Roberts R, Hall C, Nuki G. Reversible ovulatory failure associated with the development of luteinized unruptured follicles in women with inflammatory arthritis taking non-steroidal anti-inflammatory drugs. Br J Rheumatol 1996;35(5):458–62.

180. Akil M, Amos RS, Stewart P. Infertility may sometimes be associated with NSAID consumption. Br J Rheumatol 1996;35(1):76–8.

181. Mendonca LL, Khamashta MA, Nelson-Piercy C, Hunt BJ, Hughes GR. Non-steroidal anti-inflammatory drugs as a possible cause for reversible infertility. Rheumatology (Oxford) 2000;39(8):880–2.

182. Stevenson DD, Sanchez-Borges M, Szczeklik A. Classification of allergic and pseudoallergic reactions to drugs that inhibit cyclooxygenase enzymes. Ann Allergy Asthma Immunol 2001;87(3):177–80.

183. Grob M, Pichler WJ, Wuthrich B. Anaphylaxis to celecoxib. Allergy 2002;57(3):264–5.

184. Skowron F, Berard F, Bernard N, Balme B, Perrot H. Cutaneous vasculitis related to celecoxib. Dermatology 2002;204(4):305.

185. Jordan KM, Edwards CJ, Arden NK. Allergic vasculitis associated with celecoxib. Rheumatology (Oxford) 2002;41(12):1453–5.

186. Schneider F, Meziani F, Chartier C, Alt M, Jaeger A. Fatal allergic vasculitis associated with celecoxib. Lancet 2002;359(9309):852–3.

187. Wiholm BE, Shear NH, Knowles S, Shapiro L. Should celecoxib be contraindicated in patients who are allergic to sulfonamides? Drug Saf 2002;25(4):297–9.

188. Kumar NP, Wild G, Ramasamy KA, Snape J. Fatal haemorrhagic pulmonary oedema and associated angioedema after the ingestion of rofecoxib. Postgrad Med J 2002;78(921):439–40.

189. Nettis E, Di PR, Ferrannini A, Tursi A. Tolerability of rofecoxib in patients with cutaneous adverse reactions to nonsteroidal anti-inflammatory drugs. Ann Allergy Asthma Immunol 2002;88(3):331–4.

190. Levy MB, Fink JN. Anaphylaxis to celecoxib. Ann Allergy Asthma Immunol 2001;87(1):72–3.

191. Habki R, Vermeulen C, Bachmeyer C, Charoud A, Mofredj A. Choc anaphylactique au célécoxib. [Anaphylactic shock induced by celecoxib.] Ann Med Interne (Paris) 2001;152(5):355.

192. Schellenberg RR, Isserow SH. Anaphylactoid reaction to a cyclooxygenase-2 inhibitor in a patient who had a reaction to a cyclooxygenase-1 inhibitor. N Engl J Med 2001;345(25):1856.

193. Knowles S, Shapiro L, Shear NH. Should celecoxib be contraindicated in patients who are allergic to sulfonamides? Revisiting the meaning of "sulfa" allergy. Drug Saf 2001;24(4):239–47.

194. Wiholm BE. Identification of sulfonamide-like adverse drug reactions to celecoxib in the World Health Organization database. Curr Med Res Opin 2001;17(3):210–6.

195. Anonymous. COX-2 inhibitor-induced rash. Consultant 2001;41:1338.

196. Kaur C, Sarkar R, Kanwar AJ. Fixed drug eruption to rofecoxib with cross-reactivity to sulfonamides. Dermatology 2001;203(4):351.

197. Sanchez Borges M, Capriles-Hulett A, Caballero-Fonseca F, Perez CR. Tolerability to new COX-2 inhibitors in NSAID-sensitive patients with cutaneous reactions. Ann Allergy Asthma Immunol 2001;87(3):201–4.

198. Warner TD, Giuliano F, Vojnovic I, Bukasa A, Mitchell JA, Vane JR. Nonsteroid drug selectivities for cyclo-oxygenase-1 rather than cyclo-oxygenase-2 are associated with human gastrointestinal toxicity: a full in vitro analysis. Proc Natl Acad Sci USA 1999;96(13):7563–8.

199. Asero R. Tolerability of rofecoxib. Allergy 2001;56(9):916–7.

200. Berges-Gimeno MP, Camacho-Garrido E, Garcia-Rodriguez RM, Alfaya T, Martin Garcia C, Hinojosa M. Rofecoxib safe in NSAID hypersensitivity. Allergy 2001;56(10):1017–8.

201. Enrique E, Cistero-Bahima A, San Miguel-Moncin MM, Alonso R. Rofecoxib should be tried in NSAID hypersensitivity. Allergy 2000;55(11):1090.

202. Kelkar PS, Butterfield JH, Teaford HG. Urticaria and angioedema from cyclooxygenase-2 inhibitors. J Rheumatol 2001;28(11):2553–4.

203. Sawdy R, Slater D, Fisk N, Edmonds DK, Bennett P. Use of a cyclo-oxygenase type-2-selective non-steroidal anti-inflammatory agent to prevent preterm delivery. Lancet 1997;350(9073):265–6.

204. Fahey SM, Silver RM. Use of NSAIDs and COX-2 inhibitors in children with musculoskeletal disorders. J Pediatr Orthop 2003;23:794–9.

205. Pickering AE, Bridge HS, Nolan J, Stoddart PA. Double-blind, placebo-controlled analgesic study of ibuprofen or rofecoxib in combination with paracetamol for tonsillectomy in children. Br J Anaesth 2002;88:72–7.

206. Stempak D, Gammon J, Klein J, Koren G, Baruchel S. Single-dose and steady-state pharmackinetics of celocoxib in children. Clin Pharmacol Ther 2002;72:490–7.

207. Lundmark J, Gunnarsson T, Bengtsson F. A possible interaction between lithium and rofecoxib. Br J Clin Pharmacol 2002;53(4):403–4.

208. Ibrahim A, Park S, Feldman J, Karim A, Kharasch ED. Effects of parecoxib, a parenteral COX-2-specific inhibitor, on the pharmacokinetics and pharmacodynamics of propofol. Anesthesiology 2002;96(1):88–95.

209. Schwartz JI, Wong PH, Porras AG, Ebel DL, Hunt TR, Gertz BJ. Effect of rofecoxib on the pharmacokinetics of chronically administered oral contraceptives in healthy female volunteers. J Clin Pharmacol 2002;42(2):215–21.

210. Montvale NJ, Physicians' Desk Reference. Medical Economics Company, Inc; 2001:248.

211. Davies NM, McLachlan AJ, Day RO, Williams KM. Clinical pharmacokinetics and pharmacodynamics of celecoxib: a selective cyclo-oxygenase-2 inhibitor. Clin Pharmacokinet 2000;38(3):225–42.

212. Davies NM, Gudde TW, de Leeuw MA. Celecoxib: a new option in the treatment of arthropathies and familial adenomatous polyposis. Expert Opin Pharmacother 2001;2(1):139–52.

213. Rossat J, Maillard M, Nussberger J, Brunner HR, Burnier M. Renal effects of selective cyclooxygenase-2 inhibition in normotensive salt-depleted subjects. Clin Pharmacol Ther 1999;66(1):76–84.

214. Moltedo JM, Porter GA, State MW, Snyder CS. Sinus node dysfunction associated with lithium therapy in a child. Tex Heart Inst J 2002;29(3):200–2.

215. Gunja N, Graudins A, Dowsett R. Lithium toxicity: a potential interaction with celecoxib. Intern Med J 2002;32(9–10):494.

216. Lundmark J, Gunnarsson T, Bengtsson F. A possible interaction between lithium and rofecoxib. Br J Clin Pharmacol 2002;53(4):403–4.

217. Sajbel TA, Carter GW, Wiley RB. Pharmacokinetics/pharmacodynamics/pharmacometrics/drug metabolism. Pharmacotherapy 2001;21:380.

218. Bocchia M, Bertola G, Morganti D, Toscano M, Colombo E. Intossicazione da litio e uso di nimesulide. [Lithium poisoning and the use of nimesulide.] Recenti Prog Med 2001;92(7–8):462.

219. Adverse Drug Reactions Advisory Committee (ADRAC). Interaction of celecoxib and warfarin. Adv Drug React Bull 2001;20:2.

220. Med Safe Editorial Team. Interaction between COX-2 inhibitors and warfarin. Prescriber Update 2001;22:16–18.

221. Adverse Drug Reactions Advisory Committee (ADRAC). Interaction of rofecoxib and warfarin. Adv Drug React Bull 2002;21:3.

222. Savage R. Cyclo-oxygenase-2 inhibitors: when should they be used in the elderly? Drugs Aging 2005;22:185–200.

223. Battistella M, Mamdami MM, Juurlink DN, Rabeneck L, Laupacis A. Risk of upper gastrointestinal hemorrhage in warfarin users treated with nonselective NSAIDs or COX-2 inhibitors. Arch Intern Med 2005;24:158–60.

Aceclofenac

General Information

Despite claims that aceclofenac is a COX-2 selective inhibitor, experience shows that its adverse effects profile is similar to that of the non-selective NSAIDs.

Organs and Systems

Gastrointestinal

Symptoms of gastrointestinal intolerance in patients taking aceclofenac commonly require withdrawal, at a rate of 3–15% (SEDA-20, 91).

Liver

Acute hepatitis has been reported with aceclofenac (SEDA-21, 103).

Skin

Aceclofenac cream can cause erythema, itching, and a burning sensation in under 3% of patients (SEDA-20, 91). Aceclofenac can cause photosensitivity.

- After starting twice-daily topical application of a cream containing aceclofenac, a woman developed acute eczema affecting the sun-exposed areas of her legs (1).

Allergic contact dermatitis has been attributed to aceclofenac (2), as has generalized pustular psoriasis (3), and Stevens-Johnson syndrome (4).

- A 75-year-old woman who took aceclofenac for 15 days for arthritis developed erythema of the face followed by multiple target lesions with central bullae on the neck, chest, back, and palmoplantar regions. The lesions became confluent and also involved mucous membranes. She was treated with glucocorticoids and within 4 weeks the lesions had cleared completely.

Immunologic

A hypersensitivity reaction characterized by multiple purpuric lesions and reduced renal function has been described in an elderly patient (SEDA-18, 103), and there have been reports of hypersensitivity vasculitis (SEDA-20, 91; SEDA-21, 103).

References

1. Goday Bujan JJ, Garcia Alvarez-Eire GM, Martinez W, del Pozo J, Fonseca E. Photoallergic contact dermatitis from aceclofenac. Contact Dermatitis 2001;45(3):170.
2. Pitarch Bort G, de la Cuadra Oyanguren J, Torrijos Aguilar A, García-Melgares Linares M. Allergic contact dermatitis due to aceclofenac. Contact Dermatitis 2006;55(6):365-6.
3. Vergara A, Arrue I, Dominuez JD, Vanaclocha F. Generalized pustular psoriasis precipitated by aceclofenac. J Eur Acad Dermatol Venereol 2006;20(8):1028-9.
4. Ludwig C, Brinkmeier T, Frosch PJ. Exudative erythema multiforme with transition to a toxic epidermal necrolysis after taking aceclofenac (Beofenac). Dtsch Med Wochenschr 2003;128:487-90.

Acemetacin

General Information

Acemetacin is an indometacin derivative with the same adverse effects profile (SEDA-6, 94). In an open multicenter study, 187 of 280 patients had adverse effects (57% gastrointestinal); treatment had to be stopped in 7% (1). The use of acemetacin is limited and there is no justification for claims that it has advantages over existing NSAIDs.

Reference

1. Heiter A, Tausch G, Eberl R. Ergebnisse einer Langstudie mit Acemetacin bei der Behandlung von Patienten mit chronischer Polyarthritis. [Results of a long-term study with acemetacin in the therapy of patients suffering from rheumatoid arthritis.] Arzneimittelforschung 1980;30(8A):460-3.

Alclofenac

General Information

While the pattern of alclofenac toxicity resembles that of other NSAIDs, the frequency of adverse effects differs widely. Allergic reactions have been reported more frequently and skin rashes have been particularly common. Hypersensitivity reactions, including anaphylactic shock, severe generalized vasculitis, hepatotoxicity, and nephrotoxicity, have been observed. Alclofenac has therefore been withdrawn in several countries (1). Blood dyscrasias and neurological symptoms are rare.

Reference

1. Morison WL, Baughman RD, Day RM, Forbes PD, Hoenigsmann H, Krueger GG, Lebwohl M, Lew R, Naldi L, Parrish JA, Piepkorn M, Stern RS, Weinstein GD, Whitmore SE. Consensus workshop on the toxic effects of long-term PUVA therapy. Arch Dermatol 1998;134(5):595-8.

Ampiroxicam

General Information

Ampiroxicam is a piroxicam prodrug, which is completely converted to piroxicam after oral administration. Its adverse effects profile is expected to be similar to that of piroxicam. A few cases of photosensitivity have been reported (1–5).

References

1. Carty TJ, Marfat A, Moore PF, Falkner FC, Twomey TM, Weissman A. Ampiroxicam, an anti-inflammatory agent which is a prodrug of piroxicam. Agents Actions 1993;39(3-4):157-65.
2. Falkner FC, Twomey TM, Borgers AP, Garg D, Weidler D, Gerber N, Browder IW. Disposition of ampiroxicam, a prodrug of piroxicam, in man. Xenobiotica 1990;20(6):645-52.
3. Chishiki M, Kawada A, Fujioka A, Hiruma M, Ishibashi A, Banba H. Photosensitivity due to ampiroxicam. Dermatology 1997;195(4):409-10.
4. Toyohara A, Chen KR, Miyakawa S, Inada M, Ishiko A. Ampiroxicam-induced photosensitivity. Contact Dermatitis 1996;35(2):101-2.
5. Kurumaji Y. Ampiroxicam-induced photosensitivity. Contact Dermatitis 1996;34(4):298-9.

Amtolmetin guacil

General Information

Amtolmetin guacil (2-[2[1-methyl-5-(4-methylbenzoyl)-2-yl] acetamido] acetic acid 2-methoxyphenyl ester) is a non-acid prodrug of tolmetin. It has been introduced in various countries, and its launch was characterized by claims of better gastrointestinal tolerability than older compounds (1,2). Clinical and endoscopic comparative studies have been carried out in patients with various osteoarticular diseases (3–5). In most of these studies amtolmetin showed similar anti-inflammatory activity to other NSAIDs (diclofenac, flurbiprofen, ibuprofen, indometacin, naproxen) but less gastrotoxicity at endoscopic evaluation, with no difference in the incidence of gastrointestinal symptoms. Unfortunately, the clinical studies were small and of short duration, and the prognostic value of endoscopic studies with respect to severe gastrointestinal complications (bleeding, perforation, and obstruction) is debatable. It has been suggested that the mechanism of the gastric sparing effect of amtolmetin might be related to the local production of nitric oxide, which can counteract the damaging effects of prostaglandin inhibition (6,7).

A renal sparing effect has also been reported, but clinical experience with this compound is limited (8).

References

1. Marcolongo R, Frediani B, Biasi G, Minari C, Barreca C. Metanalisi sulla tollerabilità di amtolmetina guacil, un nuovo, efficace farmaco antinfiammatorio non steroideo, confrontato con FANS tradizionali. Clin Drug Invest 1999;17:89–96.
2. Caruso A, Cutuli VM, De Bernardis E, Attaguile G, Amico-Roxas M. Pharmacological properties and toxicology of MED-15, a prodrug of tolmetin. Drugs Exp Clin Res 1992;18(11–12):481–5.
3. Tavella A, Ursini G. Studio clinico sull'attivita antiinfiammatoria e sulla tollerabilita gastro-enterica di amtolmetineguacil, un nuovo FANS, in confronto a diclofenac su pazienti anziani con patologie osteoarticolari. [A clinical study on the anti-inflammatory activity and gastrointestinal tolerability of amtolmetin guacyl, a new NSAID, compared with diclofenac in aged patients with osteoarticular diseases.] Clin Ter 1997;148(11):543–8.
4. Montrone F, Santandrea S, Caruso I, Gerli R, Cesarotti ME, Frediani P, Bassani R. Amtolmetin guacyl versus piroxicam in patients with osteoarthritis. J Int Med Res 2000;28(2):91–100.
5. Bianchi Porro G, Montrone F, Lazzaroni M, Manzionna G, Caruso I. Clinical and gastroscopic evaluation of amtolmetin guacyl versus diclofenac in patients with rheumatoid arthritis. Ital J Gastroenterol Hepatol 1999;31(5):378–85.
6. Tubaro E, Belogi L, Mezzadri CM. The mechanism of action of amtolmetin guacyl, a new gastroprotective nonsteroidal anti-inflammatory drug. Eur J Pharmacol 2000;387(2):233–44.
7. Pisano C, Grandi D, Morini G, Coppelli G, Vesci L, Lo Giudice P, Pace S, Pacifici L, Longo A, Coruzzi G, Carminati P. Gastrosparing effect of new antiinflammatory drug amtolmetin guacyl in the rat: involvement of nitric oxide. Dig Dis Sci 1999;44(4):713–24.
8. Niccoli L, Bellino S, Cantini F. Renal tolerability of three commonly employed non-steroidal anti-inflammatory drugs in elderly patients with osteoarthritis. Clin Exp Rheumatol 2002;20(2):201–7.

Antrafenine

General Information

Antrafenine closely resembles glafenine and floctafenine (SED-9, 153; SEDA-7, 116; SEDA-11, 96; 1). The same adverse effects must be expected and some have been described, for example nephrotoxicity (SEDA-4, 69) (2). Gastrotoxicity is claimed to be less than with aspirin (3), again no doubt merely because it is a weak anti-inflammatory drug.

References

1. Neuman M. Antrafenine. Drugs of Today 1978;14:56.
2. Leguy P, Herve JP, Garre M, Youinou P, Leroy JP. Nephropathie aiguë tubulo-interstitielle après ingestion d'antrafénine de mécanisme apparemment non immunoallergique. [Acute tubulo-interstitial nephropathy following ingestion of antrafenine with an apparently non-immunoallergic mechanism.] Nouv Presse Méd 1981;10(16):1336.
3. Bressot C, Dechavanne M, Ville D, Meunier PJ. Effet antalgique et pertes sanguines fécales induites par l'antrafénine. [Analgesic effect and fecal blood loss induced by antrafenine. A double-blind comparison with aspirin.] Rev Rhum Mal Osteoartic 1981;48(7–9):601–4.

Azapropazone

General Information

Azapropazone is structurally related to phenylbutazone and probably shares the same adverse effects: gastrotoxicity, skin reactions, headache, vertigo, edema, and renal impairment. A review of a very large series described azapropazone adverse effects in 1724 patients (18%), causing withdrawal in 3.7%. Surprisingly, however, there were no phenylbutazone-type blood dyscrasias (SED-11, 176) (1). Azapropazone should be prescribed only for patients with active rheumatic diseases who have failed to respond to other NSAIDs (2).

Organs and Systems

Hematologic

Hemolytic anemia has been reported (SEDA-10, 79) (SEDA-12, 83). A high percentage of patients taking azapropazone had a positive direct Coombs' test, but this did not persist after treatment had been stopped for several weeks (SEDA-12, 83). Hemolytic anemia has also been described in combination with pulmonary alveolitis, which suggests an allergic or immune reaction (3). Photosensitivity is often reported: 190 reports of photosensitivity were submitted to several national drug-monitoring centers in Europe in 1985 (SEDA-10, 79) (SEDA-12, 83).

Skin

Photosensitivity is more frequent with azapropazone than with almost any other NSAID (4).

Immunologic

Patients with aspirin intolerance often also react to many other NSAIDs. Azapropazone seems to be a safe alternative in these patients, according a study that showed good tolerance of the drug in patients with aspirin intolerance (5).

Susceptibility Factors

Renal disease

Because of increases in unbound drug and reduced clearance in renal insufficiency, the dosage should be carefully adjusted in patients with renal disease (SEDA-11, 92).

Hepatic disease

Because of increases in the unbound drug and reduced clearance, the dosage should be carefully adjusted in patients with liver disease (SEDA-11, 92).

Drug–Drug Interactions

Oral anticoagulants

Azapropazone has the same pattern of interactions as phenylbutazone with oral anticoagulants (SEDA-2, 98).

Phenytoin

Azapropazone has the same pattern of interactions as phenylbutazone with phenytoin (6,7).

Tolbutamide

Azapropazone has the same pattern of interactions as phenylbutazone with tolbutamide (8).

References

1. Sondervosst M. Azapropazone. Clin Rheum Dis 1979;5:465.
2. Anonymous. CSM recommends azapropazone restriction. Scrip 1994;1957:24.
3. Albazzaz MK, Harvey JE, Hoffman JN, Siddorn JA. Alveolitis and haemolytic anaemia induced by azapropazone. BMJ (Clin Res Ed) 1986;293(6561):1537–8.
4. Olsson S, Biriell C, Boman G. Photosensitivity during treatment with azapropazone. BMJ (Clin Res Ed) 1985;291(6500):939.
5. Gutgesell C, Fuchs T. Azapropazone in aspirin intolerance. Allergy 1999;54(8):897–8.
6. Geaney DP, Carver JG, Aronson JK, Warlow CP. Interaction of azapropazone with phenytoin. BMJ (Clin Res Ed) 1982;284(6326):1373.
7. Geaney DP, Carver JG, Davies CL, Aronson JK. Pharmacokinetic investigation of the interaction of azapropazone with phenytoin. Br J Clin Pharmacol 1983;15(6):727–34.
8. Andreasen PB, Simonsen K, Brocks K, Dimo B, Bouchelouche P. Hypoglycaemia induced by azapropazone–tolbutamide interaction. Br J Clin Pharmacol 1981;12(4):581–583.

Benoxaprofen

General Information

Since benoxaprofen, like zomepirac, provided an experience from which several lessons can be learnt, it deserves to be briefly reviewed, even though it was withdrawn 10 years ago. Some newer drugs may have some of its chemical or pharmacological characteristics and, consequently, its problems. Benoxaprofen was originally launched in 1980, with claims of a favorable adverse effects profile and "unique disease-modifying properties" in rheumatoid arthritis. These claims appeared to have been based on the fact that it was a relatively more potent inhibitor of leukotriene production and a less potent inhibitor of prostaglandin synthesis than other NSAIDs. Having passed all preclinical and clinical tests and satisfied the safety requirements set by regulatory authorities in many countries (despite rejection in several on grounds of safety), benoxaprofen was then suspended by the UK Committee on Safety of Medicines in 1982, about 18 months after marketing. Shortly afterwards it was withdrawn worldwide by its manufacturers (1). Benoxaprofen was associated with a very high incidence of adverse effects, prominent effects on the skin and nails and liver reactions, which sometimes proved fatal, particularly in elderly people.

The case led to considerable regulatory and medicolegal discussions in the 10 years after withdrawal. In the USA the company was charged by the Food and Drug Administration with misbranding the drug in press statements and associated materials, which contained a misleading headline implying that the drug was harmless, even though the company was aware of a report of deaths related to the use of benoxaprofen. The company's intense marketing campaign was heavily criticized (SEDA-8) and it was noted that the recommendation of the WHO that drugs likely to be used in elderly people should be investigated in them at an early stage had certainly been disregarded in the premarketing phases. In the UK the company rejected patients' demands to establish a compensation scheme and offered instead a financial settlement that the patients rejected as inadequate. The case shows how some legal systems are inadequate for dealing with mass claims of personal injury due to drugs.

Organs and Systems

Gastrointestinal

The hope of better gastric tolerance of benoxaprofen was not fulfilled, and the incidence of this type of reaction was actually higher in elderly patients.

Liver

Fatal liver damage was observed particularly in the UK and tended to occur in elderly subjects. The complication initially presented as jaundice or raised liver enzymes (including alkaline phosphatase). Surprisingly, biochemical and histological liver changes were not consistent with major hepatocellular damage. There were three reports of primary biliary cirrhosis, but a causal relation was not proven (SEDA-12, 84).

Urinary tract

All types of kidney damage were reported, ranging from a transitory fall in glomerular filtration rate and reversible renal insufficiency (part of multisystem disease with circulating LE cells) to the nephrotic syndrome.

Skin

Cutaneous adverse effects were the most frequent problem and (together with hepatic complications) the most serious: 63% of 300 patients treated for 6 months complained of one or more adverse effects (total 259 reactions); 70% were cutaneous; photosensitivity led to withdrawal in 30% of cases. Multiple subepidermal cysts (milia) on sun-exposed skin areas and onycholysis (13% of patients) were documented. Other skin reactions included rashes, hypertrichosis, erythema multiforme, and Stevens–Johnson syndrome (2). Phototoxicity persisted for many months after withdrawal (SEDA-12, 84); although a later study on persistent photosensitivity as a sequel to benoxaprofen in 42 subjects failed to confirm the link between photosensitivity and the drug (3), this was contrary to the overwhelming experience in the field. In retrospect, it seems likely that one problem was that benoxaprofen had largely been studied during the winter months, whereas in the UK it was launched in the summer.

References

1. Anonymous. Benoxaprofen. BMJ (Clin Res Ed) 1982;285(6340):459–60.
2. Halsey JP, Cardoe N. Benoxaprofen: side-effect profile in 300 patients. BMJ (Clin Res Ed) 1982;284(6326):1365–8.
3. Frain-Bell W. A study of persistent photosensitivity as a sequel of the prior administration of the drug benoxaprofen. Br J Dermatol 1989;121(5):551–62.

Bromfenac sodium

General Information

Bromfenac sodium (2-amino-3-(4-bromo-benzoyl)-benzeneacetic acid sodium salt sesquihydrate) has a safety profile apparently similar to that of other NSAIDs (SEDA-17, 109; SEDA-21, 104). It was approved by the FDA in 1997 for short-term management of acute pain, but was withdrawn by the manufacturers in 1998.

Organs and Systems

Liver

In June 1998 bromfenac was withdrawn from the market because of postmarketing reports of severe hepatic failure, resulting in four deaths and eight liver transplants (SEDA-22, 115). Descriptions of some cases have appeared (1–4).

References

1. Moses PL, Schroeder B, Alkhatib O, Ferrentino N, Suppan T, Lidofsky SD. Severe hepatotoxicity associated with bromfenac sodium. Am J Gastroenterol 1999;94(5):1393–6.
2. Rabkin JM, Smith MJ, Orloff SL, Corless CL, Stenzel P, Olyaei AJ. Fatal fulminant hepatitis associated with bromfenac use. Ann Pharmacother 1999;33(9):945–7.
3. Hunter EB, Johnston PE, Tanner G, Pinson CW, Awad JA. Bromfenac (Duract)-associated hepatic failure requiring liver transplantation. Am J Gastroenterol 1999;94(8):2299–301.
4. Fontana RJ, McCashland TM, Benner KG, Appelman HD, Gunartanam NT, Wisecarver JL, Rabkin JM, Lee WMThe Acute Liver Failure Study Group. Acute liver failure associated with prolonged use of bromfenac leading to liver transplantation. Liver Transpl Surg 1999;5(6):480–4.

Bucloxic acid

General Information

Bucloxic acid is an NSAID that is not widely used. The usual symptoms of gastrotoxicity, nephrotoxicity, and increased blood pressure have been reported, but the major adverse effects involve skin and allergic reactions. Quincke's edema has been observed (SED-9, 152) (1) (SEDA-1, 93).

Reference

1. Penard M, Guillou M. Notre expérience de l'Esfar en cardiologie hospitalière. Ouest Med 1975;28:967.

Bufexamac

General Information

Bufexamac is intended for topical use as a cream (using iontophoresis, ultrasound, and massage). Local intolerance causes burning and irritation, attributable to components of the cream. Urticaria, folliculitis, and pyoderma can occur when occlusive dressings are used. The course of contact allergy by bufexamac was particularly protracted and refractory in most of the 24 patients observed in one hospital in 1983–1987 (1). An erythema multiforme-like rash associated with contact dermatitis has been reported (SEDA-18, 103). In children, long-term topical use of bufexamac was well tolerated with few mild local adverse effects (SEDA-20, 91).

Reference

1. Geier J, Fuchs T. Kontaktallergien durch Bufexamac. [Contact allergies caused by bufexamac.] Med Klin (Munich) 1989;84(7):333–8.

Bumadizone

General Information

Bumadizone is an NSAID that is metabolized to phenylbutazone and oxyphenbutazone.

In a study in 647 patients, about 15% had adverse effects (gastrointestinal, fluid retention, and hypersensitivity); treatment was stopped in 7% (1).

Reference

1. Du Lac Y. Banc d'essai therapeutique d'un anti-inflammatoire Eumotol. Reumatologie 1979;8:405.

Butibufen

General Information

Experience with the NSAID butibufen is limited. Only gastrointestinal adverse effects have been described (1).

Reference

1. Aparicio L. Butibufen. Drugs Today 1979;15:43.

Carprofen

General Information

The main adverse effects of the NSAID carprofen are cutaneous and hepatic. Photoreactions are being increasingly reported and its chemical similarity to benoxaprofen is worth noting (SEDA-12, 84). The photosensitivity mechanism is either toxic or allergic. Other cutaneous symptoms, such as burning, pruritus, dermatitis, and skin redness, have also been reported (1). In trials in the USA, 14% of 1500 patients had slight transient rises in liver function tests, the significance of which is unclear (SEDA-13, 79). Headache, dizziness, gastrointestinal discomfort, and dysuria have also been described (1). Asthma can be precipitated in aspirin-sensitive patients.

Susceptibility Factors

Other features of the patient

Although carprofen is reported to be well tolerated by patients with peptic ulcers taking ranitidine (2), it cannot be presumed to be without risk in patients with ulcer disease.

References

1. Jensen EM, Fossgren J, Kirchheiner B, et al. Treatment of rheumatoid arthritis with carprofen (Imadyl) or indometacin: a randomized multicentre trial. Curr Ther Res 1980; 28:882.
2. Czarnobilski Z, Bem S, Czarnobilski K, Konturek SJ. Carprofen and the therapy of gastroduodenal ulcerations by ranitidine. Hepatogastroenterology 1985;32(1):20–3.

Celecoxib

See also COX-2 inhibitors

General Information

Celecoxib is a selective COX-2 inhibitor.

Organs and Systems

Psychological, psychiatric

A 78-year-old woman had auditory hallucinations while taking celecoxib for osteoarthritis (1). Her symptoms occurred after she had taken celecoxib 200 mg bd for 48 hours and progressed over the next 8 days. Celecoxib was withdrawn and her hallucinations gradually disappeared over the next 4 days. Rechallenge with a lower dose (100 mg bd) caused recurrence.

There have been two reports of visual hallucinations in patients taking celecoxib.

- A 79-year-old woman presented to her optometrist with a 2-day history of seeing orange spots in both visual fields 2 months after starting to take celecoxib 100 mg/day (2). Physical examination and a CT scan were normal. Celecoxib was withdrawn and her symptoms resolved within 3 days.
- An 81-year-old woman took celecoxib 100 mg/day, and over the next 2 weeks developed delirium and auditory and visual hallucinations (3). Celecoxib was withdrawn and her symptoms resolved over several days. She took a few doses of rofecoxib 12.5 mg/day 6 months later without any problem. She began to take rofecoxib regularly again 2 months later, and after 1 month developed agitation, confusion, and hallucinations. Physical

examination suggested no cause of the delirium other than rofecoxib. A CT scan was negative. The rofecoxib was withdrawn, and over the next 2 days her symptoms resolved.

Auditory hallucinations have been previously reported in a patient taking celecoxib (SEDA-25, 134) but are probably uncommon.

Hematologic

A report has raised the possibility that patients with a known prothrombotic state and raised platelet thromboxane A_2 production may be at high risk of thrombosis when selective COX-2 inhibitors are used (4).

Thrombosis occurred during celecoxib therapy (400 mg/day) in four women (aged 37–56 years) with connective tissue diseases and conditions that predisposed them to thrombosis, including Raynaud's phenomenon, raised anticardiolipin antibody titers, and a previous history of thrombosis. Peripheral artery thrombosis (three patients) and pulmonary embolism (one patient) were documented after starting celecoxib. Symptoms of thrombosis began to appear within 1 week of starting celecoxib in three patients and 2 months after starting celecoxib in the fourth patient.

A causal relation between celecoxib and these thrombotic events cannot be established with certainty on the basis of the available evidence. However, the temporal relation between the start of treatment and the thrombotic event was impressive, at least in three patients, and the findings were consistent with the hypothesis that thrombosis is an adverse consequence of reduced production of systemic prostaglandin I_2 brought about by COX-2 inhibition. Reduced synthesis of prostaglandin I_2 may act in concert with other thrombotic risk factors (such as those occurring in this series of patients) to precipitate acute vascular occlusion.

Gastrointestinal

With extensive use of COX-2 inhibitors, gastrointestinal adverse reactions similar to those observed with non-selective NSAID are being increasingly observed.

- An 87-year-old man developed severe esophagitis with a chronic peptic esophageal stricture and had dysphagia and odynophagia. He had taken celecoxib for 5 months (200-400 mg/day) and endoscopy showed severe desquamative esophagitis. Celecoxib was withdrawn and he was given esomeprazole. His symptoms improved and 3 months later the esophageal mucosa had completely healing (5).

Inhibition of COX-2 in the large bowel can worsen inflammatory bowel disease and collagenous colitis has been reported.

- An 80-year-old woman who had taken celecoxib 100 mg bd for 18 months developed a collagenous colitis, with watery diarrhea, with multiple non-bloody stools each day, and crampy lower abdominal pain (6). Colonoscopy showed diffuse erythema, hyperemia, and multiple linear ulcers. Ulcer biopsies were consistent with collagenous colitis. Celecoxib was withdrawn, she was given mesalazine, and the diarrhea resolved.

Celecoxib reportedly exacerbated inflammatory bowel disease in two patients (7).

- An 80-year-old woman with ulcerative colitis started taking celecoxib for arthritic pain, and 3 days later developed abdominal pain and diarrhea. Celecoxib was withdrawn and her symptoms improved.
- A 35-year-old woman with ileal and perianal Crohn's disease took four doses of celecoxib for an orthopedic injury, and had rectal bleeding, severe abdominal pain, and worse diarrhea. Celecoxib was withdrawn and her symptoms returned to baseline within 5 days.

The possible association of NSAIDs with inflammatory bowel disease is a matter of controversy (SEDA-25, 131), and there is little clinical experience with the selective COX-2 inhibitors. Coxibs should not be prescribed for patients with chronic inflammatory bowel disease until more experience has accumulated.

Liver

A 67-year-old woman developed acute hepatocellular and cholestatic liver damage after taking celecoxib 100 mg/day for 1 week (8). Celecoxib was withdrawn and the liver function tests normalized within 2 weeks.

There have been three case reports of acute cholestatic hepatitis in patients taking celecoxib.

- A 55-year-old non-alcoholic obese woman, who was allergic to sulfa drugs, presented with a 5-day history of jaundice, malaise, and a pruritic rash that began 3 weeks after she started to take celecoxib 200 mg/day for radicular pain (9). There were marked increases in liver enzymes and bilirubin and a peripheral eosinophilia. Liver biopsy showed marked intrahepatocyte cholestasis with eosinophil-rich inflammation, consistent with a drug reaction. Her symptoms and laboratory abnormalities completely resolved after withdrawal of celecoxib but took a long time (4 months) to normalize.
- A 54-year-old woman took celecoxib 200 mg/day for sacroiliac pain (10). After 4 days her pain resolved, but she developed generalized pruritus, which resolved when celecoxib was withdrawn. A week later, the pain recurred and celecoxib was restarted; 2 days later she again developed pruritus associated with dark urine, and 5 days later jaundice and raised bilirubin and liver enzymes. Her eosinophil count was raised. On withdrawal of celecoxib her liver function tests improved and her symptoms resolved.
- A 49-year-old man with alcoholic cirrhosis developed jaundice, fatigue, and choluria after he started to take celecoxib 200 mg/day for musculoskeletal pain (11). There were increases in transaminases, alkaline phosphatase, and bilirubin (to 547 µmol/l). Liver biopsy showed cirrhosis and marked hepatocellular cholestasis. On withdrawal of celecoxib the bilirubin began to fall very slowly; 1 year later he was well, with a total bilirubin concentration of 44 µmol/l.

The histories, clinical findings, and laboratory tests in these cases all suggested celecoxib-induced acute cholestatic hepatitis. The first case suggested that a sulfonamide-like allergic reaction was the pathogenic mechanism, and the same mechanism cannot be excluded in the other two patients, as sulfonamide allergy is often ignored and is discovered only when an adverse reaction occurs. Celecoxib should not be given to patients who are allergic to sulfa drugs.

Urinary tract

As more experience accumulates it appears clear that COX-2 inhibitors have a nephrotoxic potential similar to that of the non-selective NSAIDs. Sixteen cases of tubulointerstitial nephritis were reported to the manufacturers of celecoxib between the time when it was launched in 1999 and July 2001, but the diagnosis was not confirmed in 12 of these cases (12). Most of these renal adverse reactions occur in patients with susceptibility factors associated with prostaglandin-dependent renal function (13–15).

- A 61-year-old woman with rheumatoid arthritis developed renal papillary necrosis after taken celecoxib (200 mg bd) for about 6 months. The drug history and clinical findings suggested celecoxib as the most likely cause (16).
- A 59-year-old man with type 2 diabetes mellitus developed acute allergic interstitial nephritis associated with minimal change disease after taking celecoxib (100-200 mg/day) for 1 year. The laboratory abnormalities lasted for several months after withdrawal of celecoxib and normalized only after treatment with prednisone (17).
- A 78-year-old woman developed membranous glomerulopathy after taking celecoxib (200 mg bd) for 7 months. She developed orbital and leg edema and proteinuria in the nephrotic range. Renal biopsy was consistent with membranous glomerulopathy. Celecoxib was withdrawn and she recovered rapidly and completely (18).
- A 71-year-old man developed nausea and weakness 9 months after starting to take celecoxib (100 mg bd). Tests showed acute interstitial nephritis. Celecoxib was withdrawn and he was given prednisone for 4 weeks; the serum creatinine returned to normal 1 month later (31).

As more experience accumulates it appears that celecoxib has the same adverse renal effects as other NSAIDs. Minimal-change disease with interstitial nephritis and nephritic syndrome have been described in two elderly patients taking celecoxib (19,20). However, it has been claimed that celecoxib is less nephrotoxic than conventional NSAIDs, from the results of a double-blind, randomized, placebo-controlled comparison of the effect of celecoxib, 200 mg every 12 hours to a total of 5 doses, on renal function with that of naproxen 500 mg every 12 hours to a total of 5 doses, in 28 patients with cirrhosis and ascites (21). There was a significant reduction in glomerular filtration rate and renal plasma flow in the patients who took naproxen but not in the other two groups. This suggests that short-term celecoxib does not impair renal function in patients with decompensated cirrhosis. However, further studies are needed before concluding that celecoxib is safer than other NSAIDs in such patients.

Skin

Skin reactions, including rashes, urticaria, and other allergic reactions, are not uncommon, according to data reported to the Australian Adverse Reactions Advisory Committee (22) and other reports (23–25).

Stevens–Johnson syndrome occurred in a 58-year-old man taking celecoxib (26). He recovered promptly after withdrawal. The reaction recurred 1 month later, after one dose of celecoxib.

Sweet's syndrome can be associated with several drugs. A case involving celecoxib has been reported (27).

- A 57-year-old man developed the typical cutaneous erosions and plaques of Sweet's syndrome after taking celecoxib 100 mg bd for 1 week for bursitis. Celecoxib was withdrawn and the mucocutaneous lesions began to clear. However, the bursitis recurred and he restarted celecoxib. The cutaneous lesions worsened dramatically. After withdrawal of celecoxib for the second time the lesions cleared completely.

A fixed drug eruption has been attributed to celecoxib.

- A 57-year-old woman developed a fixed drug eruption while taking celecoxib (200 mg/day for 10 days) for osteoarthritis (28). She developed an eruption or the abdomen and forearm. Both lesions subsided spontaneously but recurred on rechallenge.

Immunologic

Drug-induced lupus-like syndrome has been associated with celecoxib (29).

- A 68-year-old woman started to take celecoxib (200 mg/day) and 2 weeks later developed generalized joint pains and a micropapular skin rash associated with a malar rash. Celecoxib was withdrawn and she was given oral antihistamines and glucocorticoids, with complete resolution of the reaction within 5 days. Skin prick and patch tests with celecoxib were negative. She underwent an oral rechallenge test with increasing doses of celecoxib up to 200 mg/day over 3 days. The rash and polyarthralgia recurred. She had a weakly positive titer of antinuclear antibodies and a skin biopsy that was characteristic of lupus erythematosus. She also had a predisposing HLA-DR4 subtype. Antihistone antibodies and serial antinuclear antibodies were negative. She remained asymptomatic for 1 year of follow up.

Although the product labelling of celecoxib (Celebrex) contains a warning that patient allergic to "sulfa" drugs should avoid using this COX-2 inhibitor, which contain a sulfonamide substituent, there is evidence that cross-reactivity between sulfonamide antimicrobials and celecoxib is low (30). However, further investigations are required to confirm this, in view of a case report that suggested cross-reactivity of celecoxib with sulfamethoxazole (31).

Second-Generation Effects

Lactation

In six lactating women in the final stage of weaning, celecoxib concentrations in breast milk were low relative to concentrations in the maternal plasma, with a median milk/plasma AUC ratio of 0.18, after single dose of celecoxib 200 mg (32).

Drug Administration

Drug overdose

In cases of overdose with celecoxib reported to Texas poison control centers from 1999 to 2004 the mean dose was 701 mg, and the patient age distribution was 5 years or under—48%; 6–19 years—8%; and 20 years or over—44% (33). In 78% of cases exposure was unintentional. The final medical outcome was classified as no effect in 82% of the cases, and minor effects in 12% of the cases. Adverse effects were listed in 5% of the patients, the most common being rash (3%), drowsiness (3%), pruritus (2%), and vomiting (2%). The most frequently listed treatment was decontamination by dilution (43%) or food (32%).

Drug–Drug Interactions

Clopidogrel

Co-administration of celecoxib and clopidogrel can increase the hemorrhagic potential of clopidogrel, possibly by a pharmacokinetic interaction involving CYP2C9 (34). However, this possibility requires confirmation, as serious, sometimes fatal, hemorrhage has been reported during the postmarketing use of clopidogrel alone (35).

Lithium

An interaction of rofecoxib with lithium has been described (SEDA-27, 113) and two reports document the same type of interaction with celecoxib (36,37). Recovery was uneventful. The proposed mechanism was a celecoxib-induced reduction in renal function, causing increased serum lithium concentrations.

Warfarin

Celecoxib can potentiate the anticoagulant effects of warfarin. Although concomitant administration of celecoxib and warfarin had no significant effect on prothrombin time or the steady-state pharmacokinetics of S-warfarin or R-warfarin in 24 healthy volunteers (38), serious bleeding complications have been reported to adverse drug reactions monitoring systems (39) and in journals (40–42). These data suggest that celecoxib potentiates the anticoagulant effects of warfarin in some patients. Patients taking warfarin must be fully monitored when celecoxib is adding, changed, or withdrawn.

References

1. Lantz MS, Giambanco V. Acute onset of auditory hallucinations after initiation of celecoxib therapy. Am J Psychiatry 2000;157(6):1022–3.
2. Lund BC, Neiman RF. Visual disturbance associated with celecoxib. Pharmacotherapy 2001;21(1):114–5.
3. Macknight C, Rojas-Fernandez CH. Celecoxib- and rofecoxib-induced delirium. J Neuropsychiatry Clin Neurosci 2001;13(2):305–6.
4. Crofford LJ, Oates JC, McCune WJ, Gupta S, Kaplan MJ, Catella-Lawson F, Morrow JD, McDonagh KT, Schmaier AH. Thrombosis in patients with connective tissue diseases treated with specific cyclooxygenase 2 inhibitors. A report of four cases. Arthritis Rheum 2000; 43(8):1891–6.
5. Mantry P, Shah A, Sundarman U. Celecoxib associated esophagitis: review of gastrointestinal side effect from COX-2 inhibitors. J Clin Gastroenterol 2003;37:61–6.
6. Fucci JK, Kurella R. Collagenous colitis presenting with linear colonic ulcers in a patient taking a COX-2 nonsteroidal anti-inflammatory drug. Am J Gastroenterol 2002;97 Suppl:127.
7. Bonner GF. Exacerbation of inflammatory bowel disease associated with use of celecoxib. Am J Gastroenterol 2001;96(4):1306–8.
8. Nachimuthu S, Volfinoz L, Gopal LN. Acute liver injury induced by celecoxib. Gastroenterology 2000;118:1471.
9. Galan MV, Gordon SC, Silverman AL. Celecoxib-induced cholestatic hepatitis. Ann Intern Med 2001;134(3):254.
10. O'Beirne JP, Cairns SR. Drug Points: Cholestatic hepatitis in association with celecoxib. BMJ 2001;323(7303):23.
11. Alegria P, Lebre L, Chagas C. Celecoxib-induced cholestatic hepatotoxicity in a patient with cirrhosis. Ann Intern Med 2002;137(1):75.
12. Demke D, Zhao S, Arellano FM. Interstitial nephritis associated with celecoxib. Lancet 2001;358(9294):1726–7.
13. Graham MG. Acute renal failure related to high-dose celecoxib. Ann Intern Med 2001;135(1):69–70.
14. Pfister AK, Crisalli RJ, Carter WH. Cyclooxygenase-2 inhibition and renal function. Ann Intern Med 2001;134(11):1077author reply 1078.
15. Alkhuja S, Menkel RA, Alwarshetty M, Ibrahimbacha AM. Celecoxib-induced nonoliguric acute renal failure. Ann Pharmacother 2002;36(1):52–4.
16. Akhund L, Quinet RJ, Ishaq S. Celecoxib-related renal papillary necrosis. Arch Intern Med 2003;163:114–5.
17. Alper AB Jr, Meleg-Smith S, Krane NK. Nephrotic syndrome and interstitial nephritis associated with celecoxib. Am J Kidney Dis 2002;40:1086–90.
18. Markowitz GS, Falkowitz DC, Isom R, Zaki M, Imaizumi S, Appel GB, D'Agati D. Membranous glomerulopathy and acute interstitial nephritis following treatment with celecoxib. Clin Nephrol 2003;59:137–42.
19. Almansori M, Kovithavongs T, Qarni MU. Cyclooxygenase-2 inhibitor-associated minimal-change disease. Clin Nephrol 2005;63:381–4.
20. Sirvent AE, Enriquez R, Amoros F, Reyes A. Nephrotic syndrome associated with celecoxib {please give original Spanish title}. Nefrologia 2005;25:81–2.
21. Clària J, Kent JD, Lòpez-Parra M, Escolar G, Ruiz-Del-Arbol L, Ginès P, Jimènez W, Vucelic B, Arroyo V. Effects of celecoxib and naproxen on renal function in nonazotemic patients with cirrhosis and ascites. Hepatology 2005;42:579–87.
22. Anonymous. Celecoxib: early Australian reposting experience. Aust Adv Drug React Bull 2000;19:6.
23. Grob M, Scheidegger P, Wuthrich B. Allergic skin reaction to celecoxib. Dermatology 2000;201(4):383.

24. Crouch TE, Stafford CT. Urticaria associated with COX-2 inhibitors. Ann Allergy Asthma Immunol 2000;84:140.
25. Cummins R, Wagner-Weiner L, Paller A. Pseudoporphyria induced by celecoxib in a patient with juvenile rheumatoid arthritis. J Rheumatol 2000;27(12):2938–40.
26. Gill S, Hermolin RH. Case report of a Stevens–Johnson type reaction to celecoxib. Can J Hosp Pharm 2001;54:146.
27. Fye KH, Crowley E, Berger TG, LeBoit PE, Connolly MK. Celecoxib-induced Sweet's syndrome. J Am Acad Dermatol 2001;45(2):300–2.
28. Bandyopadhyay D. Celecoxib-induced fixed drug eruprion. Clin Exp Dermatol 2003;28:45.
29. Poza-Guedes P, Gonzales-Perez R, Canto G. Celecoxib-induced lupus-like syndrome. Rheumatology 2003;42:916–7.
30. Shapiro LE, Knowles SR, Weber E, Neuman MG, Shear NH. Safety of celecoxib in individuals allergic to sulfonamide: a pilot study. Drug Saf 2003;26:187–9.
31. Schuster C, Wüthrich B. Anaphylactic drug reaction to celecoxib and sulfamethoxazole: cross reactivity or coincidence? Allergy 2003;58:107.
32. Gardiner SJ, Doogue MP, Zhang M, Begg EJ. Quantification of infant exposure to celecoxib through breast milk. Br J Clin Pharmacol 2006;61(1):101–5.
33. Forrester MB. Celecoxib exposures reported to Texas poison control centers from 1999 to 2004. Hum Exp Toxicol 2006;25(5):261–6.
34. Fisher AA, Le Couteur DG. Intracerebral hemorrhage following possible interaction between celecoxib and clopidogrel. Ann Pharmacother 2001;35(12):1567–9.
35. Irish Medicines Board. Clopidogrel (Plavix). Newsletter National Pharmacovigilance Center 2001;2–3.
36. Slordal L, Samstad S, Bathen J, Spigset O. A life-threatening interaction between lithium and celecoxib. Br J Clin Pharmacol 2003;55:413–4.
37. Gunja N, Graudins A, Dowsett R. Lithium toxicity: a potential interaction with celecoxib. Intern Med J 2002;32:494.
38. Karim A, Tolbert D, Piergies A, Hubbard RC, Harper K, Wallemark CB, Slater M, Geis GS. Celecoxib does not significantly alter the pharmacokinetics or hypoprothrombinemic effect of warfarin in healthy subjects. J Clin Pharmacol 2000;40(6):655–63.
39. McMorran M, Morawiecka I. Celecoxib (Celebrex): 1 year later. CMAJ 2000;162(7):1044–61048–50.
40. Linder JD, Monkemuller KE, Davis JV, Wilcox CM. Cyclooxygenase-2 inhibitor celecoxib: a possible cause of gastropathy and hypoprothrombinemia. South Med J 2000;93(9):930–2.
41. Mersfelder TL, Stewart LR. Warfarin and celecoxib interaction. Ann Pharmacother 2000;34(3):325–7.
42. Haase KK, Rojas-Fernandez CH, Lane L, Frank DA. Potential interaction between celecoxib and warfarin. Ann Pharmacother 2000;34(5):666–7.

Cinmetacin

General Information

Cinmetacin is an NSAID related to indometacin. There has been little experience with its use. In one study, gastrointestinal adverse effects developed in 13 of 30 patients (1).

Reference

1. Lucietti MV, Banchieri G. Studio clinico sulla efficacia e tollerabilita di un nuovo antiflogistico non-steroideo, la cinmetacina. [Clinical study of the efficacy of and tolerance for a new nonsteroidal anti-inflammatory agent, cinmetacin.] G Clin Med 1980;61(7):545–52.

Clobuzarit

See also Non-steroidal anti-inflammatory drugs

General Information

Clobuzarit, a methylpropionic acid derivative, thought to have a penicillamine-like effect, was withdrawn from the market in the 1980s because of several reports of Stevens–Johnson syndrome (1).

Reference

1. Bird HA. Rheumatology and the pharmaceutical industry. J Rheumatol 1983;10(4):663–4.

Clometacin

General Information

The NSAID clometacin is an indometacin derivative.

Because of the risk of long-term or repeated use of clometacin, the French authorities restricted its use to prescriptions for no more than 8 days. It seems wise to recommend that it be no longer used.

Organs and Systems

Hematologic

Thrombocytopenia has been attributed to clometacin (SEDA-6, 94).

Liver

The hepatotoxic potential of clometacin was first reported in France in 1978. Since then many cases of hepatotoxic effects have been described (SEDA-7, 109). In two retrospective studies the clinical, biochemical, immunological, and histopathological features were outlined in detail (1,2). The patients had jaundice and/or hepatomegaly (90%), weakness (60%), fever (30%), and abdominal pain (20%), with or without diarrhea, nausea, and vomiting, usually presenting after long-term use or shortly after a rechallenge. The biochemical disorders were hepatocellular hepatitis and cholestatic hepatitis. High titers of antitissue antibodies and hypergammaglobulinemia were also present in most patients. Histological findings were characteristic of acute hepatitis or chronic active hepatitis. There was a high prevalence of HLA-antigen B8. These immunological features suggest an autoimmune pathogenesis.

Urinary tract

A retrospective analysis of acute renal insufficiency related to NSAID therapy in France showed that clometacin was most frequently implicated. Cases of functional renal insufficiency and interstitial nephritis with nephrotic syndrome were reported (SEDA-12, 84).

Skin

Skin eruptions, generalized pruritus, and weight loss have been reported (1).

References

1. Pariente EA, Hamoud A, Goldfain D, Latrive JP, Gislon J, Cassan P, Morin T, Staub JL, Ramain JP, Bertrand JL. Hepatites a la clometacine (Duperan). Etude retrospective de 30 cas. Un modèle d'hépatité autoimmune médicamenteuse?. [Hepatitis caused by clometacin (Duperan). Retrospective study of 30 cases. A model of autoimmune drug-induced hepatitis?.] Gastroenterol Clin Biol 1989;13(10):769–74.
2. Islam S, Mekhloufi F, Paul JM, Islam M, Johanet C, Legendre C, Degott C, Abuaf N, Homberg JC. Characteristics of clometacin-induced hepatitis with special reference to the presence of anti-actin cable antibodies. Autoimmunity 1989;2(3):213–21.

Dexibuprofen

General Information

Dexibuprofen is the dextrorotatory isomer of ibuprofen. Clinical experience is still inadequate to judge its safety profile, although there are claims that it is of comparable safety to celecoxib (1).

Pharmacokinetics

The pharmacokinetics of dexibuprofen 400 mg and ibuprofen arginate 600 mg have been compared in 24 healthy volunteers in an open, randomized, two-period, crossover study (2). Ibuprofen arginate had a 45% higher C_{max} and its t_{max} occurred 2 hours earlier, suggesting faster absorption.

Comparative studies

Dexibuprofen and celecoxib

Dexibuprofen 800 mg/day and celecoxib 200 mg/day have been compared in 148 adults with osteoarthritis of the hip in a randomized, parallel-group, double-blind trial (3). The overall incidence of adverse drug reactions was 12% with dexibuprofen and 14% with celecoxib; 8.1%

of those who took dexibuprofen and 9.5% of those who took celecoxib had gastrointestinal disorders.

Dexibuprofen and diclofenac

Oral dexibuprofen 300 mg tds and diclofenac sodium 50 mg tds have been compared in a randomized double-blind, parallel-group study for 15-days in 110 patients with painful osteoarthritis of the knee; 7.3% of the patients taking dexibuprofen and 15% of those taking diclofenac sodium dropped out because of adverse effects (4).

Dexibuprofen and ibuprofen

Dexibuprofen 200 or 400 mg tds and racemic ibuprofen 800 mg tds have been compared in a double-blind randomized trial in 178 patients with painful osteoarthritis of the hip (5). There were adverse drug reactions, mainly gastrointestinal disorders, in 13–15% of those taking dexibuprofen and 17% of those taking racemic ibuprofen.

Dexibuprofen 600 or 1200 mg/day and racemic ibuprofen 2400 mg/day have been compared in an open study for 1-year in 223 inpatients with osteoarthritis of the hip (6). The overall incidence of clinical adverse events was 15% (gastrointestinal tract 12%, nervous system 1.3%, skin 1.3%, others 0.9%).

Dexibuprofen 5 and 7 mg/kg has been compared with ibuprofen 10 mg/kg in children aged 6 months to 14 years with fever caused by upper respiratory tract infections (7). There were no significant differences in efficacy or adverse drug reactions.

Systematic reviews

In a meta-analysis of five trials and three postmarketing surveillance studies in 7133, dexibuprofen was at least as efficacious as racemic ibuprofen in rheumatoid arthritis, ankylosing spondylitis, osteoarthritis of the hip, osteoarthritis of the knee, lumbar vertebral syndrome, distortion of the ankle joint, and dysmenorrhoea (8). Racemic ibuprofen had a 30% and diclofenac a 90% higher incidence of adverse drug reactions. The incidence of adverse drug reactions in the postmarketing surveillance studies was 5.5–7.4% and withdrawals were 2.3–2.7%.

Organs and Systems

Nervous system

Meningoencephalitis has been attributed to dexibuprofen in a 22-year-old woman with systemic lupus erythematosus (9). Patients with systemic lupus erythematosus have increased susceptibility to NSAID-induced aseptic meningitis or encephalitis.

Hematologic

The effects of dexibuprofen 800 mg/day and aspirin 100 mg/day on platelet function have been studied in 12 healthy volunteers; the effects were quantitatively similar, but the effect of aspirin persisted for 24 hours after the last dose whereas platelet aggregation returned to baseline within 24 hours after the last dose of dexibuprofen (10).

Gastrointestinal

The effects of treatment with dexibuprofen, ibuprofen, and diclofenac for 2 weeks on plasma pepsinogen concentrations and the gastrointestinal mucosa have been studied in 60 patients with rheumatological diseases (11). There were no differences in plasma pepsinogen concentrations or gastrointestinal injury between the groups. Adverse events occurred with similar frequencies in the three groups (28%, 38% and 34%).

Drug-Drug Interactions

Phenytoin

Dexibuprofen has been reported to cause phenytoin toxicity, presumably by inhibiting its metabolism (12).

- A 70-year-old woman with epilepsy who had been fit-free while taking phenytoin 300 mg/day, plasma concentrations 48–64 μmol/l, was given dexibuprofen 800 mg/day and 72 hours later developed severe nystagmus, vertigo, somnolence, blurred vision, and xanthopsia. Her total plasma phenytoin concentration was 122 6 μmol/l, unbound concentration 16 μmol/l. All medications were withdrawn and 2 weeks later the phenytoin concentration had fallen to 30 μmol/l (unbound 6.4 μmol/l).

References

1. Hawel R, Klein G, Singer F, Mayrhofer F, Kahler ST. Comparison of the efficacy and tolerability of dexibuprofen and celecoxib in the treatment of osteoarthritis of the hip. Int J Clin Pharmacol Ther 2003;41:153–64.
2. Sádaba B, Campanero MA, Muñoz-Juarez MJ, Gil-Aldea I, García-Quetglas E, Esteras A, Azanza JR. A comparative study of the pharmacokinetics of ibuprofen arginate versus dexibuprofen in healthy volunteers. Eur J Clin Pharmacol 2006;62(10):849–54.
3. Hawel R, Klein G, Singer F, Mayrhofer F, Kähler ST. Comparison of the efficacy and tolerability of dexibuprofen and celecoxib in the treatment of osteoarthritis of the hip. Int J Clin Pharmacol Ther 2003;41(4):153–64.
4. Hawel R, Klein G, Mitterhuber J, Brugger A. Doppelblinde Studie zum Vergleich der Wirksamkeit und Verträglichkeit von 900 mg Dexibuprofen und 150 mg Diclofenac-Natrium bei Patienten mit schmerzhafter Gonarthrose. [Double-blind comparative study of the effectiveness and tolerance of 900 mg dexibuprofen and 150 mg diclofenac sodium in patients with painful gonarthrosis.] Wien Klin Wochenschr 1997;109(2):53–9.
5. Singer F, Mayrhofer F, Klein G, Hawel R, Kollenz CJ. Evaluation of the efficacy and dose-response relationship of dexibuprofen (S(+)-ibuprofen) in patients with osteoarthritis of the hip and comparison with racemic ibuprofen using the WOMAC osteoarthritis index. Int J Clin Pharmacol Ther 2000;38(1):15–24.
6. Mayrhofer F. Efficacy and long-term safety of dexibuprofen [S(+)-ibuprofen]: a short-term efficacy study in patients with osteoarthritis of the hip and a 1-year tolerability study in patients with rheumatic disorders. Clin Rheumatol 2001;20 Suppl 1:S22–9.
7. Yoon JS, Jeong DC, Oh JW, Lee KY, Lee HS, Koh YY, Kim JT, Kang JH, Lee JS. The effects and safety of dexibuprofen compared with ibuprofen in febrile children caused by upper respiratory tract infection. Br J Clin Pharmacol 2008;66(6):854–60.
8. Phleps W. Overview on clinical data of dexibuprofen. Clin Rheumatol 2001;20 Suppl 1:S15–21.
9. Obermoser G, Bellmann R, Pfausler B, Schmutzhard E, Sepp N. Aseptic meningo-encephalitis related to dexibuprofen use in a patient with systemic lupus erythematosus: a case report with MR findings. Lupus 2002;11(7):451–3.
10. González-Correa JA, Arrebola MM, Martín-Salido E, Muñoz-Marín J, de la Cuesta FS, De La Cruz JP. Effects of dexibuprofen on platelet function in humans: comparison with low-dose aspirin. Anesthesiology 2007;106(2):218–25.
11. Gómez BJ, Caunedo A, Redondo L, Esteban J, Sáenz-Dana M, Blasco M, Hergueta P, Rodríguez-Téllez M, Romero R, Pellicer FJ, Herrerías JM. Modification of pepsinogen I levels and their correlation with gastrointestinal injury after administration of dexibuprofen, ibuprofen or diclofenac: a randomized, open-label, controlled clinical trial. Int J Clin Pharmacol Ther 2006;44(4):154–62.
12. Llinares-Tello F, Hernández-Prats C, Pastor-Climente I, Escrivá-Moscardó S.Toxicidad neurológica aguda por probable interacción farmacocinética entre fenitoína y dexibuprofeno. [Pharmacokinetic interaction between phenytoin and dexibuprofen resulting in acute neurological toxicity.] Med Clin (Barc) 2007;128(6):239.

Dexindoprofen

General Information

The NSAID dexindoprofen has a similar adverse effect pattern to the parent drug, indoprofen. Gastrointestinal and nervous system effects and skin reactions are the most frequent (1).

Reference

1. Fornasari PA, Mattara L. Efficacia e tollerabilità del dexindoprofen in confronto con il diclofenac sodico nel trattamento di patienti osteoartrosici. [Efficacy and tolerance of dexindoprofen compared with diclofenac sodium in the treatment of osteoarthrosis patients.] Clin Ter 1985;113(2):125–33.

Dexketoprofen

General Information

Dexketoprofen is an arylpropionic acid derivative, the dextrorotatory stereoisomer of ketoprofen. The analgesic effect of ketoprofen is due to the S(+)-enantiomer (dexketoprofen), while the R(−)-enantiomer has no analgesic activity [1] but may be ulcerogenic [2]. Thus, dexketoprofen should produce equivalent analgesia to twice the dose of ketoprofen, but with less risk of gastrointestinal damage.

Pharmacokinetics

Dexketoprofen is formulated as the water-soluble salt dexketoprofen trometamol, to improve its absorption [3]. The systemic availability of oral dexketoprofen trometamol (12.5 and 25 mg) is similar to that of oral racemic ketoprofen (25 and 50 mg respectively) [4]. Dexketoprofen trometamol is rapidly absorbed, with a t_{max} of 0.25–0.75 hours compared with a t_{max} of 0.5–3 hours for the S-enantiomer after the racemic drug. Of the administered dose 70–80% is recovered in the urine during the first 12 hours, mainly as the acyl-glucuronidated parent drug. R-ketoprofen is not found in the urine after administration of dexketoprofen, confirming the absence of stereoisomeric interconversion in vivo.

Comparative studies

Dexketoprofen trometamol 25mg qds and ketorolac 10 mg qds have been compared in 115 patients with bone cancer pain in a multicenter, randomized, double-blind, parallel-group study [5]. Fewer patients withdrew for any reason, including insufficient therapeutic effect or adverse events, among those who were given dexketoprofen. A total of 54 adverse events were reported by 39 (34%) of the 115 patients. The number of patients with treatment-related adverse events was slightly lower among those who were given dexketoprofen trometamol (16%) than among those who were given ketorolac (24%). Most of the adverse events were mild or moderate in intensity, the most frequent being gastrointestinal complaints, especially constipation, vomiting, and abdominal pain; 3.5% had serious adverse events in each group. Only one of the five serious adverse events was considered to be related to the study treatment—gastrointestinal hemorrhage in one patient who received ketorolac). Six patients withdrew because of adverse events: one taking dexketoprofen died from progression of cancer and five who were given ketorolac withdrew because of gastrointestinal bleeding, diarrhea, feeling of hot/cold, erythematous rash, and abdominal pain.

Dexketoprofen trometamol 50 mg has been compared with racemic ketoprofen100 mg every 8 hours over 2 days, both given intravenously, in 252 patients with pain after hip or knee replacement surgery in a multicenter, double-blind, randomized, parallel-group study in patients with moderate to severe pain [6]. Both groups needed rescue analgesia—81% of those who received dexketoprofen and 87% of those who received ketoprofen. There were treatment-related adverse events in 16% of patients who were given dexketoprofen compared with 21% of those who were given ketoprofen.

A single intravenous dose of dexketoprofen trometamol has been compared with an intravenous infusion of metamizole (dipyrone) in 308 patients with moderate to severe pain due to renal colic. Dexketoprofen produced similar analgesia to metamizole but with a faster onset.

In a randomized, double-blind, parallel, active controlled, multicenter study in 370 out-patients with acute low back pain intramuscular dexketoprofen 25 or 50 mg bd was compared with intramuscular diclofenac 75mg bd for 2 days [7]. Five patients withdrew from the study because of adverse events (two who took dexketoprofen 25 mg, one who took dexketoprofen 50 mg, and two who took metamizole). Injections site reactions were common with dexketoprofen (19 patients in all, 9.3%) and did not occur with metamizole. Gastrointestinal disorders (abdominal pain, constipation, dyspepsia, nausea, vomiting, and dry mouth) occurred in 11 patients (5.4%). Otherwise adverse effects were uncommon and similar in the three groups. There were 10 serious adverse events in those who were given dexketoprofen; most were recurrences of renal pain and none was considered to be drug-related.

Placebo-controlled studies

Rofecoxib 50 mg and dexketoprofen trometamol 25 mg have been compared in a double-blind, randomized, placebo-controlled trial in 120 patients undergoing surgical removal of a single mandibular third molar [8]. Adverse events were mild to moderate in intensity. There were 20 adverse events in 15 subjects, six with rofecoxib, five with dexketoprofen, and four with placebo. The most frequent events were nausea and vomiting (n = 4), tiredness/drowsiness (n = 3), headache (n = 2), and feeling hot/feverish (n = 2). One patient who was given dexketoprofen reported profuse bleeding (not otherwise specified) starting 4 hours after the administration of dexketoprofen and lasting for 30 minutes. None of the reported events resulted in withdrawal from the study.

Systematic reviews

In a systematic review of trials in acute and chronic pain in 6380 patients, of whom 3381 took dexketoprofen, 35 trials were included [9]. Almost all of them were of short duration in acute conditions or recent onset pain. In all 12 randomised trials that compared dexketoprofen (any dose) with placebo dexketoprofen was statistically superior. Adverse event withdrawal rates, which are shown in Table 1, were low in postoperative pain and higher in trials of longer duration; no serious adverse events, such as gastrointestinal bleeding, myocardial infarction, or death, were reported.

Table 1. Adverse events withdrawal rates in trials involving dexketoprofen

Drug	Withdrawals due to adverse events (%) (n)	
	Dental and postsurgical pain	Other acute pain, back pain, arthritis
Placebo	2.5 (236)	no data
Dexketoprofen	1.8 (652)	3.2 (844)
Tramadol	1.4 (72)	9.7 (247)
Ketoprofen	1.3 (301)	7.9 (152)
Diclofenac	0.0 (80)	3.7 (272)
Paracetamol + opioid	0.0 (100)	1.2 (167)

Organs and Systems

Hematologic

- A previously healthy 35-year-old woman had an episode of fever, neutropenia, thrombocytopenia, and raised liver function tests 10 days after she started to take dexketoprofen trometamol [10]. Infectious and autoimmune causes of neutropenia and viral or autoimmune hepatitis were excluded. She recovered after withdrawal of dexketoprofen.

Skin

Dexketoprofen has been reported to cause photosensitivity after oral therapy [11].

- A 27-year-old woman developed contact photosensitivity after applying topical dexketoprofen trometamol for joint pains [12]. Photopatch testing for components of the gel was positive for ketoprofen trometamol only.

In another case a patient developed a cutaneous eruption in a photoexposed area 1 week after topical treatment with dexketoprofen [13]. Photopatch tests were positive for dexketoprofen, ketoprofen, and piketoprofen and a patch test was positive for piketoprofen. Control photopatch testing with dexketoprofen in 15 healthy volunteers was negative.

Other reports have appeared [14], and photoallergic contact dermatitis in patients taking dexketoprofen has also been discussed in the context of six cases [15].

Drug-Drug Interactions

Co-magaldrox

The effect of co-magaldrox (magnesium trisilicate + aluminium hydroxide) on the pharmacokinetics of dexketoprofen trometamol has been studied in a randomized, three-way, crossover study in 24 healthy volunteers who took three single doses of dexketoprofen trometamol 25 mg either fasting, after co-magaldrox, or after a high-fat breakfast [16]. Co-magaldrox, given 10 minutes before dexketoprofen trometamol did not alter its pharmacokinetics. Food significantly increased the t_{max} and significantly reduced the C_{max}. of dexketoprofen trometamol, suggesting a change in the rate of absorption, but did not alter the extent of absorption.

References

1. Barbanoj MJ, Antonijoan RM, Gich I. Clinical pharmacokinetics of dexketoprofen. Clin Pharmacokinet 2001;40:245–62.
2. Herrero JF, Romero-Sandoval EA, Gaitan G, Mazario J. Antinociception and the new COX inhibitors: research approaches and clinical perspectives. CNS Drug Rev 2003;9:227–52.
3. Barbanoj MJ, Gich I, Artigas R, Tost D, Moros C, Antonijoan RM, García ML, Mauleón D. Pharmacokinetics of dexketoprofen trometamol in healthy volunteers after single and repeated oral doses. J Clin Pharmacol 1998;38(12 Suppl):33S-40S..
4. Mauleón D, Artigas R, García ML, Carganico G. Preclinical and clinical development of dexketoprofen. Drugs 1996;52 Suppl 5:24–45.
5. Rodríguez MJ, Contreras D, Gálvez R, Castro A, Camba MA, Busquets C, Herrera J. Double-blind evaluation of short-term analgesic efficacy of orally administered dexketoprofen trometamol and ketorolac in bone cancer pain. Pain 2003;104(1-2):103–10.
6. Zippel H, Wagenitz A. Comparison of the efficacy and safety of intravenously administered dexketoprofen trometamol and ketoprofen in the management of pain after orthopaedic surgery: a multicentre, double-blind, randomised, parallel-group clinical trial. Clin Drug Investig 2006;26(9):517–28.
7. Sánchez-Carpena J, Domínguez-Hervella F, García I, Gene E, Bugarín R, Martín A, Tomás-Vecina S, García D, Serrano JA, Roman A, Mariné M, Mosteiro ML; Dexketoprofen Renal Colic Study Group. Comparison of intravenous dexketoprofen and dipyrone in acute renal colic. Eur J Clin Pharmacol 2007;63(8):751–60.
8. Jackson ID, Heidemann BH, Wilson J, Power I, Brown RD. Double-blind, randomized, placebo-controlled trial comparing rofecoxib with dexketoprofen trometamol in surgical dentistry. Br J Anaesth 2004;92(5):675–80.
9. Moore RA, Barden J. Systematic review of dexketoprofen in acute and chronic pain. BMC Clin Pharmacol 2008;8:11.
10. Zabala S, Calpe MJ, Pérez G, Lerín FJ, Mouronval L. Neutropenia, thrombocytopenia and hepatic injury associated with dexketoprofen trometamol therapy in a previously healthy 35-year-old woman. J Clin Pharm Ther 2008;33(1):79–81.
11. Asensio T, Sanchís ME, Sánchez P, Vega JM, García JC. Photocontact dermatitis because of oral dexketoprofen. Contact Dermatitis 2008;58(1):59–60.
12. Cuerda Galindo E, Goday Bujan JJ, del Pozzo Losada J, Garcia Silva J, Pena Penabad C, Fonseca E. Photocontact dermatitis due to dexketoprofen. Contact Dermatitis 2003;48:283–4.
13. López-Abad R, Paniagua MJ, Botey E, Gaig P, Rodriguez P, Richart C. Topical dexketoprofen as a cause of photocontact dermatitis. J Investig Allergol Clin Immunol 2004;14(3):247–9.
14. Valenzuela N, Puig L, Barnadas MA, Alomar A. Photocontact dermatitis due to dexketoprofen. Contact Dermatitis 2002;47(4):237.
15. Goday-Bujan JJ, Rodríguez-Lozano J, Martínez-González MC, Fonseca E. Photoallergic contact dermatitis from dexketoprofen: study of 6 cases. Contact Dermatitis 2006;55(1):59–61.
16. McEwen J, De Luca M, Casini A, Gich I, Barbanoj MJ, Tost D, Artigas R, Mauleón D. The effect of food and an antacid on the bioavailability of dexketoprofen trometamol. J Clin Pharmacol 1998;38(12 Suppl):41S–45S.

Diclofenac

General Information

The overall incidence of adverse reactions to diclofenac is about 30%, but less than 1% of patients have to have treatment withdrawn for this reason. The manufacturers' analysis of 1966 adverse effects in 987 patients over about 6 years, when over 30 million patients had been treated, provided some interesting quantitative data. Of the total number of adverse reactions, 34% were gastrointestinal and 16% hematological. Worldwide experience with diclofenac showed that the incidences of serious adverse drug reactions in phase III short-term trials (1227 patients) and long-term trials (1173 patients) in the USA were respectively as follows (1):

- peptic ulcer 0.16 and 0.34%;
- gastrointestinal bleeding 0.16 and 0.17%;
- hepatitis 0 and 0.26%;
- thrombocytopenia 0 and 0.17%.

Organs and Systems

Respiratory

Oral diclofenac caused eosinophilic pneumonitis in a 67-year-old man (2) and also during long-term topical use in a 62-year-old woman (3).

- A 62-year-old woman developed a chronic cough and bilateral infiltrates on the chest X-ray. She had been taking diclofenac emulgel for 10 years for osteoarthritis. Bronchoscopy showed eosinophilic alveolitis. After ruling out other possible causes, eosinophilic pneumonia was diagnosed. Diclofenac was withdrawn and oral glucocorticoids started. Within 7 days the bilateral pulmonary infiltrates on CT scan resolved.

Nervous system

The frequency of central nervous system adverse effects is 1–9%. Headache, dizziness, vertigo, insomnia, drowsiness, and agitation have been reported. Hallucinatory symptoms and generalized tonic-clonic seizures have also been described (SEDA-16, 109). Toxic encephalitis can be part of a general toxic reaction (4). Diclofenac provoked aseptic meningitis in patients with systemic lupus erythematosus (SEDA-17, 109).

Sensory systems

Hyperemia, burning of the eyes, eyelid allergic contact dermatitis, and conjunctivitis can occur in patients who use diclofenac eye-drops (SEDA-20, 92) (SEDA-21, 104).

Diclofenac can cause reduced corneal sensitivity, starting from 15 minutes after instillation and measurable after 1 hour (5). This corneal hypesthesia can be useful in reducing pain and discomfort in ocular inflammation and after surgery. In chronic treatment, however, the effect of diclofenac on corneal nerves can cause either increased healing time of the corneal epithelium or a neurotrophic epitheliopathy in patients with conditions that predispose to epithelial damage, such as dry eyes. In contrast, flurbiprofen, indometacin, and ketorolac tromethamine did not cause corneal hypesthesia.

Keratolysis (corneal melting) occurred after 5 days during the use of topical preservative-free diclofenac qds after laser-assisted subepithelial keratectomy in a 25-year-old man (6). There was corneal edema with

Descemet's membrane striae and epithelial microcysts and a vertical epithelial defect (1.0×2.0 mm), with 30% tissue loss in the affected area. After withdrawal of diclofenac topical dexamethasone produced improvement but not complete healing.

Electrolyte balance

Severe hyponatremia developed in an elderly woman treated with intramuscular diclofenac (SEDA-13, 80).

NSAIDs can cause hyperkalemic acidosis and should be used with caution in the presence of renal impairment (7).

- A 76-year-old woman developed quadriparesis associated with hyperkalemia after taking diclofenac 100 mg/day for 10 months for gouty arthritis. She had a metabolic acidosis with a normal anion gap and mild renal impairment. Her weakness resolved after withdrawal of diclofenac and correction of the hyperkalemia.

Mineral balance

At least three reports of severe hyponatremia have been described (SEDA-12, 85) (SEDA-13, 80) (SEDA-18, 103). In the last case the withdrawal of diclofenac and fluid restriction led to normal fluid and electrolyte balance within 10 days, despite concomitant treatment with nabumetone.

Hematologic

In an analysis of 447 adverse effects in 194 patients worldwide (8), 20 had blood abnormalities, including two cases of agranulocytosis and one of granulocytopenia. One of these patients, who was sensitive to pyrazolone, had taken a pyrazolone compound as well. Immune-mediated agranulocytosis and thrombocytopenia have been reported (SEDA-16, 110).

Reversible hemolytic anemia (SEDA-4, 69) (9), two cases of severe immune hemolytic anemia with acute renal insufficiency (SEDA-20, 92) (SEDA-22, 115), and fatal hemolytic anemia have occurred (10).

Occasionally, for unknown reasons, patients who develop either immune hemolysis or thrombocytopenia while taking diclofenac may simultaneously be sensitized to both erythrocytes and platelets.

- Two patients developed antibodies against platelets and red blood cells while taking diclofenac (11). One developed severe hemolysis and significant thrombocytopenic purpura, and the other developed thrombocytopenia but no hemolysis. Standard serological tests for antibodies against platelets and erythrocytes were carried out in the presence and absence of diclofenac and its metabolites. Both patients had a positive direct antiglobulin test and drug-dependent and/or metabolite-dependent antibodies against erythrocytes and platelets.

A systematic evaluation of 12 patients who had diclofenac-induced immune hemolysis has provided evidence that patients with diclofenac-induced immune hemolysis produce a broad spectrum of anti-diclofenac erythrocyte antibodies (12). The metabolite 4'-OH-diclofenac seems to be the most immunogenic metabolite. Nevertheless, all patients' sera samples contain a mixture of antibodies that recognize several distinguishable epitopes, which consist of different drug metabolites and a target protein on the erythrocyte surface, which appears to be the Rh complex in many, but not all, cases. However, when serum samples were processed to detect platelet antibodies to diclofenac or diclofenac metabolites, none of the 12 patients gave positive results. Additional target proteins remain to be identified.

Diclofenac can cause panmyelopathy (13). Data from the International Agranulocytosis and Aplastic Anemia Study showed an increased risk of aplastic anemia (multivariate rate-ratio 8.8) (14). Fatal aplastic anemia has also been described (SEDA-4, 69) (15), as have purpura and thrombocytopenia, although not always with certainty. Spontaneous bleeding (subcutaneous bruises, hematoma, greater wound drainage) has been associated with diclofenac (SEDA-15, 100).

Bone marrow necrosis has been attributed to diclofenac (16).

- A 26-year-old man who received 12 doses of intramuscular diclofenac 75 mg at 30-minute intervals for renal colic developed fever and bone pain 5 days later. His hemoglobin was 7.7 g/dl and there was leukopenia (1.6 x 10^9/l) and neutropenia (0.5 x 10^9/l) but no thrombocytopenia (179 x 10^9/l). Bone marrow aspiration smears showed striking necrosis and nearly absent intact hemopoietic cells; bone marrow biopsy showed bone marrow necrosis. He recovered after blood transfusion.

The authors attributed the bone marrow necrosis to cytokine release because of the large dose of diclofenac.

Gastrointestinal

Gastrointestinal adverse effects are particularly frequent, and affect some 14–25% of patients; the incidence of the most serious, peptic ulcer and bleeding were 0.16–0.34% and 0.16–0.17%, respectively (1). A prospective 12-week endoscopic study documented better gastrointestinal tolerability with diclofenac than naproxen (SEDA-20, 92). Upper gastrointestinal hemorrhage has been associated with transdermal application of diclofenac, with massive bleeding in two of four patients (SEDA-21, 104).

Perforation of the terminal ileum occurred in one patient who had taken a high dose (400 mg/day) of modified-release diclofenac (17).

Colonic stricture, similar to ileum "diaphragm" disease, developed in a patient during prolonged administration of modified-release diclofenac (18). Pseudomembranous colitis and colonic ulceration, with or without a diaphragm-like colonic stricture, have been reported (SEDA-16, 110; SEDA-17, 109). Dispersible diclofenac is a formulation from which absorption is more rapid than the usual formulation, but gastrointestinal adverse events still occur (SEDA-20, 92).

Non-specific colitis has been reported in a 69-year-old man who took modified-release diclofenac 200 mg/day (19).

Rectal administration caused adverse effects in 16% of patients (20); anorectal lesions (erosions, ulcers, stenosis of the anal margin) occurred after a relatively short period of suppository use (21).

Liver

Liver function can be impaired during diclofenac treatment, and liver damage may be more common than previously thought (SEDA-10, 83; 22). The risk is the same as with the few other NSAIDs that have been adequately studied. Biopsy-proven hepatitis with positive rechallenge and dechallenge has been described (23) and confirmed (24,25). The usual clinical presentation is acute hepatitis, but chronic active hepatitis has been described (24–27). Although recovery is usually rapid in the acute form after drug withdrawal, fatal cases have occurred (SEDA-11, 93; SEDA-12, 85; SEDA-13, 80; 28). Diclofenac-induced fulminant hepatic failure has been successfully treated with liver transplantation (29). Patients who developed combined reversible hepatorenal damage have also been reported (30–32) (SEDA-20, 91).

In a retrospective study, two-thirds of cases were detected by symptoms (jaundice, anorexia, nausea, vomiting, with or without fever) (33). The illness developed more than 5 weeks after starting diclofenac in more than 75% of patients, and within six months in 85%. Liver injury was classified as hepatocellular in 54% of patients and the histology was acute hepatocellular injury (nine patients) and chronic hepatitis (six patients). Factors affecting the susceptibility to diclofenac liver damage were sex (female) and type of disease (osteoarthritis). The mechanism of diclofenac-induced liver injury is unknown, but since the incidence is very low an idiosyncratic mechanism rather than intrinsic toxicity of the drug seems likely. In view of the rarity of hallmarks of hypersensitivity, the delayed development of injury and the delayed response to rechallenge, a metabolic effect rather than immunological idiosyncratic mechanism seems probable in most cases. The usefulness of monitoring serum enzymes is unknown, but it might be prudent to do so in the first 6 months of treatment.

Susceptibility to hepatotoxicity due to diclofenac in 24 patients has been associated with polymorphisms in the genes encoding the enzymes UGT2B7 and CYP2C8, which determine the formation of reactive diclofenac metabolites, and in ABCC2, which encodes the transporter MRP2, which contributes to the biliary excretion of the reactive metabolite (34). The UGT2B7*2 allele was eight times more common in patients with diclofenac hepatotoxicity than in controls and the ABCC2 C-24T variant was 5–6 times more common. Haplotype distributions for CYP2C8 were different in patients compared with hospital controls.

Urinary tract

Renal papillary necrosis and interstitial nephritis with the nephrotic syndrome have been documented (35,36). Other cases of the nephrotic syndrome, with or without renal insufficiency, which were apparently due to minimal-change nephropathy (which is relatively more common in NSAID users), have been reported (37,38). The unusual feature of diclofenac-associated renal interstitial mucinosis has been described (SEDA-17, 109). Functional renal insufficiency after the use of diclofenac in a patient with burns has been described (SEDA-20, 92).

Skin

Allergic skin rashes, serous bullous dermatitis with positive rechallenge, and linear IgA deposits along the basal membrane in lesional and perilesional skin have all been reported (39). A patient who developed Stevens–Johnson syndrome died (SEDA-5, 103). Contact dermatitis and a generalized maculopapular eruption caused by delayed hypersensitivity to diclofenac have been reported with topical and oral diclofenac (SEDA-18, 104). Photosensitivity after topical application has been described (SEDA-22, 115). Diclofenac triggered pemphigus vulgaris, an uncommon manifestation of NSAID toxicity (SEDA-22, 115).

Photoallergic contact dermatitis has been attributed to topical diclofenac (40).

- Contact dermatitis on the eyelids developed in a 70-year-old-woman after she had used eye-drops containing diclofenac. Patch tests were positive to both diclofenac and indometacin, suggesting possible cross-reactivity between the two compounds (41).
- Staphylococcal scalded skin syndrome developed in a 68-year-old man after he had taken diclofenac for knee arthritis subsequently diagnosed as septic arthritis due to *Staphylococcus aureus* (42).

NSAIDs can predispose to severe infections (SEDA-22, 112).

Nicolau syndrome (embolia cutis medicamentosa) is a very rare complication of intramuscular injections, in which there is extensive necrosis of the injected skin area, perhaps due to accidental intra-arterial and/or para-arterial injection; it usually occurs in children (43). Of the NSAIDs with which it has been reported, diclofenac is the most common (44–47).

Musculoskeletal

Massive rhabdomyolysis resulting in renal insufficiency with complete recovery after withdrawal has been described in a man who took diclofenac for 2 weeks (SEDA-21, 104).

Immunologic

Acute allergic reactions were reported in 48 patients, and included anaphylactic or anaphylactoid reactions and angioedema without shock. Two anaphylactic reactions, one fatal, to parenteral diclofenac have been reported (SEDA-18, 104). Hepatorenal damage (SEDA-15, 100), thrombocytopenia, and hemolytic anemia mediated by an immune mechanism have been reported (SEDA-16, 110).

Skin tests with diclofenac were not useful in diagnosing hypersensitivity in a series of 12 non-atopic patients who had severe symptoms of hypersensitivity (48). However, oral challenge in patients who had had only cutaneous symptoms was diagnostic.

Second-Generation Effects

Fertility

Three cases of infertility have been reported with diclofenac (SEDA-21, 104).

Fetotoxicity

As inhibitors of cyclo-oxygenase, NSAIDs given during pregnancy can cause adverse maternal and fetal effects (SEDA-22, 112).

- Premature closure of the ductus arteriosus occurred in a fetus who was exposed in utero to diclofenac at 34–35 weeks of gestation (49). Emergency cesarean section was performed and the baby girl required cardiorespiratory support and multiple medications. She gradually improved and further development was normal.

Susceptibility Factors

The Japanese Health Authority has sent a "Dear Doctor" letter warning against the use of diclofenac in patients with encephalitis or encephalopathy related to influenza, which may be associated with higher mortality (50).

Drug Administration

Drug administration route

Aseptic tissue necrosis after intramuscular injection (Nicolau syndrome) has been reported after accidental intra-arterial injection.

Nicolau syndrome (livedoid dermatitis) is a rare adverse reaction that occurs at the site of intramuscular injection (51). It typically causes pain around the injection site soon after injection, followed by erythema, a livedoid patch, a hemorrhagic patch, and finally necrosis of skin, subcutaneous fat, and muscle. It has commonly been reported in association with non-steroidal anti-inflammatory drugs, corticosteroids, and penicillins. In a case of Nicolau syndrome after injection of diclofenac, a large ulcer over the right buttock became infected with *Pseudomonas aeruginosa*, and there was subcutaneous fat necrosis and non-specific inflammation without evidence of malignancy or vasculitis; the lesion required repeated debridement and a partial-thickness skin graft (52). Subcutaneous injection, rather than intramuscular injection, was found to be a determining factor in this case.

During 1997–2002 the Iran pharmacovigilance center received reports of adverse reactions after intramuscular injection of diclofenac (53). An estimated 326 million injections were given; there were 73 reports of foot drop, 40 of leg paralysis, and 63 of difficulty in walking. The sites of injection were not specified.

Antirheumatic drugs are often involved in these reactions and diclofenac has also been implicated (54). Other consequences of intramuscular administration of diclofenac are asymptomatic high serum creatine kinase activity or damage to muscle, nerve, or blood vessels (SEDA-17, 109).

NSAIDs should not be injected into the gluteal muscles because of the risk of adverse effects; the lateral thigh should be preferred (55). Many injections into the buttocks that are intended to be intramuscular are actually subcutaneous, because the needle is too short to reach the muscle through a large thickness of subcutaneous fat; intramuscular NSAIDs should be given into the lateral thigh, if at all.

Necrotizing fasciitis was reported in three patients, two of whom died as a consequence of severe local reactions associated with intramuscular diclofenac (56).

If appropriately diluted and infused intravenously, diclofenac is usually well tolerated, although local venous thrombosis has been described (SEDA-17, 109).

Drug–Drug Interactions

Ciclosporin

The risk of ciclosporin-induced nephrotoxicity can be increased when NSAIDs are also used (57,58). Diclofenac in particular should be avoided, because it is more likely to cause deterioration of renal function in patients taking ciclosporin (SEDA-15, 100) (SEDA-17, 107). There is also a pharmacokinetic interaction, which may be caused by inhibition by ciclosporin of the first-pass metabolism of diclofenac (SEDA-21, 104).

In 16 healthy volunteers there were no important pharmacokinetic changes when a single dose of ciclosporin was taken during steady-state administration of aspirin, indometacin, or piroxicam, but there was an interaction with diclofenac, whose AUC was doubled in the presence of ciclosporin (59).

In patients with rheumatoid arthritis, steady-state coadministration of diclofenac with ciclosporin was associated with a significant rise in serum creatinine concentration.

Lithium

Diclofenac increases serum lithium concentrations by impairing its renal excretion (60).

Diclofenac increases serum lithium concentrations by impairing its renal excretion (62).

- The serum lithium concentration nearly doubled to 1.3 mmol/l after a 57-year-old woman started to take diclofenac (63).

Morphine

Although spinal morphine provides effective analgesia, different ways of managing and minimizing its troubling adverse effects are constantly sought. Diclofenac, a non-steroidal anti-inflammatory drug, improves the analgesia provided by epidural morphine and may allow dosage reduction. In an investigation of this drug combination, intrathecal morphine was administered either regularly or on demand to 120 women undergoing cesarean section in doses of 0.1 mg, 0.05 mg, or 0.025 mg with diclofenac 75 mg intramuscularly (64). Severe pruritus was significantly more common in those who received morphine 0.1 mg and there was a trend toward less vomiting with smaller doses. There was no respiratory depression. The results suggested that the adverse effects of intrathecal morphine are dose-dependent and that there was no advantage in using doses of morphine larger than 0.25 mg.

Quinidine

In human liver microsomes, diclofenac inhibited testosterone 6-beta-hydroxylation with characteristics that suggested that it inactivated CYP3A4 (65). Quinidine, which stimulates CYP3A4-mediated diclofenac 5-hydroxylation, did not affect the inactivation of CYP3A4 assessed by testosterone 6-beta-hydroxylation activity but accelerated the inactivation assessed by diazepam 3-hydroxylation activity.

In 30 healthy young men the pharmacokinetics of a single oral dose of quinidine 200 mg were studied before and during the daily administration of diclofenac 100 mg (a substrate of CYP2C9) (66). The clearance of quinidine by N-oxidation was reduced by diclofenac, but only by 27%. This small effect of diclofenac suggests a minor role for CYP2C9 in the metabolism of quinidine.

Triamterene

The interaction between diclofenac and triamterene causes renal impairment (61).

Interference with Diagnostic Tests

Thyroid hormone tests

Diclofenac alters thyroid hormone tests, causing a fall in total serum triiodothyronine, principally by interfering with its serum protein binding (SEDA-19, 98).

References

1. Catalano MA. Worldwide safety experience with diclofenac. Am J Med 1986;80(4B):81–7.
2. Khalil H, Molinary E, Stoller JK. Diclofenac (Voltaren)-induced eosinophilic pneumonitis. Case report and review of the literature. Arch Intern Med 1993;153(14):1649–5.
3. Kohlhaulfl M, Weber N, Morresi-Hauf A, Geiger D, Raith H, Haussinger K. Pulmonary infiltrates with blood eosinophilia in a 62-year-old patient. Internist 2003;44:1037–4.
4. Bandelot JB, Mihout B. Encephalopathie myoclonique au diclofénac. [Myoclonic encephalopathy due to diclofenac.] Nouv Presse Med 1978;7(16):1406.
5. Aragona P, Tripodi G, Spinella R, Lagana E, Ferreri G. The effects of the topical administration of non-steroidal anti-inflammatory drugs on corneal epithelium and corneal sensitivity in normal subjects. Eye 2000;14(Pt 2):206–10.

6. Zanini M, Savini G, Barboni P. Corneal melting associated with topical diclofenac use after laser-assisted subepithelial keratectomy. J Cataract Refract Surg 2006;32(9):1570–2.

7. Patel P, Mandal B, Greenway MW. Hyperkalaemic quadriparesis secondary to chronic diclofenac treatment. Postgrad Med J 2001;77(903):50–1.

8. Ciucci AG. A review of spontaneously reported adverse drug reactions with diclofenac sodium (Voltarol). Rheumatol Rehabil 1979;(Suppl 2):116–21.

9. Salama A, Gottsche B, Mueller-Eckhardt C. Autoantibodies and drug- or metabolite-dependent antibodies in patients with diclofenac-induced immune haemolysis. Br J Haematol 1991;77(4):546–9.

10. Heuft HG, Postels H, Hoppe I, Weisbach V, Zeiler T, Zingsem J, Eckstein R. Eine todlich verlaufene immunhämolytische Anämie nach Applikation von Diclofenac. [Fatal course of immune hemolytic anemia following administration of diclofenac.] Beitr Infusionsther 1990;26:412–4.

11. Meyer O, Hoffman T, Aslan T, Ahrens N, Kiesewetter H, Salama A. Diclofenac-induced antibodies against RBCs and platelets: two case reports and a concise review. Transfusion 2003;43:345–9.

12. Sachs UJ, Santoso S, Roder L, Smart E, Bein G, Kroll H. Diclofenac-induced antibodies against red blood cells are heterogeneous and recognize different epitopes. Transfusion 2004;44:1226–30.

13. Porzsolt F, Heit W, Heimpel H, Asbeck F. Panmyelopathie nach Einnahme von Diclofenac?. [Panmyelopathy after administration of diclofenac?.] Dtsch Med Wochenschr 1979;104(27):986–7.

14. The International Agranulocytosis and Aplastic Anemia Study. Risks of agranulocytosis and aplastic anemia. A first report of their relation to drug use with special reference to analgesics. JAMA 1986;256(13):1749–57.

15. Eustace S, O'Neill T, McHale S, Molony J. Fatal aplastic anaemia following prolonged diclofenac use in an elderly patient. Ir J Med Sci 1989;158(8):217.

16. Aydogdu I, Erkurt MA, Ozhan O, Kaya E, Kuku I, Yitmen E, Aydin NE. Reversible bone marrow necrosis in a patient due to overdosage of diclofenac sodium. Am J Hematol 2006;81(4):298.

17. Deakin M. Small bowel perforation associated with an excessive dose of slow release diclofenac sodium. BMJ 1988;297(6646):488–9.

18. Huber T, Ruchti C, Halter F. Nonsteroidal antiinflammatory drug-induced colonic strictures: a case report. Gastroenterology 1991;100(4):1119–22.

19. Bielsa Martín S, Porcel Pérez JM, Madroñero Vuelta AB, Planella Rubinat MJ. Colitis aguda por diclofenaco. [Acute colitis from diclofenac.] Rev Esp Enferm Dig 2006;98(3):226–7.

20. Baroni L, Comoglio T, Trombetta N, Cornelli U. Il diclofenac sodico nella terapia ambulatoriale dell'infiammazione o del dolore articolare. Ricerca multicentrica aperta condotta da 223 medici italiani. [Sodium diclofenac in the ambulatory therapy of joint inflammation and pain. Multicentric open-ended research performed by 223 Italian physicians.] Clin Ter 1982;100(4):383–99.

21. Gizzi G, Villani V, Brandi G, Paganelli GM, Di Febo G, Biasco G. Ano-rectal lesions in patients taking suppositories containing non-steroidal anti-inflammatory drugs (NSAID). Endoscopy 1990;22(3):146–8.

22. Tanner E, Wachter G, Lasarof I, Gaida P. Klinische Erfahrungen mit dem neuen Antirheumatikum Diclofenac. [Clinical experiences with the new antirheumatic diclofenac.] Z Gesamte Inn Med 1982;37(1):8–12.

23. Dunk AA, Walt RP, Jenkins WJ, Sherlock SS. Diclofenac hepatitis. BMJ (Clin Res Ed) 1982;284(6329):1605–6.

24. Iveson TJ, Ryley NG, Kelly PM, Trowell JM, McGee JO, Chapman RW. Diclofenac associated hepatitis. J Hepatol 1990;10(1):85–9.

25. Strom BL, Carson JL, Schinnar R, Sim E, Morse ML. The effect of indication on the risk of hypersensitivity reactions associated with tolmetin sodium vs other nonsteroidal anti-inflammatory drugs. J Rheumatol 1988;15(4):695–9.

26. Mazeika PK, Ford MJ. Chronic active hepatitis associated with diclofenac sodium therapy. Br J Clin Pract 1989;43(3):125–6.

27. Sallie RW, McKenzie T, Reed WD, Quinlan MF, Shilkin KB. Diclofenac hepatitis. Aust NZ J Med 1991;21(2):251–5.

28. Helfgott SM, Sandberg-Cook J, Zakim D, Nestler J. Diclofenac-associated hepatotoxicity. JAMA 1990;264(20):2660–2.

29. Jones AL, Latham T, Shallcross TM, Simpson KJ. Fulminant hepatic failure due to diclofenac treated successfully by orthotopic liver transplantation. Transplant Proc 1998;30(1):192–4.

30. Diggory P, Golding RL, Lancaster R. Renal and hepatic impairment in association with diclofenac administration. Postgrad Med J 1989;65(765):507–8.

31. Hovette P, Touze JE, Debonne JM, Delmarre B, Rogier C, Schmoor P, Aubry P. Hépatite choléstatique et insuffisance rénale aiguë au cours d'un traitement par diclofénac. [Cholestatic hepatitis and acute kidney insufficiency during treatment with diclofenac.] Ann Gastroenterol Hepatol (Paris) 1989;25(6):257–8.

32. Gray GR. Another side effect of NSAIDs. JAMA 1990;264:2677.

33. Banks AT, Zimmerman HJ, Ishak KG, Harter JG. Diclofenac-associated hepatotoxicity: analysis of 180 cases reported to the Food and Drug Administration as adverse reactions. Hepatology 1995;22(3):820–7.

34. Daly AK, Aithal GP, Leathart JB, Swainsbury RA, Dang TS, Day CP. Genetic susceptibility to diclofenac-induced hepatotoxicity: contribution of UGT2B7, CYP2C8, and ABCC2 genotypes. Gastroenterology 2007;132(1):272–81.

35. Wolters J, van Breda Vriesman PJ. Minimal change nephropathy and interstitial nephritis associated with diclofenac. Neth J Med 1985;28(8):311–4.

36. Campistol JM, Galofre J, Botey A, Torras A, Revert L. Reversible membranous nephritis associated with diclofenac. Nephrol Dial Transplant 1989;4(5):393–5.

37. Beun GD, Leunissen KM, Van Breda Vriesman PJ, Van Hooff JP, Grave W. Isolated minimal change nephropathy associated with diclofenac. BMJ (Clin Res Ed) 1987;295(6591):182–3.

38. Yinnon AM, Moreb JS, Slotki IN. Nephrotic syndrome associated with diclofenac sodium. BMJ (Clin Res Ed) 1987;295:556.

39. Gabrielsen TO, Staerfelt F, Thune PO. Drug-induced bullous dermatosis with linear IgA deposits along the basement membrane. Acta Derm Venereol 1981;61(5):439–41.

40. Kowalzick L, Ziegler H. Photoallergic contact dermatitis from topical diclofenac in Solaraze gel. Contact Dermatitis 2006;54(6):348–9.

41. Ueda K, Higashi N, Kume A, Ikushima-Fujimoto M, Ogiwara S. Allergic contact dermatitis due to diclofenac and indomethacin. Contact Dermatitis 1998;39(6):323.

42. Oono T, Kanzaki H, Yoshioka T, Arata J. Staphylococcal scalded skin syndrome in an adult. Identification of exfoliative toxin A and B genes by polymerase chain reaction. Dermatology 1997;195(3):268–70.

43. Saputo V, Bruni G. La sindrome di Nicolau da preparati di penicillina: analisi della letteratura alla ricerca di potenziali

fattori di rischio. [Nicolau syndrome caused by penicillin preparations: review of the literature in search for potential risk factors.] Pediatr Med Chir 1998;20(2):105–23.

44. Stricker BH, van Kasteren BJ. Diclofenac-induced isolated myonecrosis and the Nicolau syndrome. Ann Intern Med 1992;117(12):1058.

45. Rygnestad T, Kvam AM. Streptococcal myositis and tissue necrosis with intramuscular administration of diclofenac (Voltaren). Acta Anaesthesiol Scand 1995;39(8):1128–30.

46. Forsbach Sanchez G, Eloy Tamez H. Sindrome de nicolau por la administracion intramuscular de diclofenaco. [Nicolau syndrome caused by intramuscular administration of diclofenac.] Rev Invest Clin 1999;51(1):71.

47. Ezzedine K, Vadoud-Seyedi J, Heenen M. Nicolau syndrome following diclofenac administration. Br J Dermatol 2004;150(2):385–7.

48. del Pozo MD, Lobera T, Blasco A. Selective hypersensitivity to diclofenac. Allergy 2000;55(4):412–3.

49. Mas C, Menaham S. Premature in utero closure of the ductus arteriosus following maternal ingestion of sodium diclofenac. Aust NZ J Obstet Gynaecol 1999;39(1):106–7.

50. Anonymous. Diclofenac Dear Doctor letter issue in Japan. Scrip 2000;17:2597.

51. Hauben M, Aronson JK. Gold standards in pharmacovigilance: the use of definitive anecdotal reports of adverse drug reactions as pure gold and high-grade ore. Drug Saf 2007;30(8):645–55.

52. Lie C, Leung F, Chow SP. Nicolau syndrome following intramuscular diclofenac administration: a case report. J Orthop Surg (Hong Kong) 2006;14(1):104–7.

53. Cheraghali AM. Injectable diclofenac: a painful shot into Iran's health system. Soc Sci Med 2006;63(6):1597–601.

54. Muller-Vahl H. Aseptische Gewebsnekrose: eine schwerwiegende Komplikation nach intramuskularer Injektion. [Aseptic tissue necrosis: a severe complication after intramuscular injections.] Dtsch Med Wochenschr 1984;109(20):786–92.

55. Aronson JK. Routes of drug administration: uses and adverse effects. Part 1: Intramuscular and subcutaneous injection. Adv Drug React Bull 2009;253:971–4.

56. Pillans PI, O'Connor N. Tissue necrosis and necrotizing fasciitis after intramuscular administration of diclofenac. Ann Pharmacother 1995;29(3):264–6.

57. Deray G, Le Hoang P, Aupetit B, Achour A, Rottembourg J, Baumelou A. Enhancement of cyclosporine A nephrotoxicity by diclofenac. Clin Nephrol 1987; 27(4):213–4.

58. Harris KP, Jenkins D, Walls J. Nonsteroidal antiinflammatory drugs and cyclosporine. A potentially serious adverse interaction. Transplantation 1988;46(4):598–9.

59. Kovarik JM, Mueller EA, Gerbeau C, Tarral A, Francheteau P, Guerret M. Cyclosporine and nonsteroidal antiinflammatory drugs: exploring potential drug interactions and their implications for the treatment of rheumatoid arthritis. J Clin Pharmacol 1997;37(4):336–43.

60. Reimann IW, Frolich JC. Effects of diclofenac on lithium kinetics. Clin Pharmacol Ther 1981;30(3):348–52.

61. Weinblatt ME. Drug interactions with non steroidal anti-inflammatory drugs (NSAIDs). Scand J Rheumatol Suppl 1989;83:7–10.

62. Reimann IW, Frolich JC. Effects of diclofenac on lithium kinetics. Clin Pharmacol Ther 1981;30(3):348–52.

63. Monji A, Maekawa T, Miura T, Nishi D, Horikawa H, Nakagawa Y, Tashiro N. Interactions between lithium and non-steroidal antiinflammatory drugs. Clin Neuropharmacol 2002;25(5):241–2.

64. Cardoso MM, Carvalho JC, Amaro AR, Prado AA, Cappelli EL. Small doses of intrathecal morphine combined with systemic diclofenac for postoperative pain control after cesarean delivery. Anesth Analg 1998;86(3):538–41.

65. Masubuchi Y, Ose A, Horie T. Diclofenac-induced inactivation of CYP3A4 and its stimulation by quinidine. Drug Metab Dispos 2002;30(10):1143–8.

66. Gilliland WR. Quinidine-induced dermatomyositis-like illness. J Clin Rheumatol 1999;5:39.

Difenpiramide

General Information

Difenpiramide, a phenylacetic acid derivative, is less efficacious but has fewer adverse effects than indometacin or phenylbutazone. The most frequent reactions are in the gastrointestinal tract and skin (1). However, gastrointestinal tolerance is, as one would expect, better (2).

References

1. Jochems OB, Janbroers JM. Diphenpyramide: a review of its pharmacology and anti-inflammatory effects. Pharmatherapeutica 1986;4(7):429–41.

2. Fumagalli M, Montrone F, Vernazza M, Tirrito M, Santandrea S, Caruso I. La difenpiramide nel trattamento dell'artrite reumatoide: studio in doppio cieco a breve termine versus indometacina. [Diphenpiramide in the treatment of rheumatoid arthritis: short-time double-blind study of its comparison with indomethacin.] Clin Ter 1979;89(6):581–8.

Droxicam

General Information

Droxicam, a piroxicam prodrug, has similar adverse effects (SEDA-16, 113; 1). Because of many Spanish reports of non-fatal liver damage, according to the CPMP the Summary of Product Characteristics should state that serious hepatic damage can occur (SEDA-17, 113). Owing to its hepatotoxicity, droxicam has been withdrawn in many countries (SEDA-19, 99).

Reference

1. Jane F, Rodriguez de la Serna A. Droxicam: a pharmacological and clinical review of a new NSAID. Eur J Rheumatol Inflamm 1991;11(4):3–9.

Etodolac

General Information

Etodolac, a pyranocarboxylic acid, was first marketed in the UK in 1986. By 1988, etodolac had been reported 27 times to the UK Committee on Safety of Medicines as being suspected of causing serious adverse reactions (1). In a French postmarketing safety study in 51 355 patients taking 200–600 mg/day, 10% of patients reported a total of 6236 adverse reactions and 9% dropped out because of adverse reactions, 21 of which were judged severe (2). In another four postmarketing surveillance studies in 8334 patients with rheumatic conditions who took 200–600 mg/day of etodolac for periods ranging from 4 weeks to 1 year, 23% reported adverse events and 9% stopped taking the drug because of adverse reactions; gastrointestinal events were the most commonly reported (3).

Organs and Systems

Nervous system

Nervous system effects of etodolac include dizziness (4.4%), headache (6.0%), and tinnitus (2.6%).

Hematologic

One case of agranulocytosis, probably induced by etodolac, with the pattern common to the other NSAIDs, has been reported (4).

Gastrointestinal

Animal experiments, as well as endoscopic and ^{51}Cr blood loss studies in man, suggest that the gastric irritancy of etodolac is low (5,6), but such claims have to be regarded with the reservations expressed about all NSAIDs. Etodolac in short-term dosages of 200, 400, and 600 mg bd caused significantly less damage to both the gastric and the duodenal mucosa than aspirin 3.9 g/day (SEDA-12, 85). It had a less damaging effect on the stomach than naproxen in a short-term endoscopic study in rheumatoid arthritis (7). The most frequent adverse effects in 1379 patients in trials were gastrointestinal symptoms: 8.9% of patients had nausea, 5.8% epigastric pain, 5.7% heartburn, and 5.2% indigestion; 1.9% of patients had to be withdrawn because of these adverse effects.

Acute colitis demonstrated by endoscopy and rechallenge was reported in two patients taking etodolac for arthritis (8). Colonic strictures have been described in another report (SEDA-22, 115).

Skin

Skin rashes occur in 3% of patients who take etodolac (SEDA-12, 85).

Susceptibility Factors

Age

The safety profiles of etodolac in elderly and younger patients are similar (SEDA-19, 98).

Drug Administration

Drug formulations

The long-term treatment safety profile of a modified-release formulation of etodolac was similar to that of the standard formulation (SEDA-18, 104).

Drug dosage regimens

In 1986, the UK Drug Safety Research Unit at Southampton published a report on its prescription event monitoring study of etodolac (SEDA-13, 80). Etodolac was rated effective in only 56% of 9109 patients, and the Unit concluded that the average dosage used (400 mg/day) was too low to be effective. Consequently, the adverse reaction figures should be viewed with great caution. Indeed, at an adequate dosage they might actually be unfavorable, since in this study the rate of dyspepsia during the first month was 16 per 1000 compared with 3 per 1000 for piroxicam. After the first month, the rates were similar for etodolac and piroxicam. Few serious events were recorded: exfoliative dermatitis in one patient with psoriatic arthritis and 20 cases of hematemesis or melena.

References

1. Bem JL, Breckenridge AM, Mann RD, Rawlins MD. Review of yellow cards (1986): report to the Committee on the Safety of Medicines. Br J Clin Pharmacol 1988;26(6):679–89.
2. Benhamou CL. Large-scale open trials with etodolac (Lodine) in France: an assessment of safety. Rheumatol Int 1990;10(Suppl):29–34.
3. Serni U. Global safety of etodolac: reports from worldwide postmarketing surveillance studies. Rheumatol Int 1990;10(Suppl):23–7.
4. Cramer RL, Aboko-Cole VC, Gualtieri RJ. Agranulocytosis associated with etodolac. Ann Pharmacother 1994;28(4):458–60.
5. Jacob G, Messina M, Kennedy J, Epstein C, Sanda M, Mullane J. Minimum effective dose of etodolac for the treatment of rheumatoid arthritis. J Clin Pharmacol 1986;26(3):195–202.
6. Lanza FL, Arnold JD. Etodolac, a new nonsteroidal anti-inflammatory drug: gastrointestinal microbleeding and endoscopic studies. Clin Rheumatol 1989;8(Suppl 1):5–15.
7. Taha AS, McLaughlin S, Sturrock RD, Russell RI. Evaluation of the efficacy and comparative effects on gastric and duodenal mucosa of etodolac and naproxen in patients with rheumatoid arthritis using endoscopy. Br J Rheumatol 1989;28(4):329–32.
8. Wilcox GM, Porensky RS. Acute colitis associated with etodolac. J Clin Gastroenterol 1997;25(1):367–8.

Etoricoxib

See also COX-2 inhibitors

General Information

Etoricoxib is a selective COX-2 inhibitor.

Organs and Systems

Cardiovascular

See the monograph on COX-2 inhibitors.

Gastrointestinal

Two randomized, double-blind, placebo-controlled and non-selective NSAID-controlled studies have documented the upper gastrointestinal tract tolerability of etoricoxib [1]. In the first study, fecal blood loss was measured daily in 62 healthy volunteers taking etoricoxib (120 mg/day), ibuprofen (800 mg tds), or placebo; etoricoxib caused less fecal blood loss than placebo or ibuprofen. In the second study, the incidence of endoscopically detectable gastric/duodenal ulcers was measured in 742 patients with osteoarthritis or rheumatoid arthritis taking etoricoxib (120 mg/day), naproxen (500 mg bd), or placebo over 12 weeks. Etoricoxib caused significantly fewer ulcers and erosions than naproxen. However, there was a higher incidence of ulcers in patients taking etoricoxib relative to placebo. The real benefit to harm balance of this derivative is still unknown.

Skin

A fixed drug eruption has been attributed to etoricoxib [2].

- A 38-year-old woman developed a 1.5 cm, round, well circumscribed, erythematous patch on the right forearm 3 days after taking etoricoxib for bursitis. Over the next few days, the center of the patch blistered and necrosed and later healed with residual hyperpigmentation. She had taken various NSAIDs many times in the past, rofecoxib on more than two occasions, celecoxib for at least 1 week 2 years before, and etoricoxib once for 1 week 5 months before. She took a single tablet of etoricoxib again 2 months later, and within 2 hours noticed erythema, itching, and burning at the site of the old lesion. Over the next 3–4 hours she developed generalized itching and burning followed by intense erythema all over the body. Nikolsky's sign was negative. There was no mucosal involvement. She had neither a fever nor other constitutional symptoms. There were no systemic abnormalities on physical and routine laboratory examination. She was given systemic steroids, and although most of the symptoms and signs gradually subsided in 10 days, mild acral dusky erythema persisted for 4 weeks. The lesion over the right forearm developed a small blister and healed with a larger area of residual pigmentation. The erythema over the rest of the body resolved without residual pigmentation. A patch test with etoricoxib 10% in petrolatum 6 months later resulted in erythema and edema, double the size of the previous patch but in the same place, within 8 hours. The control area did not react.

References

1. Hunt RH, Harper S, Watson DJ, Yu C, Quan H, Lee M, Evans JK, Oxenius B. The gastrointestinal safety of the COX-2 selective inhibitor etoricoxib assessed by both endoscopy and analysis of upper gastrointestinal events. Am J Gastroenterol 2003;98:1725–33.
2. Augustine M, Sharma P, Stephen J, Jayaseelan E. Fixed drug eruption and generalised erythema following etoricoxib. Indian J Dermatol Venereol Leprol 2006;72(4):307–9.

Felbinac

General Information

Felbinac, an active metabolite of fenbufen, is used as a gel for topical treatment (1).

Organs and Systems

Skin

Felbinac can cause itching, rash, and eosinophilia (SEDA-16, 110).

Reference

1. Hosie G, Bird H. The topical NSAID felbinac versus oral NSAIDS: a critical review. Eur J Rheumatol Inflamm 1994;14(4):21–8.

Fenbufen

General Information

The profile of fenbufen is similar to the profiles of other NSAIDs (1). The dropout rate due to adverse reactions was 12–22% in different studies.

Organs and Systems

Respiratory

Fenbufen can cause a pulmonary alveolitis with rash, dry cough, breathlessness, fever, hypoxia, sometimes eosinophilia, and bilateral alveolar shadowing or infiltrates, which regress after withdrawal (SEDA-12, 85) (SEDA-13, 80) (SEDA-15, 100).

Nervous system

Headache has been reported with fenbufen (2).

Severe encephalitis, with generalized erythema and maculopapular rash on the trunk, has been reported (SEDA-19, 98).

Hematologic

Hemolytic anemia, in some cases with signs of hypersensitivity, has been reported (SEDA-14, 94). Aplastic anemia has been described in two patients (SEDA-18, 104), but both recovered fully after withdrawal.

Liver

The incidence of hepatotoxicity with fenbufen varies greatly. Changes in liver function tests were recorded in 25% patients in an early study (SEDA-4, 68), but were not confirmed later (SEDA-5, 194; SEDA-6, 96). Abnormalities in the liver function of patients with rheumatoid arthritis may be a non-specific reaction to inflammation; however, hepatotoxicity should be watched for in patients taking fenbufen.

Skin

About 5% of patients have itching, rashes, or erythema multiforme (3). Circulating immune complexes have been found (4). The UK's Committee on Safety of Medicines issued a warning about the high rate of cutaneous adverse reactions with fenbufen and noted that some are followed by severe illnesses (SEDA-13, 72; SEDA-14, 94; SEDA-15, 100). Toxic epidermal necrolysis, a life-threatening reaction, has also been reported (SEDA-6, 96) (SEDA-8, 106) and a 1981–85 review on its incidence in France identified fenbufen as the third most common NSAID, after isoxicam and oxyphenbutazone, as a causal factor (5). Another severe skin reaction with laboratory evidence of hepatotoxicity has been described (SEDA-22, 115).

Drug–Drug Interactions

Enoxacin

Many cases of epileptic seizures have been reported in Japan in patients taking a combination of fenbufen and enoxacin (SEDA-12, 85; SEDA-15, 100).

Quinolones

Fenbufen can cause convulsions, which has mainly been described in patients taking quinolone antibiotics (SEDA-18, 104).

References

1. Brogden RN, Heel RC, Speight TM, Avery GS. Fenbufen: a review of its pharmacological properties and therapeutic use in rheumatic diseases and acute pain. Drugs 1981;21(1):22.
2. Deodhar SD, Sethi R. A comparative study of fenbufen and indomethacin in patients with rheumatoid arthritis. Curr Med Res Opin 1979;6(4):263–6.
3. Peacock A, Ledingham J. Fenbufen-induced erythema multiforme. BMJ (Clin Res Ed) 1981;283(6291):582.
4. Nicolas C, Chouvet B, Cambazard F, Bernollin C, Thivolet J. Accidents cutanés lies à un nouvel anti-inflammatoire: fenbufene. [Skin lesions related to a new anti-inflammatory agent: fenbufen. Apropos of 3 clinical cases.] Ann Dermatol Venereol 1983;110(5):419–23.
5. Roujeau JC, Guillaume JC, Fabre JP, Penso D, Flechet ML, Girre JP. Toxic epidermal necrolysis (Lyell syndrome). Incidence and drug etiology in France, 1981–1985. Arch Dermatol 1990;126(1):37–42.

Fenclofenac

General Information

Fenclofenac was withdrawn in the UK after its license was not renewed because of its adverse drug reaction profile (1). Data from the UK's Committee on Safety of Medicines included records of seven deaths and 895 adverse effects in patients taking fenclofenac. Shortly afterwards it was withdrawn in all other countries in which it had been marketed.

Organs and Systems

Skin

Fenclofenac has the second highest incidence of complications and ranks first in the number and severity of skin reactions (2).

References

1. Anonymous. Fenclofenac withdrawn. Lancet 1984;2:56.
2. Weber JCP. Epidemiology of adverse reactions to non-steroidal anti-inflammatory drugs. Adv Inflam Res 1984;6:1.

Fentiazac

General Information

Fentiazac, a thiazoleacetic acid derivative, has the same adverse reactions profile as other NSAIDs. Adverse effects in as many as 56% of patients (5-56%), are even more frequent than with phenylbutazone (1).

In 40 patients with rheumatoid arthritis enrolled in a double-blind trial of fentiazac 400 mg/day or sulindac 200 mg/day for 3 months, adverse effects were reported in three patients taking fentiazac (rash, headache, epigastric pain) (2).

Organs and Systems

Nervous system

Adverse effects involving the central nervous system include headache, dizziness, mental confusion, sedation, giddiness, and blurred vision; dysesthesia and oral paresthesia have also been reported (3).

Gastrointestinal

Pyrosis, epigastric pain, nausea, constipation/diarrhea, and occult bleeding are the most frequent gastrointestinal effects of fentiazac (3). Rectal administration can cause both local and systemic adverse effects.

Liver

In one study, seven of 20 patients with rheumatoid arthritis had significant rises in aspartate transaminase and alkaline phosphatase activities (4). Reversible hepatotoxicity occurred in three of 33 patients who took fentiazac during long-term therapy (2).

References

1. Buerklin EM, Ballard IM. A double blind comparison of fentiazac and phenylbutazone in the treatment of acute tendinitis and bursitis. Curr Med Res Opin 1979;6(Suppl 2):90.
2. Bunde B, Deckers Y, Dequeker J. Fentiazac in rheumatoid arthritis: comparison with sulindac and long-term tolerance. Curr Med Res Opin 1983;8(5):310–4.
3. Teixeira MA, Da Silva AP, Lourenco I, Teixeira ML. Fentiazac in the treatment of some rheumatic disorders. Curr Med Res Opin 1979;(Suppl 2):97–106.
4. Katona G, Boudani A. Efficacy and tolerability of fentiazac in rheumatoid arthritis: double blind study versus indometacine. Curr Med Res Opin 1979;6(Suppl 2):71.

Feprazone

General Information

Feprazone is an NSAID that is related to phenylbutazone. Feprazone was withdrawn in the UK because of its adverse effects, which resemble those of phenylbutazone. It was designated as a last-resort drug by the Japanese Committee on Safety of Drugs (SEDA-12, 83).

In an 8-week trial in 2693 patients with rheumatoid arthritis and osteoarthritis, 30% reported adverse effects and 11% failed to complete the study. However, two large short-term multicenter studies in general practices in 11 000 patients in Italy reported a very low percentage (1.2–9.8%) of adverse effects (1,2).

Gastrotoxicity, nephrotoxicity, edema, headache, tinnitus, and depression have been attributed to feprazone (3).

Organs and Systems

Hematologic

Thrombocytopenia and immune complex-mediated hemolytic anemia have been reported with feprazone (SEDA-7, 108).

Skin

Skin reactions (including severe bullous dermatosis) have been attributed to feprazone (SEDA-9, 87). Contact dermatitis has been described with feprazone cream (SEDA-18, 101).

References

1. Montanari C. Large cooperative multicentric trial with feprazone in the inflammatory process of dental tissues. Curr Ther Res Clin Exp 1975;17(2):166–74.
2. Chierichetti S. Esempio di monitoraggio attivo su un farmaco: il feprazone. Emerg Med 1976;500:.
3. Sturrock R, Isaacs A, Hart FD. Feprazone compared with indomethacin in the management of rheumatoid arthritis. Practitioner 1975;215(1285):94–7.

Floctafenine

General Information

Floctafenine is a 4-aminoquinoline NSAID, closely related to antrafenine and glafenine, and its adverse effects profile is similar (1).

Organs and Systems

Urinary tract

Floctafenine has been detected in a urinary calculus (2).

Immunologic

Floctafenine has frequently been associated with anaphylactic reactions (3).

Drug Interactions

Cimetidine

Coma has been reported in a patient taking diuretics and cimetidine, who was given floctafenine (4).

Coumarin anticoagulants

Floctafenine may increase the action of coumarin anticoagulants (5).

References

1. Cheymol G, Biour M, Bruneel M, Albengres E, Hamel JD. Bilan d'une enquête nationale prospective sur les effets indesirables de la glafénine, de l'antrafénine et de la floctafénine. [Evaluation of a national prospective survey on the undesirable effects of glafenine, antrafenine and floctafenine.] Therapie 1985;40(1):45–50.
2. Moesch C, Rince M, Raby C, Leroux-Robert C. Identification d'un metabolite de la floctafénine dans un calcul urinaire. [Identification of metabolite of floctafenine in urinary calculi.] Ann Biol Clin (Paris) 1987;45(5):546–50.
3. van der Klauw MM, Wilson JH, Stricker BH. Drug-associated anaphylaxis: 20 years of reporting in The

Netherlands (1974–1994) and review of the literature. Clin Exp Allergy 1996;26(12):1355–63.
4. Pasqua P, Craxi A, Pagliara L. Floctafenine and coma in cirrhosis. Ann Intern Med 1982;96(2):253.
5. Boeijinga JK, van de Broeke RN, Jochemsen R, Breimer DD, Hoogslag MA, Jeletich-Bastiaanse A. De involved van floctafenine (Idalon) op antistollingsbehandeling met coumarinederivaten. [The effect of floctafenine (Idalon) on anticoagulant treatment with coumarin derivatives.] Ned Tijdschr Geneeskd 1981;125(47):1931–5.

Flufenamic acid and meclofenamic acid

General Information

Flufenamic acid and meclofenamic acid are anthranilic acid derivatives similar to mefenamic acid. The withdrawal rate because of adverse effects is 7–31% and is higher in long-term studies. Flufenamic acid and meclofenamic acid are not widely prescribed and so there is little evidence to show whether they have any advantages over other NSAIDs. Both have a high incidence of gastrointestinal adverse effects (30–60% of patients at recommended doses). Diarrhea affects 11–46% of patients (SEDA-4, 68; SEDA-6, 99; SEDA-7, 116; SEDA-14, 95). Thrombocytopenia with positive rechallenge has been described (1). Rashes occur in under 10% of patients. Meclofenamic acid exacerbates psoriasis in psoriatic arthropathy (2).

References

1. Rodriguez J. Thrombocytopenia associated with meclofenamate. Drug Intell Clin Pharm 1981;5(12):999.
2. Meyerhoff JO. Exacerbation of psoriasis with meclofenamate. N Engl J Med 1983;309(8):496.

Flunoxaprofen

General Information

Flunoxaprofen is an NSAID, an arylalkanoic acid derivative. Its adverse effects profile is similar to the profiles of other NSAIDs, including gastrointestinal disturbances (1).

Reference

1. Forgione A, Zanoboni A, Zanoboni-Muciaccia W, et al. Long-term tolerability of flunoxaprofen in elderly subjects with normal or impaired renal function. Curr Ther Res 1985;37:77.

Fluproquazone and proquazone

General Information

Fluproquazone and proquazone, quinazoline derivatives, are analgesics of minor importance. Gastrointestinal adverse effects are the most frequent (SEDA-4, 69; SEDA-5, 197; SEDA-10, 88). Because fluproquazone caused hepatic injury in 14% of patients in clinical trials, evaluation was halted (1).

Reference

1. Lewis JH. Hepatic toxicity of nonsteroidal anti-inflammatory drugs. Clin Pharm 1984;3(2):128–38.

Flurbiprofen

General Information

In a short-term multicenter study of flurbiprofen only 6% of patients were withdrawn because of adverse effects (1). However, in a prolonged open study in 1200 patients, more than 50% reported adverse reactions and therapy had to be withdrawn in 19% (2).

Organs and Systems

Nervous system

Nervous system effects with flurbiprofen are less common than with indometacin (3). Flurbiprofen precipitates extrapyramidal reactions, albeit rarely (SEDA-15, 101), and a parkinsonian syndrome has been reported in a predisposed patient (SEDA-15, 101).

Gastrointestinal

Flurbiprofen causes more gastrointestinal adverse effects than naproxen or ibuprofen. In a series of controlled double-blind studies, adverse reactions occurred in 27–42% of patients and were most commonly gastrointestinal in origin (18–28%) (SEDA-12, 85).

Local tolerance of flurbiprofen suppositories is often satisfactory, but discomfort, irritation, tenesmus, and diarrhea have been observed (4).

Urinary tract

Interstitial nephritis with the nephrotic syndrome and one case of renal papillary necrosis have been recorded (SEDA-12, 86) (SEDA-17, 110). Flurbiprofen can cause a membranous nephropathy (SEDA-21, 105).

Skin

There have been two reports of a dermatitis herpetiformis-like eruption in patients taking flurbiprofen (SEDA-18, 104).

Immunologic

Leukocytoclastic vasculitis caused by flurbiprofen has been observed in a patient with rheumatoid arthritis (SEDA-15, 101).

Susceptibility Factors

Age

Elderly patients seem to be particularly sensitive to and intolerant of flurbiprofen; one study reported adverse effects in 80% (SED-11, 183) (5).

Drug Administration

Drug administration route

Intramuscular flurbiprofen was effective and well tolerated in ureteric colic; local adverse effects were slight (SEDA-20, 93).

Drug–Drug Interactions

Acenocoumarol

Flurbiprofen potentiates the anticoagulant effect of acenocoumarol (SEDA-7, 112).

Furosemide

Flurbiprofen reduces the diuretic action of furosemide (6).

Quinolone antibiotics

The Japanese regulatory authority has suggested that the data sheet for flurbiprofen should include a warning that it can cause convulsions, which has mainly been described in patients taking quinolone antibiotics (SEDA-18, 104); quinolones should not be used concomitantly (SEDA-18, 104).

References

1. Benvenuti C, Longoni L. Multicentre study on effectiveness and safety of flurbiprofen versus alternative therapy in 738 rheumatic patients. Curr Ther Res 1983;34:30.
2. Sheldrake FE, Webber JM, Marsh BD. A long-term assessment of flurbiprofen. Curr Med Res Opin 1977;5(1):106–16.
3. De Moor M, Ooghe R. A double-blind comparison of flurbiprofen and indomethacin suppositories in the treatment of osteoarthrosis and rheumatoid disease. J Int Med Res 1981;9(6):495–500.
4. Huskisson EC, Woolf DL, Boyle DV, Scott J. A trial of naproxen, flurbiprofen, indometacin and placebo in the treatment of osteoarthritis. Eur J Rheumatol Inflamm 1980;2:69.
5. Innes EH. Efficacy and tolerance of flurbiprofen in the elderly using liquid and tablet formulations. Curr Med Res Opin 1977;5(1):122–6.
6. Rawles JM. Antagonism between non-steroidal anti-inflammatory drugs and diuretics. Scott Med J 1982;27(1):37–40.

Glafenine

General Information

Glafenine, an anthranilic acid derivative, has been withdrawn in much of the world (1). Until 1991 it was sold in about 70 countries (although never marketed or accepted in others), despite a long history of severe reactions (particularly anaphylaxis, fatal hepatotoxicity, and nephrotoxicity, even with normal doses). As late as 1989 the EC Committee on Proprietary Medicinal Products (CPMP) astonishingly recommended keeping glafenine on the market but controlling its distribution and monitoring adverse effects more closely (2). Firm restrictions or prohibitions nevertheless preceded or followed this recommendation in several European countries, and the CPMP finally condemned glafenine early in 1992. See also floctafenine.

Organs and Systems

Cardiovascular

A rise in blood pressure coupled with renal adverse effects has been reported. Coronary artery spasm leading to myocardial infarction was described as part of an allergic reaction with Quincke's edema (SED-11, 190) (3).

Hematologic

Acute hemolytic anemia, probably as part of an allergic reaction (SED-9, 154) (4,5), leukopenia through an unknown mechanism, and thrombocytopenic purpura with hemorrhage have been documented (6).

Liver

Liver injury has repeatedly been described in patients taking glafenine (SEDA-4, 69) (SEDA-5, 106), with fatal hepatotoxicity as part of a general toxic reaction in several cases (7). Glafenine-associated hepatic injury is characterized by a high prevalence of jaundice, a high death rate, and a predominantly hepatocellular histological pattern of liver lesions, varying from spotty panlobular, centrilobular, and submassive necrosis (acute pattern) to fibrosis and cirrhosis (chronic pattern) (8).

Biliary tract

Gallstones containing glafenic acid have been reported in a patient taking long-term therapy (SEDA-14, 95).

Urinary tract

Many nephrotoxic features have been observed in preclinical and clinical studies of glafenine in therapeutic doses and more especially in overdosage (SEDA-4, 69). Acute oliguria, anuria, increased blood urea and creatinine, proteinuria, and raised blood pressure have been repeatedly reported. Glafenine stones have been documented in five patients (9).

Musculoskeletal

Symptoms of rhabdomyolysis, associated with other disorders, occurred in two patients a few hours after glafenine (10).

Immunologic

Although rash has sometimes occurred (11), hypersensitivity reactions have been much more serious. Many acute anaphylactic reactions have been observed (SEDA-4, 69) (SEDA-6, 98) (12,13), with shock in more than 50% of cases; it was recorded in 24 of 1517 reports on the drug collected by the Pharmacovigilance Unit in Lyons, France (11). Occasional isolated fever, confirmed by rechallenge (14), is probably also of hypersensitive origin. Interstitial nephritis, hepatitis, and pulmonary hypersensitivity have been reported.

Drug–Drug Interactions

Methotrexate

An interaction of glafenine with methotrexate has been described in a patient with rheumatoid arthritis (SEDA-14, 95).

References

1. Anonymous. Withdrawal of glafenine. Lancet 1992;339:357.
2. Herxheimer A. Belgium: withdrawal of glafenine. Lancet 1991;337:102.
3. Weber S, Genevray B, Pasquier G, Chapsal J, Bonnin A, Degeorges M. Severe coronary spasm during drug-induced immediate hypersensitivity reaction. Lancet 1982;2(8302):821.
4. Mallein R, Boucherat M, Rondelet J, Fillastre JP, Mantel O. Pharmacocinétique de la glafénine chez des sujets ayant une fonction rénale normale et chez des malades atteints d'insuffisance rénale chronique. [Pharmacokinetics of glaphenine in subjects with normal renal function and in patients with chronic renal insufficiency.] Therapie 1976;31(6):739–45.
5. Grand A, Despret P. Choc anaphylactique inuit par la glafenine. [Anaphylactic shock induced by glafenine.] Nouv Presse Méd 1973;2(16):1075.
6. Bosset JF, Perriguey G, Rozenbaum A, Leconte Des Floris R. Thrombopénie aiguë récidivante après prise de glafénine: une observation. [Recurrent acute thrombopenia after glaphenine. 1 case.] Nouv Presse Méd 1979;8(19):1606.
7. Ypma RT, Festen JJ, De Bruin CD. Hepatotoxicity of glafenine. Lancet 1978;2(8087):480–1.
8. Stricker BH, Blok AP, Bronkhorst FB. Glafenine-associated hepatic injury. Analysis of 38 cases and review of the literature. Liver 1986;6(2):63–72.
9. Daudon M, Protat MF, Reveillaud RJ. Toxicité rénale de la glafénine chez l'homme: calculs rénaux et insuffisance rénale aiguë. [Renal toxicity of glafenine in man: renal stones and acute renal failure.] Ann Biol Clin (Paris) 1983;41(2):105–11.
10. Rouveix B, Benhamed S, Regnier B. Rhabdomyolyse et glafénine. [Rhabdomyolysis and glafenine.] Therapie 1984;39(1):53–4.
11. Descotes J, Lery N, Vigneau C, Loupi E, Evreux JC. Bilan des effets secondaires dus a la glafénine au Centre de Pharmacovigilance de Lyon. [Overview of glafenin side-effects from the experience of Lyon Pharmacovigilance Unit.] Therapie 1980;35(3):405–8.
12. Stricker BH, de Groot RR, Wilson JH. Anaphylaxis to glafenine. Lancet 1990;336(8720):943–4.
13. Stricker BH, de Groot RR, Wilson JH. Glafenine-associated anaphylaxis as a cause of hospital admission in The Netherlands. Eur J Clin Pharmacol 1991;40(4):367–71.
14. Garre M, Youinou P, Burtin C, Rolland J, Deraedt R. Fièvre isolée: effet secondaire singulier de la glafénine. [Isolated fever: an unusual side effect of glafenine.] Therapie 1980;35(6):752–3.

Glucametacin

General Information

Glucametacin is a glucosamide derivative of indometacin, with no advantages over indometacin and the same pattern of adverse effects, the most common of which are nausea and heartburn (1).

Reference

1. Colombo B, Carrabba M, Paresce E. Glucamethacin in the treatment of rheumatoid arthritis and arthrosis. Clin Trials J 1978;15:66.

Ibuprofen

General Information

Like other NSAIDs, ibuprofen is a potent inhibitor of prostaglandin synthesis, and many or all of its therapeutic and toxic effects are linked to this characteristic. The general impression is that it is less potent and thus less toxic than indometacin in usual doses, but it has often been used in the past in relatively low doses. In a comparative, double-blind, crossover study of ibuprofen, naproxen, fenoprofen, and tolmetin in patients with rheumatoid arthritis, ibuprofen in equieffective doses was the best tolerated; however, patients and physicians preferred naproxen (1).

There are few data on the long-term safety of NSAIDs in the treatment of juvenile rheumatoid arthritis. In a study of the adverse reactions of patients treated with long-term ibuprofen, gastrotoxicity was directly correlated with dosage and 5% withdrew early because they had gastro-intestinal bleeding, vomiting, severe rash, hearing loss, and abnormalities of liver function tests (SEDA-16, 110).

High dosages of ibuprofen for 4 years were used in 41 patients with cystic fibrosis to slow progression of lung disease and only two adverse effects (conjunctivitis and epistaxis) were drug-related (SEDA-20, 93).

General adverse reactions

Gastrointestinal adverse effects are the most frequent. They occur in up to 30% of patients and range from abdominal discomfort to serious bleeding or activation of peptic ulcer. Nervous system effects, with headache and dizziness, are very common. Severe renal impairment has not been noted. Blood dyscrasias can occur when high dosage treatment is prolonged. There is no significant general hepatotoxicity, but both the liver and the central nervous system (meningitis) can be affected as part of a hypersensitivity reaction.

Hypersensitivity reactions are uncommon, but they can be severe. Aseptic meningitis, hypotension, fever, con-junctivitis, arthralgias, and leukopenia were reported in a woman with systemic lupus erythematosus (2). Other similar patients have experienced fever with rashes, abdominal pain, headache, nausea and vomiting, signs of liver damage, and meningitis. This type of reaction seems to occur especially (but not exclusively) in patients with connective tissue diseases (SEDA-5, 105) (SEDA-10, 84) and it can be difficult to differentiate between a hyper-sensitivity reaction and a flare-up of the disease. Ibuprofen can provoke bronchospasm and anaphylaxis in asthmatics (SEDA-22, 116).

Tumor-inducing effects have not been reported.

Organs and Systems

Cardiovascular

Apart from the consequences of salt and water retention, ibuprofen does not affect myocardial or vascular function. Congestive heart failure has rarely been reported (3).

All NSAIDs can cause or aggravate hypertension and inhibit the effects of antihypertensive drugs (SEDA-22,102,SEDA-26, 116). Data from a randomized trial have suggested that ibuprofen significantly increases blood pressure in patients taking ACE inhibitors, but that celecoxib and nabumetone do not (4).

Compared with placebo, ibuprofen was associated with significantly greater increases in both systolic and diasto-lic blood pressure, whereas blood pressure increases with nabumetone and celecoxib were not significantly differ-ent to placebo. In addition, the proportion of patients with systolic blood pressure increases of clinical concern was significantly greater in those taking ibuprofen (17%) than in those taking nabumetone (5.5%), celecoxib (4.6%), or placebo (1.1%). However, the results of this study must be confirmed in a larger population of hyper-tensive patients on the basis of relevant clinical outcomes.

Pulmonary hypertension occurred in one of 169 pre-term infants who were given lysine ibuprofen (10 mg/kg

followed by 5 mg/kg after 24 and 48 hours) for closure of a patent ductus arteriosus; symptoms started within 1 hour of the second dose (5).

In a small comparison of ibuprofen and indometacin in preterm infants with patent ductus arteriosus there was no apparent difference in the rate of patent ductus arteriosus closure; ibuprofen did not impair cerebral hemodynamics or oxygenation, while indometacin impaired cerebral oxy-gen delivery (6).

Respiratory

Ibuprofen rarely provokes attacks of asthma in predis-posed individuals. There is probably cross-sensitivity with aspirin; a death was reported after an asthmatic patient with no history of aspirin sensitivity took two ibuprofen tablets (SEDA-12, 86).

Pulmonary infiltrates with eosinophilia have been described with ibuprofen (SEDA-18, 104).

Two episodes of acute pulmonary edema and progres-sive pulmonary infiltrates without eosinophilia have been reported in a man with HIV infection after ibuprofen (SEDA-18, 104).

Nervous system

Headache, vertigo, tinnitus, and insomnia are the most frequent nervous system effects, but are rarely severe. Depression and other psychotic reactions have been reported. Some nervous system reactions (meningism and meningitis, lethargy, and irritability) are thought to result from hypersensitivity (SEDA-9, 91) (SEDA-18, 104) (7). This has been confirmed by a report of aseptic meningitis with increased intrathecal IgG synthesis and evidence of immune complexes in the cerebrospinal fluid (SEDA-16, 110).

Analgesic-induced headache, not uncommon in adults, has also been described in children. One report (8) described 12 children, aged 6–16 years, who gave a history of headaches on at least 4 days a week, for 3 months to 10 years. Eleven of the children had been taking paraceta-mol, six in combination with codeine, and one was taking ibuprofen alone. They were taking at least one dose of an analgesic for each headache and eight were taking analge-sics every day. The headaches presented with increasing frequency and were related to overuse of analgesics, a typical finding in analgesic-induced headache. The analgesics were withdrawn; in six children the headaches resolved completely, another five children experienced a reduced frequency of headaches, and one resumed analgesic abuse.

The second report (9) was a retrospective study of patients seen in a pediatric headache clinic. During 8 months 98 patients were seen for headache; 46 of them suffered from daily or near daily headache and 30 were consuming analgesics daily. Follow-up information was available in 25. The average number of doses of analgesics per week they consumed was 26. The most commonly used medications were paracetamol and ibuprofen. In addition, a minority were taking combinations that con-tained aspirin, codeine, caffeine, propoxyphene, or butal-bital, or other NSAIDs. Abrupt withdrawal of all analgesics concomitant with the use of amitriptyline 10 mg/day (in 22 patients) prompted a significant reduction in the frequency and severity of headache.

Ibuprofen can cause aseptic meningitis (10), the incidence of which is increasing, mainly among patients with underlying autoimmune disorders. Recurrent meningitis mimicking bacterial meningitis occurred in two women taking ibuprofen, one with dermatomyositis and one with autoimmune thyroiditis (11). In the authors' review of 71 reported episodes of ibuprofen-related meningitis in 36 patients, 22 had an autoimmune disorder, mainly systemic lupus erythematosus, and 22 had recurrent episodes. Most of the episodes consisted of an acute meningeal syndrome with a predominance of neutrophils and raised protein in the cerebrospinal fluid in 26 patients.

Sensory systems

Ocular reactions described to date are reversible and not severe. They include blurred vision, changes in color perception, and toxic amblyopia (12).

Ibuprofen significantly correlated with high-altitude retinal hemorrhages (SEDA-17, 110).

Vortex keratopathy has been described in a woman taking oral ibuprofen (SEDA-21, 105).

Optic neuritis with a visual field defect has been associated with ibuprofen (13).

- A 41-year-old man took ibuprofen 400 mg tds for 3 weeks and developed blurred vision in his right eye and pain during eye and head movements that lasted 2 days. There was a marked reduction in visual acuity to 20/200 in the right eye, with quadrantanopia and absent visual-evoked potentials. After withdrawal of the drug and treatment with high-dose intravenous methylprednisolone and subcutaneous low-molecular-weight heparin, his vision improved to 20/70, the visual field defect vanished, and the visual-evoked potentials returned to almost normal values.

Although the authors could not rule out idiopathic optic neuritis, they thought that the absence of other susceptibility factors plus improvement after drug withdrawal suggested a toxic effect.

Psychiatric

Dementia has been attributed to ibuprofen.

- A 76-year-old man became confused and lost in familiar places and had short-term memory loss after taking ibuprofen 600 mg/ tds for osteoarthritic pain for 2 weeks (14). These symptoms continued for 2 weeks until he stopped taking ibuprofen, when his mental symptoms resolved within 1 week. Six months later he started taking ibuprofen again and within 1 week had the same symptoms. He stopped taking ibuprofen and his mental status again returned to normal.

Metabolism

An increase in serum concentrations of uric acid has been described with ibuprofen (15).

Hematologic

Ibuprofen prolongs bleeding time, although less than aspirin (16). There are reports that a daily dose of less than 1 g does not affect the bleeding time (17).

Blood dyscrasias, ranging from thrombocytopenia and granulocytopenia to agranulocytosis and fatal pancytopenia, have been reported. (SED-9, 150). Reversible pure white cell aplasia with bone marrow plasmacytosis and complement-dependent IgG antibody has been observed in one patient (18).

Fatal autoimmune hemolytic anemia has been attributed to ibuprofen in a patient who was taking other drugs (19). Reversible hemolytic anemia has been described during ibuprofen treatment, but tartrazine, the orange dye in the coating of the brand used (Motrin 400), may have been responsible (20).

Gastrointestinal blood loss due to ibuprofen can cause iron deficiency anemia.

Gastrointestinal

When ibuprofen was first introduced, its gastrointestinal tolerance was regarded as better than with other NSAIDs, especially aspirin and indometacin. However, with the use of higher doses, which were probably equipotent with the usual doses of older agents, there seemed to be no significant differences. As with other NSAIDs there is a close correlation between efficacy and adverse effects. Gastrointestinal adverse effects include a variety of symptoms, such as irritation, nausea, anorexia, vomiting, dyspepsia, heartburn, abdominal discomfort, bleeding, hematemesis, and activation of peptic ulcer; 10–30% of patients taking prescription doses (for example for rheumatic conditions) develop these adverse effects (SED-9, 150; 21). It is not possible to give a reliable estimate of the frequency when the drug is used as a self-medication analgesic in lower doses, since exact information on the complications of self-medication is rarely available and there is always likely to be a proportion of misuse (for example ingestion of higher or lower doses than recommended).

Bleeding from a Meckel's diverticulum has been described with oral ibuprofen (SEDA-17, 110).

Irritation of the rectal mucosa after ibuprofen suppositories has also been reported (22). Ulcerative proctitis has been reported in a patient with systemic lupus erythematosus (SEDA-14, 94).

Liver

The liver can be damaged by as part of a generalized hypersensitivity reaction. Toxic hepatitis with Stevens–Johnson syndrome has been ibuprofen described (23).

Ibuprofen has been rarely thought responsible for direct liver damage. A recent report has described three patients, 33–44 years old, with chronic hepatitis C infection who developed more than five-fold increases in serum liver transaminases after taking ibuprofen for musculoskeletal pain. In all three there were no associated symptoms of hepatitis, and serum transaminases normalized after ibuprofen was withdrawn (24).

Biliary tract

The vanishing bile duct syndrome has been associated with the use of ibuprofen in an atopic man, but the causal relation was not certain (25).

Another report of this rare syndrome was associated with Stevens–Johnson syndrome in a 10-year-old girl who took ibuprofen in conventional doses (up to 30 mg/kg/day) for 2 days (26). She recovered uneventfully.

Pancreas

An 18-year-old man developed acute pancreatitis immediately after an overdose of ibuprofen 51 mg/kg (27). Other causes of acute pancreatitis were excluded.

Urinary tract

Ibuprofen can cause renal impairment, ranging from an insignificant reduction to an acute fall in creatinine clearance associated with a general hypersensitivity reaction, especially in patients with systemic lupus erythematosus or acute tubular necrosis (28). The nephrotic syndrome without renal insufficiency and acute interstitial nephritis without the nephrotic syndrome have been described after self-administration of over-the-counter ibuprofen (SEDA-12, 86).

Irreversible renal insufficiency due to acute cortical necrosis triggered by severe renal hypoperfusion has been reported (SEDA-12, 86). A pharmacokinetic study showed that conversion of inactive *R*-ibuprofen to active *S*-ibuprofen was greater in patients with renal impairment than in healthy controls; this may aggravate renal insufficiency (29).

Acute deterioration in renal function can occur also in other at-risk patients, such as those with renal transplants (30,31).

Reports of acute renal insufficiency in children taking ibuprofen as an analgesic or antipyretic continue to appear (32,33). In most cases dehydration was the main precipitating cause. Ibuprofen and other NSAIDs should be avoided in dehydrated patients.

Acute papillary necrosis causing bilateral ureteric obstruction has been attributed to ibuprofen in an 8-year-old boy (34).

Skin

Rashes usually occur during general hypersensitivity. Urticarial, purpuric, and erythematous changes with pruritus have been reported (21). Bullous pemphigoid has been described after 6 months of treatment and was observed in two other patients on ibuprofen (SEDA-14, 94). Photosensitization has been attributed to ibuprofen (SEDA-17, 110). The association between ibuprofen and dermatological superinfection in children with recent *Varicella* infection has not been demonstrated in a retrospective cohort study (SEDA-22, 116).

Ibuprofen exacerbates psoriasis (SEDA-12, 86; SEDA-7, 108; SEDA-8, 102).

A fixed drug eruption has been attributed to ibuprofen (35).

- After taking ibuprofen for 2 days a 61-year-old woman developed erythema and pain affecting the tongue and oral mucosa; 2 months later she started taking ibuprofen and erythromycin, and the same lesions reappeared in the oral mucosa 24 hours later, with two new erythematosus violaceous macular lesions. Topical challenge through an occluded patch with ibuprofen 5% on the residual cutaneous lesion was positive.

Hair

Alopecia has been described in black women; normal hair growth returned after therapy was stopped (SED-11, 183) (36).

Musculoskeletal

In a case-control study in 124 655 subjects matched three to one for age and sex with 373 962 controls, there was an increased overall risk of *fractures* with ibuprofen (OR = 2.09; 95% CI = 2.00, 2.18), but not with celecoxib (OR = 0.76; 95% CI = 0.51, 1.13) (37). The effects in most cases were small. The authors suggested that falls may be one reason for the increase in fracture risk with some NSAIDs.

Immunologic

Anaphylaxis after ibuprofen was reported in a patient with asthma who was also taking zafirlukast, a leukotriene receptor antagonist (SEDA-22, 116).

A severe systemic hypersensitivity reaction (fever, rash, altered mental status, and hypotension) to oral ibuprofen in an 11-year-old boy was the first evidence of systemic lupus erythematosus; re-challenge with ibuprofen resulted in a recurrence of the previous symptoms (38).

Body temperature

Ibuprofen is commonly prescribed for a raised temperature and is well tolerated in children. Adverse effects are not common, even in overdose. Nevertheless, there have been two case reports of profound and protracted *hypothermia* after a single dose of ibuprofen in a 7-year-old girl (39) and after four doses over 3 days in a 19-month-old child (40).

Fever accompanied by nausea, vomiting, and hypotension occurred in a 68-year-old woman with Sjögren's syndrome and a leukocytoclastic vasculitis 15 minutes after a dose of ibuprofen; 3 months later she had a similar episode without hypotension and oral challenge with ibuprofen produced the same symptoms 3 hours after the last dose (41).

Susceptibility Factors

Age

The controversy over the use of ibuprofen as an antipyretic or analgesic is still open and the question of whether it is safer than paracetamol in children has not been answered (SEDA-16, 110) (SEDA-17, 110) (SEDA-19, 96).

Surgery

Despite paucity of evidence, clinicians routinely discontinue NSAIDs at least 1 week before most surgical procedures to avoid a possible risk of bleeding due to platelet dysfunction. In a prospective cohort study platelet function was tested in 11 healthy adult volunteers at baseline and after completion of a 7-day course of ibuprofen (600 mg orally every 8 hours) (42). There was platelet dysfunction after completion of the course of ibuprofen in seven of the 11 patients, which normalized by 24 hours after the last dose. These results, if confirmed, provide a rational basis for timing NSAID withdrawal before surgery.

Other features of the patient

In patients with a history of peptic ulcer or systemic lupus erythematosus the benefit-to-harm balance must be evaluated before prescribing ibuprofen. The first group is in danger of ulcer exacerbation and the second of a severe generalized hypersensitivity reaction.

Drug Administration

Drug formulations

Modified-release formulations seem to cause the same adverse effects as conventionally formulated ibuprofen (43), and four-times-daily treatment is better tolerated than twice-daily (SEDA-12, 86).

Ibuprofen lysine is more rapidly absorbed than ibuprofen free acid, but the comparative tolerability of the two formulations is not known (SEDA-20, 93).

Drug overdose

In spite of the large number of prescriptions and over-the-counter sales, acute intoxication is rare. Symptoms are usually limited to nausea and vomiting, but more severe cases of coma, acidosis, mild hypothermia, renal insufficiency, and acute papillary necrosis have been described (SEDA-12, 86) (SEDA-22, 116). Treatment is supportive (SEDA-9, 81).

A fatal overdose has been reported in a 26-year-old woman who took up to 105 g of modified-release ibuprofen (44). She presented with a reduced level of consciousness, a severe metabolic acidosis, and hemodynamic compromise, and died despite intensive supportive management, gut decontamination with multidose activated charcoal, and correction of the metabolic acidosis with sodium bicarbonate and hemofiltration. The ante-mortem blood ibuprofen concentration was 760 mg/l and the post-mortem concentrations were 518 mg/l in blood, 74 mg/kg in liver, and 116 mg/l in the gastric contents.

Drug–Drug Interactions

Aminoglycoside antibiotics

High-dose ibuprofen can slow the progression of lung disease in patients with cystic fibrosis and is usually well tolerated (SEDA-20, 93). However, transient renal insufficiency developed in four children with cystic fibrosis who were taking maintenance ibuprofen when an intravenous aminoglycoside was added to their regimen to treat an exacerbation of lung disease (45). Ibuprofen should probably be stopped during intravenous aminoglycoside therapy.

Antifungal azoles

The effects of voriconazole and fluconazole on the pharmacokinetics of S(+)-ibuprofen and R(–)-ibuprofen have been studied in 12 healthy men, who took a single oral dose of racemic ibuprofen 400 mg in a randomized order alone or 1 hour after voriconazole or fluconazole 400 mg bd on day 1 and 200 mg bd on day 2 (46). Voriconazole increased the AUC of S-ibuprofen to 205% and the C_{max} to 122%; the half-life was prolonged from 2.4 to 3.2 hours. Fluconazole increased the AUC of S-ibuprofen to 183% and the C_{max} to 116%; the half-life was prolonged from 2.4 to 3.1 hours. These effects were attributed to inhibition of CYP2C9-mediated metabolism of S-ibuprofen. Voriconazole and fluconazole had minor effects on the pharmacokinetics of R-ibuprofen. The authors recommended that the dosage of ibuprofen should be reduced when it is co-administered with voriconazole or fluconazole, especially when the initial dose of ibuprofen is high.

Antihypertensive agents

Ibuprofen interacts with antihypertensive agents, reducing their efficacy (47).

Aspirin

Patients with arthritis and vascular disease sometimes take both low-dose aspirin and other NSAIDs. However, concomitant treatment with ibuprofen can limit the cardioprotective effects of aspirin, according to the results of a study of the effects of ibuprofen, diclofenac, coxibs, and paracetamol on the antiplatelet activity of aspirin (48). The following combinations of drugs were used: aspirin (81 mg every morning) 2 hours before ibuprofen (400 mg every morning) or in the reverse order; aspirin 2 hours before rofecoxib (25 mg every morning or in the reverse order); enteric-coated aspirin 2 hours before ibuprofen (400 mg tds); and enteric-coated aspirin 2 hours before modified-release diclofenac (75 mg bd). Inhibition of the formation of serum thromboxane B2 (an index of COX-1 activity in platelets) and platelet aggregation by aspirin was blocked when a single daily dose of ibuprofen was given before aspirin, as well as when multiple daily doses of ibuprofen were given. Diclofenac, paracetamol, and rofecoxib did not affect the pharmacodynamics of aspirin. These results suggest that ibuprofen, but not diclofenac, paracetamol, or rofecoxib, antagonizes the irreversible inhibition of platelet COX-1 by aspirin and can therefore limit the cardioprotective effects of aspirin.

This hypothesis has now been supported in a study of over 7000 patients who were discharged after a first admission for cardiovascular disease between 1989 and 1997 and who took low-dose aspirin and survived for at least 1 month (49). The adjusted hazard ratios for all-cause mortality (HR = 1.93; 95% CI = 1.30, 287) and for cardiovascular mortality (HR = 1.73; CI = 1.05, 2.84) were significantly raised in patients who took ibuprofen (mean dose 1210 mg/day) in addition to the aspirin. There was no increase in hazard in patients who combined aspirin with diclofenac, which is consistent with the in vitro data. However, this study had many limitations (50), and further epidemiological studies are needed to address this potentially important interaction. In the meantime, when patients taking low-dose aspirin for cardioprotection also require long-term treatment with an NSAID, diclofenac would be preferable to ibuprofen.

Desmopressin

Hyponatremic coma induced by the concomitant use of desmopressin and ibuprofen has been reported (54).

- A 55-year-old woman with von Willebrand's disease became comatose. A brain CT scan was normal and laboratory investigations showed hyponatremia (121 mmol/l) and a low plasma osmolality (247 mosm/kg) with normal sodium excretion and urine osmolality. A diagnosis of hyponatremic coma was made. She had taken desmopressin for hemostasis plus ibuprofen for analgesia 2 days before, after a dental intervention. She was treated with water restriction and recovered fully within 24 hours.

The fact that she had previously used desmopressin several times without developing hyponatremia suggests that the effect was due to the combination of ibuprofen with vasopressin. Water intoxication and severe hyponatremia, sometimes resulting in coma and seizures, is a severe, but rare, complication of desmopressin when given alone. On the other hand, NSAIDs inhibit prostaglandin synthesis, and renal medullary prostaglandins are important regulators of urinary dilution. By inhibiting prostaglandin synthesis, NSAIDs potentiate the effect of vasopressin on water reabsorption in the renal tubules, thereby enhancing water retention. Despite these renal effects of NSAIDs and their frequent use, hyponatremia as a result of water intoxication has rarely been described with NSAIDs used alone, suggesting that additional factors are needed in order to develop symptoms of water intoxication.

Diazepam

The effect of diazepam on the pharmacokinetics of ibuprofen has been studied in eight healthy subjects, who took ibuprofen or ibuprofen plus diazepam at 10.00 or 22.00 hours in a randomized, crossover study (55). Diazepam significantly prolonged the half-life of ibuprofen at 22.00 hours but not at 10.00 hours. The mean clearance of ibuprofen was therefore reduced by diazepam at night. This time-dependent effect of diazepam on the pharmacokinetics of ibuprofen may be due to circadian variation in the pattern of protein production in the liver and/or competitive protein binding of the two drugs during the night.

Fibrates

Acute renal insufficiency occurred in one patient taking ciprofibrate 100 mg/day and ibuprofen 400 mg/day (56). Both drugs are highly protein-bound and contain propionic acid groups. Thus, ibuprofen may displace ciprofibrate.

Ginkgo biloba

Ginkgo biloba and NSAIDs both inhibit platelet aggregation, albeit by different mechanisms.

- A fatal cerebral hemorrhage occurred in an elderly patient without susceptibility factors who was taking a *Ginkgo biloba* extract (40 mg bd for more than 2.5 years) and ibuprofen (600 mg/day for 4 weeks) for osteoarthritis (57). A CT scan showed massive intracerebral bleeding.

Lithium

Ibuprofen can increase the serum lithium concentration (SEDA-13, 81) (58,59).

- A man of unspecified age developed cognitive impairment and a serum lithium concentration of 2.4 mmol/l after taking ibuprofen for shoulder pain (60).

Methotrexate

Ibuprofen can potentiate methotrexate-induced renal toxicity (51).

Pancreatic enzymes

An interaction between ibuprofen and pancreatic enzymes causing serious gastrointestinal damage has been described in animals (SEDA-21, 105).

Pemetrexed

In a randomized, crossover study in 27 patients with cancer with a creatinine clearance below 80 ml/minute, ibuprofen 400 mg was given orally every 6 hours, starting 2 days before intravenous administration of pemetrexed 500 mg/m^2 and continuing until 1 hour before the infusion (61). Ibuprofen caused a 16% reduction in the clearance of pemetrexed, a 15% increase in C_{max}, and a 20% increase in AUC, but no significant change in V_{ss}.

Phenytoin

Ibuprofen inhibits the metabolism of phenytoin (52).

Sulfonylureas

Ibuprofen (150 mg, 3 doses) for arthralgias was associated with hypoglycemia in a 72-year-old man who was taking glibenclamide 2.5 mg/day for type 2 diabetes mellitus; after the last dose he lost consciousness, and his blood glucose concentration was under 2.2 mmol/l (53).

Tacrolimus

Acute renal insufficiency has been described in concomitant treatment with tacrolimus in two liver transplant recipients (SEDA-18, 104).

Zaleplon

The interaction of zaleplon with ibuprofen has been investigated in 17 subjects (62). Healthy adult volunteers were given zaleplon 10 mg alone, ibuprofen 600 mg alone, or zaleplon 10 mg plus ibuprofen 600 mg in an open, randomized, crossover study. The adverse effects were mild and resolved without intervention. The authors concluded that there was no evidence of a significant interaction between zaleplon and ibuprofen.

References

1. Gall EP, Caperton EM, McComb JE, Messner R, Multz CV, O'Hanlan M, Willkens RF. Clinical comparison of ibuprofen, fenoprofen calcium, naproxen and tolmetin sodium in rheumatoid arthritis. J Rheumatol 1982;9(3):402–7.

2. Mandell BF, Raps EC. Severe systemic hypersensitivity reaction to ibuprofen occurring after prolonged therapy. Am J Med 1987;82(4):817–20.

3. Schooley RT, Wagley PF, Lietman PS. Edema associated with ibuprofen therapy. JAMA 1977;237(16):1716–7.

4. Palmer R, Weiss R, Zusman RM, Haig A, Flavin S, MacDonald B. Effects of nabumetone, celecoxib, and ibuprofen on blood pressure control in hypertensive patients on angiotensin converting enzyme inhibitors. Am J Hypertens 2003;16:135–9.

5. Bellini C, Campone F, Serra G. Pulmonary hypertension following L-lysine ibuprofen therapy in a preterm infant with patent ductus arteriosus. CMAJ 2006;174(13):1843–4.

6. Patel J, Marks KA, Roberts I, Azzopardi D, Edwards AD. Ibuprofen treatment of patent ductus arteriosus. Lancet 1995;346(8969):255.

7. Samuelson CO Jr, Williams HJ. Ibuprofen-associated aseptic meningitis in systemic lupus erythematosus. West J Med 1979;131(1):57–9.

8. Symon DN. Twelve cases of analgesic headache. Arch Dis Child 1998;78(6):555–6.

9. Vasconcellos E, Pina-Garza JE, Millan EJ, Warner JS. Analgesic rebound headache in children and adolescents. J Child Neurol 1998;13(9):443–7.

10. Periard D, Mayor C, Aubert V, Spertini F. Recurrent ibuprofen-induced aseptic meningitis: evidence against an antigen-specific immune response. Neurology 2006;67(3):539–40.

11. Rodríguez SC, Olguín AM, Miralles CP, Viladrich PF. Characteristics of meningitis caused by ibuprofen: report of 2 cases with recurrent episodes and review of the literature. Medicine (Baltimore) 2006;85(4):214–20.

12. Williamson J, Sturrock RD. An ophthalmic study of ibuprofen in rheumatoid conditions. Curr Med Res Opin 1976;4(2):128–31.

13. Gamulescu MA, Schalke B, Schuierer G, Gabel VP. Optic neuritis with visual field defect–possible Ibuprofen-related toxicity. Ann Pharmacother 2006;40(3):571–3.

14. Bernsetin AL, Werlin A. Pseudodementia associated with use of ibuprofen. Ann Pharmacother 2003;37:80–2.

15. Chalmers TM. Clinical experience with ibuprofen in rheumatoid arthritis. Schweiz Med Wochenschr 1971;101(8):280–2.

16. McIntyre BA, Philp RB, Inwood MJ. Effect of ibuprofen on platelet function in normal subjects and hemophiliac patients. Clin Pharmacol Ther 1978;24(5):616–21.

17. Thilo D, Nyman D, Duckert F. A study of the effect of the antirheumatic drug ibuprofen (Brufen) on patients being treated with the oral anti-coagulant phenprocoumon (Marcoumar). J Int Med Res 1974;2:276.

18. Mamus SW, Burton JD, Groat JD, Schulte DA, Lobell M, Zanjani ED. Ibuprofen-associated pure white-cell aplasia. N Engl J Med 1986;314(10):624–5.

19. Guidry JB, Ogburn CL Jr, Griffin FM Jr. Fatal autoimmune hemolytic anemia associated with ibuprofen. JAMA 1979;242(1):68–9.

20. Law IP, Wickman CJ, Harrison BR. Coombs'-positive hemolytic anemia and ibuprofen. South Med J 1979;72(6):707–10.

21. Davies EF, Avery GS. Ibuprofen: a review of its pharmacological properties and therapeutic efficacy in rheumatic disorders. Drugs 1971;2(5):416–46.

22. Caro H, Conture B, Pethilaz R, Royar JC. Etude clinique sur l'ibuprofen sous forme suppositoires. Gaz Med Fr 1976;83:372.

23. Sternlieb P, Robinson RM. Stevens–Johnson syndrome plus toxic hepatitis due to ibuprofen. NY State J Med 1978;78(8):1239–43.

24. Riley TR 3rd, Smith JP. Ibuprofen-induced hepatotoxicity in patients with chronic hepatitis C: a case series. Am J Gastroenterol 1998;93(9):1563–5.

25. Alam I, Ferrell LD, Bass NM. Vanishing bile duct syndrome temporally associated with ibuprofen use. Am J Gastroenterol 1996;91(8):1626–30.

26. Taghian M, Tran TA, Bresson-Hadni S, Menget A, Felix S, Jacquemin E. Acute vanishing bile duct syndrome after ibuprofen therapy in a child. J Pediatr 2004;145:273–6.

27. Magill P, Ridgway PF, Conlon KC, Neary P. A case of probable ibuprofen-induced acute pancreatitis. JOP 2006;7(3):311–4.

28. Fong HJ, Cohen AH. Ibuprofen-induced acute renal failure with acute tubular necrosis. Am J Nephrol 1982;2(1):28–31.

29. Chen CY, Chen CS. Stereoselective disposition of ibuprofen in patients with renal dysfunction. J Pharmacol Exp Ther 1994;268(2):590–4.

30. Moghal NE, Hulton SA, Milford DV. Care in the use of ibuprofen as an antipyretic in children. Clin Nephrol 1998;49(5):293–5.

31. Stoves J, Rosenberg K, Harnden P, Turney JH. Acute interstitial nephritis due to over-the-counter ibuprofen in a renal transplant recipient. Nephrol Dial Transplant 1998;13(1):227–8.

32. Moghal NE, Hegde S, Eastham KM. Ibuprofen and acute renal failure in a toddler. Arch Dis Child 2004;89:276–7.

33. Ulinski T, Guigonis V, Dunan O, Bensman A. Acute renal failure after treatment with non-steroidal anti-inflammatory drugs. Eur J Pediatr 2004;163:148–50.

34. Ismail M, Hegarty PK, Taghizadah A, Kumar N, Mushtaq I. Ibuprofen-induced papillary necrosis causing bilateral ureteric obstruction. J Pediatr Urol 2007;3(1):60–2.

35. Alvarez Santullano CV, Tover Flores V, De Barrio Fernández M, Tornero Molina P, Prieto Garcia A. Fixed drug eruption due to ibuprofen. Allergol Immunopathol (Madr) 2006;34(6):280–1.

36. Meyer HC. Alopecia associated with ibuprofen. JAMA 1979;242(2):142.

37. Vestergaard P, Rejnmark L, Mosekilde L. Fracture risk associated with use of nonsteroidal anti-inflammatory drugs, acetylsalicylic acid, and acetaminophen and the effects of rheumatoid arthritis and osteoarthritis. Calcif Tissue Int 2006;79(2):84–94.

38. Mou SS, Punaro L, Antón J, Luckett PM. Severe systemic hypersensitivity reaction to ibuprofen: a presentation of systemic lupus erythematosus. J Rheumatol 2006;33(1):171–2.

39. Desai PR, Sriskandan S. Hypothermia in a child secondary to ibuprofen. Arch Dis Child 200;88:87–8.

40. Malik SA, Thomson M, Taylor T. Hypothermia and ibuprofen. Electronic Letter Arch Dis Child 2003;17 Februar.

41. Gonzalo-Garijo MA, Bobadilla P. Ibuprofen-induced fever in Sjögren's syndrome. J Investig Allergol Clin Immunol 2006;16(4):266–7.

42. Goldenberg NA, Jacobs L, Manco-Johnson MJ. Duration of platelet dysfunction after a 7-day course of ibuprofen. Ann Intern Med 2005;142:506–9.

43. Fernandez L, Jacoby RK, Smith PJ, et al. Comparative trial of standard and sustained release formulations of ibuprofen in patients with osteoarthritis. Curr Med Res Opin 1982;7:610.

44. Wood DM, Monaghan J, Streete P, Jones AL, Dargan PI. Fatality after deliberate ingestion of sustained-release ibuprofen: a case report. Crit Care 2006;10(2):R4.

45. Kovesi TA, Swartz R, MacDonald N. Transient renal failure due to simultaneous ibuprofen and aminoglycoside therapy in children with cystic fibrosis. N Engl J Med 1998;338(1):65–6.

46. Hynninen VV, Olkkola KT, Leino K, Lundgren S, Neuvonen PJ, Rane A, Valtonen M, Vyyryläinen H, Laine K. Effects of the antifungals voriconazole and fluconazole on the pharmacokinetics of S-(+)- and R-(–)-ibuprofen. Antimicrob Agents Chemother 2006;50(6):1967–72.

47. Radack KL, Deck CC, Bloomfield SS. Ibuprofen interferes with the efficacy of antihypertensive drugs. A randomized, double-blind, placebo-controlled trial of ibuprofen compared with acetaminophen. Ann Intern Med 1987;107(5):628–35.

48. Catella-Lawson F, Reilly MP, Kapoor SC, Cucchiara AJ, DeMarco S, Tournier B, Vyas SN, FitzGerald GA. Cyclooxygenase inhibitors and the antiplatelet effects of aspirin. N Engl J Med 2001;345(25):1809–17.

49. MacDonald TM, Wei L. Effect of ibuprofen on cardioprotective effect of aspirin. Lancet 2003;361(9357):573–4.

50. FitzGerald GA. Parsing an enigma: the pharmacodynamics of aspirin resistance. Lancet 2003;361(9357):542–4.

51. Cassano WF. Serious methotrexate toxicity caused by interaction with ibuprofen. Am J Pediatr Hematol Oncol 1989;11(4):481–2.

52. Sandyk R. Phenytoin toxicity induced by interaction with ibuprofen. S Afr Med J 1982;62(17):592.

53. Sone H, Takahashi A, Yamada N. Ibuprofen-related hypoglycemia in a patient receiving sulfonylurea. Ann Intern Med 2001;134(4):344.

54. Garcia EB, Ruitenberg A, Madretsma GS, Hintzen RQ. Hyponatraemic coma induced by desmopressin and ibuprofen in a woman with von Willebrand's disease. Haemophilia 2003;9:232–4.

55. Bapuji AT, Rambhau D, Srinivasu P, Rao BR, Apte SS. Time dependent influence of diazepam on the pharmacokinetics of ibuprofen in man. Drug Metabol Drug Interact 1999;15(1):71–81.

56. Ramachandran S, Giles PD, Hartland A. Acute renal failure due to rhabdomyolysis in presence of concurrent ciprofibrate and ibuprofen treatment. BMJ 1997;314(7094):1593.

57. Meisel C, Johne A, Roots I. Fatal intracerebral mass bleeding associated with Ginkgo biloba and ibuprofen. Atherosclerosis 2003;167:367.

58. Ragheb M. Ibuprofen can increase serum lithium level in lithium-treated patients. J Clin Psychiatry 1987;48(4):161–3.

59. Bailey CE, Stewart JT, McElroy RA. Ibuprofen-induced lithium toxicity. South Med J 1989;82(9):1197.

60. Joseph DiGiacomo. Interview with F Flach. Risk management issues associated with psychopharmacological treatment. Essent Psychopharmacol 2001;4:137–50.

61. Sweeney CJ, Takimoto CH, Latz JE, Baker SD, Murry DJ, Krull JH, Fife K, Battiato L, Cleverly A, Chaudhary AK, Chaudhuri T, Sandler A, Mita AC, Rowinsky EK. Two drug interaction studies evaluating the pharmacokinetics and toxicity of pemetrexed when coadministered with aspirin or ibuprofen in patients with advanced cancer. Clin Cancer Res 2006;12(2):536–42.

62. Sanchez Garcia P, Carcas A, Zapater P, Rosendo J, Paty I, Leister CA, Troy SM. Absence of an interaction between ibuprofen and zaleplon. Am J Health Syst Pharm 2000;57(12):1137–41.

Ibuproxam

General Information

Ibuproxam is an NSAID that causes similar adverse effects to other NSAIDs.

Organs and Systems

Gastrointestinal

Gastrointestinal adverse effects have been reported with ibuproxam, including nausea, vomiting, occult gastrointestinal blood loss, and rectal pain (1).

Skin

Skin rashes have been reported with ibuproxam (1).

Reference

1. Scaranelli M, Delli Gatti I, Menegale G, et al. Casi di artrite reumatoide resistent al trattamento con farmaci antiflogistici non-steroidei: uso di dosi piu elevate di ibuproxam. Gaz Med Ital 1981;140:27.

Indometacin

General Information

Indometacin is the best-known and most thoroughly tested indoleacetic acid derivative. It is one of the most effective NSAIDs, and most of its toxic and therapeutic effects appear to be due to marked inhibition of prostaglandin synthesis. Because of its potency, its clinical efficacy is comparable, if not superior, to any other NSAID, but for precisely the same reason its adverse effects on the gastrointestinal tract and the nervous system inevitably limit its use. However, patients who tolerate it reasonably well are naturally not anxious to exchange it for any newer drugs with fewer problems but less potency. A meta-analysis of patients' preference in 37 crossover comparisons of indometacin with newer NSAIDs did not provide evidence of a trend to replace indometacin with newer NSAIDs (1).

Tropesin is the tropic acid ester of indometacin, and its adverse effects profile is similar to that of indometacin (SEDA-17, 113).

General adverse reactions

Adverse effects, in up to 60% of patients, are closely related to indometacin's strong anti-inflammatory potency. Gastric irritation, including ulcers, bleeding, and perforation, predominates. Nervous system complications are related to cerebral edema. Headache is common. Hematological effects are infrequently reported. Nephrotoxicity is exacerbated by pre-existing renal impairment. Ocular toxicity can follow long-term use.

Cross-reactivity with aspirin has been reported (2). The hazards of administering topical indometacin to asthmatic patients should be widely known (3).

Tumor-induced effects have not been demonstrated.

Organs and Systems

Cardiovascular

Clinical experience and reports have provided little evidence that indometacin precipitates angina or myocardial infarction. However, an individual angina-provoking effect has been documented (4), and there are grounds for believing that it can happen.

Intravenous administration of indometacin increases blood pressure, coronary vascular resistance, and myocardial oxygen demands, decreasing coronary flow. A controlled short-term study showed that indometacin increased blood pressure in patients with mild untreated essential hypertension (SEDA-17, 108). In view of the increasing use of parenteral administration, the acute hemodynamic effects of indometacin may now occur more often, especially in the elderly (5). The mechanism is poorly understood, but apparently a direct action is exerted on the resistance vessels in various regions. This is probably independent of indometacin's action on prostaglandin formation. The clinical relevance is largely unknown, but other NSAIDs should probably be prescribed for patients with occlusive vascular diseases affecting the cerebral and/or coronary vessels.

Other systemic cardiovascular adverse effects are due to salt and fluid retention and also to a reduction in the vasodilator action of circulating prostaglandins E_2 and I_2 (6).

Unlike other NSAIDs, indometacin acts as a cerebral vasoconstrictor. It reduces cerebral flow by up to 35% and the response to hypercapnia disappears (SEDA-10, 79). It also reduces blood flow in the splanchnic vascular bed, by increasing local vascular resistance, but does not impair circulation in the forearm and leg muscles.

Respiratory

Inhibition of prostaglandin synthesis explains indometacin's ability to provoke or aggravate asthma in hypersensitive patients (7). Indometacin in ophthalmic solution reportedly caused such deterioration in asthmatic patients as to require mechanical ventilation (3,8). Cross-sensitivity between indometacin and aspirin has been observed.

The risk of bronchopulmonary dysplasia has been determined in 999 infants of extremely low birth weight with and without patent ductus arteriosus who survived to a postmenstrual age of 36 weeks and who were randomized to indometacin prophylaxis or placebo (9). The incidence of bronchopulmonary dysplasia in infants with patent ductus arteriosus was 52% (55/105) after indometacin and 56% (137/246) after placebo. In contrast, rates of bronchopulmonary dysplasia in those without a patent ductus arteriosus were 43% (170/391) after indometacin prophylaxis and 30% (78/257) after placebo. There was evidence that this difference was related to poor oxygenation and edema formation in those who developed bronchopulmonary dysplasia.

Nervous system

Adverse reactions to indometacin involving the central nervous system are frequent and come second in importance only to gastrointestinal effects. They are attributed to salt and water retention. Up to 60% of patients experience headache (often migraine-like), frontal throbbing, and vertigo. Vomiting, tinnitus, ataxia, tremor, dizziness, and insomnia follow. Somnolence, confusion, hallucinations (especially in the elderly), and psychotic symptoms have been described. Coma, clonic seizures, and myoclonic spasms (SEDA-18, 101) can develop. Muscle weakness and paresthesia, that is, peripheral neuropathy, may develop in elderly patients, but recede after withdrawal (10,11).

Indometacin is used for non-invasive closure of symptomatic ductus arteriosus in the preterm infant. Intravenous administration causes an instant reduction in cerebral blood flow, increasing cerebral vascular resistance. The clinical significance for the nervous system of these hemodynamic changes is unknown (12,13), but they seem to be linked to the effects seen in the central nervous system. Advantage has been taken of this effect for reducing intracranial hypertension in patients with severe head injury (SEDA-15, 99).

Indometacin is also used in preterm infants as prophylaxis against intraventricular hemorrhage. In a prospective, randomised, placebo-controlled trial in 431 preterm neonates, low-dose indometacin prevented intraventricular hemorrhage without adverse cognitive or motor outcomes at 36 months (14).

Low-dose indometacin (0.1 mg/kg), begun in the first 24 hours of life and given every 24 hours for 6 doses, was not associated with adverse neurodevelopmental outcome at 36 months corrected age (15).

Sensory systems

Prolonged therapy can cause a number of adverse reactions in the eyes. Trivial effects are ocular discomfort, conjunctival pain, and increased ocular tension, but mydriasis, photophobia, blurred vision, diplopia, amblyopia, and loss of vision can occur. The most serious complications are retinopathy with reduced retinal sensitivity, and corneal and retinal pigmentation. They are reversible, but improvement is slow. A report on indometacin retinopathy has added more doubt than certainty to the question of the frequency and severity of retinal toxicity (SEDA-14, 93). Patients taking prolonged therapy should have regular ophthalmic examinations.

Metabolism

Indometacin reduces the area under the corticotropin (ACTH) plasma concentration–time curve after insulin in normal men, possibly because of the role of prostaglandins in the control of ACTH secretion (16).

One report has described low plasma ascorbic acid concentrations during indometacin treatment, and a case of hyperglycemia has been reported (17).

Electrolyte balance

Hyperkalemia has been reported in patients with pre-existing renal disease treated with indometacin (SEDA-4, 65; SEDA-5, 90; SEDA-6, 93) and in a patient with Bartter's syndrome receiving concomitant oral potassium chloride (SEDA-11, 92; 18). Indometacin caused a high serum potassium concentration in a young athlete (SEDA-14, 93).

Mineral balance

During indometacin therapy, urinary excretion of zinc and calcium can increase significantly (19). The clinical relevance is not known.

Fluid balance

Salt and fluid retention is an adverse effect of indometacin, although it is less important than with the pyrazolone derivatives. Indometacin can antagonize antihypertensive agents, including beta-adrenoceptor antagonists (20,21). The effect on blood pressure in normotensive patients has not been adequately studied.

Severe water intoxication caused by inappropriate ADH secretion has been described in an elderly woman taking indometacin (SEDA-17, 108).

Hematologic

Anemia caused by repetitive gastrointestinal bleeding is a relatively frequent, although indirect, hematological adverse effect.

Blood dyscrasias, sometimes fatal aplastic anemia (22), isolated granulocytopenia, and agranulocytosis have been reported (23). The International Agranulocytosis and Aplastic Anemia study showed that indometacin was significantly associated with agranulocytosis and aplastic anemia (24).

Neutropenia has been reported in a preterm male infant with a patent ductus arteriosus during treatment with indometacin; this could have been coincidence, but his mother had also previously had indometacin-associated neutropenia (25).

Since indometacin is an inhibitor of platelet aggregation, impairment of thrombocyte function is frequent, but thrombocytopenia is rare. Severe clotting defects due to inhibition of platelet aggregation in premature infants have been described (26). Postoperative bleeding is significantly more frequent in indometacin-treated patients.

Indometacin should probably not be used postoperatively in patients at increased risk of bleeding (SEDA-8, 103).

Gastrointestinal

Gastrotoxicity is the main adverse effect of indometacin, and symptoms range from abdominal discomfort to ulcer penetration and perforation (27). The phenomenon of gastric mucosal adaptation has been evoked to explain the relatively low incidence of severe adverse effects, compared with the acute gastric damage that occurs in short-term studies. In healthy volunteers, indometacin produced acute gastroduodenal damage in all cases, but resolved in almost all, despite continuing administration. The author hypothesized that the severity of mucosal damage depends on the reduction in mucosal blood flow (SEDA-16, 108; SEDA-17, 108).

Small bowel ulceration with thickening of the bowel wall and stricture formation in the terminal ileum and the ileocecal junction occurred in a patient with rheumatoid arthritis taking long-term indometacin (SEDA-12, 84). This is one reason why prolonged courses of indometacin should be avoided whenever possible, especially in elderly women.

Osmosin, a formulation that contains potassium bicarbonate and releases indometacin osmotically, was withdrawn because of reports of intestinal irritation, bleeding, perforation, and even death. These adverse effects were most probably caused by the very high local concentrations of indometacin and potassium in the lower part of the gastrointestinal tract produced by the tablet, which shifted the adverse reactions from the stomach to the intestine (SEDA-8, 103; 28).

Like other NSAIDs, a diaphragm-likesided colonic stricture has been described in a woman taking indometacin suppositories (29). Perforation of colonic diverticula has been described (30).

The use of indometacin suppositories can be associated with rectal irritation, mucosal inflammation, or necrosis with bleeding (31). The local effect on the gastric mucosa is less important than the systemic one, and suppositories do not cause fewer gastric lesions than oral formulations (32).

Both dexamethasone and indometacin can cause spontaneous intestinal perforation in very low birth weight neonates. In a retrospective case-control study in 16 such neonates and 32 controls matched by birth weight, those who received three or more doses of indometacin for ductal closure or intraventricular hemorrhage prophylaxis and three or more doses of dexamethasone (0.3 mg/kg cumulative dose over 3 days) for refractory hypotension during the first postnatal week were 10 times more likely to develop intestinal perforation (95% CI = 1.22, 76) (33).

Pancreas

Two cases of acute pancreatitis have been attributed to indometacin.

- A 56-year-old man developed acute pancreatitis after taking indometacin 150 mg/day orally for 3 weeks (34). Other causes were ruled out. He made a complete recovery after indometacin was withdrawn.
- A 71-year-old woman developed acute pancreatitis after taking indometacin for 1 month. Other causes were ruled out (35). The duct of Wirsung was dilated and the pancreas hypertrophied. An abdominal CT scan showed diffuse pancreatic necrosis with fluid collections in the anterior lateral spaces of both kidneys and in the lower omental sac. She improved spontaneously after withdrawal of indometacin.

Liver

Despite reversible changes in liver enzyme tests (36) and a fatal case of acute hepatocellular necrosis, which may have been related to indometacin, the drug is rarely hepatotoxic (37). Indometacin-associated cholestatic liver injury has been described. The reaction was not severe and recovery was rapid and uneventful (38).

Urinary tract

Indometacin nephrotoxicity is rare in patients with normal renal function, but indometacin can aggravate pre-existing renal impairment, as has been observed in patients with glomerulonephritis, nephrotic syndrome, systemic lupus erythematosus, and cirrhosis complicated by ascites (SED-8, 219; SEDA-4, 65; SEDA-7, 108; SEDA-11, 85). Severe but reversible loss of renal function in patients with systemic lupus erythematosus in the absence of active renal disease suggests that mesangial contraction in the glomerulus could significantly reduce the capillary surface area available for filtration and hence reduce the glomerular filtration rate (39,40). There is a significant reduction in the glomerular filtration rate and a concomitant drop in renal excretion of sodium and water in patients with compensated cirrhosis without ascites treated with indometacin (SEDA-18, 101).

Probable indometacin-induced renal papillary necrosis has been described in two patients with chronic juvenile arthritis (SEDA-8, 103).

Reversible acute renal insufficiency with eosinophilia has been described (41).

The harmful effect of indometacin on renal function has been used therapeutically to induce medical nephrectomy (SEDA-7, 108).

Skin

Reactions to indometacin range from urticaria and pruritus to fixed rashes, purpura, and maculopapular and morbilliform eruptions. Toxic epidermal necrolysis has also been described (42). The frequency of skin reactions is lower than with pyrazolone derivatives. There is cross-sensitivity with aspirin.

Whether indometacin exacerbates psoriasis is not certain, but one report (43) suggests that it can.

Indometacin can exacerbate dermatitis herpetiformis (SEDA-10, 81).

Musculoskeletal

Progressive destruction of large weight-bearing hip joints was first observed during long-term indometacin therapy more than 25 years ago (SEDA-11, 87; 44). In one comparison of the effects of azapropazone and indometacin, the osteoarthritic process in the hip progressed more quickly in patients treated with indometacin, no doubt a further indication of its powerful inhibitory effect on prostaglandin synthesis (45). The mechanisms responsible for the harmful effect of NSAIDs on osteoarthritic joints have been reviewed (SEDA-11, 87).

Sexual function

Inhibition of prostaglandin synthesis can cause impotence. A healthy man became impotent while taking short-term indometacin 150 mg/day (SEDA-5, 101).

Immunologic

Masking of infection and abnormal immune reactions have been reported (46). It is not clear whether this has any clinical significance.

Second-Generation Effects

Fertility

Ovulation was inhibited by indometacin at high doses in the preovulatory period (SEDA-16, 109).

Pregnancy

The use of indometacin in late pregnancy has been much debated. Because of its ability to inhibit prostaglandin synthesis it can be used to arrest premature labor for a short time, although there is no evidence that it reduces the incidence of premature delivery. The hazards of using it as a tocolytic agent seem to outweigh any theoretical advantage, since there are many reports of serious adverse neonatal effects after the treatment of preterm labor with indometacin. They include premature closure of the ductus arteriosus, pulmonary hypertension with persistent fetal circulation, fetal anuria, severe oligohydramnios, necrotizing enterocolitis, perinatal death, and severe respiratory distress syndrome resulting in oxygen dependence for several days (SED-11, 179) (47–49) (SEDA-5, 101) (SEDA-6, 93) (SEDA-7, 108) (SEDA-8, 102) (SEDA-9, 88) (SEDA-12, 84) (SEDA-15, 99) (SEDA-16, 109) (SEDA-17, 108). The risks might be linked to the duration of use, but one study provided evidence that short-term indometacin can cause closure of the ductus arteriosus, even if several weeks elapse between treatment and delivery (50).

The risks involved in longer-term use are multiple, as several studies have shown. The use of indometacin and ibuprofen for more than 72 hours in 67 women in preterm labor was significantly associated with more oligohydramnios than either ritodrine or magnesium sulfate. Oligohydramnios developed in 70% of 37 women treated with indometacin, in 27% treated with ibuprofen, and in 2 controls (51).

Pregnant women taking beta-blockers for hypertension in pregnancy should not be given indometacin, as it can raise the blood pressure (52).

Teratogenicity

Indometacin in pregnancy is probably safe, provided its use is limited to the first 32 weeks of gestation. However, a possible teratogenic effect has been ascribed to it (53).

Cerebral ischemia has been described in premature twins following maternal use of indometacin (54).

The incidence and type of cerebral lesions were studied by ultrasound in 159 preterm infants: 76 fetuses were exposed to indometacin used as a tocolytic agent; in the other 83 pregnancies, tocolysis was either not started or limited to fenoterol. The incidence of periventricular leukomalacia was increased in infants exposed to any tocolytic agent; cystic lesions occurred more often in those exposed to indometacin (55).

Oligohydramnios and renal dysgenesis developed in one identical twin exposed to early prolonged high-dose indometacin. As indometacin causes oligohydramnios and renal dysgenesis in fetal monkeys, it may also have caused the abnormalities in this patient (56).

Antenatal indometacin therapy has been extensively reviewed (SEDA-18, 102). Data from a retrospective cohort study of 57 premature infants, born between the 24th and 30th weeks of gestation, whose mothers had been treated unsuccessfully with indometacin for preterm labor, confirmed several fetal and neonatal complications (57). However, the overall results provided inconclusive or contradictory data on the benefit to harm balance of indometacin as a tocolytic agent or as treatment for hydramnios (SEDA-18, 102).

Fetotoxicity

The possible association of indometacin tocolysis with neonatal necrotizing enterocolitis has been the subject of a case-control study (58). All cases of proven necrotizing enterocolitis were ascertained and four controls for each case were randomly identified. During 18 months there were 24 cases of necrotizing enterocolitis. Indometacin as a single tocolytic agent was not associated with necrotizing enterocolitis (OR = 1.0, 95% CI = 0.2, 4.8).

The risk of premature closure of the ductus arteriosus due to indometacin used during the third trimester of pregnancy has been studied in a systematic review of studies in 217 patients exposed to indometacin and 221 to placebo; the risk of ductal closure was 15-fold higher in the group of women exposed to indometacin than in those who took either placebo or other NSAIDs (8 studies; OR = 15; 95% CI = 3.29, 69)(59). There was no significant increased risk of ductal closure in the infants of

women treated with indometacin compared with those who took other NSAIDs (4 studies; OR = 2.12; 95% CI = 0.48, 9.25). Fetal hypoxia may be important in increasing the risk of this complication (60).

Lactation

The effects of indometacin during lactation are unclear. Convulsions in a breast-fed infant were linked to indometacin in the milk (61).

Susceptibility Factors

Age

Children

Pharmacokinetic factors (slow metabolism) may underlie the marked effect of indometacin on platelet aggregation in premature infants and small children. The use of indometacin in children with patent ductus arteriosus can be followed by a severe general reaction. Nephrotoxicity, abdominal distension, hemorrhagic enteritis, and necrotizing enterocolitis have been observed (SEDA-10, 81) (26,62). No retrospective study has shown that indometacin-treated infants have a higher incidence of retrolental hyperplasia or visual problems (63). Reopening of the ductus after indometacin-induced occlusion has been described (SEDA-18, 101), but the risks of using intravenous indometacin are few and it is more efficacious and safer than ligation.

Elderly people

Elderly patients are susceptible to the adverse effects of NSAIDs on the nervous system. A psychotic reaction has been described in one elderly man taking indometacin (64) and behavioral changes in another (65).

Gastrotoxicity is more frequent in this age group. Of 125 516 residents of US nursing homes during 1992–1996, patients who received at least one prescription for aspirin (*n* = 19 101) or NSAIDs (*n* = 9777) were identified (66). NSAID exposure increased the overall gastrointestinal-event-related hospitalization rate. The rates were highest in those taking sulindac, naproxen, or indometacin.

Other features of the patient

Patients with asthma or allergic rhinitis may be hypersensitive to indometacin and can develop severe general allergic reactions, especially if they are allergic to aspirin.

Indometacin should probably not be used postoperatively in patients with an increased risk of bleeding (SEDA-8, 103), because of its anti-platelet activity.

In athletes in training for a marathon, the use of indometacin may be dangerous, since it can provoke hyperkalemia and there is a risk of serious dysrhythmias (SEDA-14, 93).

Drug Administration

Drug formulations

Indometacin in eye-drop form can cause burning sensations, pruritus, local congestion and irritation, corneal epithelial changes, and edema of the eyelids (67).

Osmosin (Indosmos)

Osmosin (Indosmos) was an osmotic pump version of indometacin, which after a brief career, was withdrawn from the market in the summer of 1982. Indometacin, as a potent NSAID, found itself at the beginning of the 1980s facing heavy competition from a series of newer drugs that were about to be introduced; all were under patent, whereas some of the indometacin patents were about to expire, which could lead to a substantial fall in prices; some of the newer drugs (notably benoxaprofen, itself soon withdrawn, and piroxicam) were suitable for use as a single daily oral dose, which provided at least a marketing advantage; several were claimed, rightly or wrongly, to be relatively well-tolerated by the stomach. One possible answer to these problems seemed to be offered by developing an osmotic pump form of indometacin; in this form, the drug could be released relatively slowly, perhaps prolonging its duration of action and improving its gastric tolerability.

In fact, the question as to whether this form of indometacin really had these advantages has never been satisfactorily settled. The literature (68–71) does not appear to have shown a reduction in gastric adverse effects, at least not if one assesses the papers in question with the critical eye that must be brought to bear on claims of this type. On the other hand, it is clear that if a drug that has a potentially irritant action on the gastrointestinal tract is put into a modified-releasing form, tolerability problems may be displaced from the stomach to the lower parts of the gastrointestinal tract.

In the course of 1982, serious suspicions arose that this was indeed happening. In August, the UK's Committee on Safety of Medicines (CSM) stated that it had received 200 reports of adverse reactions to the product, which was considered a relatively high reporting level for a new drug, though more than 400 000 prescriptions had been issued over the previous 7 months. Many of the reports were of effects traditionally associated with indometacin (such as headache and gastrointestinal problems) and these did not seem to be less frequent with the new system. Two of the reports were of intestinal perforation distal to the duodenum, an unusual site for damage by NSAIDs. The CSM remarked that the release characteristics of the system might expose certain areas of the bowel to higher concentrations of indometacin than usual. It was also noted that the formulation contained potassium bicarbonate, a known bowel irritant (28).

It subsequently became clear that a fair number of cases of intestinal irritation, bleeding, perforation, and probably even death were attributable to the new formulation, leading to the product's withdrawal in countries where it had already been introduced.

The proposed mechanism of small bowel damage due to Osmosin is that the tablets adhered to the intestinal wall (or became lodged in diverticula), resulting in much higher local concentrations of indometacin and potassium than usual.

Indometacin-farnesil

Limited early experiences with indometacin-farnesil, a lipid-soluble indometacin derivative esterified with farnesol, suggested an adverse-effects profile similar to the indometacin, even though the compound was synthesized to reduce gastrotoxicity (SEDA-17, 109).

Drug administration route

Intravenous administration (in the treatment of ureteric colic) is effective and well tolerated. However, in 90% of patients who receive slow (5 minutes) intravenous injection, hypertension, nausea, vertigo, vomiting, and peptic ulcer symptoms have been documented (72). Intravenous administration should be avoided in patients with heart failure.

Intramuscular indometacin causes few adverse effects at the site of injection (redness, pain, induration) (SEDA-8, 102) and seems to have better systemic tolerability than intravenous indometacin: 26% of 388 patients treated with indometacin 100 mg/day developed an adverse effect (gastrointestinal or nervous system-related) and 4.6% interrupted treatment (73).

Drug–Drug Interactions

ACE inhibitors

Although lisinopril in association with indometacin reduced proteinuria in a small group of patients with nephritic syndrome, the combination also caused impairment of renal function and hyperkalemia in many patients (SEDA-16, 109).

Acenocoumarol

Major bleeding occurred during combined treatment with indometacin and low doses of acenocoumarol in a patient who was homozygous for the 2C9*3 variant of CYP2C9, which is responsible for low requirements of acenocoumarol and makes dosing difficult (74).

Anti-platelet drugs

Indometacin potentiates the effect of anti-platelet drugs and anticoagulants (75).

Aspirin

Indometacin reduces the absorption of aspirin (76).

Beta-blockers

Attenuation of the hypotensive effect of propranolol and thiazide diuretics by indometacin was shown several years ago in a double-blind, placebo-controlled study of patients with essential hypertension (SEDA-6, 94). Two women with pre-eclampsia treated with pindolol and propranolol became extremely hypertensive when indometacin was added for premature contractions (52). Pregnant women taking beta-blockers for hypertension in pregnancy should not be given indometacin, as it can raise the blood pressure (52).

Cardiac glycosides

Indometacin increased plasma digoxin concentrations in premature neonates with a patent ductus arteriosus (80), but a formal study in healthy adults showed no interaction (81). It may be that pre-existing impairment of renal function is required for this interaction, but this remains to be elucidated.

Cocaine

Cocaine combined with indometacin in a 23-year-old pregnant woman at 34 weeks gestation may have caused fetal anuria and neonatal gastric hemorrhage (82).

Cyclophosphamide

Synergy between indometacin and cyclophosphamide has been advanced as the cause of a life-threatening acute water intoxication and severe hyponatremia observed in a patient with multiple myeloma and normal renal function (SEDA-15, 99).

Dipyridamole

Marked water retention has been observed during acute administration of dipyridamole in combination with indometacin (SEDA-13, 79).

Diuretics

Indometacin reduces the effect of diuretics (77). Combination of indometacin with Moduretic (co-amilozide; amiloride + hydrochlorothiazide) results in hyperkalemia (78).

Losartan

Indometacin 50 mg bd for one week did not interfere with the antihypertensive efficacy of losartan 50–100 mg/day in patients with essential hypertension, despite the fact that indometacin caused significant increases in weight and extracellular fluid volume (83). Glomerular filtration rate remained unchanged. Indometacin did not adversely influence peripheral hemodynamics. This is in contrast to the reported effects of indometacin during ACE inhibition, leading to an increase in blood pressure. It suggests that prostaglandins in part mediate vasodilatation during ACE inhibition, a mechanism that is not shared by angiotensin II antagonists. However, the result of this study is in contrast with those of several similar interaction studies with other antihypertensive agents, in which prostaglandin inhibition for 1–4 weeks caused an increase in weight combined with an increase in blood pressure. If indometacin had been given with losartan for more than 1 week, it may have produced a similar increase in blood pressure. Thus, the results of this study should not be taken as an argument against the recommendation that non-steroidal anti-inflammatory drugs should not be combined with angiotensin II antagonists, a recommendation that should be re-emphasized.

Metformin

Renal insufficiency and severe metabolic acidosis developed in a patient with diabetes mellitus taking metformin after recent treatment with indometacin (SEDA-22, 118).

Muromonab

The interaction of indometacin with the immunosuppressive agent muromonab, a monoclonal antibody to CD3, is characterized by an increased risk of encephalopathic or psychotic features (79).

Probenecid

Probenecid inhibits the tubular secretion of indometacin (SEDA-4, 66).

Interactions with indometacin have been documented through inhibition of renal tubular excretion (84,85). In 17 patients with rheumatoid arthritis, probenecid 500 mg bd improved the therapeutic response to indometacin 25 mg tds over 3 weeks (86). There were changes in the pharmacokinetics of indometacin, which the authors attributed to a reduction in the non-renal clearance of indometacin, possibly because of reduced biliary clearance.

References

1. Gotzsche PC. Patients' preference in indomethacin trials: an overview. Lancet 1989;1(8629):88–91.
2. Smith AP. Response of aspirin-allergic patients to challenge by some analgesics in common use. BMJ 1971;2(760):494–6.
3. Sheehan GJ, Kutzner MR, Chin WD. Acute asthma attack due to ophthalmic indomethacin. Ann Intern Med 1989;111(4):337–8.
4. Golding D. Angina and indomethacin. BMJ 1970;4(735):622.
5. Wennmalm A, Carlsson I, Edlund A, Eriksson S, Kaijser L, Nowak J. Central and peripheral haemodynamic effects of non-steroidal anti-inflammatory drugs in man. Arch Toxicol Suppl 1984;7:350–9.
6. Dzau VJ, Packer M, Lilly LS, Swartz SL, Hollenberg NK, Williams GH. Prostaglandins in severe congestive heart failure. Relation to activation of the renin–angiotensin system and hyponatremia. N Engl J Med 1984;310(6):347–52.
7. Szczeklik A, Gryglewski RJ, Czerniawska-Mysik G. Participation of prostaglandins in pathogenesis of aspirin-sensitive asthma. Naunyn Schmiedebergs Arch Pharmacol 1977;297(Suppl 1):S99–S110.

8. Polachek J, Shvartzman P. Acute bronchial asthma associated with the administration of ophthalmic indomethacin. Isr J Med Sci 1996;32(11):1107–9.

9. Schmidt B, Roberts RS, Fanaroff A, Davis P, Kirpalani HM, Nwaesei C, Vincer M; TIPP Investigators. Indomethacin prophylaxis, patent ductus arteriosus, and the risk of bronchopulmonary dysplasia: further analyses from the Trial of Indomethacin Prophylaxis in Preterms (TIPP). J Pediatr 2006;148(6):730–4.

10. Eade OE, Acheson ED, Cuthbert MF, Hawkes CH. Peripheral neuropathy and indomethacin. BMJ 1975;2(5962):66–7.

11. Rothermich NO. Deafness and hand tremor with indometacin. JAMA 1973;226:1471.

12. Van Bel F, Van de Bor M, Stijnen T, Baan J, Ruys JH. Cerebral blood flow velocity changes in preterm infants after a single dose of indomethacin: duration of its effect. Pediatrics 1989;84(5):802–7.

13. Edwards AD, Wyatt JS, Richardson C, Potter A, Cope M, Delpy DT, Reynolds EO. Effects of indomethacin on cerebral haemodynamics in very preterm infants. Lancet 1990;335(8704):1491–5.

14. Ment LR, Vohr B, Oh W, Scott DT, Allan WC, Westerveld M, Duncan CC, Ehrenkranz RA, Katz KH, Schneider KC, Makuch RW. Neurodevelopmental outcome at 36 months' corrected age of preterm infants in the Multicenter Indomethacin Intraventricular Hemorrhage Prevention Trial. Pediatrics 1996;98(4 Pt 1):714–8.

15. Couser RJ, Hoekstra RE, Ferrara TB, Wright GB, Cabalka AK, Connett JE. Neurodevelopmental follow-up at 36 months' corrected age of preterm infants treated with prophylactic indomethacin. Arch Pediatr Adolesc Med 2000;154(6):598–602.

16. Beirne J, Jubiz W. Effect of indomethacin on the hypothalamic–pituitary–adrenal axis in man. J Clin Endocrinol Metab 1978;47(4):713–6.

17. Thack JR, Bozeman MT. Indometacin induced hyperglycemia. J Am Acad Dermatol 1982;7:502.

18. Akbarpour F, Afrasiabi A, Vaziri ND. Severe hyperkalemia caused by indomethacin and potassium supplementation. South Med J 1985;78(6):756–7.

19. Ambanelli U, Ferraccioli GF, Serventi G, Vaona GL. Changes in serum and urinary zinc induced by ASA and indomethacin. Scand J Rheumatol 1982;11(1):63–4.

20. Durao V, Prata MM, Goncalves LM. Modification of antihypertensive effect of beta-adrenoceptor-blocking agents by inhibition of endogenous prostaglandin synthesis. Lancet 1977;2(8046):1005–7.

21. Watkins J, Abbott EC, Hensby CN, Webster J, Dollery CT. Attenuation of hypotensive effect of propranolol and thiazide diuretics by indomethacin. BMJ 1980;281(6242):702–5.

22. Menkes E, Kutas GJ. Fatal aplastic anemia following indomethacin ingestion. Can Med Assoc J 1977;117(2):118.

23. Cuthbert MF. Adverse reactions to non-steroidal antirheumatic drugs. Curr Med Res Opin 1974;2(9):600–10.

24. The International Agranulocytosis and Aplastic Anemia Study. Risks of agranulocytosis and aplastic anemia. A first report of their relation to drug use with special reference to analgesics. JAMA 1986;256(13):1749–57.

25. Bengtsson BO, Milstein JM, Sherman MP. Indomethacin-associated neutropenia with subsequent Gram-negative sepsis in a preterm infant. Cause or coincidence? J Perinatol 2006;26(6):381–3.

26. Friedman Z, Whitman V, Maisels MJ, Berman W Jr, Marks KH, Vesell ES. Indomethacin disposition and indomethacin-induced platelet dysfunction in premature infants. J Clin Pharmacol 1978;18(5-6):272–9.

27. Maclaurin BP, Richards DA, Heads D. Indomethacin-associated peptic ulceration. NZ Med J 1978;88(625):439–41.

28. Anonymous. "Osmosin" may not reduce indometacin's side effects. Scrip 1983;82:1.

29. Hooker GD, Gregor JC, Ponich TP, McLarty TD. Diaphragm-like strictures of the right colon induced by indomethacin suppositories: evidence of a systemic effect. Gastrointest Endosc 1996;44(2):199–202.

30. Coutrot S, Roland D, Barbier J, Van Der Marcq P, Alcalay M, Matuchansky C. Acute perforation of colonic diverticula associated with short-term indomethacin. Lancet 1978;2(8098):1055–6.

31. Levy N, Gaspar E. Letter: Rectal bleeding and indomethacin suppositories. Lancet 1975;1(7906):577.

32. Hansen TM, Matzen P, Madsen P. Endoscopic evaluation of the effect of indomethacin capsules and suppositories on the gastric mucosa in rheumatic patients. J Rheumatol 1984;11(4):484–7.

33. Paquette L, Friedlich P, Ramanathan R, Seri I. Concurrent use of indomethacin and dexamethasone increases the risk of spontaneous intestinal perforation in very low birth weight neonates. J Perinatol 2006;26(8):486–9.

34. Memis D, Akalin E, Yücel T. Indomethacin-induced pancreatitis: a case report. JOP 2005;6(4):344–.

35. Mahjoub W, Jarboui S, Ben Moussa M, Abdesselem MM, Zaouche A. Indomethacin-induced pancreatitis. A second case report. JOP 2006;7(3):321–.

36. Fenech FF, Bannister WH, Grech JL. Hepatitis with biliverdinaemia in association with indomethacin therapy. BMJ 1967;3(558):155–6.

37. de Kraker-Sangster M, Bronkhorst FB, Brandt KH, Boersma JW. Massale Levercelnecrose na toediening van indometacine in combinatie met aminofenazon. [Massive liver cell necrosis following administration of indomethacin in combination with aminophenzone.] Ned Tijdschr Geneeskd 1981;125(45):1828–31.

38. Cappell MS, Kozicky O, Competiello LS. Indomethacin-associated cholestasis. J Clin Gastroenterol 1988;10(4):445–7.

39. ter Borg EJ, de Jong PE, Meyer S, van Rijswijk MH, Kallenberg CG. Indomethacin and ibuprofen-induced reversible acute renal failure in a patient with systemic lupus erythematosus. Neth J Med 1987;30(3-4):181–6.

40. ter Borg EJ, de Jong PE, Meijer S, Kallenberg CG. Renal effects of indomethacin in patients with systemic lupus erythematosus. Nephron 1989;53(3):238–43.

41. Fawaz-Estrup F, Ho G Jr. Reversible acute renal failure induced by indomethacin. Arch Intern Med 1981;141(12):1670–1.

42. O'Sullivan M, Hanly JG, Molloy M. A case of toxic epidermal necrolysis secondary to indomethacin. Br J Rheumatol 1983;22(1):47–9.

43. Katayama H, Kawada A. Exacerbation of psoriasis induced by indomethacin. J Dermatol 1981;8(4):323–7.

44. Rubens-Duval A, Villiaumey J, Kaplan G, Bailly D. Surmenage et detérioration rapide de coxo-fémorales arthrosiques au cours de thérapeutiques anti-inflammatoires non corticoides. [Overworking and fast deterioration of arthrosic hips during non-steroid anti-inflammatory treatment.] Rev Rhum Mal Osteoartic 1970;37(8):535–41.

45. Rashad S, Revell P, Hemingway A, Low F, Rainsford K, Walker F. Effect of non-steroidal anti-inflammatory drugs on the course of osteoarthritis. Lancet 1989;2(8662):519–22.

46. Romanowska-Gorecka B, Oleszczak B. Maskukacy wplyw indocydu na przebieg ropnych procesow zapalnych. [Masking effect of indocin on the course of purulent inflammatory processes.] Pol Tyg Lek 1969;24(52):2019–20.

47. Grella P, Zanor P. Premature labor and indomethacin. Prostaglandins 1978;16(6):1007–17.

48. Manchester D, Margolis HS, Sheldon RE. Possible association between maternal indomethacin therapy and primary pulmonary hypertension of the newborn. Am J Obstet Gynecol 1976;126(4):467–9.

49. Levin DL, Fixler DE, Morriss FC, Tyson J. Morphologic analysis of the pulmonary vascular bed in infants exposed in utero to prostaglandin synthetase inhibitors. J Pediatr 1978;92(3):478–83.

50. Moise KJ Jr, Huhta JC, Sharif DS, Ou CN, Kirshon B, Wasserstrum N, Cano L. Indomethacin in the treatment of premature labor. Effects on the fetal ductus arteriosus. N Engl J Med 1988;319(6):327–31.

51. Hendricks SK, Smith JR, Moore DE, Brown ZA. Oligohydramnios associated with prostaglandin synthetase inhibitors in preterm labour. Br J Obstet Gynaecol 1990;97(4):312–6.

52. Schoenfeld A, Freedman S, Hod M, Ovadia Y. Antagonism of antihypertensive drug therapy in pregnancy by indomethacin? Am J Obstet Gynecol 1989;161(5):1204–5.

53. Di Battista C, Laudizi L, Tamborino G. Focomelia ed agenesia del pene in neonato Possible ruolo teratogeno di un farmaco assunto dalla madre in gravidanza. [Phocomelia and agenesis of the penis in a newborn infant. Possible teratogenic role of a drug taken by the mother during pregnancy.] Minerva Pediatr 1975;27(11):675–9.

54. Haddad J, Messer J, Casanova R, Simeoni U, Willard D. Indomethacin and ischemic brain injury in neonates. J Pediatr 1990;116(5):839–40.

55. Baerts W, Fetter WP, Hop WC, Wallenburg HC, Spritzer R, Sauer PJ. Cerebral lesions in preterm infants after tocolytic indomethacin. Dev Med Child Neurol 1990;32(10):910–8.

56. Restaino I, Kaplan BS, Kaplan P, Rosenberg HK, Witzleben C, Roberts N. Renal dysgenesis in a monozygotic twin: association with in utero exposure to indomethacin. Am J Med Genet 1991;39(3):252–7.

57. Norton ME, Merrill J, Cooper BA, Kuller JA, Clyman RI. Neonatal complications after the administration of indomethacin for preterm labor. N Engl J Med 1993;329(22):1602–7.

58. Parilla BV, Grobman WA, Holtzman RB, Thomas HA, Dooley SL. Indomethacin tocolysis and risk of necrotizing enterocolitis. Obstet Gynecol 2000;96(1):120–3.

59. Koren G, Florescu A, Costei AM, Boskovic R, Moretti ME. Nonsteroidal antiinflammatory drugs during third trimester and the risk of premature closure of the ductus arteriosus: a meta-analysis. Ann Pharmacother 2006;40(5):824–.

60. Shehata BM, Bare JB, Denton TD, Habib MN, Black JO. Premature closure of the ductus arteriosus: variable response among monozygotic twins after in utero exposure to indomethacin. Fetal Pediatr Pathol 2006;25(3):151–.

61. Eeg-Olofsson O, Malmros I, Elwin CE, Steen B. Convulsions in a breast-fed infant after maternal indomethacin. Lancet 1978;2(8082):215.

62. Harinck E, van Ertbruggen I, Senders RC, Moulaert AJ. Problems with indomethacin for ductus closure. Lancet 1977;2(8031):245.

63. Merritt TA, Bejar R, Coraza M, et al. Clinical trials of intravenous indometacin for closure of the patent ductus arteriosus. Pediatr Cardiol 1983;4(Suppl 2):71.

64. Tharumaratnam D, Bashford S, Khan SA. Indomethacin induced psychosis. Postgrad Med J 2000;76(901):736–7.

65. Mallet L, Kuyumjian J. Indomethacin-induced behavioral changes in an elderly patient with dementia. Ann Pharmacother 1998;32(2):201–3.

66. Lapane KL, Spooner JJ, Mucha L, Straus WL. Effect of nonsteroidal anti-inflammatory drug use on the rate of gastrointestinal hospitalizations among people living in long-term care. J Am Geriatr Soc 2001;49(5):577–84.

67. Pichon P, Moreau PG. Complications cornéennes par usage de collyre a l'indométacine. [Corneal complications caused by indomethacin eyedrop.] Bull Soc Ophtalmol Fr 1990;90(4):449–51.

68. Young JH, Currie WJ. "Osmosin" in general practice: preliminary report of a double-blind study in the treatment of osteoarthritis. Curr Med Res Opin 1983;8(Suppl 2):99–108.

69. Gallacchi G, Strolz F. Clinical evaluation of "Osmosin" versus piroxicam. Curr Med Res Opin 1983;8(Suppl 2):83–9.

70. Rhymer AR, Sromovsky JA, Dicenta C, Hart CB. "Osmosin": a multi-centre evaluation of a technological advance in the treatment of osteoarthritis. Curr Med Res Opin 1983;8(Suppl 2):62–71.

71. Bobrove AM, Calin A. Efficacy and tolerance of a novel precision-dose formulation of indomethacin: double-blind trials in rheumatoid arthritis and osteoarthritis. Curr Med Res Opin 1983;8(Suppl 2):55–61.

72. Galassi P, Vicentini C, Scapellato F, Laurenti C. L'impiego dell'indometacina e del metamizolo per via endovenosa nella colica renale. [Use of indomethacin and metamizole administered intravenously in renal colic. Comparative study.] Minerva Urol 1983;35(4):295–300.

73. Vincent G, Vincent H. Indocid 50 mg injectable dans la pathologie disco-vertebrale Sem Hop 1986;62:2189.

74. Zarza J. Major bleeding during combined treatment with indomethacin and low doses of acenocoumarol in a homozygous patient for 2C9*3 variant of cytochrome P-450 CYP2C9. Thromb Haemost 2003;90:161–.

75. Chan TY, Lui SF, Chung SY, Luk S, Critchley JA. Adverse interaction between warfarin and indomethacin. Drug Saf 1994;10(3):267–9.

76. Jeremy R, Towson J. Interaction between aspirin and indomethacin in the treatment of rheumatoid arthritis. Med J Aust 1970;2(3):127–9.

77. Allan SG, Knox J, Kerr F. Interaction between diuretics and indomethacin. BMJ (Clin Res Ed) 1981;283(6306):1611.

78. Mor R, Pitlik S, Rosenfeld JB. Indomethacin- and Moduretic–induced hyperkalemia. Isr J Med Sci 1983;19(6):535–7.

79. Mignat C. Clinically significant drug interactions with new immunosuppressive agents. Drug Saf 1997;16(4):267–78.

80. Schimmel MS, Inwood RJ, Eidelman AI, Eylath U. Toxic digitalis levels associated with indomethacin therapy in a neonate. Clin Pediatr (Phila) 1980;19(11):768–9.

81. Finch MB, Kelly JG, Johnston GD, McDevitt DG. Evidence against a digoxin–indomethacin interaction. Br J Clin Pharmacol 1983;16:P212–3.

82. Carlan SJ, Stromquist C, Angel JL, Harris M, O'Brien WF. Cocaine and indomethacin: fetal anuria, neonatal edema, and gastrointestinal bleeding. Obstet Gynecol 1991;78(3 Pt 2):501–3.

83. Olsen ME, Thomsen T, Hassager C, Ibsen H, Dige-Petersen H. Hemodynamic and renal effects of indomethacin in losartan-treated hypertensive individuals. Am J Hypertens 1999;12(2 Pt 1):209–16.

84. Brooks PM, Bell MA, Sturrock RD, Famaey JP, Dick WC. The clinical significance of indomethacin–probenecid interaction. Br J Clin Pharmacol 1974;1:287.

85. Sinclair H, Gibson T. Interaction between probenecid and indomethacin. Br J Rheumatol 1986;25(3):316–7.

86. Baber N, Halliday L, Sibeon R, Littler T, Orme ML. The interaction between indomethacin and probenecid. A clinical and pharmacokinetic study. Clin Pharmacol Ther 1978;24(3):298–307.

Indoprofen

General Information

Indoprofen is one of several NSAIDs that have been withdrawn because of adverse effects. The UK Licensing Authority suspended the product licence on grounds of safety in 1983, and in 1984 the Italian manufacturers decided to withdraw it from the world market. The UK decision was taken because there was a high rate of adverse drug reactions in a voluntary postmarketing surveillance study and the spontaneous adverse reaction reporting system had noted 217 serious adverse effects, mainly gastrointestinal bleeding and perforation. According to the manufacturers, the adverse effects profile in the UK did not emerge in other countries (1). A survey of adverse reactions in 6764 patients, mostly treated for 1 month or less, showed that life-threatening events were rare. A postmarketing surveillance study in 3823 osteoarthritic patients showed that serious adverse reactions were even less frequent (2).

Organs and Systems

Hematologic

The fact that indoprofen prolongs bleeding time and reduces platelet aggregation could result in indirect interactions with anticoagulants (3).

Gastrointestinal

When the UK Licensing Authority suspended the product licence the spontaneous adverse reaction reporting system had received 217 reports of serious adverse effects, mainly gastrointestinal bleeding and perforation.

Death

There were 46 deaths associated with indoprofen in three countries (UK 34, Italy 7, Germany 5), but only 11 were judged to be probably or possibly drug-related. Nine of these deaths were caused by gastrointestinal reactions.

Long-Term Effects

Tumorigenicity

The manufacturers' ultimate reason for worldwide withdrawal was the finding of carcinogenicity in long-term animal studies. To what extent the clinical events actually played a role in their decision is not clear.

References

1. Anonymous. Flosin hearing. Scrip 1984;883:14.
2. Emanueli A, Caso P, Gualtieri S, et al. Postmarketing surveillance of indoprofen. In: Proceedings, Scientific Symposium on Indoprofen in Inflammatory and Painful Conditions, Venice 1982:95.
3. Jacono A, Caso P, Gualtieri S, Raucci D, Bianchi A, Vigorito C, Bergamini N, Iadevaia V. Clinical study of

possible interactions between indoprofen and oral anticoagulants. Eur J Rheumatol Inflamm 1981;4(1):32–5.

Isoxicam

General Information

The oxicam NSAID isoxicam has a shorter half-life (30 hours) than piroxicam. However, there are large variations in half-life, clearance, and mean steady-state plasma concentrations. Except for edema, the incidence of adverse effects is unrelated to age (1).

Isoxicam was withdrawn from the market following a higher than expected number of cases of Stevens–Johnson syndrome and toxic epidermal necrolysis (SEDA-10, 88).

Organs and Systems

Gastrointestinal

The main adverse effects of isoxicam are gastrointestinal (pain, dyspepsia, nausea, vomiting, stomatitis, constipation, and occasionally peptic ulcer), which occur in up to 80% of patients.

Skin

Serious skin reactions (Stevens–Johnson syndrome and Lyell's syndrome) caused temporary withdrawal of isoxicam in several countries, even though an analysis of 1800 patients with rheumatoid arthritis or degenerative joint disease failed to confirm an increased risk (2).

References

1. Haslock I. Tolerance of isoxicam with respect to age. In: Amor B, editor. Non-steroidal Anti-inflammatory Agents in the Elderly. Basel: Eular, 1984:114.
2. Burch FX. Evaluation of the safety of isoxicam. Am J Med 1985;79(4B):28–32.

Kebuzone

General Information

Kebuzone is an NSAID that is related to phenylbutazone. Allergic reactions, gastrotoxicity, nephrotoxicity, local reactions with necrosis (1), and liver damage have been reported (SED-11, 176; 2). The Japanese authorities have asked that the package insert should indicate that this drug must be used only as a last resort when other anti-inflammatory agents and uricosuric drugs are ineffective (SEDA-12, 83).

Organs and Systems

Liver

In 20 cases of kebuzone-induced liver damage, biopsy showed hepatocellular damage with or without cholestasis, reactive hepatitis, or cholangiolitis (3). There was hepatitis with central lobular necrosis in one case. In five patients, a lymphocyte proliferation test was positive.

Skin

Nicolau syndrome (embolia cutis medicamentosa) is a very rare complication of intramuscular injections, in which there is extensive necrosis of the injected skin area, perhaps due to accidental intra-arterial and/or para-arterial injection; it usually occurs in children (4). Nicolau syndrome has been reported in three patients who had received intramuscular injections of kebuzone (5).

References

1. Capusan I, Moise IG, Maier N. Nicolaus syndrome following intramuscular injections of ketophenylbutazone (Ketazon). Dermatol Venereol 1976;21:205.
2. Porst H, Roschlau G, Schentke U, Weise L. Leberschäden durch Ketophenylbutazone (Ketazon). Dtsch Gesundheitsw 1978;33:1181.
3. Kunze KD, Porst H, Tschopel L. Morphologie und Pathogenese von Leberschäden durch Dihydralazin, Propranolol und Ketophenylbutazon. [Morphology and pathogenesis of liver injury produced by dihydralazine, propranolol and ketophenylbutazone.] Zentralbl Allg Pathol 1985;130(6):509–18.
4. Saputo V, Bruni G. La sindrome di Nicolau da preparati di penicillina: analisi della letteratura alla ricerca di potenziali fattori di rischio. [Nicolau syndrome caused by penicillin preparations: review of the literature in search for potential risk factors.] Pediatr Med Chir 1998;20(2):105–23.
5. Varga L, Asztalos L. Nicolau-szindroma ketazon injekcio utan. [Nicolau syndrome after ketazon injection.] Orv Hetil 1990;131(21):1143–6.

Ketoprofen

General Information

The spectrum of adverse effects of ketoprofen is similar to that of ibuprofen.

Ketoprofen was originally approved for over-the-counter sales in the USA by the FDA, but in the same year, in Italy, the Ministry of Health transferred two ketoprofen-containing products from non-prescription to prescription status (SEDA-20, 93). The reasons for this difference are not clear.

Organs and Systems

Respiratory

A fatal asthmatic reaction has been described (1), and severe bronchospasm with respiratory and cardiac arrest has been reported in a young man with a history of mild asthma after he took ketoprofen (2). Topical application can provoke asthma in predisposed subjects (3).

Even topical formulations of NSAIDs should be avoided in patients with a history of analgesic-induced asthma (4).

- A 74-year-old woman with a history of sinusitis, nasal polyps, and analgesic-induced asthma had a sudden life-threatening attack of asthma 2 hours after the application of a 2% ketoprofen adhesive tape. Asthma had not previously occurred when she had used a 0.3% ketoprofen adhesive patch.

Nervous system

Retention of salt and water, sometimes with reversible pseudotumor cerebri, can occur with ketoprofen (5).

Gastrointestinal

The overall frequency of adverse reactions was 15–50% in different trials; gastrotoxicity predominated, at a frequency of 6.5–42% (6–8), even after rectal administration. In some epidemiological studies, ketoprofen in prescription doses was more gastrotoxic than other NSAIDs (SEDA-18, 99).

There are very few data on the gastrointestinal toxicity of over-the-counter doses of ketoprofen. In an endoscopic short-term study in healthy subjects ketoprofen was associated with significant gastrointestinal toxicity (9). Another endoscopic study showed that the R-enantiomer of ketoprofen has less gastrointestinal toxicity than the racemic mixture or the S-enantiomer while retaining good analgesic activity (SEDA-22, 116).

Local symptoms, including rectal bleeding, can accompany treatment with ketoprofen suppositories (8.3% of patients) (6).

Liver

Hepatotoxicity has rarely been reported with ketoprofen (SEDA-17, 110).

Urinary tract

Like many other NSAIDs, ketoprofen can cause acute interstitial nephritis (10). Renal insufficiency and the nephrotic syndrome due to membranous glomerulonephritis (an unusual cause of NSAID-induced nephrotic syndrome) have been described in an elderly patient taking long-term ketoprofen (SEDA-12, 86).

As topical NSAIDs can be absorbed via the skin, they cannot be considered safe in high-risk patients, in whom all NSAIDs are contraindicated.

- A 62-year-old woman developed acute renal insufficiency after using topical ketoprofen for 5 days (11). She had several predisposing factors to NSAID-induced acute renal insufficiency, such as advanced age, chronic renal impairment due to polycystic kidney disease, and treatment with an ACE inhibitor and furosemide.

Ketoprofen use has been followed by red discoloration of urine (SEDA-16, 110).

Skin

Topical ketoprofen can cause contact dermatitis and photodermatitis, like other NSAIDs (SEDA-18, 104; SEDA-22, 116). Data from Sweden have confirmed the photosensitizing potential of topical gel formulations of ketoprofen and have included a number of reports of contact dermatitis (12). In some cases ketoprofen can be responsible for very prolonged photosensitivity after only a single application (13).

The allergenic potential of different topical NSAIDs has been determined in a retrospective observational study (14). There were 139 contact reactions, and ketoprofen was responsible for 28% of cases of allergy and 82% of cases of contact photoallergy, although it was only the third most commonly used topical NSAID, diclofenac being the first. The reporting odds ratio for ketoprofen was 3.9 (2.4, 6.4) and the proportional reporting ratio was 3.4 (2.1, 5.5), confirming the possibility of a signal.

Toxic epidermal necrolysis has been described with ketoprofen (SEDA-21, 105).

Drug Administration

Drug administration route

Studies on a modified-release formulation of ketoprofen showed a similar pattern of adverse effects to the usual formulations (SEDA-12, 86).

An injectable form of ketoprofen has acceptable tolerability (6,7), but about 4.5% of patients have local reactions.

Drug overdose

A 64-year-old woman had auditory and visual hallucinations, persecutory delusions, and slurred speech after she took an overdose of ketoprofen; her psychiatric symptoms resolved within 48 hours (15).

Drug–Drug Interactions

Aspirin

Concurrent administration of aspirin reduces ketoprofen protein binding and increases its clearance. Salicylate also reduces the metabolic conversion of ketoprofen to its conjugates and their renal elimination, and enhances its conversion to non-conjugated metabolites (16).

Co-triamterzide

Irreversible renal insufficiency has been reported in an elderly patient who took ketoprofen in combination with co-triamterzide   (triamterene + hydrochlorothiazide) (17). The interaction with triamterene is well documented (SEDA-12, 80) and co-administration with ketoprofen has proved dangerous.

Warfarin

Although data from healthy subjects indicate no interaction of ketoprofen with warfarin, severe gastrointestinal bleeding and a prolonged prothrombin time have been attributed to this combination (SEDA-13, 81).

References

1. Egede F. Fatal asthmatic reaction following ketoprofen (Orudis) (Alreumat). [A fatal asthmatic reaction following ketoprofen (Alreumat), (Orudis).] Ugeskr Laeger 1979;141(17):1151–2.
2. Schreuder G. Ketoprofen: possible idiosyncratic acute bronchospasm. Med J Aust 1990;152(6):332–3.
3. Miyairi A, Ohori K. Aspirin-induced asthma due to rubbing ketoprofen ointment. Kokyu 1990;9:110.
4. Kashiwabara K, Nakamura H. Analgesic-induced asthma caused by 2.0% ketoprofen adhesive agents, but not by 0.3% agents Intern Med 2001;40(2):124–6.
5. Larizza D, Colombo A, Lorini R, Severi F. Ketoprofen causing pseudotumor cerebri in Bartter's syndrome. N Engl J Med 1979;300(14):796.
6. Tamisier JN. Ketoprofen. Clin Rheum Dis 1979;5:381.
7. Gougeon J, Mireau-Hottin J, Gaillard F. Clinical trial of the injectable form of ketoprofen. Rheumatol Rehabil 1976;(Suppl):75–8.
8. Willans MJ, Digby JW, Topp JR, et al. Long term treatment of arthritis disease with ketoprofen (Orudis): a Canadian multicentre evaluation. Curr Ther Res 1979;25:35.
9. Lanza FL, Codispoti JR, Nelson EB. An endoscopic comparison of gastroduodenal injury with over-the-counter doses of ketoprofen and acetaminophen. Am J Gastroenterol 1998;93(7):1051–4.
10. Ducret F, Pointet P, Martin D, Villermet B. Insuffisance rénale aiguë réversible induite par le kétoprofene. [Acute reversible renal insufficiency induced by ketoprofen.] Nephrologie 1982;3(2):105–6.
11. Krummel T, Dimitrov Y, Moulin B, Hannedouche T. Drug points: Acute renal failure induced by topical ketoprofen. BMJ 2000;320(7227):93.
12. Swedish Adverse Drug Reactions Advisory Committee. Ketoprofen gel—contact dermatitis and photosensitivity. SADRAC Bull 1998;67:2.
13. Offidani A, Cellini A, Amerio P, Simonetti O, Bossi G. A case of persistent light reaction phenomenon to ketoprofen? Eur J Dermatol 2000;10(2):153–4.
14. Diaz RL, Gardeazabal J, Manrique P, Ratón JA, Urrutia I, Rodríguez-Sasiain JM, Aguirre C. Greater allergenicity of topical ketoprofen in contact dermatitis confirmed by use. Contact Dermatitis 2006;54(5):239–4.
15. Tavcar R, Dernovsek MZ, Brosch S. Ketoprofen intoxication delirium. J Clin Psychopharmacol 1999;19(1):95–6.
16. Williams RL, Upton RA, Buskin JN, Jones RM. Ketoprofen–aspirin interactions. Clin Pharmacol Ther 1981;30(2):226–31.
17. Pazmino PA, Pazmino PB. Ketoprofen-induced irreversible renal failure. Nephron 1988;50(1):70–1.

Ketorolac

General Information

Ketorolac is, like several other NSAIDs, promoted as a non-narcotic analgesic. This is merely a marketing ploy, which does not reflect any special characteristics, except that it is one of many NSAIDs that can be given parenterally. A pyrrolizine carboxylic acid derivative, it is structurally and pharmacologically related to tolmetin, zomepirac, and indometacin. The trometamol salt of ketorolac enhances its solubility and allows parenteral administration; single intramuscular injections are better tolerated than morphine.

Opinions on the safety of ketorolac in EC drug regulatory authorities are conflicting (SEDA-18, 104) (1). However, the risk of adverse effects is higher when ketorolac is used in higher doses, in elderly subjects, and for more than 5 days (SEDA-21, 105).

Other information on the benefit-to-harm balance of parenteral ketorolac tromethamine as a postoperative analgesic has been provided by three studies (SEDA-21, 105). The overall risk of gastrointestinal and operative site bleeding and acute renal insufficiency associated with parenteral ketorolac and a parenteral opiate were relatively small.

The most commonly reported symptoms are somnolence, headache, dizziness, nausea, dyspepsia, and abdominal pain. Edema, hyperkalemia, diarrhea, sweating, self-limiting wheezing, and itching have also been reported occasionally (SEDA-12, 86; SEDA-16, 110; SEDA-17, 111).

There are contrasting data on the benefit-to-harm balance of parenteral ketorolac as an analgesic (SEDA-21, 105). This prompted regulatory review of ketorolac in many countries, leading to revision of labelling, dosage recommendations, and prescribing practices. The use of ketorolac should be limited in dosage and duration; in elderly patients it should probably not be used at all. It is important for prescribers to understand that increasing the dosage of ketorolac beyond the label recommendations (60–120 mg/day for a maximum of 2–5 days) will not provide better efficacy, but will increase the risk of serious adverse reactions (2).

Organs and Systems

Sensory systems

Reversible hearing loss with tinnitus and headache were described in a woman with a predisposition to ototoxicity in end-stage renal disease (SEDA-21, 106).

Hematologic

Ketorolac prolongs bleeding time reversibly. The clinical significance of the effect of ketorolac on hemostasis in perioperative use is still imperfectly understood. Serious bleeding, either at the operative site or in the gastrointestinal tract after perioperative administration of ketorolac, has been documented in several reports (SEDA-18, 105) and in controlled studies (SEDA-20, 93).

Concomitant use of anticoagulants increases the risk of bleeding (SEDA-18, 105).

Gastrointestinal

Gastric lesions (endoscopically demonstrated erosions, ulcers, and giant duodenal or gastric ulcers) have been described in healthy volunteers (SEDA-14, 94) and patients (SEDA-18, 105) treated with parenteral ketorolac (SEDA-14, 94); gastric damage is dose-related (SEDA-17, 112). A case-control study on hospitalization for upper gastrointestinal tract bleeding and/or perforation provided further evidence of the unfavorable benefit-to-harm balance of ketorolac compared with other NSAIDs. Ketorolac was five times more gastrotoxic than all other NSAIDs. The relative risk with intramuscular ketorolac was higher than with oral ketorolac (SEDA-22, 117).

Further evidence of the unfavorable benefit-to-harm balance of ketorolac compared with other NSAIDs has been provided by another case-control study on first-time hospitalization for gastroduodenal ulcer (documented by endoscopy, radiology, surgery, or autopsy), with or without bleeding or perforation. Of all the NSAIDs used in outpatients the highest rate ratio for lesions of any degree of severity was seen with piroxicam (4.6; 95% CI = 1.4, 8.3); ketorolac ranked second highest (3.4; 95% CI = 1.4, 8.3). For patients who suffered hemorrhage or perforation, the highest rate ratio observed was for ketorolac (5.9; 95% CI = 2.1, 16) (3).

Colonic ulceration with massive bleeding has been reported in a woman who received ketorolac intramuscularly (SEDA-21, 106).

Urinary tract

There have been several reports of impaired renal function in patients taking ketorolac (SEDA-17, 112; SEDA-18, 105; SEDA-22, 117). The severity varies from slight to severe forms of renal insufficiency, which may even occur after a single dose of 30 mg. Because recent major surgery is considered a risk factor for renal insufficiency, particularly in elderly patients, the use of ketorolac, or other NSAIDs, for postoperative pain management is warranted only in carefully selected patients. Furthermore, a case report confirmed that oral ketorolac can cause acute renal insufficiency in young subjects without any predisposing factors (SEDA-21, 106).

Immunologic

Anaphylaxis and anaphylactoid reactions have been reported (SEDA-17, 112).

Second-Generation Effects

Pregnancy

As ketorolac crosses the placental barrier, it should not be used in pregnant women. When it is given to mothers during labor, it significantly inhibits platelet aggregation in the neonate (SEDA-14, 94).

Susceptibility Factors

Children undergoing tonsillectomy had a significant increase in the risk of major postoperative hemorrhage without beneficial effects, compared with opioid analgesics (SEDA-21, 106).

Several reports have documented the high risk of ketorolac in patients with a history of asthma, nasal polyposis, and sensitivity to aspirin or any other NSAID (SEDA-18, 105). Exacerbation of chronic asthma has been reported after the use of ketorolac eye-drops (SEDA-21, 106).

Drug–Drug Interactions

Lithium

Reports of lithium neurotoxicity resulting from an interaction with ketorolac have been published (SEDA-22, 117) (4).

In a pharmacokinetic study in healthy volunteers ketorolac increased the concentration of lithium in both serum and erythrocytes, which may reflect concentration of the drug in the nervous system more accurately. Ketorolac can therefore increase the risk of adverse reactions of lithium (5), as do many other NSAIDs.

Sevoflurane

Ketorolac, which can cause renal vasoconstriction by inhibiting cyclo-oxygenase, is often given to patients anesthetized with sevoflurane, which is also potentially nephrotoxic. The effect of ketorolac has been assessed in a placebo-controlled, randomized study in 30 women undergoing breast surgery with sevoflurane anesthesia (6). There were no differences in several markers of renal injury in those who did or did not receive ketorolac.

References

1. Lewis S. Ketorolac in Europe. Lancet 1994;343:784.
2. Reinhart DI. Minimising the adverse effects of ketorolac. Drug Saf 2000;22(6):487–97.
3. Menniti-Ippolito F, Maggini M, Raschetti R, Da Cas R, Traversa G, Walker AM. Ketorolac use in outpatients and gastrointestinal hospitalization: a comparison with other non-steroidal anti-inflammatory drugs in Italy. Eur J Clin Pharmacol 1998;54(5):393–7.
4. Iyer V. Ketorolac (Toradol) induced lithium toxicity. Headache 1994;34(7):442–4.
5. Cold JA, ZumBrunnen TL, Simpson MA, Augustin BG, Awad E, Jann MW. Increased lithium serum and red blood cell concentrations during ketorolac coadministration. J Clin Psychopharmacol 1998;18(1):33–7.
6. Laisalmi M, Eriksson H, Koivusalo AM, Pere P, Rosenberg P, Lindgren L. Ketorolac is not nephrotoxic in connection with sevoflurane anesthesia in patients undergoing breast surgery. Anesth Analg 2001;92(4):1058–63.

Lonazolac

General Information

Lonazolac, an arylacetic acid derivative, causes adverse effects like those of other NSAIDs. Gastrointestinal disturbances are followed in frequency by nervous system and skin reactions. The extent of gastro-intestinal blood loss is similar to that with diclofenac (1). Cholestatic hepatitis has also been reported (SEDA-8, 106).

Reference

1. Uthgenannt H, Arent H. Uber den Einfluss von 3-(4-Chlorphenyl-) 1-phenyl-1H-pyrazol-4-Essigsäure (Lonazolac-Ca), Diclofenac-Na und Indometacin auf die gastrointestinale Blutausscheidung. [Effect of 3-(4-chlorphenyl-) 1-phenyl-1H-pyrazole-4-acetic acid (lonazolac-Ca), diclofenac-Na and indomethacin on the gastrointestinal blood loss.] Wien Klin Wochenschr 1982;94(13):345–9.

Lornoxicam

General Information

Data are insufficient to indicate whether the oxicam NSAID lornoxicam is safer for the gastrointestinal tract than other oxicam derivatives (SEDA-16, 113). Headache, dizziness, and gastrointestinal symptoms are the most frequent adverse effects; clinically significant gastrointestinal events include upper gastrointestinal ulceration, with or without hemorrhage or perforation (SEDA-20, 94; SEDA-21, 107). The profile of drug interactions is similar to the profiles of other NSAIDs (SEDA-21, 108).

Organs and Systems

Gastrointestinal

Multiple small hemispheric polyps, associated with luminal narrowing, were found in the gastric antrum of a 74-year-old man who had taken lornoxicam (1). The polyps consisted of granulation tissue and immature regenerative epithelium. The authors suggested that in the hypoacidic conditions induced by nizatidine, inflammatory polyps could have arisen through rapid and excessive regeneration after gastric mucosal injury due to the NSAID. However, there was no evidence in this case of a cause-and-effect relation.

Susceptibility Factors

Genetic

Lornoxicam 8 mg bd for 2 weeks was well tolerated by subject with the Mediterranean form of G6PD deficiency (2).

Drug–Drug Interactions

Phenprocoumon

Lornoxicam altered the pharmacokinetics of the more potent *S*-isomer of phenprocoumon and to a lesser extent *R*-phenprocoumon, with a reduction in factor II and VII activity (3). In contrast, at the upper limit of the recommended doses lornoxicam did not alter the pharmacokinetics of *R*-acenocoumarol or the anticoagulant activity of acenocoumarol (4).

Warfarin

Lornoxicam increased the mean serum concentration of racemic warfarin and correspondingly increased its anticoagulant effect (5).

References

1. Hizawa K, Takeya T, Yao T, Yamamoto H, Aomi H, Nakahara T, Matsumoto T, Iida M. Gastric inflammatory polyposis after long term intermittent use of nonsteroidal anti-inflammatory drugs and histamine 2 receptor antagonists. Endoscopy 2005;37:685.
2. Perpignano G, Cacace E, Matulli C, Ruggiero V. Sicurezza terapeutica di lornoxicam in sogetti G-6-PDH carenti. Reumatismo 2003;55:45–7.
3. Masche UP, Rentsch KM, von Felten A, Meier PJ, Fattinger KE. Opposite effects of lornoxicam co-administration on phenprocoumon pharmacokinetics and pharmacodynamics. Eur J Clin Pharmacol 1999;54(11):857–64.
4. Masche UP, Rentsch KM, von Felten A, Meier PJ, Fattinger KE. No clinically relevant effect of lornoxicam intake on acenocoumarol pharmacokinetics and pharmacodynamics. Eur J Clin Pharmacol 1999;54(11):865–8.
5. Ravic M, Johnston A, Turner P, Ferber HP. A study of the interaction between lornoxicam and warfarin in healthy volunteers. Hum Exp Toxicol 1990;9(6):413–4.

Loxoprofen

General Information

Data on the safety of loxoprofen are based on an open, multicenter trial of about 4000 elderly patients in Japan (SEDA-17, 112). Adverse effects were mainly gastrointestinal, but other adverse effects, common to every NSAID, included edema, dizziness, skin rashes, pruritus, and a case of eosinophilic pneumonia and liver dysfunction (SEDA-17, 112).

Organs and Systems

Respiratory

A fatal asthmatic attack occurred in a young man with a history of asthma and nasal polyps who took loxoprofen (SEDA-18, 105).

Gastrointestinal

In a retrospective study of NSAID-induced colonic ulceration related to NSAID therapy, five of 14 patients were taking loxoprofen (1). However, this finding does not prove that loxoprofen is more ulcerogenic than other NSAIDs.

Liver

The Japanese Health Authority has tightened the hepatic warnings for loxoprofen after eight reports of serious hepatic adverse events since 1997, including two deaths (2).

Immunologic

Three cases of a type-I hypersensitivity reaction to loxoprofen, characterized by generalized urticarial rash and dyspnea, have been reported (3,4).

Drug–Drug Interactions

ACE inihibitors

Loss of consciousness due to marked bradycardia caused by severe hyperkalemia has been described in an 85-year-old woman who took loxoprofen for several days and long-term imidapril, an ACE inhibitor. The combination of an NSAID with an ACE inhibitor can produce serious adverse effects in high-risk patients (5).

References

1. Kurahara K, Matsumoto T, Iida M, Honda K, Yao T, Fujishima M. Clinical and endoscopic features of nonsteroidal anti-inflammatory drug-induced colonic ulcerations. Am J Gastroenterol 2001;96(2):473–80.
2. Anonymous. Loxoprofen hepatic warning tightened in Japan. Scrip 2000;24:2544.
3. Maeda K, Anan S, Akaboshi Y, Yoshida H. A case of urticarial drug eruption from loxoprofen sodium (Loxonin). Skin Res 1988;30(Suppl 4):44.
4. Nagaoka K, Ozaki S, Chinen Y, et al. Clinical effects of loxonin in patients of rheumatoid arthritis. Jpn Arch Intern Med 1989;36:65.
5. Kurahara K, Matsumoto T, Iida M, Honda K, Yao T, Fujishima M. Clinical and endoscopic features of nonsteroidal anti-inflammatory drug-induced colonic ulcerations. Am J Gastroenterol 2001;96(2):473–80.

Mefenamic acid

General Information

The NSAID mefenamic acid is an anthranilic acid derivative. It has been argued for more than a decade that, since there is a wide range of effective and less toxic drugs, there is no reason for continuing to prescribe mefenamic acid and related drugs (SEDA-5, 93). All the same, some of the figures have been disputed, and, strictly speaking, a comparative controlled study to estimate the incidence of the adverse effects of mefenamic acid is still needed. The main reasons for concern are particular effects that are unexpected of an NSAID, such as hemolytic anemia, and which may therefore take the user by surprise.

Organs and Systems

Nervous system

Epileptic seizures in overdosed patients may indicate a degree of nervous system toxicity. Convulsions in poisoned patients are reported to be more likely with mefenamic acid than with other compounds (1). Other nervous system reactions (such as headache) are less frequent than with the arylcarboxylic acid derivatives. Coma has also been described as a consequence of mefenamic acid overdosage (2).

Sensory systems

Hyperacusia, vertigo, and tinnitus have been described in one patient (SEDA-12, 90).

Hematologic

Several hematological disturbances have been reported, although their overall incidence is probably moderate. They include Coombs' positive hemolytic autoimmune anemia, leukopenia, thrombocytopenia, and agranulocytosis (SED-8, 223; SEDA-4, 68; 3–5). Neutropenic reactions have also been described (6). Severe neutropenia developed simultaneously with non-oliguric renal insufficiency in two elderly hypothyroid women (7).

Gastrointestinal

Gastrotoxicity due to mefenamic acid is marked. Other than the common adverse effects (nausea, anorexia, vomiting, pain, diarrhea), acute peptic ulcer, intestinal hemorrhage, hematemesis, abdominal distension, and profuse steatorrhea (SEDA-2, 97) have been reported. Mefenamic acid, unlike other NSAIDs, can provoke enteritis and colitis in patients with no known predisposing factors (8). It accelerates bowel transit in healthy volunteers (SEDA-16, 112).

Esophageal injury is a rare adverse effect of NSAIDs. The published evidence comprises only a few specific studies and a small number of single case reports regarding various NSAIDs (SEDA-15, 92). A report of esophageal ulceration associated with mefenamic acid capsules has been published (9).

- Five days before he presented with esophageal ulceration, a 35-year-old man took two capsules of mefenamic acid (total dose 500 mg) in bed with a small amount of water. The following morning he noted severe retrosternal pain, which persisted until he was seen 4 days later. Endoscopy showed a 3 cm esophageal ulcer near the aortic arch. Within a few days there was complete resolution of ulceration.

All NSAIDs should be taken while standing or sitting, rather than lying, and with about 200 ml of water.

Pancreas

Pancreatitis has been attributed to mefenamic acid (10).

Urinary tract

Mefenamic acid and other anthranilic acid derivatives are nephrotoxic. Many renal effects have been demonstrated in animals. Acute renal insufficiency, renal papillary necrosis, and non-oliguric renal insufficiency have been reported in man (11,12). Renal biopsies in renal insufficiency have shown interstitial nephritis, mesangial proliferation, and focal pedicle fusion, previously undescribed (13).

Skin

Fixed drug eruption has been described in two patients within hours of taking mefenamic acid (SEDA-12, 90). In another case, a multifocal fixed drug eruption mimicked erythema multiforme (14).

Pseudoporphyria is an infrequent adverse effect of some NSAIDs, including naproxen (SEDA-12, 87), nabumetone (SEDA-16, 111), and oxaprozin (SEDA-21, 106).

- A 22-year-old woman developed pseudoporphyria during long-term treatment with mefenamic acid for menstrual problems. After withdrawal of mefenamic acid, the skin lesions gradually disappeared, and at follow-up after 18 months she did not have any skin lesions and had minimal residual scarring (15).
- An unusual skin reaction characterized by widespread pruritic papules and nodules occurred in a 62-year-old woman who had taken long-term mefenamic acid for arthritis. The histological findings were consistent with dermatitis herpetiformis, whereas direct immunofluorescence was suggestive of atypical bullous pemphigoid or linear IgA disease. The skin eruption responded to dapsone, but an increase in the dosage of mefenamic acid caused diarrhea and steatorrhea with IgA antigliadin antibodies. A lymphocyte stimulation test with mefenamic acid was positive. Mefenamic acid was withdrawn and all her symptoms disappeared within 2 weeks (16).

Sexual function

Although mefenamic acid can be used to relieve dysmenorrhea, it can delay menstruation for several days (17).

Immunologic

Asthma and anaphylactic shock are the most dangerous acute hypersensitivity reactions. There is cross-sensitivity with other NSAIDs (18). Rash, urticaria, and pruritus accompany more serious reactions.

Susceptibility Factors

Age

The dosage of mefenamic acid that is used in preterm infants to induce closure of patent ductus arteriosus must not exceed 2 mg/kg/day in three divided doses, to avoid the danger of renal insufficiency (SEDA-19, 97). The promotion of mefenamic acid in Pakistan for fever in children, as a drug of "unsurpassed efficacy compared to [paracetamol] in fever control" and "better tolerance", has been criticized by the Medical Lobby for Appropriate Marketing. In fact, there have been no controlled comparisons of mefenamic acid with a reference drug or placebo, and its safety and efficacy have not been established in children (SEDA-19, 97).

Drug Administration

Drug overdose

Mefenamic acid overdosage is characterized by nervous system symptoms, such as generalized seizures, agitation, and confusion, sometimes progressing to coma, gastrointestinal problems (bloody diarrhea, abdominal pain, and vomiting), and renal impairment (SEDA-13, 83; SEDA-14, 95; 19).

Drug–Drug Interactions

Lithium

Mefenamic acid may have interacted with lithium in a patient with reduced renal function, causing acute symptoms of lithium toxicity (SEDA-13, 83; 20).

References

1. Prescott LF, Balali-Mood M, Critchley JA, Proudfoot AT. Avoidance of mefenamic acid in epilepsy. Lancet 1981;2(8243):418.
2. Gossinger H, Hruby K, Haubenstock A, Jung M, Zwerina N. Coma in mefenamic acid poisoning. Lancet 1982;2(8294):384.
3. Scott GL, Myles AB, Bacon PA. Autoimmune haemolytic anaemia and mefenamic acid therapy. BMJ 1968;3(617):534–5.
4. Farid NR, Johnson RJ, Low WT. Haemolytic reaction to mefenamic acid. Lancet 1971;2:382.
5. Robertson JH, Kennedy CC, Hill CM. Haemolytic anaemia associated with mefenamic acid. Ir J Med Sci 1971;140(5):226–9.
6. Euler HH, Kleine L, Herrlinger JD. Neutropenie unter Mefenaminsäure. [Neutropenia induced by mephenaminic acid.] Dtsch Med Wochenschr 1980;105(34):1192–3.
7. Handa SI, Freestone S. Mefenamic acid-induced neutropenia and renal failure in elderly females with hypothyroidism. Postgrad Med J 1990;66(777):557–9.
8. Phillips MS, Fehilly B, Stewart S, et al. Enteritis and colitis associated with mefenamic acid. BMJ (Clin Res Ed) 1983;287(6405):1626–7.
9. Katsinelos P, Dimiropoulos S, Vasiliadis T, Fotiadis G, Xiarchos P, Eugenidis N. Oesophageal ulceration associated with ingestion of mefenamic acid capsules. Eur J Gastroenterol Hepatol 1999;11(12):1431–2.
10. VanWalraven AA, Edels M, Fong S. Pancreatitis caused by mefenamic acid. Can Med Assoc J 1982;126(8):894.
11. Robertson CE, Ford MJ, Van Someren V, Dlugolecka M, Prescott LF. Mefenamic acid nephropathy. Lancet 1980;2(8188):232–3.
12. Woods KL, Michael J. Mefenamic acid nephropathy. BMJ (Clin Res Ed) 1981;282(6274):1471.
13. Jenkins DA, Harrison DJ, MacDonald MK, Winney RJ. Mefenamic acid nephropathy: an interstitial and mesangial lesion. Nephrol Dial Transplant 1988;3(2):217–20.
14. Sowden JM, Smith AG. Multifocal fixed drug eruption mimicking erythema multiforme. Clin Exp Dermatol 1990;15(5):387–8.
15. O'Hagan AH, Irvine AD, Allen GE, Walsh M. Pseudoporphyria induced by mefenamic acid. Br J Dermatol 1998;139(6):1131–2.
16. Gerbig AW, Paredes B, Hunziker T. Multiple IgA autoantibodies associated with mefenamic acid. Ann Intern Med 1998;129(7):588–9.
17. Halbert DR. Menstrual delay and dysfunctional uterine bleeding associated with antiprostaglandin therapy for dysmenorrhea. J Reprod Med 1983;28(9):592–4.
18. Szczeklik A, Gryglewski RJ, Czerniawska-Mysik G. Participation of prostaglandins in pathogenesis of aspirin-sensitive asthma. Naunyn Schmiedebergs Arch Pharmacol 1977;297(Suppl 1):S99–S110.
19. Meredith TJ, Vale JA. Non-narcotic analgesics. Problems of overdosage. Drugs 1986;32(Suppl 4):177–205.
20. Danion JM, Schmidt M, Welsch M, Imbs JL, Singer L. Interaction entre les anti-inflammatoires non steroidiens et les sels de lithium. [Interaction between non-steroidal anti-inflammatory agents and lithium salts.] Encephale 1987;13(4):255–60.

Meloxicam

General Information

Meloxicam, a COX-2 inhibitor, has been marketed in some countries and promoted as having an improved safety profile over current NSAIDs. It has a long half-life, is highly protein-bound, is metabolized to inactive compounds, and is excreted in the urine and feces. Neither hepatic insufficiency nor moderate renal dysfunction affects its pharmacokinetics, but in one study meloxicam plasma concentrations were 26% higher in patients over 65 than in younger patients.

Changes have been made to the Summary of Product Characteristics by the manufacturers of meloxicam (1), in agreement with the type of adverse drug reaction reports received by the Committee on Safety of Medicine in the UK. Warnings about gastrointestinal reactions (perforation, ulceration, and/or bleeding) and skin reactions (including erythema multiforme and Stevens–Johnson syndrome) have been strengthened (2).

Organs and Systems

Cardiovascular

The NSAIDs in Unstable Angina Treatment-2 (NUT-2) pilot study, which compared meloxicam (15 mg/day until 30 days after discharge) with aspirin plus heparin in 120 patients who had a non-ST segment elevation acute coronary syndrome, showed that patients who took meloxicam had a significant reduction in the primary composite outcome of recurrent angina, myocardial infarction, or death during their stay in the coronary care unit (3): the relative risk reduction was 61% (95% CI=23, 80). Larger trials are required to confirm the findings of this pilot study.

Respiratory

Meloxicam can be added to the long list of drugs that can cause eosinophilic pneumonia, albeit rarely.

- A 23-year-old man developed pulmonary infiltrates in both lungs and an eosinophilia after taking meloxicam 7.5 mg/day for 4 days for shoulder pain (4).

In 21 subjects with asthma and/or nasal polyps and intolerance of oral aspirin (rhinitis + bronchospasm in 13, isolated rhinitis in three, and extrabronchial reactions in five), meloxicam, cumulative dose 7.5 mg, caused a reaction in only one in a single-blind, placebo-controlled challenge (5).

Nervous system

About 7% of patients have dizziness and headache (6).

Gastrointestinal

Gastrointestinal adverse effects were the most frequently reported (in about 15–20% of patients), but their incidence was lower with meloxicam than with piroxicam, naproxen, and diclofenac in long-term double-blind studies. They were more frequent with a dosage of 15 mg/day than with 7.5 mg/day, were judged to be severe in 1.7%, and led to withdrawal in about 4% of patients. The most frequent symptoms were abdominal pain, dyspepsia, eructation, nausea, and vomiting. Upper gastrointestinal perforation, ulceration, and bleeding occurred rarely with meloxicam; the incidence was dose related and lower than with the comparators (7,8). A double-blind endoscopic microbleeding comparison of meloxicam and piroxicam in healthy volunteers showed better gastrointestinal tolerability with meloxicam. Fecal blood loss and endoscopy scores were higher in piroxicam-treated patients, and six piroxicam volunteers versus one treated with meloxicam withdrew because of severe gastrointestinal toxicity; colitis was reported in one case (9). In a few patients meloxicam suppositories can cause abdominal pain and rectal bleeding.

A large prospective comparison of meloxicam 7.5 mg/day with piroxicam 20 mg/day for a median of 28 days suggested that meloxicam has a lower propensity to cause gastroduodenal adverse events. However, serious gastrointestinal events (that is, ulceration, perforation, or bleeding), albeit rare, had similar frequencies in meloxicam and piroxicam recipients, and furthermore the difference in the incidence of adverse gastrointestinal events, although statistically significant, was clinically less relevant (10). Reports received by the Swedish Adverse Drug Reaction Advisory Committee (SADRAC) have suggested that meloxicam has a similar adverse drug reactions profile to other NSAIDs (11) and reports of gastrointestinal hemorrhage have started to appear (12).

Colitis has been described as an adverse effect of meloxicam (SEDA-20, 94).

- Ischemic colitis occurred in a 49-year-old woman 10 days after she started to take meloxicam 15 mg/day for osteoarthritis; meloxicam was withdrawn and her symptoms completely resolved within 1 week (13).

Although meloxicam is considered to be a preferential COX-2 inhibitor, its safety profile is not much different from other traditional NSAIDs, especially in high doses (14).

Liver

Acute cytolytic hepatitis has been described in a 46-year-old woman who took meloxicam for 4 days (15).

Urinary tract

Deterioration in renal function, reversible on withdrawal, was rare (0.4%) (6).

Skin

Rash, pruritus, and other skin problems occurred in about 6.5% of patients (6).

In oral challenges with two doses of meloxicam 7.5 and 15 mg in 114 patients, mean age 46 years, five developed urticaria (16).

A 49-year-old man developed *psoriasis* on two different occasions after taking meloxicam 15 mg/day for 16 days on the first occasion and 8 days after two doses on the second (17).

Reproductive system

The effects of meloxicam on ovulation have been studied in 20 fertile women, who were monitored during a baseline cycle, two treatment cycles, and a washout cycle between treatment cycles (18). Compared with placebo, meloxicam caused a 5-day delay in follicle rupture, a 56% increase in mean maximum follicle diameter, and a 34% reduction in plasma progesterone concentrations. The effects reversed during meloxicam withdrawal. The clinical relevance of these findings is not clear.

- Erythema multiforme has been reported in a 19-year-old man 8 days after he started to take meloxicam for tendonitis; withdrawal and therapy with corticosteroids resulted in complete recovery (19).

Immunologic

Meloxicam may be relatively safe when given to patients with NSAID-induced urticaria/angioedema (20,21). Of 148 NSAID-sensitive subjects with an unequivocal history of urticaria with or without angioedema, who were challenged with increasing oral doses of meloxicam (1–7 mg/day) in a single-blind placebo-controlled trial, only two had a positive test (urticaria in one and urticaria/angioedema in the other); both had chronic idiopathic urticaria (22).

Two cases of meloxicam-induced anaphylactic reactions have been reported (23).

Drug Administration

Drug administration route

Local tolerability with intramuscular administration is reportedly good (24). Serum creatine kinase activity can increase slightly. Gastrointestinal disorders, central nervous system adverse events, and skin rashes have been reported with intramuscular administration.

Drug–Drug Interactions

Lithium

In 16 subjects, meloxicam 15 mg increased plasma lithium concentrations by 21% (range −9 to 59%) and reduced total plasma lithium clearance by 18% (26).

Methotrexate

In 13 patients with rheumatoid arthritis, oral meloxicam for 1 week had no effect on the pharmacokinetics of a single dose of intravenous methotrexate 15 mg (25).

References

1. Anonymous. BI strengthens meloxicam warnings. Scrip 1998;31:2368.
2. Committee on Safety of Medicines/Medicines Control Agency. Meloxicam (Mobic): gastrointestinal and skin reactions. Curr Probl Pharmacovig 1998;24:13.
3. Altman R, Luciardi HL, Muntaner J, Del Rio F, Berman SG, Lopez R, Gonzalez C. Efficacy assessment of meloxicam, a preferential cyclooxygenase-2 inhibitor, in acute coronary syndromes without ST-segment elevation. Nonsteroidal Anti-Inflammatory Drugs in Unstable Angina Treatment (NUT-2) pilot study. Circulation 2002;106:191–5.
4. Karakatsani A, Chroneou A, Kouloris NG, Orphanidou D, Jordanoglu J. Meloxicam-induced pulmonary infiltrates with eosinophilia: a case report Rheumatology 2003;42:1112–3.
5. Bavbek S, Dursun AB, Dursun E, Eryilmaz A, Misirligil Z. Safety of meloxicam in aspirin-hypersensitive patients with asthma and/or nasal polyps. A challenge-proven study. Int Arch Allergy Immunol 2007;142(1):64–9.
6. Auvinet B, Ziller R, Appelboom T, Velicitat P. Comparison of the onset and intensity of action of intramuscular meloxicam and oral meloxicam in patients with acute sciatica. Clin Ther 1995;17(6):1078–98.
7. Huskisson EC, Ghozlan R, Kurthen R, Degner FL, Bluhmki E. A long-term study to evaluate the safety and efficacy of meloxicam therapy in patients with rheumatoid arthritis. Br J Rheumatol 1996;35(Suppl 1):29–34.
8. Hosie J, Distel M, Bluhmki E. Meloxicam in osteoarthritis: a 6-month, double-blind comparison with diclofenac sodium. Br J Rheumatol 1996;35(Suppl 1):39–43.
9. Patoia L, Santucci L, Furno P, Dionisi MS, Dell'Orso S, Romagnoli M, Sattarinia A, Marini MG. A 4-week, double-blind, parallel-group study to compare the gastrointestinal effects of meloxicam 7.5 mg, meloxicam 15 mg, piroxicam 20 mg and placebo by means of faecal blood loss, endoscopy and symptom evaluation in healthy volunteers Br J Rheumatol 1996;35(Suppl 1):61–7.
10. Dequeker J, Hawkey C, Kahan A, Steinbruck K, Alegre C, Baumelou E, Begaud B, Isomaki H, Littlejohn G, Mau J, Papazoglou S. Improvement in gastrointestinal tolerability of the selective cyclooxygenase (COX)-2 inhibitor, meloxicam, compared with piroxicam: results of the Safety and Efficacy Large-scale Evaluation of COX-inhibiting Therapies (SELECT) trial in osteoarthritis. Br J Rheumatol 1998;37(9):946–51.
11. Anonymous. Meloxicam safety similar to other NSAIDs. WHO Drug Inf 1998;12:147.
12. del Val A, Llorente MJ, Tenias JM, Lluch A. Hemorragia digestiva alta causada por meloxicam. [Upper digestive hemorrhage caused by meloxicam.] Rev Esp Enferm Dig 1998;90(6):461–2.
13. Garcia B, Ramaholimihaso F, Diebold MD, Cadiot G, Thiefin G. Ischaemic colitis in a patient taking meloxicam. Lancet 2001;357(9257):690.
14. Degner F, Richardson B. Review of gastrointestinal tolerability and safety of meloxicam. Inflammopharmacology 2001;9:71–80.
15. Staerkel P, Horsmans Y. Meloxicam-induced liver toxicity. Acta Gastroenterol Belg 1999;62(2):255–6.
16. Domingo MV, Marchuet MJ, Culla MT, Joanpere RS, Guadaño EM. Meloxicam tolerance in hypersensitivity to nonsteroidal anti-inflammatory drugs. J Investig Allergol Clin Immunol 2006;16(6):364–6.
17. Ilknur T, Fetil E, Akarsu S, Arda F, Sis B, Günes AT. Development of psoriasis after meloxicam. Eur J Dermatol 2006;16(4):444–5.
18. Bata MS, Al-Ramahi M, Salhab AS, Gharaibeh MN, Schwartz J. Delay of ovulation by meloxicam in healthy cycling volunteers: a placebo-controlled, double-blind, crossover study. J Clin Pharmacol 2006;46(8):925–32.
19. Nikas SN, Kittas G, Karamaounas N, Drosos AA. Meloxicam-induced erythema multiforme. Am J Med 1999;107(5):532–4.
20. Kosnik M, Music E, Matjaz F, Suskovic S. Relative safety of meloxicam in NSAID-intolerant patients. Allergy 1998;53(12):1231–3.
21. Quaratino D, Romano A, Di Fonso M, Papa G, Perrone MR, D'Ambrosio FP, Venuti A. Tolerability of meloxicam in patients with histories of adverse reactions to nonsteroidal anti-inflammatory drugs. Ann Allergy Asthma Immunol 2000;84(6):613–7.
22. Nettis E, Di Paola R, Ferrannini A, Tursi A. Meloxicam in hypersensitivity to NSAIDs. Allergy 2001;56(8):803–4.
23. Bavbek S, Erkekol FO, Dursun B, Misirligil Z. Meloxicam-associated anaphylactic reaction. J Investig Allergol Clin Immunol 2006;16(5):317–20.
24. Euller-Ziegler L, Velicitat P, Bluhmki E, Turck D, Scheuerer S, Combe B. Meloxicam: a review of its pharmacokinetics, efficacy and tolerability following intramuscular administration. Inflamm Res 2001;50(Suppl 1):S5–9.

25. Hubner G, Sander O, Degner FL, Turck D, Rau R. Lack of pharmacokinetic interaction of meloxicam with methotrexate in patients with rheumatoid arthritis. J Rheumatol 1997;24(5):845–51.
26. Turck D, Heinzel G, Luik G. Steady-state pharmacokinetics of lithium in healthy volunteers receiving concomitant meloxicam. Br J Clin Pharmacol 2000;50(3):197–204.

Mofebutazone

See also Non-steroidal anti-inflammatory drugs

General Information

Adverse reactions to mofebutazone are similar to those of the parent drug, phenylbutazone, and include skin reactions, including epidermal necrolysis and bullous drug eruption (1). Gastrotoxicity, hepatotoxicity, nephrotoxicity, edema, headache, and hematological adverse effects (SED-9, 145) (2) have been described.

References

1. Walchner M, Rueff F, Przybilla B. Delayed-type hypersensitivity to mofebutazone underlying a severe drug reaction. Contact Dermatitis 1997;36(1):54–5.
2. Kimura S, Shorota N. [A case report of massive bleeding from conjunctiva due to drug-induced thrombocytopenia.] Nippon Ganka Kiyo 1971;22(11):954–8.

Morniflumate

General Information

Morniflumate is an NSAID that is widely prescribed in some countries as an antipyretic analgesic in children.

Organs and Systems

Immunologic

- A 4-year-old girl developed angioedema and urticaria 30 minutes after receiving rectal morniflumate. Her signs and symptoms resolved in 48 hours. Skin prick and intradermal tests to morniflumate were negative, but rechallenge with rectal administration caused a recurrence (1).

Reference

1. Matheu V, Sierra Z, Gracia MT, Caloto M, Alcazar MM, Martinez MI, Zapatero L. Morniflumate-induced urticaria–angioedema. Allergy 1998;53(8):812–3.

Nabumetone

General Information

Nabumetone is a naproxen derivative, whose efficacy is related to its active metabolite, 6-methoxy-2-naphthylacetic acid. Not unexpectedly, a study in 2000 patients, mostly treated for more than 6 months, elicited an adverse events pattern similar to the other derivatives of this class of NSAIDs (SEDA-13, 81). Adverse effects were reported in 18% of patients and 10% stopped taking the drug because of adverse reactions. Diarrhea was the most common problem (13%) followed by abdominal pain (9.9%), dyspepsia (9.3%), nausea (7.8%), and flatulence (4.7%). Ten ulcers were detected. Nervous system reactions, skin rashes, edema, unspecified eye disorders, and liver function test abnormalities all occur (1).

A postmarketing surveillance study in 10 800 patients with osteoarthritis and rheumatoid arthritis, who were followed up at 12 months, reported that 12% of patients discontinued the drug because of adverse events; 11 serious events may have been related to nabumetone and seven of these were gastrointestinal hemorrhage (2). In 6148 patients treated with nabumetone in long-term trials, the 3-month cumulative incidence of clinically detected perforations, ulcers, and bleeding was 0.1% and the 6-month incidence was 0.2% (3).

Organs and Systems

Metabolism

Nabumetone-induced pseudoporphyria has been described (SEDA-16, 11; SEDA 22, 117), and a further five cases in four adults and a child have been reported (4–6).

Gastrointestinal

Being a non-acidic compound and a weak inhibitor of prostaglandin synthesis, nabumetone was designed as a prodrug that could be administered without causing gastric damage. This theoretical advantage still awaits confirmation. Although there was no gastrointestinal toxicity in animals, in humans gastric problems with NSAIDs are not primarily a local effect but are exerted systemically, so a metabolite formed after gastric passage could still cause gastric problems. Again, although radiochromium evaluation of gastrointestinal blood loss in healthy volunteers and endoscopic studies in patients with rheumatoid arthritis showed that nabumetone provokes less gastric damage than naproxen, the usual defects of such studies limit their clinical relevance (SEDA-13, 81). The same applies to the preliminary results of a long-term study in patients with osteoarthritis and rheumatoid arthritis, which also showed that nabumetone is less gastrotoxic than naproxen, but it was not possible to exclude the possibility that the dosage was lower than was needed for optimal efficacy (7).

Susceptibility Factors

Age

After repeated once-daily doses, nabumetone accumulates in elderly patients but not in others; it is therefore wise to reduce the dose in elderly patients.

Drug–Drug Interactions

Warfarin

Concomitant therapy with warfarin and NSAIDs is of concern, owing to the potential for increasing bleeding.

- In a 72-year-old man the concomitant use of nabumetone and warfarin led to an increased international normalized ratio and hemarthrosis (8).

Previous reports suggested a lack of interaction of nabumetone with warfarin, but close monitoring is advisable when these two drugs are co-administered.

References

1. Jenner PN, Johnson ES. Review of the experience with nabumetone in clinical trials outside of the United States. Am J Med 1987;83(4B):110–4.
2. Jenner PN. A 12-month postmarketing surveillance study of nabumetone. A preliminary report. Drugs 1990;40(Suppl 5):80–6.
3. Lipani JA, Poland M. Clinical update of the relative safety of nabumetone in long-term clinical trials. Inflammopharmacology 1995;3:351–61.
4. Antony F, Layton AM. Nabumetone-associated pseudoporphyria. Br J Dermatol 2000;142(5):1067–9.
5. Checketts SR, Morgan GJ Jr. Two cases of nabumetone induced pseudoporphyria. J Rheumatol 1999;26(12):2703–5.
6. Cron RQ, Finkel TH. Nabumetone induced pseudoporphyria in childhood. J Rheumatol 2000;27(7):1817–8.
7. Roth SH. New understandings of NSAID gastropathy. Scand J Rheumatol Suppl 1989;78:24–9.
8. Dennis VC, Thomas BK, Hanlon JE. Potentiation of oral anticoagulation and hemarthrosis associated with nabumetone. Clin Reumatol 2000;75:967–70.

Naproxen and Piproxen

General Information

Naproxen sodium, an arylalkanoic acid NSAID, was approved for over-the-counter marketing in January 1994.

The adverse effects of naproxen resemble those of ibuprofen. Any minor differences in frequency cannot be assessed with certainty. In 881 patients who had been followed for more than 3 years, only 8.9% dropped out because of adverse effects. In shorter studies, doses of up to 1.5 g/day produced no more adverse effects than lower or standard doses of other NSAIDs (1).

The safety profile of over-the-counter naproxen has been adequately evaluated, and the incidence of adverse events was similar to the incidence with placebo, ibuprofen, and paracetamol. There were no serious adverse reactions in these studies (SEDA-20, 93).

A comparative case-cohort study on the risk of gastrointestinal tract bleeding associated with naproxen or ibuprofen showed a low incidence of upper gastrointestinal tract bleeding with both drugs, but low-dose naproxen put patients at increased risk of gastrointestinal bleeding compared with low-dose ibuprofen (2). If properly advised, patients can use the over-the-counter formulations without serious risks; patients taking NSAIDs must swallow their tablets with large amounts of water while standing, at least 1 hour before retiring.

The safety and efficacy of NSAIDs for the relief of symptoms of the common cold have been insufficiently studied. Naproxen did not alter virus shedding or the serum-neutralizing antibody response in healthy young adults with experimental rhinovirus colds but had some beneficial effect on symptoms (SEDA-17, 113).

The fact that its half-life is unchanged in renal insufficiency can be therapeutically useful (3).

Piproxen

Piproxen is a piperazine derivative of naproxen; its adverse effects profile is similar to that of naproxen (4).

Organs and Systems

Respiratory

Eosinophilic interstitial pneumonitis has been reported (5); the incidence is greater with naproxen than ibuprofen, as shown by an FDA survey (SEDA-17, 112).

Exacerbation of asthma in sensitive patients is rare, but has been reported with naproxen (6–8).

Nervous system

Peripheral neuropathy has been reported in a patient with psoriatic arthropathy taking naproxen and hydroxychloroquine (SEDA-12, 87).

Aseptic meningitis has been attributed to naproxen in a healthy young man taking it for neck pain (SEDA-14, 95).

Worsening of parkinsonian symptoms has been described with naproxen (SEDA-19, 99).

Sensory systems

Eyes

Blurred vision, ocular discomfort, and lenticular and corneal changes were observed in a long-term study (1).

Ears

Hearing loss and tinnitus (sudden, bilateral, and permanent) have been associated with naproxen (9).

Psychological, psychiatric

Abnormalities in cognitive capacity and altered behavior have been described in elderly patients taking naproxen (SEDA-8, 107) (10).

Hematologic

Fatal aplastic anemia was reported in a patient taking naproxen as the only drug for 4 months (11). Cases of Coombs' positive and Coombs' negative autoimmune hemolytic anemia (12), agranulocytosis (SEDA-13, 82), and thrombocytopenia (SEDA-15, 102) have also been reported.

- Three men, aged 56, 57, and 71 years developed extensive purpuric hemorrhages involving their legs ($n = 3$), arms ($n = 2$), and abdomen ($n = 1$) 10–20 days after having taken naproxen 250 mg tds for musculoskeletal disorders (13). One patient also had gastrointestinal bleeding. They all had severe thrombocytopenia (platelet counts below $3 \times 10^9/l$). Naproxen was withdrawn and prednisone started. The platelet counts normalized within a week. The prednisone was withdrawn and the thrombocytopenia did not recur during follow up. Analysis of their sera showed the presence of IgG antibodies that recognized normal platelets in the presence of the metabolite naproxen glucuronide.

Gastrointestinal

By December 1995 the FDA had received 81 reports of esophageal symptoms and 7 had esophageal ulcers. No hemorrhages were reported (SEDA-22, 117).

Naproxen-induced gastrotoxicity has been reported with varying frequency (SED-9, 152) (1).

There were no differences in the incidence of middle and distal duodenum lesions (14). Esophageal ulceration with bleeding was reported in an elderly woman with esophageal dysmotility (SEDA-17, 112). Esophageal symptoms and esophageal ulcers were reported with naproxen sodium tablets (as opposed to capsules) for over-the-counter use (SEDA-22, 111). Naproxen did not cause reflux and had no significant effect on motility in healthy subjects (15).

Local adverse effects of naproxen suppositories include edema, erythema, and bleeding, which are usually mild.

Acute eosinophilic colitis has been described; it resolved rapidly when naproxen was withdrawn (16).

Liver

Abnormal liver function tests (SED-9, 152) (17) and hepatic injury have been associated with naproxen (18), but no definite cause–effect relation has been established.

Pancreas

Acute pancreatitis has been described in two young women taking naproxen for dysmenorrhea (SEDA-18, 105; (SEDA-20, 93)

- A 20-year-old man took 10 tablets of naproxen sodium 550 mg. He developed mild upper abdominal pain and had raised activities of serum amylase 1050 IU/l (25–125

IU/l) and lipase 151 IU/l (8–78 IU/l) (19). There was no evidence of hypercalcemia or hyperlipidemia and a viral screen was negative. He denied alcohol consumption and there was no family history of pancreatitis. Abdominal ultrasound and a CT scan showed a homogeneous pancreas and a normal gall-bladder and biliary tree. The symptoms resolved within a day, but the laboratory findings persisted for 3 days.

Urinary tract

Interstitial nephritis, with rises in serum urea and creatinine, which fell after withdrawal, has been described after treatment for 3 months in adults (20) and in a young boy (SEDA-16, 111).

Oliguric renal insufficiency with the nephrotic syndrome and active interstitial nephritis has been described in a young woman with systemic lupus erythematosus taking intermittent long-term naproxen (SEDA-15, 102).

- A marathon runner, who had taken naproxen until 36 hours before the race, developed acute oliguric renal insufficiency that required hemodialysis 2 days afterwards (SEDA-12, 87).

The kidney can be affected in generalized hypersensitivity reactions to naproxen (3).

Skin

Acne has been reported in a woman with primary dysmenorrhea (21).

The skin can be affected in the course of generalized allergic reactions (22).

Bullous photodermatitis resembling porphyria cutanea tarda has been described in patients taking long-term treatment (SEDA-12, 87).

Hair loss can be induced by naproxen (SEDA-15, 102).

A photodermatitis, defined as pseudoporphyria, has been reported in 21 children with juvenile rheumatoid arthritis and one with systemic lupus erythematosus after prolonged treatment with naproxen (23) and in another four children with juvenile rheumatoid arthritis (24). This effect is rare, but since naproxen is widely used in juvenile rheumatoid arthritis, it is worth mentioning.

- Linear IgA bullous dermatosis occurred in a 69-year-old man (25). Long-term corticosteroid treatment caused gradual resolution.

Lichen planus has been described in 55 patients taking naproxen; in 42 it was of the eruptive type (26). In 25 patients no other drugs had been used; 12 had taken naproxen with other drugs that have been associated with lichen planus; 18 had taken naproxen with drugs that had not been previously associated with lichen planus. New lesions did not occur after withdrawal of naproxen.

Sexual function

Impotence and failure to ejaculate have been described, the latter with positive rechallenge(27).

In women, naproxen, like other NSAIDs, can interfere with menstruation; two young women had interrupted menstrual blood flow after taking the drug (SEDA-15, 102).

At high doses in mid-cycle, naproxen can inhibit ovulation and cause the so-called luteinized unruptured follicle syndrome (SEDA-16, 111).

Immunologic

Generalized reactions (28) include cutaneous necrotizing vasculitis (SEDA-5, 106) (SEDA-17, 113), nephritis, paralytic ileus, and angiitis with cutaneous, muscular, articular, and renal involvement (21).

- A leukocytoclastic vasculitis occurred in a 62-year-old woman with skin, peripheral nerve, and renal involvement (29). Long-term corticosteroid treatment caused gradually resolution.
- Exercise-induced anaphylaxis in a girl who had been taking naproxen for 3 weeks was confirmed by rechallenge (SEDA-21, 106).

Second-Generation Effects

Teratogenicity

Renal tubular dysgenesis, a rare, lethal, autosomal recessive disorder characterized by short poorly differentiated proximal convoluted tubules associated with oligohydramnios, Potter sequence, and neonatal death from respiratory failure, has been reported after in utero exposure to naproxen sodium; the glomeruli were not as crowded as is usually seen in this condition (30). However, a cause-and-effect association in this case cannot be assumed.

Fetotoxicity

Pulmonary hypertension and severe protracted hypoxemia occurred in babies born to mothers who took naproxen to delay delivery (31). The babies also had disorders of blood clotting, renal function, and bilirubin metabolism. Necroscopy showed subarachnoid hemorrhage, gastric ulcers, and closed ductus arteriosus.

Susceptibility Factors

Age

In an analysis of nine double-blind, controlled studies, adverse reactions to naproxen in older and in younger subjects had similar incidences (32).

Drug Administration

Drug formulations

The suspension and modified-release tablets produce the usual pattern of adverse effects (SEDA-15, 101), although an enteric-coated formulation of naproxen in patients intolerant of NSAIDs caused fewer gastrointestinal adverse effects (SEDA-19, 99).

Drug overdose

Nothing more serious than nausea and indigestion have been reported after 25 g of naproxen (33), whereas 35 g caused an epileptic fit (34). Metabolic acidosis, loss of consciousness, seizures, and apnea have been reported after the ingestion of more than 10 g (35).

Drug–Drug Interactions

Diuretics

Naproxen reduces the actions of diuretics (SEDA-8, 107).

Lithium

There were no significant changes in serum lithium concentrations in 12 men taking over-the-counter doses of naproxen (220 mg tds) or paracetamol (650 mg qds) for 5 days (38).

Methotrexate

Methotrexate alters naproxen kinetics and vice versa (36).

Methyldopa

Naproxen reduces the actions of methyldopa (SEDA- 8, 107).

Prebenecid

Naproxen inhibits the metabolism and renal excretion of probenecid, prolonging its half-life (37).

Propranolol

Naproxen reduces the actions of propranolol (SEDA-8, 107).

References

1. Segre E. Long term experience with naproxen: open labeled cohort survey of nearly 900 rheumatoid arthritis and osteoarthritis patients. Curr Ther Res 1980;28:47.
2. Strom BL, Schinnar R, Bilker WB, Feldman H, Farrar JT, Carson JL. Gastrointestinal tract bleeding associated with naproxen sodium vs ibuprofen. Arch Intern Med 1997;157(22):2626–31.
3. Anttila M, Haataja M, Kasanen A. Pharmacokinetics of naproxen in subjects with normal and impaired renal function. Eur J Clin Pharmacol 1980;18(3):263–8.
4. Gualdi A, Arancio V, Bonollo L. Il piproxen nella terapia delle sindromi reumatiche extrarticolari. Gazz Med Ital Arch Sci Med 1986;145:417.
5. Nader DA, Schillaci RF. Pulmonary infiltrates with eosinophilia due to naproxen. Chest 1983;83(2):280–2.
6. Szczeklik A, Gryglewski RJ, Czerniawska-Mysik G, Pieton R. Asthmatic attacks induced in aspirin-sensitive patients by diclofenac and naproxen. BMJ 1977;2(6081):231–2.
7. Salberg DJ, Simon MR. Severe asthma induced by naproxen—a case report and review of the literature. Ann Allergy 1980;45(6):372–5.

8. Lewis RV. Severe asthma after naproxen. Lancet 1987;1(8544):1270.

9. Chapman P. Naproxen and sudden hearing loss. J Laryngol Otol 1982;96(2):163–6.

10. Wysenbeek AJ, Klein Z, Nakar S, Mane R. Assessment of cognitive function in elderly patients treated with naproxen. A prospective study. Clin Exp Rheumatol 1988;6(4):399–400.

11. Arnold R, Heimpel H. Aplastic anaemia after naproxen? Lancet 1980;1(8163):321.

12. Lo TCN, Martin MA. Autoimmune hemolytic anemia associated with naproxen suppositories. BMJ (Clin Res Ed) 1986;292:1430.

13. Bougie D, Aster R. Immune thrombocytopenia resulting from sensitivity to metabolites of naproxen and acetaminophen. Blood 2001;97(12):3846–50.

14. Aabakken L, Bjornbeth BA, Hofstad B, Olaussen B, Larsen S, Osnes M. Comparison of the gastrointestinal side effects of naproxen formulated as plain tablets, enteric-coated tablets, or enteric-coated granules in capsules. Scand J Gastroenterol Suppl 1989;163:65–73.

15. Scheiman JM, Patel PM, Henson EK, Nostrant TT. Effect of naproxen on gastroesophageal reflux and esophageal function: a randomized, double-blind, placebo-controlled study. Am J Gastroenterol 1995;90(5):754–7.

16. Bridges AJ, Marshall JB, Diaz-Arias AA. Acute eosinophilic colitis and hypersensitivity reaction associated with naproxen therapy. Am J Med 1990;89(4):526–7.

17. Frenger W, Morbach HJ. Klinische Untersuchung von Naproxen, von allem mit Bezug auf seine Verträglichkeit. [Clinical trial with naproxen, with particular consideration to tolerance.] Scand J Rheumatol 1973;(Suppl 2):137–9.

18. Victorino RM, Silveira JC, Baptista A, de Moura MC. Jaundice associated with naproxen. Postgrad Med J 1980;56(655):368–70.

19. Aygencel G, Akbuga B, Keles A. Acute pancreatitis following naproxen intake. Eur J Emerg Med 2006;13(6):372.

20. Cartwright KC, Trotter TL, Cohen ML. Naproxen nephrotoxicity. Ariz Med 1979;36(2):124–6.

21. Hamann GO. Severe, primary dysmenorrhea treated with naproxen. A prospective, double-blind, crossover investigation. Prostaglandins 1980;19(5):651–7.

22. Plouvier B, Gosselin B, Hatron PY, Plouvier-Carrez J, Devulder B. Vasculopathie allergique systémique induite par le naproxen. [Systemic allergic vasculopathy after naproxen.] Ann Med Interne (Paris) 1979;130(3):173–6.

23. Levy ML, Barron KS, Eichenfield A, Honig PJ. Naproxen-induced pseudoporphyria: a distinctive photodermatitis. J Pediatr 1990;117(4):660–4.

24. Girschick HJ, Hamm H, Ganser G, Huppertz HI. Naproxen-induced pseudoporphyria: appearance of new skin lesions after discontinuation of treatment. Scand J Rheumatol 1995;24(2):108–11.

25. Bouldin MB, Clowers-Webb HE, Davis JL, McEvoy MT, Davis MD. Naproxen-associated linear IgA bullous dermatosis: case report and review. Mayo Clin Proc 2000;75(9):967–70.

26. Güneş AT, Fetil E, Ilknur T, Birgin B, Ozkan S. Naproxen-induced lichen planus: report of 55 cases. Int J Dermatol 2006;45(6):709–12.

27. Wei N, Hood JC. Naproxen and ejaculatory dysfunction. Ann Intern Med 1980;93(6):933.

28. Grennan DM, Jolly J, Holloway LJ, Palmer DG. Vasculitis in a patient receiving naproxen. NZ Med J 1979;89(628):48–9.

29. Schapira D, Balbir-Gurman A, Nahir AM. Naproxen-induced leukocytoclastic vasculitis. Clin Rheumatol 2000;19(3):242–4.

30. Koklu E, Gurgoze M, Akgun H, Ozturk MA, Poyrazoglu MH. Renal tubular dysgenesis with atypical histology and in-utero exposure to naproxen sodium. Ann Trop Paediatr 2006;26(3):241–5.

31. Wilkinson AR, Aynsley-Green A, Mitchell MD. Persistent pulmonary hypertension and abnormal prostaglandin E levels in preterm infants after maternal treatment with naproxen. Arch Dis Child 1979;54(12):942–5.

32. Geczy M, Peltier L, Wolbach R. Naproxen tolerability in the elderly: a summary report. J Rheumatol 1987;14(2):348–54.

33. Fredell EW, Strand LJ. Naproxen overdose. JAMA 1977;238(9):938.

34. Court H, Volans GN. Poisoning after overdose with non-steroidal anti-inflammatory drugs. Adverse Drug React Acute Poisoning Rev 1984;3(1):1–21.

35. Martinez R, Smith DW, Frankel LR. Severe metabolic acidosis after acute naproxen sodium ingestion. Ann Emerg Med 1989;18(10):1102–4.

36. Wallace CA, Smith AL, Sherry DD. Pilot investigation of naproxen/methotrexate interaction in patients with juvenile rheumatoid arthritis. J Rheumatol 1993;20(10):1764–8.

37. Runkel R, Mroszczak E, Chaplin M, Sevelius H, Segre E. Naproxen–probenecid interaction. Clin Pharmacol Ther 1978;24(6):706–13.

38. Levin GM, Grum C, Eisele G. Effect of over-the-counter dosages of naproxen sodium and acetaminophen on plasma lithium concentrations in normal volunteers. J Clin Psychopharmacol 1998;18(3):237–40.

Niflumic acid

General Information

The three atoms of fluoride in the niflumic acid molecule may be critically implicated in its adverse effects. However, as niflumic acid has been on the market in many countries for more than a decade, fluoride-induced adverse effects are probably very rare, and they are clinically relevant only if therapy is very prolonged. There are no adequate prospective studies of the comparative advantages and disadvantages of niflumic acid.

Organs and Systems

Nervous system

Headache is a common adverse effect of niflumic acid (SED-8, 223).

Hematologic

A patient with agranulocytosis and a positive lymphocytic stimulation test recovered after withdrawal (1).

Gastrointestinal

Niflumic acid has the same gastrointestinal adverse effects profile as other anthranilic acids (SED-8, 223).

Liver

Hepatic damage has rarely been reported (SEDA-1, 90). Fatal icteric hepatitis occurred in a patient taking niflumic acid and paracetamol (SEDA-13, 83).

Urinary tract

Nephrotoxic effects have often been reported with niflumic acid, although whether this really indicates a relatively high potential for renal toxicity is an open question. Water retention with edema, oliguria, proteinuria, and increases in urea and creatinine concentrations have been described (SED-8, 223; 2).

Seven children taking niflumic acid for ear, nose, and throat disorders for 1-5 days developed acute renal insufficiency due to immune interstitial nephritis; oedema, oliguria, or anuria occurred at 3–6 days (2). There were signs of hypersensitivity (fever, skin rash, eosinophilia, and/or increased IgE) in all cases, leukocyturia in five, and hematuria in six. Renal biopsy showed interstitial lesions with infiltrates of lymphocytes, eosinophils, and plasma cells, but no tubular cell necrosis. In two patients renal insufficiency was irreversible despite the use of methylprednisolone.

Musculoskeletal

Niflumic acid can provoke rhabdomyolysis (SEDA-14, 95).

There are several accounts of skeletal fluorosis attributable solely to chronic intoxication with fluoride as a result of long-term use of the drug (up to 11 years) (SEDA-6, 99). As each capsule of niflumic acid contains 50.5 mg of fluoride, daily intake could be up to 0.30 g. The skeletal fluorosis was asymptomatic and was discovered only by routine radiology. Homogeneous osteosclerosis was in all cases greatest in the axial skeleton. Urinary fluoride concentrations were high and associated with hypocalcemia, hypocalciuria, and increased serum alkaline phosphatase activity. Bone biopsies showed increased trabecular bone volume, suggesting bone fluorosis. Persistent fluoride ingestion leads to a high bone fluoride content, since fluoride is trapped at the site in the apatite mineral lattice that is normally occupied by the hydroxyl group (3). Exactly how fluoride causes changes in bone structure and why osteocondensation is unevenly distributed is not known. It is not clear whether osteoid stimulation increases bone fragility (4). In view of the dangers of fluoride accumulation in renal insufficiency, niflumic acid should not be given in this condition (5).

References

1. Szczeklik A, Gryglewski RJ, Czerniawska-Mysik G. Clinical patterns of hypersensitivity to nonsteroidal anti-inflammatory drugs and their pathogenesis. J Allergy Clin Immunol 1977;60(5):276–84.
2. Lantz B, Cochat P, Bouchet JL, Fischbach M. Short-term niflumic-acid-induced acute renal failure in children. Nephrol Dial Transplant 1994;9(9):1234–9.
3. Haynes RC Jr, Murad F. Agents affecting calcification, calcium parathyroid hormone, calcitonin, vitamin D and other compounds. In: Goodman LS, Gilman A, editors. The Pharmacological Basis of Therapeutics. 6th ed.. New York: MacMillan, 1980:1545.
4. Stevens RM. Chronic fluorosis. BMJ (Clin Res Ed) 1981;282(6265):741–2.
5. Anonymous. Fluoride osteosis with niflumic acid. Prescrire Int 2003;12(63):18.

Nimesulide

General Information

Nimesulide is a selective COX-2 inhibitor. Data from a postmarketing survey on short-term nimesulide treatment of osteoarthritis in 22 938 outpatients confirmed that its adverse effects profile is similar to the profiles of other NSAIDs (SEDA-16, 114). Evidence that nimesulide is well tolerated in aspirin-sensitive asthmatic patients requires confirmation in more extensive well-conducted studies (SEDA-18, 107).

Organs and Systems

Nervous system

Nervous system adverse effects (nervousness, vertigo) have been reported with nimesulide (1).

Hematologic

Thrombocytopenia in an HIV-positive patient treated with nimesulide regressed rapidly when the drug was withdrawn (SEDA-14, 96).

Thrombocytopenia with oligohydramios occurred during pregnancy with premature labor in a woman taking nimesulide (2).

Mouth and teeth

A fixed drug eruption occurred in the mouth of a young woman who had taken nimesulide (SEDA-17, 114).

Gastrointestinal

Gastrointestinal symptoms (pyrosis, pain, nausea) can occur (1), but in a short-term endoscopic study nimesulide caused less gastric damage than indometacin (SEDA-15, 104).

Liver

Many cases of liver toxicity have been reported with nimesulide.

Consequent concern about its benefit to harm balance has prompted its withdrawal from the market in some countries.

From estimates of patient exposure and data from spontaneous reports received from the Spanish pharmacovigilance system (3), nimesulide was associated with a higher risk of hepatotoxicity than other NSAIDs.

However, these data were in contrast to those from an epidemiological study conducted in Italy, one of the countries with the highest prevalence of nimesulide prescription (4). The study was a retrospective cohort and nested case-control study in 400 000 individuals from the Umbria region admitted to hospital for acute non-viral hepatitis and who had received at least one prescription for an NSAID between 1997 and 2001. Nimesulide was the most commonly prescribed NSAID, with 551 000 prescriptions. Of the 176 cases of hepatotoxicity included in the final analysis, 42 occurred during current use of the NSAID, giving an increased risk of hepatotoxicity compared with past use of an NSAID (RR=1.4; 95% CI=1, 2.1?. This ratio was increased among elderly patients. In current users of nimesulide the RRs for all hepatopathies and more severe liver injury were 1.3 (0.7, 2.3) and 1.9 (1.1, 3.8) respectively. Fulminant hepatitis was not observed. This study has therefore confirmed that hepatotoxicity is a rare class effect of NSAIDs. Despite the fact that data from spontaneous reports suggest an increased risk of hepatic injury with nimesulide, this retrospective study showed that the risk of liver injury in patients taking nimesulide and other NSAIDs is small.

Following a Community-wide review of nimesulide, the CPMP concluded that it has a favourable benefit to harm balance and that marketing authorization should be maintained (5). However, the CPMP recommended that systemic use of nimesulide be restricted to the treatment of acute pain. Patients using nimesulide must be monitored for possible hepatotoxicity and the drug should be withdrawn if laboratory or clinical findings suggest liver toxicity.

Of five patients, two died as a result of fulminant hepatic failure while taking nimesulide (6).

Six cases of acute hepatitis occurred in four patients during the first 10 weeks of treatment, and in two after 15 weeks of therapy (7). They were represented by jaundice ($n = 5$), itching ($n = 2$), weakness ($n = 3$), and anorexia, nausea, and vomiting ($n = 2$). Increases in liver enzymes varied from 1.5 to over 30 times the upper limit of the reference range. Liver biopsy showed centrilobular or panlobular bridging necrosis in the four women and intrahepatic cholestasis in the two men. Complete recovery of normal liver function tests ensued at follow-up after interruption of nimesulide therapy.

- Fulminant hepatic failure due to massive hepatic necrosis occurred in a 58-year-old woman who took nimesulide for a few weeks for osteoarthritis (8). In the months before, she had received a first short course of the drug, apparently without problems. When she resumed - nimesulide therapy she complained of non-specific symptoms, including nausea, and appeared jaundiced. The drug was withdrawn and liver transplantation was performed, but she died of multiorgan failure.

The previous exposure may have sensitized the patient with accelerated liver injury on re-exposure.

Several other reports of the potential hepatotoxicity of nimesulide have appeared (SEDA-25, 135; 9–11). A wide range of types of liver damage have been documented (12). Some patients have required liver transplantation (13) and deaths have occurred (14). The pathogenic mechanism of these unpredictable, sometimes severe, reactions is uncertain (15,16). In some countries nimesulide has been withdrawn from the market or its use has been restricted.

Liver failure requiring liver transplant in patients taking nimesulide has also been associated with hemolytic anemia (17)

In some cases the hepatitis is severe (SEDA-23, 121). In one case fatal hepatitis occurred after 8 months of treatment (18) and in another treatment for 5 days precipitated fulminant hepatitis (19).

The Portuguese Pharmacy and Medicines Institute suspended the pediatric formulation of nimesulide in March 1999 (20). This decision was made because of reports of serious adverse drug reactions, including liver damage, in children taking the drug. Nimesulide should be withdrawn immediately if abnormal liver function tests develop, and rechallenge must be avoided. However, it is not yet clear if the potential for hepatotoxicity of this drug is similar or greater to that found with other NSAIDs (21).

Urinary tract

Acute oliguric renal insufficiency caused by interstitial nephritis was attributed to nimesulide in a 68-year-old woman with diffuse arteriosclerosis but normal renal function (SEDA-22, 119).

A series of 11 spontaneously reported cases in which renal impairment was associated with the use of nimesulide has been described (22). The adverse events were represented by acute renal insufficiency ($n = 2$), acute deterioration of chronic renal insufficiency ($n = 3$), fluid retention ($n = 4$), and oliguria and macrohematuria ($n = 1$ each). The patients had a median age of 57 (range 17–81) years and six had some predisposing condition (chronic renal insufficiency, heart failure, diabetes, use of diuretics) to NSAID-induced functional renal impairment. Apart from one patient, nimesulide was taken for a very short time (less than 8 days). A favorable outcome ensued after withdrawal of therapy in all patients. The acute deterioration of renal function described in these patients pointed to hemodynamically mediated renal impairment in all cases, with the exception of one man in whom interstitial nephritis was suspected.

Skin

Reported cutaneous effects of nimesulide include rash and itching (1) and toxic epidermal necrolysis (SEDA-22, 119).

Second-Generation Effects

Fetotoxicity

Various types of nephrotoxicity have been described with nimesulide (SEDA-22, 119; SEDA-23, 121). Two reports have illustrated the potential danger of using it as a tocolytic (23) or during late pregnancy (24). In both cases, maternal ingestion of nimesulide was accompanied by irreversible neonatal renal insufficiency. In the second case, renal biopsy showed abnormal tubular differentiation and signs of tubulointerstitial nephritis. The mechanism of this adverse reaction is not known, but it is probably related to fetal COX-2 inhibition. COX-2 is fundamental for nephrogenesis, and is upregulated in fetal membranes and myometrium at parturition.

A report has confirmed the potential danger of using nimesulide as a tocolytic agent (SEDA 24, 123). Nimesulide (100 mg bd) was prescribed for postoperative preterm labor prophylaxis, and severe oligohydramnios was identified 3 weeks later (25). After withdrawal the amniotic fluid volume returned to normal over 2 weeks. There were no adverse neonatal renal effects.

References

1. Biscarini L, Patoia L, Del Favero A. Nimesulide-a new non-steroidal anti-inflammatory agent. Drugs Today 1988;24:23.
2. Paternoster DM, Snijders D, Manganelli F, Torrisi A, Bracciante R. Anhydramnios and maternal thrombocytopenia after prolonged use of nimesulide. Eur J Obstet Gynecol Reprod Biol 2003;108:97–8.
3. Macia MA, Carvajal A, Del Pozo JG, Vera E, Del Pino A. Hepatotoxicity associated with nimesulide: data from the Spanish Pharmacovigilance System. Clin Pharmacol Ther 2002;72:596–7.
4. Traversa G, Bianchi C, Da Cas R, Abraha I, Menniti-Ippolito F, Venegoni M. Cohort study of hepatotoxicity associated with nimesulide and other steroidal anti-inflammatory drugs. BMJ 2003;327:18–22.
5. Anonymous. Nimesulide-containing products have a favorable risk-benefit profile. Reactions 2003;963:2.
6. Figueras A, Estevez F, Laporte JR. New drugs, new adverse drug reactions, and bibliographic databases. Lancet 1999;353(9162):1447–8.
7. Van Steenbergen W, Peeters P, De Bondt J, Staessen D, Buscher H, Laporta T, Roskams T, Desmet V. Nimesulide-induced acute hepatitis: evidence from six cases. J Hepatol 1998;29(1):135–41.
8. McCormick PA, Kennedy F, Curry M, Traynor O. COX 2 inhibitor and fulminant hepatic failure. Lancet 1999;353(9146):40–1.
9. Sbeit W, Krivoy N, Shiller M, Farah R, Cohen HI, Struminger L, Reshef R. Nimesulide-induced acute hepatitis. Ann Pharmacother 2001;35(9):1049–52.
10. Dumortier J, Borel I, Delafosse B, Vial T, Scoazec JY, Boillot O. Transplantation hépatique pour hépatite subfulminante après prise de nimésulide. [Subfulminant hepatitis associated with nimesulide treatment requiring liver transplantation.] Gastroenterol Clin Biol 2002;26(4):415–6.
11. Ferreiro C, Vivas S, Jorquera F, Dominguez AB, Espinel J, Munoz F, Herrera A, Fernandez MJ, Olcoz JL, Ortiz de Urbina J. Hepatitis toxica por nimesulida, presentacion de un nuevo caso y revision de la bibliografia. [Toxic hepatitis caused by nimesulide, presentation of a new case and review of the literature.] Gastroenterol Hepatol 2000;23(9):428–30.
12. Macia MA, Carvajal A, del Pozo JG, Vera E, del Pino A. Hepatotoxicity associated with nimesulide: data from the Spanish Pharmacovigilance System. Clin Pharmacol Ther 2002;72(5):596–7.
13. Rodrigo L, de Francisco R, Perez-Pariente JM, Cadahia V, Tojo R, Rodriguez M, Lucena MI, Andrade RJ. Nimesulide-induced severe hemolytic anemia and acute liver failure leading to liver transplantation. Scand J Gastroenterol 2002;37(11):1341–3.
14. Merlani G, Fox M, Oehen HP, Cathomas G, Renner EL, Fattinger K, Schneemann M, Kullak-Ublick GA. Fatal hepatotoxicity secondary to nimesulide. Eur J Clin Pharmacol 2001;57(4):321–6.
15. Boelsterli UA. Mechanisms of NSAID-induced hepatotoxicity: focus on nimesulide. Drug Saf 2002;25(9):633–48.
16. Rainsford KD. Relationship of nimesulide safety to its pharmacokinetics: assessment of adverse reactions. Rheumatology (Oxford) 1999;38(Suppl 1):4–10.
17. Rodrigo L, De Francisco R, Perez-Pariente JM, Cadahia V, Tojo R, Rodriguez M, Lucena MI, Andrade RJ. Nimesulide-induced severe hemolytic anemia and acute liver failure leading to liver transplantation. Scand J Gastroenterol 2002;37:1341–3.
18. Andrade RJ, Lucena MI, Fernandez MC, Gonzalez M. Fatal hepatitis associated with nimesulide. J Hepatol 2000;32(1):174.
19. Schattner A, Sokolovskaya N, Cohen J. Fatal hepatitis and renal failure during treatment with nimesulide. J Intern Med 2000;247(1):153–5.
20. Tolman KG. Hepatotoxicity of non-narcotic analgesics. Am J Med 1998;105(1B):S13–9.
21. Anonymous. Portugal suspends paediatric nimesulide. Scrip 1999;20:2431.
22. Leone R, Conforti A, Ghiotto E, Moretti U, Valvo E, Velo GP. Nimesulide and renal impairment. Eur J Clin Pharmacol 1999;55(2):151–4.
23. Peruzzi L, Gianoglio B, Porcellini MG, Coppo R. Neonatal end-stage renal failure associated with maternal ingestion of cyclo-oxygenase-type-1 [Sic] selective inhibitor nimesulide as tocolytic. Lancet 1999;354(9190):1615.
24. Balasubramaniam J. Nimesulide and neonatal renal failure. Lancet 2000;355(9203):575.
25. Holmes RP, Stone PR. Severe oligohydramnios induced by cyclooxygenase-2 inhibitor nimesulide. Obstet Gynecol 2000;96(5 Pt 2):810–1.

Nitronaproxen

General Information

Nitronaproxen, naproxen nitroxybutylester, is a naproxen derivative with similar anti-inflammatory activity to naproxen, but with less gastrointestinal toxicity by virtue of nitric oxide donation (1). It was originally being developed by a company called NicOx in partnership with AstraZeneca, but the latter wihtdrew in 2003 and NicOx reacquired the rights to the compound.

Organs and Systems

Gastrointestinal

In a small, short term, crossover, endoscopic study in healthy volunteers, nitronaproxen caused less gastrointestinal damage than naproxen (2). However, no firm conclusions can be made and confirmation is required in large, prospective, comparative trials.

Oxametacin

General Information

The adverse reactions pattern of oxametacin is similar to that of indometacin. In one study, 17% of 771 patients taking oxametacin had adverse effects, which led to withdrawal of treatment in 87. Gastrointestinal adverse effects accounted for 60% and nervous system reactions (headache, dizziness) for 31% (3).

References

1. Anonymous. Nitronaproxen: AZD 3582, HCT 3012, naproxen nitroxybutylester, NO-naproxen. Drugs RD 2006;7(4):262–6.
2. Hawkey CJ, Jones JI, Atherton CT, Skelly MM, Bebb JR, Fagerholm U, Jonzon B, Karlsson P, Bjarnason IT. Gastrointestinal safety of AZD3582, a cyclooxygenase inhibiting nitrioxide donator: proof of concept study in humans. Gut 2003;52:1537–42.
3. Demay F, De Sy J. A new non-steroidal anti-imflammatory (NSAID) in current rheumatological practice (oxamethacin). Curr Ther Res 1982;31:113.

Oxaprozin

General Information

In controlled studies, oxaprozin caused adverse effects in 23–58% of patients (1). It was considered better than aspirin and similar to other NSAIDs in long-term studies (2). However, treatment had to be interrupted owing to adverse effects in 8–31% of patients.

Organs and Systems

Nervous system

Headache, dizziness, vertigo, and tinnitus are less frequent with oxaprozin than with indometacin or aspirin (3,4).

Metabolism

Drug-induced pseudoporphyria has been ascribed to oxaprozin (SEDA-21, 106).

Liver

There were minor rises in transaminase activity in 10–20% of patients taking oxaprozin. Liver function should be monitored, especially during the first 6 months of therapy. Fulminant hepatitis has been reported (5).

Urinary tract

Of 847 patients with different rheumatic diseases who took oxaprozin daily for up to 1 year, 6% developed significant rises in blood urea nitrogen or creatinine, but a severe adverse renal effect occurred in only one patient (SEDA-12, 87). Oxaprozin can cause membranous nephropathy with nephrotic syndrome (SEDA-21, 106).

Skin

Under 5% of patients taking oxaprozin develop rashes. Some have phototoxic reactions (SEDA-12, 87).

Toxic epidermal necrolysis occurred in a 71-year-old man after treatment with oxaprozin for shoulder pain (6).

Immunologic

Life-threatening respiratory distress, facial edema, and lethargy occurred in a woman with a history of severe asthma and aspirin allergy (SEDA-22, 118).

Susceptibility Factors

Age

Older patients are more likely to have gastrointestinal and nephrotoxic reactions to oxaprozin. In this respect, it differs little from other NSAIDs.

Drug–Drug Interactions

Cimetidine

The clinical significance of the reduced renal clearance of oxaprozin when it is given concomitantly with cimetidine is not clear (SEDA-12, 87).

Ranitidine

The clinical significance of the reduced renal clearance of oxaprozin when it is given concomitantly with ranitidine is not clear (SEDA-12, 87).

References

1. Hubsher JA, Ballard IM, Walker BR, Gold JA. A multicentre double-blind comparison of oxaprozin aspirin therapy on rheumatoid arthritis. J Int Med Res 1979;7(1):69–76.
2. Jamar R, Dequeker J. Oxaprozin versus aspirin in rheumatoid arthritis: a double-blind trial. Curr Med Res Opin 1978;5(6):433–8.
3. Kolodny AL, Klipper AR, Harris BK, et al. The efficacy and safety of single daily doses of oxaprozin in the treatment of osteoarthritis: a comparison with aspirin. Semin Arthritis Rheum 1986;15:72.
4. Barber JV, Collins RL, Kitridou RC, et al. The efficacy and safety of single daily doses of oxaprozin in the treatment of rheumatoid arthritis: a comparison with aspirin. Semin Arthritis Rheum 1986;15:90.
5. Purdum PP 3rd, Shelden SL, Boyd JW, Shiffman ML. Oxaprozin-induced fulminant hepatitis. Ann Pharmacother 1994;28(10):1159–61.
6. Carucci JA, Cohen DE. Toxic epidermal necrolysis following treatment with oxaprozin. Int J Dermatol 1999;38(3):233–4.

Oxyphenbutazone

General Information

Oxyphenbutazone is a parahydroxylated analogue of phenylbutazone, and is one of its active metabolites. It has the same spectrum of activity, therapeutic uses, interactions, dangers, and contraindications. In April 1985, Ciba-Geigy decided to stop sales of systemic dosage forms of oxyphenbutazone worldwide. They stated that they had reached this decision because a survey had shown that although the recommended limitations on the use of phenylbutazone had been widely respected, the same could not be said of oxyphenbutazone. Evidence that oxyphenbutazone was more likely to cause death due to bone marrow failure than phenylbutazone (1) was provided by data from the UK's Committee on Safety of Medicines. Furthermore, according to Ciba-Geigy's reassessment in January 1984, deaths per million prescriptions of oxyphenbutazone were 5.5 (USA) to 12.8 (UK) compared with phenylbutazone (3.8–7.6 deaths per million prescriptions) (SEDA-9, 87).

Reference

1. Anonymous. Phenylbutazone and oxyphenbutazone: time to call a halt. Drug Ther Bull 1984;22(2):5–6.

Parecoxib

See also COX-2 inhibitors

General Information

Parecoxib sodium is an injectable COX-2 inhibitor developed for the treatment of acute pain. It is a prodrug of a sulfonamide-based COX-2 inhibitor, valdecoxib, a potent anti-inflammatory and analgesic drug. The published information on this compound is inadequate to draw any conclusion about its tolerability. Single-dose and multiple-dose studies have not shown any safety problems compared with placebo (1–4). In small short-term endoscopic studies parecoxib was much better tolerated than the non-selective NSAID ketorolac (5,6). However, it should be noted that valdecoxib was withdrawn in 2005 (7).

Organs and Systems

Cardiovascular

See COX-2 inhibitors

Respiratory

Non-selective NSAIDs are more likely to precipitate bronchoconstriction than COX-2 inhibitors (SEDA-26, 119). However, there has been a recent report of two patients who developed severe, life-threatening bronchospasm soon after receiving parenteral parecoxib (8). Both had a history of mild asthma. This suggests that COX-2 inhibitors are not without risk and should be used with great caution, especially in patients with asthma.

Urinary tract

The effects of intravenous parecoxib 40 mg on renal function have been studied in 75 elderly patients undergoing orthopedic surgery in a randomized placebo-controlled study (9). During the first 2 hours after the dose, creatinine clearance fell from 125 to 86, whereas there were no effects in groups who were given placebo or paracetamol.

References

1. Sorbera LA, Leeson PA, Castaner J, Castaner RM. Valdecoxib and parecoxib sodium. Analgesic, antiarthritic, cyclooxygenase inhibitor. Drugs Future 2001;26:133–40.
2. Cheer SM, Goa KL. Parecoxib (parecoxib sodium). Drugs 2001;61(8):1133–41.
3. Karim A, Laurent A, Slater ME, Kuss ME, Qian J, Crosby-Sessoms SL, Hubbard RC. A pharmacokinetic study of intramuscular (i.m.) parecoxib sodium in normal subjects J Clin Pharmacol 2001;41(10):1111–9.
4. Daniels SE, Grossman EH, Kuss ME, Talwalker S, Hubbard RC. A double-blind, randomized comparison of intramuscularly and intravenously administered parecoxib sodium versus ketorolac and placebo in a post-oral surgery pain model. Clin Ther 2001;23(7):1018–31.
5. Stoltz RR, Harris SI, Kuss ME, LeComte D, Talwalker S, Dhadda S, Hubbard RC. Upper GI mucosal effects of parecoxib sodium in healthy elderly subjects. Am J Gastroenterol 2002;97(1):65–71.
6. Harris SI, Kuss M, Hubbard RC, Goldstein JL. Upper gastrointestinal safety evaluation of parecoxib sodium, a new parenteral cyclooxygenase-2-specific inhibitor, compared with ketorolac, naproxen, and placebo. Clin Ther 2001;23(9):1422–8.
7. Cotter J, Woolterton E. New restriction on celecoxib (Celebrex) use and the withdrawal of valdecoxib (Bextra). CMAJ 2005;172(10):1299.
8. Looney Y, O'Shea A, O'Dwyer R. Severe bronchospasm after parenteral parecoxib: cyclooxygenase-2 inhibitors: not the answer yet. Anesthesiology 2005; 102: 473–5.
9. Koppert W, Frötsch K, Huzurudin N, Böswald W, Griessinger N, Weisbach V, Schmieder RE, Schüttler J. The effects of paracetamol and parecoxib on kidney function in elderly patients undergoing orthopedic surgery. Anesth Analg 2006;103(5):1170–6.

Phenylbutazone

General Information

Phenylbutazone was originally a solubilizing agent for aminopyrine and was first used to treat rheumatoid arthritis and allied disorders in 1949. Phenylbutazone and its related compounds were used worldwide until the early 1980s when, following growing concern about their safety, Ciba-Geigy published its own international assessment on phenylbutazone (Butazolidine) and oxyphenbutazone (Tanderil), which summarized reports on 1182 deaths associated with them from their initial use until 1982 (SEDA-9, 85). The report showed that the percentage of serious unwanted effects was high for both drugs, and in both cases the most frequent problems were dermatological and hematological, closely followed by gastrointestinal disorders.

Since 1983 phenylbutazone and oxyphenbutazone have been removed from the market in many countries or have been limited to specific indications. In 1985, Ciba-Geigy decided to stop sales of systemic dosage forms of oxyphenbutazone worldwide and to reduce the indications for phenylbutazone (SEDA-9, 85) (SEDA-10, 78). Nevertheless, phenylbutazone is still to be found in many places. Phenylbutazone and its congeners are now used only for ankylosing spondylitis and sometimes for acute gout, psoriatic arthritis, and active rheumatoid arthritis in patients who have not responded to other therapy, including other NSAIDs. For other indications, less toxic alternatives suffice (1,2).

All combinations of butazone derivatives and a corticosteroid have been removed from the market, even in Germany, one of the most lenient countries in the regulation of phenylbutazone use.

Significant adverse effects can affect up to 40% of patients (3).

Pyrazinobutazone is pyrazine phenylbutazone, which is metabolized to phenylbutazone (4).

General adverse effects

Most of the adverse effects of phenylbutazone are on the gastrointestinal system; they include symptoms ranging from gastric irritation to ulcer perforation and bleeding. Salt and water retention leads to edema, which is undesirable in older patients, and even to congestive heart failure. Hematological adverse effects include blood dyscrasias, lymphadenopathy, and agranulocytosis. Hepatotoxicity and nephrotoxicity occur (5). Headache is common, but other nervous system effects are mild. Acute poisoning can be successfully treated by hemoperfusion (6). Hypersensitivity reactions can be very severe (7); asthma and systemic lupus erythematosus have been reported. Tumor-inducing effects have not been reported.

Organs and Systems

Cardiovascular

Salt and water retention (see the section on Fluid balance in this monograph) are particularly dangerous for patients with impaired cardiac function. Hypertension due to increased plasma volume readily occurs.

Respiratory

Left ventricular failure can result in pleural effusions. Asthma can be provoked. Cross-reactivity with aspirin has been noted (8). A picture resembling allergic alveolitis has been described (9).

Nervous system

Therapeutic doses of phenylbutazone can be followed by headache, dizziness, and vertigo (10). Overdose can cause coma and convulsions (11).

Sensory systems

Phenylbutazone can damage the eyes. Conjunctivitis, damage to the cornea with vascularization and scarring, adhesion of the lids to the eyeballs, amblyopia, retinal hemorrhage, and even blindness have been reported (12).

Psychological, psychiatric

Psychomotor reactions to phenylbutazone when driving have been reported (13).

Endocrine

Because of interference with iodine uptake, hypothyroidism and goiter can result (14). The condition is reversible, but an obstructive syndrome due to thyroid enlargement has been observed (14).

Fluid balance

As many as 10% of patients show signs of salt and fluid retention and edema (7). Increased intravascular fluid volume is responsible for dilution anemia and increasing cardiac load (SED-8, 216). There is still no explanation for the water-retaining effect, but it might reflect increased production of antidiuretic hormone.

Hematologic

Phenylbutazone causes blood dyscrasias (SED-8, 213; SEDA-2, 92; 7,15). The most serious adverse effect is aplastic anemia which, according to Swedish and British sources, ends fatally in almost 50% of cases (15,16,17). More than 1100 deaths are on record with the principal manufacturer (SEDA-8, Essay).

Specific anti-platelet antibodies can cause thrombocytopenic purpura (18), which can be fatal. The increased risk of leukemia after phenylbutazone could be secondary to bone marrow depression (SED-9, 143; 19).

Agranulocytosis and liver injury have been described in a patient with Reiter's syndrome who took pyrazinobutazone for 6 weeks (20). Other causes of agranulocytosis and hepatic damage were excluded and a lymphocyte transformation test showed significant lymphocyte proliferation in response to pyrazinobutazone.

Gastrointestinal

A potent gastric and intestinal irritant, phenylbutazone can cause ulcers and bleeding. In one study in 1975, when the drug was widely used, 19% of 241 cases had acute gastrointestinal bleeding due to phenylbutazone (21). According to the UK's Committee on Safety of Medicines, 120 of 1967 adverse reactions attributed to phenylbutazone and its metabolite oxyphenbutazone involved gastrointestinal bleeding, and 32 ended fatally (22). The risk of developing a peptic ulcer during phenylbutazone therapy is estimated at 1–3% (SED-8, 214). Perforation has also been repeatedly observed (21,23). Other adverse effects are nausea, vomiting, abdominal pain, heartburn, diarrhea, and abdominal discomfort.

Even rectal and enteric-coated formulations can cause adverse reactions in the upper gastrointestinal tract. In one double-blind, crossover trial, plain naproxen caused fewer gastrointestinal adverse effects than enteric-coated phenylbutazone (Butacote) (24).

Phenylbutazone suppositories can cause rectal irritation, with mucosal defects, severe hemorrhagic proctitis (25), perforation of the large bowel, and necrotizing colitis (26).

Gastrointestinal toxicity has been reported in a patient treated short-term with pyrazinobutazone (27).

Liver

Hepatotoxicity has been clearly documented (28). Phenylbutazone causes three types of liver damage through three separate pathogenic mechanisms:

1. acute hepatic necrosis after overdosage, related to the hepatotoxicity of phenylbutazone and/or its metabolites;
2. mild hepatocellular damage (with or without cholestasis) and granulomas (sometimes also found at extrahepatic sites, with varying degrees of steatosis); these changes are the result of hypersusceptibility and possibly a certain degree of toxicity;
3. more pronounced hepatocellular damage with cholestasis but without granulomas; toxicity plays a more important role than hypersusceptibility.

Concomitant treatment with other hepatotoxic agents can predispose to phenylbutazone-induced liver toxicity.

Urinary tract

Although adverse renal effects can occur with any NSAID, phenylbutazone-induced nephrotoxicity has mainly been reported when the drug was taken in association with other anti-inflammatory agents (SED-8, 215) or when taken alone in a high dose (29).

Skin

Skin eruptions, Quincke's edema, and even epidermal necrolysis (SEDA-5, 100) (30,31) can develop during or after phenylbutazone therapy.

Considerable local irritation and pain at the site of injection are sometimes followed by necrosis. Sterile abscess formation has also been reported (32).

Long-Term Effects

Mutagenicity

Phenylbutazone infusion for 10 days induced chromosomal abnormalities in patients with rheumatoid arthritis (33), although the significance of this finding is not clear.

Second-Generation Effects

Lactation

If phenylbutazone is taken during lactation, only small amounts are found in the milk (34).

Susceptibility Factors

Age

The risk of adverse reactions to phenylbutazone increases with age (SED-8, 213) (17).

Other features of the patient

The specific risks of salt and water retention in cardiac and renal disease have already been mentioned. The potential for ulcerogenic activity should be kept in mind if phenylbutazone is given to a patient with a history of peptic ulceration. Patients who are hypersensitive to other drugs (especially aspirin) should be carefully monitored when taking phenylbutazone.

Drug Administration

Drug overdose

Acute intoxication with phenylbutazone is dominated by metabolic acidosis, which can progress to coma, seizures, hypotension, shock, and oliguria. Kidney and liver reactions, acute bone marrow depression, and acute perforation of peptic ulcer have all been described (5,11,35).

Drug–Drug Interactions

Antihypertensive agents

Inhibition of the effect of antihypertensive agents by phenylbutazone can probably be explained by salt and water retention (36).

Aspirin

Phenylbutazone interferes with the tubular excretion of aspirin (3).

Coumarin anticoagulants

Phenylbutazone displaces warfarin from binding sites on serum albumin, temporarily increasing its effects before the clearance of warfarin increases because of an increase in the unbound fraction (37). If that were the only mechanism, this interaction would not be important. However, phenylbutazone also inhibits the metabolism of *S*-warfarin and induces the metabolism of *R*-warfarin (38); the half-life of racemic warfarin is unchanged, but because the *S* isomer is more potent than the *R* isomer, the action of warfarin is potentiated (SED-9, 144) (36,39).

Oral hypoglycemic drugs

Phenylbutazone can potentiate the hypoglycemic effects of the sulfonylureas acetohexamide (40), chlorpropamide (41), tolbutamide (42), and glibenclamide (43). One mechanism of this interaction is interference with tubular excretion (3).

Penicillins

Phenylbutazone interferes with the tubular excretion of penicillins (3).

Phenytoin

Phenylbutazone can reduce the clearance of phenytoin by inhibiting CYP2C9 (44).

Sulfinpyrazone

Sulfinpyrazone has a biphasic interaction with phenylbutazone (enhancement followed by antagonism).

Sulfonamides

Phenylbutazone can displace sulfonamides from protein-binding sites (SED-9, 144) (45).

Interference with Diagnostic Tests

Thyroid function tests

Phenylbutazone inhibits thyroid uptake of iodine and/or competes for protein-binding sites with thyroxine (SED-9, 145) (46,47), and can thus interfere with the use of thyroid function tests.

References

1. Anonymous. BGA "loose" Butazone Coombs warning. Scrip 1985;974:8.
2. Anonymous. Mofebuzone restriction explained. Scrip 1985;965:1.
3. In: Martindale: The Extra Pharmacopoeia. 28th ed.. London: The Pharmaceutical Press, 1983:273.
4. von Bruchhausen V, Lohmann H, O'svath J. The pharmacokinetic profile of pyrazinobutazone in man. Arzneimittelforschung 1978;28(12):2337–43.
5. Prescott LF, Critchley JA, Balali-Mood M. Phenylbutazone overdosage: abnormal metabolism associated with hepatic and renal damage. BMJ 1980;281(6248):1106–7.
6. Berlinger WG, Spector R, Flanigan MJ, Johnson GF, Groh MR. Hemoperfusion for phenylbutazone poisoning. Ann Intern Med 1982;96(3):334–5.
7. Adverse Drug Reactions Advisory Committee. Phenylbutazone. Med J Aust 1979;2:553.
8. Szczeklik A, Gryglewski RJ, Czerniawska-Mysik G. Relationship of inhibition of prostaglandin biosynthesis by analgesics to asthma attacks in aspirin-sensitive patients. BMJ 1975;1(5949):67–9.
9. Thurston JG, Marks P, Trapnell D. Lung changes associated with phenylbutazone treatment. BMJ 1976;2(6049):1422–3.
10. Rechenberg HK. In: Phenylbutazone. London: Edward Arnold Ltd, 1962:113–20 125–5, 131.
11. Anvik T. Akutt forgittning med fenylbutazon. [Acute poisoning with phenylbutazone.] Tidsskr Nor Laegeforen 1970;90(2):95–7.
12. Willetts GS. Ocular side-effects of drugs. Br J Ophthalmol 1969;53(4):252–62.
13. Linnoila M, Seppalla M, Mattila MJ. Acute effect of antipyretic analgesics alone or in combination with alcohol on human psychomotor skills related to driving. Br J Clin Pharmacol 1974;1:477.
14. Schwarzmann E, Quast M. Kasuistische Betrachtungen zur Phenylbutazon-Struma. Dtsch Gesundheitsw 1973;28:1417.
15. Bottiger LE, Westerholm B. Drug-induced blood dyscrasias in Sweden. BMJ 1973;3(5875):339–43.
16. Bottiger LE. Phenylbutazone, oxyphenbutazone and aplastic anaemia. BMJ 1977;2(6081):265.
17. Inman WH. Study of fatal bone marrow depression with special reference to phenylbutazone and oxyphenbutazone. BMJ 1977;1(6075):1500–5.
18. Davidson C, Manohitharajah SM. Drug-induced antiplatelet antibodies. BMJ 1973;3(5879):545.
19. Hartwich G, Lutz H. Leukämieentstehung nach benzol und phenylbutazon. [Leukemia origin after benzene and phenylbutazone.] Verh Dtsch Ges Inn Med 1973;79:394–6.
20. Maria VA, da Silva JA, Victorino RM. Agranulocytosis and liver damage associated with pyrazinobutazone with evidence for an immunological mechanism. J Rheumatol 1989;16(11):1484–5.
21. Schwenke W, Schwenke G, Willgeroth C. Die grosse obere Gastrointestinalblutung unter besonderer Berucksichtigung der akuten Magenschleimhäutlasionen durch Medikamente. Z Gesamte Inn Med Ihre Grenzgeb 1975;30:198.
22. Cuthbert MF. Adverse reactions to non-steroidal antirheumatic drugs. Curr Med Res Opin 1974;2(9):600–10.
23. Schwabe H. Magenperforation und Blutung nach langeren Gaben von Antirheumatika. 2. [Stomach perforation and hemorrhage after long-term administration of antirheumatic agents.] Z Allgemeinmed 1975;51(25):1097–8.
24. Ansell BM, Major G, Liyanage SP, Gumpel JM, Seifert MH, Mathews JA, Engler C. A comparative study of Butacote and Naprosyn in ankylosing spondylitis. Ann Rheum Dis 1978;37(5):436–9.
25. Cheli R, Ciancamerla G. Proctiti emorragiche da medicamenti locali. [Hemorrhagic proctitis due to local drugs.] Minerva Gastroenterol 1974;20(2):56.
26. Liaras H, Neidhardt JH, Tairraz JP, Lesbros F, Guelpa G. Les entérites et colites aiguës nécrosantes: essai nosologique et pathogenique—étude clinique: à propos de 8 cas. [Acute necrosing colitis and enteritis. Nosologic and pathogenic attempt. Clinical study (apropos of 8 cases).] J Chir (Paris) 1968;96(6):501–18.
27. Ritschard T, Filippini L. Nebenwirkungen nichtsteroidaler Antirheumatika auf den unteren Intestinaltrakt. [Side effects of non-steroidal antirheumatic agents on the lower intestinal tract.] Dtsch Med Wochenschr 1986;111(41):1561–4.
28. Benjamin SB, Ishak KG, Zimmerman HJ, Grushka A. Phenylbutazone liver injury: a clinical-pathologic survey of 23 cases and review of the literature. Hepatology 1981;1(3):255–63.
29. Wigley RA. The New Zealand experience. Aust NZ J Med 1976;6(Suppl 1):37–44.
30. Eischbeck R, Huhle G, Stiller D, Zucker G. Durch immunologische in vitro Untersuchungen gesicherte hochgradige Phenylbutazon Uberempfindlichkeit bei einem Fall von Morbus Lyell. Dtsch Gesundheitsw 1975;30:2331.
31. Zurcher K, Krebs A. Nebenwirkungen interner Arzneimittel auf die Haut unter besonderer Berudcksichtigung neuerer

Medikamente. [Cutaneous side effects of systemic drugs with special reference to recently introduced medicaments. I.] Dermatologica 1970;141(2):119–29.

32. Hadida A, Groulier P. Nécrose de la fesse après une injection de phénylbutazone. Marseille Chir 1968;20:270.

33. Vormittag W, Kolarz G. Chromosomenuntersuchungen vor und nach Infusionstherapie mit Phenylbutazon. [Chromosome studies before and after phenylbutazone infusion therapy.] Arzneimittelforschung 1979;29(8):1163–8.

34. Strobel E, Herrmann B. [On the problem of the passage of oxyphenbutazone into the fetal circulation and maternal milk.]Arzneimittelforschung 1962;12:302–5.

35. Farber D, Liel E. Phenylbutazon-Vergiftung in Kindesalter. Tadgl Prax 1968;9:231.

36. Polak F. Die hemmende Wirkung von Phenylbutazon auf die durch einige Antihypertonika hervorgerufene Blutdrucksenkung bei Hypertonikern. [The inhibitory effect of phenylbutazone on lowered blood pressure produced by antihypertensives in hypertensive patients.] Z Gesamte Inn Med 1967;22(12):375–6.

37. Lewis RJ, Trager WF, Chan KK, Breckenridge A, Orme M, Roland M, Schary W. Warfarin. Stereochemical aspects of its metabolism and the interaction with phenylbutazone. J Clin Invest 1974;53(6):1607–17.

38. O'Reilly RA, Goulart DA. Comparative interaction of sulfinpyrazone and phenylbutazone with racemic warfarin: alteration in vivo of free fraction of plasma warfarin. J Pharmacol Exp Ther 1981;219(3):691–4.

39. Aggeler PM, O'Reilly RA, Leong L, Kowitz PE. Potentiation of anticoagulant effect of warfarin by phenylbutazone. N Engl J Med 1967;276(9):496–501.

40. Field JB, Ohta M, Boyle C, Remer A. Potentiation of acetohexamide hypoglycemia by phenylbutazone. N Engl J Med 1967;277(17):889–94.

41. Shah SJ, Bhandarkar SD, Satoskar RS. Drug interaction between chlorpropamide and non-steroidal anti-inflammatory drugs, ibuprofen and phenylbutazone. Int J Clin Pharmacol Ther Toxicol 1984;22(9):470–2.

42. Szita M, Gachalyi B, Tornyossy M, Kaldor A. Interaction of phenylbutazone and tolbutamide in man. Int J Clin Pharmacol Ther Toxicol 1980;18(9):378–80.

43. Schulz E, Koch K, Schmidt FH. [Potentiation of the hypoglycemic effect of sulfonylurea derivatives by drugs. II. Pharmacokinetics and metabolism of glibenclamide (HB 419) in presence of phenylbutazone.]Eur J Clin Pharmacol 1971;4(1):32–7.

44. Levy RH. Cytochrome P450 isozymes and antiepileptic drug interactions. Epilepsia 1995;36(Suppl 5):S8–S13.

45. Wardell WM. Drug displacement from protein binding: source of the sulphadoxine liberated by phenylbutazone. Br J Pharmacol 1971;43(2):325–34.

46. Aly FW, Hadam W, Kallee E, Kloss G. Veränderungen des freien Thyroxins unter kurzfristiger Phenylbutazon-Behandlung. Nucl -Med (Stuttg) 1970;(Suppl):195–8.

47. Bartha KG. Iodine kinetics of the organism under the influence of phenylbutazone. Acta Med Acad Sci Hung 1971;28(3):271–7.

Piketoprofen

General Information

Piketoprofen is an NSAID that has been used topically as the hydrochloride salt.

Organs and Systems

Skin

A photoallergic contact dermatitis followed topical administration of piketoprofen in a 46-year-old man after 3 days; photopatch testing for piketoprofen was positive (1).

Reference

1. Bujan JJ, Morante JM, Guemes MG, Del Pozo Losada J, Capdevila EF. Photoallergic contact dermatitis from piketoprofen. Contact Dermatitis 2000;43(5):315.

Pipebuzone

General Information

Pipebuzone is a combination of phenylbutazone with piperazine, produced in an unsuccessful attempt to improve the tolerance of phenylbutazone. Typical phenylbutazone reactions (abdominal, hematological, renal, allergic, and rectal irritation from suppositories) were common (SED-9, 145; 1–3).

References

1. Poulain D. Bilan de l'utilisation de l'élarzone dausse en chirurgie gynécologique et obstétricale. A propos de 228 cas. Arch Med Ouest 1976;8:117.

2. Chovelon R, Hovasse BM. Expérimentation de l'élarzonedausse, nouvel antiinflammatoire, dans les affectations des voies respiratoires chez les personnes âgées. Med Int Pol 1975;10:179.

3. Pelissier P, Colas IJ, Beaulieux J. Expérimentation de l'élarzone dausse dans un service de chirurgie vasculaire. J Méd Lyon 1974;55:709.

Pirazolac

General Information

Pirazolac, a pyrazoloacetic acid derivative, caused heartburn, upper abdominal pain, cutaneous adverse effects (rashes, exacerbation of pre-existing eczema), and eosinophilia in early clinical studies (1). In two comparative studies it was withdrawn in 15–20% of patients, that is more often than the comparator NSAIDs (indometacin, sulindac) (SEDA-16, 111).

Reference

1. Symmons D, Clark B, Panayi G, Geddawi M. Differential dosing study of pirazolac, a new non-steroidal anti-inflammatory agent, in patients with rheumatoid arthritis. Curr Med Res Opin 1985;9(8):542–7.

Piroxicam

General Information

Piroxicam was the first of the oxicam compounds, and is by far the most widely used. It is an inhibitor of prostaglandin synthesis and platelet aggregation. Its long half-life (36–48 hours) allows it to be given in a single daily dose. Adverse effects data from 46 trials in 3827 patients, 2716 on short-term treatment (less than 12 weeks), have been reviewed (SEDA-6, 1; 1). In 20 controlled trials in 816 patients, adverse effects occurred in 27%, causing withdrawal in 2.2%. However, an uncontrolled study registered adverse effects in only 16% of patients. Allowing for all analyses and reviews, the overall adverse effects profile of piroxicam seems to be qualitatively the same as that of other NSAIDs, with gastrointestinal complaints at the top of the list.

Reactions involving the gastrointestinal system occur in up to 40% of patients. The approximately 1% incidence of peptic ulcer appears to be dose-related, as it rises to 7% in patients who take dosages higher than 20 mg/day for several weeks (2). Nervous system reactions are the second most frequent types of adverse effect. Changes in laboratory findings (creatinine, aspartate transaminase, alanine transaminase) are frequent, but they have little clinical relevance. Hypersensitivity reactions do not seem to be a problem with piroxicam treatment, although skin or mucosal reactions have been reported. Shock has been described. Tumor-inducing effects have not been reported.

Cinnoxicam is the cinnamate ester of piroxicam; its adverse effects are similar. Gastrointestinal effects (81%), nervous system effects (4%), and cutaneous effects (4%) were most common in a multicenter postmarketing surveillance study of 2969 patients; 12% had adverse effects (SEDA-16, 113). Cinnoxicam cream can cause itchy erythema, edema, vesicles, and exudation (SEDA-20, 94).

Organs and Systems

Respiratory

In two cases piroxicam caused pulmonary infiltrates and eosinophilia (SEDA-19, 99).

Nervous system

Adverse effects in about 11% of patients include headache, dizziness, drowsiness, fatigue, and sweating (3).

Sensory systems

Eyes
Blurred vision and burning eyes have been described with piroxicam (SEDA-5, 107).

Ears
Permanent sensorineural hearing loss and tinnitus have been described with piroxicam (4).

Electrolyte balance

Severe hyponatremia, characterized by increasing confusion and disorientation, has been reported (SEDA-13, 83).

Hyperkalemia has often been linked to prolonged use of piroxicam, especially in the elderly (SEDA-8, 110) (SEDA-10, 87).

Hematologic

Piroxicam can cause thrombocytopenia, including a case of thrombocytopenic purpura due to an immunological mechanism (SEDA-13, 83). As an inhibitor of prostaglandin synthesis, piroxicam also inhibits platelet aggregation and prolongs bleeding time.

Leukopenia has been reported; the leukocyte count returned to normal after withdrawal (5). Agranulocytosis in a woman who took piroxicam for 3 days disappeared rapidly after withdrawal (SEDA-14, 95).

Aplastic anemia, which resolved fully after withdrawal, has been described (SEDA-17, 114).

Gastrointestinal

Gastrointestinal effects are the most frequent adverse effects of piroxicam. Although epigastric distress, nausea, abdominal pain, constipation, flatulence, and diarrhea have all been reported, they rarely interfere with treatment.

Esophageal lesions have been recorded in young healthy volunteers taking piroxicam (6).

An unusual case of gastrocolic fistula occurred in an old man who had taken piroxicam for 2 months (7).

Peptic ulceration and gastrointestinal bleeding were recorded in 1–1.4% of patients taking piroxicam 20 mg/day, and the incidence of ulceration increased to 6.9% at a dosage of 40 mg/day. A comparative study of gastrointestinal blood loss after aspirin 972 mg qds for 4 days versus different doses of piroxicam (20 mg od, 5 mg qds, and 10 mg qds) showed that piroxicam did not increase fecal blood loss, whereas aspirin did. Gastroscopic evidence of irritation was also greater with aspirin (8). The debate on the ulcerogenicity and relative safety of piroxicam continues, as new reports are published (SEDA-10, 85; SEDA-11, 97; SEDA-12, 91). As the perfect epidemiological study has yet not been carried out, the only thing that can be said is that piroxicam's ulcerogenicity increases with dosage and that 20 mg/day constitutes high-dose therapy, especially in elderly women.

Piroxicam can cause diaphragm-like strictures of the intestinal tract (9).

- A 65 year-old woman who had taken piroxicam for the previous 3 years presented with frequent episodes of abdominal bloating and cramping, sometimes associated with nausea and vomiting, and loss of weight. Small bowel examination showed several mid-ileal strictures associated with proximal dilated bowel.

Liver

Transient rises in aspartate transaminase and alanine transaminase can occur (10). Biopsy-proven hepatitis was noted in one patient who was also taking other medications (SEDA-5, 107). Cases of acute hepatitis have been described. Two elderly women developed acute hepatocellular injury, which progressed to fatal subacute hepatic necrosis (SEDA-12, 93; 11,12).

Pancreas

Acute pancreatitis has been reported in a patient taking piroxicam (13).

Urinary tract

Piroxicam reduces renal blood flow by inhibition of renal prostaglandins. It can cause transient and probably insignificant rises in urea or blood urea nitrogen, without increases in serum creatinine concentrations. Renal function should be monitored during long-term therapy and piroxicam should be avoided in renal insufficiency. An occasional patient develops edema and dysuria.

Hematuria with purpuric rash and Henoch–Schönlein purpura have been described (14).

Fatal acute renal insufficiency due to diffuse interstitial nephritis has been described in a young man (SEDA-14, 95).

Skin

Minor, often transient, rashes are relatively common, as with other NSAIDs. Light-induced skin eruptions have been reported to national ADR monitoring centers in several countries and generally occur only 1–6 days after the start of therapy. They are characterized by pruritic, papulo-vesicular, or bullous eruptions, usually restricted to exposed areas. Clinical, histological, and provocation studies are not conclusive in distinguishing the eruptions as photoallergic or phototoxic (SEDA-13, 76) (SEDA-15, 103) (15). Cross-reactivity between thiosalicylic acid and piroxicam supports the hypothesis that piroxicam-induced photosensitive reactions have a photoallergic mechanism and occur soon after starting therapy when patients have previously been sensitized to thiosalicylate (SEDA-16, 113) (16). The wide range of adverse skin effects include several types of rashes, urticaria, vasculitis, and life-threatening reactions (toxic epidermal necrolysis, erythema multiforme, and pemphigus) (SEDA-8, 110) (SEDA-11, 192) (SEDA-13, 77). Fixed drug eruptions have also been described (SEDA-16, 113).

- After piroxicam intake and sun exposure a patient with Sjögren's syndrome developed the typical cutaneous lesions and serological markers of systemic lupus erythematosus, despite drug withdrawal (17).

The risk of the life-threatening adverse reactions such as Stevens–Johnson syndrome and toxic epidermal necrolysis associated with NSAIDs has been quantified in an analysis of three large data sources: first, an international case-control study of severe skin reactions (SCAR study); secondly, a population-based registry in Germany; thirdly, the spontaneous reporting system of the US Food and Drug Administration (FDA) (18).

In the SCAR study the oxicams were associated with the greatest increase in risk of Stevens–Johnson syndrome and toxic epidermal necrolysis, with a selective risk of 34 (95% CI=11, 105). When the risk for only recent use was compared with that for long term use (over 8 weeks), the relative risk of Stevens-Johnson syndrome and toxic epidermal necrolysis associated with oxicams was significantly increased. The German data registry confirmed these findings. The numbers of spontaneous reports of Stevens–Johnson syndrome and toxic epidermal necrolysis to the FDA were similar for piroxicam and other NSAIDs (diflunisal, etodolac, oxaprozin, sulindac). The authors concluded that the absolute risks of Stevens–Johnson syndrome and toxic epidermal necrolysis associated with NSAIDs are low.

Susceptibility Factors

Renal disease

Reduced piroxicam excretion increases the risk of gastrointestinal adverse effects. Most reports of these effects refer to elderly women, since impaired renal function in the elderly can lower excretion of the drug by 33%. Dosages should be as low as possible, and certainly not above 20 mg/day in these patients.

Drug Administration

Drug formulations

The adverse effects profile of suppositories, soluble tablet formulations, and standard capsules are similar (SEDA-13, 83). A parenteral formulation of piroxicam caused somnolence more often than diclofenac in a double-blind study, but diclofenac provoked more gastric discomfort and nausea than piroxicam. Local adverse effects of both drugs were pain, burning, and induration at the site of injection (SEDA-15, 103).

In an attempt to reduce gastric toxicity, piroxicam has been complexed with cyclodextrins. In healthy volunteers piroxicam beta-cyclodextrin is less toxic than either piroxicam or indometacin; gastrointestinal adverse effects were the most frequent (SEDA-16, 113).

A fast-dissolving form of piroxicam that can be taken under the tongue infrequently causes local adverse effects, including stomatitis, mucosal erythema, and dysesthesia (SEDA-20, 95).

Drug–Drug Interactions

Azithromycin

In 66 patients undergoing oral surgery, treatment with azithromycin impaired the periodontal disposition of piroxicam (22).

Furosemide

Furosemide natriuresis and kaliuresis can be reduced by short-term treatment with piroxicam in hypertensive patients with impaired renal function (SEDA-16, 113).

Lithium

Piroxicam can increase the risk of lithium toxicity (19–21).

Phenazone

The half-life of phenazone (antipyrine) was prolonged and its metabolic clearance significantly reduced in proportion to the dose of piroxicam administered to healthy young volunteers (SEDA-16, 113).

References

1. Pitts NE. Ubersicht udber die mit Piroxicam in klinischen Untersuchungen gewonnenen Erfahrungen. Aktuel Rheumatol 1980;5:53.
2. Pisko EJ, Rahaman MA, Turner RA, et al. Long term efficacy and safety of piroxicam in the treatment of rheumatoid arthritis. Curr Ther Res 1980;27:852.
3. Dessain P, Estabrooks TF, Gordon AJ. Piroxicam in the treatment of osteoarthrosis: a multicentre study in general practice involving 1218 patients. J Int Med Res 1979;7(5):335–43.
4. Vernick DM, Kelly JH. Sudden hearing loss associated with piroxicam. Am J Otol 1986;7(2):97–8.
5. Box J, Box P, Turner R, Pisko E. Piroxicam and rheumatoid arthritis: a double blind 16-week study comparing piroxicam and phenylbutazone. In: Piroxicam, International Congress and Symposium Series No. 1Royal Soceity of Medicine, 1978:1545.
6. Santucci L, Patoia L, Fiorucci S, Farroni F, Favero D, Morelli A. Oesophageal lesions during treatment with piroxicam. BMJ 1990;300(6730):1018.
7. Carver N, Wedgwood KR, Ralphs DN. Iatrogenic gastrocolic fistula associated with non-steroidal anti-inflammatory drug administration. Br J Clin Pract 1990;44(12):759–61.
8. Bianchine JR, Procter RR, Thomas FB. Piroxicam, aspirin, and gastrointestinal blood loss. Clin Pharmacol Ther 1982;32(2):247–52.
9. Abrahamian GA, Polhamus CD, Muskat P, Karulf RE. Diaphragm-like strictures of the ileum associated with NSAID use: a rare complication. South Med J 1998;91(4):395–7.
10. Blackburn WD Jr, Prupas HM, Silverfield JC, Poiley JE, Caldwell JR, Collins RL, Miller MJ, Sikes DH, Kaplan H, Fleischmann R, et al. Tenidap in rheumatoid arthritis. A 24-week double-blind comparison with hydroxychloroquine-plus-piroxicam, and piroxicam alone. Arthritis Rheum 1995;38(10):1447–56.
11. Planas R, De Leon R, Quer JC, Barranco C, Bruguera M, Gassull MA. Fatal submassive necrosis of the liver associated with piroxicam. Am J Gastroenterol 1990;85(4):468–70.
12. Honein K, Attali P, Pelletier G, Ink O. Hépatite aiguë due au piroxicam: un nouveau cas. [Acute hepatitis due to piroxicam: a new case.] Gastroenterol Clin Biol 1988;12(1):79.
13. Heluwaert F, Pofelski J, Germain E, Roblin X. Pancréatite aiguë au piroxicam. [Piroxicam and acute pancreatitis.] Gastroenterol Clin Biol 2006;30(4):635–6.
14. Goebel KM, Mueller-Brodmann W. Reversible overt nephropathy with Henoch–Schönlein purpura due to piroxicam. BMJ (Clin Res Ed) 1982;284(6312):311–2.
15. Ljunggren B. The piroxicam enigma. Photodermatol 1989;6(4):151–3.
16. Mammen L, Schmidt CP. Photosensitivity reactions: a case report involving NSAIDs. Am Fam Physician 1995;52(2):575–9.
17. Roura M, Lopez-Gil F, Umbert P. Systemic lupus erythematosus exacerbated by piroxicam. Dermatologica 1991;182(1):56–8.
18. Mockenhaupt M, Kelly JP, Kaufman D, Stern RS. SCAR Study Group. The risk of Stevens-Johnson syndrome and toxic epidermal necrolysis associated with nonsteroidal anti-inflammatory drugs: a multinational perspective. J Rheumatol 2003;30:2234–40.
19. Kerry RJ, Owen G, Michaelson S. Possible toxic interaction between lithium and piroxicam. Lancet 1983;1(8321):418–9.
20. Nadarajah J, Stein GS. Piroxicam induced lithium toxicity. Ann Rheum Dis 1985;44(7):502.
21. Walbridge DG, Bazire SR. An interaction between lithium carbonate and piroxicam presenting as lithium toxicity. Br J Psychiatry 1985;147:206–7.
22. Malizia T, Batoni G, Ghelardi E, Baschiera F, Graziani F, Blandizzi C, Gabriele M, Campa M, Del Tacca M, Senesi S. Interaction between piroxicam and azithromycin during distribution to human periodontal tissues. J Periodontol 2001;72(9):1151–6.

Pirprofen

General Information

In an open, non-comparative trial in 1506 patients, the adverse effects of pirprofen were mainly gastrointestinal, and consisted mostly of epigastric pain. There were single cases of an attack of asthma, iron deficiency anemia, leukopenia, and an increase in serum transaminases to more than 10 times normal (1). In a long-term trial, 9.7% of over 3000 patients stopped treatment because of poor tolerability. The manufacturers decided to discontinue marketing it worldwide, saying that this was a commercial decision (SEDA-16, 111).

Organs and Systems

Liver

Laboratory signs of hepatic damage were documented in 37 patients, including three cases of hepatitis (2); pirprofen can definitely be considered hepatotoxic.

References

1. Daubresse AJ. Pirprofen for the treatment of rheumatic disorders and post-traumatic lesions. Acta Ther 1984;10:97.
2. Salliere D, Alcalay M. Rangasil en traitement prolongé. Rheumatologie 1986;38:131.

Pranoprofen

General Information

Pranoprofen is an arylalkanoic acid NSAID (1).

Respiratory

Acute eosinophilic pneumonia has been attributed to pranoprofen in a 48-year-old man (2).

Gastrointestinal

Multiple small bowel ulcers and massive bleeding occurred in a patient taking oral pranoprofen and rectal indometacin (SEDA-17, 113).

Urinary tract

Hemolytic urenic syndrome has been reported in a 25-year-old woman on two separate occasions (3).

References

1. Yoshio I, Iwata A, Isobe M, Takamatsu R, Higashi M. [The pharmacokinetics of pranoprofen in humans.]Yakugaku Zasshi 1990;110(7):509–15.
2. Fujimori K, Shimatsu Y, Suzuki E, Gejyo F, Arakawa M. [Pranoprofen-induced lung injury manifesting as acute eosimophilic pneumonia.]Nihon Kokyuki Gakkai Zasshi 1999;37(5):401–5.
3. Okura H, Hino M, Nishiki S, Kono K, Hasegawa T, Nakamae H, Ohta K, Yamane T, Takubo T, Tatsumi N. [Recurrent hemolytic uremic syndrome induced by pranoprofen.]Rinsho Ketsueki 1999;40(8):663–6.

Proglumetacin

General Information

Proglumetacin, an indoleacetic acid derivative, is particularly associated with gastrointestinal adverse effects: in different trials 18–41% of patients had adverse effects, but not to the extent that they interfered with treatment. Comparisons of proglumetacin with indometacin and oxyphenbutazone showed that it is equally effective and usually better tolerated (SEDA-5, 103). In an uncontrolled, open, multicenter, short-term study in patients with cervical or low back pain treated with proglumetacin, the most frequent adverse effects were gastrointestinal, while adverse effects on the nervous system were rare (1).

Reference

1. Ginsberg F, Lefebvre D. A large, open-label study of proglumetacin in the treatment of patients with cervical and low-back pain. Curr Ther Res Clin Exp 1995;56:1237–46.

Rofecoxib

See also COX-2 inhibitors

General Information

Rofecoxib is a selective inhibitor of COX-2. Although it was originally introduced with the expectation that it would be safer than conventional NSAIDs, because of less gastrointestinal bleeding, the benefit to harm balance is now considered to be unfavorable during long-term treatment, mainly because of an increased risk of cardiovascular disease (heart attacks and strokes; see the monograph on COX-2 inhibitors), and it has been voluntarily withdrawn by its manufacturers.

Observational studies

The results of a post-marketing Prescription Event Monitoring study have better defined the safety profile of rofecoxib as used in general practice in England (1). Questionnaires requesting clinical event data were sent to prescribing physicians between February and November 2000. They identified 15 268 patients, mean age 62 years, 67% women. The commonest indication was osteoarthritis (24%). Dyspepsia and nausea were the most frequently reported adverse events. During treatment or within 1 month of withdrawal, 110 serious gastrointestinal events were reported, including 76 upper gastrointestinal tract bleeds/peptic ulcers and one perforated colon. Other events were: thromboembolism (n=101), acute renal insufficiency (n=3), Stevens-Johnson syndrome (n=1), severe anaphylaxis (n=1), and angioedema (n=1).

Organs and Systems

Cardiovascular

See also COX-2 inhibitors

Hypertensive patients taking rofecoxib are more likely to require an increase in their antihypertensive drug dosages (2) than those taking celecoxib: OR=1.68 (95% CI=1.09, 2.6).

Nervous system

Aseptic meningitis is a rare adverse effect of non-selective NSAIDs in patients with or without connective tissue disease or rheumatological disease. Rofecoxib has been implicated in five patients (four women and one man), in each case occurring within 12 days of the start of rofecoxib therapy (3). The clinical presentations and cerebrospinal fluid findings were typical of aseptic meningitis. One patient had rheumatoid arthritis. After drug withdrawal and recovery, two consecutive rechallenges in one patient led to relapses.

- A 28-year-old woman with a history of Sjögren's syndrome who had aseptic meningitis from two different non-selective NSAIDs (naproxen and ibuprofen) had similar symptoms 2 years later, after taking rofecoxib 25 mg/day for 1 week for joint pain. She improved significantly 2 days after rofecoxib was withdrawn (4).

Sensory systems

Visual impairment associated with rofecoxib and other coxibs may be more frequent than has previously been thought and may be under-recognised (SEDA-28, 129). There have been three reports of central retinal vein occlusion after starting rofecoxib or after a dosage increase (5).

- A 72-year-old woman took rofecoxib 25 mg/day for rheumatoid arthritis for 6 months. She then increased the dose to 50 mg/day and 3 days later she had sudden deterioration of vision in her right eye due to central retinal vein occlusion.
- A 69-year-old woman had severe deterioration of vision in her right eye 24 hours after starting to take rofecoxib 25 mg/day for osteoarthritis. Ophthalmic examination showed severe intraretinal hemorrhage and retinal vein occlusion.
- A 47-year-old man started to take rofecoxib for hip pain. A week later he had temporary blotches in his right eye. He stopped treatment but started rofecoxib again 1 month later, after which his vision progressively deteriorated. Ophthalmic examination showed central retinal vein occlusion.

All three patients stopped taking rofecoxib. About 1 year later visual acuity in the first two had improved.

Psychiatric

Acute psychotic syndromes have been reported in two patients taking rofecoxib, one with visual hallucinations and one with auditory hallucinations (6).

Hematologic

Thrombocytopenia has been attributed to rofecoxib.
- A 66-year-old man took rofecoxib 12.5 mg/day for 5 days before stopping because of purpura; 3 days later he developed a disseminated petechial rash and epistaxis (7). His platelet count was 1×10^9/l. Rofecoxib was withdrawn but he required treatment with prednisone, immunoglobulin, and plasmapheresis owing to the severity of the hemorrhagic event. The platelet count slowly returned to normal.

Mouth

There have been three reports of oral lesions attributed to rofecoxib (8).

- A 72-year-old woman, who had taken rofecoxib 50 mg/day for rheumatoid arthritis for 4 weeks, developed atrophic erosive lesions on her right buccal mucosa. Rofecoxib was withdrawn and within 15 days the lesions had resolved. Six months later she again took rofecoxib and the same mucosal lesions appeared at the same site. Rofecoxib was again withdrawn and the buccal lesions resolved. There was no recurrence 8 months later.
- An 83-year-old woman, who had taken rofecoxib 50 mg/day for osteoarthritis for 6 weeks developed erosive lesions on the left side of her tongue and floor of her mouth. Rofecoxib was withdrawn and the lesions resolved completely within 10 days. There was no recurrence 1 year later.
- A 67-year-old woman, who had taken rofecoxib 25 mg/day for osteoarthritis for 16 months, developed severe erosive oral lesions with pseudomembranes. Topical triamcinolone was ineffective. Rofecoxib was replaced by meloxicam and 2 weeks later her symptoms had eased markedly.

Gastrointestinal

Rofecoxib has been studied in patients with inflammatory bowel disease and an associated peripheral arthropathy and/or arthritis in an uncontrolled study in 32 patients, of whom 26 took 25mg/day and six took 12.5 mg/day (9). Three patients had to be withdrawn because of gastrointestinal complaints. There was no exacerbation of the inflammatory bowel disease and in 32 patients the arthralgia was thought to have responded.

In a small phase II study rofecoxib did not increase the antitumor activity of chemotherapy in the treatment of metastatic colorectal cancer, and resulted in increased gastrointestinal toxicity (10).

Contrasting data on the safety of rofecoxib in patients with pre-existing primary inflammatory bowel disease have been reported. In one study in 32 patients rofecoxib did not exacerbate inflammatory bowel disease (SEDA 28, 132), but in isolated cases inhibition of COX-2 in the large bowel worsened inflammatory bowel disease, as has again been reported in three patients exposed to rofecoxib—two patients developed inflammatory bowel disease de novo and one had exacerbation of pre-existing disease (11).

- A 42-year-old man developed abdominal pain and diarrhea with 15 loose bowel movements per day after taking rofecoxib 25 mg/day for 3 days. Rofecoxib was withdrawn but over the next few weeks his symptoms improved only partially. Colonoscopy showed focal shallow ulceration with adherent exudate. Biopsy showed active colitis with a focal erosion involving the transverse colon. Colonoscopy at 4 months showed resolution of the inflammatory changes, but a biopsy still showed patchy active ileitis with focal erosions in the transverse colon. Normal bowel function gradually returned and the abdominal pain resolved.
- A 65-year-old woman developed a change in bowel habit and rectal bleeding after taking aspirin for 5 days, ibuprofen for 2 days, and then rofecoxib (dosage not stated) for 10 days. While taking rofecoxib she developed loose bowel movements with small amounts of bright red blood. Rofecoxib was withdrawn and her symptoms resolved completely. Colonoscopy after 12 days showed segmental inflammatory changes with serpiginous ulceration. Biopsy showed active colitis with erosions, cryptitis, and crypt abscesses.
- A 52-year-old man with a 14-month history of inflammatory bowel disease, currently in remission, took

rofecoxib 50 mg/day for 5 days and developed abdominal cramp and loose stools with bright red blood. Colonoscopy showed focal ulceration of the cecum and descending colon. Biopsy showed patchy acute cryptitis and active colitis with ulceration. Rofecoxib was withdrawn and his symptoms resolved.

These observations suggest that extreme caution should be taken when prescribing rofecoxib for patients with inflammatory bowel disease. Furthermore, patients who develop symptoms of diarrhea and abdominal pain should be monitored carefully for possible inflammatory bowel disease.

Liver

Two cases of severe hepatotoxicity have been reported in patients, a man and woman, both aged 44 years, soon after exposure to rofecoxib (12). There was cholestasis and abnormal liver biochemistry and in both cases, liver histology was compatible with drug-induced hepatotoxicity. There was rapid clinical and biochemical improvement after withdrawal of rofecoxib.

Urinary tract

The pattern of nephrotoxicity of rofecoxib is similar to that with non-selective NSAIDs. There have been reports of acute interstitial nephritis (13)and acute renal insufficiency (14,15), particularly in patients with predisposing conditions, such as chronic renal insufficiency, renal transplantation, heart disease, liver cirrhosis, and dehydration (16–19). COX-2 inhibitors should be used with great caution, if at all, in patients with medical problems that are associated with prostaglandin-dependent renal function. From this point of view they do not differ from traditional NSAIDs (20).

- Rofecoxib 12.5 mg bd for arthritic pain was associated with biopsy-proven acute tubulointerstitial nephritis in a 67-year-old woman.

Skin

Two women developed neutrophilic dermatosis (Sweet's syndrome) while taking rofecoxib (21).

- A 31-year-old woman with Crohn's disease started to take rofecoxib 50 mg/day for joint pain and 1 week later developed multiple tender erythematous nodules on her legs. Some had central pustules and some were ulcerated. She stopped taking rofecoxib. Biopsy of a nodule showed infiltration of neutrophils into the surrounding derma and a central area of abscess formation. Ten days later her lesions were less indurated and the ulcerated lesion had stopped draining and 5 weeks later her lesions had resolved.
- A 30-year-old woman with rheumatoid arthritis started to develop multiple tender subcutaneous nodules over both her legs within 2 weeks of starting to take rofecoxib (50 mg/day) for joint pain. After 1 month the lesions had progressed to focal areas of ulceration with purulent drainage. A biopsy showed neutrophilic dermatitis, consistent with pyoderma gangrenosum.

Rofecoxib was withdrawn and her lesions resolved in 4 weeks.

Non-selective NSAIDs have been reported to exacerbate psoriasis.

- A 46-year-old woman developed severe psoriasis 5 days after starting to take rofecoxib 25 mg/day for a neck strain. She had had a similar reaction while taking diclofenac. In both cases remission did not occur until several months after withdrawal (22).

This report, and others involving non-selective NSAIDs, adds strength to the likelihood of an association between all types of NSAIDs and exacerbation of psoriasis.

Severe cutaneous vasculitis has been described in two patients taking rofecoxib (23,24).

- A 63-year-old woman developed Stevens–Johnson syndrome while taking rofecoxib for arthralgia. Despite early withdrawal she developed serious corneal and conjunctival complications (25).

Immunologic

Rofecoxib has been implicated in a case of combined interstitial nephritis and acute hepatitis (26).

- A 62-year-old man who had taken rofecoxib for 6 months, developed malaise, anorexia, weight loss, pruritus, jaundice, and upper quadrant abdominal discomfort. His liver function tests were abnormal: serum bilirubin 240 µmol/l (reference range < 20), γ - glutamyl transferase 98 units/l (< 60), alkaline phosphatase 218 units/l (< 150). A liver biopsy was consistent with drug-induced hepatic damage. He was treated with ursodeoxycholic acid, but his cholestasis deteriorated. Over the next few days his renal function also worsened (serum creatinine 540 µmol/l) and urinalysis showed heavy proteinuria. He needed hemodialysis for 6 weeks. A renal biopsy was consistent with drug-induced acute interstitial nephritis and acute tubular necrosis. He was given a glucocorticoid and his renal and liver function recovered after 3 months.

Isolated severe acute cholestatic and cytolytic hepatitis has previously been attributed to rofecoxib (27).

Drug–Drug Interactions

Methotrexate

Methotrexate is often prescribed for the management of rheumatoid arthritis, and some NSAIDs have been reported to interact with it, causing increased plasma methotrexate concentrations, associated with impaired renal function. The safety of concurrent rofecoxib and oral methotrexate has been studied for 3 weeks in 25 patients with rheumatoid arthritis (28). Rofecoxib 12.5–50 mg/day had no effect on the plasma concentrations or renal clearance of methotrexate, but supratherapeutic doses of rofecoxib (75 and 250 mg) caused a significant increase in the plasma methotrexate AUC and reduced its renal clearance.

Tizanidine

In a randomized, double-blind, two-phase crossover study, nine healthy subjects took placebo or rofecoxib 25 mg/day for 4 days and then took tizanidine 4 mg (29). Rofecoxib increased the AUC of tizanidine 14-fold (95% CI = 8, 16), the C_{max} 6-fold (4.8, 7.3), and the half-life from 1.6 to 3.0 hours. Rofecoxib increased several-fold the tizanidine/M_3 and tizanidine/M_4 ratios in plasma and urine and the tizanidine/M_5, tizanidine/M_9, and tizanidine/M_{10} ratios in urine (the M_i being different metabolites of tizanidine). Rofecoxib markedly increased the blood pressure-lowering and sedative effects of tizanidine. It also increased the plasma caffeine/paraxanthine ratio 2.4-fold (95% CI = 1.4, 3.4) and this ratio correlated with the tizanidine/metabolite ratios. The authors attributed these effects to inhibition of CYP1A2 by rofecoxib.

Warfarin

Significant increases in International Normalized Ratio (INR) have been reported in patients who took rofecoxib and warfarin; in some, the increase in INR was accompanied by a bleeding event (30,31). Careful monitoring of the INR in patients taking warfarin and concomitant rofecoxib is mandatory.

References

1. Layton D, Riley J, Wilton LV, Shakir SA. Safety profile of rofecoxib as used in general practice in England: results of a prescription-event monitoring study. Br J Clin Pharmacol 2003;55:166–74.
2. Nietert PJ, Ornstein SM, Dickerson LM, Rothenberg RJ. Comparison of changes in blood pressure measurments and antihypertensive therapy in older, hypertensive, ambulatory care patients prescribed celecoxib or rofecoxib. Pharmacotherapy 2003;23:1416–23.
3. Bonnel RA, Villalba ML, Karwoski CB, Beitz J. Aseptic meningitis associated with rofecoxib. Arch Intern Med 2002;162(6):713–5.
4. Ashwath ML, Katner HP. Recurrent aseptic meningitis due to different non-steroidal anti-inflammatory drugs including rofecoxib. Postgrad Med J 2003;79:295–6.
5. Meyer CH, Schmidt JC, Rodrigues EB, Mennel S. Risk of retinal vein occlusions in patients treated with rofecoxib (Vioxx). Ophthalmogica 2005;219:243–7.
6. Sabolek M, Unrath A, Sperfeld AD, Connemann BJ, Kassubek J. Psychotische Storung unter Rofecoxib. [Rofecoxib-induced psychosis.] Psychiatr Prax 2007;34(4):200–2.
7. Kentos A, Robin V, Lambermont M, Jurdan M, Pignarelli M, Feremans W. Probable rofecoxib-induced thrombocytopenia. Rheumatology 2003;42:699–700.
8. Bagàan JV, Thongprasom K, Scully C. Adverse oral reactions associated with the COX-2 inhibitor rofecoxib. Oral Dis 2004;10:401–3.
9. Reinisch W, Miehsler W, Dejaco C, Harrer M, Waldhoer T, Lichtenberger C, Vogelsang H. An open-label trial of the selective cyclo-oxygenase-2 inhibitor, rofecoxib in inflammatory bowel disease-associated peripheral arthritis and arthralgia. Aliment Pharmacol Ther 2003;17:1371–80.
10. Becerra CR, Frenkel EP, Ashfaq R, Gaynor RB. Increased toxicity and lack of efficacy of rofecoxib in combination with chemotherapy for treatment of metastatic colerectal cancer: a phase II study. Int J Cancer 2003;105:868–72.
11. Wilcox GM, Mattia AR. Rofecoxib and inflammatory bowel disease: clinical and pathologic observations. J Clin Gastroeneterol 2005;39:142–3.
12. Yan B, Leung Y, Urbanski SJ, Myers RP. Rofecoxib-induced hepatotoxicity: a forgotten complication of the coxibs. Can J Gastroenterol 2006;20(5):351–5.
13. Alim N, Peterson L, Zimmerman SW, Updike S. Rofecoxib-induced acute interstitial nephritis. Am J Kidney Dis 2003;41:720–1.
14. Morales E, Mucksavage JJ. Cyclooxygenase-2 inhibitor-associated acute renal failure: case report with rofecoxib and review of the literature. Pharmacotherapy 2002;22:1317–21.
15. Reinhold SW, Fischereder M, Reigger GA, Kramer BK. Acute renal failure after administration of a single dose of a highly selective COX-2 inhibitor. Clin Nephrol 2003;60:295–6.
16. Woywodt A, Schwarz A, Mengel M, Haller H, Zeidler H, Kohler L. Nephrotoxicity of selective COX-2 inhibitors. J Rheumatol 2001;28(9):2133–5.
17. Ofran Y, Bursztyn M, Ackerman Z. Rofecoxib-induced renal dysfunction in a patient with compensated cirrhosis and heart failure. Am J Gastroenterol 2001;96(6):1941.
18. Wahba AL, Soper C. Acute, anuric renal failure associated with two doses of a cyclooxygenase-2 inhibitor. Nephron 2001;89(2):239.
19. Meador R, Kolasinski S. Acute renal failure can occur with inappropriate use of a coxib. J Clin Rheumatol 2001;7:413–4.
20. Rocha JL, Fernandez-Alonso J. Acute tubulointerstitial nephritis associated with the selective COX-2 enzyme inhibitor, rofecoxib. Lancet 2001;357(9272):1946–7.
21. Smith KJ, Skelton H. Acute onset of neutrophilic dermatosis after therapy with COX-2-specific inhibitor. Int J Dermatol 2003;42:389–93.
22. Clark DW, Coulter DM. Psoriasis associated with rofecoxib. Arch Dermatol 2003;139:1223.
23. Lillicrap MS, Merry P. Cutaneous vasculitis associated with rofecoxib. Rheumatology 2003;42:1267–8.
24. Palop-Larrea V, Melchor-Penella MA, Ortega-Monzo C, Martinez Mir I. Leukocytoclastic vasculitis related to rofecoxib. Ann Pharmacother 2003;37:1731–2.
25. Goldberg D, Panigrahi D, Barazi M, Abelson M, Butrus S. A case of rofecoxib-associated Stevens–Johnson syndrome with corneal and conjunctival changes. Cornea 2004;23:736–7.
26. Haider M, Gain E, Khadem G, Pilmore H, Yun K, Jayasinghe N, Walker R. Simultaneous presentation of rofecoxib-induced acute hepatitis and acute interstitial nephritis. Intern Med J 2005;35:370–2.
27. Ouar S, Bellaïche G, Belloc J, Tordjman G, Ley G, Slama JL. Severe acute cholestatic and cytolytic hepatitis induced by rofecoxib. Gastroenterol Clin Biol 2005;29:471–2.
28. Schwartz JI, Agrawal NG, Wong PH, Bachmann KA, Porras AG, Miller JL, Ebel DL, Sack MR, Holmes GB, Redfern JS, Gertz BJ. Lack of pharmacokinetic interaction between rofecoxib and methotrexate in rheumatoid arthritis patients. J Clin Pharmacol 2001;41(10):1120–30.
29. Backman JT, Karjalainen MJ, Neuvonen M, Laitila J, Neuvonen PJ. Rofecoxib is a potent inhibitor of cytochrome P450 1A2: studies with tizanidine and caffeine in healthy subjects. Br J Clin Pharmacol 2006;62(3):345–57.
30. Anonymous. Interaction of rofecoxib with warfarin. Aust Adv Drug React Bull 2002;21:3.
31. Stading JA, Skrabal MZ, Faulkner MA. Seven cases of interaction between warfarin and cyclooxygenase-2 inhibitors. Am J Health Syst Pharm 2001;58(21):2076–80.

Romazarit

General Information

Romazarit, a slow-acting drug for use in rheumatoid arthritis, was well tolerated in pharmacokinetic studies. It is structurally similar to clobuzarit, which was withdrawn because of four possible cases of Stevens–Johnson syndrome (SEDA-17, 114).

In a double-blind placebo-controlled study in 224 patients with rheumatoid arthritis romazarit 200 mg or 450 mg bd for up to 24 weeks reduced the rate of progress of the disease. Adverse effects were not reported (1). In a double-blind placebo-controlled in 24 patients with rheumatoid arthritis romazarit 100 mg tds, 350 mg bd, or 350 mg tds was associated with adverse events that were mainly trival and similar in incidence to placebo (2).

References

1. Holford NH, Williams PE, Muirhead GJ, Mitchell A, York A. Population pharmacodynamics of romazarit. Br J Clin Pharmacol 1995;39(3):313–20.
2. Williams PE, Bird HA, Minty S, Helliwell PS, Muirhead GJ, Bentley J, York A. A pharmacokinetic and tolerance study of romazarit in patients with rheumatoid arthritis. Biopharm Drug Dispos 1992;13(2):119–29.

Sulfamazone

General Information

Sulfamazone is a pyrazolone derivative. It causes benign intracranial hypertension in children (SEDA-5, 100; 1).

Reference

1. Laverda AM, Casara GL, Furlannt M, et al. Ipertensione endocranica acuta benigna da sulfafenazone. Riv Ital Pediatr 1981;7:83.

Sulindac

General Information

There is still no firm evidence that by acting through an active metabolite, sulindac has any distinct advantage over other members of the group of NSAIDs that are related to indometacin. However, its good tolerance in elderly patients has been stressed (1). Its pattern of adverse effects is similar to that of indometacin (2), with an incidence ranging from 17 (3) to 50% (4). Sulindac causes fewer gastrointestinal adverse effects than aspirin, but in some studies the incidence equalled that of ibuprofen (5), fenoprofen (6), and indometacin (7).

Organs and Systems

Cardiovascular

Several cardiac abnormalities have been reported, including congestive heart failure, dysrhythmias, and palpitation (8).

Respiratory

Pulmonary infiltrates were described in a woman with osteoarthritis who had been taking sulindac for 6 months (9).

Nervous system

Adverse effects on the nervous system were found in 2.5–6.5% of patients in one study (4). Dizziness, drowsiness and headache, somnolence, vertigo, insomnia, and blurred vision, that is all adverse effects described with indometacin, have been observed. Acute reversible encephalopathy with rash and fever has been described.

Like other NSAIDs, sulindac can cause aseptic meningitis in patients with systemic lupus erythematosus (SEDA-7, 109). Recurrent aseptic meningitis, described in a patient with no underlying connective tissue disease who had tolerated other NSAIDs, suggested immunological hypersensitivity to sulindac (10).

Psychological, psychiatric

Psychiatric symptoms, bizarre behavior, and paranoia have been attributed to sulindac (11).

Electrolyte balance

The risk of severe hyperkalemia with sulindac has been documented in a series of four cases (12).

Hematologic

Agranulocytosis (probably due to toxicity rather than hypersusceptibility) can be caused by sulindac (13), as can bone marrow aplasia (14) and severe thrombocytopenia (15,16), which may be the consequence of autoimmune platelet destruction in the presence of sulindac or its metabolite (SEDA-7, 109). Immune-mediated hemolytic anemia with a positive direct antiglobulin test has been reported (SEDA-18, 103).

Aplastic anemia in a woman with osteoarthritis taking sulindac relapsed 3 years later during therapy with fenbufen, suggesting that extreme caution should be exercised before giving NSAIDs to a patient with a history of NSAID-related aplastic anemia (17).

Gastrointestinal

Sulindac can cause all of the gastrointestinal adverse effects that are associated with indometacin, from dyspepsia to peptic ulcer. Nausea and abdominal pain are the most frequent, followed by constipation (18).

Surprisingly, a study in healthy volunteers showed no gastroscopic mucosal damage after 7 days (19). This recalls past papers showing a lack of mucosal damage in short-term therapy, even with NSAIDs known to be gastrotoxic. A giant esophageal ulcer has been described (20). A preterm neonate developed fatal hemorrhagic gastritis with oral sulindac (21).

Ulcers in an ileal pouch with chronic bleeding have been described (22).

Sulindac reduces the number and size of rectal and colon polyps (23) and colon-mucosal synthesis of prostaglandin E_2 and 6-keto-prostaglandin $F_{1\alpha}$ is markedly reduced in patients taking sulindac. As this occurs concomitantly with the regression of polyps, it supports the hypothesis that prostaglandins are implicated in the regulation of colonic polyp growth (24). These observations have been confirmed in two other studies. Low-dose rectal sulindac produced complete adenoma remission in 87% of 15 colectomized patients with familial adenomatous polyposis. Polyp number and size fell significantly in 22 patients who took sulindac 150 mg bd for 3 months (25). After rectal administration of sulindac two patients had histologically proven mild gastritis (26).

Liver

Sulindac can cause toxic hepatitis, and several cases, some with positive rechallenge, have been described (27,28). A retrospective cohort study with secondary case-control analysis suggested that sulindac has a higher incidence of acute liver damage than all other NSAIDs, although the calculated risk is very low (27 per 100 000 prescriptions) (29). Liver function impairment is generally mild and reversible. Analysis of spontaneous reports to the FDA and the Danish Committee on ADRs (SEDA-18, 103) has confirmed these data.

Abdominal pain, nausea, high fever with chills, icterus, high liver enzyme activities, and hepatomegaly are characteristic and are probably caused by hypersensitivity. The occurrence of fever, rash, and/or eosinophilia in 35–55% of patients seems to confirm a hypersensitivity mechanism (SEDA-18, 103).

Cholestatic jaundice (30) and acute cholangitis in combination with acute pancreatitis (SEDA-13, 79) have been described.

Pancreas

There are several reports of pancreatitis associated with sulindac (SEDA-4, 66; SEDA-7, 109). Symptoms resembling acute pancreatitis appeared after 3–90 days. Rechallenge was positive in one case (31). Acute cholangitis in combination with acute pancreatitis has been described (SEDA-13, 79).

Urinary tract

Sulindac may be less likely to cause renal toxicity than other NSAIDs (32), at least when it is used in low dosages, but there is some disagreement on this point (33–35), and five cases of nephrotic syndrome and renal insufficiency have been described (36,37).

Analysis of small renal and biliary stones has shown that sulindac or its metabolite was present in the material (SEDA-15, 99), and the labeling of sulindac was revised in 1989 to warn physicians of this phenomenon. However, despite the presence of sulindac or its metabolites in some renal stones, patients taking long-term sulindac are not at risk of an increased incidence of renal stone formation compared with those taking other NSAIDs (38).

Skin

The Stevens–Johnson syndrome has been reported in women who all recovered after the drug was withdrawn and corticosteroids given (SEDA-6, 95). Toxic epidermal necrolysis has also been reported (39–41).

A reaction like lupus pernio, with purple discoloration, swelling, red papules, and desquamation of the distal parts of several toes, which resolved after drug suspension and recurred after resumption, has been observed (42), as have subcutaneous fat necrosis (SEDA-11, 92), and fixed drug reaction (SEDA-12, 84).

Immunologic

Several types of proven or suspected hypersensitivity have already been mentioned, for example in connection with the liver, but the exact mechanism of a particular adverse effect has not always been clear. One case of fever, pharyngitis, cervical lymphadenopathy, leukopenia, liver abnormalities, proteinuria, pulmonary infiltrates, and abdominal pain has been described. Another patient who previously took sulindac without problems developed pruritus, dyspnea, perioral edema, and lethargy after taking a single dose of sulindac 150 mg.

Pneumonitis is probably part of a general hypersensitivity reaction (SEDA-6, 94; 9,43).

An anaphylactic reaction has been described (44). Sulindac is also thought to have been responsible for a severe multisystem reaction (possibly again anaphylactic) involving the cardiovascular, hepatic, pulmonary, and hematological systems in a patient with quiescent systemic lupus erythematosus (45).

Second-Generation Effects

Fetotoxicity

The use of oral sulindac for closure of patent ductus arteriosus has been evaluated in a prospective comparison with intravenous indometacin. Sulindac promoted ductal constriction without compromising renal function in preterm infants, but its use was associated with severe gastrointestinal complications (46).

Susceptibility Factors

Patients with sodium depletion are at risk of developing hyponatremia with all NSAIDs. Sulindac also provoked hyponatremia in an elderly patient taking a salt-restricted diet (47).

Drug Administration

Drug overdose

Agranulocytosis of short duration was described after an overdose of sulindac 12 g (48). Eight cases of sulindac overdose have been reported to the UK National Poisons Information Service; all the patients remained asymptomatic (SEDA-9, 89).

Drug–Drug Interactions

Furosemide

Data on sulindac inhibition of the diuretic effect of furosemide are contradictory (49).

Lithium

Unlike other NSAIDs, sulindac does not seem to interact with lithium (SEDA-10, 82). However, in one case it may have increased serum lithium concentrations in a 23-year-old man and a 27-year-old woman (to 2.0 and 1.7 mmol/l respectively) (50).

Propranolol

Like indometacin, sulindac interacted with propranolol and a thiazide diuretic in a hypertensive patient (SEDA-6, 95).

Thiazide diuretics

Like indometacin, sulindac interacted with propranolol and a thiazide diuretic in a hypertensive patient (SEDA-6, 95).

Topical dimethylsulfoxide

Two cases of peripheral neuropathy attributed to a combination of oral sulindac and topical dimethylsulfoxide have been reported (SEDA-9, 89).

Warfarin

Potentiation of warfarin effects by sulindac has been reported (51).

References

1. Davis P. Comparative efficacy and tolerance of sulindac (Clinoril) in geriatric and nongeriatric patients. Curr Ther Res 1985;37:945.
2. Anonymous. Clinoril adverse reactions. FDA Drug Bull 1979;9(5):29.
3. Delcambre B. The sulindac profile—use of sulindac in hospital and private practice: multicentre study in general practice. Eur J Rheumatol Inflamm 1978;1:47.
4. Bordier P, Knutz DD. Sulindac: clinical results of treatment of osteoarthritis. Eur J Rheumatol Inflamm 1978;1:27.
5. Andrade L, Fernandez A. Sulindac in the treatment of osteoarthritis: a double blind 8 week study comparing sulindac with ibuprofen and 96 weeks of long term therapy. Eur J Rheumatol Inflamm 1978;1:36.
6. Durance RA, Jacobi RK, Thompson M, Whittington JR. A multicentre comparative analgesic study of fenoprofen and sulindac in rheumatoid arthritis. Curr Ther Res 1979;26:79.
7. Calin A, Britton M. Sulindac in ankylosing spondylitis. Double-blind evaluation of sulindac and indomethacin. JAMA 1979;242(17):1885–6.
8. Anonymous. Clinoril sulindac: cardiac abnormalities. ADR Highlights 1979;July 3.
9. Takimoto CH, Lynch D, Stulbarg MS. Pulmonary infiltrates associated with sulindac therapy. Chest 1990;97(1):230–2.
10. Greenberg GN. Recurrent sulindac-induced aseptic meningitis in a patient tolerant to other nonsteroidal anti-inflammatory drugs. South Med J 1988;81(11):1463–4.
11. Kruis R, Barger R. Paranoid psychosis with sulindac. JAMA 1980;243(14):1420.
12. Nesher G, Zimran A, Hershko C. Hyperkalemia associated with sulindac therapy. J Rheumatol 1986;13(6):1084–5.
13. Romeril KR, Duke DS, Hollings PE. Sulindac induced agranulocytosis and bone marrow culture. Lancet 1981;2(8245):523.
14. Miller JL. Marrow aplasia and sulindac. Ann Intern Med 1980;92(1):129.
15. Stambaugh JE Jr, Gordon RL, Geller R. Leukopenia and thrombocytopenia secondary to clinoril therapy. Lancet 1980;2(8194):594.
16. Rosenbaum JT. Thrombocytopenia associated with sulindac. Arthritis Rheum 1981;24(5):753–4.
17. Andrews R, Russell N. Aplastic anaemia associated with a non-steroidal anti-inflammatory drug: relapse after exposure to another such drug. BMJ 1990;301(6742):38.
18. Anonymous. Sulindac (Clinoril)—a new drug for arthritis. Med Lett Drugs Ther 1979;21(1):1–2.
19. Graham DY, Smith JL, Holmes GI, Davies RO. Nonsteroidal anti-inflammatory effect of sulindac sulfoxide and sulfide on gastric mucosa. Clin Pharmacol Ther 1985;38(1):65–70.
20. Levine MS, Rothstein RD, Laufer I. Giant esophageal ulcer due to Clinoril. Am J Roentgenol 1991;156(5):955–6.
21. Ng PC, So KW, Fok TF, To KF, Wong W, Liu K. Fatal haemorrhagic gastritis associated with oral sulindac treatment for patent ductus arteriosus. Acta Paediatr 1996;85(7):884–6.
22. Bertoni G, Sassatelli R, Bedogni G, Nigrisoli E. Sulindac-associated ulcerative pouchitis in familial adenomatous polyposis. Am J Gastroenterol 1996;91(11):2431–2.
23. Rigau J, Pique JM, Rubio E, Planas R, Tarrech JM, Bordas JM. Effects of long-term sulindac therapy on colonic polyposis. Ann Intern Med 1991;115(12):952–4.
24. Smalley WE, DuBois RN. Colorectal cancer and nonsteroidal anti-inflammatory drugs. Adv Pharmacol 1997;39:1–20.
25. Giardiello FM, Offerhaus JA, Tersmette AC, Hylind LM, Krush AJ, Brensinger JD, Booker SV, Hamilton SR. Sulindac induced regression of colorectal adenomas in familial adenomatous polyposis: evaluation of predictive factors. Gut 1996;38(4):578–81.
26. Winde G, Schmid KW, Schlegel W, Fischer R, Osswald H, Bunte H. Complete reversion and prevention of rectal adenomas in colectomized patients with familial adenomatous polyposis by rectal low-dose sulindac maintenance treatment. Advantages of a low-dose nonsteroidal anti-inflammatory drug regimen in reversing adenomas exceeding 33 months. Dis Colon Rectum 1995;38(8):813–30.
27. Kaul A, Reddy JC, Fagman E, Smith GF. Hepatitis associated with use of sulindac in a child. J Pediatr 1981;99(4):650–1.
28. Smith FE, Lindberg PJ. Life-threatening hypersensitivity to sulindac. JAMA 1980;244(3):269–70.

29. Garcia Rodriguez LA, Williams R, Derby LE, Dean AD, Jick H. Acute liver injury associated with nonsteroidal anti-inflammatory drugs and the role of risk factors. Arch Intern Med 1994;154(3):311–6.

30. Giroux Y, Moreau M, Kass TG. Cholestatic jaundice caused by sulindac. Can J Surg 1982;25(3):334–5.

31. Lilly EL. Pancreatitis after administration of sulindac. JAMA 1981;246(23):2680.

32. Bunning RD, Barth WF. Sulindac. A potentially renal-sparing nonsteroidal anti-inflammatory drug. JAMA 1982;248(21):2864–7.

33. Dunn MJ, Simonson M, Davidson EW, Scharschmidt LA, Sedor JR. Nonsteroidal anti-inflammatory drugs and renal function. J Clin Pharmacol 1988;28(6):524–9.

34. Stillman MT, Schlesinger PA. Nonsteroidal anti-inflammatory drug nephrotoxicity. Should we be concerned? Arch Intern Med 1990;150(2):268–70.

35. Whelton A, Stout RL, Spilman PS, Klassen DK. Renal effects of ibuprofen, piroxicam, and sulindac in patients with asymptomatic renal failure. A prospective, randomized, crossover comparison. Ann Intern Med 1990;112(8):568–76.

36. Champion de Crespigny PJ, Becker GJ, Ihle BU, Walter NM, Wright CA, Kincaid-Smith P. Renal failure and nephrotic syndrome associated with sulindac. Clin Nephrol 1988;30(1):52–5.

37. Pagniez D, Gosset D, Hardouin P, Noel C, Delvallez L, Dequiedt P. Evolution vers la hyalinose segmentaire et focale d'un syndrome néphrotique à lésions glomérulaires minimes chez une patiente traitée par le sulindac. [Development toward segmental and focal hyalinosis of a nephrotic syndrome with minimal glomerular lesions in a patient treated with sulindac.] Nephrologie 1988;9(2):90–1.

38. Ito S, Hasegawa H, Nozawa S, Murasawa A, Nakano M, Arakawa M. Sulindac usage may not be associated with an increased incidence of renal stone formation in patients with rheumatoid arthritis. J Rheumatol 1999;9:119–21.

39. Breton JC, Pibouin M, Allain H, et al. Toxic epidermal necrolysis induced by sulindac. Therapie 1985;40:67.

40. Small RE, Garnett WR. Sulindac-induced toxic epidermal necrolysis. Clin Pharm 1988;7(10):766–71.

41. Hovde O. Sulindakindusert toksisk epidermal nekrolyse. [Sulindac-induced toxic epidermal necrolysis.] Tidsskr Nor Laegeforen 1990;110(19):2537–8.

42. Reinertsen JL. Unusual pernio-like reaction to sulindac. Arthritis Rheum 1981;24(9):1215.

43. Fein M. Sulindac and pneumonitis. Ann Intern Med 1981;95(2):245.

44. Burrish GF, Kaatz BL. Sulindac-induced anaphylaxis. Ann Emerg Med 1981;10(3):154–5.

45. Hyson CP, Kazakoff MA. A severe multisystem reaction to sulindac. Arch Intern Med 1991;151(2):387–8.

46. Ng PC, So KW, Fok TF, Yam MC, Wong MY, Wong W. Comparing sulindac with indomethacin for closure of ductus arteriosus in preterm infants. J Paediatr Child Health 1997;33(4):324–8.

47. Chamontin B, Fille A, Salva P, Salvador M. L'inhibition sélective des prostaglandines existe-t-elle? A propos d'une hyponatrémie sous sulindac. [Does selective inhibition of prostaglandins exist? Apropos of hyponatrémia with sulindac.] Presse Méd 1988;17(40):2140–1.

48. Gross GE. Granulocytosis and a sulindac overdose. Ann Intern Med 1982;96(6 Pt 1):793–4.

49. Brater DC, Anderson S, Baird B, Campbell WB. Effects of ibuprofen, naproxen, and sulindac on prostaglandins in men. Kidney Int 1985;27(1):66–73.

50. Jones MT, Stoner SC. Increased lithium concentrations reported in patients treated with sulindac. J Clin Psychiatry 2000;61(7):527–8.

51. Ross JR, Beeley L. Sulindac, prothrombin time, and anticoagulants. Lancet 1979;2(8151):1075.

Suprofen

General Information

Suprofen, alpha-methyl-4-(2-thienylcarbonyl)-phenylacetic acid, was specifically promoted as a non-narcotic analgesic for many painful conditions, and was withdrawn from the market worldwide in 1987. It caused an unusual clinical syndrome of acute flank pain and nephrotoxicity (SEDA-12, 89). It is still available as a 1% ointment in some countries.

Organs and Systems

Urinary tract

The pathogenesis of suprofen nephrotoxicity in young healthy volunteers involved a transient reduction in renal plasma flow and glomerular filtration rate, possibly due to intratubular precipitation of uric acid (1).

Skin

Suprofen ointment can cause photodermatitis (SEDA-17, 113).

Susceptibility Factors

A case-control study identified as susceptibility factors for adverse effects of suprofen male sex, hay fever and asthma, exercise, and alcohol consumption (2).

References

1. Abraham PA, Halstenson CE, Opsahl JA, Matzke GR, Keane WF. Suprofen-induced uricosuria. A potential mechanism for acute nephropathy and flank pain. Am J Nephrol 1988;8(2):90–5.

2. Strom BL, West SL, Sim E, Carson JL. The epidemiology of the acute flank pain syndrome from suprofen. Clin Pharmacol Ther 1989;46(6):693–9.

Suxibuzone

General Information

Suxibuzone, a derivative of phenylbutazone, is an NSAID that has been used topically. Skin reactions, gastrotoxicity, nephrotoxicity, headache, and vertigo have been noted. The carcinogenic potential of suxibuzone in animals has attracted attention (1) and put an end to sales in some countries.

Reference

1. Anonymous. Other action on suxibuzone. Scrip 1982;669:14.

Talniflumate

See also Non-steroidal anti-inflammatory drugs

General Information

Talniflumate is an inhibitor of calcium-activated chloride channels, which has been developed to treat mucous hypersecretion (1). It is a phthalidyl ester of pyridinecarboxylic acid, related to niflumic acid.

Organs and Systems

Gastrointestinal

Gastrointestinal effects are the most frequent adverse effects of talniflumate (2).

References

1. Donnelly LE, Rogers DF. Therapy for chronic obstructive pulmonary disease in the 21st century. Drugs 2003;63(19):1973–98.
2. Torriani H. Talniflumate. Drugs Today 1983;19:97.

Tenidap sodium

General Information

Tenidap sodium, an antirheumatic drug, combines the clinical and pharmacological properties of NSAIDs with those of a disease-modifying agent. Data from clinical studies have been reviewed (SEDA-19, 100).

Pfizer abandoned tenidap sodium for use in rheumatoid arthritis after a non-approval letter from the FDA was issued because of unresolved questions about its safety. The decision related only to the 120 mg dose. The FDA's Arthritis Drugs Advisory Committee also voted against approving tenidap sodium for osteoarthritis.

Organs and Systems

Nervous system

The adverse effects of tenidap sodium include headache (3.8%) (1).

Hematologic

Acute eosinophilic pneumonia has been described in a man with osteoarthritis taking tenidap sodium (2).

Gastrointestinal

As expected with a cyclo-oxygenase inhibitor, the adverse effects most frequently reported by patients taking tenidap sodium were gastrointestinal; serious gastrointestinal events occurred in 2.1% (1).

Liver

Increases in serum transaminases can occur, and severe abnormalities in liver function tests have been reported (1,3–5).

Urinary tract

Proteinuria, by an unknown mechanism, is a frequent adverse effect of tenidap sodium (13%), but is reversible and non-progressive in the long term, and with no evidence of deteriorating renal function (1,6).

Skin

The adverse effects of tenidap sodium include alopecia (3.2%) (1).

Drug–Drug Interactions

ACE inhibitors

Tenidap sodium reduces the antihypertensive effects of ACE inhibitors (7).

Diuretics

Tenidap sodium reduces the antihypertensive effects of diuretics (7).

Lithium

Tenidap sodium interacts with lithium, reducing its renal clearance and increasing steady-state lithium concentrations; the dosage of lithium should be reduced to avoid toxicity (7,8).

Phenytoin

Tenidap sodium displaces phenytoin from plasma albumin binding sites by about 25% (9).

Warfarin

Tenidap sodium interacts with warfarin by displacing it from plasma albumin, although there may be another mechanism; the dosage of warfarin may need to be reduced to avoid toxicity (7,10).

References

1. Breedveld F. Tenidap: a novel cytokine-modulating antirheumatic drug for the treatment of rheumatoid arthritis. Scand J Rheumatol Suppl 1994;100:31–44.
2. Martinez BM, Domingo P. Acute eosinophilic pneumonia associated with tenidap. BMJ 1997;314(7077):349.
3. Anonymous. Hepatic monitoring for tenidap. Scrip 1995;2073:21.

4. Blackburn WD Jr, Prupas HM, Silverfield JC, Poiley JE, Caldwell JR, Collins RL, Miller MJ, Sikes DH, Kaplan H, Fleischmann R, et al. Tenidap in rheumatoid arthritis. A 24-week double-blind comparison with hydroxychloroquine-plus-piroxicam, and piroxicam alone. Arthritis Rheum 1995;38(10):1447–56.
5. Wylie G, Appelboom T, Bolten W, Breedveld FC, Feely J, Leeming MR, Le Loet X, Manthorpe R, Marcolongo R, Smolen J. A comparative study of tenidap, a cytokine-modulating anti-rheumatic drug, and diclofenac in rheumatoid arthritis: a 24-week analysis of a 1-year clinical trial. Br J Rheumatol 1995;34(6):554–63.
6. Martel-Pelletier J, Quinissi H, Cloutier JM, Pellettier JP. Tenidap effectively reduces cytochine synthesis and expression by human rheumatoid arthritis synovium. Arth Rheum 1994;37:.
7. Pullar T. The pharmacokinetics of tenidap sodium: introduction. Br J Clin Pharmacol 1995;39(Suppl 1):S1–2.
8. Apseloff G, Wilner KD, von Deutsch DA, Gerber N. Tenidap sodium decreases renal clearance and increases steady-state concentrations of lithium in healthy volunteers. Br J Clin Pharmacol 1995;39(Suppl 1):S25–8.
9. Blum RA, Schentag JJ, Gardner MJ, Wilner KD. The effect of tenidap sodium on the disposition and plasma protein binding of phenytoin in healthy male volunteers. Br J Clin Pharmacol 1995;39(Suppl 1):S35–8.
10. Apseloff G, Wilner KD, Gerber N. Effect of tenidap sodium on the pharmacodynamics and plasma protein binding of warfarin in healthy volunteers. Br J Clin Pharmacol 1995;39(Suppl 1):S29–33.

Tenoxicam

General Information

Tenoxicam is a piroxicam analogue with a half-life of 75 hours. Whether the differences in pharmacokinetics in elderly patients have any clinical significance is unknown (SEDA-12, 93).

The pattern of adverse effects is similar to that of piroxicam, but tenoxicam causes slightly fewer serious gastrointestinal effects (1). Fecal blood loss is lower than with aspirin (SEDA-8, 111). A large, multicenter, hospital-based study confirmed that tenoxicam and piroxicam had similar tolerance ratings: 13% of patients had severe adverse effects, most often gastrointestinal (melena, hematemesis, rectal bleeding, exacerbation of ulcerative colitis) and serious rashes (SEDA-15, 103). Gastrointestinal adverse effects are more frequent with higher doses (2).

In an open, non-comparative study in 1267 patients, performed to test tenoxicam safety in general practice, the most common adverse reactions were gastrointestinal (11%), central and peripheral nervous system disorders (2.8%), and skin reactions (2.5%) (3). Patients who take long-term tenoxicam are at low risk of nephrotoxicity. The prevalence of urinary system adverse effects was 0.07% in trials that included 67 000 patients (4).

Other adverse effects include phototoxic dermatitis, thrombocytopenia, edema of the legs, pruritus, and hypersalivation (SEDA-12, 93).

Organs and Systems

Respiratory

Tenoxicam can provoke severe bronchoconstriction and nasal obstruction in aspirin-sensitive asthmatic patients (SEDA-12, 93).

Liver

Mild chronic drug-induced hepatitis has been attributed to tenoxicam (SEDA-21, 108).

Biliary tract

Cholestatic cholangitis accompanied by toxic epidermal necrolysis and prolonged ductopenia has been described in a 36-year-old man who took tenoxicam 20 mg/day for 7 days (5). He improved initially, but at follow-up at 1 and 3 years his cholestatic enzymes were still raised and liver biopsies showed ductopenia, suggesting vanishing bile duct syndrome.

Skin

Three cases of toxic epidermal necrolysis (Lyell's syndrome) have been described in patients taking tenoxicam (SEDA-17, 114).

A fixed drug eruption with cross-sensitivity to droxicam and tenoxicam has been reported (SEDA-18, 107), but tenoxicam may not cross-react in patients with photosensitivity to piroxicam (SEDA-18, 107).

Drug Administration

Drug administration route

Tenoxicam can be given intravenously, but phlebitis and pain at the injection site occur, albeit rarely (SEDA-19, 99).

References

1. Bird HA. International experience with tenoxicam: a review. Scand J Rheumatol Suppl 1988;73:22–7.
2. Gonzalez JP, Todd PA. Tenoxicam. A preliminary review of its pharmacodynamic and pharmacokinetic properties, and therapeutic efficacy. Drugs 1987;34(3):289–310.
3. Caughey D, Waterworth RF. A study of the safety of tenoxicam in general practice. NZ Med J 1989;102(879):582–3.
4. Heintz RC. Tenoxicam and renal function. Drug Saf 1995;12(2):110–9.
5. Trak-Smayra V, Cazals-Hatem D, Asselah T, Duchatelle V, Degott C. Prolonged cholestasis and ductopenia with tenoxicam. J Hepatol 2003;39:125–8.

Tiaprofenic acid

General Information

Data are available on the incidence of adverse effects of this drug (1–3). A review of published studies showed that about 13–15% of patients have adverse effects. The withdrawal rate because of unwanted reactions was 3.2–12% in short-term studies and 4% in one long-term trial. Adverse effects involved the gastrointestinal tract in 8–12% of patients, the central nervous system in 1–10% and the skin (rash, sweating, and itching) in 1–4%. Cutaneous photosensitivity and edema have also been reported.

The adverse effects profile does not differ from that of other propionic acid derivatives and includes the whole spectrum of gastrointestinal adverse reactions usually found with NSAIDs (SED-10, 166; SEDA-10, 84; 4). The claim of good tolerance and gastric protection, based on animal data, which the company extrapolated to humans, has not been confirmed by appropriate clinical studies (SEDA-12, 89).

Organs and Systems

Urinary tract

Although many NSAIDs have rarely been reported to be responsible for increased urinary frequency and dysuria, and never for severe cystitis, tiaprofenic acid causes severe cystitis (SEDA-18, 106; SEDA-20; 94; SEDA-21, 107; 5,6).

If this complication occurs, the drug should be withdrawn immediately (7). A report has given some data on the frequency with which tiaprofenic acid cystitis-related disorders were reported to the UK's Committee on Safety of Medicines. Between 1981 and 1996, 770 adverse drug reactions involving 221 patients were reported. A peak in the reporting of cystitis was noted in 1994, when tiaprofenic acid product information was changed and advice was sent to UK doctors warning about cystitis-related disorders. This peak was followed by a fall in the number of reports, but it is not clear if this was due to reduced drug usage or also to a fall in the reporting rate of such adverse reactions (8).

References

1. Anonymous. The side effects of tiaprofenic acid. Reactions 1985;118:11.
2. Rave O, Penth B. Arzneimittelsicherheit bei Antirheumatika: Ergebnisse einer Breitenprufung mit Tiaprofensaure an 20,947 Patienten. Med Welt 1984;35:1587.
3. Poletto B. Tiaprofenic acid. Clin Rheum Dis 1984;10(2):333–51.
4. Anonymous. Tiaprofenic acid (Surgam) — a major claim is dropped. Drug Ther Bull 1983;21(13):49–50.
5. Crew JP, Donat R, Roskell D, Fellows GJ. Bilateral ureteric obstruction secondary to the prolonged use of tiaprofenic acid. Br J Clin Pract 1997;51(1):59–60.
6. Crawford ML, Waller PC, Wood SM. Severe cystitis associated with tiaprofenic acid. Br J Urol 1997;79(4):578–84.
7. Drake MJ, Nixon PM, Crew JP. Drug-induced bladder and urinary disorders. Incidence, prevention and management. Drug Saf 1998;19(1):45–55.
8. Brown EG, Waller PC, Sallie BA. Tiaprofenic acid and severe cystitis. Postgrad Med J 1998;74(873):443–4.

Timegadine

General Information

Timegadine, a guanidine derivative, inhibits cyclo-oxygenase, lipoxygenase, and phospholipase activity. Reported adverse effects are skin rashes, oral lesions, epigastric pain, nausea, dysuria, dizziness, vertigo, and sleep disturbances. Liver enzyme changes and pneumonitis have also been described (1–4).

References

1. Egsmose C, Lund B, Andersen RB. Timegadine: more than a non-steroidal for the treatment of rheumatoid arthritis. A controlled, double-blind study. Scand J Rheumatol 1988;17(2):103–11.
2. Mbuyi-Muamba JM, Dequeker J. A comparative trial of timegadine and D-penicillamine in rheumatoid arthritis. Clin Rheumatol 1983;2(4):369–74.
3. Caruso I, Fumagalli M, Montrone F, Greco M, Boccassini L. Timegadine: long-term open study in rheumatoid arthritis. Clin Rheumatol 1983;2(4):363–7.
4. Berry H, Bloom B, Fernandes L, Morris M. Comparison of timegadine and naproxen in rheumatoid arthritis. A placebo controlled trial. Clin Rheumatol 1983;2(4):357–61.

Tolfenamic acid

General Information

The main adverse effects of tolfenamic acid (particularly nephrotoxicity) are similar to those of the other anthranilic acid derivatives. However, dysuria has been reported more often and confirmed by rechallenge (SEDA-4, 68). Skin disorders are frequent (40% of all reported effects), and fixed drug eruption has occurred (SEDA-18, 107). Diarrhea (10%) and upper gastrointestinal symptoms (including dyspepsia, nausea, vomiting, gastric pain, and ulcer) (6%) are common (SEDA-19, 98). Hepatitis has been described with positive rechallenge. Six patients with pulmonary infiltrates, possibly caused by tolfenamic acid, were reported to the Finnish National Centre for Adverse Drug Reaction Monitoring over a 12-year period. In some patients with hemolytic anemia, a positive Coombs' test and antinuclear antibodies suggested an immunological mechanism (SEDA-13, 83).

Organs and Systems

Electrolyte balance

Hyperkalemia has been attributed to tolfenamic acid (1).

- A hemodialysis patient with nephritic syndrome and diabetic end-stage renal disease developed severe hyperkalemia with muscle paresis after taking tolfenamic acid 300 mg/day for chronic headache. Five days after starting treatment he reported pain and tenderness affecting the muscles of his back and lower extremities. He had hyponatremia and severe hyperkalemia. During the following days he developed increasing weakness and became unable to move his head and limbs. Tolfenamic acid was withdrawn and aggressive treatment and repeated hemodialysis started, leading to complete recovery in a few days.

In this case, end-stage renal disease with nephrotic syndrome and insulin-dependent diabetes mellitus were predisposing factors to the development of hyperkalemia, but a possible role of accumulated tolfenamic acid metabolites could not be excluded. Patients with severe renal insufficiency should not receive NSAIDs.

Reference

1. Nielsen EH. Hyperkalaemic muscle paresis—side-effect of prostaglandin inhibition in a haemodialysis patient. Nephrol Dial Transplant 1999;14(2):480–2.

Tolmetin

General Information

In 32 207 patients taking part in a short (1–4 weeks) postmarketing study of tolmetin, adverse effects occurred in 12%, and led to withdrawal in 3.6% (1). Tolerability was similar to that of naproxen, indometacin (SEDA-7, 114), and ibuprofen (SED-9, 152) (2). In another retrospective study in patients treated for 1 year or more with tolmetin, 64% reported generally mild transitory adverse effects. In controlled studies, about 10% of patients withdrew owing to adverse effects (3). In another study of 25 000 prescription records (4), tolmetin caused adverse reactions severe enough to merit hospitalization in only two cases (drug fever and membranous glomerulopathy).

Organs and Systems

Cardiovascular

Increased blood pressure can occur after long-term treatment with tolmetin (5).

Nervous system

The usual adverse reactions of NSAIDs on the nervous system have been attributed to tolmetin (SEDA-6, 98). One woman developed aseptic meningitis, similar to that seen with ibuprofen (6).

Sensory systems

Hearing loss has been documented (SED-9, 152) (7).

Hematologic

Acute reversible thrombocytopenic purpura and tolmetin-related antibodies have been reported in a patient with a history of multiple allergies; rechallenge was positive (8). Peripheral blood eosinophilia has also been found (SEDA-6, 98).

Gastrointestinal

Gastrointestinal adverse effects occurred in 31% of patients taking tolmetin and peptic ulceration in 2% (3). In older patients, the percentage of peptic ulceration and gastrointestinal bleeding was somewhat higher (9).

Urinary tract

Reversible renal insufficiency and acute interstitial nephritis have been reported. Nephrotic syndrome was attributed to tolmetin, but a firm causal relation was not established (10). Nephrotic syndrome has also been described in a 16-year-old girl after she had taken tolmetin for 6 months (SEDA-16, 122).

Immunologic

From early on, the high incidence of hypersensitivity reactions with tolmetin was striking, for example in spontaneous adverse reaction reports. However, the high incidence was not confirmed in a retrospective comparative review (SEDA-6, 98; SEDA-7, 134; 11). Several factors can explain the discrepancy. For example, patients covered by the review may have persisted with treatment, since they did not experience such reactions.

Multiorgan failure

Fatal multisystem toxicity including both renal and hepatic failure, with microvesicular fatty change in the liver, has been reported with tolmetin in a young woman (12).

Drug–Drug Interactions

Warfarin

Tolmetin combined with warfarin can markedly prolong the prothrombin time and cause bleeding (SEDA-13, 82).

References

1. Sarchi C, Cioffi T, Bertelletti D, Guslandi M. Tolmetin sodium in clinical practice: a survey of 32,207 treated patients. J Int Med Res 1981;9(6):482–9.

2. Brogden RN, Heel RC, Speight TM, Avery GS. Tolmetin: a review of its pharmacological properties and therapeutic efficacy in rheumatic diseases. Drugs 1978;15(6):429–50.
3. Reid RT, Levin J, Ricca LR, et al. Tolmetin sodium in the treatment of osteoarthrtis: an analysis of 725 patients with a year or more of therapy. Curr Ther Res 1982;28:173.
4. Jick H, Jick SS, Hunter JR, Walker AM. Follow-up study of tolmetin users. Pharmacotherapy 1989;9(2):91–4.
5. Maibach E. European experiences with tolmetin in the treatment of rheumatic diseases. Curr Ther Res Clin Exp 1976;19(3):350–62.
6. Ruppert GB, Barth WF. Tolmetin-induced aseptic meningitis. JAMA 1981;245(1):67–8.
7. Brown JH, Hull J, Biundo JJ. Results of a one-year trial of tolmetin in patients with rheumatoid arthritis. J Clin Pharmacol 1975;15(5–6):455–63.
8. Stefanini M, Nassif RI. Acute thrombocytopenic purpura traced to tolmetin-related antibody. Va Med 1982;109(3):171–5.
9. O'Brien WM. Long-term efficacy and safety of tolmetin sodium in treatment of geriatric patients with rheumatoid arthritis and osteoarthritis: a retrospective study. J Clin Pharmacol 1983;23(7):309–23.
10. Chatterjee GP. Nephrotic syndrome induced by tolmetin. JAMA 1981;246(14):1589.
11. Strom BL, Carson JL, Schinnar R, Sim E, Morse ML. The effect of indication on the risk of hypersensitivity reactions associated with tolmetin sodium vs other nonsteroidal anti-inflammatory drugs. J Rheumatol 1988;15(4):695–9.
12. Shaw GR, Anderson WR. Multisystem failure and hepatic microvesicular fatty metamorphosis associated with tolmetin ingestion. Arch Pathol Lab Med 1991;115(8):818–21.

Tribuzone

General Information

The usual adverse effects of NSAIDs have been observed with tribuzone, namely gastric effects, fluid retention, and headache (SED-9, 145; 1).

Reference

1. Pavelka K, Vojtisek O, Bremova A, Kaukova D, Handlova D. A new pyrazolidine derivative—Benetazone Spofa—in short- and medium-term treatment of rheumatoid arthritis. (Double-blind comparative study with phenylbutazone). Int J Clin Pharmacol Biopharm 1976;14(1):20–8.

Valdecoxib

See also COX-2 inhibitors

General Information

Valdecoxib is a COX-2 inhibitor

Organs and Systems

Cardiovascular

See also COX-2 inhibitors

Despite claims from the results of a meta-analysis conducted by its manufacturer that valdecoxib appears to be associated with significantly fewer adverse gastrointestinal events that non-selective NSAIDs (1), its marketing authorization has been suspended in many countries because of an increased risk of serious cardiovascular outcomes (2) found in two randomized placebo-controlled trials in high-risk patients (SEDA-29, 122).

Urinary tract

Acute anuric renal insufficiency has been described with NSAIDs and can also occur with coxibs (SEDA-26, 125).

- A 31-year-old woman with pyelonephritis developed acute anuric renal insufficiency while taking valdecoxib for back pain and needed hemodialysis (3). No susceptibility factor for acute renal insufficiency was identified.

Skin

Various serious skin reactions to valdecoxib have been described in publications and/or reported to drug control agencies, including exanthematous skin eruptions, purpura, and systemic allergic contact dermatitis (4,5,6).

Toxic epidermal necrolysis has been attributed to valdecoxib (7).

- A 55-year-old woman developed toxic epidermal necrolysis while taking valdecoxib (dosage not stated) for knee pain. She had previously had an allergic reaction to a sulfonamide antibacterial cream. Eight days after starting to take valdecoxib, she developed a diffuse erythematous rash and fever. Valdecoxib was withdrawn, but her reaction worsened and she was transferred to a burns unit with lesions consistent with toxic epidermal necrolysis, with complete skin and hair loss, and received wound care for 12 days. At 5 months follow-up she still had leg pain and complete hair loss.

Valdecoxib has been associated with rare cases of serious skin reactions and of hypersensitivity reactions in patients with or without a history of allergic reactions to sulfonamides and should not be given to patients with such a history (8).

Musculoskeletal

Exacerbation of pre-existing carpal tunnel syndrome has been attributed to valdecoxib (9).

- A 40-year old patient had worsening of carpal tunnel syndrome after a single dose of valdecoxib 40 mg for a knee contusion. Valdecoxib was switched to ibuprofen and within 12 hours the symptoms resolved.

Valdecoxib-associated edema may have aggravated pre-existing carpal tunnel syndrome.

Table 1 Demographic data (%) in a series of 328 episodes of overdose with valdecoxib

Feature	Isolated cases	Non-isolated cases
Women	58	69
Aged under 6 years	53	47
Aged over 20 years	71	29
Intentional overdose	84	67
Management outside health-care facilities	84	26
Outcome no effect	92	35

Drug Administration

Drug overdose

In a survey of 328 cases of overdose with valdecoxib reported to six Texas poison centers, comparisons were made between isolated and non-isolated cases with respect to various demographic and clinical factors (10). The results are shown in Table 1.

References

1. Eisen GM, Goldstein JL, Hanna DB, Rublee DA. Meta-analysis: upper gastrointestinal tolerability of valdecoxib, a cyclooxygenase-2-specific inhibitor, compared with nonspecific nonsteroidal anti-inflammatory drugs among patients with osteoarthritis and rheumatoid arthritis. Aliment Pharmacol Ther 2005;21:591-8.
2. Ray A, Griffin MR, Stein CM. Cardiovascular toxicity of valdecoxib. N Engl J Med 2004;351:2767.
3. Muhlfeld AS, Gloege J. Cox-2 inhibitors induced anuric renal failure in a previously healthy young woman. Clin Nephrol 2005;63:221-4.
4. Talhari C, Lauceviciute U, Enderlein E, Ruzicka T, Homey B. Cox-2-selective inhibitor valdecoxib induces severe allergic skin reactions. J Allergy Clin Immunol 2005;115:1089-90.
5. Knowles SR, Phillips EJ, Wong G, Shera NH. Serious dermatologic reaction associated with valdecoxib: report of two cases. J Am Acad Dermatol 2004;51:1028-9.
6. Jaeger C, Jappe U. Valdecoxib. Valdecoxib-induced systemic contact dermatitis confirmed by positive patch test. Contact Dermatitis 2005;52:47-8.
7. Glasser DL, Burroughs SH. Valdecoxib-induced toxic epidermal necrolysis in a patient allergic to sulfa drugs. Pharmacotherapy 2003;23:551-3.
8. Anonymous. A "Dear Healthcare Professional" letter regarding important safety information for valdecoxib. Reactions 2003;937:2.
9. Ruppen W, Schüpfer GK. Exacerbation of carpal tunnel syndrome under treatment with valdecoxib. Anesth Analg 2005;100:1215-6.
10. Forrester MB. Valdecoxib exposures reported to Texas poison centers during 2002–2004. J Toxicol Environ Health A 2006;69(10):899-905.

Zidometacin

General Information

Zidometacin differs from indometacin in having an azido group in the *para*-position, where indometacin has a benzyl group. It appears to be less ulcerogenic in animals. However, epigastric pain, burning, and nausea have been experienced by patients taking zidometacin (1).

Reference

1. Friez L. Preliminary clinical experience with zidometacin. Acta Ther 1985;11:109.

Zomepirac

General Information

Although zomepirac is a pyrrole-acetic acid compound closely related to tolmetin, it was originally claimed to be a new type of analgesic drug. Its history is not unlike that of benoxaprofen. In 1982, because of the severity and frequency of hypersensitivity reactions, it was withdrawn voluntarily by the manufacturers worldwide on a temporary basis (1). It has not been relaunched.

The overall incidence of its adverse effects, according to numerous reviews (SEDA-7, 114), is similar to or somewhat higher than with other NSAIDs. After single oral doses 36% of 496 patients had some adverse effects. The percentage was even higher (43%; 458 of 1079 patients) during short-term therapy (2 weeks). Owing to adverse reactions, 3.5% of patients dropped out. When it was given over 2–3 weeks, 65–70% patients had adverse effects, but the discontinuation rate was similar to or lower than that of other NSAIDs (2,3). Only the most important adverse effects are presented here.

Organs and Systems

Gastrointestinal

Adverse effects of zomepirac on the gastrointestinal tract were the most frequent reason for interruption of treatment. They increase with duration of administration. Nausea, vomiting, dyspepsia, discomfort, abdominal pain, and diarrhea or constipation have been recorded, as have stomatitis and tongue pain (4).

Zomepirac 300 mg/day increases fecal blood loss, but less than aspirin.

Urinary tract

In five patients with prior normal renal function, zomepirac caused acute renal insufficiency, with varying degrees of uremia, proteinuria, and oliguria (5). All recovered either after withdrawal or with prednisone therapy. In another case renal biopsy showed a tubulointerstitial nephritis (6).

Immunologic

The manufacturers received 1100 reports of allergic reactions in the first 2 years after launch. Fatal anaphylactic and anaphylactoid reactions have been reported: 10% of all reports on anaphylactic reactions in the USA named zomepirac, making it second only to the much older drug tolmetin. Hypersensitivity reactions are characterized by hypotension, bronchospasm, and serious respiratory distress, with or without oropharyngeal edema. Type-III allergic reactions have also been described.

Long-Term Effects

Drug dependence

Suspicions based on cluster reports that zomepirac may be addictive have not been confirmed (7).

References

1. World Health Organization. Zomepirac (United States of America). PHA (DIA) 1983;83.3.8.
2. Ruoff GE, Andelman SY, Cannella JJ. Long-term safety of zomepirac: a double-blind comparison with aspirin in patients with osteoarthritis. J Clin Pharmacol 1980;20(5-6 Pt 2):377–84.
3. McMillen JI, Urbaniak JR, Boas R. Treatment of chronic orthopedic pain with zomepirac. J Clin Pharmacol 1980;20(5-6 Pt 2):385–91.
4. Bates LH, Triplett WC, Berry ER, Weddle RA. Stomatitis associated with zomepirac. JAMA 1982;247(4):461–2.
5. Miller FC, Schorr WJ, Lacher JW. Zomepirac-induced renal failure. Arch Intern Med 1983;143(6):1171–3.
6. McCarthy JT, Schwartz GL, Blair TJ, Pierides AM, Van den Berg CJ. Reversible nonoliguric acute renal failure associated with zomepirac therapy. Mayo Clin Proc 1982;57(6):351–4.
7. Mendelis PS. Abuse potential associated with nonsteroidal anti-inflammatory drugs. ADR Highlights 1982;82:.

GLUCOCORTICOIDS AND DISEASE – MODIFYING ANTIRHEUMATIC DRUGS

Adalimumab

General Information

Adalimumab, a fully human monoclonal antibody, is the third commercially available TNF alfa antagonist for patients with rheumatoid arthritis for whom previous treatment with disease-modifying antirheumatic drugs has failed. Double-blind, placebo-controlled comparisons of adalimumab alone or combined with disease-modifying antirheumatic drugs showed no significant differences in the incidence of serious adverse effects and infections, but more frequent injection-site reactions with adalimumab (1,2,3).

Adalimumab has been approved alone or in combination with methotrexate for the treatment of rheumatoid arthritis in the EU and USA; approval for the treatment of psoriasis, psoriatic arthritis, and ankylosing spondylitis is expected in the near future (4). Adverse effects that have been reported in trials include worsening or initiation of congestive heart failure, raised transaminases, medically significant cytopenias, including pancytopenia, and a lupus-like syndrome. Other adverse effects include asthma (5), paresthesia in the leg and foot drop (6), and severe oral epithelial dysplasia (7). Adalimumab increases the risk of rare serious infections two-fold, and it should not be used during periods of active infection. Its most notable infectious complication is reactivation of tuberculosis and screening is recommended. Deep fungal and other serious and atypical infections can also be promoted.

Placebo-controlled studies

In a multicenter, randomized, double-blind, placebo-controlled study of subcutaneous adalimumab 40 mg every other week for 24 weeks, those who received adalimumab reported more adverse events (75% versus 60%), but there was no statistically significant difference in the incidence of infections; most adverse events were mild or moderate in intensity (8).

Organs and Systems

Respiratory

Pulmonary granulomas with caseating necrosis, but no evidence of mycobacteria or other infectious agents, were attributed to adalimumab in a 73-year-old man (9). That pulmonary lesions persisted for more than 1 year after withdrawal made interpretation difficult.

Respiratory

Adalimumab-associated pulmonary fibrosis can occur in patients with rheumatoid arthritis.

- A 67-year-old man with rheumatoid arthritis developed a non-productive cough and progressive dyspnea after being given subcutaneous adalimumab 40 mg every 2 weeks for 2 months. A CT scan showed extensive pulmonary fibrosis, with ground-glass lesions, honeycombing, and traction atelectasis. The dose of prednisone was increased to 90 mg/day, antibiotics were withdrawn, and 2 months later he was discharged in satisfactory condition (10).

- A 76-year-old woman with severe rheumatoid arthritis and no respiratory symptoms was given adalimumab instead of sulfasalazine and hydroxycholoroquine. There was marked symptomatic improvement in her arthritis, but within 2.5 months she developed progressive shortness of breath. A CT scan showed extensive confluent reticular and honeycomb shadowing basally and posteriorly. Methotrexate and adalimumab were both withdrawn and she was given oral prednisolone. Her symptoms improved and she was discharged to receive home oxygen therapy (11).

A patient receiving adalimumab developed fatal exacerbation of fibrosing alveolitis associated with systemic sclerosis (12).

- A 74-year-old woman with severe Raynaud's syndrome, sclerodactyly, pulmonary fibrosis, abnormal esophageal peristalsis, and severe polyarthritis taking azathioprine was given adalimumab. After 7 months she developed respiratory failure and fever (39.3°C). A CT angiogram showed lesions with extensive ground glass opacities. She was treated with oxygen, diuretics, azithromycin, and methylprednisolone 1 g/day for 3 days, followed by prednisone 1 mg/kg/day and azathioprine. Adalimumab was withdrawn, but 3 months later her pulmonary function worsened and she died 2 months later from respiratory distress without infection.

Sensory systems

Optic neuritis has been attributed to adalimumab (13).

- A 55-year-old man with psoriatic arthritis and hyperlipidemia developed reduced central vision in his right eye; there was no pain on eye movement and there were no other visual or somatic complaints. Because the psoriatic rash was severe and associated with arthropathy in the wrists and fingers, he received adalimumab injections 40 mg twice weekly over 4 months. After 3.5 months he noted visual loss. The best corrected visual acuity in the affected eye was 20/30 and there was a subtle right afferent pupillary defect. After treatment with methylprednisolone he recovered completely.

Hematologic

Reversible neutropenia has been associated with adalimumab (14).

- A 53-year-old woman with rheumatoid arthritis taking many drugs, including NSAIDs, glucocorticoids, hydroxychloroquine, methotrexate, and etanercept, had a poor response and was given adalimumab. She developed a neutropenia—1.5×10^9/l neutrophils and 3.8×10^9/l lymphocytes, of which 12% had typical large granular lymphocyte morphology. After withdrawal of adalimumab the neutropenia recovered within 3 weeks.

Urinary tract

A 64-year-old man developed nephrotic syndrome with membranous glomerulopathy on renal biopsy 1 year after starting to take adalimumab (15). Although proteinuria resolved spontaneously after adalimumab withdrawal and recurred on rechallenge, the case was complicated by simultaneous reduction of the prednisone dosage before each episode of proteinuria.

Skin

New-onset psoriasis can develop during TNF-α inhibitor treatment (16,17). Nine patients with rheumatoid arthritis who were treated with different types of TNF-α antagonists unexpectedly developed either new-onset or worsened psoriatic skin lesions (18).

- A 54-year-old woman with rheumatoid arthritis was given adalimumab and after 10 months developed hyperkeratotic skin lesions consistent with guttate psoriasis; with conservative management her rash resolved completely.
- A 64-year-old woman with rheumatoid arthritis was given adalimumab and 3 months later developed erythema at the injection site. After 18 months she developed a symmetrical psoriatic rash, with stable plaques involving the neck and elbows and thickening of the toenails. Histological examination showed psoriasiform dermatitis. She was given topical glucocorticoids. Adalimumab was continued and the rash improved significantly.
- A 49-year-old man with ankylosing spondylitis was given infliximab and after 8 months developed an erythematosus pustular rash over his back, histologically pustular psoriasis. The lesions resolved when the dose of methotrexate was increased.
- A 68-year-old woman with plaque psoriasis and inflammatory arthritis was given infliximab and developed a new variant of psoriasis affecting her axillae and groins; she responded to topical treatments.

Eosinophilic cellulitis (Wells' syndrome) has been attributed to adalimumab (19).

- A 72-year-old woman with rheumatoid arthritis was given adalimumab and 6–8 hours after the first injection developed a mild reaction at the injection site; 4 hours after a second injection 2 weeks later she developed chest discomfort, fever, rigor, fatigue, and a 10 x 9 cm violaceous plaque. Skin biopsy showed eosinophilic cellulitis (Wells' syndrome). She was given glucocorticoids and her other medications were withdrawn.

Alopecia areata can occur during treatment with adalimumab (20) (cf. efalizumab and infliximab below).

- A 23-year-old woman with a 2-year history of patchy hair loss due to alopecia areata was given topical dexamethasone; the alopecia resolved within 4 months. She was given adalimumab for rheumatoid arthritis and the alopecia areata recurred and developed into alopecia totalis. Topical dexamethasone was ineffective.

An urticarial eruption occurred in a patient with psoriasis treated with adalimumab (21).

- A 41-year-old woman with psoriasis was given adalimumab. She had an injection site reaction with each injection, followed by a pruritic urticarial eruption, primarily on her neck and arms. She required no treatment for the eruption, which became less severe with each injection. Her psoriasis responded dramatically to adalimumab.

A 63-year-old woman developed an erythema multiforme-like eruption after the sixth injection of adalimumab; the lesions disappeared after withdrawal (22).

Immunologic

According to the package insert of adalimumab, the rate of positive antinuclear antibodies was 12% compared with 7% in placebo groups. There was only one case of lupus-like syndrome, reversible on adalimumab withdrawal, among 2334 treated patients. The immunogenicity of adalimumab has been assessed in 15 patients with highly active rheumatoid arthritis (23). Four were treated with adalimumab as monotherapy and 11 with concomitant DMARDs. Anti-adalimumab antibodies were detected in four patients without concomitant DMARDs and in nine of the others. Five of seven patients with adverse drug reactions and all nine patients with lack of efficacy had antibodies. Two antibody-positive patients developed a rash. These results suggest that adalimumab, in spite of its fully human sequences, is immunogenic and induces antibody formation in a large number of patients.

Severe hypersensitivity reactions to adalimumab have not been documented, and it was supposed to be safe in patients previously intolerant to infliximab. Adalimumab was successfully used in a 22-year-old woman who had had a severe anaphylactic-like reaction to infliximab (24). Apart from injection site reactions, there was good tolerance to adalimumab in seven patients with a history of immediate or delayed hypersensitivity reactions to infliximab, and only one had a pruritic rash after each injection of adalimumab (25). One additional patient with infliximab-associated lupus also tolerated adalimumab uneventfully. The previous therapeutic response obtained with infliximab seemed to be unaffected in these patients.

Infection risk

See also Etanercept and Infliximab

Data from randomized controlled trials of adalimumab, open extensions, and two phase IIIb open trials have been analysed and postmarketing spontaneous reports of adverse events in the USA collected after FDA approval of adalimumab on 31 December 2002 [26]. As of 15 April 2005, the rheumatoid arthritis clinical trial safety database covered 10 050 patients, representing 12 506 patient-years of exposure. The rate of serious infections, 5.1/100 patient-years, was comparable to that reported on 31 August 2002 (4.9/100 patient-years), and to the rate in published reports from patients who have not received anti-tumour necrosis factor therapy. After implementation of tuberculosis screening in clinical trials, the rate of tuberculosis fell, but there were 34 cases in this analysis (0.27/100 patient-years). The standardized incidence ratio for lymphoma was 3.19 (95% CI = 1.78, 5.26), consistent with the observed increased incidence in patients with rheumatoid arthritis. As of 30 June 2005, there were an estimated 78 522 patient-years of exposure to adalimumab in the US postmarketing period. Seventeen cases of tuberculosis were spontaneously reported (0.02/100 patient-years) from the USA. Rates of other postmarketing events of interest, such as congestive heart failure, systemic lupus erythematosus, opportunistic infections, blood dyscrasias, lymphomas, and demyelinating disease, supported observations from clinical trials.

Two cases of infectious complications associated with the use of adalimumab in patients with rheumatoid arthritis have been reported.

- A 61-year-old man with rheumatoid arthritis developed tonsillar tuberculosis after 8 months of adalimumab treatment despite a prophylactic antituberculosis regimen correctly used after an initial screening positive for tuberculosis [27].
- A 70-year-old man died from fulminant pneumonia with candidal colonies after he had received his third injection of adalimumab together with methotrexate and prednisolone for rheumatoid arthritis [28].

Visceral leishmaniasis has been reported in a patient with rheumatoid arthritis treated with adalimumab (29).

- A 69-year-old woman with rheumatoid arthritis received adalimumab (40 mg every other week) plus methotrexate 7.5 mg weekly and prednisone 5 mg/day . After 2 years she developed an intermittent daily fever (maximum 38.5°C) and severe weakness. Her CRP was 2400 mg/l and she had a pancytopenia. A CT scan did not show any localized infection. Giemsa-stained smears from a bone marrow aspirate showed *Leishmania* parasites. She was given intravenous amphotericin B and 2 weeks later PCR for *Leishmania* in the blood no longer showed parasites.

In a double-blind, placebo controlled study of the addition of adalimumab (20 mg every week or 40 mg every other week) to methotrexate in 619 patients there was a significantly higher incidence of serious infections requiring hospitalization or intravenous antibiotics in patients taking adalimumab (3.8%) than in those taking placebo (0.5%) (30). The highest incidence (5.3%) was in those who took adalimumab 40 mg every other week, and tuberculosis, histoplasmosis, and herpes encephalitis (one case each) were observed only in this group. Overall, there were 13 cases of tuberculosis, mostly within the first 8 months of treatment, during 4870 patient-years of trials with adalimumab, but eight occurred in phase I and II trials with doses higher than those currently used. Recommendations regarding the risk of tuberculosis are therefore similar to those for infliximab.

- A 61-year-old man with rheumatoid arthritis receiving adalimumab developed a sore throat (31). Screening for tuberculosis using PPD was positive, and isoniazid was prescribed prophylactically for 6 months. After taking adalimumab for 8 months he developed tonsillar enlargement and nodular pulmonary lesions. Histopathological and microbial investigations established the diagnosis of tonsillar tuberculosis.

Long-Term Effects

Tumorigenicity

According to the Australian Adverse Drug Reactions Advisory Committee (ADRAC), TNF-α antagonists may predispose patients to an increased risk of malignancy or accelerate its development (32). Since 2000, ADRAC has received 319 reports involving infliximab, etanercept, and adalimumab. The more serious reports were as follows: malignant melanoma (3 reports), tuberculosis (n = 4), lymphoma (n = 5), anaphylaxis (n = 9), sepsis (n = 10), lupus or lupus-like syndrome (n = 22), and pneumonia/lower respiratory tract infections (n = 23). The Australian Product Information has advised caution when considering these drugs in patients with a history of malignancy, or when considering continued treatment in those who develop a malignancy.

The extent to which TNF-α antagonists increase the risk of serious malignancies has been assessed in patients with rheumatoid arthritis by meta-analysis to derive estimates of sparse harmful events occurring in randomized trials of TNF-α antagonists. From a systematic literature search (EMBASE, MEDLINE, Cochrane Library, and electronic abstract databases, annual scientific meetings of both the European League Against Rheumatism and the American College of Rheumatology, interviews of the manufacturers of the two licensed anti-TNF antibodies, and randomized placebo-controlled trials of infliximab and adalimumab), nine trials met the inclusion criteria; 3493 patients received anti-TNF antibody treatment and 1512 patients received placebo (33). The pooled odds ratio for malignancy was 3.3 (95% CI = 1.2, 9.1). Malignancies were significantly more common in patients taking higher doses than in patients who received lower doses of TNF-α antibody antagonists. For patients treated with TNF-α antagonists in the included trials, the number needed to treat for harm (NNT_H) was 154 (95% CI = 91, 500) for one additional malignancy during 6–12 months.

A meta-analysis of randomized clinical trials of infliximab and adalimumab, has found an increased risk of serious infections and malignancies. The malignancy rates were not higher than the expected rate in the general population, although they were increased compared with the randomized concurrent controls (34).

Promotion of lymphoma is a rare adverse effect of adalimumab. There has been a report of follicular mucinosis associated with mycosis fungoides in a patient taking adalimumab (35). Non-Hodgkin's lymphoma in a 70-year-old man was attributed to adalimumab, but he had also taken long-term glucocorticoids and methotrexate (36). During clinical trials, 10 of 2468 patients taking adalimumab developed lymphoma (1.8 were expected), but it is not yet known whether adalimumab per se increases the risk of lymphoma in patients with active rheumatoid arthritis.

Drug-Administration

Drug dosage regimens

The efficacy and safety of subcutaneous adalimumab has been analysed in patients with moderate to severe Crohn's disease (37). Patients received open induction therapy with adalimumab 80 mg in week 0 and 40 mg in week 2. In week 4 they were stratified by response (a reduction in the Crohn's Disease Activity Index of at least 70 points from baseline) and randomized to double-blind treatment with placebo, adalimumab 40 mg every other week, or adalimumab 40 mg weekly for 56 weeks. More patients receiving placebo withdrew because of an adverse event (13%) than those who received adalimumab (4.7% and 6.9% in the weekly and every other week groups respectively). Among patients who responded to adalimumab, both adalimumab regimens were significantly more effective than placebo in maintaining remission.

Drug administration route

Adalimumab is available for subcutaneous administration in two single-use injection devices, which provide bioequivalent amounts of adalimumab: a ready-to-use prefilled syringe and an integrated disposable delivery system, the autoinjection Pen. Although patients who require long-term subcutaneous administration of medications generally prefer pens, there are no data on preferences and pain in the use of biologics in patients with chronic inflammatory diseases. Injection-site pain, overall tolerability, and patient preferences for two different adalimumab delivery systems have been studied in 52 patients with rheumatoid arthritis (mean age 54 years; 32 women, 20 men) in a phase II, multicenter, open, single-arm, sequential trial (38). Patients self-administered a standard dose of subcutaneous adalimumab 40 mg every other week during each of three monitored clinical visits: visit 1 (syringe), visits 2 and 3 (pen). At each visit they rated their pain on an 11-point scale (0 = none to 10 = pain as bad as it could be) immediately and 15–30 minutes after the injection and gave their impressions of and preferences for each delivery system. Adverse events were recorded throughout the study and 70 days after the final dose. Forty patients reported that the pen was less painful than the syringe, four found the syringe to be less painful, and eight had no preference. Injection-pain scores were significantly lower from visit 1 to visit 2 and from visit 1 to visit 3. In all, 46 patients preferred the pen, three preferred the syringe, and three had no preference. Patients evaluated the pen as being easier to use (94%), more convenient (92%), requiring less time to inject (83%), and safer (89%).

References

1. Furst DE, Schiff MH, Fleischmann RM, Strand V, Birbara CA, Compagnone D, Fischkoff SA, Chartash EK. Adalimumab, a fully human anti tumor necrosis factor-alfa monoclonal antibody, and concomitant standard antirheumatic therapy for the treatment of rheumatoid arthritis: results of STAR (Safety Trial of Adalimumab in Rheumatoid Arthritis). J Rheumatol 2003;30:2563–7.
2. Van de Putte LB, Atkins C, Malaise M, Sany J, Russell AS, Van Riel PL, Settas L, Bijlsma JW, Todesco S, Dougados M, Nash P, Emery P, Walter N, Kaul M, Fischkoff S, Kupper H. Efficacy and safety of adalimumab as monotherapy in patients with rheumatoid arthritis for whom previous disease modifying antirheumatic drug treatment has failed. Ann Rheum Dis 2004;63:508–16.
3. Weinblatt ME, Keystone EC, Furst DE, Moreland LW, Weisman MH, Birbara CA, Teoh LA, Fischkoff SA, Chartash EK. Adalimumab, a fully human anti-tumor necrosis factor alfa monoclonal antibody, for the treatment of rheumatoid arthritis in patients taking concomitant methotrexate: the ARMADA trial. Arthritis Rheum 2003;48:35–45.
4. Scheinfeld N. Adalimumab: a review of side effects. Expert Opin Drug Saf 2005;4(4):637-41..
5. Bennett AN, Wong M, Zain A, Panayi G, Kirkham B. Adalimumab-induced asthma. Rheumatol (Oxf) 2005;44(9):1199-200..
6. Berthelot CN, George SJ, Hsu S. Distal lower extremity paresthesia and foot drop developing during adalimumab therapy. J Am Acad Dermatol 2005;53(5 Suppl 1):S260–2.
7. Leão JC, Duarte A, Gueiros LA, Carvalho AA, Barrett AW, Scully C, Porter S. Severe oral epithelial dysplasia in a patient receiving adalimumab therapy. J Oral Pathol Med 2005;34(7):447–8.
8. van der Heijde D, Kivitz A, Schiff MH, Sieper J, Dijkmans BA, Braun J, Dougados M, Reveille JD, Wong RL, Kupper H, Davis JC Jr; ATLAS Study Group. Efficacy and safety of adalimumab in patients with ankylosing spondylitis: results of a multicenter, randomized, double-blind, placebo-controlled trial. Arthritis Rheum 2006;54(7):2136–46.
9. Vavricka SR, Wettstein T, Speich R, Gaspert A, Bachli EB. Pulmonary granulomas after tumour necrosis factor alfa antagonist therapy. Thorax 2003;58:278–9.
10. Schoe A, van der Laan-Baalbergen NE, Huizinga TW, Breedveld FC, van Laar JM. Pulmonary fibrosis in a patient with rheumatoid arthritis treated with adalimumab. Arthritis Rheum 2006;55(1):157–9.
11. Huggett MT, Armstrong R. Adalimumab-associated pulmonary fibrosis. Rheumatology (Oxford) 2006;45(10):1312–3.
12. Allanore Y, Devos-François G, Caramella C, Boumier P, Jounieaux V, Kahan A. Fatal exacerbation of fibrosing alveolitis associated with systemic sclerosis in a patient treated with adalimumab. Ann Rheum Dis 2006;65(6):834–5.
13. Chung JH, Van Stavern GP, Frohman LP, Turbin RE. Adalimumab-associated optic neuritis. J Neurol Sci. 2006;244(1-2):133–6.
14. Theodoridou A, Kartsios C, Yiannaki E, Markala D, Settas L. Reversible T-large granular lymphocyte expansion and neutropenia associated with adalimumab therapy. Rheumatol Int 2006;27(2):201–2.
15. Den Broeder AA, Assmann KJ, Van Riel PL, Wetzels JF. Nephrotic syndrome as a complication of anti-TNFalfa in a patient with rheumatoid arthritis. Neth J Med 2003;61:137–41.

16. Matthews C, Rogers S, FitzGerald O. Development of new-onset psoriasis while on anti-TNFalpha treatment. Ann Rheum Dis 2006;65(11):1529–30.

17. Aslanidis S, Pyrpasopoulou A, Leontsini M, Zamboulis C. Anti-TNF-alpha-induced psoriasis: case report of an unusual adverse event. Int J Dermatol 2006;45(8):982–3.

18. Kary S, Worm M, Audring H, Huscher D, Renelt M, Sörensen H, Ständer E, Maass U, Lee H, Sterry W, Burmester GR. New onset or exacerbation of psoriatic skin lesions in patients with definite rheumatoid arthritis receiving tumour necrosis factor alpha antagonists. Ann Rheum Dis 2006;65(3):405–7.

19. Boura P, Sarantopoulos A, Lefaki I, Skendros P, Papadopoulos P. Eosinophilic cellulitis (Wells' syndrome) as a cutaneous reaction to the administration of adalimumab. Ann Rheum Dis 2006;65(6):839–40.

20. Garcia Bartels N, Lee HH, Worm M, Burmester GR, Sterry W, Blume-Peytavi U. Development of alopecia areata universalis in a patient receiving adalimumab. Arch Dermatol 2006;142(12):1654–5.

21. George SJ, Anderson HL, Hsu S. Adalimumab-induced urticaria. Dermatol Online J 2006;12(2):4.

22. Beuthien W, Mellinghoff HU, Von Kempis J. Skin reaction to adalimumab. Arthritis Rheum 2004;50:1690–2.

23. Bender NK, Heilig CE, Dröll B, Wohlgemuth J, Armbruster FP, Heilig B. Immunogenicity, efficacy and adverse events of adalimumab in RA patients. Rheumatol Int 2007;27(3):269–74.

24. Stallmach A, Giese T, Schmidt C, Meuer SC, Zeuzem SS. Severe anaphylactic reaction to infliximab: successful treatment with adalimumab. Report of a case. Eur J Gastroenterol Hepatol 2004;16:627–30.

25. Youdim A, Vasiliauskas EA, Targan SR, Papadakis KA, Ippoliti A, Dubinsky MC, Lechago J, Paavola J, Loane J, Lee SK, Gaiennie J, Smith K, Do J, Abreu MT. A pilot study of adalimumab in infliximab-allergic patients. Inflamm Bowel Dis 2004;10:333–8.

26. Schiff MH, Burmester GR, Kent JD, Pangan AL, Kupper H, Fitzpatrick SB, Donovan C. Safety analyses of adalimumab (HUMIRA) in global clinical trials and US postmarketing surveillance of patients with rheumatoid arthritis. Ann Rheum Dis 2006;65(7): 889–94.

27. Efde MN, Houtman PM, Spoorenberg JP, Jansen TL. Tonsillar tuberculosis in a rheumatoid arthritis patient receiving anti-TNFalpha (adalimumab) treatment. Neth J Med 2005;63:112–4.

28. Molloy E, Ramakrishnan S, Murphy E, Barry M. Morbidity and mortality in rheumatoid patients during treatment with adalimumab and infliximab. Rheumatology 2004;43:522–3.

29. Bassetti M, Pizzorni C, Gradoni L, Del Bono V, Cutolo M, Viscoli C. Visceral leishmaniasis infection in a rheumatoid arthritis patient treated with adalimumab. Rheumatology (Oxford) 2006;45(11):1446–8.

30. Keystone EC, Kavanaugh AF, Sharp JT, Tannenbaum H, Hua Y, Teoh LS, Fischkoff SA, Chartash EK. Radiographic, clinical, and functional outcomes of treatment with adalimumab (a human anti-tumor necrosis factor monoclonal antibody) in patients with active rheumatoid arthritis receiving concomitant methotrexate therapy: a randomized, placebo-controlled, 52-week trial. Arthritis Rheum 2004;50:1400–11.

31. Efde MN, Houtman PM, Spoorenberg JP, Jansen TL. Tonsillar tuberculosis in a rheumatoid arthritis patient receiving anti-TNFalpha (adalimumab) treatment. Neth J Med 2005;63(3):112–4.

32. Anonymous. Tumor necrosis factor (TNF)-α inhibitors. Increased risk of malignancy. WHO Pharm Newslett 2007;1:5.

33. Bongartz T, Sutton AJ, Sweeting MJ, Buchan I, Matteson EL, Montori V. Anti-TNF antibody therapy in rheumatoid arthritis and the risk of serious infections and malignancies: systematic review and meta-analysis of rare harmful effects in randomized controlled trials. JAMA 2006;295(19):2275-85. Erratum: 2006;295(21):2482.

34. Kunzlberger B, Pieck C, Altmeyer P, Stucker M. Risk of serious infections and malignancies with anti-TNF antibody therapy in rheumatoid arthritis. JAMA 2006;296:1410–3.

35. Dalle S, Balme B, Berger F, Hayette S, Thomas L. Mycosis fungoides-associated follicular mucinosis under adalimumab. Br J Dermatol 2005;153(1):207–8.

36. Ziakas PD, Giannouli S, Tzioufas AG, Voulgarelis M. Lymphoma development in a patient receiving anti-TNF therapy. Haematologica 2003;88:ECR25.

37. Colombel JF, Sandborn WJ, Rutgeerts P, Enns R, Hanauer SB, Panaccione R, Schreiber S, Byczkowski D, Li J, Kent JD, Pollack PF. Adalimumab for maintenance of clinical response and remission in patients with Crohn's disease: the CHARM trial. Gastroenterology 2007;132(1):52–65.

38. Kivitz A, Cohen S, Dowd JE, Edwards W, Thakker S, Wellborne FR, Renz CL, Segurado OG. Clinical assessment of pain, tolerability, and preference of an autoinjection pen versus a prefilled syringe for patient self-administration of the fully human, monoclonal antibody adalimumab: the TOUCH trial. Clin Ther 2006;28(10):1619–29.

Alefacept

General Information

Alefacept is a bioengineered fusion protein of soluble lymphocyte function antigen (LFA-3) with Fc fragments of IgG1. It blocks the LFA-3/CD2 interaction necessary for activation and proliferation of memory effector T cells by binding to CD2 expressed on the surface of the T cell. It has been used in the treatment of psoriasis and psoriatic arthritis. There has also been a small pilot study of it use in rheumatoid arthritis (1). Its uses and efficacy have been reviewed (2,3).

The reported adverse effects of alefacept are generally minor and include headache, nasopharyngitis, rhinitis, influenza, upper respiratory tract infections, pruritus, arthralgias, fatigue, nausea, accidental injury, and increases in liver enzymes (4). A few patients develop antibodies against alefacept.

Observational studies

In an open study in 11 patients with active psoriatic arthritis who were given alefacept for 12 weeks the most common adverse effects that were probably or definitely associated with the drug were a flu-like syndrome (54%) and infections (18%) (5). There were two severe adverse events, which were both judged to be unrelated to alefacept.

Placebo-controlled studies

In a randomized, double-blind, placebo-controlled trial in 185 patients with psoriatic arthritis aged 18–70 years alefacept 15 mg or placebo was given intramuscularly once a week for 12 weeks in combination with methotrexate, followed by 12 weeks of observation during which only methotrexate was continued (6). Back pain and a raised alanine transaminase activity were more common than in those given placebo. Adverse events led to withdrawal of treatment in two patients taking alefacept, one because of worsening and one because of increased transaminase activities to 3–5 times the upper limit of normal; in the latter the transaminases returned to normal after withdrawal of alefacept. There were serious adverse events in two patients who received alefacept (metrorrhagia, rectocele, and emphysema) and in three who received placebo (intervertebral disc protrusion, non-infectious gastroenteritis, and breast cancer). Most of the recorded adverse events were mild to moderate in intensity and none of the serious events was attributed to the drug. There were no opportunistic infections or malignancies.

Systematic reviews

In a systematic review of double-blind, randomized, controlled trials of alefacept (n = 3), efalizumab (n = 5), etanercept (n = 4), and infliximab (n = 4); in patients with psoriasis the relative risks of one or more adverse events in were significantly increased compared with placebo:

- alefacept: RR = 1.09; NNT_H = 15;
- efalizumab: RR = 1.15; NNT_H = 9;
- infliximab: RR = 1.18; NNT_H = 9

Serious adverse events were increased in a sensitivity analysis of four efalizumab trials (n = 2443; RR = 1.92; NNT_H = 60) (7).

Organs and Systems

Hematologic

Because of its pharmacological action, the CD4+ count is reduced by alefacept. It has therefore been suggested that the CD4+ count should be monitored regularly to ensure that it does not fall below 250 x 10^6/l (8); however, the usefulness of doing this has not been demonstrated (9).

Long-Term Effects

Tumorigenicity

Lymphoproliferative disorders are more common in individuals taking immunosuppressive drugs, and mycosis fungoides has been reported in a 72-year-old patient with a psoriasiform dermatitis taking alefacept (10). The authors suggested that alefacept should be used with caution in patients with known mycosis fungoides or an unclassified atypical lymphocytic infiltrate of the skin.

Drug Administration

Drug administration route

In two open studies in healthy men a single dose of alefacept 0.15 mg/kg was given as a 30-secong intravenous bolus (n = 12), 0.04 mg/kg intramuscularly (n = 8), or 0.04 mg/kg as a 30-minute intravenous infusion (n = 8) (11). The intramuscular availability was about 60%. The half-life was about 12 days.

In a randomized, open, crossover comparison of subcutaneous and intramuscular alefacept 15 mg in 50 healthy volunteers, the systemic availabilities were similar (12).

References

1. Schneider M, Stahl H-D, Podrebarac T, Braun J. Tolerability and safety of combination methotrexate and alefacept in rheumatoid arthritis: results of a pilot study. Arthritis Rheum 2004;12:S654.
2. Hodak E, David M. Alefacept: a review of the literature and practical guidelines for management. Dermatol Ther 2004;17(5):383–92.
3. Krueger GG. Current concepts and review of alefacept in the treatment of psoriasis. Dermatol Clin 2004;22(4):407–26, viii.
4. Scheinfeld N. Alefacept: a safety profile. Expert Opin Drug Saf 2005;4(6):975–85.
5. Kraan MC, van Kuijk AW, Dinant HJ, Goedkoop AY, Smeets TJ, de Rie MA, Dijkmans BA, Vaishnaw AK, Bos JD, Tak PP. Alefacept treatment in psoriatic arthritis: reduction of the effector T cell population in peripheral blood and synovial tissue is associated with improvement of clinical signs of arthritis. Arthritis Rheum 2002;46(10):2776–84.
6. Mease PJ, Gladman DD, Keystone EC; Alefacept in Psoriatic Arthritis Study Group. Alefacept in combination with methotrexate for the treatment of psoriatic arthritis: results of a randomized, double-blind, placebo-controlled study. Arthritis Rheum 2006;54(5):1638–45.
7. Brimhall AK, King LN, Licciardone JC, Jacobe H, Menter A. Safety and efficacy of alefacept, efalizumab, etanercept and infliximab in treating moderate to severe plaque psoriasis: a meta-analysis of randomized controlled trials. Br J Dermatol 2008;159(2):274–85.
8. Papp KA. Monitoring patients treated with efalizumab or alefacept. Curr Probl Dermatol 2009;38:95–106.
9. Scheinfeld N. Alefacept: its safety profile, off-label uses, and potential as part of combination therapies for psoriasis. J Dermatolog Treat 2007;18(4):197–208.
10. Schmidt A, Robbins J, Zic J. Transformed mycosis fungoides developing after treatment with alefacept. J Am Acad Dermatol 2005;2:355–6.
11. Vaishnaw AK, TenHoor CN. Pharmacokinetics, biologic activity, and tolerability of alefacept by intravenous and intramuscular administration. J Pharmacokinet Pharmacodyn 2002;29(5-6):415–26.
12. Sweetser MT, Woodworth J, Swan S, Ticho B. Results of a randomized open-label crossover study of the bioequivalence of subcutaneous versus intramuscular administration of alefacept. Dermatol Online J 2006 30;12(3):1.

Anakinra

General Information

Anakinra is an interleukin-1 receptor antagonist. It has been used to treat rheumatoid arthritis (1,2). It has been tried in graft-versus-host disease, but without success (3). According to published trial data, moderate injection site reactions were the primary adverse effect and required treatment withdrawal in under 5% of patients. An erythematous rash was seldom observed. Although a few patients have developed antibodies to anakinra, these have not so far been associated with lack of efficacy or allergic skin reactions.

Placebo-controlled studies

In 1414 patients with rheumatoid arthritis of varying severity and various co-morbid conditions randomized to receive anakinra 100 mg/day (n=1116) or placebo (n=283) the rate of serious adverse events and malignancies after 6 months of treatment was similar in the two groups (4). Serious infectious episodes occurred more often in the treated group (2.1%) than in the placebo group (0.4%), but the difference was not statistically significant. Unusual or opportunistic infections were not identified. Mild-to-moderate *injection-site reactions* were the most commonly reported adverse effects attributed to anakinra (73%).

Organs and Systems

Gastrointestinal

Acute exacerbation of Crohn's disease has been attributed to anakinra (5).

- A 40-year-old with a previous history of chronic intermittent diarrhea had worsening arthralgia and fever, increased diarrhea, and abdominal pain within 3-4 days of anakinra 100 mg/day for rheumatoid arthritis. Most of the symptoms abated after withdrawal, but promptly reappeared on rechallenge. Further investigations were consistent with a diagnosis of Crohn's disease.

Skin

Metastatic malignant melanoma occurred in a patient taking anakinra (6).

- A 61-year-old man with rheumatoid arthritis was given anakinra 100mg/day and 3 years later a biopsy of a pigmented skin lesion behind his right ear showed a malignant melanoma with metastases in several cervical lymph nodes and in the right parotid gland. The stage was T3a, N3, M1.

Infection risk

Anakinra 100 mg/day has been compared with placebo in 1346 patients with rheumatoid arthritis in a 6-month, randomized, double-blind study. The most frequent adverse events were injection site reactions (122 events/100 patient-years), rheumatoid arthritis progression (68 events/100 patient-years), and upper respiratory infections (26 events/100 patient-years) (7). The exposure adjusted event rate of serious infections was higher in patients treated with anakinra for 0–3 years (5.4 events/100 patient-years) than for controls during the blinded phase (1.7 events/100 patient-years). However, if the patient was not receiving corticosteroid treatment at baseline, the serious infection rate was substantially lower (2.9 event/100 patient-years).

Anakinra was suspected to favor the development of an abscess in the forearm in a 38-year-old diabetic man who underwent local surgery (8).

Septicemia with *Staphylococcus aureus*, group B and G beta-hemolytic streptococci, and *Escherichia coli* has been reported in a 66-year-old woman 2 months after anakinra was added to prednisolone for rheumatoid arthritis (9).

Drug–Drug Interactions

Etanercept

Regulatory agencies have issued an important postmarketing warning of an increased risk of serious infections and neutropenia in patients who receive concomitant anakinra and etanercept (10). This warning was based on an analysis of a randomized clinical trial in 242 patients with rheumatoid arthritis, in which 7% of patients receiving concomitant treatment had serious infections, compared with none in those treated with etanercept alone. Concurrent administration of these two drugs was therefore not recommended.

References

1. Cohen SB. The use of anakinra, an interleukin-1 receptor antagonist, in the treatment of rheumatoid arthritis. Rheum Dis Clin North Am 2004;30(2):365–80.
2. Bresnihan B. The safety and efficacy of interleukin-1 receptor antagonist in the treatment of rheumatoid arthritis. Semin Arthritis Rheum 2001;30(5 Suppl 2):17–20.
3. Antin JH, Weisdorf D, Neuberg D, Nicklow R, Clouthier S, Lee SJ, Alyea E, McGarigle C, Blazar BR, Sonis S, Soiffer RJ, Ferrara JL. Interleukin-1 blockade does not prevent acute graft-versus-host disease: results of a randomized, double-blind, placebo-controlled trial of interleukin-1 receptor antagonist in allogeneic bone marrow transplantation. Blood 2002;100(10):3479–82.
4. Fleischmann RM, Schechtman J, Bennett R, Handel ML, Burmester GR, Tesser J, Modafferi D, Poulakos J, Sun G. Anakinra, a recombinant human interleukin-1 receptor antagonist (r-metHuIL-1ra), in patients with rheumatoid arthritis: a large, international, multicenter, placebo-controlled trial. Arthritis Rheum 2003;48:927–34.

5. Carter JD, Valeriano J, Vasey JB. Crohn disease worsened by anakinra administration. J Clin Rheumatol 2003;9:276–7.
6. Wendling D, Aubin F. Metastatic malignant melanoma in a patient taking interleukin-1 receptor antagonist. Joint Bone Spine 2006;73(3):333–4.
7. Fleischmann RM, Tesser J, Schiff MH, Schechtman J, Burmester GR, Bennett R, Modafferi D, Zhou L, Bell D, Appleton B. Safety of extended treatment with anakinra in patients with rheumatoid arthritis. Ann Rheum Dis 2006;65(8):1006–12.
8. Gaulke R. Unterarmphlegmone unter Anakinra (interleukin-1-receptor-antagonist). Z Rheumatol 2003;62:566–9.
9. Turesson C, Riesbeck K. Septicemia with Staphylococcus aureus, beta-hemolytic streptococci group B and G, and Escherichia coli in a patient with rheumatoid arthritis treated with a recombinant human interleukin 1 receptor antagonist (anakinra). J Rheumatol 2004;31:1876.
10. EMEA/31631/02 Public Statement. Increased risk of serious infection and neutropenia in patients treated concurrently with Kineret (anakinra) and Enbrel (etanercept). http://www.emea.eu.int/pdfs/human/press/pus/3163102en.pdf.

Azathioprine [and mercaptopurine]

General Information

Azathioprine, 6-mercaptopurine, and 6-thioguanine are thiopurines. Azathioprine is a prodrug of mercaptopurine and thioguanine is an active metabolite. Thioguanine is covered in a separate monograph.

Azathioprine, a prodrug converted to 6-mercaptopurine, is widely used as a post-transplant immunosuppressant and in various autoimmune or chronic inflammatory disorders, such as rheumatoid arthritis, dermatomyositis, systemic lupus erythematosus, skin diseases, and inflammatory bowel diseases.

Adverse effects usually occur during the first two months of treatment, do not correlate with the daily dose, and result in treatment withdrawal in 14–18% of patients, mainly because of bone marrow suppression, gastrointestinal symptoms, hypersensitivity reactions, and infections (1–3). Immediate or long-term adverse effects are of particular concern outside the field of immunosuppression where other treatment options are frequently available, but in any field of use the adverse effects of these drugs weigh heavily.

Observational studies

In a follow-up study of 157 patients receiving azathioprine or mercaptopurine for Crohn's disease, the long-term risks (mainly hematological toxicity and malignancies) over 4 years of treatment were deemed to outweigh the therapeutic benefit (4). In contrast to these findings, both drugs were considered efficacious and reasonably safe in patients with inflammatory bowel disease, provided that patients are carefully selected and regularly investigated for bone marrow toxicity (5). Similar opinions were

expressed regarding renal transplant patients. Conversion from ciclosporin to azathioprine in selected and carefully monitored patients had beneficial effects, by improving renal function, reducing cardiovascular risk factors, and reducing financial costs, without increasing the incidence of chronic rejection and graft loss (6).

Experience in children with juvenile chronic arthritis or chronic inflammatory bowel disease has also accumulated, and the toxicity profile of azathioprine or mercaptopurine appears to be very similar to that previously found in the adult population (SEDA-21, 381; SEDA-22, 410).

The "azathioprine hypersensitivity syndrome"

The complex of azathioprine-associated multisystemic adverse effects is referred to by the misnomer "azathioprine hypersensitivity syndrome." This well-characterized reaction has been described in numerous case reports and includes various symptoms which can occur separately or concomitantly; they comprise fever and rigors, arthralgia, myalgia, leukocytosis, cutaneous reactions, gastrointestinal disturbances, hypotension, liver injury, pancreatitis, interstitial nephritis, pneumonitis, and pulmonary hemorrhage (SED-13, 1121; SEDA-20, 341; SEDA-21, 381; SEDA-22, 410) (7). Isolated fever and rigors are sometimes observed, and severe renal and cardiac toxicity or leukocytoclastic cutaneous vasculitis are infrequent. Symptoms usually occur within the first 6 weeks of treatment and can mimic sepsis. The initial febrile reaction is often misdiagnosed as infectious, and could be associated with acute exacerbation of the underlying disease, for example myasthenia gravis (SEDA-21, 381; SEDA-22, 410). Hypersensitivity associated with reversible interstitial nephritis can also be mistaken for an acute rejection episode (8). This syndrome should therefore be promptly recognized to avoid unnecessary and costly investigations, and further recurrence on azathioprine rechallenge.

Organs and Systems

Respiratory

Although azathioprine-associated pulmonary toxicity mostly occurs as part of the azathioprine hypersensitivity reaction, isolated interstitial pneumonitis has been reported in a 13-year-old girl with autoimmune chronic active hepatitis (9).

It can resolve after drug withdrawal (10).

- A 40-year-old man took azathioprine for 10 years for extensive ulcerative colitis. He then developed fever, cough, and catarrhal signs. Opportunistic infections were ruled out. Chest X-ray, a CT scan, and a lung biopsy showed interstitial inflammation. Azathioprine was withdrawn and he was given steroids; the pulmonary infiltrates gradually resolved.

Acute upper airway edema has been observed after a single dose of azathioprine (11).

- A 57-year-old woman with a history of several drug allergies underwent renal transplantation for end-stage polycystic kidney disease and 1 hour later was given intravenous azathioprine 400 mg. She developed profound hypotension and bradycardia within 30 minutes, reversed by sympathomimetics. Shortly after extubation, she had severe breathing difficulties with loss of consciousness. Laryngoscopy showed massive swelling of the tongue and upper airways. Later, while still taking glucocorticoids, she was rechallenged with azathioprine and had milder hypotension and edema of the airways.

Even if no clear mechanism can account for this adverse effect, positive rechallenge strongly suggested that azathioprine was the culprit.

Nervous system

Neuritis multiplex occurred in a patient taking azathioprine for autoimmune hepatitis and resolved after conversion to cyclophosphamide (12).

- A 37-year-old woman with autoimmune hepatitis taking azathioprine and prednisolone developed a left-sided hemisensory deficit followed by right foot drop and bilateral paraesthesia in the ulnar nerve territory. An MRI scan and cerebral panangiography suggested cerebral vasculitis. Neurological investigations and electromyography showed neuritis multiplex probably due to vasculitis. There were serum autoantibodies to extractable nuclear antigens. Azathioprine was withdrawn and oral cyclophosphamide 150 mg/day introduced. Almost complete motoric remission was achieved after 3 months, but sensation remained reduced in the right peroneal nerve distribution.

Azathioprine can cause a posterior leukoencephalopathy (13).

- A patient was given azathioprine for systemic lupus erythematosus and after 3 weeks developed a posterior leukoencephalopathy with headache, tonic–clonic seizures, loss of consciousness, bilateral loss of vision, and hypertension. A CT scan showed hypodense lesions in both bilateral occipital lobes, mainly in the white matter. The symptoms and follow-up MRI scan improved after control of hypertension and withdrawal of azathioprine.

Neuromuscular function

In two patients azathioprine caused profound muscular weakness, resulting in an inability to perform simple tasks, such as lifting even light objects, sitting upright, and walking a few steps (14). Withdrawal of azathioprine resulted in prompt improvement, and rechallenge led to recurrence of similar symptoms within hours.

Psychiatric

Azathioprine has been associated with psychiatric adverse events (15).

- A 13-year-old boy with Wegener's granulomatosis developed incapacitating obsessive–compulsive symptoms and severe panic attacks 4 weeks after switching from cyclophosphamide to azathioprine. He had obsessions about dying, committing suicide, and harming others, obsessive negative thoughts about himself and others, compulsive behavior, severe panic attacks more than once a day, and sleep disturbances. He was given fluvoxamine 100 mg/day, but 18 months later the symptoms suddenly disappeared, 3 weeks after he switched from azathioprine to methotrexate. In the next 4 years, he had no relapse.

Psychiatric adverse effects have not previously been reported with azathioprine. Neither does the database of the WHO Uppsala Monitoring Centre mention obsessive–compulsive symptoms or panic attacks as a possible adverse effect of azathioprine. However, the time course in this case and the absence of symptoms before and after azathioprine therapy suggest a causal relation. It is possible that the combination of subtle cerebral dysfunction as a result of the vasculitis and the use of azathioprine may have caused the symptoms in this patient.

Endocrine

Hyperprolactinemia has been attributed to azathioprine (16).

- A 24-year-old woman, with a 3-year history of psoriasis, in the last trimester of her first pregnancy developed autoimmune thrombocytic purpura, which resolved after delivery. After 1 year, her liver function tests rose to 10 times normal values, associated with fatigue, weakness, and splenomegaly. Fine-needle liver aspiration showed autoimmune hepatitis. Her transaminases normalized with a glucocorticoid. She was then given azathioprine 50 mg/day instead of the glucocorticoid. After 1 month, her liver function tests rose about seven-fold and her prolactin concentrations by three-fold. She was again given a glucocorticoid and the azathioprine was continued. Six weeks later she was in remission, but her prolactin concentration was still high. There was no galactorrhea or amenorrhea, and the hyperprolactinemia was thought to have been be caused by azathioprine.

Hematologic

Hematological toxicity is the most commonly reported severe adverse effect of azathioprine, and is marked by predominant leukopenia, thrombocytopenia, and pancytopenia (SED-13, 1120). In a 27-year survey of 739 patients treated with azathioprine 2 mg/kg for inflammatory bowel disease, dosage reduction or withdrawal of the drug because of bone marrow toxicity was necessary in 37 patients (5%) (17). There was moderate or severe leukopenia in 3.8% of patients; in three patients pancytopenia resulted in severe sepsis or death.

Leukopenia is the most serious adverse effect of azathioprine in patients with inflammatory bowel disease (18). It is variable and unpredictable and occurs 2 weeks to 11 years after the start of treatment (median 9 months); most cases recover 1 month after withdrawal.

The short-term and long-term toxicity of mercaptopurine has been investigated in 410 patients with inflammatory bowel disease treated for 20 years. There was significant leukopenia (3.5×10^9/l or less) in 11% (19).

Dual therapy with ciclosporin and prednisone has been compared with triple therapy with ciclosporin, prednisone, and azathioprine in a randomized trial in 250 renal transplant patients (20). Patients in the triple therapy group had less frequent severe episodes of acute rejection and more frequent episodes of leukopenia than the double therapy group (28% versus 4%). There were no other differences in the adverse effects profiles, in particular the incidence of infectious complications.

Macrocytic anemia and isolated thrombocytopenia without severe clinical consequences have sometimes been observed. Pure red cell aplasia can occur, but the few relevant reports concern only isolated instances involving renal transplant patients (21,22). The facts in one patient suggested that parvovirus B19 infection resulting from the immunosuppressive effects of azathioprine should also be considered as a possible indirect cause (23). Although blood cell disorders usually occur in the first 4 weeks of treatment, strict and regular surveillance of blood cell counts continuing for as long as treatment is maintained is usually recommended, since delayed hematological toxicity remains possible.

Megaloblastic change occurs in 16-82% of bone marrow aspirates, but long-term use of azathioprine rarely causes severe anemia. In addition, azathioprine can cause refractory pure red cell aplasia, particularly after kidney transplantation (24). Refractory anemia was reported in a patient with 17p– syndrome after heart transplantation (25).

Among patients receiving mycophenolate mofetil or azathioprine the latter had lower hemoglobin concentrations after 1 and 6 months; mean corpuscular hemoglobin concentrations were also lower at 1 week and 1 months after transplantation but were comparable at 6 months (26).

- Immune hemolytic anemia has been reported in a 67-year-old man taking mercaptopurine for chronic myelomonocytic leukemia (27). Serology showed a positive direct antiglobulin test and confirmed the presence of mercaptopurine drug-dependent antibodies. He improved and the direct antiglobulin test was no longer positive 20 days after mercaptopurine withdrawal.

Azathioprine can cause pancytopenia and subsequent myelodysplasia or secondary leukemia. Complex genetic alterations involving chromosome 7 are characteristic.

- A 49-year-old woman with multiple sclerosis received azathioprine for 5 years (cumulative dose 45 g) (28). She developed fatigue and a sinus tachycardia. She had a pancytopenia with a normochromic anemia (hemoglobin 6.2 g/dl), a mild leukopenia (leukocyte count 3.5×10^9/l), and thrombocytopenia (platelet count 22×10^9/l) requiring platelet transfusion. A bone marrow aspirate showed dysplasia of all three lineages, with reduced thrombopoiesis and ineffective erythropoiesis. Cytogenetic analysis showed a complex aberrant clone, including loss of the critically deleted

regions in 5q31 and 7q31, as well as structural changes in 12p. Refractory cytopenia with multilineage dysplasia was diagnosed according to the WHO classification of myelodysplastic syndromes. Allogeneic sibling transplantation was planned, but she developed a spontaneous recurrent subdural hematoma and died due to persistent bleeding refractory to platelet transfusion.

Aplastic anemia due to azathioprine therapy after corneal transplantation has reportedly caused bilateral macular hemorrhage (29).

- A 38-year-old man underwent therapeutic penetrating keratoplasty for non-healing fungal keratitis in his left eye. Although the infection was controlled, he underwent a second corneal transplantation after 2 years. Since there was corneal vascularization in three quadrants, he was given oral azathioprine postoperatively. Four months later he developed gastrointestinal bleeding and a sudden reduction in vision in both eyes. His platelet count was less than 30×10^9/l, his hemoglobin 4.1 g/dl, and a bone marrow aspirate was hypocellular. There were macular hemorrhages in both eyes. The hemorrhages resolved within 2 months.

Gastrointestinal

Gastrointestinal disturbances with nausea, vomiting, and diarrhea are frequent in patients taking azathioprine or mercaptopurine. Diarrhea may be isolated or part of the azathioprine hypersensitivity syndrome. In two patients with azathioprine-induced diarrhea proven by positive rechallenge, the period of sensitization ranged from 1 week to 1 year (30).

In two cases, azathioprine caused severe gastrointestinal symptoms that could have been easily confused with an acute exacerbation of the underlying inflammatory bowel disease (31).

- A 32-year-old man with ulcerative colitis improved with prednisolone, mesalazine, and antibiotics. The dose of prednisolone was reduced and the disease flared up again. He was therefore given azathioprine and an increased dose of prednisolone, with rapid clinical improvement. After 3 weeks, he reported increasing abdominal pain, worse diarrhea, and weight loss of 3 kg. He stopped taking azathioprine and the pain improved. Because of progressive disease and active pancolitis at colonoscopy, he was given high-dose prednisolone, mesalazine, and ciprofloxacin, without improvement. He was therefore given intravenous azathioprine, but developed devastating diarrhea and weight loss of more than 6 kg in 24 hours, his CRP rose from 5 to 305 µg/ml, and he developed hypovolemic shock. He recovered after treatment with parenteral nutrition for 7 days.
- A 50-year-old woman with Crohn's disease and active disease throughout the colon was given prednisolone, mesalazine, and azathioprine 50 mg/day. After 3 weeks, the dose of azathioprine was increased to 100 mg/day, but she developed nausea, severe diarrhea, and abdominal tenderness. The symptoms subsided after

azathioprine was withdrawn. She was then given mercaptopurine, without significant adverse effects.

Azathioprine can cause severe small-bowel villous atrophy, diarrhea, and malabsorption, reversible after withdrawal.

- A 20-year-old man with autoimmune hepatitis developed severe small-bowel villous atrophy and chronic diarrhea after taking azathioprine 50 mg/day (32). The diarrhea was unresponsive to oral pancreatic enzymes or a gluten-free diet, and severe malabsorption required parenteral nutrition for more than 1.5 years, until the association with azathioprine was identified. Within 2 weeks after withdrawal, the diarrhea resolved completely and parenteral nutrition was discontinued. Mucosal biopsies before and 4 months after azathioprine withdrawal showed complete reversal of severe duodenal villous atrophy and marked up-regulation of mucosal dipeptidyl peptidase IV and PepT1 messenger RNA. The patient subsequently maintained normal liver function tests on low-dose prednisone alone, with normal stools and stable nutritional status for more than 4 years.

Liver

Thiopurines can cause liver damage, and the incidence varies in different studies. Although rarely severe, any increase in liver enzyme activity justifies careful and regular monitoring of liver function and the results may be a reason for withdrawing treatment (SED-8, 1118; 33). In a retrospective study, hepatitis was found in 21 (2%) of 1035 renal transplant patients, and it was suggested that hepatitis B or C infection increases the risk of azathioprine hepatotoxicity (34). In 29 cardiac transplant recipients who had had probable azathioprine-induced liver dysfunction, cyclophosphamide was given, with improvement of liver enzyme activities and no increase in the rate of graft rejection or significant changes in the doses of other immunosuppressive drugs (35).

Hepatotoxicity, defined as alanine transaminase or alkaline phosphatase activities greater than twice the upper normal limit, was studied in 161 patients with inflammatory bowel disease over a median follow-up of 271 days (36). There was abnormal liver function in 21 patients (13%), hepatotoxicity in 16 (10 %) after a median of 85 days, and thiopurines were withdrawn in five patients because of hepatotoxicity.

Azathioprine can cause reversible cholestasis (37), perhaps due to bile duct injury (38).

Direct hepatocellular injury with acute cytolytic hepatitis has been reported rarely (SEDA-21, 381).

In one patient, azathioprine-induced lymphoma with massive liver infiltration was the probable cause of fulminant hepatic failure (SEDA-21, 381).

Other histological features that have been described include lesions of the hepatic venous system (peliosis hepatis, sinusoidal dilatation, perivenous fibrosis, and nodular regenerative hyperplasia) and these can be associated with portal hypertension (SEDA-16, 520; SED-13, 1120; 33). Particularly severe and potentially fatal veno-

occlusive liver disease has been reported in patients with renal and allogeneic bone marrow transplants taking chronic treatment (SEDA-12, 386; 39), but complete histological reversal can be observed (SEDA-20, 341).

- In a 33-year-old man azathioprine-induced veno-occlusive disease was treated with a transjugular intrahepatic portosystemic shunt over 26 months, with progressive worsening 15 months after renal transplantation (40).

Four patients with renal transplants developed hepatic veno-occlusive disease after immunosuppression with azathioprine. The diagnosis was based on typical histopathological findings: perivenular fibrosis, trilobular sinusoidal dilatation and congestion, and perisinusoidal fibrosis. The patients presented with severe progressive portal hypertension followed by fulminant liver failure and death. The disease was associated with cytomegalovirus infection, and it was not related to the dose of azathioprine (39). Veno-occlusive liver disease has also been described shortly after liver transplantation (41,42). A history of acute liver rejection affecting the hepatic veins was supposedly a contributing factor in these patients, and the presence of non-inflammatory small hepatic vein lesions was a possible early indicator of hepatotoxicity. Liver biopsy should therefore be considered in liver recipients who have biological features of hepatitis, so that treatment can be withdrawn rapidly if necessary.

Azathioprine allergy can be associated with biochemical hepatitis and a normal liver biopsy, apart form marked lipofuscin deposition (43). These findings, combined with patchy isotope uptake on technetium scintigraphy, are suggestive of focal hepatocellular necrosis.

It has been suggested that there is an increased risk of azathioprine-induced liver damage in renal transplant patients with chronic viral hepatitis (SEDA-20, 341; SEDA-23, 402).

- Fatal fibrosing cholestatic hepatitis has been reported in a 63-year-old cardiac transplant patient with acquired post-transplant hepatitis C virus infection whose immunosuppressive regimen included azathioprine (44). Histology showed several features of azathioprine hepatotoxicity, namely veno-subocclusive lesions and nodular regenerative diffuse hyperplasia, suggesting a pathogenic role of azathioprine.

In 79 renal transplant patients with chronic viral hepatitis, azathioprine maintenance treatment ($n = 34$) was associated with a poorer outcome than in 45 patients who discontinued azathioprine (45). Cirrhosis was more frequent in the first group (six versus one), and more patients died with a functioning graft (14 versus two), mostly because of liver dysfunction ($n = 5$) or infection ($n = 6$). These results suggest that azathioprine further accelerates the course of the liver disease in these patients.

Nodular regenerative hyperplasia of the liver can occur with any of the purine analogues (azathioprine, 6-mercaptopurine, and 6-thioguanine) (46). It has been described in four patients with inflammatory bowel disease taking azathioprine (47). All had either abnormal liver function tests and/or a low platelet count. The biochemical and hematological abnormalities resolved after azathioprine withdrawal. Male sex was a major susceptibility factor. In another series, two patients taking azathioprine developed nodular regenerative hyperplasia; both were heterozygous for the TPMT*3A mutation (48).

- A 50-year-old woman with nodular sclerosis developed azathioprine-induced hepatotoxicity within the first weeks of treatment (49), the usual time-course. Positive rechallenge confirmed the role of azathioprine.

However, delayed occurrence of hepatitis is also possible.

- Canalicular cholestasis with portal fibrosis and ductal proliferation has been reported after 24 years of azathioprine in a 57-year-old woman with myasthenia gravis (50).

An unusual diffuse liver disease with sinusoidal dilatation (SEDA-11, 392) has been described.

In vitro, glycyrrhizic acid and liquorice had a protective effect against azathioprine hepatotoxicity; glycyrrhizic acid protected human hepatocytes from intracellular glutathione depletion on exposure to 1 μm azathioprine (51). In another in vitro study a novel glutathione transferase (GST)-dependent pathway in the biotransformation of azathioprine was described (52). Glutathione transferases A1-1, A2-2, and M1-1, all abundantly expressed in human liver, had the highest activity among the 14 isoenzymes tested. The uncatalysed reaction of azathioprine with glutathione was less than 1% of the glutathione transferase-catalysed biotransformation. GST M1-1 is polymorphic, with a frequently occurring null allele, and GST A1-1 and GST A2-2 are variably expressed in humans, implying significant differences in the rate of mercaptopurine production from azathioprine. Individuals who expressing high GST activity are predisposed to adverse reactions to azathioprine, both by promoting excessively high concentrations of mercaptopurine and its toxic metabolites and by depleting cellular glutathione.

Pancreas

Pancreatitis due to azathioprine or mercaptopurine has usually been reported as part of the hypersensitivity syndrome (SEDA-16, 520; SEDA-20, 341). It has mostly been observed in patients with inflammatory bowel disease, and required withdrawal of treatment in 1.3% of patients with Crohn's disease (3). Pancreatitis was not dose-related within the therapeutic range of doses and often recurred in patients who were rechallenged with either drug (SEDA-20, 341; 53). Fatal hemorrhagic pancreatitis occurred in one patient, but a role of concomitant drugs was also possible (SEDA-20, 341). Pancreatitis or hyperamylasemia were not significantly different in renal transplant patients randomly assigned to receive azathioprine or ciclosporin, and other causative factors were found in most patients with pancreatitis (54).

In a review of definite or probable drug-associated pancreatitis spontaneously reported to the Dutch adverse drug reactions system during 1977–98, azathioprine was the suspected drug in four of 34 patients, two of whom had positive rechallenge (55). Although most of the carefully described reports of azathioprine-induced pancreatitis were found in patients with inflammatory bowel disease, transplant recipients can also suffer this complication.

- Over a year after renal transplantation, a 48-year-old man, who took azathioprine, ciclosporin, and prednisolone, developed acute necrotizing pancreatitis (56). Improvement was obtained after azathioprine withdrawal, but he again took azathioprine and had similar symptoms within 30 hours after a single dose.
- Pancreatitis has been reported after a progressive increase in dose of 6-thioguanine in a 10-year-old infant (57). She had had two previous episodes of pancreatitis after mercaptopurine.

In Denmark, 1317 patients redeemed a total of 15 811 prescriptions for azathioprine during 1991 and 2000. The incidence rate for acute pancreatitis was one per 659 treatment year. The risk increased with presence of gallstone disease, alcohol-related diseases, inflammatory bowel disease, and the use of glucocorticoids. Thus, the relative risk of acute pancreatitis is increased in azathioprine users (58).

Azathioprine-associated acute pancreatitis is strongly associated with Crohn's disease and occurs less commonly with other underlying conditions (59). The incidence of acute pancreatitis was 4.9% in 224 patients with Crohn's disease, 1.5% in 129 with autoimmune hepatitis, 0.5% in 388 with kidney transplants, and 0.4% in 254 with liver transplants.

The chemical structure of 6-thioguanine, which results from the metabolism of azathioprine/mercaptopurine, is very similar to that of mercaptopurine. Therefore, a history of previous adverse effects with mercaptopurine should be anticipated in patients considered for 6-thioguanine treatment.

Urinary tract

A woman with Wegener's granulomatosis progressed to renal failure within 10 days of starting azathioprine for vasculitis (60). A renal biopsy showed acute tubulointerstitial nephritis and no active glomerulonephritis.

Skin

Rashes or other allergic-type cutaneous reactions are usually noted during the azathioprine hypersensitivity syndrome. Isolated but convincing reports point to the occurrence of vasculitis with microscopic polyarteritis (SEDA-21, 381) and Sweet's syndrome, which recurred after subsequent azathioprine exposure (SEDA-22, 410).

Pellagra with a photosensitivity-like rash and skin peeling syndrome has also been noted (SEDA-21, 381).

A febrile diffuse skin eruption occurred in a patient taking azathioprine and a glucocorticoid (61).

- A 53-year-old man with moderately active ulcerative colitis developed a febrile diffuse skin eruption after taking a glucocorticoid and azathioprine for a few days. Azathioprine was withdrawn. Skin biopsies showed features typical of Sweet's syndrome (neutrophilic dermatosis). The eruption gradually improved and there was complete regression after further glucocorticoid treatment.

Musculoskeletal

Severe myalgia and symmetrical polyarthritis are sometimes reported in patients taking azathioprine. Eight cases of azathioprine-associated arthritis were identified in the WHO Drug Monitoring Database, including six cases with a typical hypersensitivity syndrome and two cases in whom joint involvement was the only reported symptom (62). Rhabdomyolysis has also been reported as a possible feature of the azathioprine hypersensitivity syndrome (SEDA-20, 341).

In two patients with Crohn's disease, azathioprine was suspected to have caused severe gait disorders with an inability to walk (63). Within 1 month of treatment, both had joint pains or diffuse arthralgias that were the presumed cause of pseudoparalysis of the legs. In one patient other causes were carefully ruled out and similar symptoms recurred shortly after azathioprine was re-introduced.

The risk of fractures has been studied in a case-control study in 124 655 patients. Azathioprine was associated with an increase in overall risk of fractures, but not spine, hip, or forearm fractures (64). Methotrexate and ciclosporin were not associated with a risk of fractures. This association might be related to the underlying disease for which azathioprine was being used.

Reproductive system

Sperm function has been studied in ejaculates from 37 immunocompromised kidney transplant recipients (20 taking tacrolimus and prednisolone, 17 ciclosporin, azathioprine, and prednisolone) compared with 15 healthy fertile men; there were no significant differences (65).

Immunologic

The distinction between relapse of the treated disease, systemic sepsis, and acute azathioprine allergy can be difficult, as has been shown in three patients with vasculitic disorders (66).

Allergic reactions to azathioprine were recorded in 2% of patients with Crohn's disease taking azathioprine (3), and there was no evidence to suggest that the incidence depended on the underlying disease. The more rapid recurrence and/or the severity of symptoms following rechallenge were in keeping with a putative immune-mediated reaction, but no immunological mechanism has been conclusively demonstrated (SED-13, 1121) (67,68). In one patient, progressively rising doses of azathioprine were successfully administered, despite positive skin prick tests (SEDA-21, 382). Anaphylactic shock has been occasionally reported (69). Delayed contact hypersensitivity with a positive patch test was described in a pharmaceutical handler of azathioprine (70).

In 410 patients with inflammatory bowel disease treated with mercaptopurine for 20 years, the incidence of early drug-related allergic reactions was 3.9% (19).

Two patients with azathioprine hypersensitivity both had vasculitis with anti-neutrophil cytoplasmic antibodies (ANCA), each mimicking a relapse of vasculitis or a septic complication of immunosuppression (71).

A hypersensitivity reaction to azathioprine was also described in a patient with a demyelinating polyneuropathy (72).

Shock due to a hypersensitivity response to azathioprine is unpredictable and uncommon and can be fatal. It has been reported in a 46-year-old Caucasian man who rechallenged himself with azathioprine after having withdrawn it because of a persistent fever up to 40°C, nausea, and vomiting (73).

Desensitization to either mercaptopurine or azathioprine is often successful with the same or the other drug (19,74,75,76).

Desensitization has been successfully performed in isolated patients (77), and this has been more extensively addressed in a retrospective analysis of the charts of patients treated for inflammatory bowel disease (78). Of 591 patients observed over a 28-year period, 16 (2.7%) developed allergic reactions, which mostly consisted of fever ($n = 14$), joint pains ($n = 6$), or severe back pain ($n = 5$). Symptoms commonly appeared within 1 month and lasted 5 days on average. All nine patients rechallenged with mercaptopurine had similar but less severe symptoms. Further rechallenge with azathioprine in six of these patients caused symptoms in five of them. Careful desensitization with mercaptopurine or azathioprine was attempted in five patients, and resulted in tolerance and therapeutic success in four. The last patient, who had a previous history of mercaptopurine-induced sepsis-like syndrome with renal insufficiency, had a similar reaction only after one-quarter of the dose of azathioprine. This study suggests that a direct switch from mercaptopurine to the parent drug azathioprine cannot be recommended in patients who developed allergic reactions to mercaptopurine, and that desensitization should not be attempted in patients with previous life-threatening hypersensitivity reactions.

A genetic predisposition is suspected, with a possible association between the hypersensitivity syndrome and the Bw4 and Bw6 phenotypes (SED-13, 1121). Mercaptopurine has sometimes been re-administered safely after a severe hypersensitivity reaction to azathioprine (79), suggesting a major role for the imidazole moiety of azathioprine. However, typical allergic reactions to mercaptopurine can also occur (SEDA-21, 381).

Infection risk

Infections, in particular bacterial and viral (cytomegalovirus, *Herpes simplex* virus, Epstein–Barr virus), and also protozoal and fungal infections, are major causes of morbidity and mortality in the post-transplantation period, whatever the immunosuppressive regimen used (80–82). Based on an analysis of medical and autopsy records, infections were found to be the cause of death in 70% of transplant patients, with bacteria (50%) or fungi (29%) the most common pathogens (83).

The frequency, course, and severity of *Herpes zoster* infection have been retrospectively evaluated in a sample of 550 patients treated with 6-mercaptopurine for inflammatory bowel disease (84). Twelve patients aged 14–73 years developed shingles after an average of 921 days, an incidence that was about two-fold higher than in the general population. Only three patients were still taking glucocorticoids at the time of onset of the shingles, and leukopenia was not associated with the occurrence of the infection. In nine patients, the course of the infection was 7–71 days and was uncomplicated. Two patients had more severe symptoms and suffered from postherpetic neuralgia. The last patient, a 14-year-old boy, had a brief episode of *H. zoster* during initial treatment and had *H. zoster* encephalitis at the age of 23 years, 16 months after 6-mercaptopurine had been restarted. From this report, it appears that 6-mercaptopurine can be restarted after brief discontinuation in patients who are expected to benefit from it.

- Fatal Epstein–Barr virus-associated hemophagocytic syndrome was reported in a young man taking azathioprine and prednisone for Crohn's disease (85).

Donor-specific blood transfusion in the preparation for transplantation was complicated by a higher incidence of cytomegalovirus infection in patients receiving azathioprine (86).

Immunosuppression can lead to infections caused by *Salmonella enteritidis* (87).

- A 56-year-old man with systemic lupus erythematosus took azathioprine and prednisolone and developed a urinary tract infection followed by bacteremia and epididymo-orchitis. Both urine and blood cultures yielded *Salmonella enteritidis* strains, which were typed by pulsed-field gel electrophoresis and were genotypically identical.

Disseminated *Varicella zoster* infection is rare among patients with inflammatory bowel disease, despite the frequent use of azathioprine.

- An 18-year-old woman developed severe *Varicella zoster* pneumonia 9 months after starting to take azathioprine for Crohn's disease. She recovered after prompt treatment with aciclovir and withdrawal of azathioprine (88).

In 410 patients with inflammatory bowel disease, infectious complications occurred at different times during treatment with mercaptopurine in 14%, including pneumonia in 3.9% and *Herpes zoster* in 3% (19).

Long-Term Effects

Drug withdrawal

In clinical trials, azathioprine is withdrawn in 0–15% of patients because of adverse effects. In patients with Crohn's disease, azathioprine was preliminary withdrawn

in 15 of 50 patients because of adverse events that were probably related to azathioprine in 11 cases (89). The rate of azathioprine withdrawal differs between various indications (59). Azathioprine withdrawal due to drug-related toxicity was significantly higher in patients with rheumatoid arthritis (78/317), ulcerative colitis (20/94), and Crohn's disease (52/224) compared with systemic lupus erythematosus (5/73), Wegener's granulomatosis (6/85), autoimmune hepatitis (8/129), after liver transplantation (17/254), and after kidney transplantation (22/388).

Tumorigenicity

Because of the varied indications for azathioprine and mercaptopurine, it is difficult to determine whether there is an increased incidence of cancer specifically related to prolonged drug exposure. Data from the Cincinnati Transplant Tumor Registry, published in 1993, helped to define comprehensively the characteristics of neoplasms observed in organ transplant recipients (90). Skin and lip cancers were the most common, and non-Hodgkin's lymphomas represent the majority of lymphoproliferative disorders, with an incidence some 30- to 50-fold higher than in controls. An excess of Kaposi's sarcomas, carcinomas of the vulva and perineum, hepatobiliary tumors, and various sarcomas has also been reported. In contrast, the incidence of common neoplasms encountered in the general population is not increased. In renal transplant patients, the actuarial cumulative risk of cancer was 14–18% at 10 years and 40–50% at 20 years (91,92). Skin cancers accounted for about half of the cases. Very similar figures were found in later studies (SEDA-20, 341).

While there is no doubt that the incidence of malignancies is increased in the transplant population, there have been controversies as to which factors (duration of treatment, total dosage, the degree of immunosuppression, or the type of immunosuppressive regimens) are the most relevant in determining risk. Partial or complete regression of lymphoproliferative disorders and Kaposi's sarcomas after reduction of immunosuppressive therapy argues strongly for the role of the degree of immunosuppression (90). The incidence of cancer was also significantly higher in renal transplant patients taking triple therapy regimens compared with dual therapy (93). Similarly, aggressive immunosuppressive therapy may account for the higher incidence of lymphomas in patients with cardiac versus renal allografts.

In a large multicenter study in more than 52 000 kidney or heart transplant patients between 1983 and 1991, the rate of non-Hodgkin's lymphomas in the first post-transplantation year was 0.2% in kidney and 1.2% in heart recipients, and fell substantially thereafter (94). Initial immunosuppression with azathioprine and ciclosporin and prophylactic treatment with antilymphocyte antibodies or muromonab were associated with a significantly increased incidence of non-Hodgkin's lymphomas compared with other immunosuppressive regimens, which confirmed the major role of the level of immunosuppression. Later studies confirmed that immunosuppression per se rather than a single agent is responsible for the increased risk of cancer (SEDA-20, 340). Finally, the most striking difference between conventional and modern immunosuppressive regimens, including ciclosporin, was the average time to the appearance of tumors, in particular skin cancers and lymphomas, which was shorter in ciclosporin-treated patients (95,96). There was an increased incidence of non-Hodgkin's lymphomas in patients receiving long-term azathioprine and prednisolone for rheumatoid disease, although the latent period was longer than in other patients, perhaps reflecting a different pathogenesis (97).

Multiple factors with complex interactions are involved in the observed pattern and increased incidence of neoplasms. They include severely depressed immunity with an impaired immune surveillance against various carcinogens, the activation of several oncogenic viruses, and a possible mutagenic effect of the drugs. Viruses, such as papillomavirus, cytomegalovirus, and Epstein–Barr virus, are believed to play an important role in the development of several post-transplant cancers. From a theoretical point of view, the use of antiviral drugs active against herpes viruses, which are commonly implicated as co-factors, can be expected to produce a reduction in the incidence of post-transplant lymphoproliferative disorders.

Long-term treatment with azathioprine has been associated with transitional carcinoma of the bladder and non-Hodgkin's lymphoma in a single case (98).

- A 59-year-old man who had had a testicular non-Hodgkin's lymphoma for 9 years, developed diplopia and ptosis due to myasthenia gravis with antibodies to the acetylcholine receptor. He was given pyridostigmine and prednisolone. After 6 months he developed pernicious anemia, and he was given vitamin B_{12} injections. An attempt to reduce the dose of prednisolone failed, and he was therefore given azathioprine and the dose of prednisone was progressively reduced. Two years later he developed a transitional carcinoma of the bladder (pTa g1), which was removed by transurethral resection. Seven years later he developed a swollen tender right testis due to a B cell lymphoma. He tolerated chemotherapy (CHOP) poorly and died 2 months later.

In renal transplant recipients, premalignant dysplastic keratotic lesions increased in frequency by 6.8% per year after the first 3.5 years after transplantation, and were ultimately observed in all 167 patients within 16 years of transplantation (99). No relation with sun exposure or skin type was found. The great majority of these patients were taking prednisolone and azathioprine, but azathioprine was considered as the main causative factor, possibly due to a carcinogenic effect rather than to immunosuppression itself.

Several isolated reports and epidemiological studies have addressed the risk of cancer in non-transplant patients treated with azathioprine. Promptly reversible Epstein–Barr virus-associated lymphomas have been reported as single cases, as have reports of acute myeloid leukemia with 7q deletion, rapidly aggressive squamous cell carcinomas, soft tissue carcinomas, or fatal Merkel cell carcinomas in patients taking long-term azathioprine

maintenance (SED-13, 1122; SEDA-20, 342; SEDA-21, 382; SEDA-22, 410). Although epidemiological studies allow a more accurate estimate, conflicting results have emerged and there is as yet no definite evidence that azathioprine actually increases the risk of cancer.

The etiology of diffuse large B cell lymphomas is unknown. Epstein–Barr-virus may be involved and patients with immunodeficiencies are primarily affected (100). Two further cases have been reported (101).

- A 39-year-old woman developed an Epstein–Barr virus-associated diffuse large B cell lymphoma of the plasmablastic subtype in the maxillary alveolar ridge in the region of teeth 11 and 21 after 24 years of immunosuppressive therapy with azathioprine for myasthenia gravis.
- A 56-year-old man developed an Epstein–Barr virus-associated diffuse large B cell lymphoma of immunoblastic variant in the right maxillary edentulous alveolar ridge in the posterior region 7 weeks after cardiac transplantation and immunosuppressive therapy with azathioprine and ciclosporin. There was a soft painless swelling measuring 1.5 x 0.5 x 0.5 cm with central ulceration. The tumor was excised followed by local radiotherapy and did not recur during 15-years of follow up.

The demonstration of Epstein–Barr virus in the tumor cells in both of these cases underlines the involvement of this virus in the pathogenesis of oral diffuse large B cell lymphoma arising in the setting of immunodeficiency. These tumors may disseminate early.

The risk of lymphoma may be increased by about four-fold in patients with inflammatory bowel disease taking thiopurines, as a result of the medications, the severity of the underlying disease, or a combination of the two (102).

Over 20 years, lymphoma developed in three of 410 patients with inflammatory bowel disease taking mercaptopurine; however, this incidence was not greater than in the overall population of patients with inflammatory bowel disease (19).

An increased risk of non-Hodgkin's lymphomas, possibly related to treatment duration, has been found in patients with rheumatoid arthritis (103). There was no evidence that azathioprine increased the overall incidence of any cancer in 259 patients with rheumatoid arthritis on immunosuppressive treatment (azathioprine in 223) and matched for age and sex (but not for disease duration and severity) with unexposed patients (104). However, death more often resulted from malignancies in those taking azathioprine.

In another study of inflammatory bowel disease, no overall increased incidence of cancer was noted after a median of 9 years follow-up in 755 patients who had taken less than 2 mg/kg/day of azathioprine over a median period of 12.5 years (105). Only colorectal cancers (mostly adenocarcinoma) were more frequent, but their incidence was also increased in chronic inflammatory bowel diseases. More specifically, there was no excess of non-Hodgkin's lymphoma, but the power of the study to detect an increased risk of this disorder was low.

Another group of investigators has estimated that the potential long-term risk of malignancies outweighs the therapeutic benefit, but this conclusion was based on the follow-up of only 157 patients treated for Crohn's disease (4).

In 626 patients with inflammatory bowel disease who had taken azathioprine for a mean duration of 27 months (mean follow-up 6.9 years), there was no increased risk of cancer (colorectal or other) (106).

In a case-control study using a database of 1191 patients with multiple sclerosis, 23 cancers (17 solid tumors, two skin tumors, and four hemopoietic cancers) were found. The relative risk of cancer was 1.3 in patients treated for less than 5 years, 2.0 in those treated for 5–10 years, and 4.4 in those treated for more than 10 years; however, none of these later changes was significant (107). Nevertheless, there was a significant association for cumulative dosages in excess of 600 g. Taken together, these results suggest a low risk of cancer in non-transplant patients, but they cannot exclude a possible dose-related increase in risk during long-term treatment.

Skin carcinoma (predominantly squamous-cell carcinoma), cancer of the lip, Kaposi's sarcoma, and carcinoma of the cervix and anus are reported to be more common following azathioprine than in the general population (108).

The incidence of secondary myelodysplastic syndromes associated with a poor prognosis is increased in patients taking azathioprine for non-malignant disorders. In a retrospective analysis of 317 patients with multiple sclerosis there was one case of myelodysplastic syndrome (cumulative dose 627 g) in a young patient and two further malignancies (cumulative doses 27 g and 54 g) in those who had taken azathioprine (n = 81; 3.7%). In those who had not taken azathioprine (n = 236) there were five malignancies (2.1%) (109). Three other cases of myelodysplastic syndromes have been reported after long-term azathioprine therapy in multiple sclerosis. The cases suggest a time- and dose-dependent risk of myelodysplastic syndromes during long-term therapy.

- A woman with relapsing-remitting multiple sclerosis took oral azathioprine for 4 years and subsequently switched to interferon-beta1a (110). After 5 years, she developed a leukopenia, which resolved after interferon was withdrawn. She was given copolymer-1 instead, but. recurrent pancytopenia subsequently led to a diagnosis of myelodysplastic syndrome with deletion of the long arm of chromosome 5. Within several months,which is unusually rapid for this subtype, the myelodysplasia progressed to secondary acute myeloid leukemia. •

Azathioprine may have caused the chromosomal deletion and myelodysplasia in this case.

Of 439 children who received mercaptopurine as part of their maintenance therapy for acute lymphoblastic leukemia five developed secondary myelodysplasia or acute myeloid leukemia 23–53 months after diagnosis, a consequence that was attributed to mercaptopurine (111). These five patients had significantly lower TPMT activity, and two were classified as heterozygous for TPMT deficiency on genotype analysis. Although the number of evaluable patients was small, the suggestion was that a subset of patients with low TMPT activity might have an increased leukemogenic risk when exposed to mercaptopurine with other cytotoxic agents. Whether these findings can be extrapolated to patients without cancers is not known.

There are concerns about whether azathioprine could predispose to malignancies other than lymphomas in patients with inflammatory bowel disease.

- A 39-year-old non-smoker with Crohn's disease who had taken azathioprine for 3 years with developed a lingual ulcer (112). A biopsy showed a squamous cell carcinoma, a tumor that has not previously been associated with Crohn's disease.
- An invasive cancer of the cervix has been reported in a woman with Crohn's disease treated by mercaptopurine (113).

A colon cancer developed after introduction of azathioprine (114).

Of 550 patients with inflammatory bowel disease treated for a mean of 8 years, 25 (4.5%) developed a malignancy, with an overall incidence of 2.7 neoplasms per 1000 years of follow-up (115). The numbers of the most commonly observed cancers, such as bowel cancers (n = 8), breast cancers (n = 3), or single cases of other cancers, did not seem to be higher than expected in the general population or in the inflammatory bowel disease population. Although mercaptopurine was suspected in two cases of testicular carcinoma, two cases of lymphoma, and one case of leukemia, the authors emphasized the small risk of malignancies compared with the beneficial results of mercaptopurine in inflammatory bowel disease.

Second-Generation Effects

Pregnancy

The use of azathioprine in women of reproductive age at time of conception and during pregnancy has been reviewed (116).

Even though azathioprine is teratogenic in animals, human experience allows no firm conclusions, being limited to single case reports of birth defects after first trimester exposure to azathioprine. More convincingly, there was no evidence of increased risk or of a specific pattern of congenital anomalies among hundreds of infants born to azathioprine-treated transplant patients (117–119), but large series with adequate long-term follow-up are still lacking. The absence of inosinate pyrophosphorylase, an enzyme that converts azathioprine to its active metabolites, in the fetus was suggested to account for these reassuring data. Other potential risks, that is miscarriages or stillbirths, were also within the normal range, and intrauterine growth retardation did not appear to be specifically related to azathioprine use. Potential neonatal consequences of maternal azathioprine maintenance during the whole pregnancy should be borne in mind, in view of isolated reports of immunohematological immunosuppression, pancytopenia, cytomegalovirus infection, and chromosome aberrations. Unfortunately, the extent of this risk has not been carefully evaluated.

The placenta forms a relative barrier to azathioprine and its metabolites, and intrauterine exposure to the metabolite 6-thioguanine can be minimized by careful monitoring of the mother during pregnancy. This has been confirmed in three patients with autoimmune diseases who took azathioprine throughout their pregnancies (120). The thiopurine metabolites (6-thioguaninenucleotides and 6-methylmercaptopurine were measured in the erythrocytes of the mother and infant directly after delivery. The erythrocyte concentration of thioguanine nucleotides was slightly lower in the infant than the mother and methylmercaptopurine could not be detected in the infant.

Teratogenicity

Maternal azathioprine treatment during pregnancy is clearly teratogenic in animals, but the mechanisms are not known. A large number of reports have described the outcome of pregnancies following the use of immunosuppressant drugs, in particular in renal transplant patients, and hundreds of pregnancies have been analysed (117). The largest experience is that derived from the National Transplantation Pregnancy Registry which has been built up in the USA since 1991 (118). This registry has accumulated data on more than 900 pregnancies, of which 83% followed kidney transplantation. Overall, the immunosuppressant drug regimens commonly used in transplant patients (azathioprine or ciclosporin) do not appear to increase the overall risk of congenital malformations or produce a specific pattern of malformation. Risk factors associated with adverse pregnancy outcomes included a short time interval between transplantation and pregnancy (that is less than 1–2 years), graft dysfunction before or during pregnancy, and hypertension (121).

Possible long-term effects of in utero exposure to immunosuppressants are still seldom investigated. There have been no reports that physical and mental development or renal function are altered. In one study, there were changes in T lymphocyte development in seven children born to mothers who had taken azathioprine or ciclosporin, but immune function assays were normal, suggesting that development of the fetal immune system was not affected (122).

In 27 clinical series, the frequency of congenital anomalies among infants of patients who took azathioprine after renal transplantation ranged from 0 to 11% (123).

The consequences of paternal mercaptopurine exposure on the outcome of pregnancies have been retrospectively studied in 57 men with inflammatory bowel disease: 23 men had fathered 50 pregnancies and had taken mercaptopurine before conception; of these, 13 pregnancies were conceived within 3 months of paternal mercaptopurine use (group 1A) and 37 pregnancies were conceived at least 3 months after paternal mercaptopurine withdrawal (group 1B); the other 34 men, who fathered 90 pregnancies, had not been exposed to mercaptopurine before conception (group II) (124). Of the 140 conceptions, two resulted in congenital anomalies in group 1A, whereas there were no congenital anomalies in the other groups. One child had a missing thumb, and the other had acrania

with multiple digital and limb abnormalities. The overall number of complications (spontaneous abortion and congenital anomalies) was significantly higher in group 1A (4/13) compared with both group IB (1/37) and group II (2/90). Although the retrospective nature of this study and the limited number of evaluable patients precluded any definitive conclusion, the observed congenital anomalies were similar to those found in the offspring of female rabbits treated with mercaptopurine during pregnancy, and suggested that paternal mercaptopurine treatment should ideally be discontinued at least 3 months before planned conception.

Pregnancies in patients with inflammatory bowel disease were analysed to determine whether the patient had taken mercaptopurine before or at the time of conception; they were compared with pregnant women with inflammatory bowel disease who had their pregnancies before taking mercaptopurine (125). There was no statistical difference in conception failures (defined as spontaneous abortion), abortion secondary to a birth defect, major congenital malformations, neoplasia, or infections among patients taking mercaptopurine compared with controls (RR=0.85; 95% CI=0.47, 1.55). The authors concluded that the use of mercaptopurine before or at conception or during pregnancy appears to be safe and that withdrawal before and during pregnancy is not indicated.

The risk of adverse birth outcomes in 11 women who took up prescriptions for azathioprine or mercaptopurine during pregnancy was examined in a Danish cohort study (126). To examine the risk of congenital malformations, nine pregnancies exposed up to 30 days before conception or during the first trimester were included. To examine perinatal mortality, the frequency of premature births, and low birth weight, 10 pregnancies exposed during the entire pregnancy were included. Outcomes were compared with those of 19 418 pregnancies in which no drugs were prescribed. Of the exposed women, 55% had inflammatory bowel disease and 45% other diseases. Adjusted odds ratios were 6.7 (95%CI=1.4, 32) for congenital malformations, 20 (2.5, 161) for perinatal mortality, 6.6 (1.7, 26) for premature births, and 3.8 (0.4, 33) for low birth weight. In conclusion, children born to women treated with azathioprine or mercaptopurine during pregnancy had increased risks of congenital malformations, perinatal mortality, and premature birth. However, more data are needed to determine whether the associations are causal or occur through confounding.

Whereas neutropenia and immune deficiencies can affect neonates born to transplant patients, the exact role of azathioprine is difficult to establish. A report has suggested that such effects should also be expected in neonates born to patients taking azathioprine for other conditions (127).

- A 27-year-old woman, who took azathioprine (125 mg/day) and mesalazine (3 g/day) during her whole pregnancy, delivered a normal boy who had febrile respiratory distress after 36 hours. Chest X-ray showed interstitial pneumonitis and thymus hypoplasia. There was severe neutropenia (20×10^6/l), lymphopenia

$(24 \times 10^6/l)$, and hypogammaglobulinemia. His clinical condition improved over the next 26 days with immunoglobulin treatment and antibiotics, but B lymphocytes and IgM were still undetectable.

Fetotoxicity

Out of 57 249 pregnancies, 54 were fathered by men who had filled a prescription for azathioprine or mercaptopurine before conception (128,129). There were congenital abnormalities in four children (7.4%) compared with 2334 of 57 195 children whose fathers had not taken azathioprine (4.1%), but the odds ratio was not statistically significant. All four congenital abnormalities occurred in boys and consisted of polysyndactyly, esophageal atresia, hydronephrosis with megaloureter, and a ventricular septal defect.

Immune function was studied in nine babies from six mothers taking ciclosporin (n = 2), azathioprine (n = 1), and dexamethasone (n = 3) during pregnancy compared with 14 babies from mothers with similar diseases not taking immunosuppressive drugs (130). The children were tested at a mean age of 11 (1–17) months. Only a minor proportion of children displayed low values for age, mainly IgA and IgG2. Blood counts, IgA, IgG, IgM, and IgG subclasses, and lymphocyte subpopulations did not differ significantly, and all the children responded satisfactorily to hepatitis B immunization. Prenatal exposure to immunosuppressive drugs had no profound effect on the developing immune system.

Azathioprine/mercaptopurine was not associated with poor pregnancy outcomes in 101 women with inflammatory bowel disease (131).

Lactation

Because very few data on breastfed infants from azathioprine-treated mothers are available, breast-feeding is not recommended owing to the potential risk of immunosuppression, growth retardation, and carcinogenesis.

Lactation

However, infant exposure to the metabolites 6-thioguanine and 6-methylmercaptopurine nucleotides has been determined during maternal use of azathioprine (1.2–2.1 mg/kg/day) in four breast-feeding women and their infants (132). All the women had the wild type TPMT genotype. Maternal thioguanine and methylmercaptopurine concentrations were 234–291 and 284–1178 pmol/8 x 10^8 erythrocytes, comparable to those associated with improved therapeutic outcomes. Neither metabolite was detected in any of the infants. Thus, azathioprine may be safe during breastfeeding in patients with wild-type TPMT genotype taking normal doses.

Susceptibility Factors

Genetic

TPMT deficiency

The complex metabolism of azathioprine and mercaptopurine is subject to a pharmacogenetic polymorphism that is relevant to the degree of efficacy and toxicity attained in a given individual. Thiopurine methyltransferase (TPMT) is one of the key enzymes regulating the catabolism of thiopurine drugs to inactive products. Owing to an inherited autosomal codominant trait, a significant number of patients have intermediate (11%) to low or undetectable (0.3-0.6%) TPMT activity (133), 134,135. These patients produce larger amounts of the active 6-thioguanine nucleotides and may therefore be unusually sensitive to commonly used dosages and an increased risk of myelotoxicity (SED-13, 1120; SEDA-21, 381).

In individuals with low TPMT activity, toxicity can be avoided by carefully titrating the dose (136).

Monitoring azathioprine therapy by measuring erythrocyte 6-thioguanine concentrations and TPMT activity is thought to ensure optimal immunosuppressive effects and to reduce the likelihood of hematological toxicity (137,138). A range of optimal concentrations has been defined, as has an association of metabolite concentrations with medication-induced toxicity and the genotype of TPMT (139) Low or completely absent erythrocyte TPMT activity and high concentrations of erythrocyte 6-thioguanine metabolites have been found in patients with severe azathioprine-induced bone marrow toxicity, as compared to those without bone marrow toxicity (140,141). However, intracellular concentrations of thiopurine nucleotides alone did not always correlate with hematological toxicity (142). In patients in whom TPMT deficiency was not clearly demonstrated, low lymphocyte 5'-nucleotidase activity and xanthine oxidase deficiency or other factors have been postulated as possible causes of hemotoxicity, suggesting that bone marrow toxicity is probably multifactorial (141,143,144). Although not all investigators recommend systematic pretreatment screening for purine enzyme activities, evidence of deficiency of purine enzymes could well be sought when early bone marrow toxicity occurs.

- A woman underwent azathioprine therapy without prior knowledge of TPMT status. Pancytopenia developed over several months. TPMT activity was low at 16 nmol 6-methyl-thioguanine/g Hb/hour, that is within the reference range associated with heterozygosity for TPMT mutant alleles. Three months later, TPMT activity was 2 nmol 6-methyl-thioguanine/g Hb/hour, consistent with deficient TPMT activity (homozygosity for TPMT mutant alleles). Retrospectively, it was realized that the patient had received erythrocyte and platelet transfusions 6 days before TPMT activity was first measured.

Genotypes

Allelic polymorphisms in the TPMT gene predict the activity of the enzyme; 1 in 10 of the population are heterozygous and have about 50% of normal activity, while 1 in 300 are completely deficient. These individuals are at high risk of severe myelosuppression. Conversely, individuals with very high TPMT activity are hypermethylators, in whom a beneficial clinical response is less likely. Prior knowledge of TPMT status avoids exposure of individuals with zero TPMT to potentially fatal treatment with azathioprine or mercaptopurine and provides one of the best examples of predictive pharmacogenetics in therapeutics (145). Patients with low or deficient TPMT activity are at risk of severe complications and even death, and determination of TPMT is recommended before azathioprine therapy. However, caution must be taken in interpreting TPMT activity in patients who have recently been transfused. Deficient TPMT activity might be missed after erythrocyte or platelet transfusions from patients with normal TPMT activity (146).

TPMT genotypes were analysed in 111 patients with rheumatoid arthritis including 40 patients taking azathioprine; TPMT3A [G(460)→A, A(719)→G], the most common mutant allele, was detected in seven of 111 patients (6.3%). Azathioprine was withdrawn in six patients because of adverse effects and in 26 patients because of lack of efficacy. Three patients with moderate adverse effects were homozygous for the wild type TPMT allele, and the other three, who developed severe nausea and vomiting, were TPMT3A carriers. Absence of response, probably due to the low-dose scheme used, was the major cause of azathioprine withdrawal. TPMT genotyping may allow the use of high doses of azathioprine in patients with normal TPMT alleles to improve efficacy (147).

Azathioprine-induced fatal myelosuppression has been reported in a kidney recipient who carried heterozygous TPMT*1/*3C (148).

Adverse effects related to TPMT enzyme activity and genotype were analysed in 50 patients with inflammatory bowel disease and azathioprine- or mercaptopurine-related adverse effects. The TPMT genotype *1/*3 was detected in five patients, genotype *3/*3 in one, and the wild type genotype *1/*1 in 44. The patient with genotype *3/*3 had severe pancytopenia. In the control group, three of 50 patients had genotype *1/*3 and the rest genotype *1/*1. There was no significant correlation between TPMT mutations and adverse reactions, and most patients with reactions did not have gene mutations (149).

In dialysed patients, TPMT phenotype and genotype (*2, *3A, and *3C variant alleles), determined by hplc, PCR-RFLP, and allele-specific PCR, were significantly correlated (150). Median TPMT activity was 31 (12, 46) nmol of methylmercaptopurine/g of hemoglobin/hour. Heterozygous patients (12%) had significantly lower mean TPMT activity than wild homozygotes (17 versus 32). TPMT activities in heterozygous and wild-type homozygous patients did not overlap. TPMT activity after hemodialysis and TPMT genotyping were convergent in dialysed patients, so both methods can be used to identify patients with lower TPMT activity before azathioprine therapy after renal transplantation.

The pattern and frequency of the main mutant TPMT alleles (TPMT*2, *3A, *3B, and *3C) were similar in 122 transplant patients taking azathioprine and 210 healthy subjects (151). TPMT heterozygosity was associated with significant reductions in hematological indices and a significant reduction in ciclosporin plasma concentrations in the first year after renal transplantation.

Measurement techniques

TPMT activity has been studied by a rapid genetic PCR-RFLP screening test for the most prevalent mutant TPMT*3A and TPMT*3C alleles, which result in reduced TPMT enzyme activity (152). Of 871 Caucasians, 8.6% carried the TPMT*3A allele and 0.23% were heterozygous for the TPMT*3C allele, which is in accord with previously reported allele frequencies.

A non-radioactive method that uses hplc with ion-trap mass detection has been developed to measure the activities of TPMT in erythrocytes and inosine 5′-monophosphate dehydrogenase (IMPDH) in peripheral blood mononuclear cells (153).

In a retrospective analysis of 106 patients with inflammatory bowel disease, to evaluate the importance of TPMT activity in the management of azathioprine therapy in inflammatory bowel disease, the relation between inherited variations in TPMT enzyme activity and azathioprine toxicity was confirmed (154).

In 3291 patients receiving azathioprine, 10% had a low TPMT activity and 15 (1 in 220 or 0.46%) had no detectable enzymatic activity at all (155), slightly more common than has been reported in other studies (1 in 300). This makes the economics of screening, to avoid myelosuppression in patients receiving azathioprine, attractive.

Of 78 patients treated with azathioprine for systemic lupus erythematosus, 10 developed azathioprine-associated reversible neutropenia (156). Only one of these patients was homozygous for TPMT deficiency, but he had the most severe episode (aplastic anemia).

In one study, 14 of 33 patients with rheumatoid arthritis had severe adverse effects (mostly gastrointestinal toxicity, flu-like reactions or fever, pancytopenia, and hepatotoxicity) within 1–8 weeks after azathioprine was started (157). The adverse effects subsided after withdrawal in all patients, but all eight patients who were rechallenged developed the same adverse effect. A baseline reduction in TPMT activity was significantly associated with the occurrence of these adverse effects in seven of eight patients, with a relative risk of 3.1 (95% CI = 1.6–6.2) compared with patients with high TPMT activity (seven of 25 patients). Another prospective evaluation in 67 patients with rheumatic disorders showed that TPMT genotype analysis is useful in identifying patients at risk of azathioprine toxicity (158). Treatment duration was significantly longer in patients with the wild-type TPMP alleles than in those with mutant alleles, and that was due to the early occurrence of leukopenia in the latter.

In 22 children with renal transplants, high erythrocyte TPMT activity, measured 1 month after transplantation, correlated positively with rejection episodes during the first 3 months, and this was probably due to more rapid azathioprine catabolism (159). As suggested in a study of 180 patients with acute lymphoblastic leukemia, determination of genetic polymorphisms in TMPT can be useful in predicting potential toxicity and in optimizing the determination of an appropriate dose in patients who are homozygous or heterozygous for TMPT deficiency (160).

In 30 heart transplant patients taking azathioprine, the myelosuppressive effects of azathioprine/mercaptopurine were predicted by systematic genotypic screening of thiopurine methyltransferase deficiency (161). However, myelosuppression can also be observed in patients without the thiopurine methyltransferase mutation. Of 41 patients with leukopenia or thrombocytopenia taking azathioprine/mercaptopurine for Crohn's disease, four were classified as low methylators, seven as intermediate methylators, and 30 as high methylators by genotypic analysis (162). Thus, only 27% of the patients had the typical mutations associated with enzyme deficiency and a risk of myelosuppression. The delay in bone marrow toxicity was shorter in the four homozygous patients (median 1 month) than in the others (median 3–4 months). Many other causes, including viral infections, associated drugs, or another azathioprine/mercaptopurine metabolic pathway, were suggested to account for most of the cases of late hemotoxicity. This confirmed that continuous hematological monitoring is required, even in patients with no thiopurine methyltransferase mutations.

Clinical studies

The relation between TPMT activity and the incidence of adverse effects has been studied in 788 patients with inflammatory bowel disease taking azathioprine (163). Erythrocyte TPMT activity was measured radiochemically. The mean TPMT activity was 19 (range 9–34) U/ml. No patient had low activity (<5), 7.1% had intermediate activity (5–14), and 93% had high activity (>14). Adverse effects were reported in 74 patients (19%), the most frequent being gastrointestinal intolerance (9.1%) and myelotoxicity (4.3%). No patient with adverse effects had low TPMT activity. However, mean TPMT activity was significantly lower in those with adverse effects (17 versus 19 U/ml). Moreover, the probability of myelotoxicity in the high TPMT group was only 3.5%, compared with 14% in the TPMT intermediate group (OR = 4.5; 95% CI = 1.37, 15).

Of patients with Crohn's disease (n = 33) or ulcerative colitis (n = 27) taking a thiopurine in a daily target dose at week 3 of 2.5 mg/kg of azathioprine or 1.25 mg/kg of mercaptopurine, 27 completed the study per protocol, 33 withdrew because of thiopurine-related adverse events (n = 27), early protocol violation (n = 5), or TPMT deficiency (n = 1) (164). Of the patients with adverse effects 67% tolerated long term-treatment with a lower dose of azathioprine (median 1.32 mg/kg). TPMT activity did not change during the 20 week course of the study but there was a significant reduction in TPMT gene expression. Patients with methylthioinosine monophosphate

concentrations over 11 450 pmol/8 x 10^8 erythrocytes during steady state at week 5 had an increased risk of myelotoxicity (OR = 45). TPMT enzyme activity was not induced during thiopurine treatment, but TPMT gene expression fell. The development of different types of toxicity was unpredictable, but measurement of methylthioinosine monophosphate early in the steady state phase helped to identify patients at risk of myelotoxicity.

The frequency of TPMT deficiency has been assessed in 86 patients with autoimmune hepatitis taking azathioprine 50-150 mg/day compared with 89 similarly treated but untested patients (165). There was low TPMT activity (11, range 3.5–15, U/ml erythrocytes) in 13 tested patients. Azathioprine intolerance occurred as often in patients with normal or above normal enzyme activity as in patients with below normal activity (12% versus 15%). The frequency of complications was similar in the two groups (9 versus 13%). In this study routine screening of TPMT-activity did not identify individual patients at risk of azathioprine toxicity during conventional low dose therapy.

In another study on patients with autoimmune hepatitis, azathioprine toxicity was predicted by the stage of fibrosis but not by TPMT genotype or activity (166).

TPMT activity has been studied prospectively in 139 patients (35 men, 104 women) with systemic lupus erythematosus (n = 38), progressive systemic sclerosis (n = 13), Wegener's granulomatosis (n = 4), rheumatoid arthritis (n = 5), and other chronic inflammatory diseases (n = 79) (167). Of 96 patients who took azathioprine, there were minor adverse effects in 11 (sickness, rash, and cholestasis) and severe adverse effects (bone marrow toxicity) in seven. Below a cut-off value of TPMT activity of 12 nmol/ml erythrocytes/hour, adverse effects were significantly more frequent.

ITPase deficiency

Adverse drug reactions to azathioprine occur in 15–28% of patients, but often cannot be explained by TPMT deficiency. Inosine triphosphate pyrophosphatase (ITPase) is an enzyme that catalyses the pyrophosphohydrolysis of ITP to IMP. ITPase deficiency is a clinically benign autosomal recessive condition characterized by the abnormal accumulation of ITP in erythrocytes (168). Mercaptopurine is activated through a 6-thio-IMP intermediate, and in patients deficient in ITPase there will be accumulation of 6-thio-ITP, which is potentially toxic. It is thought that deficiency of ITPase may predict adverse reactions to therapy with mercaptopurine and azathioprine (169) and that alternative immunosuppressive drugs, particularly thioguanine, should be considered for azathioprine-intolerant patients with ITPase deficiency. However, this was not confirmed in relation to the ITPA 94C>A polymorphism in a meta-analysis of six studies in 751 patients (170).

Genotypes

The frequencies of ITPA polymorphisms have been studied in 100 healthy Japanese individuals (160). The allele frequency of the 94C→A variant was 0.135 (Caucasian allele frequency = 0.06). The IV2 + 21A→C polymorphism was not found (Caucasian allele frequency = 0.13). Allele frequencies of the 138G→A, 561G→A, and 708G→A polymorphisms were 0.57, 0.18, and 0.06 respectively, similar to the allele frequencies in Caucasians, with the exception of the 138G→A polymorphism (171).

An hplc procedure has been developed to investigate the inosine triphosphate pyrophosphatase (ITPA) phenotype and phenotype–genotype correlation and a novel IVS2 + 68T>C mutation was found (172).

Clinical studies

The association between polymorphism in the ITPA gene and adverse drug reactions to azathioprine has been studied in 62 patients with inflammatory bowel disease who had adverse reactions to azathioprine (173). The patients were genotyped for ITPA 94C→A and IVS2 plus 21A→C polymorphisms, and TPMT*3A, TPMT*3C, and TPMT*2 polymorphisms. Genotype frequencies were compared with the frequencies in a consecutive control series (n = 68) treated with azathioprine without adverse effects. The ITPA 94C→A allele was significantly associated with adverse drug reactions (OR = 4.2; 95% CI = 1.6, 12). There were significant associations for flu-like symptoms (OR = 4.7; 95% CI = 1.2, 18), rash (OR = 10; 95% CI = 4.7, 63), and pancreatitis (OR = 6.2; CI = 1.1-33). Heterozygous TPMT genotypes did not predict adverse drug reactions but were significantly associated with a subgroup of patients who had nausea and vomiting as the predominant adverse reaction to azathioprine (OR = 5.5; 95% CI = 1.4, 22).

In a 6-month prospective study in 71 patients with Crohn's disease taking azathioprine, early drop-out within 2 weeks was associated with the ITPA polymorphism 94C→A and low TPMT activity (<10 nmol/ml of erythrocytes/hour) (174). High-risk individuals, defined by the 94C→A polymorphism or low TPMT activity, were significantly more likely to drop out at any stage. Drop-outs attributed to azathioprine-related adverse effects (n = 16) were significantly associated with the 94C→A polymorphism. A time-to-event analysis over the 24-week study period showed a significant association between the time to drop-out and carriage of the ITPA 94C>A mutant allele.

ITPA genotypes (94C>A, IVS2+21A>C) and TPMT genotypes (238G>C, 460G>A, and 719A>G) have been assessed in 262 patients with inflammatory bowel disease (159 women, 103 men; 67 patients with ulcerative colitis and 195 patients with Crohn's disease) taking azathioprine and correlated with the development of leukopenia and hepatotoxicity (175). There was leukopenia (leukocyte count < 3.0 x 10^9/l) in 4.6%. Mutant ITPA 94C>A and TPMT alleles were significantly more common in those with leukopenia than in those without (17% and 5.4%, respectively for ITPA 94C>A, and 21% and 4% respectively for TPMT). Moreover, the ITPA 94C>A and TPMT mutations predicted leukopenia: ITPA 94C>A OR = 3.50 (95% CI = 1.12, 10); TPMT OR = 6.32 (2.14, 18). Neither TPMT nor ITPA genotypes predicted hepatotoxicity.

The ITPA 94C→A, TPMT*2, and TPMT*3 polymorphisms were determined in azathioprine-intolerant (n = 73) and azathioprine-tolerant (n = 74) patients. In contrast to the studies described above, this study showed no significant association between the ITPA94C→A genotype and any adverse effects (OR = 1.0, 95% CI = 0.4, 2.9), flu-like symptoms (OR = 1.5, 95%CI = 0.4, 6.5), rash (no ITPA 94C→A polymorphism identified), or pancreatitis (no ITPA 94C→A polymorphism identified) (176).

Drug Administration

Drug dosage regimens

About 40% of patients with inflammatory bowel disease fail to respond to azathioprine 2 mg/kg/day. An increase in dose had no therapeutic benefit in 17 of 40 patients who had been unresponsive to azathioprine 2 mg/kg/day for at least 3 months; dosages over 2.5 mg/kg/day were less likely to be efficacious and were associated with a substantial risk of adverse reactions (177).

Drug–Drug Interactions

Allopurinol

Allopurinol inhibits xanthine oxidase, which is involved in the inactivation of azathioprine and mercaptopurine, and bone marrow suppression is a well-known complication of the concomitant use of allopurinol and azathioprine (SEDA-16, 114; SEDA-20, 342). Concomitant administration can result in life-threatening neutropenia unless the dose of allopurinol is reduced by about 75% (178) (179). However, compliance with these above guidelines was observed in only 58% of 24 patients with heart or lung transplants (180). In addition, although adequate azathioprine dosage reduction reduces the incidence of cytopenias, the risk persists even after the first month of the combination.

Because of the possible risks of reduced immunosuppression if the dose of azathioprine is reduced when allopurinol is given, cyclic urate oxidase can be given instead, as has been shown in six hyperuricemic transplant patients treated with azathioprine (181).

Aminosalicylates

In vitro studies have suggested that sulfasalazine and other aminosalicylates can inhibit TPMT activity, predisposing to an increased risk of bone marrow suppression in patients taking azathioprine or mercaptopurine. This was not clinically substantiated until an extensively investigated case was reported of leukopenia and anemia in a patient treated with both olsalazine and mercaptopurine (SEDA-21, 382). A further inhibiting effect of olsalazine was suggested in this patient, who had a relatively low baseline TPMT activity.

In 16 patients with Crohn's disease taking a stable dose of azathioprine, plus sulfasalazine or mesalazine, mean 6-thioguanine nucleotide concentrations fell significantly over 3 months; withdrawal of the aminosalicylates had no effect on the clinical and biological evolution of Crohn's disease in these patients (182).

Coumarin anticoagulants

Azathioprine or mercaptopurine have been sometimes involved in reduced warfarin and acenocoumarol activity, and increased warfarin dosages may be necessary (183). Similar findings were found in a patient taking maintenance phenprocoumon (SEDA-21, 382).

- Two patients required an approximate three-fold increase in the weekly anticoagulant dosage while taking azathioprine or mercaptopurine (184,185).

A pharmacokinetic interaction is the most likely cause, but the mechanism (impaired absorption or enhanced anticoagulant metabolism) is unknown.

Infliximab

The interaction of infliximab with azathioprine has been studied in 32 patients with Crohn's disease (186). The mean concentration of 6-tioguanine nucleotide was comparable before and 3 months after the first infusion, but there was a significant increase within 1-3 weeks after the first infusion. In parallel, there was a significant fall in leukocyte count and an increase in mean corpuscular volume. These changes normalized 3 months after infusion. An increase in 6-tioguanine nucleotide concentration of more than 400 pmol/8×10^8 erythrocytes was strongly related to good tolerance and a favourable response to infliximab, with a predictive value of 100%.

Isotretinoin

The combination of isotretinoin and azathioprine was reported to have a synergistic effect on the occurrence of curly hair in three transplant patients with ciclosporin-induced acne (SEDA-20, 342).

Methotrexate

In 43 patients with rheumatoid arthritis, methotrexate was thought to have increased the risk of the azathioprine-induced hypersensitivity syndrome (187).

Warfarin

An interaction between warfarin and azathioprine resulted in increased warfarin requirements (188).

- A 67-year-old woman took warfarin for recurrent deep vein thrombosis associated with systemic lupus erythematosus. Azathioprine 150 mg/day was introduced for its steroid-sparing effect and the dose of warfarin was titrated to a mean dose of 60–75 mg/week (8.5–10.5 mg/dayover the next 18 months. Her dose of azathioprine was then increased to 200 mg/day, after which subtherapeutic international normalized ratios required an increase in the dose of warfarin to a mean of 130 mg/week (18.5 mg/day). Subsequent withdrawal of azathioprine resulted in a dramatic increase in her INR (from 1.8 to 14.0 4 weeks after withdrawal).

An interaction between warfarin and azathioprine has been reported in seven other reports. The evidence suggests a clinically important inhibitory effect of azathioprine on warfarin and calls for close monitoring of the INR when doses of azathioprine are altered during concurrent administration of warfarin.

Interference with Diagnostic Tests

Erythrocyte sedimentation rate and C-reactive protein

Erythrocyte sedimentation rate (ESR) and C-reactive protein (CRP) concentrations are widely used as markers of inflammation. There was an unexplained discordance between ESR and CRP in children with asymptomatic inflammatory bowel disease taking azathioprine or mercaptopurine. The ESR was persistently raised in 11 of 120 children but the CRP was normal and there was no clinical evidence of active disease (189).

Diagnosis of Adverse Drug Reactions

Azathioprine-induced drug eruption occurred in two patients with systemic scleroderma and polymyositis (190). One presented with Stevens–Johnson syndrome and the other had systemic papular erythema. Stimulation indices of the drug-induced lymphocyte stimulation test (DLST) for azathioprine in these patients were as high as 2180% and 430%, while healthy volunteers had values under 120% without non-specific suppression of lymphocyte proliferation. Other drugs used simultaneously were ruled out by patch and challenge tests. DLST might therefore be useful in testing for azathioprine allergy.

Management of Adverse Drug Reactions

Desensitization has been successfully used in patients previously intolerant to azathioprine (191). All had inflammatory bowel disease. Azathioprine was started at a low dose and thereafter gradually increased to a therapeutic dose. Nine of 14 patients were able to tolerate a full dose; the rest had recurrent adverse effects and were offered alternative treatment.

References

1. Savolainen HA, Kautiainen H, Isomaki H, Aho K, Verronen P. Azathioprine in patients with juvenile chronic arthritis: a longterm followup study. J Rheumatol 1997;24(12):2444–50.
2. Kirschner BS. Safety of azathioprine and 6-mercaptopurine in pediatric patients with inflammatory bowel disease. Gastroenterology 1998;115(4):813–21.
3. Pearson DC, May GR, Fick GH, Sutherland LR. Azathioprine and 6-mercaptopurine in Crohn disease. A meta-analysis. Ann Intern Med 1995;123(2):132–42.
4. Bouhnik Y, Lemann M, Mary JY, Scemama G, Tai R, Matuchansky C, Modigliani R, Rambaud JC. Long-term follow-up of patients with Crohn's disease treated with

azathioprine or 6-mercaptopurine. Lancet 1996;347(8996): 215–9.

5. Sandborn WJ. A review of immune modifier therapy for inflammatory bowel disease: azathioprine, 6-mercaptopurine, cyclosporine, and methotrexate. Am J Gastroenterol 1996;91(3):423–33.

6. Hollander AAMJ, Van der Woude FJ. Efficacy and tolerability of conversion from cyclosporin to azathioprine after kidney transplantation. A review of the evidence. BioDrugs 1998;9:197–210.

7. Saway PA, Heck LW, Bonner JR, Kirklin JK. Azathioprine hypersensitivity. Case report and review of the literature. Am J Med 1988;84(5):960–4.

8. Parnham AP, Dittmer I, Mathieson PW, McIver A, Dudley C. Acute allergic reactions associated with azathioprine. Lancet 1996;348(9026):542–3.

9. Perreaux F, Zenaty D, Capron F, Trioche P, Odievre M, Labrune P. Azathioprine-induced lung toxicity and efficacy of cyclosporin A in a young girl with type 2 autoimmune hepatitis. J Pediatr Gastroenterol Nutr 2000;31(2):190–2.

10. Nagy F, Molnár T, Makula E, Kiss I, Milassin P, Zöllei E, Tiszlavicz L, Lonovics J. Azathioprin okozta interstitialis pneumonitis. [Azathioprine-associated interstitial pneumonitis.] Orv Hetil 2006;147(6):259–62.

11. Jungling AS, Shangraw RE. Massive airway edema after azathioprine. Anesthesiology 2000;92(3):888–90.

12. Luth S, Birklein F, Schramm C, Herkel J, Hennes E, Muller-Forell W, Galle PR, Lohse AW. Multiplex neuritis in a patient with autoimmune hepatitis: a case report. World J Gastroenterol 2006;12(33):5396–8.

13. Foocharoen C, Tiamkao S, Srinakarin J, Chamadol N, Sawanyawisuth K. Reversible posterior leukoencephalopathy caused by azathioprine in systemic lupus erythematosus. J Med Assoc Thai 2006;89(7):1029–32.

14. Karhadkar AS, Schwartz HJ, Arora M, Dutta SK. Severe muscular weakness: an unusual adverse effect of azathioprine therapy. J Clin Gastroenterol 2006;40(7):626–8.

15. van der HJ, Duyx J, de Langen JJ, van Royen A. Probable psychiatric side effects of azathioprine. Psychosom Med 2005;67(3):508.

16. Uygur-Bayramicli O, Aydin D, Ak O, Karadayi N. Hyperprolactinemia caused by azathioprine. J Clin Gastroenterol 2003;36:79–80.

17. Connell WR, Kamm MA, Ritchie JK, Lennard-Jones JE. Bone marrow toxicity caused by azathioprine in inflammatory bowel disease: 27 years of experience. Gut 1993; 34(8):1081–5.

18. Cunliffe RN, Scott BB. Review article: monitoring for drug side-effects in inflammatory bowel disease. Aliment Pharmacol Ther 2002;16(4):647–62.

19. Warman JI, Korelitz BI, Fleisher MR, Janardhanam R. Cumulative experience with short- and long-term toxicity to 6-mercaptopurine in the treatment of Crohn's disease and ulcerative colitis. J Clin Gastroenterol 2003;37:220–5.

20. Amenabar JJ, Gomez-Ullate P, Garcia-Lopez FJ, Aurrecoechea B, Garcia-Erauzkin G, Lampreabe I. A randomized trial comparing cyclosporine and steroids with cyclosporine, azathioprine, and steroids in cadaveric renal transplantation. Transplantation 1998;65(5):653–61.

21. Creemers GJ, van Boven WP, Lowenberg B, van der Heul C. Azathioprine-associated pure red cell aplasia. J Intern Med 1993;233(1):85–7.

22. Pruijt JF, Haanen JB, Hollander AA, den Ottolander GJ. Azathioprine-induced pure red-cell aplasia. Nephrol Dial Transplant 1996;11(7):1371–3.

23. Higashida K, Kobayashi K, Sugita K, Karakida N, Nakagomi Y, Sawanobori E, Sata Y, Aihara M, Amemiya S, Nakazawa S. Pure red blood cell aplasia during azathioprine therapy associated with parvovirus B19 infection. Pediatr Infect Dis J 1997;16(11):1093–5.

24. Agrawal A, Parrott NR, Riad HN, Augustine T. Azathioprine-induced pure red cell aplasia: case report and review. Transplant Proc 2004;36(9):2689–91.

25. Depil S, Lepelley P, Soenen V, Preudhomme C, Lai JL, Broly F, Quesnel B. A case of refractory anemia with 17p– syndrome following azathioprine treatment for heart transplantation. Leukemia 2004;18(4):878.

26. Khosroshahi HT, Asghari A, Estakhr R, Baiaz B, Ardalan MR, Shoja MM. Effects of azathioprine and mycophenolate mofetil-immunosuppressive regimens on the erythropoietic system of renal transplant recipients. Transplant Proc 2006;38(7):2077–9.

27. Pujol M, Fernandez F, Sancho JM, Ribera JM, Milla F, Feliu E. Immune hemolytic anemia induced by 6-mercaptopurine. Transfusion 2000;40(1):75–6.

28. Willerding-Mollmann S, Wilkens L, Schlegelberger B, Kaiser U. Azathioprin-assoziiertes myelodysplastisches Syndrom mit zytogenetischen Aberrationen. [Azathioprine-associated myelodysplastic syndrome with cytogenetic aberrations.] Dtsch Med Wochenschr 2004;129(22):1246–8.

29. Sudhir RR, Rao SK, Shanmugam MP, Padmanabhan P. Bilateral macular hemorrhage caused by azathioprine-induced aplastic anemia in a corneal graft recipient. Cornea 2002;21(7):712–4.

30. Santiago M. Diarrhoea secondary to azathioprine in two patients with SLE. Lupus 1999;8(7):565.

31. Marbet U, Schmid I. Severe life-threatening diarrhea caused by azathioprine but not by 6-mercaptopurine. Digestion 2001;63(2):139–42.

32. Ziegler TR, Fernandez-Estivariz C, Gu LH, Fried MW, Leader LM. Severe villus atrophy and chronic malabsorption induced by azathioprine. Gastroenterology 2003;124:1950–7.

33. Kowdley KV, Keeffe EB. Hepatotoxicity of transplant immunosuppressive agents. Gastroenterol Clin North Am 1995;24(4):991–1001.

34. Pol S, Cavalcanti R, Carnot F, Legendre C, Driss F, Chaix ML, Thervet E, Chkoff N, Brechot C, Berthelot P, Kreis H. Azathioprine hepatitis in kidney transplant recipients. A predisposing role of chronic viral hepatitis. Transplantation 1996;61(12):1774–6.

35. Wagoner LE, Olsen SL, Bristow MR, O'Connell JB, Taylor DO, Lappe DL, Renlund DG. Cyclophosphamide as an alternative to azathioprine in cardiac transplant recipients with suspected azathioprine-induced hepatotoxicity. Transplantation 1993;56(6):1415–8.

36. Bastida G, Nos P, Aguas M, Beltrán B, Rubín A, Dasí F, Ponce J. Incidence, risk factors and clinical course of thiopurine-induced liver injury in patients with inflammatory bowel disease. Aliment Pharmacol Ther 2005;22(9):775–82.

37. Ramalho HJ, Terra EG, Cartapatti E, Barberato JB, Alves VA, Gayotto LC, Abbud-Filho M. Hepatotoxicity of azathioprine in renal transplant recipients. Transplant Proc 1989;21(1 Pt 2):1716–7.

38. Horsmans Y, Rahier J, Geubel AP. Reversible cholestasis with bile duct injury following azathioprine therapy. A case report. Liver 1991;11(2):89–93.

39. Read AE, Wiesner RH, LaBrecque DR, Tifft JG, Mullen KD, Sheer RL, Petrelli M, Ricanati ES, McCullough AJ. Hepatic veno-occlusive disease associated

with renal transplantation and azathioprine therapy. Ann Intern Med 1986;104(5):651–5.

40. Azoulay D, Castaing D, Lemoine A, Samuel D, Majno P, Reynes M, Charpentier B, Bismuth H. Successful treatment of severe azathioprine-induced hepatic veno-occlusive disease in a kidney-transplanted patient with transjugular intrahepatic portosystemic shunt. Clin Nephrol 1998;50(2):118–22.

41. Mion F, Cloix P, Boillot O, Gille D, Bouvier R, Paliard P, Berger F. Maladie veino-occlusive après transplantation hépatique. Association d'un rejet aiguë cellulaire et de la toxicité de l'azathioprine. [Veno-occlusive disease after liver transplantation. Association of acute cellular rejection and toxicity of azathioprine.] Gastroenterol Clin Biol 1993;17(11):863–7.

42. Sterneck M, Wiesner R, Ascher N, Roberts J, Ferrell L, Ludwig J, Lake J. Azathioprine hepatotoxicity after liver transplantation. Hepatology 1991;14(5):806–10.

43. Cooper C, Cotton DW, Minihane N, Cawley MI. Azathioprine hypersensitivity manifesting as acute focal hepatocellular necrosis. J R Soc Med 1986;79(3):171–3.

44. Delgado J, Munoz de Bustillo E, Ibarrola C, Colina F, Morales JM, Rodriguez E, Aguado JM, Fuertes A, Gomez MA. Hepatitis C virus-related fibrosing cholestatic hepatitis after cardiac transplantation: is azathioprine a contributory factor? J Heart Lung Transplant 1999;18(6):607–10.

45. David-Neto E, da Fonseca JA, de Paula FJ, Nahas WC, Sabbaga E, Ianhez LE. Is azathioprine harmful to chronic viral hepatitis in renal transplantation? A long-term study on azathioprine withdrawal. Transplant Proc 1999;31(1–2):1149–50.

46. Seiderer J, Zech CJ, Diebold J, Schoenberg SO, Brand S, Tillack C, Göke B, Ochsenkühn T. Nodular regenerative hyperplasia: a reversible entity associated with azathioprine therapy. Eur J Gastroenterol Hepatol 2006;18(5):553–5.

47. Daniel F, Cadranel JF, Seksik P, Cazier A, Duong Van Huyen JP, Ziol M, Coutarel P, Loison P, Jian R, Marteau P. Azathioprine induced nodular regenerative hyperplasia in IBD patients. Gastroenterol Clin Biol 2005;29(5):600–3.

48. Breen DP, Marinaki AM, Arenas M, Hayes PC. Pharmacogenetic association with adverse drug reactions to azathioprine immunosuppressive therapy following liver transplantation. Liver Transpl 2005;11(7):826–33.

49. Eaton VS, Casanova JM, Kupa A. Azathioprine hepatotoxicity confirmed by rechallenge. Aust J Hosp Pharm 2000;30:58–9.

50. Muszkat M, Pappo O, Caraco Y, Haviv YS. Hepatocanalicular cholestasis after 24 years of azathioprine administration for myasthenia gravis. Clin Drug Invest 2000;19:75–8.

51. Wu YT, Shen C, Yin J, Yu JP, Meng Q. Azathioprine hepatotoxicity and the protective effect of liquorice and glycyrrhizic acid. Phytother Res 2006;20(8):640–5.

52. Eklund BI, Moberg M, Bergquist J, Mannervik B. Divergent activities of human glutathione transferases in the bioactivation of azathioprine. Mol Pharmacol 2006;70(2):747–54.

53. Present DH, Meltzer SJ, Krumholz MP, Wolke A, Korelitz BI. 6-Mercaptopurine in the management of inflammatory bowel disease: short- and long-term toxicity. Ann Intern Med 1989;111(8):641–9.

54. Frick TW, Fryd DS, Goodale RL, Simmons RL, Sutherland DE, Najarian JS. Lack of association between azathioprine and acute pancreatitis in renal transplantation patients. Lancet 1991;337(8735):251–2.

55. Eland IA, van Puijenbroek EP, Sturkenboom MJ, Wilson JH, Stricker BH. Drug-associated acute pancreatitis: twenty-one years of spontaneous reporting in The Netherlands. Am J Gastroenterol 1999;94(9):2417–22.

56. Siwach V, Bansal V, Kumar A, Rao Ch U, Sharma A, Minz M. Post-renal transplant azathioprine-induced pancreatitis. Nephrol Dial Transplant 1999;14(10):2495–8.

57. Bisschop D, Germain ML, Munzer M, Trenque T. Thioguanine, pancréatotoxicité?. [Thioguanine, pancreatotoxicity?.] Therapie 2001;56(1):67–9.

58. Floyd A, Pedersen L, Nielsen GL, Thorlacius-Ussing O, Sorensen HT. Risk of acute pancreatitis in users of azathioprine: a population-based case-control study. Am J Gastroenterol 2003;98:1305–8.

59. Weersma RK, Peters FT, Oostenbrug LE, van den Berg AP, van Haastert M, Ploeg RJ, Posthumus MD, Homan van der Heide JJ, Jansen PL, van Dullemen HM. Increased incidence of azathioprine-induced pancreatitis in Crohn's disease compared with other diseases. Aliment Pharmacol Ther 2004;20(8):843–50..

60. Bir K, Herzenberg AM, Carette S. Azathioprine induced acute interstitial nephritis as the cause of rapidly progressive renal failure in a patient with Wegener's granulomatosis. J Rheumatol 2006;33(1):185–7..

61. Paoluzi OA, Crispino P, Amantea A, Pica R, Iacopini F, Consolazio A, Di Palma V, Rivera M, Paoluzi P. Diffuse febrile dermatosis in a patient with active ulcerative colitis under treatment with steroids and azathioprine: a case of Sweet's syndrome. Case report and review of literature. Dig Liver Dis 2004;36(5):361–6..

62. Pillans PI, Tooke AF, Bateman ED, Ainslie GM. Acute polyarthritis associated with azathioprine for interstitial lung disease. Respir Med 1995;89(1):63–4.

63. Bellaiche G, Cosnes J, Nouts A, Ley G, Slama JL. Troubles de la marche secondaires à la prise d'azathioprine chez 2 malades ayant une maladie de Crohn. [Gait disorders secondary to azathioprine treatment in 2 patients with Crohn's disease.] Gastroenterol Clin Biol 1999;23(4):533–4.

64. Vestergaard P, Rejnmark L, Mosekilde L. Methotrexate, azathioprine, cyclosporine, and risk of fracture. Calcif Tissue Int 2006;79(2):69–75.

65. Cao ZG, Liu JH, Zhu YP, Zhou SW, Qi L, Dong XC, Wu B, Lin ZB. [Effects of different immunodepressants on the sperm parameters of kidney transplant recipients.] Zhonghua Nan Ke Xue 2006;12(5):405–7.

66. Stratton JD, Farrington K. Relapse of vasculitis, sepsis, or azathioprine allergy? Nephrol Dial Transplant 1998;13(11):2927–8.

67. Jeurissen ME, Boerbooms AM, van de Putte LB, Kruijsen MW. Azathioprine induced fever, chills, rash, and hepatotoxicity in rheumatoid arthritis. Ann Rheum Dis 1990;49(1):25–7.

68. Meys E, Devogelaer JP, Geubel A, Rahier J, Nagant de Deuxchaisnes C. Fever, hepatitis and acute interstitial nephritis in a patient with rheumatoid arthritis. Concurrent manifestations of azathioprine hypersensitivity. J Rheumatol 1992;19(5):807–9.

69. Jones JJ, Ashworth J. Azathioprine-induced shock in dermatology patients. J Am Acad Dermatol 1993;29(5 Pt 1):795–6.

70. Burden AD, Beck MH. Contact hypersensitivity to azathioprine. Contact Dermatitis 1992;27(5):329–30.

71. Sinico RA, Sabadini E, Borlandelli S, Cosci P, Di Toma L, Imbasciati E. Azathioprine hypersensitivity: report of two cases and review of the literature. J Nephrol 2003;16:272–6.

72. Hinrichs R, Schneider LA, Ozdemir C, Staib G, Scharffetter- Kochanek K. Azathioprine hypersensitivity in a patient with peripheral demyelinating polyneuropathy. Br J Dermatol 2003;148:1076–7.

73. Demirtas-Ertan G, Rowshani AT, ten Berge IJ. Azathioprine-induced shock in a patient suffering from undifferentiated erosive oligoarthritis. Neth J Med 2006;64(4):124–6.

74. Korelitz BI, Zlatanic J, Goel F, Fuller S. Allergic reactions to 6-mercaptopurine during treatment of inflammatory bowel disease. J Clin Gastroenterol 1999;28:341–4.

75. Schmitt K, Pfeiffer U, Stiehrle HE, Thuermann PA. Absence of azathioprine hypersensitivity after administration of its active metabolite 6-mercaptopurine. Acta Dermatol Venereol 2000;80:147–8.

76. Dominguez Ortega J, Robledo T, Martinez-Cocera C, Alonso A, Cimarra M, Chamorro M, Plaza A. Desensitization to azathioprine. J Invest Allergol Clin Immunol 1999;9:337–8.

77. Dominguez Ortega J, Robledo T, Martinez-Cocera C, Alonso A, Cimarra M, Chamorro M, Plaza A. Desensitization to azathioprine. J Investig Allergol Clin Immunol 1999;9(5):337–8.

78. Korelitz BI, Zlatanic J, Goel F, Fuller S. Allergic reactions to 6-mercaptopurine during treatment of inflammatory bowel disease. J Clin Gastroenterol 1999;28(4):341–4.

79. Godeau B, Paul M, Autegarden JE, Leynadier F, Astier A, Schaeffer A. Hypersensitivity to azathioprine mimicking gastroenteritis. Absence of recurrence with 6-mercaptopurine. Gastroenterol Clin Biol 1995;19(1):117–9.

80. Garcia VD, Keitel E, Almeida P, Santos AF, Becker M, Goldani JC. Morbidity after renal transplantation: role of bacterial infection. Transplant Proc 1995;27(2):1825–6.

81. Wade JJ, Rolando N, Hayllar K, Philpott-Howard J, Casewell MW, Williams R. Bacterial and fungal infections after liver transplantation: an analysis of 284 patients. Hepatology 1995;21(5):1328–36.

82. Singh N, Yu VL. Infections in organ transplant recipients. Curr Opin Infect Dis 1996;9:223–9.

83. Reis MA, Costa RS, Ferraz AS. Causes of death in renal transplant recipients: a study of 102 autopsies from 1968 to 1991. J R Soc Med 1995;88(1):24–7.

84. Korelitz BI, Fuller SR, Warman JI, Goldberg MD. Shingles during the course of treatment with 6-mercaptopurine for inflammatory bowel disease. Am J Gastroenterol 1999;94(2):424–6.

85. Posthuma EF, Westendorp RG, van der Sluys Veer A, Kluin-Nelemans JC, Kluin PM, Lamers CB. Fatal infectious mononucleosis: a severe complication in the treatment of Crohn's disease with azathioprine. Gut 1995;36(2):311–3.

86. Suassuna JH, Machado RD, Sampaio JC, Leite LL, Villela LH, Ruzany F, Souza ER, Moraes JR. Active cytomegalovirus infection in hemodialysis patients receiving donor-specific blood transfusions under azathioprine coverage. Transplantation 1993;56(6):1552–4.

87. Al Obeid K, Al Khalifan NN, Jamal W, Kehinde EO, Rotimi VO. Epididymo-orchitis and testicular abscess caused by Salmonella enteritidis in immunocompromised patients in Kuwait. Med Princ Pract 2006;15(4):305–8.

88. Lemyze M, Tavernier JY, Chevalon B, Lamblin C. Severe varicella zoster pneumonia during the course of treatment with azathioprine for Crohn's disease. Rev Mal Respir 2003;20:773–6.

89. de Jong DJ, Goullet M, Naber TH. Side effects of azathioprine in patients with Crohn's disease. Eur J Gastroenterol Hepatol 2004;16(2):207–12.

90. Penn I. Tumors after renal and cardiac transplantation. Hematol Oncol Clin North Am 1993;7(2):431–45.

91. Gaya SB, Rees AJ, Lechler RI, Williams G, Mason PD. Malignant disease in patients with long-term renal transplants. Transplantation 1995;59(12):1705–9.

92. London NJ, Farmery SM, Will EJ, Davison AM, Lodge JP. Risk of neoplasia in renal transplant patients. Lancet 1995;346(8972):403–6.

93. Kehinde EO, Petermann A, Morgan JD, Butt ZA, Donnelly PK, Veitch PS, Bell PR. Triple therapy and incidence of de novo cancer in renal transplant recipients. Br J Surg 1994;81(7):985–6.

94. Opelz G, Henderson R. Incidence of non-Hodgkin lymphoma in kidney and heart transplant recipients. Lancet 1993;342(8886–8887):1514–6.

95. Gruber SA, Gillingham K, Sothern RB, Stephanian E, Matas AJ, Dunn DL. De novo cancer in cyclosporine-treated and non-cyclosporine-treated adult primary renal allograft recipients. Clin Transplant 1994;8(4):388–95.

96. Hiesse C, Kriaa F, Rieu P, Larue JR, Benoit G, Bellamy J, Blanchet P, Charpentier B. Incidence and type of malignancies occurring after renal transplantation in conventionally and cyclosporine-treated recipients: analysis of a 20-year period in 1600 patients. Transplant Proc 1995;27(1):972–4.

97. Pitt PI, Sultan AH, Malone M, Andrews V, Hamilton EB. Association between azathioprine therapy and lymphoma in rheumatoid disease. J R Soc Med 1987;80(7):428–9.

98. Barthelmes L, Thomas KJ, Seale JR. Prostatic involvement of a testicular lymphoma in a patient with myasthenia gravis on long-term azathioprine. Leuk Lymphoma 2002;43(12):2425–6.

99. Taylor AE, Shuster S. Skin cancer after renal transplantation: the causal role of azathioprine. Acta Dermatol Venereol 1992;72(2):115–9.

100. Moss AC, Farrell RJ. Lymphoma risk with azathioprine/6-MP therapy—read beyond the headlines. Gastroenterology 2006;130(4):1363–4.

101. Rhinow K, Schirmer I, Loddenkemper C, Anagnostopoulos I, Stein H, Reichart PA. Orale Epstein-Barr-Virus-assoziierte diffuse grosszellige B-Zell-Lymphome bei HIV-negativen immunsupprimierten Patienten. [Oral EBV-associated diffuse large B-cell lymphomas in HIV-negative immunocompromised patients.] Mund Kiefer Gesichtschir 2006;10(3):155–61.

102. McGovern DP, Jewell DP. Risks and benefits of azathioprine therapy. Gut 2005;54(8):1055–9.

103. Silman AJ, Petrie J, Hazleman B, Evans SJ. Lymphoproliferative cancer and other malignancy in patients with rheumatoid arthritis treated with azathioprine: a 20 year follow up study. Ann Rheum Dis 1988;47(12):988–92.

104. Jones M, Symmons D, Finn J, Wolfe F. Does exposure to immunosuppressive therapy increase the 10 year malignancy and mortality risks in rheumatoid arthritis? A matched cohort study. Br J Rheumatol 1996;35(8):738–45.

105. Connell WR, Kamm MA, Dickson M, Balkwill AM, Ritchie JK, Lennard-Jones JE. Long-term neoplasia risk after azathioprine treatment in inflammatory bowel disease. Lancet 1994;343(8908):1249–52.

106. Fraser AG, Orchard TR, Robinson EM, Jewell DP. Long-term risk of malignancy after treatment of inflammatory bowel disease with azathioprine. Aliment Pharmacol Ther 2002;16(7):1225–32.

107. Confavreux C, Saddier P, Grimaud J, Moreau T, Adeleine P, Aimard G. Risk of cancer from azathioprine therapy in multiple sclerosis: a case-control study. Neurology 1996;46(6):1607–12.

108. Penn I. Cancers in cyclosporine-treated vs azathioprine-treated patients. Transplant Proc 1996;28(2):876–8.

109. Putzki N, Knipp S, Ramczykowski T, Vago S, Germing U, Diener HC, Limmroth V. Secondary myelodysplastic

syndrome following long-term treatment with azathioprine in patients with multiple sclerosis. Mult Scler 2006;12(3):363–6.

110. Then Bergh F, Niklas A, Strauss A, von Ahsen N, Niederwieser D, Schwarz J, Wagner A, Al-Ali HK. Rapid progression of myelodysplastic syndrome to acute myeloid leukemia on sequential azathioprine, IFN-beta and copolymer-1 in a patient with multiple sclerosis. Acta Haematol 2006;116(3):207–10.

111. Bo J, Schroder H, Kristinsson J, Madsen B, Szumlanski C, Weinshilboum R, Andersen JB, Schmiegelow K. Possible carcinogenic effect of 6-mercaptopurine on bone marrow stem cells: relation to thiopurine metabolism. Cancer 1999;86(6):1080–6.

112. Li AC, Warnakulasuriya S, Thompson RP. Neoplasia of the tongue in a patient with Crohn's disease treated with azathioprine: case report. Eur J Gastroenterol Hepatol 2003;15:185–7.

113. Alvarez Delgado A, Perez Garcia ML, Fradejas Salazar PM, de la Coba Ortiz C, Rodriguez Perez A. Invasive cancer of the cervix in a patient undergoing chronic treatment with 6-mercaptopurine for Crohn's disease. Gastroenterol Hepatol 2003;26:52–3.

114. Sasaki J, Kawamura YJ, Konishi F, Tosha T. Colitic cancer developed after introduction of azathioprine. Dig Dis Sci 2004;49(10):1727–9.

115. Korelitz BI, Mirsky FJ, Fleisher MR, Warman JI, Wisch N, Gleim GW. Malignant neoplasms subsequent to treatment of inflammatory bowel disease with 6-mercaptopurine. Am J Gastroenterol 1999;94(11):3248–53.

116. Vroom F, de Walle HE, van de Laar MA, Brouwers JR, de Jong-van den Berg LT. Disease-modifying antirheumatic drugs in pregnancy: current status and implications for the future. Drug Saf 2006;29(10):845–63.

117. Ramsey-Goldman R, Schilling E. Immunosuppressive drug use during pregnancy. Rheum Dis Clin North Am 1997;23(1):149–67.

118. Armenti VT, Moritz MJ, Davison JM. Drug safety issues in pregnancy following transplantation and immunosuppression: effects and outcomes. Drug Saf 1998;19(3):219–32.

119. Cararach V, Carmona F, Monleon FJ, Andreu J. Pregnancy after renal transplantation: 25 years experience in Spain. Br J Obstet Gynaecol 1993;100(2):122–5.

120. de Boer NK, Jarbandhan SV, de Graaf P, Mulder CJ, van Elburg RM, van Bodegraven AA. Azathioprine use during pregnancy: unexpected intrauterine exposure to metabolites. Am J Gastroenterol 2006;101(6):1390–2.

121. Armenti VT, Ahlswede BA, Moritz MJ, Jarrell BE. National Transplantation Pregnancy Registry: analysis of pregnancy outcomes of female kidney recipients with relation to time interval from transplant to conception. Transplant Proc 1993;25(1 Pt 2):1036–7.

122. Pilarski LM, Yacyshyn BR, Lazarovits AI. Analysis of peripheral blood lymphocyte populations and immune function from children exposed to cyclosporine or to azathioprine in utero. Transplantation 1994;57(1):133–44.

123. Polifka JE, Friedman JM. Teratogen update: azathioprine and 6-mercaptopurine. Teratology 2002;65(5):240–61.

124. Rajapakse RO, Korelitz BI, Zlatanic J, Baiocco PJ, Gleim GW. Outcome of pregnancies when fathers are treated with 6-mercaptopurine for inflammatory bowel disease. Am J Gastroenterol 2000;95(3):684–8.

125. Francella A, Dyan A, Bodian C, Rubin P, Chapman M, Present DH. The safety of 6-mercaptopurine for childbearing patients with inflammatory bowel disease: a retrospective cohort study. Gastroenterology 2003;124:9–17.

126. Norgard B, Pedersen L, Fonager K, Rasmussen SN, Sorensen HT. Azathioprine, mercaptopurine and birth outcome: a population-based cohort study. Aliment Pharmacol Ther 2003;17:827–34.

127. Cissoko H, Jonville-Bera AP, Lenain H, Riviere MF, Saugier J, Casanova JL, Autret-Leca E. Agranulocytose et déficit immunitaire transitoires après expostition ftale à l'azathioprine et mésalazine. [Agranulocytosis and transitory immune deficiency after fetal exposure to azathioprine and mesalazine.] Arch Pediatr 1999;6(10):1136–7.

128. Cohen RD. Sperm, sex, and 6-MP: the perception on conception. Gastroenterology 2004;127(4):1263–4.

129. Norgard B, Pedersen L, Jacobsen J, Rasmussen SN, Sorensen HT. The risk of congenital abnormalities in children fathered by men treated with azathioprine or mercaptopurine before conception. Aliment Pharmacol Ther 2004;19(6):679–85.

130. Cimaz R, Meregalli E, Biggioggero M, Borghi O, Tincani A, Motta M, Airo P, Meroni PL. Alterations in the immune system of children from mothers treated with immunosuppressive agents during pregnancy. Toxicol Lett 2004;149(1-3):155–62.

131. Moskovitz DN, Bodian C, Chapman ML, Marion JF, Rubin PH, Scherl E, Present DH. The effect on the fetus of medications used to treat pregnant inflammatory bowel-disease patients. Am J Gastroenterol 2004;99(4):656–61..

132. Gardiner SJ, Gearry RB, Roberts RL, Zhang M, Barclay ML, Begg EJ. Exposure to thiopurine drugs through breast milk is low based on metabolite concentrations in mother-infant pairs. Br J Clin Pharmacol 2006;62(4):453–6.

133. Cuffari C, Hunt S, Bayless T. Utilisation of erythrocyte 6-thioguanine metabolite levels to optimise azathioprine therapy in patients with inflammatory bowel disease. Gut 2001;48(5):642–6.

134. Gardiner SJ, Gearry RB, Barclay ML, Begg EJ. Two cases of thiopurine methyltransferase (TPMT) deficiency—a lucky save and a near miss with azathioprine. Br J Clin Pharmacol 2006;62(4):473–6.

135. Gardiner SJ, Begg EJ. Pharmacogenetics, drug-metabolizing enzymes, and clinical practice. Pharmacol Rev 2006;58(3):521–90.

136. Kaskas BA, Louis E, Hindorf U, Schaeffeler E, Deflandre J, Graepler F, Schmiegelow K, Gregor M, Zanger UM, Eichelbaum M, Schwab M. Safe treatment of thiopurine S-methyltransferase deficient Crohn's disease patients with azathioprine. Gut 2003;52:140–2.

137. Bergan S. Optimisation of azathioprine immunosuppression after organ transplantation by pharmacological measurements. BioDrugs 1997;8:446–56.

138. Meggitt SJ, Reynolds NJ. Azathioprine for atopic dermatitis. Clin Exp Dermatol 2001;26(5):369–75.

139. Seidman EG. Clinical use and practical application of TPMT enzyme and 6-mercaptopurine metabolite monitoring in IBD. Rev Gastroenterol Disord 2003;3 Suppl 1:S30–8.

140. Schutz E, Gummert J, Mohr FW, Armstrong VW, Oellerich M. Azathioprine myelotoxicity related to elevated 6-thioguanine nucleotides in heart transplantation. Transplant Proc 1995;27(1):1298–300.

141. Kerstens PJ, Stolk JN, De Abreu RA, Lambooy LH, van de Putte LB, Boerbooms AA. Azathioprine-related bone marrow toxicity and low activities of purine enzymes in patients with rheumatoid arthritis. Arthritis Rheum 1995;38(1):142–5.

142. Boulieu R, Lenoir A, Bertocchi M, Mornex JF. Intracellular thiopurine nucleotides and azathioprine myelotoxicity in organ transplant patients. Br J Clin Pharmacol 1997;43(1):116–8.

143. Soria-Royer C, Legendre C, Mircheva J, Premel S, Beaune P, Kreis H. Thiopurine-methyl-transferase activity to assess azathioprine myelotoxicity in renal transplant recipients. Lancet 1993;341(8860):1593–4.

144. Serre-Debeauvais F, Bayle F, Amirou M, Bechtel Y, Boujet C, Vialtel P, Bessard G. Hématotoxicité de l'azathioprine à déterminisme génétique aggravé par un déficit en xanthine oxydase chez une transplantée rénale. [Hematotoxicity caused by azathioprine genetically determined and aggravated by xanthine oxidase deficiency in a patient following renal transplantation.] Presse Méd 1995;24(21):987–8.

145. Sanderson J, Ansari A, Marinaki T, Duley J. Thiopurine methyltransferase: should it be measured before commencing thiopurine drug therapy? Ann Clin Biochem 2004;41(Pt 4):294–302.

146. Ford L, Prout C, Gaffney D, Berg J. Whose TPMT activity is it anyway? Ann Clin Biochem 2004;41(Pt 6):498–500.

147. Corominas H, Domenech M, Laiz A, Gich I, Geli C, Diaz C, De Cuevillas F, Moreno M, Vazquez G, Baiget M. Is thiopurine methyltransferase genetic polymorphism a major factor for withdrawal of azathioprine in rheumatoid arthritis patients? Rheumatol (Oxf) 2003;42:40–5.

148. Tassaneeyakul W, Srimarthpirom S, Reungjui S, Chansung K, Romphruk A, Tassaneeyakul W. Azathioprine-induced fatal myelosuppression in a renal-transplant recipient who carried heterozygous TPMT*1/*3C. Transplantation 2003;76:265–6.

149. Gearry RB, Barclay ML, Burt MJ, Collett JA, Chapman BA, Roberts RL, Kennedy MA. Thiopurine S-methyltransferase (TPMT) genotype does not predict adverse drug reactions to thiopurine drugs in patients with inflammatory bowel disease. Aliment Pharmacol Ther 2003;18:395–400.

150. Chrzanowska M, Kurzawski M, Drozdzik M, Mazik M, Oko A, Czekalski S. Thiopurine S-methyltransferase phenotype-genotype correlation in hemodialyzed patients. Pharmacol Rep 2006;58(6):973-8..

151. Song DK, Zhao J, Zhang LR. TPMT genotype and its clinical implication in renal transplant recipients with azathioprine treatment. J Clin Pharm Ther 2006;31(6):627–35.

152. Oender K, Lanschuetzer CM, Laimer M, Klausegger A, Paulweber B, Kofler B, Hintner H, Bauer JW. Introducing a fast and simple PCR-RFLP analysis for the detection of mutant thiopurine S-methyltransferase alleles TPMT*3A and TPMT*3C. J Eur Acad Dermatol Venereol 2006;20(4):396-400..

153. Kalsi K, Marinaki AM, Yacoub MH, Smolenski RT. HPLC/tandem ion trap mass detector methods for determination of inosine monophosphate dehydrogenase (IMPDH) and thiopurine methyltransferase (TPMT). Nucleosides Nucleotides Nucleic Acids 2006;25(9-11):1241–4.

154. Ansari A, Hassan C, Duley J, Marinaki A, Shobowale-Bakre EM, Seed P, Meenan J, Yim A, Sanderson J. Thiopurine methyltransferase activity and the use of azathioprine in inflammatory bowel disease. Aliment Pharmacol Ther 2002;16(10):1743–50.

155. Holme SA, Duley JA, Sanderson J, Routledge PA, Anstey AV. Erythrocyte thiopurine methyl transferase assessment prior to azathioprine use in the UK. QJM 2002;95(7):439–44.

156. Naughton MA, Battaglia E, O'Brien S, Walport MJ, Botto M. Identification of thiopurine methyltransferase (TPMT) polymorphisms cannot predict myelosuppression in systemic lupus erythematosus patients taking azathioprine. Rheumatology (Oxford) 1999;38(7):640–4.

157. Stolk JN, Boerbooms AM, de Abreu RA, de Koning DG, van Beusekom HJ, Muller WH, van de Putte LB. Reduced thiopurine methyltransferase activity and development of side effects of azathioprine treatment in patients with rheumatoid arthritis. Arthritis Rheum 1998;41(10):1858–66.

158. Black AJ, McLeod HL, Capell HA, Powrie RH, Matowe LK, Pritchard SC, Collie-Duguid ES, Reid DM. Thiopurine methyltransferase genotype predicts therapy-limiting severe toxicity from azathioprine. Ann Intern Med 1998;129(9):716–8.

159. Dervieux T, Medard Y, Baudouin V, Maisin A, Zhang D, Broly F, Loirat C, Jacqz-Aigrain E. Thiopurine methyltransferase activity and its relationship to the occurrence of rejection episodes in paediatric renal transplant recipients treated with azathioprine. Br J Clin Pharmacol 1999;48(6):793–800.

160. Relling MV, Hancock ML, Rivera GK, Sandlund JT, Ribeiro RC, Krynetski EY, Pui CH, Evans WE. Mercaptopurine therapy intolerance and heterozygosity at the thiopurine S-methyltransferase gene locus. J Natl Cancer Inst 1999;91(23):2001–8.

161. Sebbag L, Boucher P, Davelu P, Boissonnat P, Champsaur G, Ninet J, Dureau G, Obadia JF, Vallon JJ, Delaye J. Thiopurine S-methyltransferase gene polymorphism is predictive of azathioprine-induced myelosuppression in heart transplant recipients. Transplantation 2000;69(7):1524–7.

162. Colombel JF, Ferrari N, Debuysere H, Marteau P, Gendre JP, Bonaz B, Soule JC, Modigliani R, Touze Y, Catala P, Libersa C, Broly F. Genotypic analysis of thiopurine S-methyltransferase in patients with Crohn's disease and severe myelosuppression during azathioprine therapy. Gastroenterology 2000;118(6):1025–30.

163. Gisbert JP, Nino P, Rodrigo L, Cara C, Guijarro LG. Thiopurine methyltransferase (TPMT) activity and adverse effects of azathioprine in inflammatory bowel disease: long-term follow-up study of 394 patients. Am J Gastroenterol 2006;101(12):2769–76.

164. Hindorf U, Lindqvist M, Peterson C, Söderkvist P, Ström M, Hjortswang H, Pousette A, Almer S. Pharmacogenetics during standardised initiation of thiopurine treatment in inflammatory bowel disease. Gut 2006;55(10):1423–31.

165. Czaja AJ, Carpenter HA. Thiopurine methyltransferase deficiency and azathioprine intolerance in autoimmune hepatitis. Dig Dis Sci 2006;51(5):968–75.

166. Heneghan MA, Allan ML, Bornstein JD, Muir AJ, Tendler DA. Utility of thiopurine methyltransferase genotyping and phenotyping, and measurement of azathioprine metabolites in the management of patients with autoimmune hepatitis. J Hepatol 2006;45(4):584–91.

167. Schedel J, Gödde A, Schütz E, Bongartz TA, Lang B, Schölmerich J, Müller-Ladner U. Impact of thiopurine methyltransferase activity and 6-thioguanine nucleotide concentrations in patients with chronic inflammatory diseases. Ann N Y Acad Sci 2006;1069:477–91.

168. Marinaki AM, Sumi S, Arenas M, Fairbanks L, Harihara S, Shimizu K, Ueta A, Duley JA. Allele frequency of inosine triphosphate pyrophosphatase gene polymorphisms in a Japanese population. Nucleosides Nucleotides Nucleic Acids 2004;23(8-9):1399–401.

169. Marinaki AM, Ansari A, Duley JA, Arenas M, Sumi S, Lewis CM, Shobowale-Bakre el-M, Escuredo E, Fairbanks LD, Sanderson JD. Adverse drug reactions to azathioprine therapy are associated with polymorphism in the gene

encoding inosine triphosphate pyrophosphatase (ITPase). Pharmacogenetics 2004;14(3):181–7.

170. Van Dieren JM, Hansen BE, Kuipers EJ, Nieuwenhuis EE, Van der Woude CJ. Meta-analysis: inosine triphosphate pyrophosphatase polymorphisms and thiopurine toxicity in the treatment of inflammatory bowel disease. Aliment Pharmacol Ther 2007;26(5):643–52.

171. Sumi S, Marinaki AM, Arenas M, Fairbanks L, Shobowale-Bakre M, Rees DC, Thein SL, Ansari A, Sanderson J, De Abreu RA, Simmonds HA, Duley JA. Genetic basis of inosine triphosphate pyrophosphohydrolase deficiency. Hum Genet. 2002;111(4-5):360–7.

172. Shipkova M, Lorenz K, Oellerich M, Wieland E, von Ahsen N. Measurement of erythrocyte inosine triphosphate pyrophosphohydrolase (ITPA) activity by HPLC and correlation of ITPA genotype-phenotype in a Caucasian population. Clin Chem 2006;52(2):240–7.

173. Marinaki AM, Duley JA, Arenas M, Ansari A, Sumi S, Lewis CM, Shobowale-Bakre M, Fairbanks LD, Sanderson J. Mutation in the ITPA gene predicts intolerance to azathioprine. Nucleosides Nucleotides Nucleic Acids 2004;23(8-9):1393–7.

174. von Ahsen N, Armstrong VW, Behrens C, von Tirpitz C, Stallmach A, Herfarth H, Stein J, Bias P, Adler G, Shipkova M, Oellerich M, Kruis W, Reinshagen M, Schütz E. Association of inosine triphosphatase 94C>A and thiopurine S-methyltransferase deficiency with adverse events and study drop-outs under azathioprine therapy in a prospective Crohn disease study. Clin Chem 2005;51(12):2282–8.

175. Zelinkova Z, Derijks LJ, Stokkers PC, Vogels EW, van Kampen AH, Curvers WL, Cohn D, van Deventer SJ, Hommes DW. Inosine triphosphate pyrophosphatase and thiopurine s-methyltransferase genotypes relationship to azathioprine-induced myelosuppression. Clin Gastroenterol Hepatol 2006;4(1):44–9.

176. Gearry RB, Roberts RL, Barclay ML, Kennedy MA. Lack of association between the ITPA 94C→A polymorphism and adverse effects from azathioprine. Pharmacogenetics 2004;14(11):779–81.

177. Rayner CK, Hart AL, Hayward CM, Emmanuel AV, Kamm MA. Azathioprine dose escalation in inflammatory bowel disease. Aliment Pharmacol Ther 2004;20(1):65–71.

178. Russmann S, Lauterburg B. Lebensbedrohliche Nebenwirkungen der Gichtbehandlung. [Life-threatening adverse effects of pharmacologic antihyperuricemic therapy.] Ther Umsch 2004;61(9):575–7.

179. Seidel W. Panzytopenie unter kombinierter Behandlung mit Azathioprin und Allopurinol. [Pancytopenia from combination therapy with azathioprine and allopurinol.] Z Rheumatol 2004;63(5):425–7.

180. Cummins D, Sekar M, Halil O, Banner N. Myelosuppression associated with azathioprine–allopurinol interaction after heart and lung transplantation. Transplantation 1996;61(11):1661–2.

181. Ippoliti G, Negri M, Campana C, Vigano M. Urate oxidase in hyperuricemic heart transplant recipients treated with azathioprine. Transplantation 1997;63(9):1370–1.

182. Dewit O, Vanheuverzwyn R, Desager JP, Horsmans Y. Interaction between azathioprine and aminosalicylates: an in vivo study in patients with Crohn's disease. Aliment Pharmacol Ther 2002;16(1):79–85.

183. Singleton JD, Conyers L. Warfarin and azathioprine: an important drug interaction. Am J Med 1992;92(2):217.

184. Fernandez MA, Regadera A, Aznar J. Acenocoumarol and 6-mercaptopurine: an important drug interaction. Haematologica 1999;84(7):664–5.

185. Rotenberg M, Levy Y, Shoenfeld Y, Almog S, Ezra D. Effect of azathioprine on the anticoagulant activity of warfarin. Ann Pharmacother 2000;34(1):120–2.

186. Roblin X, Serre-Debeauvais F, Phelip JM, Bessard G, Bonaz B. Drug interaction between infliximab and azathioprine in patients with Crohn's disease. Aliment Pharmacol Ther 2003;18:917–25.

187. Blanco R, Martinez-Taboada VM, Gonzalez-Gay MA, Armona J, Fernandez-Sueiro JL, Gonzalez-Vela MC, Rodriguez-Valverde V. Acute febrile toxic reaction in patients with refractory rheumatoid arthritis who are receiving combined therapy with methotrexate and azathioprine. Arthritis Rheum 1996;39(6):1016–20.

188. Ng HJ, Crowther MA. Azathioprine and inhibition of the anticoagulant effect of warfarin: evidence from a case report and a literature review. Am J Geriatr Pharmacother 2006;4(1):75–7.

189. Barnes BH, Borowitz SM, Saulsbury FT, Hellems M, Sutphen JL. Discordant erythrocyte sedimentation rate and C-reactive protein in children with inflammatory bowel disease taking azathioprine or 6-mercaptopurine. J Pediatr Gastroenterol Nutr 2004;38(5):509–12.

190. Mori H, Yamanaka K, Kaketa M, Tamada K, Hakamada A, Isoda K, Yamanishi K, Mizutani H. Drug eruption caused by azathioprine: value of using the drug-induced lymphocytes stimulation test for diagnosis. J Dermatol 2004;31(9):731–6.

191. Green CJ, Mee AS. Re-introduction of azathioprine in previously intolerant patients. Eur J Gastroenterol Hepatol 2006;18(1):17–19.

Bucillamine

General Information

Bucillamine (mercaptomethylpropanoylcysteine) is chemically related to penicillamine and is also used in rheumatoid arthritis. Most of the information on bucillamine comes from Japan, its country of origin (1).

The patterns of adverse reactions to sulfhydryl compounds that are used in rheumatoid arthritis (bucillamine, pyritinol, and tiopronin) show remarkable similarities to those of penicillamine (SED-12, 548; 2).

Comparative studies

In a retrospective 12-month review of the medical records of 348 patients with rheumatoid arthritis (ACR classification) bucillamine and methotrexate were compared (3). There were 74 adverse events in 71 patients; none was life-threatening. Rashes were the most common (47%) followed by proteinuria (25%). One patient had nephrotic syndrome for about 6 months; bucillamine was withdrawn and the patient made a good recovery. Other adverse events were stomatitis, glossitis, cough, and raised transaminase activities. Rashes mainly occurred in the first 3 months of use, while proteinuria often developed after a longer interval. The authors concluded that the effectiveness of bucillamine can usually be judged within 3 months of use and that it is indicated in the treatment of rheumatoid arthritis of moderate severity, either before or after methotrexate.

Organs and Systems

Respiratory

In 10 patients with bucillamine-associated interstitial pneumonitis, the HLA antigen DR4 was present in all 10 and a positive lymphocyte stimulation test was found in three of the six patients tested (4).

Nervous system

Myasthenia gravis has been reported during the use of bucillamine (5). However, since the disease persisted after withdrawal, the role of the drug was uncertain.

Sensory systems

A change in taste has been attributed to bucillamine in a single case, without further specification (1).

Hematologic

Among 36 Korean patients with rheumatoid arthritis agranulocytosis with high fever developed in one after 3-week use of bucillamine (dose not specified) (6).

Gastrointestinal

Stomatitis, nausea, anorexia, and epigastric discomfort are common during the use of bucillamine (6).

Hemorrhagic gastritis has been reported in a single case, without further specification (1).

Liver

Increased aminotransferase activities were found in about 5% of patients using bucillamine for rheumatoid arthritis (1,6).

Urinary tract

Proteinuria occurs in about 7% of patients using bucillamine (1). Less often, nephrotic syndrome can develop (6–10). Microscopically there is membranous glomerulonephritis, with diffuse fine granular precipitation of IgG and C3 around the capillary walls, electron-dense deposits at the subepithelial side of the basement membrane and effacement of foot processes.

Skin

Bucillamine causes skin reactions in about 5% of patients (11). Rashes and pruritus are frequent and eosinophilia can occur (1,6).

Bullous pemphigoid has been attributed to bucillamine 200 mg/day (11). The mouth, pharynx, larynx, and conjunctiva were involved, as well as the skin on the chest, abdomen, and axilla. Indirect immunofluorescence showed circulating antibodies against the basement membrane.

There have been reports of bucillamine-associated pemphigus.

- A 57-year-old woman developed a generalized itchy rash 9 months after she started to take bucillamine (12). A skin biopsy showed spongiosis, lymphocytic infiltration in the epidermis, and intercellular deposition of IgG.
- Another patient had a pemphigus foliaceus-like eruption on three different occasions, in association with penicillamine, auranofin, and bucillamine (13).

A patient taking bucillamine developed an eruption that had features of both pemphigus foliaceus and pemphigus vulgaris and was associated with glomerulonephritis (14).

- A 62-year-old man with rheumatoid arthritis developed a rash on the neck, chest, and legs after taking oral bucillamine (dose not specified) for 6 months. The lesions were of two different types: small pigmented, vesicular, erythematous macules, similar to those of pemphigus foliaceus, and skin erosions, as seen in pemphigus vulgaris. There was no mucosal involvement. Serology was positive for antinuclear antibodies (1:320, nucleolar type). A biopsy showed acantholysis in the granular, spinous, and suprabasal layers. Direct immunofluorescence showed intercellular deposits of IgG and C3 throughout the epidermis, but not in the basement membrane. Indirect immunofluorescence of donor skin showed IgG reactivity in the nuclei of keratinocytes. An enzyme-linked immunoadsorbent assay (ELISA), using baculovirus-expressed recombinant desmogleins as antigen, was positive and indifferent to circulating anti-Dsg1 and anti-Dsg3 antibodies. This patient also had the nephrotic syndrome (proteinuria 8.7 g/day, total serum protein 59 g/l, serum total cholesterol 10.2 mmol/l), probably also due to bucillamine. A renal biopsy was consistent with membranous glomerulonephritis. The skin lesions improved within 1 month of bucillamine withdrawal, but full recovery of both cutaneous and renal injury was achieved only after the use of prednisone, 40 mg/day for 2 weeks.

In 13 patients with the peculiar yellow nail syndrome, bucillamine was the suspected cause in 7 (15).

Reproductive system

Gigantism of the breasts, probably induced by bucillamine, has been reported (16).

- After attempts with chrysotherapy and lobenzarit, a 24-year-old woman was given bucillamine 300 mg/day and a glucocorticoid, predonine, for rheumatoid arthritis. After 10 months she noticed bilateral breast enlargement, which over 6 months progressed to extreme proportions, the left breast ultimately reaching as far as her pubis. The skin of the breasts was thin and erythematous, with marked dilatation of the superficial veins. The nipple areola complexes were elongated and poorly defined from the surrounding skin. There were no abnormalities of prolactin, sex hormones, growth hormone, or TSH (but the values were not stated). Bilateral total mastectomy was performed and the nipple-areola complexes were removed from the resected tissue and grafted on to the breasts after insertion of a tissue expander. The breast tissue removed from the right side weighed 5 kg and that from the left side 7 kg. Histologically there was increased fibrosis and duct dilatation and no malignancy.

This effect, attributed here to bucillamine, is a rare but well-established adverse effect of penicillamine. Although the patient had also taken isoniazid for pulmonary tuberculosis, that was unlikely to have played a part, since the breast enlargement started earlier and progressed after the isoniazid had been withdrawn.

References

1. Takahashi C, Murasawi A, Nakazono K, Yoshida K, Sekiguchi H, Kikuchi M. An open clinical study of bucillamine in uncontrollable rheumatoid arthritis. Int J Immunother 1991;7:95–8.
2. Jaffe IA. Adverse effects profile of sulfhydryl compounds in man. Am J Med 1986;80(3):471–6.
3. Sekiguchi N, Kameda H, Amano K, Takeuchi T. Efficacy and safety of bucillamine, a D-penicillamine analogue, in patients with active rheumatoid arthritis. Mod Rheumatol 2006;16(2):85–91.
4. Negishi M, Kaga S, Kasama T, Hashimoto M, Fukushima T, Yamagata N, Tabata M, Kobayashi K, Ide H, Takahashi T. [Lung injury associated with bucillamine therapy.]Ryumachi 1992;32(2):135–9.
5. Fujiyama J, Tokimura Y, Ijichi S, Arimura K, Matsuda T, Osame M. Bucillamine may induce myasthenia gravis. Jpn J Med 1991;30(1):101–2.
6. Kim SY, Lee IH, Bae SC, Yoo DH. Preliminary trial of the efficacy of bucillamine in Korean patients with rheumatoid arthritis. Clin Drug Invest 1995;9:284–90.
7. Yoshida A, Morozumi K, Suganuma T, Aoki J, Sugito K, Koyama K, Oikawa T, Fujinimi T, Matsumoto Y. [Clinicopathological study of nephropathy in patients with rheumatoid arthritis.]Ryumachi 1991;31(1):14–21.
8. Kawano M, Nomura H, Iwainaka Y, Nakashima A, Koni I, Tofuku Y, Takeda R. [Bucillamine-associated membranous nephropathy in a patient with rheumatoid arthritis.]Nippon Jinzo Gakkai Shi 1990;32(7):817–21.
9. Yoshida A, Morozumi K, Suganuma T, Sugito K, Ikeda M, Oikawa T, Fujinami T, Takeda A, Koyama K. Clinicopathological findings of bucillamine-induced nephrotic syndrome in patients with rheumatoid arthritis. Am J Nephrol 1991;11(4):284–8.
10. Baba N, Nomura T, Sakemi T, Uchida M, Watanabe T. [Membranous glomerulonephritis probably related to bucillamine therapy in two patients with rheumatoid arthritis.]Nippon Jinzo Gakkai Shi 1991;33(6):629–34.
11. Yamaguchi R, Oryu F, Hidano A. A case of bullous pemphigoid induced by tiobutarit (D-penicillamine analogue). J Dermatol 1989;16(4):308–11.
12. Amasaki Y, Sagawa A, Atsumi T, Jodo S, Nakabayashi T, Watanabe I, Mukai M, Fujisaku A, Nakagawa S, Kobayashi H. [A case of rheumatoid arthritis developing pemphigus-like skin lesion during treatment with bucillamine.]Ryumachi 1991;31(5):528–34.
13. Takashima T, Tani M. Antirheumatics-induced pemphigus foliaceus-like lesions. Hihu 1990;32:205–8.
14. Moreland LW, Russell AS, Paulus HE. Management of rheumatoid arthritis: the historical context. J Rheumatol 2001;28(6):1431–52.
15. Ichikawa Y, Shimizu H, Arimori S. "Yellow nail syndrome" and rheumatoid arthritis. Tokai J Exp Clin Med 1991;16(5–6):203–9.
16. Sakai Y, Wakamatsu S, Ono K, Kumagai N. Gigantomastia induced by bucillamine. Ann Plast Surg 2002;49(2):193–5.

Chloroquine and hydroxychloroquine

General Information

Chloroquine is rapidly and almost completely absorbed from the intestinal tract, peak serum concentrations being reached in 1–6 hours (average 3 hours). It is extensively distributed and redistribution follows. It is slowly metabolized by side-chain de-ethylation. The half-life is 30–60 days. Elimination is mainly via the kidney. Malnutrition can slow down the rate of metabolism.

Comparative studies

Amodiaquine and chloroquine have been compared in an open, randomized trial in uncomplicated falciparum malaria in Nigerian children (1). The doses were amodiaquine (n = 104) 10 mg/kg/day for 3 days and chloroquine (n = 106) 10 mg/kg/day for 3 days. After 28 days, the cure rate was significantly higher with amodiaquine than chloroquine (95% versus 58%). The rates of adverse events, most commonly pruritus (10%) and gastrointestinal disturbances (3%), were similar in the two groups. Cross-resistance between the two aminoquinolines is common, and there are concerns regarding toxicity of amodiaquine with repeated use.

General adverse effects

There are relatively few adverse effects at the doses of chloroquine that are used for malaria prophylaxis and standard treatment doses. However, the use of higher doses than those recommended, for example because of problems with resistance, can cause problems. Infants are very easily overdosed (SEDA-16, 302). In the treatment of rheumatoid arthritis and lupus erythematosus, larger doses are used, often for long periods of time, and with this use the incidence of adverse effects is high. Neuromyopathy, neuritis, myopathy, and cardiac myopathy can cause serious problems. Retinopathy can lead to blindness. Chloroquine has a long half-life and accumulates in the tissues, including the brain. Concentrations in the brain can have a bearing on mental status and psychotic syndromes. Chloroquine interferes with the action of several enzymes, including alcohol dehydrogenase, and blocks the sulfhydryl–disulfide interchange reaction. Allergic reactions are generally limited to rashes and pruritus.

Organs and Systems

Cardiovascular

Electrocardiographic changes, comprising altered T waves and prolongation of the QT interval, are not uncommon during high-dose treatment with chloroquine. The clinical significance of this is uncertain. With chronic intoxication, a varying degree of atrioventricular block can be seen; first-degree right bundle branch block and total atrioventricular block have been described. Symptoms depend on the severity of the effects: syncope, Stokes–Adams attacks, and signs of cardiac failure can occur. Acute intoxication can cause cardiovascular collapse and/or respiratory failure. Cardiac complications can prove fatal in both chronic and acute intoxication.

Third-degree atrioventricular conduction defects have been reported in two patients with rheumatoid arthritis after prolonged administration of chloroquine (2,3).

Torsade de pointes following chronic use of hydroxychloroquine has been reported (4).

- A 67-year-old woman with systemic lupus erythematosus and asthma who had taken prednisolone 15 mg/day, long-acting theophylline 200 mg/day, and hydroxychloroquine 200 mg/day for 1 year developed sudden loss of consciousness and generalized rigidity. Moments later she regained consciousness with no residual symptoms, but the episode recurred several times. She had a past history of cirrhosis and hepatitis B virus-related hepatoma with portal vein thrombosis, an old myocardial infarction, and a small ventricular septal defect. An electrocardiogram showed multiple ventricular extra beats and she had another syncopal attack, with documented torsade de pointes. After defibrillation and lidocaine 100 mg her cardiac rhythm reverted to normal with a prolonged QT interval (600 msec). Cardiac enzymes were not raised. Hydroxychloroquine was suspected as the cause of ventricular tachycardia and was withdrawn. She was given intravenous magnesium sulfate 1 g followed by isoprenaline 2 micrograms/minute. After 4 days the ventricular dysrhythmia subsided but the QT interval was still prolonged (500-530 msec). After 3 weeks the ventricular dysrhythmias abated.

It is not clear in this case whether congenital long QT interval could have contributed. Chronic use of hydroxychloroquine in rheumatic diseases should be weighed against the risk of potentially lethal cardiac dysrhythmias.

Intravenous administration can result in dysrhythmias and cardiac arrest; the speed of administration is relevant, but also the concentration reached: deaths have been recorded with blood concentrations of 1 µg/ml; concentrations after a 300 mg dose are usually 50–100 µg/ml (SEDA-13, 803).

Long-term chloroquine can caouse cardiac complications, such as conduction disorders and cardiomyopathy (restrictive or hypertrophic), by structural alteration of the interventricular septum (5). Thirteen cases of cardiactoxicity associated with long-term chloroquine and hydroxychloroquine have been reported in patients with systemic autoimmune diseases. The cumulative doses were 600–2281 g for chloroquine and 292–4380 g for hydroxychloroquine.

- A 64-year-old woman with systemic lupus erythematosus took chloroquine for 7 years (cumulative dose 1000 g). She developed syncope, and the electrocardiogram showed complete heart block; a permanent pacemaker was inserted. The next year she presented with biventricular cardiac failure, skin hyperpigmentation, proximal muscle weakness, and chloroquine retinopathy. Coronary angiography was normal. An echocardiogram showed a restrictive cardiomyopathy. A skeletal muscle biopsy was characteristic of chloroquine myopathy. Chloroquine was withdrawn and she improved rapidly with diuretic therapy.
- Chloroquine cardiomyopathy occurred during long-term (7 years) treatment for rheumatoid polyarthritis in a 42-year-old woman, who had an isolated acute severe conduction defect, confirmed by histological study with electron microscopy (6).
- A 50-year-old woman took chloroquine for 6 years for rheumatoid arthritis and developed a restrictive cardiomyopathy, which required heart transplantation (7).

Regular cardiac evaluation should be considered for those who have taken a cumulative chloroquine dose of 1000 g, particularly elderly patients.

More than one mechanism may underlie the cardiac adverse effects of chloroquine. Severe hypokalemia after a single large dose of chloroquine has been documented, and some studies show a correlation between plasma potassium concentrations and the severity of the cardiac effects (8).

Light and electron microscopic abnormalities were found on endomyocardial biopsy in two patients with cardiac failure. The first had taken hydroxychloroquine 200 mg/day for 10 years, then 400 mg/day for a further 6 years; the second had taken hydroxychloroquine 400 mg/day for 2 years (SEDA-13, 239). A similar case was reported after the use of 250 mg/day for 25 years (SEDA-18, 286).

Respiratory

Respiratory collapse can occur with acute overdosage.

Acute pneumonitis probably due to chloroquine has been described (9).

- A 41-year-old man with chronic discoid lupus erythematosus was given chloroquine 150 mg bd for 10 days followed by 150 mg/day. After 2 weeks he developed fever, a diffuse papular rash, dyspnea, and sputum. A chest X-ray showed peripheral pulmonary infiltrates. He improved on withdrawal of chloroquine and treatment with cefpiramide and roxithromycin. No organism was isolated. A subsequent oral challenge with chloroquine provoked a similar reaction.

Nervous system

The incidence of serious nervous system events among patients taking chloroquine for less than a year has been estimated as one in 13 600.

Chloroquine, especially in higher doses, can cause a marked neuromyopathy, characterized by slowly progressive weakness of insidious onset. In many cases this weakness first affects the proximal muscles of the legs. Reduction in nerve conduction time and electromyographic abnormalities typical of both neuropathic and myopathic changes can be found. Histologically there is a vacuolar myopathy. Neuromyopathy is a rare adverse effect and is usually limited to patients taking 250–750 mg/day for prolonged periods. The symptoms can be accompanied by other manifestations of chloroquine toxicity (SEDA-11, 583). An 80-year-old woman developed symptoms after taking chloroquine 300 mg/day for 6 months (10), once more demonstrating that a standard dosage can be too much for elderly people.

A spastic pyramidal tract syndrome of the legs has been reported. In young children the features of an extrapyramidal syndrome include abnormal eye movements, trismus, torticollis, and torsion dystonia.

Chloroquine can cause seizures in patients with epilepsy. The mechanism is uncertain, but it may include reductions in inhibitory neurotransmitters and pharmacokinetic interactions that alter anticonvulsant concentrations. Tonic–clonic convulsions were reported in four patients in whom chloroquine was part of a prophylactic regimen. Antiepileptic treatment was required to control the seizures. None had further seizures after withdrawal of the antimalarial drugs (11).

Chloroquine and desethylchloroquine concentrations have been studied in 109 Kenyan children during the first 24 hours of admission to hospital with cerebral malaria (12). Of the 109 children 100 had received chloroquine before admission. Blood chloroquine and desethylchloroquine concentrations were no higher in children who had seizures than in those who did not, suggesting that chloroquine does not play an important role in the development of seizures in malaria.

- A 59-year-old woman had a generalized convulsion 24 hours after returning from a trip to Vietnam (13). She had a history of partial complex seizures (controlled with carbamazepine) due to a previous ruptured cerebral aneurysm. For the preceding 3 weeks she had been taking chloroquine 100 mg/day and proguanil 200 mg/day. A blood film was negative for malaria. A CT scan of the brain showed changes compatible with the previous hemorrhage. She was successfully treated with clobazam (dose not stated) until withdrawal of chemoprophylaxis.

The interaction between chloroquine and carbamazepine was not examined. Chloroquine should not be given to adults with a history of epilepsy.

Neuromuscular function

Severe neuromyopathy has been reported in patients taking chloroquine (SEDA-21, 295).

Chloroquine-induced neuromyopathy is a complication of chloroquine treatment of autoimmune disorders or long-term use of chloroquine as a prophylactic antimalarial drug (14).

Sensory systems

Eyes

Chloroquine and its congeners can cause two typical effects in the eye, a keratopathy and a specific retinopathy. Both of these effects are associated with the administration of the drug over longer periods of time.

Keratopathy

Chloroquine-induced keratopathy is limited to the corneal epithelium, where high concentrations of the drug are readily demonstrable. Slit lamp examination shows a series of punctate opacities scattered diffusely over the cornea; these are sometimes seen as lines just below the center of the cornea, while thicker yellow lines may be seen in the stroma. The keratopathy is often asymptomatic, fewer than 50% of patients having complaints. The commonest symptoms are the appearance of halos around lights and photophobia. Keratopathy can appear after 1–2 months of treatment, but dosages of under 250 mg/day usually do not cause it. Dust exposure can lead to similar changes. The incidence of keratopathy is high, occurring in 30–70% of patients treated with higher dosages of chloroquine. The condition is usually reversible on withdrawal and does not seem to involve a threat to vision (SEDA-13, 805). There are differences in incidence between chloroquine and hydroxychloroquine. In a survey of 1500 patients, 95% of the patients taking chloroquine had corneal deposition of the drug, while less than 10% of patients taking hydroxychloroquine showed any corneal changes (SEDA-16, 303).

Retinopathy

The retinopathy encountered with the prolonged use of chloroquine or related drugs is a much more serious adverse effect and can lead to irreversible damage to the retina and loss of vision. However, it is not possible to predict in which patients and in what proportion of patients an early retinopathy will progress to blindness. The typical picture is that of the "bull's eye," an intact foveal area surrounded by a depigmented ring, the whole lesion being enclosed in a scattered hyperpigmented area. At this stage the retinal vessels are contracted, there are changes in the peripheral retinal pigment epithelium, and the optic disk is atrophic. In the early stages there are changes in the macular retinal pigment epithelium. However, the picture is not always clear, and peripheral retinal changes may appear as the first sign. Another sign may be unilateral paramacular retinal edema. The macular changes and the "bull's eye" are occasionally seen in patients who have never been treated with chloroquine or related drugs (SED-13, 805). Retinopathy can occur after chloroquine antimalarial chemoprophylaxis for less than 10 years: the lowest reported total dose was 110 g (15). A case of hydroxychloroquine-induced retinopathy in a 45-year-old woman with systemic lupus erythematosus has illustrated that maculopathy can be associated with other 4-aminoquinolines (16).

The resulting functional defects are varied: difficulty in reading, scotomas, defective color vision, photophobia, light flashes, and a reduction in visual acuity. Symptoms do not parallel the retinal changes. By the time that visual acuity has become impaired, irreversible changes will have taken place.

Testing of visual acuity, central fields (with or without the use of red targets), contrast sensitivity, dark adaptation, and color vision provides no early indication of chloroquine retinopathy. Careful ophthalmoscopic examination of the macula can be a sensitive index when visual acuity remains intact. More sophisticated tests, such as the measurement of the critical flicker fusion frequency and the Amsler grid test (detection of small peripheral scotoma), can be useful. It is important to trace, if at all possible, the results of a pretreatment ophthalmological examination after dilatation of the pupils, thus reducing the possibility of confusing senile degenerative changes with chloroquine-induced abnormalities.

Despite the fact that the retinopathy has been known for many years, it is still not clear why certain patients develop these changes while others do not. There is a clear relation to daily dosage: the retinopathy is rarely seen with daily doses below 250 mg of chloroquine or 400 mg of hydroxychloroquine; the daily dose seems to be more important than the total dose. Nevertheless, cases of retinopathy have been described after the use of small doses for relatively short periods of time, while prolonged treatment and total doses of a kilogram or more have been used in many other patients without any evidence of macular changes. In the published cases there is usually no information about other treatments given previously or concomitantly. More cases are seen in older people. Patients with lupus erythematosus are more susceptible than patients with rheumatoid arthritis. The presence of nephropathy increases the likelihood of retinopathy, as does the concomitant use of probenecid. Exposure to sunlight may be of importance, since light amplifies the risk of retinopathy. The retinopathic changes are probably connected with the concentrating capacity of the melanin-containing epithelium. Chloroquine inhibits the incorporation of amino acids into the retinal pigment epithelium.

Little is yet known about the development of the retinopathy after withdrawal of treatment. Retinal changes in the early stages are probably reversible if the drug is withdrawn, and progression of a severe maculopathy to blindness seems to be less frequent than feared. In 1650 patients with 6/6 vision and relative scotomas there was no further decline in visual acuity after drug withdrawal, but 63% of patients who presented with absolute scotomas lost further vision over a median period of 6 years. This suggests that withdrawal of chloroquine at an early stage halts progression of the disease (SEDA-17, 327).

Three patients with chloroquine retinopathy have been studied with multifocal electroretinography (17). All three had been taking chloroquine for rheumatological diseases and all had electroretinographic changes that were more sensitive than full field electroretinography. It may be that multifocal electroretinography will be a useful technique in the assessment of suspected cases of subtle chloroquine retinopathy.

The need for routine ophthalmological testing of all patients who take chloroquine is under discussion, an obvious element being the cost/benefit ratio. The best current opinion seems to be that at doses not exceeding 6.5 mg/kg/day of hydroxychloroquine, given for not longer than 10 years and with periodic checking of renal and hepatic function, the likelihood of retinal damage is negligible and ophthalmological follow-up is not required (SEDA-16, 303) (SEDA-17, 327). However, patients taking chloroquine or higher doses of hydroxychloroquine should be checked.

Other adverse effects on the eyes
Rhegmatogenous retinal detachment and bitemporal hemianopsia have both been seen in association with chloroquine retinopathy. Bilateral edema of the optic nerve occurred in a woman who took chloroquine 200 mg/day for 2.5 months. Diplopia and impaired accommodation (characterized by difficulty in changing focus quickly from near to far vision and vice versa) also affect a minority of patients (SEDA-13, 806).

Ears
Ototoxicity has been mentioned occasionally over the years; tinnitus and deafness can occur in relation to high doses; symptoms described after injection of chloroquine phosphate include a case of cochlear vestibular dysfunction in a child (18). However, there is insufficient evidence to attribute ototoxicity to chloroquine in humans, except as a rare individualized phenomenon. In guinea pigs given chloroquine 25 mg/kg/day intraperitoneally, one of the first signs of intoxication was ototoxicity (SEDA-11, 586).

- Unilateral sensorineural hearing loss occurred in a 7-year-old girl with idiopathic pulmonary hemosiderosis after she had taken hydroxychloroquine 100 mg bd for 2 years (19).

Taste
Disturbances of taste and smell have been attributed to chloroquine (20).

Psychological, psychiatric

Many mental changes attributed to chloroquine have been described, notably agitation, aggressiveness, confusion, personality changes, psychotic symptoms, and depression. Acute mania has also been recognized (SEDA-18, 287). The mental changes can develop slowly and insidiously. Subtle symptoms, such as fluctuating impairment of thought, memory, and perception, can be early signs, but may also be the only signs. The symptoms may be connected with the long half-life of chloroquine and its accumulation, leading to high tissue concentrations (SEDA-11, 583). Chloroquine also inhibits glutamate dehydrogenase activity and can reduce concentrations of the inhibitory transmitter GABA.

In some cases with psychosis after the administration of recommended doses, symptoms developed after the patients had taken a total of 1.0–10.5 g of the drug, the time of onset of behavioral changes varying from 2 hours to 40 days. Most cases occurred during the first week and lasted from 2 days to 8 weeks (SEDA-11, 583).

When severe psychosis occurs after treatment with chloroquine and hydroxychloroquine it it is usually during treatment for malaria, but it can follow treatment for connective tissue disorders. Hallucinations have been reported after hydroxychloroquine treatment for erosive lichen planus (21).

- A 75-year-old woman was given hydroxychloroquine 400 mg/day for erosive lichen planus in conjunction with topical glucocorticoids and a short course of oral methylprednisolone 0.5 mg/kg/day. After 10 days she became disoriented in time and place, followed by feelings of depersonalization and kinesthetic hallucinations, preceded by nightmares. She stopped taking hydroxychloroquine 1 week later and the hallucinations progressively disappeared. She recovered her normal mental state within 1 month and had not relapsed 2 years later.

The potential for severe psychiatric adverse events must always be considered in patients taking long-term chloroquine and hydroxychloroquinine. The onset may be a few hours to many days after the start of therapy and it can occur in a patient without a preceding history of mental illness. The mechanism is unknown. Recovery is rapid and occurs within days of stopping treatment.

Transient global amnesia occurred in a healthy 62-year-old man, 3 hours after he took 300 mg chloroquine. Recovery was spontaneous after some hours (SEDA-16, 302).

In one center, toxic psychosis was reported in four children over a period of 18 months (SEDA-16, 302). The children presented with acute delirium, marked restlessness, outbursts of increased motor activity, mental inaccessibility, and insomnia. One child seemed to have visual hallucinations. In each case, chloroquine had been administered intramuscularly because of fever. The dosages were not recorded. The children returned to normal within 2 weeks.

Metabolism

Hypoglycemia was reported in a fatal chloroquine intoxication in a 32-year-old black Zambian male (SEDA-13, 240). Hypoglycemia has also been seen in patients, especially children, with cerebral malaria (SEDA-13, 240). Further studies have shown that the hypoglycemia in these African children was usually present before the antimalarial drugs had been started; in a study in Gambia hypoglycemia occurred after treatment with the drug had been started, although it was not necessarily connected with the treatment (SEDA-13, 240). Convulsions were more common in hypoglycemic children. This commonly unrecognized complication contributes to morbidity and mortality in cerebral *Plasmodium falciparum* malaria. Hypoglycemia is amenable to treatment with intravenous dextrose or glucose, which may help to prevent brain damage (SEDA-13, 804).

- A 16-year-old girl was treated empirically with chloroquine (total 450 mg of chloroquine base) for fever, had no malarial parasites in the peripheral blood smear, but had severe hypoglycemia of 1.5 mmol/l (27 mg/dl) (22).

This suggests that therapeutic doses of chloroquine can cause hypoglycemia even in the absence of malaria.

Although hydroxychloroquine has been used to treat porphyria cutanea tarda (23), there are reports that it can also worsen porphyria (24,25).

Electrolyte balance

Severe hypokalemia after a single large dose of chloroquine has been documented, and some studies show a correlation between plasma potassium concentrations and the severity of the cardiac effects. In a retrospective study of 191 consecutive patients who had taken an overdose of chloroquine (mean blood chloroquine concentration 20 µmol/l; usual target concentration up to 6 µmol/l), the mean plasma potassium concentration was 3.0 mmol/l (0.8) and was significantly lower in those who died than in those who survived (8). Plasma potassium varied directly with the systolic blood pressure and inversely with the QRS and QT intervals. Plasma potassium varied inversely with the blood chloroquine.

Hematologic

Chloroquine inhibits myelopoiesis in vitro at therapeutic concentrations and higher. In a special test procedure, a short-lasting anti-aggregating effect could be seen with chloroquine concentrations of 3.2–32 µg/ml (SEDA-16, 303). These effects have clinical consequences. Chloroquine and related aminoquinolines have reportedly caused blood dyscrasias at antimalarial doses. Leukopenia, agranulocytosis, and the occasional case of thrombocytopenia have been reported (SEDA-13, 804) (26). There is some evidence that myelosuppression is dose-dependent. This is in line with the hypothesis that 4-aminoquinoline therapy merely accentuates the cytopenia linked to other forms of bone marrow damage (SEDA-11, 584) (SEDA-16, 302).

Some studies have pointed to inhibitory effects of chloroquine on platelet aggregability. In an investigation, this aspect of chloroquine was studied in vitro in a medium containing ADP, collagen, and ristocetin. There was a highly significant effect at chloroquine concentrations of 3.2–32 µg/ml. However, there were no significant differences in platelet responses to ADP or collagen 2 or 6 hours after adding chloroquine, compared with pre-drug values. The investigators believed that these data provided no cause for concern in using chloroquine for malaria prophylaxis in patients with impaired hemostasis (SEDA-16, 303).

Chloroquine can cause methemoglobinemia, especially in enzyme-deficient subjects. An exceptionally severe case of methemoglobinema has been reported (22).

- A 16-year-old girl treated empirically for fever with chloroquine (total 450 mg of chloroquine base) developed cyanosis, jaundice, and altered consciousness. She had a moderate hemolytic anemia (hemoglobin 13.3 g/dl), severe methemoglobinema (70%), and hypoglycemia (1.5 mmol/l; 27 mg/dl). No malarial parasites were found, a Coomb's test was negative, and erythrocyte glucose-6-phosphate dehydrogenase (G6PD) activity was normal. NADPH methemoglobin reductase was not evaluated. Other causes, such as exposure to nitro-compounds, solvents, or drugs other than chloroquine were excluded. She was treated with methylthioninium (methylene blue) and the methemoglobinemia resolved over the next few days.

This girl also had hypoglycemia (see Metabolism above).

Mouth and teeth

Pigmentation of the palate can occur as a part of a more generalized pigmentation in patients taking chloroquine (27).

Several patients seen with chloroquine retinopathy in Accra have been observed to present with depigmented patches in the skin of the face. This may be associated with a greyish pigmentation of the mucosa of the hard palate. Two such cases are reported here to illustrate the condition. Stomatitis with buccal ulceration has occasionally been mentioned (SEDA-11, 584).

Gastrointestinal

Gastrointestinal discomfort is not unusual in patients receiving chloroquine, and diarrhea can occur. Changes in intestinal motility may be to blame; intramuscular injection of chloroquine caused a shortened orofecal time in the five cases in which this was measured. Overdosage can cause vomiting.

Liver

Hepatotoxicity, which is uncommon with either chloroquine or proguanil, has been reported after the use of a fixed-dose combination of chloroquine and proguanil (28).

• A day before visiting the Indian subcontinent a 50-year-old French Caucasian woman began a course of a fixed-dose combination of proguanil (200 mg) + chloroquine (100 mg), one tablet daily for chemoprophylaxis. Four days later she developed vomiting, discolored stools, dark urine, and general fatigue. The chloroquine + proguanil was stopped immediately. A week later she developed severe nausea, headache, and conjunctival hemorrhages. There was no abdominal pain, fever, or rash. She had abnormal liver function tests, with aspartate transaminase activity of 335 U/l (reference range œ35 U/l), alanine transaminase activity of 660 U/l (œ41 U/l), and alkaline phosphatase activity of 744 U/l (60–279 U/l). Total bilirubin was 616 (34–222) µmol/l and direct bilirubin was 393 (17–68) µmol/l. There were bile salts and increased bile pigments in the urine. An abdominal scan was unremarkable and serology for hepatitis A, B, and C was negative. Liver biopsy was not performed. She had no known susceptibility factors for liver disease. She had previously taken chloroquine + proguanil in 1998, 2002, and 2003 and recalled experiencing severe abdominal discomfort on the last occasion. Her symptoms improved after withdrawal of chloroquine + proguanil and her liver function tests gradually returned to normal.

The temporal relation between drug therapy and the appearance of symptoms suggested an adverse reaction to chloroquine + proguanil. The abnormal liver function tests, negative tests for hepatitis, the absence of fever, and the resolution of symptoms after withdrawal all suggested a causal relation. The exact mechanism is not known but it could have been an allergic reaction after sensitization from previous exposures.

Urinary tract

Chloroquine-induced kidney damage has occasionally been reported. A remarkably well-documented case report further elucidates this adverse drug reaction.

• A 46-year-old woman with impaired renal function (glomerular filtration rate of 23?26 ml/minute/1.7m^2, serum creatinine 186 µmol/l (2.1 mg/dl) took chloroquine 155 mg/day for Sjögren's syndrome (29). After 5 months, her serum creatinine had increased to 339 µmol/l (2.7 mg/dl) and after 11 months to 442 µmol/l (5 mg/dl) with a glomerular filtration rate of 8 ml/minute/1.7m^2. Light microscopy of a kidney biopsy showed vascular parenchymal atrophy with accumulation of colloid material in atrophic tubules. Electron microscopy showed osmiophilic lamellated bodies mainly in podocytes and to a lesser degree in glomerular and vascular endothelial and vascular smooth muscle cells. Fabry's disease was ruled out based on normal activity of alpha-galactosidase A. Because the histopathological findings resembled those seen in chloroquine-induced myopathy/cardiomyopathy, chloroquine was withdrawn and 9 months later, her glomerular filtration rate was 19 ml/minute/1.7m^2 and serum creatinine 221 µmol/l (2.5 mg/dl), close to baseline values.

Skin

Skin lesions and eruptions of different types have been attributed to chloroquine, including occasional cases of epidermal necrolysis (30).

The most common dermatological adverse event associated with chloroquine is skin discomfort (often called pruritus). It is much more common in people with darker skins and has been ascribed to chloroquine binding to increased melanin concentrations in the skin. In a pharmacokinetic study, the ratio of AUC$_{0-48}$ for chloroquine and its major metabolite desethylchloroquine was significantly higher in the plasma and urine of 18 patients with chloroquine-induced pruritus than in that of 18 patients without (31). These results imply that differences in metabolism and higher chloroquine concentrations may be partly responsible for chloroquine-induced pruritus.

Pruritus begins about 10 hours after the start of treatment, with a maximum intensity at about 24 hours. These times correspond to maximum serum concentrations of chloroquine and its metabolites after oral ingestion. In many cases, the itch is confined to the palms of the hands and the soles of the feet. In a study in Nigeria, the incidence of pruritus was 60–75%; the itch was considered unbearable in 40%, and 30% refused further chloroquine (32). In a second study, there was an even higher incidence. In a study elsewhere, the incidence of pruritus was 27% (SEDA-16, 304). Not surprisingly, pruritus is a major cause of non-adherence to treatment, and it may contribute largely to the emergence and spread of resistant *P. falciparum* (SEDA-16, 304). Pruritus is more often seen in black-skinned than in white-skinned people in Africa, a difference that has been ascribed to the binding of chloroquine to melanin, and hence a racial predisposition. No such reports have come from America (SEDA-11, 584; SEDA-16, 303; SEDA-17, 327; SEDA-18, 288). Antihistamine treatment can have a preventive effect on pruritus. Other treatments that have been mentioned include prednisone and niacin, but the results were not impressive (33).

A few cases of psoriasis, or severe exacerbation of psoriasis shortly after the start of treatment, have been reported (SEDA-13, 804; SEDA-16, 304; SEDA-17, 327).

Photosensitivity and photoallergic dermatitis have been seen, particularly during prolonged therapy with high doses.

Blue–black pigmentation involving the palate and facial, pretibial, and subungual areas occurs rarely, but it has been associated with retinopathy (SEDA-11, 584). The nail bed can turn blue–brown and the nail itself may develop longitudinal stripes and show a blue–grey fluorescence (SEDA-11, 584).

- A 44-year-old Hispanic woman developed depigmented patches on her chest, shoulders, forearms, back, and shins 1 month after switching from hydroxychloroquine to chloroquine 500 mg/day for cutaneous discoid lupus erythematosus (34). Chloroquine was immediately withdrawn, and within 2 months spontaneous re-pigmentation occurred in most of the depigmented patches.

A near fatal case of Stevens–Johnson syndrome has been reported (35).

- A 32-year old woman weighing 61kg developed painful skin blisters and erosions accompanied by fever and myalgia. The symptoms started on the third day after a course of oral chloroquine (Tablets Lariago, chloroquine phosphate 500 mg, Ipca Laboratories, Mumbai, India); two tablets initially, one tablet after 6 hours, and one tablet/day for 2 days. Her symptoms began with erythematous itchy papular eruptions on the trunk and then progressed to involve the face, limbs, and mucous membranes of the mouth. She had difficulty in swallowing because of painful erosions of the mouth and oropharynx. There was conjunctivitis but no visual impairment. Bullae continued to appear on the trunk and limbs and a purpuric rash on the trunk. She responded well to intravenous fluids, antibiotics to prevent secondary infection, and hydrocortisone.

Chloroquine can cause vitiligo (SEDA-17, 327).
Fatal toxic epidermal necrolysis has been associated with hydroxychloroquine (36).

- A 39-year-old woman with rheumatoid arthritis took hydroxychloroquine 200 mg bd for painful synovitis, in addition to meloxicam, co-dydramol, and Gaviscon. She inadvertently took twice the prescribed dose of hydroxychloroquine, but stopped it after 2 weeks because of nausea. The next day she developed a widespread blotchy erythema and 2 weeks later was admitted to hospital with clinical and histological toxic epidermal necrolysis and deteriorated rapidly with multiorgan failure; she died 1 week later.

There have been only a few isolated reports of Stevens–Johnson syndrome associated with hydroxychloroquine. A clear temporal relation to the start of treatment with hydroxychloroquine has been documented in a patient with rheumatoid arthritis (37).

An increased frequency of skin reactions to hydroxychloroquine was noted in 11 patients (seven of whom had systemic lupus erythematosus, two discoid lupus, and two a lupus-like syndrome) when a coloring agent (sunshine yellow E110) was removed from the formulation; the authors were unable to explain this unexpected finding (38).

There have been four case reports of photosensitivity associated with hydroxychloroquine (39) which has an estimated incidence of about 10 per 1000 patient-years (40).

- A 49-year-old man developed severe cutaneous necrotizing vasculitis after 13 days of treatment with a combination of chloroquine 100 mg and proguanil 200 mg/day (41). He had taken no other drugs. The lesions consisted of diffuse painful purpuric and extensive necrotizing plaques on the upper and lower limbs, mainly on the hands and feet, maculopapular erythema on the trunk, and petechial maculae on the hard palate. His temperature was normal and he had no organomegaly. Laboratory findings were normal, except for a eosinophilia of 0.72×10^9/l and a C-reactive protein of 133 mg/l. Chloroquine and proguanil were withdrawn and his condition normalized within 3 weeks. Skin tests 3 month later were positive for chloroquine, but negative for quinine and the biguanide derivatives proguanil and metformin.

Pemphigus has been attributed to chloroquine and hydroxychloroquine (42).

- A 52-year-old woman abruptly developed generalized blisters 2 weeks after starting to take hydoxychloroquine for rheumatoid arthritis. The eruption consisted of pruritic bullae and erosions on the head, trunk, limbs, and oral mucosa. She also had scattered urticarial lesions. She had had a previous similar but mild reaction following chloroquine therapy, which had cleared when the drug was withdrawn. Biopsy confirmed the diagnosis of pemphigus vulgaris with suprabasal slitting.

Drug-induced pemphigus is mainly caused by drugs containing a thiol (-SH) group, such as penicillamine, captopril, piroxicam, and ampicillin, or drugs with an active amide group, such as penicillin. In contrast, chloroquine and hydroxychloroquine are 4-aminoquinolines.

A bullous skin eruption induced by radiotherapy after the use of chloroquine has been described (43).

- A 12-year-old girl with a diffuse pontine glioma was treated with radiotherapy and developed a high-grade fever with chills. Although the blood smear was negative for malaria she was treated empirically with chloroquine 500 mg, 250 mg 6 hours later, and 250 mg/day for 2 days. On day 3 she developed localized bullous eruptions over the site of irradiation, which peeled in 6-7 hours leaving a patch of fulminant moist desquamation. The skin surrounding the patch was severely erythematous. Radiotherapy was withheld and she was treated with topical amniotic membrane and gentian violet. One week later the fever had cleared and the desquamation had almost healed. Radiotherapy was restarted and completed uneventfully.

The combination of heat, chloroquine, and radiotherapy appears to have enhanced an aggressive skin reaction in this patient. Caution is recommended when using chloroquine in patients receiving radiotherapy.

Musculoskeletal

Chloroquine and hydroxychloroquine occasionally cause a myopathy associated with muscle weakness, reduced or absent tendon reflexes, and raised creatine kinase activity; it usually develops gradually after 5?7 months of treatment. The muscle biopsy findings have been described in detail: atrophic muscle fibers, muscle fiber necrosis with vacuolar degradation, vacuoles staining positive with acid phosphatase with a granular pattern, autophagic vacuoles, and cytosomes with electron-dense curvilinear profiles on electron microscopy (44).

Severe vacuolar myopathy has been reported with hydroxychloroquine (45).

- A 51-year-old man with a mantle cell carcinoma was initially treated with cyclophosphamide, doxorubicin, vincristine, and prednisolone and obtained remission for 2 years. His lymphoma recurred and he was given rituximab, with a poor response. He subsequently received a bone marrow graft from his son. Despite complete remission he developed graft-versus-host disease with scleroderma and fascial involvement. He was given various drugs for graft-versus-host disease, including mycophenolate mofetil, tacrolimus, prednisolone, 2'-deoxycoformycin, and hydroxychloroquine. His condition was moderately sensitive to prednisolone in doses of 60–120 mg/day. While taking prednisolone and tacrolimus he was given hydroxychloroquine 400 mg bd. He then developed progressive debilitating limb and respiratory muscle weakness. Glucocorticoids were suspected of causing this and were tapered, but without much effect, and he gradually became too weak to walk. The serum creatine kinase activity was normal and acetylcholine receptor antibodies were negative. Electromyography showed a severe, non-irritable myopathy and a sensory motor axonal polyneuropathy. Muscle biopsy showed a necrotizing, vacuolar myopathy, with many fibers containing autophagic and red-rimmed vacuoles, consistent with an amphiphilic drug-induced myopathy. Following withdrawal of hydroxychloroquine, his strength and function improved

considerably. Later prednisolone and tacrolimus were reintroduced and he made a good recovery.

Nails

Chloroquine can turn the nail bed blue–brown and the nail itself can develop longitudinal stripes and show a blue–grey fluorescence (SEDA-11, 584).

Immunologic

- Allergic contact dermatitis, which progressed to generalized dermatitis and conjunctivitis, followed later by severe asthma, occurred in a 60-year-old worker in the pharmaceutical industry after exposure to hydroxychloroquine (46). Patch-testing showed delayed sensitivity to hydroxychloroquine. Equivalent tests in five healthy volunteers were negative. The patch test reactions were pustular, and a biopsy was interpreted as multiform contact dermatitis. Bronchial exposure to hydroxychloroquine dust produced delayed bronchial obstruction over the next 20 hours, progressing to fever and generalized erythema (hematogenous contact dermatitis).

Infection risk

An acute gluteal abscess after an injection of chloroquine has been reported (47).

A 24 year-old woman who had been pregnant for 24 weeks developed a fever, sweating, headache, and pain in the region where she had received an injection of chloroquine 9 days before. She was febrile (38.9°C). Chest examination was normal and the spleen was not palpable. She had a right gluteal abscess, which was later drained under general anesthesia. She was given ampicillin/cloxacillin, 500 mg intravenously at first and then orally for 7 days. *Staphylococcus aureus* sensitive to ampicillin/cloxacillin was isolated. She made uneventful recovery and delivered a live 2.9 kg baby.

Long-Term Effects

Drug tolerance

Chloroquine-resistant falciparum malaria was first reported in 1960. As of 1996, chloroquine resistance became widespread throughout the world and in many areas there is multidrug resistance. Preventive administration of drugs such as chloroquine, primaquine, and pyrimethamine, as well as the use of various sulfonamide mixtures and combinations of sulfonamides with trimethoprim, has progressively lost its usefulness. Currently, hardly half a century after the therapeutic breakthroughs occurred, quinine is once more one of the most valuable drugs in the treatment of malaria and there is a desperate need for other effective drugs.

Alongside the well-known development of resistance by *P. falciparum* to chloroquine, the emergence of chloroquine-resistant *Plasmodium vivax* is now clear (SEDA-13, 801). An increased frequency of cerebral malaria appears to coincide with the growing emergence of the chloroquine-resistant strains in Francophone Africa.

Second-Generation Effects

Pregnancy

Chloroquine inactivates DNA, and crosses the placenta in animals. Caution has generally been advised with respect to the use of chloroquine and related compounds during pregnancy, but except for one (perhaps coincidental) case, there have been no reports of complications to mother or child from treatment with chloroquine during pregnancy (SEDA-14, 239; SEDA-17, 326).

An observational comparison in a rural Ghanaian hospital of 2083 pregnant women and 3084 historical controls showed no serious adverse events with chloroquine chemoprophylaxis (300 mg/week), but a high rate of pruritus (48). There was a decrease in anemia in pregnancy but no increase in perinatal mortality or birth weight in the chloroquine-treated mothers, although this was only in comparison with historical controls.

Teratogenicity

In 133 consecutive pregnancies in 90 women who took 200 mg hydroxychloroquine twice a day (n = 122) or once a day (n = 11) the same number of pregnancies resulted in live births as in 70 consecutive pregnancies in 53 women with similar disorders who did not take hydroxychloroquine (49). Pregnancy outcomes and the results of follow-up examination of the children were comparable.

Susceptibility Factors

Genetic factors

Mutations in the ABCR gene (a photoreceptor-specific ATP-binding cassette transporter gene) have been associated with Stargardt disease, which has some features similar to chloroquine-induced retinopathy. In a case-control study of eight cases of chloroquine-induced retinopathy, five of the eight cases had mis-sense mutations in the ABCR gene, two of which have been associated with Stargardt disease (50). It may be that polymorphisms in the ABCR gene predispose to chloroquine-induced retinopathy.

Age

Small children have usually been considered as being relatively more sensitive to the effects of overdosage, but it has been calculated that on a mg/kg body weight basis, adults are in fact equally sensitive. Young children seem to be truly more susceptible to gastric irritation. Patients with a history of mania or epilepsy should be careful in taking chloroquine (10). The hypoxemic effects of chloroquine, reflecting cardiac and respiratory toxicity, pose a particular problem in the newborn, in whom existing malarial infection may not become clinically manifest until some months after birth (SEDA-16, 302).

Compared with adults, mortality in children after acute chloroquine poisoning is extremely high. Although the clinical presentation is mostly similar to that in adults (apnea, seizures, cardiac dysrhythmias), a single 300 mg chloroquine tablet was enough to kill a 12-month-old female infant (SEDA-16, 302).

Other features of the patient

Skin reactions to hydroxychloroquine occur more often in patients with dermatomyositis than in patients with systemic lupus erythematosus, as has been shown in a retrospective, age-, sex-, and race-matched case-control study in 78 patients (51). Twelve of 39 patients with dermatomyositis developed a skin reaction to hydroxychloroquine, compared with only one of 39 patients with lupus erythematosus.

Drug Administration

Drug formulations

Chloroquine has a bitter taste, which can deter children from taking it, so a sweet effervescent formulation of chloroquine phosphate has been compared with chloroquine tablets in a pharmacodynamic study (52). However, sweet-tasting medications carry a risk of accidental overdose in children.

Drug administration route

If given intravenously, chloroquine should be diluted and infused slowly, since rapid injection causes toxic concentrations. Toxicity and even death have been reported after intramuscular administration of larger doses; this is probably connected with rapid absorption in such cases (SEDA-17, 327).

Drug overdose

Acute intoxication, either accidental or in attempted suicide, can cause headache, drowsiness, vision disturbance, vomiting and diarrhea, cardiovascular collapse, and respiratory failure. Deaths have been recorded at blood concentrations of 1 µg/ml (SEDA-11, 586; 53,54). Compared with adults, mortality in children after acute chloroquine poisoning is extremely high. Although the clinical presentation is mostly similar to that in adults (apnea, seizures, cardiac dysrhythmias), a single 300 mg chloroquine tablet was enough to kill a 12-month-old female infant (SEDA-16, 302).

Deaths from chloroquine overdose have been reported with doses as low as 2–3 g in adults, and the death rate is as high as 25%. The effects of chloroquine overdose include cardiac effects (such as dysrhythmias, reduced myocardial contractility, and hypotension) and central nervous system complications (such as confusion, coma, and seizures).

There have been three reports of chloroquine overdose, two from Oman (55) and one from the Netherlands (56). The two reports from Oman were similar to previously published reports of chloroquine overdose associated with cardiac dysfunction, confusion, and coma; both patients had standard treatment with activated charcoal, diazepam infusions, and positive inotropic drugs, and both survived. The single case report from the Netherlands gave pharmacokinetic measurements performed before, during, and after hemoperfusion. This showed that hemoperfusion extracted very little chloroquine and was unlikely to be of any use in chloroquine overdose, as would be expected from the high protein binding and large volume of distribution of chloroquine.

In Zimbabwe, 544 cases of poisoning by a single agent were identified in a retrospective hospital record review (57). Antimalarial drugs accounted for the largest proportion of admissions (53%), and chloroquine accounted for 96% of these (279 cases). The median length of hospital stay in those who took chloroquine was significantly shorter (1 versus 2 days) and more patients took chloroquine deliberately (80% versus 69%). The mortality rate from chloroquine poisoning was significantly higher than from poisoning with other drugs (5.7% versus 0.7%).

Overdose with hydroxychloroquine is far less common than with chloroquine. Three of eight patients died (58). Life-threatening symptoms, such as hypotension, conduction disturbances, and hypokalemia can occur within 30 minutes of ingestion and are similar to those seen in chloroquine overdose. The lethal plasma concentration of hydroxychloroquine is not well established. Therapeutic drug concentrations are usually less than 1 μmol/l. Serious toxicity has been reported at plasma concentrations of 2.1–29 μmol/l.

Massive hydroxychloroquine overdose has been reported (59).

- A 17-year-old girl took 22 g of hydroxychloroquine in a suicide attempt. She developed hypotension, life-threatening ventricular dysrhythmias, and mild hypokalemia. She was managed with saline infusion and dopamine for hypotension, gastric lavage and activated charcoal for decontamination, and lidocaine, magnesium sulfate and defibrillation for pulseless ventricular tachycardia. Potassium replacement and bicarbonate replacement were performed. She survived without sequelae.

Management of hydroxychloroquine overdose is similar to that of chloroquine overdose, including the use of charcoal for drug adsorption, quick treatment of hypotension, continuous cardiac monitoring, and the treatment of dysrhythmias, diazepam for seizures and sedation, early intubation and mechanical ventilation, and potassium replacement for severe hypokalemia.

Drug–Drug Interactions

Amlodipine

Syncope occurred in a hypertensive 48-year-old man who took oral chloroquine sulfate (total 600 mg base) while also taking amlodipine 5 mg/day (60). Chloroquine and amlodipine both cause vasodilatation, perhaps by release of nitric oxide, and the syncope in this case was probably due to a synergistic mechanism. Malaria itself can also provoke orthostatic reactions, which may be why syncope

is not a reported adverse effect of chloroquine. However, in this patient malaria had been excluded.

Antibiotics

Studies of chloroquine used in combination with antibiotics showed an antagonistic effect with penicillin but a synergistic effect with chlortetracycline. Urinary tests after single doses of ampicillin 1 g and chloroquine 1 g showed a significant reduction in the systemic availability of the ampicillin.

Chlorphenamine

Chlorphenamine enhances the efficacy of chloroquine in acute uncomplicated falciparum malaria, but the disposition of chloroquine in these circumstances is unpredictable. Chloroquine (25 mg/kg) was given orally over 3 days in combination with chlorphenamine to Nigerian children with parasitemia (61). The peak whole blood chloroquine concentration was increased and the time to peak concentration shortened. In small trials there seemed to be an increase in QT interval with this combination, but less than with halofantrine (62). However, in other studies, the addition of chlorphenamine to chloroquine did not amplify the cardiac effects of chloroquine (62).

Ciclosporin

Chloroquine can increase ciclosporin blood concentrations (63).

Cimetidine

Cimetidine enhanced the susceptibility of *P. falciparum* to chloroquine in vitro in 60% of isolates (64).

Digoxin

The pharmacokinetic interaction of quinidine with digoxin also occurs with quinine and hydroxychloroquine (65).

Fansidar (sulfadoxine + pyrimethamine)

The combined use of Fansidar (sulfadoxine + pyrimethamine) with chloroquine has been reported to result in more severe adverse reactions (66). However, an increased risk has not been reported in recent studies (67).

Halofantrine

There is an increased risk of dysrhythmias, including torsade de pointes, when halofantrine is combined with quinine/quinidine or chloroquine and any other drug that prolongs the QT interval (68).

Insulin

There may be an interaction of chloroquine with insulin. An oral glucose load given to healthy subjects and to patients with non-insulin-dependent diabetes mellitus, before and during a short course of chloroquine, showed a small but significant reduction in fasting blood glucose concentration in the control group and improvement in glucose tolerance in the patients (SEDA-12, 240). The response seems to reflect reduced degradation of insulin rather than increased pancreatic output.

Quinine

Chloroquine antagonizes the action of quinine against *P. falciparum* in vivo. However, no such evidence of antagonism was found in a study in which Malawian children with cerebral malaria were treated with quinine. There was no difference in survival and rate of recovery in patients who had also been given chloroquine compared with those who had not (SEDA-13, 816).

Thyroxine

A marked increase in serum TSH occurred in the same patient on two occasions after several weeks of antimalarial prophylaxis with chloroquine and proguanil, the likely mechanism being enzyme induction and increased thyroxine catabolism (SEDA-22, 469).

Vaccines

Chloroquine 300 mg/week adversely affected the antibody response to human diploid-cell rabies vaccine administered concurrently. The mean rabies-neutralizing antibody titer was significantly reduced on each day of testing (SEDA-13, 806) (9). In contrast, retrospective studies of the response to pneumococcal polysaccharide in patients with systemic lupus erythematosus taking chloroquine or hydroxychloroquine, and of the response to tetanus–measles–meningococcal vaccine in a region of Nigeria where malaria is endemic, did not show an effect on antibody production. However, it was pointed out that the altered immune status of patients with systemic lupus erythematosus makes it difficult to compare their response to that of young healthy adults receiving rabies vaccine. Illness and nutritional state could have influenced the findings in the Nigerian study (SEDA-13, 807) (69).

Verapamil

Verapamil completely reversed pre-existing in vitro resistance to chloroquine to below the cut-off point of 70 nmol/l (64).

Smoking Drug-s Interactions

Antimalarial drugs (chloroquine, hydroxychloroquine, or quinacrine) were given to 36 patients with cutaneous lupus, of whom 17 were smokers and 19 non-smokers (9). The median number of cigarettes smoked was one pack/day, with a median duration of 12.5 years. There was a reduction in the efficacy of antimalarial therapy in the smokers. Patients with cutaneous lupus should therefore be encouraged to stop smoking and consideration may be given to increasing the doses of antimalarial drugs in smokers with refractory cutaneous lupus before starting a cytotoxic agent.

Monitoring Therapy

Susceptibility factors for the development of toxic retinopathy with hydroxychloroquine include high daily doses, long duration of treatment, concomitant liver or kidney disease, and age over 60 years. Constant monitoring for retinal toxicity is therefore vital for the prevention of this potentially irreversible severe adverse effect. However, most methods for monitoring retinal toxicity, such as Amsler grid testing, color vision testing, and static perimetry, are subjective. Multifocal electronic retinography is a more objective test and offers multidimensional visualization of the retina. In a longitudinal study of 12 patients who had multifocal electronic retinography at baseline and at 12–24 months, serial recordings of retinal amplitudes and peak latencies showed that patients taking hydroxychloroquine had reduced retinal function while those who stopped taking it had improved retinal function (70). Multifocal electronic retinography therefore offers the possibility of detecting early changes in retinal function in patients taking hydroxychloroquine.

References

1. Sowunmi A, Ayede AI, Falade AG, Ndikum VN, Sowunmi CO, Adedeji AA, Falade CO, Happi TC, Oduola AM. Randomized comparison of chloroquine and amodiaquine in the treatment of acute, uncomplicated, *Plasmodium falciparum* malaria in children. Ann Trop Med Parasitol 2001;95(6):549–58.
2. Veinot JP, Mai KT, Zarychanski R. Chloroquine related cardiac toxicity. J Rheumatol 1998;25(6):1221–5.
3. Guedira N, Hajjaj-Hassouni N, Srairi JE, el Hassani S, Fellat R, Benomar M. Third-degree atrioventricular block in a patient under chloroquine therapy. Rev Rhum Engl Ed 1998;65(1):58–62.
4. Chen CY, Wang FL, Lin CC. Chronic hydroxychloroquine use associated with QT prolongation and refractory ventricular arrhythmia. Clin Toxicol 2006;44:173–5..
5. Cervera A, Espinosa G, Font J, Ingelmo M. Cardiac toxicity secondary to long term treatment with chloroquine. Ann Rheum Dis 2001;60(3):301.
6. Charlier P, Cochand-Priollet B, Polivka M, Goldgran-Toledano D, Leenhardt A. Cardiomyopathie a la chloroquine revelée par un bloc auriculo-ventriculaire complete. A propos d'une observation. [Chloroquine cardiomyopathy revealed by complete atrio-ventricular block. A case report.] Arch Mal Coeur Vaiss 2002;95(9):833–7.
7. Freihage JH, Patel NC, Jacobs WR, Picken M, Fresco R, Malinowska K, Pisani BA, Mendez JC, Lichtenberg RC, Foy BK, Bakhos M, Mullen GM. Heart transplantation in a patient with chloroquine-induced cardiomyopathy. J Heart Lung Transpl 2004;23(2):252–5.
8. Clemessy JL, Favier C, Borron SW, Hantson PE, Vicaut E, Baud FJ. Hypokalaemia related to acute chloroquine ingestion. Lancet 1995;346(8979):877–80.
9. Mitja K, Izidor K, Music E. Chloroquin-induzierte arzneimitteltoxische Alveolitis. [Chloroquine-induced drug hypersensitivity alveolitis.] Pneumologie 2000;54(9):395–7.
10. Blaison G, Tranchant C, Mohr M, Roth T, Warter JM. Les complications neuromusculaires des traitements par la chloroquine. Sem Hop Paris 1990;66:2425–8.

11. Fish DR, Espir ML. Convulsions associated with prophylactic antimalarial drugs: implications for people with epilepsy. BMJ 1988;297(6647):526–7.

12. Crawley J, Kokwaro G, Ouma D, Watkins W, Marsh K. Chloroquine is not a risk factor for seizures in childhood cerebral malaria. Trop Med Int Health 2000;5(12):860–4.

13. Guilloton L, Burckard E, Fresse S, Drouet A, Felten D. Crise epileptique apres chimioprophylaxie antipalustre par chloroquine. [Epileptic crisis after antimalaria chemoprophylaxis with chloroquine.] Presse Méd 2001;30(35):1745.

14. Wasay M, Wolfe GI, Herrold JM, Burns DK, Barohn RJ. Chloroquine myopathy and neuropathy with elevated CSF protein. Neurology 1998;51(4):1226–7.

15. Bertagnolio S, Tacconelli E, Camilli G, Tumbarello M. Case report: retinopathy after malaria prophylaxis with chloroquine. Am J Trop Med Hyg 2001;65(5):637–8.

16. Warner AE. Early hydroxychloroquine macular toxicity. Arthritis Rheum 2001;44(8):1959–61.

17. Kellner U, Kraus H, Foerster MH. Multifocal ERG in chloroquine retinopathy: regional variance of retinal dysfunction. Graefes Arch Clin Exp Ophthalmol 2000;238(1):94–7.

18. Mukherjee DK. Chloroquine ototoxicity—a reversible phenomenon? J Laryngol Otol 1979;93(8):809–15.

19. Coutinho MB, Duarte I. Hydroxychloroquine ototoxicity in a child with idiopathic pulmonary haemosiderosis. Int J Pediatr Otorhinolaryngol 2002;62(1):53–7.

20. Weber JC, Alt M, Blaison G, Welsch M, Martin T, Pasquali JL. Modifications du gout et de l'odorat imputables a l'hydroxychloroquine. [Changes in taste and smell caused by hydroxychloroquine.] Presse Méd 1996;25(5):213.

21. Ferraro V, Mantoux F, Denis K, Lay-Macagno M-A, Ortonne J-P, Lacour J-P. Hallucinations au cours d'un traitement par hydroxychloroquine. Ann Dermatol Venereol 2004;131:471–3.

22. Sharma N, Varma S. Unusual life-threatening adverse drug effects with chloroquine in a young girl. J Postgrad Med 2003;49:187.

23. Petersen CS, Thomsen K. High-dose hydroxychloroquine treatment of porphyria cutanea tarda. J Am Acad Dermatol 1992;26(4):614–9.

24. Kutz DC, Bridges AJ. Bullous rash and brown urine in a systemic lupus erythematosus patient treated with hydroxychloroquine. Arthritis Rheum 1995;38(3):440–3.

25. Baler GR. Porphyria precipitated by hydroxychloroquine treatment of systemic lupus erythematosus. Cutis 1976;17(1):96–8.

26. Don PC, Kahn TA, Bickers DR. Chloroquine-induced neutropenia in a patient with dermatomyositis. J Am Acad Dermatol 1987;16(3 Pt 1):629–30.

27. Wielgo-Polanin R, Largace L, Gautron E, Diquet B, Lainé-Cessac P. Hepatotoxicity associated with the use of a fixed combination of chloroquine and proguanil. Int J Antimicrob Agents 2005;26 (2):176–8.

28. Bentsi-Enchill KO. Pigmentary skin changes associated with ocular chloroquine toxicity in Ghana. Trop Geogr Med 1980;32(3):216–20.

29. Muller Hocker J, Schmid H, Weiss M, Dendorfer U, Braun GS. Chloroquine-induced phospholipidosis of the kidney mimicking Fabry's disease: case report and review of the literature. Hum Pathol 2003;34:285–9.

30. Boffa MJ, Chalmers RJ. Toxic epidermal necrolysis due to chloroquine phosphate. Br J Dermatol 1994;131(3):444–5.

31. Onyeji CO, Ogunbona FA. Pharmacokinetic aspects of chloroquine-induced pruritus: influence of dose and evidence for varied extent of metabolism of the drug. Eur J Pharm Sci 2001;13(2):195–201.

32. Osifo NG. Chloroquine-induced pruritus among patients with malaria. Arch Dermatol 1984;120(1):80–2.

33. Ajayi AA, Akinleye AO, Udoh SJ, Ajayi OO, Oyelese O, Ijaware CO. The effects of prednisolone and niacin on chloroquine-induced pruritus in malaria. Eur J Clin Pharmacol 1991;41(4):383–5.

34. Martin Garcia RF, del R Camacho N, Sanchez JL. Chloroquine-induced, vitiligo-like depigmentation. J Am Acad Dermatol 2003;48:981–3.

35. Beedimani RS, Rambhimaiah S. Oral chloroquine induced Stevens–Johnson syndrome. Ind J Pharmacol 2004;36(2):101.

36. Murphy M, Carmichael AJ. Fatal toxic epidermal necrolysis associated with hydroxychloroquine. Clin Exp Dermatol 2001;26(5):457–8.

37. Leckie MJ, Rees RG. Stevens–Johnson syndrome in association with hydroxychloroquine treatment for rheumatoid arthritis. Rheumatology (Oxford) 2002;41(4):473–4.

38. Salido M, Joven B, D'Cruz DP, Khamashta MA, Hughes GR. Increased cutaneous reactions to hydroxychloroquine (Plaquenil) possibly associated with formulation change: comment on the letter by Alarcon. Arthritis Rheum 2002;46(12):3392–6.

39. Metayer I, Balguerie X, Courville P, Lauret P, Joly P. Toxidermies photo-induites parl'hydroxychloroquine: 4 cas. [Photodermatosis induced by hydroxychloroquine: 4 cases.] Ann Dermatol Venereol 2001;128(6–7):729–31.

40. Singh G, Fries JF, Williams CA, Zatarain E, Spitz P, Bloch DA. Toxicity profiles of disease modifying antirheumatic drugs in rheumatoid arthritis. J Rheumatol 1991;18(2):188–94.

41. Luong MS, Bessis D, Raison Peyron N, Pinzani V, Guilhou JJ, Guillot B. Severe mucocutaneous necrotizing vasculitis associated with the combination of chloroquine and proguanil. Acta Dermatol Venereol 2003;83:141.

42. Ghaffarpour G, Jalali MHA, Yaghmaii B, Mazloomi S, Soltani-Arabshahi R. Chloroquine/hydoxychloroquine-induced pemphigus. Int Soc Dermatol 2006;45:1261–3.

43. Rustogi A, Munshi A, Jalali R. Unexpected skin reaction induced by radiotherapy after chloroquine use. Lancet Oncol 2006;7:608–9.

44. Richter JG, Becker A, Ostendorf B, Specker C, Stoll G, Neuen-Jacob E, Schneider M. Differential diagnosis of high serum creatine kinase levels in systemic lupus erythematosus. Rheumatol Int 2003;23:319–23.

45. Bolaños-Meade J, Zhou L, Hoke A, Corse A, Vogelsang G, Wagner KR. Hydroxychloroquine causes severe vacuolar myopathy in a patient with chronic graft-versus-host disease. Am J Hematol 2005;78:306–9.

46. Meier H, Elsner P, Wuthrich B. Berufsbedingtes kontaktekzem und Asthma bronchiale bei ungewohnlicher allergischer Reaktion vona Spattyp auf Hydroxychloroquin. [Occupationally-induced contact dermatitis and bronchial asthma in a unusual delayed reaction to hydroxychloroquine.] Hautarzt 1999;50(9):665–9.

47. Adam I, Elbashir MI. Acute gluteal abscess due to chloroquine injection in Sudanese pregnant woman. Saudi Med J 2004;25(7):963–4.

48. Geelhoed DW, Visser LE, Addae V, Asare K, Schagen van Leeuwen JH, van Roosmalen J. Malaria prophylaxis and the reduction of anemia at childbirth. Int J Gynaecol Obstet 2001;74(2):133–8.

49. Costedoat-Chalumeau N, Amoura Z, Duhaut P, Huong du LT, Sebbough D, Wechsler B, Vauthier D, Denjoy I, Lupoglazoff JM, Piette JC. Safety of hydroxychloroquine in pregnant patients with connective tissue diseases: a study

of one hundred thirty-three cases compared with a control group. Arthritis Rheum 2003;48:3207–11.

50. Shroyer NF, Lewis RA, Lupski JR. Analysis of the ABCR (ABCA4) gene in 4-aminoquinoline retinopathy: is retinal toxicity by chloroquine and hydroxychloroquine related to Stargardt disease? Am J Ophthalmol 2001; 131(6):761–6.

51. Pelle MT, Callen JP. Adverse cutaneous reactions to hydroxychloroquine are more common in patients with dermatomyositis than in patients with cutaneous lupus erythematosus. Arch Dermatol 2002;138(9):1231–3.

52. Yanze MF, Duru C, Jacob M, Bastide JM, Lankeuh M. Rapid therapeutic response onset of a new pharmaceutical form of chloroquine phosphate 300 mg: effervescent tablets Trop Med Int Health 2001;6(3):196–201.

53. Bochner F, Carruthers G, Kampmann J, Steiner J. Handbook of Clinical PharmacologyBoston, MA: Little Brown;. 1978.

54. Di Maio VJ, Henry LD. Chloroquine poisoning. South Med J 1974;67(9):1031–5.

55. Reddy VG, Sinna S. Chloroquine poisoning: report of two cases. Acta Anaesthesiol Scand 2000;44(8):1017–20.

56. Boereboom FT, Ververs FF, Meulenbelt J, van Dijk A. Hemoperfusion is ineffectual in severe chloroquine poisoning. Crit Care Med 2000;28(9):3346–50.

57. Ball DE, Tagwireyi D, Nhachi CF. Chloroquine poisoning in Zimbabwe: a toxicoepidemiological study. J Appl Toxicol 2002;22(5):311–5.

58. Marquardt K, Albertson TE. Treatment of hydroxychloroquine overdose. Am J Emerg Med 2001;19(5):420–4.

59. Yanturali S, Aksay E, Demir OF, Atilla R. Massive hydroxychloroquine overdose. Acta Anaesthesiol Scand 2004;48:379–81.

60. Ajayi AA, Adigun AQ. Syncope following oral chloroquine administration in a hypertensive patient controlled on amlodipine. Br J Clin Pharmacol 2002;53(4):404–5.

61. Okonkwo CA, Coker HA, Agomo PU, Ogunbanwo JA, Mafe AG, Agomo CO, Afolabi BM. Effect of chlorpheniramine on the pharmacokinetics of and response to chloroquine of Nigerian children with falciparum malaria. Trans R Soc Trop Med Hyg 1999;93(3):306–11.

62. Sowunmi A, Fehintola FA, Ogundahunsi OA, Ofi AB, Happi TC, Oduola AM. Comparative cardiac effects of halofantrine and chloroquine plus chlorpheniramine in children with acute uncomplicated falciparum malaria. Trans R Soc Trop Med Hyg 1999;93(1):78–83.

63. Guiserix J, Aizel A. Interactions ciclosporine–chloroquine. [Cyclosporine–chloroquine interactions.] Presse Méd 1996;25(26):1214.

64. Ndifor AM, Howells RE, Bray PG, Ngu JL, Ward SA. Enhancement of drug susceptibility in *Plasmodium falciparum* in vitro and *Plasmodium berghei* in vivo by mixed-function oxidase inhibitors. Antimicrob Agents Chemother 1993;37(6):1318–23.

65. Leden I. Digoxin–hydroxychloroquine interaction? Acta Med Scand 1982;211(5):411–2.

66. Rombo L, Stenbeck J, Lobel HO, Campbell CC, Papaioanou M, Miller KD. Does chloroquine contribute to the risk of serious adverse reactions to Fansidar? Lancet 1985;2(8467):1298–9.

67. Rahman M, Rahman R, Bangali M, Das S, Talukder MR, Ringwald P. Efficacy of combined chloroquine and sulfadoxine–pyrimethamine in uncomplicated *Plasmodium falciparum* malaria in Bangladesh. Trans R Soc Trop Med Hyg 2004;98(7):438–41.

68. Simooya OO, Sijumbil G, Lennard MS, Tucker GT. Halofantrine and chloroquine inhibit CYP2D6 activity in healthy Zambians. Br J Clin Pharmacol 1998;45(3):315–7.

69. Van der Straeten C, Klippel JH. Antimalarials and pneumococcal immunization. N Engl J Med 1986;315(11): 712–3.

70. Lai TYY, Chan W-M, Li H, Lai RYK, Lam DSC. Multifocal retinographic changes in patients receiving hydroxychloroquine therapy. Am J Ophthamol 2005;140(5):794–808.

Ciclosporin

General Information

Ciclosporin is an immunosuppressant drug that primarily inhibits T cell activation, therefore down-regulating the T cell responses that mediate graft rejection. Myelotoxic effects are therefore not expected. Ciclosporin has also been used in a wide range of chronic inflammatory or autoimmune diseases.

Considerable efforts have been devoted to defining the optimal dose to ensure minimal toxicity while retaining efficacy. In transplant patients, the daily maintenance dose is 2–6 mg/kg/day. In non-transplant patients, daily doses of 2.5 mg/kg up to a maximum of 4 mg/kg are usually recommended.

In renal transplantation, ciclosporin maintenance monotherapy can be effectively achieved in a subset of patients with the aim of reducing adverse effects associated with glucocorticoids or azathioprine, but this should be carefully balanced against the risks of acute or chronic allograft rejection. This approach was again emphasized, based on data from 100 adults and a review of the most recent literature (1). According to the authors, clinical predictors of successful ciclosporin maintenance therapy included compliant patients over 25 years old with a donor age younger than 40 years, patients with later azathioprine withdrawal, patients with serum creatinine concentrations of 125 μmol/l or less, patients without a history of rejection (or one rejection episode responding favorably to glucocorticoids), and patients who have successfully discontinued glucocorticoids 6 months before.

Comparative studies

Although the pattern of long-term toxicity of ciclosporin and tacrolimus is remarkably similar for most serious adverse effects (particularly nephrotoxicity), a higher incidence of several minor adverse effects with ciclosporin, namely hirsutism, gingivitis or gum hyperplasia, has been thought to underlie a moderate but significant decrease in the quality of life with ciclosporin compared with tacrolimus (2).

General adverse effects

As regards long-term toxicity, particularly nephrotoxicity, and frequent drug interactions, the benefit-to-harm balance of ciclosporin is still debatable. Whereas the adverse effects have generally been deemed acceptable, although occasionally treatment-limiting in patients with rheumatoid arthritis given low-dose ciclosporin rather than conventional antirheumatic drugs, conflicting opinions have been expressed on the acceptability of the risks in patients with psoriasis (SEDA-20, 343).

Of 20 patients with chronic idiopathic thrombocytopenic purpura refractory to glucocorticoids or splenectomy treated with ciclosporin, six withdrew owing to toxicity (3). The target blood concentration range was identical to that aimed at in the first 3 months after kidney transplantation. The most common adverse effects were hypertension, headache, and severe myalgia.

The antileukemic effect of ciclosporin has been harnessed in the treatment of cytopenias associated with chronic lymphatic leukemia. In 31 patients the most common adverse effect was a raised serum creatinine concentration of grade 2 or worse in six patients (19%); three patients developed opportunistic infections (4).

In patients taking ciclosporin or tacrolimus, drug-induced hirsutism, gingival hyperplasia, acne, alopecia, or Cushingoid facies were reported in 80% of surveyed kidney recipients. Hirsutism (94%) and gingival hyperplasia (51%) occurred more often in patients taking ciclosporin, while alopecia (30%) soccurred more often in patients taking tacrolimus (5). For every condition the incidence of physical changes reported by the patients significantly exceeded the observations by the professionals; however, 84% of affected patients reported feeling "happy to endure" these changes "for the sake of having a transplant." They also reported emotional and social effects due to physical changes, an outcome that was underestimated by transplant professionals.

Drug interactions with ciclosporin have been comprehensively reviewed (6).

Organs and Systems

Cardiovascular

Compared with azathioprine, hypertension has been considered one of the main long-term risks in patients taking ciclosporin, with major concerns about the post-transplantion increase in cardiovascular morbidity and mortality. However, there are many susceptibility factors for cardiovascular disease in transplant patients (7), and it is difficult to take into account their complex interplay. Ciclosporin-associated hypertension appears to be dose-related, and higher whole-blood ciclosporin concentrations were found during the preceding months in patients who had thromboembolic complications compared with patients who did not (8).

De novo or aggravated hypertension is very common in patients taking ciclosporin, with the highest incidence in cases of heart transplant (71–100%) and the lowest incidence in bone marrow transplant recipients (33–60%) (9). In addition, 30–45% of patients with psoriasis, rheumatoid arthritis, or uveitis had hypertension, suggesting that ciclosporin is a significant cause of hypertension in organ transplantation. Ciclosporin-associated hypertension can cause acute vascular injury, with microangiopathic hemolysis, encephalopathy, seizures, and intracranial hemorrhage.

In 3365 adults with a functioning graft after the first year, the prevalence of hypertension increased progressively and significantly during follow-up (10). The presence of arterial hypertension at 1 year was significantly associated with recipient sex (male), donor age (under 60 years), immunosuppressive therapy (ciclosporin), serum creatinine, and year of transplantation. Arterial hypertension was not associated with graft survival or cardiovascular mortality. The prevalence and severity of hypertension was significantly lower in patients treated with tacrolimus than with ciclosporin.

Calcineurin inhibitors potentially contribute to the risk of cardiovascular events through the development of new-onset diabetes mellitus, hypertension, and hyperlipidemia. Trials have consistently shown a higher incidence of new-onset diabetes mellitus with tacrolimus, which has been borne out in large-scale registry analyses. However, the risk of hypertension is about 5% higher with ciclosporin than tacrolimus, as is the risk of hyperlipidemia (11).

The incidence, clinical features, consequences, and management of ciclosporin-induced hypertension have been reviewed (12). The prevalence was 29–54% in non-transplant patients and 65–100% in heart and liver transplant patients also taking glucocorticoids. Disturbed circadian rhythm with a loss of nocturnal blood pressure fall was the main characteristic, and patients therefore had higher risks of left ventricular hypertrophy, cerebrovascular damage, microalbuminuria, and other target organ damage.

The pathophysiology of ciclosporin-induced hypertension is complex and not yet fully elucidated. Increased systemic vascular resistance subsequent to altered vascular endothelium function, renal vasoconstriction with reduced glomerular filtration and sodium-water retention, and/or increased activity of the sympathetic nervous system were suggested, while only a minor role or none was attributed to the renin–angiotensin system (13). However, hypertension often occurs before changes in renal function or sodium balance can be demonstrated, and ciclosporin nephrotoxicity alone does not explain ciclosporin-associated hypertension (9,14).

It has been suggested that the increase in blood pressure induced by calcineurin inhibitors is mediated by excitation of the sympathetic nervous system. In 24 renal transplant patients who were randomly assigned to either withdrawal or continuation of ciclosporin, mean arterial pressure fell significantly during withdrawal but not during continued therapy (15). Muscle sympathetic nerve activity and plasma noradrenaline concentrations did not change in either group, and graft function remained stable.

The effects of antihypertensive agents have been evaluated in patients taking ciclosporin. Collectively, dihydropyridine calcium channel blockers that do not affect ciclosporin blood concentrations substantially or at all (felodipine, isradipine, and nifedipine) are usually considered to be the drugs of choice. However, the risk of gingival hyperplasia with nifedipine, which ciclosporin also causes, should be borne in mind. Combination therapy with angiotensin-converting enzyme inhibitors or beta-blockers, or the use of other calcium channel blockers (verapamil or diltiazem) should also be considered, but careful monitoring of ciclosporin blood concentrations is recommended with the latter because they inhibit ciclosporin metabolism.

Major cardiovascular risk factors have been analysed and the risk of coronary artery disease estimated in a comparative 6-month study of microemulsified ciclosporin (n = 271) versus tacrolimus (n = 286) concomitant with azathioprine and glucocorticoids (16). The primary endpoints were the incidence of and time to acute rejection. Blood pressure, serum cholesterol, HDL cholesterol, triglycerides, and blood glucose were measured at baseline and at months 1, 3, and 6. The 10-year risk of coronary heart disease was estimated according to the Framingham risk algorithm. Tacrolimus lowered serum cholesterol and mean arterial blood pressure, but in a higher summary measure of blood glucose than ciclosporin. Serum triglycerides were not different between tacrolimus and ciclosporin. The mean 10-year coronary artery disease risk estimate was significantly lowered in men who took tacrolimus, but was unchanged in women.

Ischemic heart disease after renal transplantation has been reported to be three to four times higher than in the general population. The records of recipients of cadaveric kidneys between January 1985 and November 1999 have been reviewed in a multicenter study in Spain (17). All received ciclosporin and steroids with or without azathioprine as initial therapy. There were 163 with ischemic heart disease and 362 control patients without ischemic heart disease. Of the patients with ischemic heart disease after transplantation, 38% had the cardiac event during the first 12 months; 29 had previously been known to have ischemic heart disease, but all were asymptomatic at the time of transplantation. After transplantation 21 revascularization procedures were performed, eight during the first year and 13 thereafter. At the time the study was performed, 28% of the patients had lost the graft and 17% (86/525) had died; 34% (55/163) from the ischemic heart disease group and 8.6% (31/362) from the control group. Death was related to ischemic heart disease in 66% of the patients with ischemic heart disease. Donor age was higher in the patients with ischemic heart disease than in the controls, as were hypercholesterolemia and hypertriglyceridemia after transplantation. Graft function was similar in the two groups, measured by serum creatinine. Multivariate analysis showed that age at transplantation increased the risk of ischemic heart disease by 5% per year. Men had a more than two-fold higher risk of ischemic heart disease than women. Body weight was associated with a 2% increased risk of ischemic heart disease. Other independent predictors were a previous history of cardiovascular disease and hypercholesterolemia before transplantation.

A possible role of ciclosporin in the exacerbation or development of Raynaud's disease has been suggested on one occasion; such an effect could be linked to endothelial damage or changes in platelet function (18).

Erythromelalgia is a symptom complex of painful inflammatory vasodilatation of the extremities, often regarded as the inverse of Raynaud's phenomenon. It is usually idiopathic or due to thrombocythemia, and rarely caused by calcium channel blockers.

- A 37 year old man took ciclosporin 150 mg/day for psoriasis and after 4 weeks developed marked erythema, edema, and tenderness over the fingers and toes (19). His symptoms increased with warmth and were partly relieved by cold compresses. His full blood count, serum biochemistry, urine analysis, and collagen profile were normal. Ciclosporin was withdrawn and the lesions regressed within 1 week but recurred when ciclosporin was restarted.

The association between the risk of thrombotic microangiopathy and the use of the combinations ciclosporin + mycophenolate mofetil, ciclosporin + sirolimus, tacrolimus + mycophenolate mofetil, and tacrolimus + sirolimus has been studied in 368 kidney or kidney-pancreas transplant recipients (20). Biopsy-proven thrombotic microangiopathy was detected in 13 patients in the absence of vascular rejection. The incidence of thrombotic microangiopathy was highest with ciclosporin + sirolimus (21%). The relative risk of thrombotic microangiopathy was 16 (95% CI = 4.3, 61) for ciclosporin + sirolimus compared with tacrolimus + mycophenolate mofetil. Ciclosporin + sirolimus was the only regimen that had concomitant pro-necrotic and anti-angiogenic effects on arterial endothelial cells. This suggests that ciclosporin + sirolimus causes thrombotic microangiopathy through dual effects on endothelial cell death and repair.

A capillary leak syndrome with subsequent pulmonary edema has also been reported after intravenous ciclosporin (SEDA-21, 383).

Infusion phlebitis has been attributed to intravenous ciclosporin (21).

- A 28-year-old man with ulcerative colitis had acute recurrent infusion phlebitis during administration of intravenous ciclosporin following intravenous hydrocortisone. The intravenous catheter and its site needed to be replaced repeatedly during treatment, which eventually led to complete remission of the ulcerative colitis. After 8 months, he was still in remission, with no permanent signs of damage to the phlebitic veins.

Respiratory

Adult respiratory distress syndrome has been described after intravenous ciclosporin. It was thought that a high concentration of the drug in the pulmonary vasculature due to administration through a central vein was responsible for capillary leakage, but in one patient the pulmonary capillary leak resolved rapidly when the intravenous ciclosporin was changed to oral (22). This suggested that Cremophor (polyoxyethylated castor oil), the solvent for parenteral ciclosporin, was responsible. However, there has been a report of an adult who developed respiratory distress syndrome in association with oral ciclosporin given after renal transplantation (23).

Hypersensitivity pneumonitis has been attributed to ciclosporin (24).

- A 35-year-old woman taking glibenclamide and mesalazine for Crohn's colitis was given ciclosporin for severe disease exacerbation. Within 6 weeks, she developed arthralgia and moderate thrombocytopenia, and ciclosporin was discontinued. Acute fever (41°C) and dyspnea were noted several days later, and a chest X-ray showed diffuse bilateral infiltrates. Bronchoalveolar lavage showed neutrophil preponderance and plasma cells, and a lung biopsy strongly suggested an acute hypersensitivity pneumonitis. All her symptoms subsided after a short course of prednisolone and oxygen.

Both the absence of an infectious cause and the rapid improvement without withdrawal of other drugs suggested that ciclosporin was the likely cause.

Nervous system

Incidence

Neurological adverse effects of ciclosporin have been reported in up to 39% of all transplant patients. Most are mild. The most frequent is a fine tremor, the mechanism of which is not known. From many case reports or studies in transplant patients, the pattern of ciclosporin neurotoxicity ranges from common and mild to moderate symptoms, such as headaches, tremors, paresthesia, restlessness, mood changes, sleep disturbances, confusion, agitation, and visual hallucinations, to rare but severe or life-threatening disorders, including acute psychotic episodes, cerebellar disorders, cortical blindness (permanent in one report), spasticity or paralysis of the limbs, catatonia, speech disorders or mutism, chorea, seizures, leukoencephalopathy, and coma (SED-13, 1124; SEDA-16, 516; SEDA-17, 520; SEDA-20, 343; SEDA-21, 383; 25–27).

A 19% incidence of central nervous system toxicity with ciclosporin has been reported in pediatric renal transplantation patients; the symptoms included seizures, drowsiness, confusion, hallucinations, visual disturbances, and mental changes (28).

Neurological symptoms were observed in 12–25% of liver-transplant patients and in 29% of bone marrow transplant patients, but severe neurotoxicity occurred only in about 1% (26,27,29). They usually appeared within the first month of treatment, but were sometimes delayed (27). Particular attention should be paid to prompt recognition of severe neurotoxicity, because abnormalities of the white matter can occur. Patients usually improved rapidly after temporary ciclosporin withdrawal or dosage reduction, and tacrolimus has sometimes been used successfully instead (SEDA-21, 383; 18). However, recurrence of seizures and persistent electroencephalographic abnormalities were found in 46 and 70% of pediatric transplant patients respectively who had had ciclosporin acute encephalopathy and

seizure syndrome and who were followed-up for 49 months (30).

Mechanisms

Although the role of many other factors should be considered when neurological symptoms occur in transplant recipients, isolated reports of neurotoxicity in non-transplanted patients are in keeping with a causal role of ciclosporin. There are many susceptibility factors in ciclosporin neurotoxicity. Blood ciclosporin concentrations are sometimes raised, but severe neurological symptoms have been observed in some patients with concentrations in the usual target range (26). Other possible susceptibility factors for ciclosporin neurotoxicity include hypocholesterolemia, hypomagnesemia, aluminium overload, concomitant high-dose glucocorticoid therapy, hypertension, and concomitant microangiopathic hemolytic anemia (SED-13, 1124; SEDA-21, 383). Acute graft-versus-host disease or HLA-mismatched and unrelated donor transplants were also potential susceptibility factors in recipients of bone marrow transplants (SEDA-22, 383; 19).

Ciclosporin-induced vasculopathy, with endothelial injury and derangement of the blood–brain barrier, is the postulated mechanism of neurological damage. Transient cerebral perfusion abnormalities, demonstrable in SPECT scans of the brain, have been suggested as a reliable indicator of ciclosporin neurotoxicity (SEDA-20, 344). Clinical symptoms as well as CT and/or MRI scans were very similar to those observed in hypertensive encephalopathy, with predominant and reversible white-matter occipital lesions (31). There was complete neurological recovery in most patients after blood pressure was normalized, and deaths due to intracranial hemorrhage are reported only exceptionally.

There is still debate about whether ciclosporin crosses the blood–brain barrier and enters the cerebrospinal fluid. Ciclosporin could not be identified in cerebrospinal fluid from 14 patients with liver transplants who had various neurological complications (32). Ciclosporin metabolites were measurable in the cerebrospinal fluid in only four patients, who had evidence of acute renal insufficiency, cholestasis, and raised blood concentrations of ciclosporin metabolites but identical ciclosporin parent drug blood concentrations compared with 10 patients with undetectable concentrations of ciclosporin metabolites in the cerebrospinal fluid. Ciclosporin metabolites enter the cerebrospinal fluid, and direct neurotoxicity is therefore possible in at least some patients with renal or hepatic dysfunction.

Endogenous ligands for ciclosporin and tacrolimus, known as immunophilins, are found in very high concentrations in the basal ganglia, and ciclosporin can alter dopamine phosphorylation in the medium-sized neurons in the striatum. Changes in basal ganglia glucose metabolism have been studied in a patient with severe ciclosporin-related tremor (33).

- A 37-year-old man received ciclosporin after bone marrow transplantation for chronic myelogenous leukemia. Soon afterwards he developed a severe tremor, which persisted despite dosage reduction. A brain MRI scan was normal. After 22 months he developed a personality change. A high resolution PET scan showed symmetrical increases in ^{18}F-deoxyglucose uptake in both caudate and putamen.

These results confirm that ciclosporin can modulate dopaminergic transmission in the striatum, presumably by inhibition of calcineurin.

- A 16-year-old girl with end-stage renal insufficiency underwent successful renal transplantation and was given ciclosporin on day 1 (34). On day 10 she complained of tinnitus and tremor and had a right facial nerve palsy. An MRI scan showed areas of increased signal in the white matter of the periventricular region. The dose of ciclosporin was reduced, since no other cause could be determined. Her tremor and tinnitus resolved, but the facial nerve palsy persisted. She was given tacrolimus, but the tremor and tinnitus recurred. She was then given mycophenolate mofetil and prednisone, and the tremor and tinnitus disappeared, although the facial nerve palsy persisted. The MRI scan 3 months later was normal.

The serum magnesium concentration was below the reference range in this case, which may have favored the development of neurotoxicity.

Susceptibility factors

A retrospective study identified a significantly higher incidence of central nervous system symptoms in patients with Behçet's disease (35). Headache, fever, paralysis, ataxia, dysarthria, or disturbed consciousness occurred in 12 of 47 ciclosporin-treated patients compared with nine of 270 patients not treated or taking other drugs. CT and/or MRI scans were abnormal in all 12. As the clinical findings were very similar to the neurological effects of Behçet's disease, it was suggested that ciclosporin can promote the development of neurological complications in this population.

Ciclosporin neurotoxicity is particularly frequent in liver and bone marrow transplant patients, who usually recover after temporary dosage reduction or withdrawal. However, a fatal outcome has been reported (36).

- A 54-year-old man was given ciclosporin and methotrexate after allogeneic bone marrow transplantation. He noted blurred vision during several days and became confused 11 weeks after transplantation. Generalized tonic-clonic seizures occurred the day after and he was given phenytoin and antibiotics. His neurological condition deteriorated during the next 5 days, despite ciclosporin withdrawal, and he died from respiratory failure. Postmortem examination showed white matter edema and astrocyte injury without demyelination.

After liver transplantation, 13 of 142 recipients ciclosporin and methylprednisolone (9.2%) had neurological symptoms, including five with central pontine myelinolysis and eight with cerebral hemorrhages or infarcts (37). Factors that were associated with central pontine

myelinolysis were hyponatremia, a rapid rise in serum sodium concentration, a postoperative increase in plasma osmolality, duration of operation, and high ciclosporin concentrations.

Clinical reports

Adverse nervous system effects of ciclosporin sometimes cause seizures.

- A ten-year-old boy with beta-thalassemia underwent autologous stem cell transplantation followed by ciclosporin 1 mg/kg/day (38). The trough ciclosporin concentration on day 14 was 392 ng/ml and the patient subsequently had a generalized tonic-clonic seizure. Ciclosporin was withdrawn, phenytoin was started, and the patient recovered. Six weeks later, a control brain MRI scan showed nearly complete resolution of multifocal high signal abnormalities on T2-weighted sequences in the cortex and subcortical white matter.
- A 58-year-old man with severe chronic obstructive pulmonary disease underwent bilateral lung transplantation with allografts from a cytomegalovirus seropositive donor; the recipient was seronegative (39). Immunosuppression was maintained with ciclosporin, prednisone, and mycophenolate mofetil. The dose of ciclosporin was adjusted to achieve blood concentrations of 350–400 ng/ml. On postoperative day 2 he had a generalized tonic–clonic seizure, when the ciclosporin concentration was 52 ng/ml; he responded to lorazepam and valproic acid. On day 10 he was given intravenous ganciclovir for prophylaxis against cytomegalovirus. By day 12 he was drowsy and unable to move his limbs. He had bilateral ptosis with intact extraocular muscles. His motor strength in the arms and legs was 0/5, with absent deep tendon reflexes. There was a five-fold increase in CSF protein with no white cells or red cells; bacterial and viral cultures of the CSF, blood, and broncheoalveolar fluid were negative, including PCR for cytomegalovirus. Electromyography and nerve-conduction studies showed a length-dependent, symmetrical, sensorimotor polyneuropathy with axonal features but no demyelination. An MRI scan of the cervical spinal cord was normal. Plasma exchange with albumin (30 ml/kg) every other day for a total of 7 sessions was undertaken and ciclosporin was replaced with tacrolimus. After the first plasmapheresis his strength improved to 2/5 in the arms and 3/5 in the legs. Over the next several weeks he continued to have steady neurological improvement.
- A 16-year-old man with chronic autoimmune hepatitis received a cadaveric orthotopic liver transplant and immunosuppression with prednisone, ciclosporin, and mycophenolate mofetil. Postoperatively he developed had generalized tonic–clonic seizures. His blood pressure was normal and electroencephalography was inconclusive. The cerebrospinal fluid was clear, with 25 cells, a protein concentration of 2 g/l, and a glucose concentration of 3.3 mmol/l. Cultures were negative. The blood ciclosporin concentration was 405 ng/ml. An MRI scan showed changes compatible with a reversible posterior leukencephalopathy. Ciclosporin was replaced with tacrolimus and he recovered.

Three patients underwent hemopoietic stem cell transplantation for thalassemia. Prophylaxis of graft-versus-host disease included ciclosporin, prednisolone, and methotrexate. All developed status epilepticus with cortical signal alterations mainly in the occipital regions on T2-weighted MRI. The neurological symptoms and radiographic findings completely disappeared without withdrawing ciclosporin. Children with thalassemia receiving busulfan or cyclophosphamide as a preparative regimen seem to be especially susceptible to ciclosporin-associated seizures (40).

In one series of 367 adult and pediatric liver recipients there were 17 cases of new-onset seizures (41). However, information on the immunosuppressants they were taking was scanty: three were reported as having ciclosporin toxicity and three as having tacrolimus (FK506) toxicity. The causes were neurotoxicity due to immunosuppressive therapy (n = 6), cerebrovascular disease (n = 4), severe metabolic derangements by sepsis or rejection (n = 3), hyperglycemia (n = 1), brain edema due to fulminant hepatic failure (n = 1), and unknown (n = 2). Seizures recurred in 15 patients, including nine on the same day. The incidence of death or persistent vegetative state in those with seizures was almost 10 times higher than in those without (53% versus 5.7%). The prognosis in patients with seizures due to cerebrovascular disease and severe metabolic derangement due to sepsis or rejection was poorer than in patients with seizures caused by drug neurotoxicity. The eight surviving patients were free of seizures for a follow-up period of 43 (16–58) months.

Reversible cortical blindness is a rare manifestation of ciclosporin toxicity and occurred in a lung transplant recipient (42).

Tremor has been studied in patients with severe liver disease without hepatic encephalopathy and after liver transplantation, comparing ciclosporin (n = 29) and tacrolimus (n = 6) (43). Compared with controls the patients had significant postural hand tremor before and after liver transplantation. The mean tremor amplitude increased after liver transplantation during treatment with both ciclosporin and tacrolimus. At higher ciclosporin plasma concentrations there was a reduction in the dominant tremor frequency with weight load and an increase in tremor amplitude, suggesting enhanced physiological or toxic tremor.

Severe headache is an uncommon adverse effect of ciclosporin (44).

- A 66-year-old woman with no history of headache or adverse drug reactions developed membranous glomerulonephritis and autoimmune non-central neutropenia. She was given ciclosporin microemulsion 2.5 mg/kg/day. Whole blood ciclosporin concentrations were within the target range. After 5 days she reported a severe, disabling, holocranial headache. A CT scan was normal and other causes of headache were ruled out. The headache subsided when ciclosporin was withdrawn.

Pseudotumor cerebri caused bilateral disk edema with cerebrospinal hypertension in a child treated with ciclosporin (45).

- An 11-year-old boy with recurrent tubulointerstitial nephritis associated with uveitis (TINU syndrome) was treated with ciclosporin to induce sustained remission. Ciclosporin was introduced as a steroid-sparing drug because of extreme obesity (BMI 32 kg/m^2). Although he did not complain of any symptoms, eye inspection after 7 months showed bilateral disk edema with retinal bleeding and he developed cerebrospinal hypertension. Pseudotumor cerebri was diagnosed by measuring the intracranial pressure (31 cm H$_2$O) and normal CT and MRI scans. Ciclosporin was withdrawn, and treatment with mycophenolate mofetil led to resolution within 12 weeks.
- A 67-year-old woman taking ciclosporin developed rapidly progressive sensorimotor changes a few months after kidney transplantation (46). The symptoms improved after ciclosporin withdrawal. Other causes were ruled out.

After liver transplantation, a patient developed a chronic inflammatory demyelinating polyradiculoneuropathy while taking ciclosporin + prednisolone (47). Treatment with intravenous immunoglobulin significantly improved the neuropathy.

Ciclosporin can cause leukoencephalopathy in organ transplant recipients (48).

- A 43-year-old man with a history of chronic renal insufficiency of unkown cause received a cadaveric kidney transplant and immunsuppression with antithymocyte-globulin, mycophenolate mofetil, ciclosporin, and prednisone. Four months later, he developed pneumonia and received fluorquinolones for 14 days. His blood ciclosporin concentration was 659 ng/ml. 10 days after discharge, he had a headache, meningism, and a bilateral sixth nerve palsy. The cerebrospinal fluid was clear with 270 cells, including 60% polymorphonuclear leukocytes and 40% mononuclear cells and a glucose concentration of 3 mmol/l. There was no evidence of infection, but ceftriacone, vancomycin, ampicillin, and ganciclovir were given empirically. An MRI scan showed many hypersignals in the subcortical white matter, particularly in the broadcast crown and semioval centers. Ciclosporin was withdrawn, with complete clinical improvement.
- A 50-year-old man with end-stage renal disease due to mesangiocapillary glomerulonephritis received a cadaveric kidney transplant and immunosuppression with azathioprine and prednisone. Because of gouty arthritis azathioprine was replaced by ciclosporin before treatment with allopurinol. Two weeks later he developed confusion, irritability, and personality changes. The blood ciclosporin concentration was 547 ng/ml. An MRI scan showed changes compatible with a leukencephalopathy. He recovered quickly when mycophenolate mofetil replaced ciclosporin.

In kidney transplant recipients and children with kidney diseases, there were 20 cases (13 boys and 7 girls, aged 2–18 years) of the posterior reversible encephalopathy syndrome (49). Of 177 kidney transplant recipients, six of 127 patients who were given ciclosporin and four of 50 patients who were given tacrolimus developed the syndrome after transplantation. Seven had idiopathic nephrotic syndrome (all treated with ciclosporin), two had acute poststreptococcal glomerulonephritis, and one had diffuse mesangial sclerosis. The symptoms varied from headache to status epilepticus. All the patients had hypertension and had cerebellar lesions on CT or MRI scans. With the exception of one patient with a delayed diagnosis and a patient with developmental delay before transplantation, all recovered clinically and radiologically within 10 weeks, with optimal control of hypertension and seizures, as well as withdrawal of the calcineurin-inhibitors.

In three children with posterior reversible encephalopathy associated with tacrolimus (n = 2) or ciclosporin (n = 1), electroencephalography showed continuous focal rhythmic activity, which normalized after the clinical effects had resolved (50).

Most studies have focused on the central nervous system adverse effects of ciclosporin, and there have been few reports of peripheral neuropathy.

- In two patients, ciclosporin was suggested as a possible cause of an entrapment neuropathy, and surgery was required in both (51).

However, the report did not provide sufficient evidence to assess the causal relation fully.

- Another patient developed a symmetric polyneuropathy with flaccid paraplegia while her ciclosporin serum concentrations were about twice normal (52). Electromyography showed features of axonal degeneration in the peripheral nerves and neurological symptoms improved on ciclosporin dosage reduction.

Migraine associated with ciclosporin is sometimes resistant to classical treatment and the consequences can be even more severe.

- Three young adult renal transplant patients, including two with a previous history of moderate migraine, had severe attacks of unilateral throbbing migraine associated with vomiting during ciclosporin treatment (53). In two patients, vomiting was severe enough to reduce compliance with the immunosuppressive regimen, and both subsequently lost their grafts. The same sequence of events was again observed after retransplantation.

Substitution by tacrolimus may be beneficial in such cases.

Severe ciclosporin neurotoxicity has mostly been reported in transplant patients, but should also be considered in non-transplanted patients.

- An 87-year-old patient with resistant nodular prurigo was successfully treated with ciclosporin (3 mg/kg/day) and prednisone (10 mg/day) (54). Bilateral numbness and distal limb weakness developed after 18 months. Clinical examination, electromyography, and nerve conduction studies confirmed a diffuse axonal neuropathy which rapidly progressed over the next 2 months. Ciclosporin alone was withdrawn and complete remission was observed within 3 months.

Unfortunately, ciclosporin blood concentrations and renal function at the time of diagnosis were not reported.

Very severe or fatal neurotoxicity has been reported in isolated patients only.

- Based on postmortem findings in a 32-year-old woman who died with an acute encephalopathy (55) and another report of two patients investigated with transcranial Doppler ultrasound and MRI for symptoms of ciclosporin neurotoxicity (56), vascular changes with vasospasm and dissection of the vascular intima strongly suggest that vasculopathy is a possible mechanism of ciclosporin-induced encephalopathy.

Prolonged confusion is a recognized complication of ciclosporin, and can be due to non-convulsive status epilepticus (57). Three patients who developed neurotoxicity following treatment with ciclosporin manifested with generalized tonic-clonic seizures and dysarthria. The plasma ciclosporin concentration in these patients increased as the neurological signs appeared, and the signs resolved quickly after dosage reduction (58). Tonic-clonic seizures have been reported in a child taking ciclosporin (59).

- A 13-year-old boy with severe Crohn's disease developed hematochezia and required blood transfusion. He was given ciclosporin on day 22 because of persistent rectal bleeding and diarrhea, despite high-dose intravenous glucocorticoids. After 6 days he developed multiple episodes of generalized tonic-clonic seizures, with MRI findings typical but not pathognomonic of ciclosporin: prominent meningeal enhancement, bifrontal, bitemporal, biparietal, and bioccipital cortical and subcortical white matter high-signal changes, and swelling of the gyri, which obliterated the sulci.

This case illustrates that severe ciclosporin neurotoxicity can develop in patients with predisposing factors, such as hypomagnesemia, hypocholesterolemia, hypertension, and glucocorticoid therapy.

Sensory systems

Controversial reports of ocular symptoms have been published in patients taking oral ciclosporin, with ptosis and diplopia attributed to unilateral or bilateral sixth nerve palsies in four patients (who had also taken ganciclovir), and nystagmus in one patient (SEDA-21, 383). Peripheral optic neuropathy, with visual loss, nystagmus, and ophthalmoplegia, has also been reported (60). Acute cerebral cortical blindness complicating ciclosporin therapy in a 5-year-old girl (61) and transient cortical blindness and occipital seizures with visual impairment (62,63) have also been reported in association with ciclosporin.

Bilateral optic disc edema is sometimes associated with ciclosporin given for bone marrow transplantation, but unilateral papilledema with otherwise asymptomatic raised intracranial pressure can occur (64). Eight cases of optic disc edema have been reported in bone marrow transplant patients taking ciclosporin. In two of the patients there were other possible explanations, but in all cases withdrawal of ciclosporin resulted in resolution of the papilledema (65).

Ciclosporin eye-drops have been used after keratoplasty, in high-risk cases, to prevent graft rejection and to treat severe vernal conjunctivitis, keratoconjunctivitis sicca, and various immune-related corneal disorders. Despite its severe adverse effects after systemic use, topical ciclosporin can generally be used without serious adverse reactions (66,67).

Ciclosporin oil-in-water emulsion has been used in the local treatment of moderate to severe dry eye disease. Chronic dry eye disease results from inflammation mediated by cytokines and receptors for autoimmune antibodies in the lacrimal glands. It affects the lacrimal gland acini and ducts, leading to abnormalities in the tear film, and ultimately disrupting the homeostasis of the ocular surface. Topical ciclosporin reduces the cell-mediated inflammatory response associated with inflammatory ocular surface diseases.

In two large, randomized controlled trials in 977 patients, the adverse effects associated with ciclosporin ophthalmic emulsion for the treatment of dry eye disease were minimal and consisted mostly of mild ocular burning and stinging (68). However, topical application of ciclosporin eye-drops was the suspected cause of severe visual loss with bilateral white corneal deposits in a 45-year-old patient with dry eye syndrome caused by graft-versus-host disease (69). Infrared spectroscopy and X-ray analysis suggested that the deposits contained ciclosporin. A reduction in tear clearance and compromised epithelial barrier function caused by the concomitant use of oxybuprocaine may have precipitated this adverse effect.

The efficacy, safety, tolerability, and optimal dose of ciclosporin eye-drops have been studied in a randomized, double-masked, vehicle-controlled multicenter trial in 162 patients with keratoconjunctivitis sicca with or without Sjögren's disease and refractory to conventional treatment (70). Ciclosporin ophthalmic emulsion 0.05, 0.1, 0.2, or 0.4%, or the vehicle alone was instilled twice daily into both eyes for 12 weeks, followed by a 4-week observation period. There was no clear dose–response relation; ciclosporin 0.1% emulsion produced the most consistent improvement in objective and subjective endpoints and ciclosporin 0.05% gave the most consistent improvement in symptoms. The vehicle also performed well, perhaps because of its long residence time on the ocular surface. There were no significant adverse effects, no microbial overgrowth, and no residence time of the vehicle emulsion on the ocular surface. All treatments were well tolerated and the highest ciclosporin blood concentration detected was 0.16 ng/ml.

To study the efficacy and safety of ciclosporin 0.05 and 0.1% ophthalmic emulsions and their vehicle in patients with moderate to severe dry eye disease, two identical multicenter, randomized, double-masked, vehicle-controlled trials have been performed in 877 patients for 6 months (68). More than 76% completed the course. Ciclosporin 0.05 or 0.1% eye-drops gave significantly greater improvement than the vehicle in two objective signs of dry eye disease (corneal staining and Schirmer values). Ciclosporin 0.05% also gave significantly greater improvement in three subjective measures (blurred vision, need for concomitant artificial tears, and the physician's evaluation of global response to treatment). There was no dose–response effect and there were no topical or systemic adverse findings.

Corneal deposition of ciclosporin can occur (69).

- A 45-year-old woman with dry eye syndrome caused by graft-versus-host disease after bone marrow transplantation for acute leukemia was given systemic ciclosporin and topical 0.1% sodium hyaluronate, 0.3% ofloxacin, 0.1% fluorometholone, and isotonic saline. She was also given 0.4% oxybuprocaine for the relief of severe ocular pain. The bilateral corneal epithelial defects persisted even after the application of punctal plugs, and 2% ciclosporin in olive oil was added as eye-drops three times a day bilaterally. Five days later she complained of severe visual loss in association with bilateral corneal opacities, which covered the pupil and the punctal plugs bilaterally. As she did not agree to keratectomy, infrared spectroscopy and X-ray analysis were conducted on the deposits on the plugs. The spectroscopic pattern and X-ray analysis showed that the deposits had the properties of ciclosporin.

As the corneal deposits did not abate after withdrawal of the ciclosporin eye-drops, the systemic ciclosporin as well as its topical use may have contributed to the deposits. One should be aware that precipitation of ciclosporin on a compromised cornea can lead to severe visual impairment.

Ocular opsoclonus responded to a reduction in the dose of ciclosporin in a liver transplant recipient (71).

- A 17-year-old Caucasian woman underwent liver transplantation for immunological cirrhosis and chronic cellular rejection. She developed ocular symptoms 8 days after transplantation. She also developed a reversible posterior leukoencephalopathy. The ciclosporin trough concentration was 412 ng/ml. The ocular symptoms improved 21 days after reduction of the ciclosporin trough concentration.

This rare condition usually occurs in patients with brain stem encephalitis, neoplasms of the mesencephalon, paraneoplastic syndromes, or intoxication.

Psychiatric

In a comparison of ciclosporin and tacrolimus, 45 of 128 patients developed complications attributed to immunosuppression (tacrolimus 36 patients; ciclosporin 7 patients) (72). There was no difference between the type of immunosuppression and the presence of neuropsychiatric complications. Patients with hepatitis C had a higher prevalence of psychiatric disorders, including *depression*, than other patients with different types of liver diseases.

Endocrine

Life-threatening hypothyroidism associated with ciclosporin was reported in a patient treated with reduced-intensity hemopoietic stem cell transplantation for metastatic renal-cell carcinoma (73).

- A 26 year old woman with metastatic renal cell carcinoma underwent reduced-intensity hemopoietic stem cell transplantation after having had a right nephrectomy, pelvic radiotherapy, interferon, and conditioning with busulfan, fludarabine, and antithymocyte globulin. Ciclosporin 3 mg/kg was added and graft-versus-host disease occurred on day 54 after ciclosporin was tapered. Ciclosporin 2 mg/kg was restarted intravenously and she developed malaise and hepatorenal dysfunction. The symptoms resolved after withdrawal of ciclosporin on day 62. One week later, ciclosporin 2 mg/kg was given orally and she developed fatigue, lethargy, and paralytic ileus. Thyroid-stimulating hormone, free triiodothyronine, and free thyroxine were undetectable; thyroid function had previously been normal. A thyrotropin-releasing hormone test showed secondary hypothalamic dysfunction.

The authors suggested that ciclosporin had suppressed the hypothalamic-pituitary axis.

Metabolism

Diabetes mellitus

Diabetes mellitus after transplantation is recognized as an important adverse effect of immunosuppressants, and has been extensively reviewed (74). In one study the use of ciclosporin in immunosuppressive regimens was not associated with diabetes mellitus after transplantation (10–20%) (75).

However, other studies have shown an increased risk. Tacrolimus + sirolimus, tacrolimus + mycophenolate mofetil, and ciclosporin + sirolimus have been compared in recipients of their first kidney transplant (76). One-year patient and graft survival did not differ. Ciclosporin + sirolimus was associated with a higher incidence of post-transplant diabetes mellitus, more antihyperlipidemic drug therapy, increased serum creatinine concentrations, reduced creatinine clearance, and more frequent protocol discontinuation.

The effect of long-term ciclosporin on glucose metabolism was analysed in heart transplant recipients who developed post-transplant hyperglycemia, 102 with impaired glycemic control and 20 with clinical diabetes (77). There was a significant negative correlation between ciclosporin concentration and insulin in both groups, a significant negative correlation between ciclosporin concentration and proinsulin, C-peptide blood concentration in those with impaired glycemic control and a significant positive correlation between ciclosporin and glucose blood concentration in both groups.

The incidence of diabetes mellitus has been investigated in a prospective multicenter study at 24 months after kidney transplantation in 1276 patients taking tacrolimus, mycophenolate mofetil, and steroids and in 507 patients taking ciclosporin, mycophenolate mofetil, and steroids (78). Significantly more of the patients who were taking tacrolimus (74/161, 46%) needed insulin than those who were taking ciclosporin (14/50, 28%). By multivariate Cox regression analysis, age over 60 years, a BMI over 30 kg/m», and immunosuppression with tacrolimus were associated with diabetes mellitus after transplantation.

Hyperlipidemia

Ciclosporin is potentially more toxic in patients with altered LDL concentrations or a low total serum cholesterol (79). Ciclosporin therapy itself significantly raises plasma lipoprotein concentrations by increasing the total serum cholesterol; this is due to an increase in LDL cholesterol, demonstrated in a prospective, double-blind, randomized, placebo-controlled trial in 36 men with amyotrophic lateral sclerosis (80). In 22 patients there were significant increases in mean serum triglycerides and cholesterol 2 weeks after they started to take low-dose ciclosporin (81). Hypertriglyceridemia developed in seven patients taking ciclosporin 2.0–7.5 mg/kg/day for psoriasis during the first month of therapy; the values were greater than the upper limit in age- and sex-matched controls (82).

The pathology of hyperlipidemia after transplantation is multifactorial, but it is clearly dose-dependently related to immunosuppressive therapy (83). This results in cardiovascular disease, which is one of the most common causes of morbidity and mortality in long-term survivors of organ transplantation (84). Hyperlipidemia can also cause renal atheroma, resulting in graft rejection. The possible impact of ciclosporin on lipids includes an increase in total cholesterol, LDL cholesterol, and apolipoprotein B concentrations, and a reduction in HDL cholesterol (SED-13, 1124). The influence of ciclosporin on lipoprotein(a) concentrations has been debated (SEDA-21, 383; 85). Post-transplant hyperlipidemia is multifactorial and can be affected by impaired renal function, diuretics and beta-blockers, increased age, and female sex. A combination of lipid-lowering drugs and optimization of immunosuppressive regimens compatible with long-term allograft survival is probably required to reduce post-transplantation hyperlipidemia.

Whereas azathioprine is considered to play no role, glucocorticoid use correlates positively with increased serum cholesterol concentrations. It is uncertain whether these lipid changes reflect primarily an effect of ciclosporin alone or an additive/synergistic effect of the drug plus glucocorticoids. Ciclosporin has been considered as a possible independent susceptibility factor by several investigators, but others were unable to find an association between hyperlipidemia and ciclosporin (SEDA-20, 344). There was indirect evidence for a causal role of ciclosporin in several studies; hyperlipidemia developed in non-transplant patients taking ciclosporin alone; there was a transient reduction in hyperlipidemia after ciclosporin withdrawal; there was a significant correlation between ciclosporin blood concentrations and lipid abnormalities; and there was a higher incidence of lipid abnormalities in patients taking ciclosporin alone compared with patients taking azathioprine and prednisolone (SED-8, 1131; SEDA-17, 524; SEDA-21, 383; 83,86). Other studies have provided striking evidence that hyperlipidemia is more frequent in patients taking ciclosporin than in those taking tacrolimus, with more patients classified as having high cholesterol concentrations in the ciclosporin group or a significant fall in total cholesterol or LDL cholesterol in patients switched from ciclosporin to tacrolimus (87,88). Although the glucocorticoid-sparing effect of tacrolimus may account for these differences, the concept that the glucocorticoid dose is a confounding factor has been disputed (SEDA-22, 412). Whether these differences translate to a higher risk of cardiovascular complications in patients taking ciclosporin has not been carefully assessed. The treatment of hyperlipidemia in transplant patients may represent a major dilemma, because of several drug interactions, with an increased risk of myopathy and rhabdomyolysis after the combined use of ciclosporin and several lipid-lowering drugs.

Of 295 patients after renal transplantation, 76 were given tacrolimus and 126 ciclosporin (89). Lipid concentrations were similar in the two groups at day 0. However, 12 months later, total cholesterol and LDL cholesterol were significantly higher in those who were taking ciclosporin; triglyceride concentrations were similar in the two groups.

Hyperuricemia

Significant hyperuricemia has been observed in as many as 80% of patients taking ciclosporin (90). In one series, hyperuricemia occurred in 72% of male and 82% of female patients taking ciclosporin after cardiac transplantation; there was also an increased incidence of gouty arthritis in these patients (91). Episodes of gout developed mostly in men taking diuretics, but the incidence was lower than in the hyperuricemic population. In renal transplant patients, the incidence of gout was 5–24% and tophi sometimes developed rapidly after the onset of gout (92). The potential mechanisms of hyperuricemia include reduced renal function and impaired tubular secretion of acid uric, with hypertension and diuretics as confounding factors (SEDA-21, 383).

In 32 children (median age 14 years), all of whom received triple immunosuppressive therapy (ciclosporin or tacrolimus, azathioprine or mycophenolate mofetil, and prednisone), 47% had hyperuricemia, with uric-acid concentrations above the age-related reference range; 55% were taking ciclosporin, 30% tacrolimus (93). Plasma uric acid concentrations did not differ among patients taking ciclosporin or tacrolimus. There was only one case of gout, 7,9 years after renal transplantation in a 15-year-old boy who also taking furosemide.

Nutrition

Higher plasma homocysteine concentrations, which may contribute to atherosclerosis, have been found in patients taking ciclosporin, compared with both transplant patients not taking ciclosporin and non-transplant patients with renal insufficiency (SEDA-20, 344).

Electrolyte balance

Mild and uncomplicated hyperkalemia is commonly observed in patients taking ciclosporin and is generally prevented by a low potassium diet. A reduction in distal nephron potassium secretion and tubular flow rate, with insensitivity to exogenous mineralocorticoids, and leakage of cellular potassium into the extracellular fluid are possible mechanisms (SED-13, 1124; 94).

Drug-related potassium-channel syndrome is a rare disorder that can occur after the administration of drugs that open K_{ATP} channels, such as ciclosporin, nicorandil, or isoflurane. It can cause severe life-threatening complications, including hyperkalemia and cardiovascular disturbances. Administration of the K_{ATP} channel blocker glibenclamide can promptly reverse these abnormalities (95).

Mineral balance

Hypomagnesemia and hypercalcemia occur infrequently during ciclosporin treatment (SED-13, 1124).

- In a 43-year-old renal transplant patient, hypomagnesemia was associated with muscle weakness and a near four-fold increase in serum creatine kinase activity (96). Both disorders resolved after magnesium supplementation, and ciclosporin was continued.

Renal magnesium wasting occurred in 24% of a series of renal transplant patients taking ciclosporin; other indicators of renal function were normal (97,98).

Hypomagnesemia in the early post-transplant period has been cited as a possible risk factor for acute ciclosporin neurotoxicity. Ciclosporin-induced sustained magnesium depletion has been investigated in 109 ciclosporin-treated patients with renal transplants who had been stable for more than 6 months (99). Total and ionized plasma magnesium concentrations were significantly lower than in 21 healthy volunteers and in 15 patients with renal transplants who were not taking ciclosporin. Ciclosporin-treated patients who were also taking hypoglycemic drugs had lower plasma magnesium concentrations, but patients taking diuretics did not.

Hematologic

Anemia is common after liver transplantation. Serum erythropoietin concentrations were measured in patients treated with ciclosporin and tacrolimus before and after liver transplantation (100). At 14 months after liver transplantation (ciclosporin n = 14, tacrolimus n = 21) mean erythropoietin concentrations were significantly lower after than before transplantation and in those who received ciclosporin the erythropoietin concentration was significant lower than in those who received tacrolimus.

A very few cases of ciclosporin-induced immune hemolytic anemia have been reported (SED-13, 1125; 101,102), but a direct causal relation with ciclosporin is difficult to establish. Ciclosporin-induced hypercoagulability was suggested in patients with aplastic anemia (SEDA-20, 344). Higher whole-blood ciclosporin concentrations were found during the preceding months in patients who experienced thromboembolic complications compared with patients who had not.

Ciclosporin-associated thrombotic microangiopathy occurs in 3–14% of patients with a renal transplant and can cause allograft loss. Renal impairment, reflected by an increase in serum creatinine concentration, is often the only change found, and hemolysis is not always present. Plasmapheresis has been used to treat this complication (103).

- A 47-year-old multiparous Hispanic woman received a living-unrelated kidney transplant for end-stage renal disease secondary to polycystic kidney disease. On the day of transplantation she received intravenous daclizumab 1 mg/kg plus methylprednisolone 300 mg and mycophenolate mofetil 3 g/day, and on day 3 ciclosporin emulsion 4 mg/kg/day. On day 8 she developed thrombotic microangiopathy without evidence of rejection. Ciclosporin was withdrawn. Plasmapheresis with fresh frozen plasma was started. Daclizumab on day 14 was postponed for 24 hours and plasmapheresis was stopped to avoid clearance of daclizumab. Thereafter she was given tacrolimus, without recurrence of hemolysis.

Mouth

Ciclosporin-induced gingival hyperplasia was noted in the early 1980s, and subsequent studies investigated the prevalence and pathophysiology of this adverse effect (SED-13, 1127). The reported incidence was 7–70%, and clinically significant gingival overgrowth, that is to say requiring treatment or surgical excision, affected about 30% of patients within the first 6 months of treatment (104). Clinical and histological features are similar to those associated with phenytoin or nifedipine. Compared with control specimens, ultrastructural gingival examinations in patients taking ciclosporin showed many fibroblasts, abundant amorphous substance, and marked plasma cell infiltration (105). Although an imbalance between the production and removal of collagen is supposed to account for gingival hyperplasia, the mechanism of ciclosporin-induced gingival overgrowth has not yet been clearly established. Possible local lymphocyte resistance to ciclosporin resulting in an increasing number of several inflammatory cells in the gingival lamina propria and ciclosporin-induced inhibition of prostaglandin I_2 synthesis have also been suggested (106,107).

There are many susceptibility factors for ciclosporin-induced gingival hyperplasia. The duration of treatment and the cumulative dose during the first 6 months play a major role. Accordingly, reduction of the ciclosporin dose can lessen the risk, and the use of lower doses is thought to reduce the overall incidence (108,109). There is also a positive correlation between the degree of gingival hyperplasia and changes in renal function (110). There are conflicting findings regarding the effects of blood concentrations on the incidence of gingival hyperplasia, and no clear relation between saliva and blood ciclosporin concentrations has been found. Lower age correlated significantly with the presence of gingival hyperplasia and children under 6 years of age are more susceptible to the complication in severe form (108,111). Male sex is a predisposing factor, a finding supported by the report of an increased androgen metabolism in gingival hyperplasia induced by ciclosporin (112). There has been also speculation concerning genetic differences in the susceptibility to develop these changes (SEDA-21, 384; 104). Finally, the combination of ciclosporin and nifedipine is additive with an increased prevalence and/or severity of gingival hyperplasia (SED-13, 1127; 76,77,112–114). As several other calcium channel blockers can produce gingival overgrowth, more frequent gingival hyperplasia should be expected, at least theoretically, when these drugs are combined with ciclosporin.

It is not yet clearly established whether bacterial plaque, gingival bleeding index, or inflammation are the cause or result of gingival hyperplasia. Certainly, poor oral health with subsequent local inflammation appears to be a contributing factor. Consequently, careful dental hygiene with plaque control is often sufficient to improve or resolve hyperplasia, but surgical treatment is sometimes necessary. Preliminary case reports have suggested that azithromycin or metronidazole can improve ciclosporin-induced gingival hyperplasia (SEDA-19, 350). This has been confirmed for azithromycin, with no indication that ciclosporin blood concentrations are modified during a short course of azithromycin (SEDA-22, 414).

In 18 renal transplant patients taking ciclosporin azithromycin 500 mg/day for 3 consecutive days reduced gingival hyperplasia (115). Thus, involvement of microorganisms is implicated in the pathogenesis of ciclosporin-induced gingival overgrowth. *Chlamydia pneumoniae* IgG and IgM antibody titers were measured by microimmunofluorescence in the sera of kidney recipients with (n = 11) and without (n = 89) gingival overgrowth (116). *Chlamydia pneumoniae* IgM titers were raised in five of 11 patients with gingival overgrowth and in none without gingival overgrowth. *Chlamydia pneumoniae*-specific DNA was found in 10 of 11 gingival overgrowth tissue samples before azithromycin therapy, which effectively reduced both gingival overgrowth and *Chlamydia pneumoniae* IgM titers. *Chlamydia pneumoniae* infection is highly prevalent in ciclosporin-induced gingival overgrowth. The infection can persist over a long period in residual gingival overgrowth despite short-term azithromycin therapy.

Ciclosporin can also less commonly cause lip enlargement, leading to a poor body image, low self-esteem, and non-adherence to therapy, especially in older children and adolescents. Two pediatric kidney recipients developed marked lip hypertrophy as a consequence of ciclosporin treatment; it resolved after conversion to tacrolimus (117).

Gastrointestinal

Gastrointestinal symptoms due to ciclosporin are usually mild and transient. In rheumatoid arthritis, gastrointestinal intolerance has been reported in 50% of patients, being the main cause for withdrawal of ciclosporin in 8% (118). Whereas worsening colitis did not occur in patients with inflammatory bowel disease, ciclosporin was involved in the development of acute colitis in isolated reports (SED-13, 1125).

Ciclosporin-induced achalasia-like esophageal dysmotility occurred in a liver transplant recipient (119).

- A 59 year old liver recipient took ciclosporin 250 mg/day, azathioprine 75 mg/day, and prednisolone, with pantoprazole 40 mg/day as ulcer prophylaxis. Dysphagia and retrosternal pain occurred 3 months after transplantation. The symptoms gradually worsened, with vomiting and severe dysphagia for liquids. Esophageal manometry showed achalasia, with inadequate relaxation of the lower sphincter. Immunosuppression was converted from ciclosporin to tacrolimus resulting in amelioration of the esophageal symptoms.

Peptic ulcer disease is a common complication among kidney transplant recipients, with significant morbidity and mortality. After kidney transplantation, 181 of 465 patients (39%) had at least one episode of peptic ulcer disease, including gastritis, gastric ulcer, duodenal ulcer, esophagitis, duodenitis, and esophageal ulceration (120). Most of the patients were taking a glucocorticoid + ciclosporin and 156 were taking mycophenolate mofetil. Methylprednisolone pulse therapy (OR = 3.95, 95% CI = 3.15, 18) and a history of pre-transplant peptic ulcer disease (OR = 7.60, 95% CI = 1.21, 13) were independent risk factors for post-transplant peptic ulcer disease by multivariate analysis. Antiulcer prophylaxis is recommended during the use of high-dose glucocorticoids after kidney transplantation, especially in recipients with a history of peptic ulcer disease.

Liver

There was at least one episode of hepatotoxicity in 228 of 466 patients (49%) with renal transplants who took ciclosporin; 110 (48%) had hyperalbuminemia, 108 (47%) a raised aspartate transaminase, and 167 (59%) a raised alkaline phosphatase (121). Ciclosporin dosage reduction resulted in resolution of hepatotoxicity in 185 patients (81%), while 32 (14%) had recurrent or persistent liver function abnormalities. Eleven (2.4%) developed biliary calculous disease. The serum ciclosporin concentration was high among the patients with hepatotoxicity. Pharmacokinetic studies showed an increased AUC in the patients with hepatotoxicity, probably due to reduced drug clearance.

Concomitant caspofungin + ciclosporin can cause transiently increased serum transaminase activities. There were rises in serum alanine transaminase and aspartate transaminase in 14 of 40 patients taking concomitant therapy for 18 (1–290) days (122). The rises were at least possibly drug-related in five cases, and two patients discontinued therapy because of hepatotoxicity.

A causal association has been shown between the hepatotoxicity of ciclosporin and cold ischemic liver damage that can occur during preservation before liver transplantation (123). This presents a problem when ciclosporin is used after liver transplantation. In more than 1000 patients there was an incidence of mild reversible hepatotoxicity of 40% in patients taking 5-fluorouracil and levamisole as adjuvants for more than 1 year; the incidence of mild hepatotoxicity in those taking levamisole alone and amongst those receiving no treatment at all was the same, a little over 16% (124).

Experiments with isolated human hepatocytes have shown that ciclosporin competitively inhibits the uptake of cholate and glycocholate bile acids; the biological features of ciclosporin-associated hepatotoxicity are therefore mostly those of cholestasis, with reduced bile excretion (125). The presence of underlying chronic viral hepatitis can increase the severity of ciclosporin-induced cholestasis (126).

Ciclosporin can cause cholestasis and cellular necrosis by an inhibitory effect on hepatocyte membrane transport proteins at both sinusoidal and canalicular levels. It induces oxidative stress by accumulation of various free radicals. Ademetionine (S-adenosylmethionine) is a naturally occurring substance that is involved in liver detoxification processes. The efficacy of ademetionine in the treatment and prevention of ciclosporin-induced cholestasis has been studied in 72 men with psoriasis (127). The patients who were given ciclosporin plus ademetionine had low plasma and erythrocyte concentrations of oxidants and high concentrations of antioxidants. The authors concluded that ademetionine may protect the liver against hepatotoxic substances such as ciclosporin.

A possible consequence of bile acid abnormalities and cholestasis associated with ciclosporin is the development of cholelithiasis in liver transplant patients when the donor has pre-existing susceptibility for cholesterol gallstone formation or abnormalities of bile composition.

- A young patient who received a liver from a 78-year-old donor subsequently developed cholesterol gallstones (SEDA-21, 383).

In a retrospective study in 50 consecutive patients who received both parenteral nutrition and glucocorticoids, with or without the addition of ciclosporin, at some stage in their management, there was no evidence that ciclosporin caused more liver dysfunction than that associated with parenteral nutrition (128).

Urinary tract

The renal toxicity of ciclosporin has been described as being an adverse effect of the drug on the compensatory mechanisms of the kidney, without effects on proximal tubular function (urea and sodium reabsorption) (129). A rise in serum creatinine concentration may be adequate to identify acute-onset ciclosporin nephrotoxicity, but it is not suitable for identification of chronic, late-onset ciclosporin nephrotoxicity (130).

It has been described in recipients of solid organs and in patients treated for autoimmune diseases (131).

Presentation
Acute renal impairment
Acute ciclosporin-induced nephrotoxicity, causing reduced renal function, develops within the first month, and includes a dose-related rise in serum creatinine concentrations and hyperkalemia. Fatal acute tubular necrosis has also been noted after very high intravenous doses (SEDA-19, 345). Although it is clinically often difficult to differentiate from acute allograft rejection in renal transplant patients, the alteration in renal function promptly resolves on ciclosporin withdrawal or dosage reduction, and initial acute renal insufficiency is not clearly associated with the development of subsequent chronic renal dysfunction (132). Several conditions, such as pre-existing hypovolemia, concomitant diuretic treatment, or renal artery stenosis, are susceptibility factors. Hypothyroidism was thought to be involved in one patient (133), and the transplanted kidney itself rather than interindividual differences between recipients was thought to play a role (SEDA-21, 384).

Hemolytic–uremic syndrome and thrombotic microangiopathy

Hemolytic–uremic syndrome, with histological findings of thrombotic microangiopathy and possible evolution to graft loss or death, is another instance of very severe acute nephrotoxicity (SED-13, 1125). It usually occurs at between the second and fourth weeks after transplant, with associated fever, thrombocytopenia, erythrocyte fragmentation, neurotoxicity, and renal impairment. Uncommon clinical features have been reported.

- In two women, hemolytic–uremic syndrome was apparently revealed by an episode of severe acute depression (134).
- In another patient, a single injection of ciclosporin may have induced the development of fibrin thrombi seen in the perioperative graft biopsy (135). Later on, she was confirmed to have clinical and biological features of hemolytic–uremic syndrome, which reversed after ciclosporin withdrawal.

Hemolyti–uremic syndrome has also been reported during ciclosporin treatment for Behçet's disease (SEDA-21, 384). Both early and delayed hemolytic–uremic syndrome can occur after transplantation, and its actual incidence may have been underestimated. Thrombotic microangiopathy with clinical features of hemolytic–uremic syndrome was found in 3.5–5% of renal transplant patients (136,137). Graft loss was mostly found in patients who developed hemolytic–uremic syndrome early after transplantation, and the clinical distinction from acute rejection can be very difficult. Hemolytic–uremic syndrome does not recur after initial withdrawal and further ciclosporin reintroduction, once renal function has normalized, or even despite ciclosporin maintenance with dosage reduction (SED-13, 1125) (SEDA-20, 345). In some cases, the patient was successfully switched to tacrolimus, and only one case of hemolytic–uremic syndrome with recurrence on ciclosporin rechallenge has been reported (SEDA-21, 384). In contrast, both ciclosporin and tacrolimus were significant susceptibility factors for recurrence of hemolytic–uremic syndrome in patients who had undergone renal transplantation for end-stage renal disease (138).

The factors that contribute to the development of thrombotic microangiopathy have been retrospectively investigated in 50 of 188 patients with kidney or kidney + pancreas allografts who underwent graft biopsies and in 19 control patients who had never had renal graft dysfunction or a biopsy (139). There were definite histological features of thrombotic microangiopathy 4 days to 6 years after transplantation in 26 patients, of whom 24 were taking ciclosporin and two were taking tacrolimus, showing that this complication can occur at any time after transplantation. Eight patients had graft loss, but only two had associated systemic evidence of microangiopathy, that is thrombocytopenia and intravascular hemolysis, suggesting that thrombotic microangiopathy should be considered in any patients with renal graft dysfunction, even if there are no suggestive systemic symptoms. Although the more frequent use of the microemulsion form of ciclosporin (Neoral) in patients with confirmed

thrombotic microangiopathy than in controls suggested a possible role of this formulation, this issue remains to be further investigated, because the number of evaluable patients was small. None of the other investigated variables (age, sex, race, living-related or cadaveric donor status, the degree of HLA mismatch, the type of allograft, or the incidence of urinary tract infections after transplantation) was significantly associated with the occurrence of thrombotic microangiopathy compared with patients without thrombotic microangiopathy. Finally, the most successful strategy was a switch from ciclosporin to tacrolimus, which resulted in normalization of graft function in 81% of these patients.

Chronic renal insufficiency

Chronic renal impairment, as first reported in cardiac transplant patients (140), is of major concern, because of possible irreversible renal dysfunction. A considerable amount of work has subsequently accumulated on the development of progressive renal dysfunction in patients receiving long-term ciclosporin for organ transplantation or chronic inflammatory disease (SED-13, 1125; SEDA-20, 345; SEDA-21, 384; SEDA-22, 413), and there have been several comprehensive reviews (141–144). About one-third of all patients have increased serum creatinine concentrations and reduced glomerular filtration rate during ciclosporin maintenance therapy. The histopathological features of chronic nephropathy consist mostly of non-specific tubular atrophy and interstitial fibrosis (145); arteriolar lesions are considered very suggestive of ciclosporin nephrotoxicity. The prevalence of renal damage due to ciclosporin has fallen considerably since the use of lower doses. Arteriolopathy sometimes improves after reducing or withdrawing ciclosporin. Morphological features in patients with autoimmune diseases are non-specific, and include a wide range of lesions, mostly characterized by tubulointerstitial changes and arteriolopathy. There is no significant correlation between histological findings and ciclosporin dose. Severe histological lesions can be identified in some patients with normal renal function (146); the severity of tubulointerstitial lesions has been deemed to be a better index than the glomerular filtration rate for predicting the occurrence of chronic nephropathy, but in one study there was no correlation between histological renal findings and various measures of renal function (147).

Because the possibility of irreversible renal dysfunction is a major problem in ciclosporin maintenance in both transplant and non-transplant patients, this issue continues to receive attention. Even though many studies have been performed, the long-term prognosis is a source of conflicting opinions, and the initial assumption that long-term use of ciclosporin will sooner or later cause irreversible chronic nephropathy is hotly debated. It is still unclear to what extent long-term ciclosporin contributes to progressive renal insufficiency and whether chronic ciclosporin nephropathy is irreversible or improves after dosage reduction. A retrospective analysis of more than 12 000 renal transplant patients showed that long-term maintenance with a glucocorticoid-free ciclosporin regimen (ciclosporin alone or with azathioprine) significantly increased renal graft and patient survival, compared with patients taking other immunosuppressive regimens (148). This allowed the use of higher doses of ciclosporin without increasing the frequency of nephrotoxicity. In contrast, several investigators have considered a change to a ciclosporin-free regimen in 40% of patients, because of progressive renal deterioration with histological signs of nephrotoxicity (149). The incidence of end-stage renal insufficiency requiring dialysis or renal transplantation ranges from 1% in renal transplant patients to 3–6% in heart-transplant patients (150–153). Nevertheless, several investigators have shown that despite an initial reduction in renal function, serum creatinine concentrations stabilized with no strong evidence of progressive nephropathy after several years of surveillance in various organ transplant patients (132,151,154–156).

The potential long-term consequences of ciclosporin nephrotoxicity constitute a major disadvantage in nontransplant patients. Renal function was assessed 7 years after the end of a 1-year ciclosporin treatment period in 36 young patients from a randomized, placebo-controlled trial of ciclosporin in diabetes mellitus, 19 taking ciclosporin, and 17 taking placebo (157). Blood pressure did not differ between the groups. Compared with baseline values, urinary albumin excretion rate was significantly higher and estimated glomerular filtration rate significantly lower with ciclosporin. The results in the placebo group showed no change or increases. In addition, there was progression to micro- or macro-albuminuria in four patients taking ciclosporin, and two of five patients who underwent renal biopsy had arteriolar hyalinosis. It is not known whether these changes will translate to an increased risk of nephropathy, but they suggest that ciclosporin might enhance it. Of 91 consecutive patients with renal transplants with a minimum graft survival of 1 year who were followed for 7–8 years, 65% had stable renal function despite ciclosporin serum concentrations of 200–250 ng/ml (158). In addition, none of the 26 patients with worsening renal function had features of ciclosporin nephrotoxicity on renal biopsy.

Frequency
In a meta-analysis of 18 trials involving ciclosporin doses below 10 mg/kg/day for at least 2 months in autoimmune diseases, the weighted percentage increase in serum creatinine concentrations was 17% in ciclosporin-treated patients and 1.7% in controls (159). The corrected risk difference for an increase of more than 50% of pretreatment serum creatinine concentrations between the two groups was 21% (95% CI = 12, 30) (159). This meta-analysis did not fully consider the long-term outcome, but clinical and histological evidence of sustained or progressive ciclosporin nephropathy in this population continues to accumulate. Unfortunately, some of the findings are discordant (146,160–169).

In a retrospective study of 106 patients following renal transplantation who had been treated with ciclosporin, 85% were hypertensive compared with 54% of patients taking azathioprine (170). Renal function was significantly better in hypertensive patients treated with nifedipine than with other antihypertensive medication (beta-blockers and vasodilators), and it was similar to that of normotensive patients treated with ciclosporin.

Pathophysiology
The pathogenesis of chronic ciclosporin nephrotoxicity is not fully understood (144). Intrarenal afferent arteriolar vasoconstriction may play an important part, particularly in acute nephrotoxicity (171), in which a marked reduction in renal blood flow associated with an increase in renal vascular resistance, probably due to postglomerular vasoconstriction, has been demonstrated (172,173). The supposed mechanism is primarily an imbalance between several regulatory mechanisms of renal vasodilatation and vasoconstriction, leading to increased renal vasoconstriction, and the explanations that have been proposed include activation of the renin–angiotensin system, prostaglandin inhibition, and sympathetic nervous system activation (174). However, it is unclear whether a continuous increase in renal vascular resistance can account for chronic renal dysfunction in patients taking long-term ciclosporin. There are many possible mediators of renal vasoconstriction, for example nitric oxide, the renin–angiotensin and kallikrein–kinin systems, endothelin-1 release, and stimulation of sympathetic nervous system activity. A major effect of ciclosporin is to promote calcium accumulation in the mitochondrial matrix, which in turn reduces ATP synthesis (175). The main morphological abnormality that has been demonstrated in the kidneys of patients taking long-term ciclosporin is interstitial fibrosis. Vascular lesions, predominantly arteriolar, with arterial intimal fibrosis have been noted in renal biopsies from patients with chronic ciclosporin nephrotoxicity (176).

Renal morphology has been studied in 17 patients who received ciclosporin for sight-threatening uveitis. Most had not received other potentially nephrotoxic drugs. Variable interstitial fibrosis, frequently associated with tubular atrophy, was noted in all 17. The extent of the pathological changes did not correlate with the age, treatment duration, or average cumulative dose (177). Ciclosporin nephrotoxicity mimics the histological features of acute allograft rejection and tubular necrosis. It is important to be able to distinguish clinically between ciclosporin toxicity on the one hand (necessitating a reduction in dose) and rejection (requiring an increase in dose) on the other.

The long-term effects of ciclosporin on renal function in 11 liver transplant recipients were evaluated over a follow-up period of 6–26 months (174). Immediately postoperatively, glomerular filtration rate (GFR) and effective renal plasma flow (ERPF) fell by 60%, subsequently settling at 45–60% of normal. There were additional toxic effects on renal tubular function. Histopathological findings were mild to moderate; notably, arterial and arteriolar nephrosclerosis. Renal function improved as the dose of ciclosporin was reduced, despite continued administration of the drug. This suggests a persistent, potentially reversible, functional component to chronic ciclosporin nephrotoxicity.

The biochemical basis of nephrotoxicity due to calcineurin inhibitors and their interaction with inhibitors of mTOR, such as tacrolimus is still poorly understood. However, there is evidence that nephrotoxicity is caused by drug-induced mitochondrial dysfunction and that inhibitors of mTOR enhance the negative effects of calcineurin inhibitors on cell energy metabolism (178).

Although the pathogenesis of ciclosporin nephrotoxicity is not completely defined, there is evidence that suggests a role of reactive oxygen species. In numerous in vivo and in vitro experiments ciclosporin caused renal insufficiency and increased the synthesis of reactive oxygen species, thromboxane, and lipid peroxidation products in the kidney. Furthermore, it modified the expression and activity of several renal enzymes (cyclooxygenase, superoxide dismutase, catalase, and glutathione-peroxidase). Antioxidant nutrients (for example vitamins E and C) can neutralize some of the effects that ciclosporin produces in the kidney (179). Thus, vitamin E inhibited the synthesis of reactive oxygen species and thromboxane and the lipid peroxidation process induced by ciclosporin. Antioxidants can also improve renal function and histological damage produced by ciclosporin. Although there are few data in humans taking ciclosporin, it is possibility that antioxidants also neutralize ciclosporin nephrotoxicity and LDL oxidation. Thus, antioxidant nutrients could have a therapeutic role in transplant patients taking ciclosporin.

The respective roles of organ preservation and ciclosporin in the pathogenesis of post-transplant renal damage have been studied in an in vitro model that simulates the hypothermic kidney preserved before surgery in Collins' solution and exposed after transplantation to ciclosporin (180). The results showed that preservation sensitizes the kidney to ciclosporin injury, which is consistent with clinical experience (181). If the preserved kidney cells were given a period of repair before administration of ciclosporin, further injury did not happen. In animal experiments, prolonged cold preservation causes progressive deterioration in the renal cortical microcirculation; concentration of ciclosporin in the renal cortex of hypoperfused kidneys markedly potentiates the vascular damage caused by cold preservation (170).

Ciclosporin-induced renal hypoperfusion was detected by quantitative cine-loop color Doppler imaging after kidney transplantation in 22 patients (182). They were taking ciclosporin + mycophenolate mofetil + prednisolone (n = 7), tacrolimus + mycophenolate mofetil + prednisolone (n = 7), or ciclopsorin + a calcium channel blocker (n = 8). The mean effect occurred 1.1 hours after ciclosporin dosing and was prevented by calcium channel blockers. Main renal artery velocities, resistive index, and small vessel perfusion were unchanged, suggesting that medium-sized arteries mediated vasoconstriction. In contrast, tacrolimus did not alter renal vascularity.

Ciclosporin-induced nephrotoxicity has been studied in prospective protocol kidney biopsies (n = 888) from 99 patients taken regularly for 10 years after kidney transplantation (183). The most sensitive histological marker of ciclosporin-induced nephrotoxicity was arteriolar hyalinosis. Structural nephrotoxicity occurred in two phases, with different clinical and histological characteristics. The acute phase occurred with a median onset of 6 months after kidney transplantation, was usually reversible, and was associated with functional nephrotoxicity, high ciclosporin blood concentrations, and mild arteriolar hyalinosis. The chronic phase persisted over several biopsies and occurred at a median onset of 3 years. It was associated with lower ciclosporin doses and trough concentrations, was largely irreversible, and was accompanied by severe arteriolar hyalinosis and progressive glomerulosclerosis. These pathological changes exacerbated chronic allograft nephropathy and strategies to ameliorate or avoid nephrotoxicity are therefore urgently needed.

Chronic interstitial fibrosis is an adverse prognostic feature of chronic allograft nephropathy. It has been analysed in protocol kidney biopsies (n = 959) obtained regularly for 10 years after kidney transplantation (184). There was substantial interstitial fibrosis within 1 year after kidney transplantation, with maximum intensity within the first 3 months as a result of early ischemia–reperfusion injury and acute, subacute, or persistent interstitial inflammation. Ciclosporin increased the risk of interstitial fibrosis compared with tacrolimus, and mycophenolate mofetil was protective compared with azathioprine.

Large-scale studies with long periods of follow-up have emphasized the major role of graft arteriopathy (chronic graft rejection) rather than chronic ciclosporin nephrotoxicity as the primary cause of graft failure (150,155,185). Severe ciclosporin nephropathy was the cause of renal transplant failure in less than 1% of patients.

Susceptibility factors and prediction

Many factors have been postulated as being relevant to ciclosporin nephrotoxicity. Whereas in several studies initial high doses of ciclosporin increased the risk of chronic nephrotoxicity (154,160), others suggested that patients maintained on relatively high ciclosporin concentrations had no more chance than others of developing toxic nephropathy (155). Neither the daily dose nor the duration of ciclosporin treatment reasonably predicts the risk of chronic renal insufficiency. Chronic renal dysfunction can be observed, despite the maintenance of ciclosporin blood concentrations below 400 ng/ml. However, age, sustained hypertension, hypertriglyceridemia, low HDL cholesterol concentrations, and recurrent episodes of severe acute nephrotoxicity increase susceptibility to chronic ciclosporin nephrotoxicity (161,186).

From a prospective study in 36 heart transplant patients with stable renal function for at least 6 months after transplantation, it was suggested that high urinary retinol-binding protein concentrations may indicate tubulointerstitial damage and therefore detect patients who are at risk of ciclosporin nephrotoxicity (187). At the start of the study, 13 patients had high urinary retinol-binding protein concentrations and 23 had normal concentrations. After 5 years of follow-up, five of the 13 patients developed end-stage renal insufficiency requiring dialysis, whereas none of the 23 other patients had terminal renal insufficiency. Although these data await confirmation, the authors suggested that ciclosporin dosage reduction should be considered in patients with high urinary retinol-binding protein concentrations, in order to limit renal damage.

Ciclosporin can cause tubulointerstitial lesions, the pathogenesis of which is unclear. In 37 patients, the duration of ciclosporin treatment and of heavy proteinuria were independent risk factors for ciclosporin-induced tubulointerstitial disease (188).

P glycoprotein contributes substantially to ciclosporin nephrotoxicity. The TT genotype at the ABCB1 3435C→T polymorphism is associated with reduced expression of P glycoprotein in renal tissue and has been implicated as a susceptibility factor for ciclosporin nephrotoxicity. Ciclosporin nephrotoxicity in 18 of 97 patients completely recovered after switching to a calcineurin inhibitor-free regimen (189). The P glycoprotein low expressor genotype 3435TT in the kidney donors, but not in the recipients, was over-represented in the cases of ciclosporin nephrotoxicity. Ciclosporin dosage, trough concentrations, and the concentration per dose ratio were not different between the groups. In a multivariate model that included several other non-genetic covariates, only the donor's ABCB1 3435TT genotype was strongly associated with ciclosporin nephrotoxicity.

Comparative studies
The effect of microemulsion ciclosporin and tacrolimus on the development of renal allograft fibrosis has been evaluated in a randomized trial in 102 kidney recipients randomized to either microemulsion ciclosporin 15 mg/kg/day (trough concentration range 200–300 ng/ml) or tacrolimus 0.2 mg/kg/day (trough concentration range 8-15 ng/ml) in conjunction with glucocorticoids, or at a lower dose (ciclosporin 7 mg/kg/day and tacrolimus 0.1 mg/kg/day), with the addition of azathioprine for recipients of non-heart-beating kidneys (190). There was a significant increase in allograft interstitial fibrosis in the patients who used microemulsion ciclosporin compared with tacrolimus. There was no significant difference in the demographic characteristics between the patients or in the incidence of acute rejection (ciclosporin 36% versus tacrolimus 35%) or glucocorticoid-resistant rejection (both 10%). The incidence of insulin resistance was higher with tacrolimus, but this was not significant. Ciclosporin was associated with significant increases in total cholesterol and low-density lipoprotein concentrations, which persisted throughout the study.

In 44 patients randomized 3 months after kidney transplantation to ciclosporin + sirolimus + prednisolone (group I) or to sirolimus + prednisolone (group II), baseline graft biopsy showed a higher degree of renal damage in group II (191). At 1 year after transplantation, chronic allograft nephropathy was diagnosed in 55% of the patients, of whom 64% were in group I and 36% in group II. Lesions of chronic allograft nephropathy were scored as moderate to severe in 90% of group I patients but only 32% of group II patients. There was a vascular score greater than or equal to 2 in 90% of group I patients

and in 38% of group II patients. Group I patients had significantly worse kidney graft function (serum creatinine 177 versus 115 µmol/l). The authors suggested that early withdrawal of ciclosporin is a safe option that allows significant reduction of chronic histological damage, particularly vascular injury, to cadaveric kidney allografts.

Kidney recipients (n = 31) with biopsy-confirmed chronic allograft nephropathy were prospectively randomized to receive a 40% ciclosporin dosage reduction either with sirolimus 2 mg/day (n = 16) or without (control, n = 15) (192). Sirolimus did not improve functional, molecular, or histological outcomes in patients with chronic allograft nephropathy after ciclosporin dosage reduction.

Management
The possible risk of precipitating end-stage renal insufficiency should not be regarded as a major limitation to ciclosporin treatment in organ-transplant patients, and no matter how defective our knowledge of the susceptibility factors is, attempts must be made to prevent or manage ciclosporin nephrotoxicity. Delaying the introduction of ciclosporin until post-transplant renal function has returned to normal and reducing the dose of ciclosporin when increases in serum creatinine concentrations are more than 30% above baseline values are measures that may well reduce the risk of acute nephrotoxicity. In the long term, switching patients from ciclosporin to azathioprine, reducing ciclosporin doses, or even electively withdrawing ciclosporin have been suggested as helpful measures, but they should be regarded cautiously and set against the risk of rejection (193–197). Once-daily dosing of ciclosporin in the morning improves glomerular filtration rate and renal blood flow compared with half the dose taken twice daily (198). Despite evidence for a very similar profile of nephrotoxicity, conversion from ciclosporin to tacrolimus has been used successfully (SEDA-20, 347).

Withdrawal of ciclosporin increases the risk of rejection, but improves renal function and other forms of ciclosporin-related toxicity. Improvement has also been observed after ciclosporin dosage reduction without an increased risk of acute rejection. Chronic allograft deterioration improved after conversion from ciclosporin to mycophenolate mofetil. Promising results of complete ciclosporin avoidance after kidney transplantation need to be confirmed in larger trials with a longer follow-up (199).

Finally, several drugs have been investigated in experimental and clinical studies to prevent ciclosporin nephrotoxicity. Calcium channel blockers, such as nifedipine, diltiazem, or verapamil, have repeatedly been proposed as reliable adjunctive drugs to minimize the long-term nephrotoxic effects of ciclosporin in renal transplant patients. Among anti-ischemic drugs, trimetazidine might be a good choice, because it prevents the loss of ATP synthesis caused by ciclosporin in rat kidney cells. S-15176 and S-16950 are trimetazidine derivatives that antagonize the mitochondrial toxicity of ciclosporin without changing its immunosuppressive effects.

Viewing the evidence as a whole, it appears that the use of lower doses of ciclosporin is probably the most important factor accounting for the fact that the majority of patients on long-term ciclosporin do not today have evidence of progressive nephrotoxicity.

Skin

Mild flushing often occurs during ciclosporin treatment, but more severe extensive erythema is uncommon.

- Recurrent episodes of diffuse flushing of the arms, the face, and the trunk reportedly occurred about 2 hours after each dose of ciclosporin in a 24-year-old man who had received a renal transplant 6 years before (200). These episodes were noted from the beginning of treatment, but worsened after he changed to Neoral, the microemulsion form of ciclosporin, and completely resolved after ciclosporin was replaced by tacrolimus.

Ciclosporin sometimes causes chronic inflammatory dermatitis, and there have been two reports of four male transplant recipients who developed clinical and histopathological features of keloid acne of the posterior scalp or neck (201,202). *Staphylococcus aureus* infection was identified in three. Ciclosporin-induced hypertrichosis was suggested as a possible cause, with local bacterial infection and immunosuppression as trigger factors.

- Multiple, large epidermoid cysts have been described in a 23-year-old man taking ciclosporin (203).

Acute generalized pustular psoriasis occurred 1 week after ciclosporin withdrawal in a 32-year-old woman who had taken ciclosporin for 12 weeks for chronic plaque psoriasis (204). This is in keeping with a similar phenomenon sometimes observed after glucocorticoid withdrawal.

Coarsening of facial features and a possibly more frequent occurrence of acne vulgaris and keratosis pilaris have been described in children taking ciclosporin (SED-8, 1125) (205). In 19 children who took ciclosporin and prednisone after renal transplantion, there was coarsening of facial features with thickening of the nares, lips, and ears, puffiness of the cheeks, prominence of the supraorbital ridges, and mandibular prognathism; this was found in all the children who had been treated for 6 months (206). Although the concurrent use of glucocorticoids may play a role in the development of acne, resolution of severe acne was in one reported case attained only after ciclosporin withdrawal (SEDA-20, 345). Convincing but anecdotal evidence of the worsening of subcutaneous sarcoidosis has been reported (SEDA-22, 384).

Pseudoporphyria is a generic term that is used to describe photoaggravated bullous dermatoses similar to those of porphyria cutanea tarda (207).

- A 50-year-old man with a history of chronic hepatitis C, alcoholism, and liver transplantation, taking ciclosporin, developed tender blisters and erosions on the backs of both hands. Skin biopsy was consistent with porphyria cutanea tarda. Urinary excretion of δ-aminolevulinic acid, porphobilinogen, uroporphyrins, hepatocarboxyporphyrin, and hexacarboxylporphyrin were within normal limits. Coproporphyrin and total porphyrin concentrations were raised. Ciclosporin was switched to tacrolimus and the blisters resolved within 3 weeks. Nevertheless, liver function progressively worsened.

Folliculodystrophy has been attributed to ciclosporin (208).

- A 34-year-old female kidney transplant recipient taking ciclosporin developed an infiltrated appearance to the skin with abundant flesh-colored, follicular papules predominantly affecting the ears, nose, and surrounding areas of the face, but also the trunk and extremities.

Ciclosporin-induced hemangiomas occurred in a patient with psoriatic arthropathy (209).

- A 35-year-old man with psoriatic arthropathy was given first methotrexate and methylprednisolone and then ciclosporin in increasing doses starting at 2.3 mg/kg/day and increasing to 4.0 mg/kg/day when remission of arthritis was achieved. Gingival hyperplasia resolved after dosage reduction to 3 mg/kg/day. Three years later he developed two raised purple, hard, painless nodules 5 mm in diameter. Histology showed a vascular lesion without any features of hemangioma. During the next 2 months new nodules appeared on the limbs. The dose of ciclosporin was reduced but the nodules persisted and ciclosporin was withdrawn. Over the next few months the nodules got smaller and finally disappeared, leaving small depigmented areas.

Sebaceous glands

Ciclosporin can cause sebaceous gland hyperplasia and hyperplastic folliculitis (210,211).
Juxtaclavicular beaded lines are unique malformation of sebaceous glands or a variant of sebaceous hyperplasia.

- A 63-year-old man developed small, asymptomatic, linear papules over the neck and clavicles. He had taken prednisone and ciclosporin for 30 months after kidney transplantation (212). A skin biopsy showed sebaceous hyperplasia.

The pathogenesis of juxtaclavicular beaded lines is unclear. Some authors have reported a prevalence of 16% in heart transplant patients, but only in men. Because ciclosporin is highly lipophilic, it has many adverse effects associated with alterations of pilosebaceous follicles, such as hypertrichosis and acne. In this case the authors postulated that the combined effect of prednisone and ciclosporin may have induced sebaceous gland hyperplasia.

Hair

Widespread hypertrichosis is one of the most common complications of ciclosporin, and distichiasis (accessory eyelashes) has been reported in one patient (SEDA-20, 345). Ciclosporin-associated soft tissue proliferation with an abnormal hyperplastic reaction has been suggested to account for the development of hyperplastic pseudofolliculitis barbae (213).

Alopecia areata or alopecia totalis has been noted in isolated cases (SEDA-21, 384).

A white-headed man noted progressive darkening of the hair while taking ciclosporin (214).

Nails

Several nail changes (excess granulation tissue or ingrowing toenails) have been attributed to ciclosporin (SED-13, 1127).

- Marked pitting with Mees' lines (homogeneous transverse white lines in the nail plates) in the fingernails, a disorder that has not been previously reported, was attributed to ciclosporin-associated kidney dysfunction in a 41-year-old man who inadvertently took ciclosporin 300 mg/day for psoriasis (215).

Musculoskeletal

Muscles

Muscle disorders attributed to ciclosporin have been mostly described in anecdotal case reports (SED-14, 1291). In an analysis of published or spontaneous case reports, the manufacturers found 29 cases of muscle disorders in patients taking ciclosporin; the complications fell into two categories (216). Myopathic symptoms, that is myalgia and muscle weakness without rhabdomyolysis, were reported in 0.17% of patients and abated after dose reduction or treatment withdrawal. Rhabdomyolysis occurred in under 0.05% of patients and was mostly observed in patients taking other drugs, such as lovastatin or colchicine.

This topic has been re-analysed in a systematic review of published papers, in which relevant information from a total of 34 patients was identified (217). All but two patients were also taking concomitant drugs known to affect the muscles, among which glucocorticoids, simvastatin, lovastatin, colchicine, and pyrazinamide were the most frequently cited. Ciclosporin is therefore difficult to implicate in most patients, but at least one case with positive ciclosporin re-administration supported a causative role. The clinical picture was non-specific, with myalgia, cramps, and muscle weakness, sometimes associated with raised serum creatine kinase activity, and heterogeneous histopathology. Finally, skeletal muscle abnormalities have rarely been described in patients without muscle symptoms.

- A 61-year-old man with incomplete Behçet's disease developed weakness and muscle pain. He had not responded fully to colchicine and ciclosporin was added (218). About 1 year later he noticed weakness of the proximal limb muscles. Within 3 months, he developed progressive severe generalized muscle pain and numbness in his hands. There were rises in serum muscle enzymes, creatinine, and hepatic transaminases. Electromyography and nerve conduction studies suggested a myopathy and a mild polyneuropathy. Colchicine was withdrawn, but the severe muscle pain continued. The dose of ciclosporin was then reduced

and 7 days later the weakness and muscle pain disappeared and the laboratory findings improved markedly.

This clinical course suggested that the pathogenesis of neuromyopathy in this case was closely related to either colchicine or ciclosporin.

Myositis occurred in a kidney recipient taking ciclosporin, mycophenolate mofetil, and prednisolone (219).

- A 60-year-old man developed acute polymyositis 4 weeks after receiving a complete HLA mismatch cadaveric renal transplant. Immunosuppression consisted of ciclosporin, mycophenolate mofetil, and prednisolone. The patient developed severe symmetrical proximal muscle weakness associated with a rise in serum creatine kinase to 46 800 U/l. Electromyography confirmed the myopathic changes and muscle biopsy showed extensive muscle fiber necrosis with an inflammatory infiltrate. Viral studies were negative. Prompt initiation of high-dose glucocorticoid therapy led to clinical and biochemical recovery.

This rare complication following kidney transplantation is most commonly the result of drug-mediated myotoxicity.

- A 33-year-old man with severe psoriasis, poorly controlled with calcipotriol, corticosteroids, tar and dithranol, and acitretin was given ciclosporin 3mg/kg/day. After 5 months his blood pressure started to increase and the dose of ciclosporin was reduced to 1.5 mg/kg/day (220). He then began to have severe pain in his legs and back and was having difficulty getting out of bed or chair and in raising his arms above his head. He had severe proximal muscle weakness in his shoulders and pelvis. Peripheral muscle power was good. There were no sensory abnormalities and his cranial nerves were normal. Electromyography confirmed myopathic changes, with an excess of short-duration action potentials. Ciclosporin was withdrawn and within 7 days his pain and weakness began to improve. A quadriceps muscle biopsy 2 weeks after the withdrawal of ciclosporin showed no evidence of mitochondrial abnormalities or type II fibre atrophy. After months his muscle strength was normal.

Bone and joints

Ciclosporin is increasingly cited as a possible cause of severe bone and joint pain (221). Acute bilateral deep bone pain, mostly involving the legs, has been retrospectively identified in 19% of patients taking ciclosporin, with the highest prevalence in renal transplant recipients (222). In addition, about half of the patients with osteonecrosis had a history of episodic bone pains. Another study showed features of acute bone marrow edema on MRI in six patients who had bone pain, including one patient who further developed avascular necrosis (SEDA-21, 385). Calcium channel blockers dramatically improved bone pain in prospectively evaluated transplant patients, suggesting a possible vascular etiology (222).

Before kidney transplantation 31 of 82 patients (38%) had joint pain and 17 of 82 (21%) after transplantation

(223). Six (7.3%) and three (3.7%) patients developed arthritis before and after transplantation. Joint pain significantly correlated with serum ciclosporin concentrations over 200 ng/ml.

Osteopenia is another potential adverse effect after renal transplantation, but the possible contribution of ciclosporin to bone loss and subsequent osteoporosis is controversial (SEDA-19, 350; SEDA-20, 345). Moreover, ciclosporin did not appear to have a negative influence on post-transplantation growth in prepubertal children (224).

Both ciclosporin and tacrolimus cause increased bone turnover and significant reductions in bone mass, more marked with tacrolimus (FK506). As most transplantation regimens include glucocorticoids, the individual effects of ciclosporin and tacrolimus are uncertain. As tacrolimus is the more potent immunosuppressant, theoretically, its use after transplantation should allow reduction in glucocorticoid doses, which would be associated with higher bone mineral density. Preliminary data suggest that there is a lower rate of vertebral fractures in patients taking tacrolimus compared with those taking ciclosporin. In 18 men who underwent liver transplantation and took ciclosporin and seven patients who took tacrolimus, bone mineral density in the lumbar spine and proximal femur was prospectively measured before and at 6, 12, and 24 months after transplantation (225). Serum concentrations of parathyroid hormone and 25-hydroxycolecalciferol were determined at the same time. Although the two groups had the same pattern of rapid early bone loss, tacrolimus was associated with lower doses of glucocorticoids and a trend to faster lumbar bone mass recovery. This may have a favorable effect on long-term bone mass evolution, especially in the femoral neck.

Bone metabolism has been studied in rats who were fed a powdered diet containing or lacking ciclosporin for 8–30 days (226). Analyses were performed on days 8, 16, and 30. There was a reduction in bone volume in the rats who were fed ciclosporin after day 16. Histology showed that the number of osteoblasts and osteoclasts on the surface of trabecular bone in the ciclosporin-treated group had increased significantly. Plasma parathormone and osteocalcin concentrations were also significantly higher. However, in a clinical study ciclosporin was not associated with an increased risk of fractures (see under azathioprine below).

Breasts

Benign mammary hyperplasia occurs in 0.7% of women taking ciclosporin (227). The mechanism is poorly understood, but it may be related to trophic effects in the breast through ciclosporin receptors on fibroblasts (228), to an effect of ciclosporin on the hypothalamic-pituitary axis (229), or to antagonism at prolactin receptor sites on B and T (230,231).

It has also been suggested that ciclosporin acts on breast fibroblasts by humoral mechanisms and a direct action (168).

Bilateral fibroadenomas were detected in four female kidney recipients taking ciclosporin (232). Symptomatic giant fibroadenomas required bilateral mammoplasty in one patient, while the size of the breasts significantly regressed in three patients after conversion to tacrolimus. Awareness of the association between ciclosporin and fibroadenomas in transplant patients might avoid unnecessary surgical procedures (232,233).

Multiple or bilateral fibroadenomas were detected in 13 of 29 ciclosporin-treated female kidney recipients (age under 55 years), while all 10 female recipients taking glucocorticoids and azathioprine had no abnormal breast findings (168). Serum estradiol concentrations were raised in the women with fibroadenomas compared with those with normal breasts, and the FSH concentration was lower.

In another series, 22 breast fibroadenomas were detected in 10 of 486 female kidney recipients taking ciclosporin and prednisolone (234). These 10 patients were compared with 100 women with fibroadenomas who had never undergone transplantation or immunosuppressive therapy. After kidney transplantation, eight patients had multiple fibroadenomas (mean diameter 4.2 cm), and seven were affected bilaterally. The histopathological features of the lesions were generally typical of fibroadenomas, but some were more typical of malignant lesions. The 100 control patients had 146 fibroadenomas. There were multiple lesions (mean diameter 2.1 cm) in 33 patients and 12 were affected bilaterally. Fibroadenomas in female ciclosporin-treated kidney recipients tend to occur multiply and bilaterally and to be of larger diameter than in control patients. The fibroadenomas also had some imaging features that differed from those of typical fibroadenomas; sonographically, the lesions were relatively highly echogenic and had a lower longitudinal to anteroposterior diameter ratio than those in the control group. The control group included 100 women with fibroadenomas who had never undergone organ transplantation or immunosuppressive therapy.

Fibroadenomata are the most common solid breast masses in young women. Between 1997 and 2000, five women who had had transplant surgery and who were taking ciclosporin developed new breast masses, which were histologically confirmed to be fibroadenomata (235).

Immunologic

Anaphylactoid reactions can occur with intravenous ciclosporin, sometimes after the first dose. Reported symptoms included pruritic rash, respiratory symptoms, chest pain, and, rarely, cardiopulmonary arrest. The presence of Cremophor EL, polyoxyethylated castor oil used as a solvent, is likely to account for this life-threatening reaction. The mechanism is still unclear, and results of skin tests were available in only three of 22 previously published patients.

In a report of an anaphylactic reaction, positive intradermal tests suggested a possible IgE-mediated reaction, most probably directed against Cremophor EL, as the patient subsequently tolerated the corn-oil-based soft gelatin formulation (236).

During a Phase I/II trial of high-dose intravenous ciclosporin, there was a high incidence of anaphylactoid reactions associated with improper mixing during preparation of the infusions, perhaps due to large initial bolus infusions of the vehicle, Cremophor EL (237).

Infection risk

Infections, in particular bacterial and viral (cytomegalovirus, *Herpes simplex* virus, Epstein–Barr virus), and also protozoal and fungal infections, are major causes of morbidity and mortality after transplantation, whatever the immunosuppressive regimen used (238–240). Based on an analysis of medical and autopsy records, infections were found to be the cause of death in 70% of transplant patients, with bacteria (50%) or fungi (29%) the most common pathogens (241).

- A patient with severe aplastic anemia developed hepatitis B virus reactivation on recovery from lymphopenia after ciclosporin and antithymocyte globulin therapy (242).

The phenomenon observed in this case supports the prevailing notion that hepatitis B flare-up in hepatitis B virus carriers after chemotherapy is caused by an immune-mediated mechanism. Pre-emptive therapy with lamivudine is recommended in SAA/HBsAg(+) patients who receive ciclosporin and antithymocyte globulin.

- A man with severe aplastic anemia and chronic hepatitis B virus infection (HbsAg(+), HBeAg(+), HBV-DNA wild-type) received ciclosporin and antithymocyte globulin (242). The patient developed lymphopenia over 1 and 2.5 months in response to antithymocyte globulin infusion and ciclosporin. Serum alanine transaminase activity normalized during lymphopenia, but serum hepatitis B viral load increased. The alanine transaminase rose again when his peripheral lymphocyte count recovered. Lamivudine normalized the raised alanine transaminase and suppressed viral replication.

Cryptococcus albidus, a non-neoformans species of the genus *Cryptococcus*, is generally regarded as a rare cause of disease. Previously, this organism has been isolated as a pathogen in only 14 cases, but disseminated *Cryptococcus albidus* infection has been reported in a renal transplant recipient (243).

- A 23-year-old male renal transplant recipient taking ciclosporin and prednisolone developed a dry cough, fever, and progressive dyspnea. After 11 days his respiratory status deteriorated dramatically and he developed acute respiratory distress syndrome (ARDS) and fulminant septic shock. A week later tender macules on both of his shins coalesced to form erythematous patches. *Cryptococcus albidus* was isolated by skin biopsy and tissue culture. Thereafter, the patient was successfully treated with fluconazole monotherapy.

Body temperature

Recurrent episodes of fever, which disappeared after ciclosporin withdrawal, have only been reported in one patient (SEDA-22, 414).

Long-Term Effects

Mutagenicity

An increase in chromosomal abnormalities correlated with serum ciclosporin concentrations in one study (244).

Tumorigenicity

Because of the varied indications for azathioprine and mercaptopurine, it is difficult to determine whether there is an increased incidence of cancer specifically related to prolonged drug exposure. Data from the Cincinnati Transplant Tumor Registry, published in 1993, helped to define comprehensively the characteristics of neoplasms observed in organ transplant recipients (245). Skin and lip cancers were the most common, and non-Hodgkin's lymphomas represent the majority of lymphoproliferative disorders, with an incidence some 30- to 50-fold higher than in controls. There is also an excess of Kaposi's sarcomas (246), carcinomas of the vulva and perineum, hepatobiliary tumors, various sarcomas, and renal cell carcinomas (247–249). In one case, complete regression of Kaposi's sarcoma followed withdrawal of ciclosporin (250). In contrast, the incidence of common neoplasms encountered in the general population is not increased. In renal transplant patients, the actuarial cumulative risk of cancer was 14–18% at 10 years and 40–50% at 20 years (251,252). Skin cancers accounted for about half of the cases. Very similar figures were found in later studies (SEDA-20, 341).

In patients with transplanted organs ciclosporin is associated with a small but significant risk of Epstein–Barr virus-associated lymphoproliferative disorders.

- A 61-year-old woman developed an anaplastic CD30+ cutaneous T cell lymphoma while taking ciclosporin for recalcitrant psoriasis (253). Two months after withdrawal the lymphoma resolved clinically and histologically. Three years later extracutaneous involvement of the lymphoma was detected.

It is not clear in this case whether the association between ciclosporin and the lymphoma was casual.

The association between Epstein–Barr virus and lymphoma in patients taking immunosuppressive drugs has been well described. Recently, an Epstein–Barr virus-negative lymphoma developed in a ciclosporin-treated patient with refractory anemia (254).

- A 70-year-old man developed pancytopenia. Bone marrow examination confirmed the diagnosis of refractory anemia. Ciclosporin 3.3 mg/kg/day was begun. He complained of epigastralgia 21 months later, and gastric endoscopic examination showed an ulcer with a cleaved bank. Biopsy showed a diffuse large B cell lymphoma without Epstein–Barr virus analysed by in situ hybridization. Ciclosporin was withdrawn and gastrectomy was performed 31 days later. Histologically, there were no abnormal B cells in the resected stomach. The spontaneous remission observed after withdrawal of ciclosporin treatment suggests that immunosuppressive therapy can be a pathogenic factor in a subset of Epstein–Barr virus-negative lymphomas.

- A 39-year-old man with atopic eczema was given ciclosporin for an exacerbation, which responded well (255). After 2 years he developed a large ulcerated erythematous nodule, a CD30+ lymphoma of the skin. Ciclosporin was withdrawn and the lesion resolved within 2 months.

Of all transplant-related lymphomas 15% are of T cell origin and are unrelated to Epstein–Barr virus infection. Cutaneous T cell lymphomas are rare and carry a good prognosis, with a 90%, 4-year survival rate. Regression is often observed when immunosuppression is withdrawn or reduced.

While there is no doubt that the incidence of malignancies is increased in the transplant population, there has been controversy as to which factors (namely duration of treatment, total dosage, the degree of immunosuppression, or the type of immunosuppressive regimens) are the most relevant in determining risk. Partial or complete regression of lymphoproliferative disorders and Kaposi's sarcomas after reduction of immunosuppressive therapy argues strongly for the role of the degree of immunosuppression (244). The incidence of cancer was also significantly higher in renal transplant patients taking triple therapy regimens compared with dual therapy (256). Similarly, aggressive immunosuppressive therapy may account for the higher incidence of lymphomas in patients with cardiac versus renal allografts.

In a large, multicenter study in more than 52 000 kidney or heart transplant patients between 1983 and 1991, the rate of non-Hodgkin's lymphomas in the first post-transplantation year was 0.2% in kidney and 1.2% in heart recipients, and fell substantially thereafter (257). Initial immunosuppression with azathioprine and ciclosporin, and prophylactic treatment with antilymphocyte antibodies or muromonab was associated with a significantly increased incidence of non-Hodgkin's lymphomas compared with other immunosuppressive regimens, which confirmed the major role of the level of immunosuppression. Later studies confirmed that immunosuppression per se rather than a single agent is responsible for the increased risk of cancer (SEDA-20, 340). Finally, the most striking difference between conventional and modern immunosuppressive regimens, including ciclosporin, was the average time to the appearance of tumors, in particular skin cancers and lymphomas, which was shorter in ciclosporin-treated patients (258,259).

Multiple factors with complex interactions are involved in the observed pattern and increased incidence of neoplasms. They include severely depressed immunity with an impaired immune surveillance against various carcinogens, the activation of several oncogenic viruses, and a possible mutagenic effect of the drugs. Viruses, such as papillomavirus, cytomegalovirus, and Epstein–Barr virus, are believed to play an important role in the development of several post-transplant cancers. From a theoretical point of view, the use of antiviral drugs active against herpes viruses which are commonly implicated as co-factors can be expected to produce a reduction in the incidence of post-transplant lymphoproliferative disorders.

The molecular effects that lead to the genesis of de novo malignancies during ciclosporin therapy are inhibition of DNA repair, synthesis of TGF-beta, induction of apoptosis of activated T cells, and inhibition of apoptosis through the inhibition of the opening of the mitochondrial permeability transition pore. Ciclosporin can promote the genesis and spread of cancer, not only because of immunosuppression but also because of its ability to facilitate the accumulation of DNA mutations, to reduce the clearance of altered cells, and to transform cancer cells into aggressive cancer cells (260).

In an in vitro and in vivo experiment, ciclosporin promoted tumor growth by a direct cellular effect (261). This was suggested to be due to increased synthesis of transforming growth factor beta (TGF beta); anti-TGF beta antibodies blocked the increased spread of cancer cells. The clinical relevance of these data awaits further careful clinical confirmation. Continuing analysis of clinical experience has not provided clear evidence for a ciclosporin-specific effect and has instead supported an immunosuppressive effect (262).

Ciclosporin-associated soft tissue proliferation with an abnormal hyperplastic reaction has been suggested to account for the development of eruptive angiomatosis (263).

A ciclosporin-treated kidney recipient developed a melanoma metastasis in the allograft (264).

- A 57-year-old female recipient of a cadaveric renal allograft took ciclosporin, azathioprine, and prednisone. The graft displayed normal renal function for 10 months after transplantation. However, she then developed multiple, large, rapidly growing skin nodules over the lower abdomen. There was metastatic melanoma within the graft and two focal points of melanoma within the skin lesions. She reverted to hemodialysis and received chemotherapy and interferon A, but failed to respond and died 11 days after nephrectomy.

Ciclosporin is effective in the treatment of psoriasis, but is associated with an increased risk of non-melanoma skin cancer, mainly squamous cell carcinoma, when patients have been previously exposed to psoralen-ultraviolet A (PUVA). However, the incidence of non-skin malignancies is not significantly different than in the general population (265). In contrast to transplant recipients, patients with autoimmune diseases tend to use lower doses of ciclosporin for shorter times. The current evidence suggests that the risk of cancer is not increased when ciclosporin is used in dermatological doses for less than 2 years in healthy patients who are not taking other immunosuppressants. Nevertheless, two patients developed an explosive basal cell carcinoma and keratoacanthoma within 3 months after starting to take ciclosporin for psoriasis (266). Neither had a history of skin cancer or had received PUVA therapy or additional immunosuppressive drugs.

For the association between ciclosporin and breast fibroadenomata see above under Breast.

Second-Generation Effects

Pregnancy

Pregnancies in women who took ciclosporin resulted in live neonates in 68%; half were premature while the other half were of low birth weights (267). Reduced renal graft function during pregnancy was associated with greater risks of neonates of lower birth weights and graft loss. In another study, a ciclosporin-based regimen was associated with more frequent miscarriage, preterm birth and intrauterine growth retardation, compared with previous experience (268).

It has been suggested that ciclosporin is more likely to induce maternal renal dysfunction or pre-eclampsia than tacrolimus, but this view was based on a comparison involving only a small number of patients (SEDA-22, 414).

- A woman had fulminant glucocorticoid-refractory ulcerative colitis during pregnancy and refused ciclosporin (269). After emergency cesarean section, she was given intravenous ciclosporin and 2 days later developed severe hypertension with hypertensive encephalopathy and seizures.

Ciclosporin in therapeutic concentrations after renal transplantation inhibits bile salt excretion pump function in rats and humans. Obstetric cholestasis leading to fetal distress and therefore to premature delivery has been reported (270).

Teratogenicity

Maternal azathioprine treatment during pregnancy is clearly teratogenic in animals, but the mechanisms are not known. A large number of reports have described the outcome of pregnancies following the use of immunosuppressant drugs, in particular in renal transplant patients, and hundreds of pregnancies have been analysed (271). The largest experience is that derived from the National Transplantation Pregnancy Registry which has been built up in the USA since 1991 (272). This registry has accumulated data on more than 900 pregnancies, of which 83% followed kidney transplantation and in this and other studies there was no difference in the rate of malformations when comparing ciclosporin with other immunosuppressive regimens (267,268,273). Ectopic pregnancies and miscarriages seemed to occur at a similar rate as in the general population. The most common complications were frequent prematurity and more frequent intrauterine growth retardation with low birthweight. Risk factors associated with adverse pregnancy outcomes included a short time interval between transplantation and pregnancy (that is less than 1–2 years), graft dysfunction before or during pregnancy, and hypertension (274).

There have been no reports that physical and mental development or renal function are altered. In one study, there were changes in T lymphocyte development in seven children born to mothers who had taken azathioprine or ciclosporin, but immune function assays were normal (275). Thus, development of the fetal immune system is not affected by ciclosporin (276).

Renal function in 14 children born to women with transplants treated throughout pregnancy with a ciclosporin-based regimen has been extensively investigated at a mean of 2.6 years after delivery (277). No renal function abnormalities were found. In particular, glomerular filtration rate was within the reference range. Renal function was found to be normal in 22 children evaluated after a mean of 39 months after birth (278), and no adverse effects on the immune function were identified in the few infants examined in this respect (275).

In a meta-analysis of the effects of exposure to ciclosporin during pregnancy, 15 studies (total 410 patients; 6 studies with control groups who were not given ciclosporin) met inclusion criteria for malformations, 10 for preterm delivery, and five for low birth weight (279). Ciclosporin did not appear to be a major human teratogen, but was associated with increased rates of prematurity.

Lactation

Ciclosporin is excreted into human breast milk and because of potential immunosuppression, breastfeeding is usually regarded as contraindicated. Reassuring reports are now however available (SEDA-21, 385). After follow-up for 12–36 months in seven breast-fed infants (duration 4–12 months) whose mothers were treated with ciclosporin, none of them experienced renal or other long-term adverse consequences (280). Although ciclosporin concentrations measured in breast milk from six mothers were close to those measured in blood samples, it was calculated that the infants ingested less than 300 µg/day, and ciclosporin was not detectable in random blood samples.

Susceptibility Factors

Genetic

African-American kidney transplant recipients have poorer long-term clinical outcomes and graft survival than Caucasian patients (281). Ethnic differences in the pharmacokinetics of immunosuppressants are potentially a key factor. Ciclosporin, tacrolimus, sirolimus, and everolimus all have ethnic-specific differences in systemic availability and/or dose-adjusted systemic exposure. The oral systemic availability of these drugs in African-Americans was 20–50% lower than in Caucasians or non-African-Americans, leading to higher dosage requirements in African-Americans to maintain similar average concentrations. All four drugs undergo extensive metabolism and are substrates for CYP3A4 and CYP3A5 as well as MDR1.

Hepatitis infection

Although the use of immunosuppression is controversial in hepatitis C positive patients (282) (283), there was no difference between tacrolimus and ciclosporin in hepatitis

C positive patients in a randomized controlled trial of tacrolimus versus microemulsified ciclosporin in liver transplantation (284).

Drug Administration

Drug formulations

In an attempt to overcome the poor and unpredictable absorption of the standard oral formulation, a microemulsion-based formulation (Neoral) has been developed. The benefit-to-harm balance of conversion from the standard to the microemulsion formulation have been discussed at length and guidelines for conversion have been proposed (285).

From the results of a retrospective study of 227 liver transplant patients who took Neoral as the primary immunosuppressant, it was suggested that this formulation may reduce the risk of severe neurotoxicity (286). Mild-to-moderate symptoms, that is headache ($n = 24$), mild hand tremor ($n = 13$), and paresthesia ($n = 5$), were the most frequent, whereas generalized seizures were reported in only two patients.

In one large study in 1097 patients, there was a significantly higher incidence of neurological complications, gastrointestinal disturbances, and increased serum creatinine concentrations during the first month of treatment with Neoral, compared with conventional ciclosporin (287). However, a meta-analysis showed that the adverse events profile was similar with the two formulations, while primary immunosuppression with Neoral produced significant benefit in terms of a lower incidence of rejection (288). In particular, in liver transplant patients treated with Neoral from the start, the incidence of adverse events was halved. All the same, because dosage adjustments were often required and often hazardous, owing to the risk of adverse effects and transplant rejection, other investigators concluded that switching to Neoral may be of little benefit, at least in previously stable liver transplant patients (289).

As the data from this meta-analysis were subject to many potential biases, the same authors reanalysed their results, taking into account only randomized, prospective studies (290). The incidence of adverse effects was higher with Sandimmune in open-label studies (840 patients) and higher with Neoral in blinded studies (3006 patients). In accordance with other investigators, these authors concluded that de novo immunosuppression with Neoral is beneficial, without significant differences in the incidence of adverse effects, whereas conversion from Sandimmune to Neoral in previously stable patients is associated with significantly more adverse effects with Neoral.

Drug dosage regimens

Several authors were unable to find convincing evidence that ciclosporin specifically increases the risk of tumors in transplant patients compared with previously used immunosuppressive regimens, and some even suggested a possibly lower incidence in ciclosporin-treated patients

(258,259,291). However, in analyses from Japan and France (3454 patients), the average time that elapsed until the occurrence of cancer was significantly shorter in patients treated with ciclosporin compared with those taking conventional immunosuppressive treatment, that is 43–452 months versus 92–96 months (292,293). In addition, French authors found a higher cumulative risk of cancer after 10 years in ciclosporin-treated patients (14 versus 8.4%), and this was mostly due to an increased incidence of skin carcinomas (292). Other significant risk factors included age, a shorter duration of pretransplant dialysis and the combination with azathioprine treatment. The occurrence of cancer in ciclosporin-treated patients is thought to be dose-related, and one study found a significantly higher frequency of cancer in the normal than in the low-dose group (294). These positive findings were limited by the more frequent occurrence of acute rejection in the low-dose group.

Long-term ciclosporin also carries the risk of malignancies in non-transplant patients, and the overall incidence of lymphoma was estimated to be 0.14% among 3700 patients treated for autoimmune disease (295). However, the available studies are again conflicting. They are mostly based on a limited number of patients or a short duration of follow-up. Patients with rheumatoid arthritis receiving ciclosporin had an increased relative risk of malignancies compared with those given glucocorticoids, but it was similar to the risk in patients treated with disease-modifying antirheumatic drugs (296). Another study showed no increased risk of malignancies in ciclosporin-treated patients compared with controls who had never received ciclosporin (297). The spontaneous occurrence of cancers unrelated to the treatment cannot be excluded, and an increased risk of lymphomas has been repeatedly found in patients with rheumatoid arthritis. In patients with psoriasis and as compared to the expected incidence rate of cancer in this population, the relative risk of malignancies was 5.6 (95% CI = 3.9, 8.0) in a cohort of 1223 ciclosporin-treated patients (298). This was comparable to the increased risk of cancer in patients treated with other immunosuppressants.

Ciclosporin is commonly administered twice daily. A comparison of once and twice daily dosing after kidney transplantation (n = 54) showed higher AUCs with once daily dosing than with twice daily dosing, but there were no differences in survival and rejection rates (299). Once daily dosing tended to be associated with lower mean serum creatinine at 1 year after transplantation.

Drug overdose

Experience with ciclosporin overdose has been reviewed by the manufacturers using published data or cases spontaneously reported (300). Accidental overdose was the most common, with doses of 20–400 mg/kg. In adults, no serious clinical consequences were observed with doses up to 100 mg/kg, and there were only minor clinical or biological effects (transient hypertension, tachycardia, headache, gastrointestinal symptoms, or slight increases in serum creatinine concentrations). However, life-threatening reactions occurred in three neonates, of whom one died after severe metabolic acidosis and renal insufficiency. Subchronic ciclosporin overdose over 8 days did not appear to cause any additional risk (301).

Taken together, the available data suggest that the acute toxicity of ciclosporin is low in adults, but that more severe intoxication could be expected in neonates. However, two reports, including one fatal case, have shown that accidental intoxication sometimes produces severe complications in adults (302,303).

- A 29-year-old man received a double lung transplantation for end-stage cystic fibrosis. After uneventful surgery, he was accidentally given ten times the intended dose of ciclosporin (30 instead of 3 mg/kg) and 18 hours later became anuric. His blood ciclosporin concentration was 4100 ng/ml. Hemodialysis was required for 6 weeks. A renal biopsy 7 weeks later showed typical features of acute tubular necrosis and lesions that resembled chronic nephrotoxicity. Renal function was still abnormal when he died from another cause 14 weeks after the accidental overdose.
- A 51-year-old man underwent double lung transplantation for pulmonary fibrosis, accidentally received an infusion of ciclosporin 30 mg/hour instead of 3 mg/hour, and 3 hours later had bilateral reactive mydriasis and absence of tendon reflexes. A CT brain scan showed diffuse cerebral edema, and massive intracranial hypertension rapidly developed. He died 5 hours later from brainstem compression, and pathological examination showed diffuse cerebral edema with neuronal necrosis.

The first of these cases suggested that acute renal dysfunction secondary to acute overdose can lead to renal sequelae. In the second patient, an isolated neurotoxic effect of ciclosporin was suggested because no predisposing factor except overdose was identified.

Drug–Drug Interactions

Acetazolamide

The interaction of ciclosporin with acetazolamide was previously supported by a single case report only. In three further patients, the addition of acetazolamide produced a near seven-fold increase in ciclosporin blood concentrations within 3 days (304).

Aciclovir

In an analysis of changes in ciclosporin clearance and systemic availability obtained from the medical records of 100 transplant patients, aciclovir altered ciclosporin pharmacokinetics (305).

The coadministration of ciclosporin with drugs with nephrotoxic effects carries a risk of increased renal dysfunction. Although a possible enhancement of nephrotoxicity has been suggested in patients also taking aciclovir (306), there were no such findings in a retrospective analysis of a double-blind study (307).

Aminoglycoside antibiotics

Severe nephrotoxicity has been reported in three renal transplant patients who received ciclosporin and gentamicin, and in others receiving both drugs before surgical procedures, even though toxic serum concentrations of either drug were not reached (308).

Amisulpride

The antipsychotic drug amisulpride is a substrate of P glycoprotein. Co-administration of ciclosporin in rats resulted in a larger and significantly longer antipsychotic effect, with higher amisulpride AUC in serum and brain; renal clearance was not affected (309). amisulpride is not metabolized by rat liver and so this interaction was probably caused by inhibition of P glycoprotein.

Angiotensin receptor blockers

In an analysis of changes in ciclosporin clearance and systemic availability obtained from the medical records of 100 transplant patients, losartan and valsartan altered ciclosporin pharmacokinetics (305).

Antiretroviral drugs

Reduced clearance of ciclosporin has been attributed to antiretroviral drugs (310).

- A 45-year-old man taking lamivudine, tenofovir, enfuvirtide, and amprenavir boosted with ritonavir was stable and underwent orthotopic liver transplantation from a cadaveric donor. Immunosuppression was induced with ciclosporin and steroids. The dosage of ciclosporin was 200–350 mg bd with ciclosporin blood concentrations of 200–300 ng/ml. Antiretroviral therapy was restarted and the ciclosporin trough concentration rose to more than 1000 ng/ml. The dosage of ciclosporin had to be reduced to 25 mg bd.
- A 43-year-old man with HIV infection taking tenofovir, lamivudine, and fosamprenavir was stable and underwent orthotopic liver transplantation. Immunosuppression was started using ciclosporin 250–350 mg bd to maintain blood concentrations at 300–400 ng/ml. On day 12 HAART was resumed with fosamprenavir 1400 mg bd, lamivudine, and tenofovir. After 48 hours, the ciclosporin concentration rose from 400 to 600 ng/ml. The dosage of ciclosporin had to be reduced to 100 mg bd.

The authors concluded that the combination of amprenavir + ritonavir had a greater effect on ciclosporin clearance than fosamprenavir.

Highly active antiretroviral therapy (HAART) improves life expectancy in HIV-infected patients. With ritonavir-boosted HAART, ciclosporin concentrations showed markedly altered absorption/elimination characteristics, with more or less constant blood concentrations throughout the dosing interval and prolongation of the half-life up to 38 hours (311). Daily ciclosporin doses were reduced to 5–20% of the individual standard doses given before initiation of ritonavir to obtain an equivalent ciclosporin AUC.

Bisphosphonates

In an analysis of changes in ciclosporin clearance and systemic availability obtained from the medical records of 100 transplant patients, alendronic acid altered ciclosporin pharmacokinetics (305).

Calcium channel blockers

A large amount of data has accumulated on the effects of various calcium channel blockers on ciclosporin metabolism or a possible renal protective effect. Diltiazem, nicardipine, or verapamil inhibit ciclosporin metabolism, and this has been investigated as a potential beneficial combination for ciclosporin-sparing effects, particularly for diltiazem or verapamil (312,313). Any change in the formulation of calcium channel blockers in patients previously stabilized should be undertaken cautiously because unpredictable changes in ciclosporin concentrations can occur (314). In contrast, nifedipine, isradipine, or felodipine do not significantly affect ciclosporin pharmacokinetics (SED-13, 1129). Results obtained with amlodipine are conflicting; some studies have shown no effect, while others indicate an increase of up to 40% in ciclosporin blood concentrations (SEDA-19, 351; SEDA-20, 345). Co-administration of calcium channel blockers is also regarded as a valuable option in the treatment of ciclosporin-induced hypertension, or to prevent ciclosporin nephrotoxicity.

There are conflicting results from studies on the protective role of calcium channel blockers in patients taking ciclosporin in regard to blood pressure and preservation of renal graft function. In a multicenter, randomized, placebo-controlled study in 131 de novo recipients of cadaveric renal allografts, lacidipine improved graft function from 1 year onwards, but had no effect on acute rejection rate, trough blood ciclosporin concentrations, blood pressure, number of antihypertensive drugs, hospitalization rate, or rate of adverse events (315).

The combination of ciclosporin with nifedipine produces an additive on gingival hyperplasia, with an increased prevalence and/or severity (SED-13, 1127) in both children (109,113) and adults (76,80,82). In contrast, verapamil had no significant additional effects on the prevalence or severity of ciclosporin-induced gingival overgrowth (SEDA-21, 385).

Chloramphenicol

Chloramphenicol was suspected of causing a dramatic increase in ciclosporin blood concentrations in a single patient (316). However, multiple concomitant confounding factors made this interaction purely speculative.

Clindamycin

In two lung-transplant patients aged 39 and 48 years, blood ciclosporin concentrations fell after the addition of oral clindamycin (1.8 g/day), and both patients required temporary increases in daily ciclosporin dose until clindamycin withdrawal (317).

Colchicine

The combination of colchicine with ciclosporin increases the risk of myopathy. In a retrospective study of 221 renal transplant patients, five of 10 patients who took both drugs developed acute or chronic proximal myopathy, whereas none of the 30 controls matched for age, sex, transplant duration, ciclosporin use, and cumulative dose of glucocorticoids had similar symptoms (318).

Multiorgan failure has been described in cases of colchicine poisoning and in patients after taking usual doses of colchicine during ciclosporin therapy after kidney transplantation.

- A renal transplant recipient developed multiorgan failure after taking appropriate doses of colchicine in combination with ciclosporin (319). An interaction between colchicine and ciclosporin was postulated, but ciclosporin toxicity was excluded because of low ciclosporin blood trough concentrations before and throughout the episode, in the presence of relatively stable renal function.

Cytotoxic drugs

High-dose chemotherapy with cyclophosphamide, vincristine, prednisolone, and intrathecal methotrexate given for post-transplant lymphoproliferative disease was suggested to have favored the occurrence of acute ciclosporin neurotoxicity (headache, fever, seizures, and visual agnosia) in a 9-year-old cardiac transplant patient (320). Ciclosporin serum concentrations were normal and a further similar episode occurred on ciclosporin readministration.

In 27 patients, ciclosporin caused a marked increase in the AUC of idarubicin and its main metabolite idarubicinol, perhaps due to inhibition of the multidrug transporter P-glycoprotein (321).

There was a dramatic increase in the systemic availability of paclitaxel when ciclosporin was administered concomitantly (322) and in a phase I study of the pharmacokinetics of twice-daily oral paclitaxel 60–160 mg/m^2 in 15 patients in combination with ciclosporin (15 mg/kg) there was a seven-fold increase in the systemic exposure to paclitaxel; the plasma concentration increased from negligible to therapeutic concentrations (323). The inhibitory effect of ciclosporin on the gastrointestinal multidrug transporter P-glycoprotein was suggested to account for these interactions.

Several studies have shown that ciclosporin reduces the clearance or increases the AUC of dactinomycin, etoposide, mitoxantrone, and vincristine (5,324).

Digoxin

In an analysis of changes in ciclosporin clearance and systemic availability obtained from the medical records of 100 transplant patients, digoxin increased ciclosporin systemic availability (305).

Doxorubicin

High-dose ciclosporin increased the AUC of doxorubicin and doxorubicinol and produced greater doxorubicin-related myelotoxicity (325).

Etoposide

Ciclosporin inhibits P glycoprotein and increases the cytotoxicity of some anticancer drugs, including etoposide. In rats, ciclosporin caused higher tissue concentrations of etoposide as a direct consequence of higher plasma concentrations resulting from a reduced clearance of etoposide rather than as a consequence of changes in the tissue distribution of etoposide (326).

Fibrates

A possible synergistic risk of muscle disorders should be considered in patients taking ciclosporin with fibric acid derivatives (SEDA-19, 351).

Fluoroquinolones

Although ciprofloxacin was initially thought to increase ciclosporin blood concentrations and enhance ciclosporin nephrotoxicity, no definite evidence to support this interaction has been found (327). A norfloxacin-induced increase in ciclosporin blood concentrations has been reported in children (5,248), while ofloxacin did not appear to alter ciclosporin metabolism (329).

Foscarnet

Foscarnet (330), but not ganciclovir (331), has also been involved in reversible renal insufficiency after concomitant use with ciclosporin.

Grapefruit juice

Following the observation that grapefruit juice ingestion can increase the systemic bioavailability of ciclosporin, there was considerable interest in its possible use to reduce ciclosporin doses (SEDA-19, 351). However, this has been strongly criticized and considered hazardous because of large interindividual variability and the commercial availability of different formulations of grapefruit juice with potentially different effects on ciclosporin pharmacokinetics (332).

Histamine H₂ receptor antagonists

The available data on a possible interaction between histamine H_2 receptor antagonists and ciclosporin are inconclusive. Whereas neither cimetidine nor ranitidine significantly altered ciclosporin pharmacokinetics, there was an increase in serum creatinine concentration in patients taking both ciclosporin and cimetidine, but not ranitidine. The clinical significance of this interaction is probably limited, and it has been attributed to competition of cimetidine with creatinine for tubular secretion (333).

HMG-CoA reductase inhibitors

Dosages of statins should be reduced in patients taking ciclosporin, because of pharmacodynamic and pharmacokinetic interactions.

Pharmacodynamic interactions

Patients taking ciclosporin with conventional dosages of lovastatin or simvastatin can develop acute muscle toxicity (SED-14, 1296) (SEDA-19, 351). Among 110 ciclosporin-treated patients with heart transplants, four of 18 patients taking simvastatin 20 mg/day developed rhabdomyolysis, whereas none of the patients taking simvastatin 10 mg/day (26 patients) or pravastatin 20 mg/day (66 patients) had similar symptoms (334). Inhibition of CYP3A by ciclosporin was the most likely mechanism. In another study, there was a five-fold higher AUC of lovastatin (10 mg/day for 10 days) in 16 patients taking ciclosporin compared with 13 patients not taking ciclosporin (335).

- The addition of atorvastatin (10 mg/day) to a multidrug regimen including ciclosporin in a 40-year-old patient with a renal transplant resulted in rhabdomyolysis within 2 months (336).

Similar interactions are expected with other HMG-CoA reductase inhibitors such as cerivastatin and rosuvastatin.

Pharmacokinetic interactions

Plasma concentrations of lovastatin- or simvastatin-active metabolites were increased in several patients and in a pharmacokinetic study, suggesting that ciclosporin can inhibit their metabolism (337–339). Lower doses of lovastatin and simvastatin can be safely administered (340). Fluvastatin or pravastatin may offer some advantages, as no significant drug interactions have been documented with ciclosporin, at least for pravastatin (341).

From an analysis of changes in ciclosporin clearance and systemic availability obtained from the medical records of 100 transplant patients, atorvastatin, fluvastatin, pravastatin, and simvastatin were found to affect ciclosporin pharmacokinetics (305).

In a study of the safety and efficacy of simvastatin in hyperlipidemia after renal transplantation in 15 patients, the C_{max} and AUC of simvastatin were increased seven-fold by ciclosporin (342). In contrast, in 17 patients, tacrolimus had no effect. Although there were no complications, such as myopathy or rhabdomyolysis, creatine kinase activity must be monitored during co-administration of simvastatin and ciclosporin.

Ciclosporin produced a three- to five-fold increase in the plasma concentrations of cerivastatin and its metabolites in 12 patients with renal transplants who took cerivastatin 0.2 mg/day for 7 days compared with a single dose in 12 healthy controls (343).

Atorvastatin is metabolized by the same pathway as ciclosporin. In stable liver transplant recipients, atorvastatin co-administration increased ciclosporin AUC by 9% (range 0–21%) (344). There were no other significant changes in ciclosporin pharmacokinetics. One patient developed a two-fold increase in transaminases after 2 weeks of atorvastatin therapy.

- A 53-year-old renal transplant recipient taking ciclosporin, azathioprine, and prednisone developed rhabdomyolysis within 32 days of starting to take simvastatin (345). She had profound muscle pain and weakness, with a rise in serum creatine kinase to 60 000 IU/l and serum creatinine to 147 μmol/l. Simvastatin was withdrawn and the dose of ciclosporin reduced, and 10 days later she was asymptomatic, with serum creatine kinase 67 IU/l and serum creatinine within the reference range.

The mechanism of this interaction does not seem to be solely inhibition of CYP3A4; it probably also partly results from inhibition of statin transport in the liver (388). The suggested mechanism of the interaction of cerivastatin with ciclosporin is inhibition of transporter-mediated uptake of the statin in the liver, which is partly mediated by an organic anion transporting polypeptide-2 (346). Ciclosporin inhibits CYP3A4, P-glycoprotein, organic anion transporting polypeptide 1B1 (OATP1B1), and some other hepatic transporters. Gemfibrozil and its glucuronide inhibit CYP2C8 and OATP1B1. These effects explain the increased plasma statin concentrations and the increased risk of muscle toxicity when these drugs are co-administered with statins (347).

Hypericum perforatum (St. John's wort, Clusiaceae)

Hypericum perforatum (St. John's wort), which is used for mild depression, is an inducer of cytochrome P-450. It caused a rapid dramatic fall in ciclosporin blood concentrations, resulting in acute heart transplant rejection in two patients aged 61 and 63 years (348). It produces an average 50% reduction in ciclosporin blood concentrations (349). At least three other case reports have clearly confirmed that St. John's wort is dangerous in transplant patients, because it produced a rapid and dramatic reduction in blood ciclosporin concentration and resulted in acute organ rejection in two patients (350–352).

- A 44-year-old black woman with a living-related renal transplant had an acute rejection within 3 months and was given muromonab but was from then on stable. She was later given oral ciclosporin (Neoral 2 mg/kg bd), mycophenolate mofetil 1000 mg bd, and prednisolone 7.5 mg/day. Over 6 months her ciclosporin blood concentrations were consistently below the target concentration of 200 ng/ml. It was then discovered that she had also been taking 2–3 tablets/day of St. John's wort (Your Life, Leiner Health Products, Carson CA, 300 mg standardized to 0.3% hypericin). The St. John's wort was withdrawn and her blood ciclosporin concentrations reached the target within 2 weeks.
- A 29-year-old white woman with cadaveric kidney and pancreas transplants had two early rejection episodes but then stabilized on ciclosporin 100 mg bd and prednisolone 5 mg/day. Her blood ciclosporin concentration was consistently 200–350 ng/ml. She then started to take St. John's wort and over the next 30 days her blood ciclosporin concentration fell to 155 ng/ml and 3 weeks later to 97 ng/ml. Her serum creatinine rose to 1.3 mg/dl (115 μmol/l) and her serum amylase rose from a

baseline of 60–90 to 314 U/l; this was associated with abdominal pain. Renal biopsy confirmed acute rejection, which was treated. She subsequently developed chronic rejection, confirmed by renal biopsy.

The effects of a *Hypericum* extract 600 mg/day for 14 days on the pharmacokinetics and metabolism of ciclosporin have been investigated in an open study in 11 patients after kidney transplantation taking regular ciclosporin (353). After 2 weeks dose-corrected AUC_{0-12}, C_{max}, and C_{min} of ciclosporin fell significantly by 46%, 42%, and 41% respectively. Ciclosporin doses were increased from a median of 2.7 mg/kg/day at baseline to 4.2 mg/kg/day at day 15, and the first dose adjustment was required only 3 days after the start of treatment with St John's wort. Dose-corrected AUCs of the metabolites AM1, AM1c, and AM4N fell significantly by 59%, 61%, and 23% compared with baseline. The AUCs of AM9 and AM19 were unchanged. After the increase in ciclosporin dose, the AUC of AM9, AM19, and AM4N increased by 47, 51, and 20% and the C_{max} by 57, 90, and 43% respectively. These substantial alterations in the kinetics of the metabolites of ciclosporin caused by St John's wort could affect the toxicity of ciclosporin.

St John's wort (*Hypericum perforatum*) lowers the blood concentrations of ciclosporin and tacrolimus by inducing P glycoprotein and/or CYP3A4 (354). It has been suggested that hyperforin is the active compound that produces these interactions, and formulations containing high and low amounts of hyperforin have been studied in patient with kidney transplants (355). The $AUC_{0?12}$ of ciclosporin was 45% lower with high-hyperforin St John's wort co-medication than low-hyperforin St John's wort. The dose-corrected $AUC_{0?12}$ of ciclosporin fell significantly from baseline by 52% after 2 weeks of co-medication with high-hyperforin St John's wort. The peak plasma concentration and the concentration at the end of a dosing interval were similarly affected, with 43% and 55% reductions. In addition, a 65% increase in daily ciclosporin dose was required during high-hyperforin St John's wort treatment. In contrast, co-administration of low-hyperforin St John's wort did not significantly affect ciclosporin pharmacokinetics and did not require ciclosporin dose adjustments compared with baseline.

Data from 35 double-blind randomized trials showed that dropout and adverse effects rates in patients taking hypericum extracts were similar to placebo, lower than with older antidepressants, and slightly lower than with selective serotonin reuptake inhibitors (356). Dropout rates due to adverse effects in 17 observational studies including 35 562 patients were 0–5.7%. Interactions or serious adverse effects were not reported in any study.

An interaction of ciclosporin with a herbal tea containing St John's wort (*Hypericum perforatum*) has been reported (357).

Imidazoles

Among the imidazole derivatives, numerous case reports or studies have shown that ketoconazole, fluconazole, and itraconazole can inhibit ciclosporin metabolism and increase blood ciclosporin concentrations (358).

Itraconazole

After kidney transplantation, eight patients took itraconazole solution 400 mg/day over about 3 months in combination with ciclosporin (359). A 48% reduction in the mean total daily dose of ciclosporin was necessary to maintain target ciclosporin trough concentrations.

Ketoconazole

Ketoconazole, which is undoubtedly the most potent inhibitor, has been used to reduce the dose, and therefore the cost or adverse effects, of ciclosporin (360–362). There was also a beneficial effect on the rate of rejection or infection. In contrast, interactions with metronidazole and miconazole have only been described in isolated case histories (SEDA-19, 351) (5).

Voriconazole

The antifungal triazole voriconazole can interact with ciclosporin by inhibiting hepatic CYP450 metabolism. Ciclosporin trough concentrations should therefore be carefully monitored to allow dosage adjustment during and after concomitant voriconazole administration (363).

- A 14-year-old girl who was taking ciclosporin after bone marrow transplantation also took voriconazole as secondary antifungal prophylaxis. Temporary withdrawal of voriconazole because of worsening liver function tests resulted in a sudden fall in ciclosporin trough blood concentrations, which returned to baseline after normalization of the liver function tests and re-introduction of voriconazole.

In a double-blind, randomized, placebo-controlled study in renal transplant patients taking ciclosporin, voriconazole increased the mean ciclosporin AUC 1.7-fold (364). The authors therefore recommend halving the dose of ciclosporin in these patients and carefully monitoring ciclosporin blood concentrations.

Imipenem/cilastatin

In contrast to what has previously been stated, there was no significant increase in the frequency of seizures among 77 patients with bone marrow transplants who were taking ciclosporin alone (three seizures), 45 patients taking ciclosporin plus imipenem/cilastatin (two seizures), and 44 patients taking imipenem/cilastatin alone (no seizures) (365).

Inducers, inhibitors, or substrates of CYP3A

Ciclosporin is absorbed to a variable extent from the gastrointestinal tract and almost completely metabolized in both the liver and small intestine by CYP3A, which metabolizes a large number of drugs. Inducers, inhibitors, or substrates of CYP3A therefore have the potential to interact with ciclosporin. In addition, ciclosporin has wide pharmacokinetic variability and a narrow therapeutic index. Conversely, ciclosporin can inhibit the hepatic metabolism of other drugs that share the same CYP3A metabolic pathway.

Drugs that increase the systemic availability of ciclosporin do not always have negative effects, and several ciclosporin-sparing agents have indeed been used for the purpose of improving efficacy while reducing the cost of treatment. However, use of such combinations should be balanced against their potential risks (366).

Table 1 lists some drugs that have proven or possible clinically relevant drug interactions with ciclosporin.

Irinotecan

In 37 patients with fluorouracil-refractory metastatic colorectal cancer, irinotecan clearance was reduced from 13 to 5.8 l/h/m^2 and AUC$_{0-tn}$ was increased 2.2-fold by coadministration of ciclosporin 5 mg/kg bd for 3 days; the AUCs of the irinotecan metabolites SN38 and SN38G were increased 2.2-fold and 2.3-fold respectively (367).

Ciclosporin allowed an increase in the dose of irinotecan from 25 to 72 mg/m^2/week, and the addition of phenobarbital allowed an increase in dose to 144 mg/m^2 (368). Dose-limiting adverse effects were neutropenia and diarrhea. Irinotecan was well tolerated at the recommended phase II dose of 120 mg/m^2, with a 6% prevalence of grade 4 neutropenia and an 18% prevalence of grade 3 diarrhea. Ciclosporin increased the AUC of the metabolite 7-ethyl-10-hydroxycamptothecin (SN-38) by 23% to 630% and reduced irinotecan clearance by 39% to 64% when compared with historical controls. Phenobarbital increased irinotecan clearance by 27% and reduced the AUC of SN-38 by 75% compared with patients treated with ciclosporin alone.

Ketamine

Various neurological symptoms have been reported in liver transplant recipients taking ciclosporin. However, seizures in the perioperative period can be due to other factors. Many anesthetics have been reported to have both proconvulsant and anticonvulsant properties. Perioperative seizures occurred after liver transplantation in a child who was taking ciclosporin and who was given ketamine (369).

- A 6-year-old boy weighing 12 kg underwent living related left lateral segment liver transplantation for cryptogenic cirrhosis with portal hypertension. Immunosuppression consisted of microemulsion ciclosporin 10 mg/kg/day, azathioprine, and prednisolone. One month after transplantation, the transaminase activities rose, without derangement of other liver function tests. He was cheerful and spontaneously breathing with a respiratory rate of 18/minute (oxygen saturation 98–100% on air), accepting oral feeding, moving around, and febrile. For liver biopsy he was given intravenous ketamine 7 mg/kg and intramuscular glycopyrrolate 0.01 mg/kg. He developed generalized tonic–clonic seizures, which were treated with intravenous midazolam 1 mg and thiopental 60 mg. A CT scan on the day after the event did not show any abnormality.

In this case ketamine was given 2 hours after the last dose of ciclosporin, close to its t_{max}. Caution is therefore recommended when ketamine is given to patients who are taking ciclosporin.

Table 1 A summary of major interactions with ciclosporin

Pharmacokinetic	Pharmacodynamic
Anticonvulsants	**Increased risk of**
Carbamazepine*	**nephrotoxicity**
Phenobarbital*	ACE inhibitors
Phenytoin*	Aciclovir (see text)
Primidone*	Aminoglycosides
Antidepressants	Amphotericin
Fluoxetine (unproven; see text)	Co-trimoxazole
Fluvoxamine	Diuretics
Nefazodone	Foscarnet (see text)
St. John's wort	Melphalan
Antimicrobial drugs	Nafcillin (see text)
Antifungal drugs	NSAIDs (unproven, see
Ketoconazole, fluconazole,	text)
itraconazole, metronidazole	**Increased risk of muscle**
Chloramphenicol (unproven)	**toxicity (see text)**
Clindamycin*	Colchicine
Fluoroquinolones	Fibric acid derivatives
Griseofulvin*	HMG CoA reductase
Macrolides or related drugs	inhibitors (statins)
(see text)	Pyrazinamide (SEDA-20,
Clarithromycin, erythromycin,	346)
josamycin, midecamycin,	**Increased risk of gingival**
miocamycin, pristinamycin	**hyperplasia**
Protease inhibitors	Nifedipine
Ritonavir, saquinavir	**Increased risk of**
Pyrazinamide*	**neurotoxicity**
Quinupristin/dalfopristin	Imipenem/cilastatin
(SEDA-21, 386)	**Increased risk of**
Rifamycins*	**hepatotoxicity**
Sulfadiazine*	Androgens
Terbinafine* (SEDA-21, 386)	Norethandrolone,
Cardiovascular drugs	oxymetholone
Amiodarone	Parenteral nutrition (see
Calcium channel blockers	text)
Amlodipine, diltiazem,	**Increased risk of**
nicardipine, verapamil	**hyperkalemia**
Carvedilol (SEDA-22, 415)	Potassium salts
Clonidine	Potassium-sparing diuretics
Propafenone	
Hypoglycemic drugs	
Glibenclamide	
Glipizide	
Troglitazone*	
Miscellaneous drugs	
Acetazolamide	
Allopurinol	
Bezafibrate	
Bile acid resin*	
Chloroquine	
Danazol	
Glucocorticoids	
Grapefruit juice	
Modafinil*	
Muromonab (SEDA-21, 386)	
Octreotide*	
Oral contraceptives (unproven)	
Orlistat*	
Probucol*	
Sulfasalazine*	
Sulfinpyrazone*	
Tacrolimus	
Ticlopidine*	
Vitamin E (water-soluble) (SEDA-20, 346)	

*These drugs reportedly reduce ciclosporin blood concentrations; the rest increase them

Macrolide antibiotics

Erythromycin increases ciclosporin blood concentrations, and increased serum creatinine concentrations have been consistently demonstrated; isolated reports have also suggested possible interactions with clarithromycin, josamycin, midecamycin, or pristinamycin (SEDA-21, 385) (370). A two-fold increase in ciclosporin concentrations has been reported in patients receiving miocamycin. In contrast, spiramycin or roxithromycin did not significantly affect ciclosporin concentrations, and a single report involving azithromycin (SEDA-19, 351) was not substantiated by several prospective studies.

Methoxsalen

Methoxsalen causes a clinically significant interaction with ciclosporin in some susceptible individuals; the reasons for this susceptibility and its clinical implications have not been established (371).

Mycophenolate mofetil

The interaction of ciclosporin with mycophenolate mofetil was investigated in 52 renal transplant patients taking triple therapy (ciclosporin, mycophenolate mofetil, and prednisone), who continued taking the same treatment ($n = 19$) or underwent elective ciclosporin withdrawal ($n = 19$) or prednisolone withdrawal ($n = 14$) 6 months after transplantation (372). Median mycophenolate mofetil trough concentrations 3 months later were about two-fold higher in patients who had discontinued ciclosporin compared with patients who continued to take triple therapy and patients who had discontinued prednisone. No clear mechanism readily explains these changes.

Nefazodone

Nefazodone can alter blood ciclosporin concentrations (373,374). In one case there was nearly a 10-fold increase in whole-blood ciclosporin concentrations in a cardiac transplant patient shortly after the addition of nefazodone (375).

NSAIDs

Based on the theoretical possibility of additive nephrotoxic effects, the combined use of NSAIDs with ciclosporin is expected to reduce renal function and therefore to increase ciclosporin-induced nephrotoxicity.

- In an 8-year-old girl with rheumatoid arthritis, the combination of ciclosporin with NSAIDs (indometacin and diclofenac) was suggested to have caused biopsy-proven, non-specific colitis, because her symptoms occurred only when the combination was used (376).

From several studies performed in healthy volunteers, repeated doses of diclofenac, aspirin, indometacin, or piroxicam did not significantly alter ciclosporin single-dose pharmacokinetics, but the AUC of diclofenac was increased by ciclosporin (377). In a further study of 20 patients with rheumatoid arthritis who took ciclosporin for 4 weeks, there was a two-fold increase in diclofenac AUC, and a small but significant increase in serum creatinine concentrations (378). Changes in renal function were easily managed by dosage titration of both drugs. In another study of 32 patients who received a 4-week course of paracetamol, indometacin, ketoprofen, or sulindac, changes in the calculated creatinine clearance were minimal (379). There were no striking differences among different NSAIDs. Taken together, the results of these studies and previous findings suggested that the clinical relevance of this interaction is limited.

Orlistat

Orlistat reduces plasma ciclosporin concentrations.

- A 29-year-old woman with increased body weight after renal transplantation was unable to adhere to a low-fat diet and took orlistat, which gave her severe diarrhea (380). Her plasma ciclosporin concentrations fell to subtherapeutic, even though she took the orlistat 2 hours before the ciclosporin and even though the daily dose of orlistat was reduced to 240 mg/day.
- There was a two-fold reduction in blood ciclosporin concentrations 2 weeks after orlistat was given to a 61-year-old patient with a heart transplant (381).
- An overweight 56-year-old man with type II diabetes on peritoneal dialysis took orlistat for some months until he received a living-unrelated kidney transplant (382). Despite oral ciclosporin for 48 hours before transplantation and much larger doses after, it was very difficult to achieve adequate ciclosporin blood concentrations for the first week. After he opened his bowels on day 7 and had been given intravenous ciclosporin for 3 days, adequate ciclosporin blood concentrations were achieved and then maintained with conventional oral doses.

Orlistat may reduce blood ciclosporin concentrations by interfering with its absorption in the small intestine (384), although the effect may be mediated indirectly by via reduced fat absorption rather than a direct drug-drug interaction (384). Co-administration of orlistat with ciclosporin is not recommended. However, if concomitant use is unavoidable, ciclosporin blood concentrations should be monitored more often, both after the addition of orlistat and on withdrawal.

The FDA has received six reports of subtherapeutic blood ciclosporin concentrations soon after transplant recipients started to take orlistat (385). Reduced absorption of ciclosporin is the most likely mechanism (386,387) by reduction in fat absorption rather than by a direct drug–drug interaction.

There are also reports that both probucol and orlistat can reduce the systemic availability of ciclosporin (388).

Oxycodone

In an analysis of changes in ciclosporin clearance and systemic availability obtained from the medical records of 100 transplant patients, oxycodone reduced ciclosporin systemic availability (305).

Parenteral nutrition

Cholestasis from other causes can increase the accumulation of ciclosporin or its metabolites, which in turn worsens hepatic cholestasis. This mechanism has been suggested in patients with bowel diseases who experienced an aggravation of hyperbilirubinemia or an increased incidence of hepatotoxicity from the combination of total parenteral nutrition and ciclosporin (SEDA-19, 348) (389).

Protease inhibitors

Interactions of ciclosporin with protease inhibitors should be expected, particularly with ritonavir, a potent inhibitor of CYP3A.

- Despite a prophylactic reduction in the dose of ciclosporin (100 mg/day) before antiretroviral treatment, a 40-year-old woman had an acute increase in ciclosporin trough concentrations (over 1000 ng/ml) and serum creatinine concentration (from 84 to 228 µmol/l) after taking zidovudine (600 mg/day), saquinavir (800 mg/day), and ritonavir (800 mg/day) for 11 days (390). Despite ciclosporin withdrawal, ciclosporin and creatinine blood concentrations remained high for over 10 days until triple drug therapy was withdrawn. Ritonavir was the most likely suspect.

A reciprocal interaction between ciclosporin and saquinavir has been reported in an HIV-positive kidney transplant patient (391). Whereas ciclosporin concentrations were previously acceptable, there was a three-fold increase in ciclosporin trough concentrations after 3 days of saquinavir (3600 mg/day). In addition, the saquinavir AUC was four times higher than that usually observed in patients taking similar dosages.

Proton pump inhibitors

Conflicting data have emerged on the interaction of omeprazole with ciclosporin, with isolated case reports suggesting that omeprazole can increase or reduce ciclosporin concentrations, whereas no effect of omeprazole was demonstrated in a controlled trial (392–394).

Quinidine

In an analysis of changes in ciclosporin clearance and systemic availability obtained from the medical records of 100 transplant patients, digoxin increased ciclosporin systemic availability (305).

Selective serotonin reuptake inhibitors

Fluvoxamine and fluoxetine have been involved in isolated cases of increased blood ciclosporin concentrations, but fluoxetine was not confirmed to affect ciclosporin concentrations significantly in 13 patients (SEDA-20, 345; SEDA-22, 385–386). In an analysis of changes in ciclosporin clearance and systemic availability obtained from the medical records of 100 transplant patients, sertraline altered ciclosporin pharmacokinetics (305).

Sevelamer

The interaction of sevelamer, a new calcium-free phosphate binder, and ciclosporin has been studied (395,396). After kidney transplantation in 10 adults and eight children sevelamer had no significant effect on ciclosporin AUC, C_{max}, or t_{max}. The AUC of the ciclosporin metabolite AM1 fell by 30% and C_{max} by 25% after 4 days of sevelamer treatment. In contrast, mycophenolic acid concentrations were significantly reduced by a mean of 25% (AUC) and 30% (C_{max}) after a single dose of sevelamer (397).

Sibutramine

An interaction of ciclosporin with sibutramine has been reported (398). Like ciclosporin, sibutramine is metabolized by CYP3A4, and a competitive inhibitory interaction is suggested.

Sirolimus

Sirolimus and ciclosporin are used together after kidney transplantation. Both are taken orally and have common intestinal and hepatic metabolism and intestinal transport mechanisms. There is therefore the potential for pharmacokinetic drug interactions. In an open, randomized, crossover study in 15 healthy men and six women the systemic availability of a single oral dose of sirolimus 10 mg was markedly increased by microemulsion ciclosporin 300 mg taken at the same time (399). C_{max}, t_{max}, and AUC increased 116%, 92%, and 230% respectively. However, when sirolimus was taken 4 hours after ciclosporin, the increases in sirolimus C_{max}, t_{max}, and AUC were only 37%, 58%, and 80% respectively. Ciclosporin did not affect the half-life or mean residence time. The systemic availability of ciclosporin was not altered. The authors concluded that ciclosporin markedly increases the systemic availability of sirolimus, perhaps due to a large intestinal and hepatic first-pass effect.

Sulfasalazine

In a 51-year-old woman with a renal transplant who had been stable for the past 13.5 months with ciclosporin (9.6 mg/kg) and sulfasalazine (1.5 g/day) for ulcerative colitis, sulfasalazine withdrawal resulted in an almost two-fold increase in ciclosporin blood concentrations over the next 10 days (400).

Sulfinpyrazone

In 120 heart transplant patients, sulfinpyrazone (200 mg/day) for ciclosporin-associated hyperuricemia was associated with lowered blood ciclosporin concentrations despite an increase in the daily dose (401). The authors cited evidence (402) that sulfinpyrazone induces ciclosporin metabolism.

Sulfonylureas

Both glipizide and glibenclamide increase ciclosporin concentrations significantly (403).

Ticlopidine

Although there was no interaction between ciclosporin and ticlopidine in a pharmacokinetic study, a 64-year-old patient with a renal transplant had a reduction in the concentration:dose ratio of ciclosporin after each of two successive courses of ticlopidine (404).

Troglitazone

Case reports and a retrospective evaluation of seven renal transplant patients showed that troglitazone can increase ciclosporin metabolism with a subsequent reduction of 15–45% in ciclosporin trough concentrations (405). The interaction of ciclosporin with troglitazone has been confirmed in four heart transplant patients with a 30–60% fall in ciclosporin concentrations within days of taking troglitazone 200 mg/day (406).

Vitamins

Supplementation with vitamin C 500–1000 mg/day and vitamin E 300 mg/day reduced the trough concentrations of ciclosporin in a single-blind, crossover, randomized, placebo-controlled study in 10 renal transplant recipients (407) and in a double-blind, placebo-controlled study in 56 renal transplant recipients (408). Although this could have led to transplant rejection, in fact glomerular filtration rate improved significantly and serum creatinine concentrations fell slightly. Changes in vitamin C and vitamin E concentrations did not correlate with changes in ciclosporin trough concentrations or changes in serum creatinine concentrations. The mechanism of this effect is not known.

Management of Adverse Drug Reactions

Switching from ciclosporin to tacrolimus is an alternative strategy in kidney transplant patients with chronic allograft dysfunction or ciclosporin intolerance, particularly since tacrolimus may be less nephrotoxic than ciclosporin and may prolong transplant function despite ciclosporin failure. Tacrolimus replaced ciclosporin-based immunosuppression in 133 transplant patients (114 kidney, 15 kidney–pancreas, 4 pancreas after kidney) who had progressive loss of renal function (71%) or ciclosporin intolerance (29%) not responding to ciclosporin dosage reduction (409). Tacrolimus was begun in an oral dosage of 0.1 mg/kg bd and was adjusted to trough concentrations of 6–10 ng/ml. Tacrolimus was well tolerated but needed to be withdrawn in 23 cases—21 graft failures, one case of diabetes, and one case of clinical intolerance. Differential creatininemia fell significantly and tacrolimus improved symptoms of ciclosporin intolerance in all cases. Blood urea, creatinine clearance, blood total cholesterol, and triglycerides improved significantly, and the number of hypertensive patients was unchanged. During follow-up, four patients died, one had acute rejection, and 21 transplants failed. Graft failure was significantly more frequent in patients with advanced renal impairment before tacrolimus.

Monitoring Therapy

Ciclosporin pharmacokinetics vary considerably between patients, and even in an individual patient from time to time, with changes in the clinical condition and treatment, particularly with administration of other drugs (401). Inadequate exposure to ciclosporin is a key factor in acute rejection and contributes to the development of chronic rejection and graft failure. Monitoring of ciclosporin concentrations is widely adopted as an accurate and practical measure of drug exposure (411).

In an open, randomized, parallel-group study in 307 patients, ciclosporin blood concentrations measured 2 hours after a dose were compared with conventional trough ciclosporin blood concentrations (412). The traditional predose blood concentration did not correlate well with drug exposure, and the 2-hour concentration was superior in preventing acute rejection. This is important, because data derived from the database of the United Network for Organ Sharing Scientific Liver Transplant Registry has shown that moderate and more severe grades of rejection are associated with poor graft function and outcome in liver transplant recipients.

Of 53 bone marrow transplant recipients in whom ciclosporin was used to suppress graft-versus-host disease, 63% developed acute nephrotoxicity (413). These patients had significantly higher plasma ciclosporin concentrations during the first month after transplantation than those who did not develop acute nephrotoxicity, even though they received the same cumulative dose. Children received a higher cumulative dose, but their plasma concentrations did not differ significantly from the adults, and they suffered less nephrotoxicity.

Although a correlation between early post-transplantation whole-blood concentrations of ciclosporin and the occurrence of ciclosporin-induced toxicity has been suggested, blood concentrations in most patients are in the target range, and the identification of patients susceptible to adverse effects has yet to be achieved (414).

The use of 2-hour peak ciclosporin blood concentrations has been recommended as an alternative to trough concentration monitoring after kidney transplantation and liver transplantation (415). In 928 analyses after 313 heart transplants, the 2-hour concentration correlated better with ciclosporin dose, renal function, and rejection profile, and had less variability between patients than the trough concentration.

Trough concentration-adjusted mycophenolate mofetil therapy has been studied in combination with tacrolimus (n = 30) or ciclosporin (n = 30) after heart transplantation (416). Target blood trough concentrations were tacrolimus 10–15 ng/ml, ciclosporin 100–300 ng/ml, and mycophenolic acid 1.5–4.0 μg/ml. Glucocorticoids were withdrawn within 6 months after heart transplantation. Tacrolimus + mycophenolate mofetil resulted in a significantly lower incidence of acute rejection than ciclosporin + mycophenolate mofetil, despite similar survival rates. Patients taking tacrolimus required a significantly lower dose of mycophenolate mofetil to achieve target mycophenolic acid blood concentrations compared with ciclosporin.

The single-dose and steady-state pharmacokinetics of a ciclosporin microemulsion formulation have been studied in six Chinese heart transplant recipients who also took everolimus, methylprednisolone, and rabbit antithymocyte globulin (417). The authors concluded that trough blood concentrations may be best for monitoring ciclosporin therapy.

References

1. Touchard G, Verove C, Bridoux F, Bauwen F. Cyclosporin maintenance monotherapy after renal transplantation. What factors predict success? BioDrugs 1999;12:91–113.
2. Shield CF III, McGrath MM, Goss TF. Assessment of health-related quality of life in kidney transplant patients receiving tacrolimus (FK506)-based versus cyclosporine-based immunosuppression. FK506 Kidney Transplant Study Group. Transplantation 1997;64(12):1738–43.
3. Kappers-Klunne MC, van't Veer MB. Cyclosporin A for the treatment of patients with chronic idiopathic thrombocytopenic purpura refractory to corticosteroids or splenectomy. Br J Haematol 2001;114(1):121–5.
4. Cortes J, O'Brien S, Loscertales J, Kantarjian H, Giles F, Thomas D, Koller C, Keating M. Cyclosporin A for the treatment of cytopenia associated with chronic lymphocytic leukemia. Cancer 2001;92(8):2016–22.
5. Peters TG, Spinola KN, West JC, Aeder MI, Danovitch GM, Klintmalm GB, Gorman KJ, Gordon JA, Kincaid CH, First MR. Differences in patient and transplant professional perceptions of immunosuppression-induced cosmetic side effects. Transplantation 2004;78(4):537–43.
6. Campana C, Regazzi MB, Buggia I, Molinaro M. Clinically significant drug interactions with cyclosporin. An update. Clin Pharmacokinet 1996;30(2):141–79.
7. Kasiske BL, Guijarro C, Massy ZA, Wiederkehr MR, Ma JZ. Cardiovascular disease after renal transplantation. J Am Soc Nephrol 1996;7(1):158–65.
8. Kronenberg F, Lhotta K, Konigsrainer A, Konig P. Renal artery thromboembolism and immunosuppressive therapy. Nephron 1996;72(1):101.
9. Textor SC, Canzanello VJ, Taler SJ, Wilson DJ, Schwartz LL, Augustine JE, Raymer JM, Romero JC, Wiesner RH, Krom RA, et al. Cyclosporine-induced hypertension after transplantation. Mayo Clin Proc 1994;69(12):1182–93.
10. Campistol JM, Romero R, Paul J, Gutierrez-Dalmau A. Epidemiology of arterial hypertension in renal transplant patients: changes over the last decade. Nephrol Dial Transplant 2004;19 Suppl 3:iii62–iii66.
11. Jardine AG. Assessing the relative risk of cardiovascular disease among renal transplant patients receiving tacrolimus or cyclosporine. Transpl Int 2005;18(4):379–84.
12. Taler SJ, Textor SC, Canzanello VJ, Schwartz L. Cyclosporin-induced hypertension: incidence, pathogenesis and management. Drug Saf 1999;20(5):437–49.
13. Ventura HO, Mehra MR, Stapleton DD, Smart FW. Cyclosporine-induced hypertension in cardiac transplantation. Med Clin North Am 1997;81(6):1347–57.
14. Sturrock ND, Lang CC, Struthers AD. Cyclosporin-induced hypertension precedes renal dysfunction and sodium retention in man. J Hypertens 1993;11(11):1209–1216.
15. Hausberg M, Lang D, Levers A, Suwelack B, Kisters K, Tokmak F, Barenbrock M, Kosch M. Sympathetic nerve

activity in renal transplant patients before and after withdrawal of cyclosporine. J Hypertens 2006;24(5):957–64.

16. Kramer BK, Zulke C, Kammerl MC, Schmidt C, Hengstenberg C, Fischereder M, Marienhagen J; European Tacrolimus vs. Cyclosporine Microemulsion Renal Transplantation Study Group. Cardiovascular risk factors and estimated risk for CAD in a randomized trial comparing calcineurin inhibitors in renal transplantation. Am J Transplant 2003;3:982–7.

17. Marcén R, Morales JM, Arias M, Fernández-Juárez G, Fernández-Fresnedo G, Andrés A, Rodrigo E, Pascual J, Domínguez B, Ortuño J. Ischemic heart disease after renal transplantation in patients on cyclosporine in Spain. J Am Soc Nephrol 2006;17(12 Suppl 3):S286–90.

18. Davenport A. The effect of renal transplantation and treatment with cyclosporin A on the prevalence of Raynaud's phenomenon. Clin Transplant 1993;7:4–8.

19. Thami GP, Bhalla M. Erythromelalgia induced by possible calcium channel blockade by ciclosporin. BMJ 2003;326:910.

20. Fortin MC, Raymond MA, Madore F, Fugere JA, Paquet M, St Louis G, Hebert MJ. Increased risk of thrombotic microangiopathy in patients receiving a cyclosporin–sirolimus combination. Am J Transplant 2004;4(6):946–52.

21. Rottenberg Y, Fridlender ZG. Recurrent infusion phlebitis induced by cyclosporine. Ann Pharmacother 2004;38(12):2071–3.

22. Blaauw AA, Leunissen KM, Cheriex EC, Wolters J, Kootstra G, Van Hooff JP. Disappearance of pulmonary capillary leak syndrome when intravenous cyclosporine is replaced by oral cyclosporine. Transplantation 1987;43(5):758–9.

23. Carbone L, Appel GB, Benvenisty AI, Cohen DJ, Kunis CL, Hardy MA. Adult respiratory distress syndrome associated with oral cyclosporine. Transplantation 1987;43(5):767–8.

24. Roelofs PM, Klinkhamer PJ, Gooszen HC. Hypersensitivity pneumonitis probably caused by cyclosporine. A case report. Respir Med 1998;92(12):1368–70.

25. Hauben M. Cyclosporine neurotoxicity. Pharmacotherapy 1996;16(4):576–83.

26. Wijdicks EF, Wiesner RH, Krom RA. Neurotoxicity in liver transplant recipients with cyclosporine immunosuppression. Neurology 1995;45(11):1962–4.

27. Erer B, Polchi P, Lucarelli G, Angelucci E, Baronciani D, Galimberti M, Giardini C, Gaziev D, Maiello A. CsA-associated neurotoxicity and ineffective prophylaxis with clonazepam in patients transplanted for thalassemia major: analysis of risk factors. Bone Marrow Transplant 1996;18(1):157–62.

28. Bohlin AB, Berg U, Englund M, Malm G, Persson A, Tibell A, Tyden G. Central nervous system complications in children treated with ciclosporin after renal transplantation. Child Nephrol Urol 1990;10(4):225–30.

29. de Groen PC, Aksamit AJ, Rakela J, Forbes GS, Krom RA. Central nervous system toxicity after liver transplantation. The role of cyclosporine and cholesterol. N Engl J Med 1987;317(14):861–6.

30. Gleeson JG, duPlessis AJ, Barnes PD, Riviello JJ Jr. Cyclosporin A acute encephalopathy and seizure syndrome in childhood: clinical features and risk of seizure recurrence. J Child Neurol 1998;13(7):336–44.

31. Schwartz RB, Bravo SM, Klufas RA, Hsu L, Barnes PD, Robson CD, Antin JH. Cyclosporine neurotoxicity and its relationship to hypertensive encephalopathy: CT and MR findings in 16 cases. Am J Roentgenol 1995;165(3):627–31.

32. Bronster DJ, Chodoff L, Yonover P, Sheiner PA. Cyclosporine levels in cerebrospinal fluid after liver transplantation. Transplantation 1999;68(9):1410–3.

33. Meyer MA. Elevated basal ganglia glucose metabolism in cyclosporine neurotoxicity: a positron emission tomography imaging study. J Neuroimaging 2002;12(1):92–3.

34. Ozkaya O, Kalman S, Bakkaloglu S, Buyan N, Soylemezoglu O. Cyclosporine-associated facial paralysis in a child with renal transplant. Pediatr Nephrol 2002;17(7):544–6.

35. Kotake S, Higashi K, Yoshikawa K, Sasamoto Y, Okamoto T, Matsuda H. Central nervous system symptoms in patients with Behçet disease receiving cyclosporine therapy. Ophthalmology 1999;106(3):586–9.

36. Gopal AK, Thorning DR, Back AL. Fatal outcome due to cyclosporine neurotoxicity with associated pathological findings. Bone Marrow Transplant 1999;23(2):191–3.

37. Yu J, Zheng SS, Liang TB, Shen Y, Wang WL, Ke QH. Possible causes of central pontine myelinolysis after liver transplantation. World J Gastroenterol 2004;10(17):2540–3.

38. Patel B, Kerridge I. Cyclosporin neurotoxicity. Br J Haematol 2003;123:755.

39. Falk JA, Cordova FC, Popescu A, Tatarian G, Criner GJ. Treatment of Guillain-Barre syndrome induced by cyclosporine in a lung transplant patient. J Heart Lung Transplant 2006;25(1):140–3.

40. Zakrzewski JL. Cyclosporin A-associated status epilepticus related to hematopoietic stem cell transplantation for thalassemia. Pediatr Hematol Oncol 2003;20:481–6.

41. Choi EJ, Kang JK, Lee SA, Kim KH, Lee SG, Andermann F. New-onset seizures after liver transplantation: clinical implications and prognosis in survivors. Eur Neurol 2004;52(4):230–6.

42. Knower MT, Pethke SD, Valentine VG. Reversible cortical blindness after lung transplantation. South Med J 2003;96:606–12.

43. Paul F, Muller J, Christe W, Steinmuller T, Poewe W, Wissel J. Postural hand tremor before and following liver transplantation and immunosuppression with cyclosporine or tacrolimus in patients without clinical signs of hepatic encephalopathy. Clin Transplant 2004;18(4):429–33.

44. Borras BJ, Enriquez R, Amoros AF, Navarro RA, Conesa G, V, Gonzalez DM. Cefalea asociada a ciclosporina en un paciente con glomerulonefritis membranosa. [Headache associated with ciclosporine in a patient with membranous glomerulonephritis.] Farm Hosp 2004;28(6):454–7.

45. Buscher R, Vij O, Hudde T, Hoyer PF, Vester U. Pseudotumor cerebri following cyclosporine A treatment in a boy with tubulointerstitial nephritis associated with uveitis. Pediatr Nephrol 2004;19(5):558–60.

46. Guennoc AM, Corcia P, Al Najjar A, Bergemer-Fouquet AM, Lebranchu Y, de Toffol B, Autret A. Neuromyopathie toxique induite par la ciclosporine. Rev Neurol (Paris) 2005;161(2):221–3.

47. Echaniz-Laguna A, Battaglia F, Ellero B, Mohr M, Jaeck D. Chronic inflammatory demyelinating polyradiculoneuropathy in patients with liver transplantation. Muscle Nerve 2004;30(4):501–4.

48. Munoz R, Espinoza M, Espinoza O, Andrade A, Bravo E, Gonzalez F. Cyclosporine-associated leukoencephalopathy in organ transplant recipients: experience of three clinical cases. Transplant Proc 2006;38(3):921–3.

49. Ishikura K, Ikeda M, Hamasaki Y, Hataya H, Shishido S, Asanuma H, Nishimura G, Hiramoto R, Honda M.Posterior reversible encephalopathy syndrome in

children: its high prevalence and more extensive imaging findings. Am J Kidney Dis 2006;48(2):231–8.

50. Natsume J, Sofue A, Yamada A, Kato K. Electroencephalographic (EEG) findings in posterior reversible encephalopathy associated with immunosuppressants. J Child Neurol 2006;21(7):620–3.

51. Kaito K, Kobayashi M, Otsubo H, Ogasawara Y, Sekita T, Shimada T, Hosoya T. Cyclosporine and entrapment neuropathy. Report of two cases. Acta Haematol 1998;100(3):159.

52. Terrovitis IV, Nanas SN, Rombos AK, Tolis G, Nanas JN. Reversible symmetric polyneuropathy with paraplegia after heart transplantation. Transplantation 1998;65(10):1394–5.

53. Maghrabi K, Bohlega S. Cyclosporine-induced migraine with severe vomiting causing loss of renal graft. Clin Neurol Neurosurg 1998;100(3):224–7.

54. Braun R, Arechalde A, French LE. Reversible ascending motor neuropathy as a side effect of systemic treatment with ciclosporine for nodular prurigo. Dermatology 1999;199(4):372–3.

55. Koide T, Yamada M, Takahashi T, Igarashi S, Masuko M, Furukawa T, Kuroha T, Koike T, Sato M, Tanaka R, Tsuji S, Takahashi H. Cyclosporine A-associated fatal central nervous system angiopathy in a bone marrow transplant recipient: an autopsy case. Acta Neuropathol (Berl) 2000;99(6):680–4.

56. Shbarou RM, Chao NJ, Morgenlander JC. Cyclosporin A-related cerebral vasculopathy. Bone Marrow Transplant 2000;26(7):801–4.

57. Delpont E, Thomas P, Gugenheim J, Chichmanian RM, Mahagne MH, Suisse G, Dolisi C. Syndrome confusionnel prolongé au cours d'un traitement par ciclosporine: etat de mal à expression confusionnelle? [Prolonged confusion syndrome in the course of cyclosporine treatment: a state of confusion?] Neurophysiol Clin 1990;20(3):207–15.

58. Labar B, Bogdanic V, Plavsic F, Francetic I, Dobric I, Kastelan A, Grgicevic D, Vrtar M, Grgic-Markulin L, Balabanic-Kamauf B, et al. Cyclosporin neurotoxicity in patients treated with allogeneic bone marrow transplantation. Biomed Pharmacother 1986;40(4):148–50.

59. Rosencrantz R, Moon A, Raynes H, Spivak W. Cyclosporine-Induced neurotoxicity during treatment of Crohn's disease: lack of correlation with previously reported risk factors. Am J Gastroenterol 2001;96(9):2778–82.

60. Porges Y, Blumen S, Fireman Z, Sternberg A, Zamir D. Cyclosporine-induced optic neuropathy, ophthalmoplegia, and nystagmus in a patient with Crohn disease. Am J Ophthalmol 1998;126(4):607–9.

61. Rubin AM, Kang H. Cerebral blindness and encephalopathy with cyclosporin A toxicity. Neurology 1987;37(6):1072–6.

62. Rubin AM. Transient cortical blindness and occipital seizures with cyclosporine toxicity. Transplantation 1989;47(3):572–3.

63. Wilson SE, de Groen PC, Aksamit AJ, Wiesner RH, Garrity JA, Krom RA. Cyclosporin A-induced reversible cortical blindness. J Clin Neuroophthalmol 1988;8(4):215–20.

64. Saito J, Kami M, Taniguchi F, Kanda Y, Takeda N, Mitani K, Hirai H, Araie M, Fujino Y. Unilateral papilledema after bone marrow transplantation. Bone Marrow Transplant 1999;23(9):963–5.

65. Avery R, Jabs DA, Wingard JR, Vogelsang G, Saral R, Santos G. Optic disc edema after bone marrow transplantation. Possible role of cyclosporine toxicity. Ophthalmology 1991;98(8):1294–301.

66. BenEzra D, Pe'er J, Brodsky M, Cohen E. Cyclosporine eyedrops for the treatment of severe vernal keratoconjunctivitis. Am J Ophthalmol 1986;101(3):278–82.

67. Zierhut M, Thiel HJ, Weidle EG, Waetjen R, Pleyer U. Topical treatment of severe corneal ulcers with cyclosporin A. Graefes Arch Clin Exp Ophthalmol 1989;227(1):30–5.

68. Sall K, Stevenson OD, Mundorf TK, Reis BL. Two multicenter, randomized studies of the efficacy and safety of cyclosporine ophthalmic emulsion in moderate to severe dry eye disease. CsA Phase 3 Study Group. Ophthalmology 2000;107(4):631–9.

69. Kachi S, Hirano K, Takesue Y, Miura M. Unusual corneal deposit after the topical use of cyclosporine as eyedrops. Am J Ophthalmol 2000;130(5):667–9.

70. Stevenson D, Tauber J, Reis BL. Efficacy and safety of cyclosporin A ophthalmic emulsion in the treatment of moderate-to-severe dry eye disease: a dose-ranging, randomized trial. The Cyclosporin A Phase 2 Study Group. Ophthalmology 2000;107(5):967–74.

71. Marchiori PE, Mies S, Scaff M. Cyclosporine A-induced ocular opsoclonus and reversible leukoencephalopathy after orthotopic liver transplantation: brief report. Clin Neuropharmacol 2004;27(4):195–7.

72. Tombazzi CR, Waters B, Shokouh-Amiri MH, Vera SR, Riely CA. Neuropsychiatric complications after liver transplantation: role of immunosuppression and hepatitis C. Dig Dis Sci 2006;51(6):1079–81.

73. Imataki O, Kim SW, Kojima R, Hori A, Hamaki T, Sakiyama M, Murashige N, Satoh M, Kami M, Makimoto A, Takaue Y. Life-threatening hypothyroidism associated with administration of cyclosporine in a patient treated with reduced-intensity hematopoietic stem-cell transplantation for metastatic renal-cell carcinoma. Transplantation 2003;75:898–907.

74. Jindal RM, Sidner RA, Milgrom ML. Post-transplant diabetes mellitus. The role of immunosuppression. Drug Saf 1997;16(4):242–57.

75. Copstein LA, Zelmanovitz T, Goncalves LF, Manfro RC. Posttransplant patients: diabetes mellitus in cyclosporine-treated renal allograft a case-control study. Transplant Proc 2004;36(4):882–3.

76. Ciancio G, Burke GW, Gaynor JJ, Mattiazzi A, Roth D, Kupin W, Nicolas M, Ruiz P, Rosen A, Miller J. A randomized long-term trial of tacrolimus/sirolimus versus tacrolimus/mycophenolate mofetil versus cyclosporine (NEORAL)/sirolimus in renal transplantation. II. Survival, function, and protocol compliance at 1 year. Transplantation 2004;77(2):252–8.

77. Zielinska T, Zakliczynski M, Szewczyk M, Zielinska-Kukla A, Foremny J, Kalarus Z, Religia Z, Zembala M. Influence of long term cyclosporine therapy on insulin and its precursors secretion in patients after heart transplantation. Ann Transplant 2003;8:10–12.

78. Marcén R, Morales JM, del Castillo D, Campistol JM, Serón D, Valdés F, Anaya F, Andrés A, Arias M, Bustamante J, Capdevila L, Escuin F, Gil-Vernet S, Gonzalez-Molina M, Lampreave I, Oppenheimer F, Pallardó L; Spanish Renal Forum. Posttransplant diabetes mellitus in renal allograft recipients: a prospective multicenter study at 2 years. Transplant Proc 2006;38(10):3530–2.

79. Raine AE, Carter R, Mann JI, Morris PJ. Adverse effect of cyclosporin on plasma cholesterol in renal transplant recipients. Nephrol Dial Transplant 1988;3(4):458–63.

80. Ballantyne CM, Podet EJ, Patsch WP, Harati Y, Appel V, Gotto AM Jr, Young JB. Effects of cyclosporine therapy on plasma lipoprotein levels. JAMA 1989;262(1):53–6.

81. Stiller MJ, Pak GH, Kenny C, Jondreau L, Davis I, Wachsman S, Shupack JL. Elevation of fasting serum lipids in patients treated with low-dose cyclosporine for severe plaque-type psoriasis. An assessment of clinical significance when viewed as a risk factor for cardiovascular disease. J Am Acad Dermatol 1992;27(3):434–8.

82. Grossman RM, Delaney RJ, Brinton EA, Carter DM, Gottlieb AB. Hypertriglyceridemia in patients with psoriasis treated with cyclosporine. J Am Acad Dermatol 1991;25(4):648–51.

83. Hricik DE. Posttransplant hyperlipidemia: the treatment dilemma. Am J Kidney Dis 1994;23(5):766–71.

84. Massy ZA. Hyperlipidemia and cardiovascular disease after organ transplantation. Transplantation 2001;72(Suppl 6):S13–5.

85. Webb AT, Reaveley DA, O'Donnell M, O'Connor B, Seed M, Brown EA. Does cyclosporin increase lipoprotein(a) concentrations in renal transplant recipients? Lancet 1993;341(8840):268–70Hunt BJ, Parratt R, Rose M, Yacoub M. Does cyclosporin affect lipoprotein(a) concentrations? Lancet 1994;343(8889):119–20(see also).

86. Kuster GM, Drexel H, Bleisch JA, Rentsch K, Pei P, Binswanger U, Amann FW. Relation of cyclosporine blood levels to adverse effects on lipoproteins. Transplantation 1994;57(10):1479–83.

87. Claesson K, Mayer AD, Squifflet JP, Grabensee B, Eigler FW, Behrend M, Vanrenterghem Y, van Hooff J, Morales JM, Johnson RW, Buchholz B, Land W, Forsythe JL, Neumayer HH, Ericzon BG, Muhlbacher F. Lipoprotein patterns in renal transplant patients: a comparison between FK 506 and cyclosporine A patients. Transplant Proc 1998;30(4):1292–4.

88. McCune TR, Thacker LR II, Peters TG, Mulloy L, Rohr MS, Adams PA, Yium J, Light JA, Pruett T, Gaber AO, Selman SH, Jonsson J, Hayes JM, Wright FH Jr, Armata T, Blanton J, Burdick JF. Effects of tacrolimus on hyperlipidemia after successful renal transplantation: a Southeastern Organ Procurement Foundation multicenter clinical study. Transplantation 1998;65(1):87–92.

89. Deleuze S, Garrigue V, Delmas S, Chong G, Swarcz I, Cristol JP, Mourad G. New onset dyslipidemia after renal transplantation: is there a difference between tacrolimus and cyclosporine? Transplant Proc 2006;38(7):2311–3.

90. Lin HY, Rocher LL, McQuillan MA, Schmaltz S, Palella TD, Fox IH. Cyclosporine-induced hyperuricemia and gout. N Engl J Med 1989;321(5):287–92.

91. Burack DA, Griffith BP, Thompson ME, Kahl LE. Hyperuricemia and gout among heart transplant recipients receiving cyclosporine. Am J Med 1992;92(2):141–6.

92. Ben Hmida M, Hachicha J, Bahloul Z, Kaddour N, Kharrat M, Jarraya F, Jarraya A. Cyclosporine-induced hyperuricemia and gout in renal transplants. Transplant Proc 1995;27(5):2722–4.

93. Sparta G, Kemper MJ, Neuhaus TJ. Hyperuricemia and gout following pediatric renal transplantation. Pediatr Nephrol 2006;21(12):1884–8.

94. Laine J, Holmberg C. Renal and adrenal mechanisms in cyclosporine-induced hyperkalaemia after renal transplantation. Eur J Clin Invest 1995;25(9):670–6.

95. Singer M, Coluzzi F, O'Brien A, Clapp LH. Reversal of life-threatening, drug-related potassium-channel syndrome by glibenclamide. Lancet 2005;365(9474):1873–5.

96. Cavdar C, Sifil A, Sanli E, Gulay H, Camsari T. Hypomagnesemia and mild rhabdomyolysis in living related donor renal transplant recipient treated with cyclosporine A. Scand J Urol Nephrol 1998;32(6):415–7.

97. Scoble JE, Freestone A, Varghese Z, Fernando ON, Sweny P, Moorhead JF. Cyclosporin-induced renal magnesium leak in renal transplant patients. Nephrol Dial Transplant 1990;5(9):812–5.

98. Nozue T, Kobayashi A, Kodama T, Uemasu F, Endoh H, Sako A, Takagi Y. Pathogenesis of cyclosporine-induced hypomagnesemia. J Pediatr 1992;120(4 Pt 1):638–40.

99. Vannini SD, Mazzola BL, Rodoni L, Truttmann AC, Wermuth B, Bianchetti MG, Ferrari P. Permanently reduced plasma ionized magnesium among renal transplant recipients on cyclosporine. Transpl Int 1999;12(4):244–9.

100. Bardet V, Junior AP, Coste J, Lecoq-Lafon C, Chouzenoux S, Bernard D, Soubrane O, Lacombe C, Calmus Y, Conti F. Impaired erythropoietin production in liver transplant recipients: the role of calcineurin inhibitors. Liver Transpl 2006;12(11):1649–54.

101. Faure JL, Causse X, Bergeret A, Meyer F, Neidecker J, Paliard P. Cyclosporine induced hemolytic anemia in a liver transplant patient. Transplant Proc 1989;21(1 Pt 2):2242–3.

102. Rougier JP, Viron B, Ronco P, Khayat R, Michel C, Mignon F. Autoimmune haemolytic anaemia after ABO-match, ABDR full match kidney transplantation. Nephrol Dial Transplant 1994;9(6):693–7.

103. Trimarchi H, Freixas E, Rabinovich O, Schropp J, Pereyra H, Bullorsky E. Cyclosporine-associated thrombotic microangiopathy during daclizumab induction: a suggested therapeutic approach. Nephron 2001;87(4):361–4.

104. Seymour RA. Drug-induced gingival overgrowth. Adverse Drug React Toxicol Rev 1993;12(4):215–32.

105. Mariani G, Calastrini C, Carinci F, Marzola R, Calura G. Ultrastructural features of cyclosporine A-induced gingival hyperplasia. J Periodontol 1993;64(11):1092–7.

106. O'Valle F, Mesa FL, Gomez-Morales M, Aguilar D, Caracuel MD, Medina-Cano MT, Andujar M, Lopez-Hidalgo J, Garcia del Moral R. Immunohistochemical study of 30 cases of cyclosporin A-induced gingival overgrowth. J Periodontol 1994;65(7):724–30.

107. Nell A, Matejka M, Solar P, Ulm C, Sinzinger H. Evidence that cyclosporine inhibits periodontal prostaglandin I2 synthesis. J Periodontal Res 1996;31(2):131–4.

108. Thomason JM, Seymour RA, Ellis JS, Kelly PJ, Parry G, Dark J, Idle JR. Iatrogenic gingival overgrowth in cardiac transplantation. J Periodontol 1995;66(8):742–6.

109. Wondimu B, Dahllof G, Berg U, Modeer T. Cyclosporin-A-induced gingival overgrowth in renal transplant children. Scand J Dent Res 1993;101(5):282–6.

110. Wondimu B, Berg U, Modeer T. Renal function in cyclosporine-treated pediatric renal transplant recipients in relation to gingival overgrowth. Transplantation 1997;64(1):92–6.

111. Kilpatrick NM, Weintraub RG, Lucas JO, Shipp A, Byrt T, Wilkinson JL. Gingival overgrowth in pediatric heart and heart-lung transplant recipients. J Heart Lung Transplant 1997;16(12):1231–7.

112. Sooriyamoorthy M, Gower DB, Eley BM. Androgen metabolism in gingival hyperplasia induced by nifedipine and cyclosporin. J Periodontal Res 1990;25(1):25–30.

113. Bokenkamp A, Bohnhorst B, Beier C, Albers N, Offner G, Brodehl J. Nifedipine aggravates cyclosporine A-induced gingival hyperplasia. Pediatr Nephrol 1994;8(2):181–5.

114. Thomason JM, Seymour RA, Rice N. The prevalence and severity of cyclosporin and nifedipine-induced gingival overgrowth. J Clin Periodontol 1993;20(1):37–40.

115. Tokgoz B, Sari HI, Yildiz O, Aslan S, Sipahioglu M, Okten T, Oymak O, Utas C. Effects of azithromycin on cyclosporine-induced gingival hyperplasia in renal transplant patients. Transplant Proc 2004;36(9):2699–702.

116. Worm HC, Wirnsberger GH, Mauric A, Holzer H. High prevalence of Chlamydia pneumoniae infection in cyclosporin A-induced post-transplant gingival overgrowth tissue

and evidence for the possibility of persistent infection despite short-term treatment with azithromycin. Nephrol Dial Transplant 2004;19(7):1890–4.

117. Cansick JC, Hulton SA. Lip hypertrophy secondary to cyclosporin treatment. Pediatr Nephrol 2003;18:710–11.

118. Landewe RB, Goei The HS, van Rijthoven AW, Rietveld JR, Breedveld FC, Dijkmans BA. Cyclosporine in common clinical practice: an estimation of the benefit/risk ratio in patients with rheumatoid arthritis. J Rheumatol 1994;21(9):1631–6.

119. Koch R, Zoller H, Graziadei I, Propst A, Vogel W. Cyclosporine A-induced achalasia-like esophageal motility disorder in a liver transplant recipient: successful conversion to tacrolimus. Transplantation 2003;76:744–5.

120. Chen KJ, Chen CH, Cheng CH, Wu MJ, Shu KH. Risk factors for peptic ulcer disease in renal transplant patients—11 years of experience from a single center. Clin Nephrol 2004;62(1):14–20.

121. Lorber MI, Van Buren CT, Flechner SM, Williams C, Kahan BD. Hepatobiliary and pancreatic complications of cyclosporine therapy in 466 renal transplant recipients. Transplantation 1987;43(1):35–40.

122. Marr KA, Hachem R, Papanicolaou G, Somani J, Arduino JM, Lipka CJ, Ngai AL, Kartsonis N, Chodakewitz J, Sable C. Retrospective study of the hepatic safety profile of patients concomitantly treated with caspofungin and cyclosporin A. Transpl Infect Dis 2004;6(3):110–6.

123. Harihara Y, Sanjo K, Idezuki Y. Cyclosporine hepatotoxicity and cold ischemia liver damage. Transplant Proc 1992;24(5):1984.

124. Moertel CG, Fleming TR, Macdonald JS, Haller DG, Laurie JA. Hepatic toxicity associated with fluorouracil plus levamisole adjuvant therapy. J Clin Oncol 1993;11(12):2386–90.

125. Kowdley KV, Keeffe EB. Hepatotoxicity of transplant immunosuppressive agents. Gastroenterol Clin North Am 1995;24(4):991–1001.

126. Myara A, Cadranel JF, Dorent R, Lunel F, Bouvier E, Gerhardt M, Bernard B, Ghoussoub JJ, Cabrol A, Gandjbakhch I, Opolon P, Trivin F. Cyclosporin A-mediated cholestasis in patients with chronic hepatitis after heart transplantation. Eur J Gastroenterol Hepatol 1996;8(3):267–71.

127. Neri S, Signorelli SS, Ierna D, Mauceri B, Abate G, Bordonaro F, Cilio D, Malaguarnera M. Role of admethionine (S-adenosylmethionine) in cyclosporin-induced cholestasis. Clin Drug Invest 2002;22:191–5.

128. Chicharro M, Guarner L, Vilaseca J, Planas M, Malagelada J. Does cyclosporin A worsen liver function in patients with inflammatory bowel disease and total parenteral nutrition? Rev Esp Enferm Dig 2000;92(2):68–77.

129. Laskow DA, Curtis JJ, Luke RG, Julian BA, Jones P, Deierhoi MH, Barber WH, Diethelm AG. Cyclosporine-induced changes in glomerular filtration rate and urea excretion. Am J Med 1990;88(5):497–502.

130. Mobb GE, Veitch PS, Bell PR. Are serum creatinine levels adequate to identify the onset of chronic cyclosporine A nephrotoxicity? Transplant Proc 1990;22(4):1708–10.

131. Burdmann EA, Andoh TF, Yu L, Bennett WM. Cyclosporine nephrotoxicity. Semin Nephrol 2003;23:465–76.

132. Greenberg A, Thompson ME, Griffith BJ, Hardesty RL, Kormos RL, el-Shahawy MA, Janosky JE, Puschett JB. Cyclosporine nephrotoxicity in cardiac allograft patients—a seven-year follow-up. Transplantation 1990;50(4):589–593.

133. Leong SO, Lye WC, Tan CC, Lee EJ. Acute cyclosporine A nephrotoxicity in a renal allograft recipient with hypothyroidism. Am J Kidney Dis 1995;25(3):503–5.

134. van der Molen LR, van Son WJ, Tegzess AM, Stegeman CA. Severe vital depression as the presenting feature of cyclosporin-A-associated thrombotic microangiopathy. Nephrol Dial Transplant 1999;14(4):998–1000.

135. Kohli HS, Sud K, Jha V, Gupta KL, Minz M, Joshi K, Sakhuja V. Cyclosporin-induced haemolytic–uraemic syndrome presenting as primary graft dysfunction. Nephrol Dial Transplant 1998;13(11):2940–2.

136. Wiener Y, Nakhleh RE, Lee MW, Escobar FS, Venkat KK, Kupin WL, Mozes MF. Prognostic factors and early resumption of cyclosporin A in renal allograft recipients with thrombotic microangiopathy and hemolytic uremic syndrome. Clin Transplant 1997;11(3):157–62.

137. Bren AF, Kandus A, Buturovic J, Koselj M, Kaplan Pavlovcic S, Ponikvar R, Kovac D, Lindic J, Vizjak A, Ferluga D. Cyclosporine-related hemolytic–uremic syndrome in kidney graft recipients: clinical and histomorphologic evaluation. Transplant Proc 1998;30(4):1201–3.

138. Ducloux D, Rebibou JM, Semhoun-Ducloux S, Jamali M, Fournier V, Bresson-Vautrin C, Chalopin JM. Recurrence of hemolytic–uremic syndrome in renal transplant recipients: a meta-analysis. Transplantation 1998;65(10):1405–7.

139. Zarifian A, Meleg-Smith S, O'donovan R, Tesi RJ, Batuman V. Cyclosporine-associated thrombotic microangiopathy in renal allografts. Kidney Int 1999;55(6):2457–66.

140. Myers BD, Ross J, Newton L, Luetscher J, Perlroth M. Cyclosporine-associated chronic nephropathy. N Engl J Med 1984;311(11):699–705.

141. Bennett WM, DeMattos A, Meyer MM, Andoh T, Barry JM. Chronic cyclosporine nephropathy: the Achilles' heel of immunosuppressive therapy. Kidney Int 1996;50(4):1089–100.

142. Mihatsch MJ, Ryffel B, Gudat F. The differential diagnosis between rejection and cyclosporine toxicity. Kidney Int Suppl 1995;52:S63–9.

143. Shihab FS. Cyclosporine nephropathy: pathophysiology and clinical impact. Semin Nephrol 1996;16(6):536–47.

144. Ader JL, Rostaing L. Cyclosporin nephrotoxicity: pathophysiology and comparison with FK-506. Curr Opin Nephrol Hypertens 1998;7(5):539–45.

145. Mihatsch MJ, Antonovych T, Bohman SO, Habib R, Helmchen U, Noel LH, Olsen S, Sibley RK, Kemeny E, Feutren G. Cyclosporin A nephropathy: standardization of the evaluation of kidney biopsies. Clin Nephrol 1994;41(1):23–32.

146. Habib R, Niaudet P. Comparison between pre- and post-treatment renal biopsies in children receiving ciclosporin for idiopathic nephrosis. Clin Nephrol 1994;42(3):141–6.

147. Jacobson SH, Jaremko G, Duraj FF, Wilczek HE. Renal fibrosis in cyclosporin A-treated renal allograft recipients: morphological findings in relation to renal hemodynamics. Transpl Int 1996;9(5):492–8.

148. Opelz G. Effect of the maintenance immunosuppressive drug regimen on kidney transplant outcome. Transplantation 1994;58(4):443–6.

149. Thiel G, Bock A, Spondlin M, Brunner FP, Mihatsch M, Rufli T, Landmann J. Long-term benefits and risks of cyclosporin A (Sandimmun)—an analysis at 10 years. Transplant Proc 1994;26(5):2493–8.

150. Mihatsch MJ, Morozumi K, Strom EH, Ryffel B, Gudat F, Thiel G. Renal transplant morphology after long-term therapy with cyclosporine. Transplant Proc 1995;27(1):39–42.

151. Gonwa TA, Klintmalm GB, Levy M, Jennings LS, Goldstein RM, Husberg BS. Impact of pretransplant renal function on survival after liver transplantation. Transplantation 1995;59(3):361–5.

152. Kuo PC, Luikart H, Busse-Henry S, Hunt SA, Valantine HA, Stinson EB, Oyer PE, Scandling JD, Alfrey EJ, Dafoe DC. Clinical outcome of interval cadaveric renal transplantation in cardiac allograft recipients. Clin Transplant 1995;9(2):92–7.

153. Goldstein DJ, Zuech N, Sehgal V, Weinberg AD, Drusin R, Cohen D. Cyclosporine-associated end-stage nephropathy after cardiac transplantation: incidence and progression. Transplantation 1997;63(5):664–8.

154. Almond PS, Gillingham KJ, Sibley R, Moss A, Melin M, Leventhal J, Manivel C, Kyriakides P, Payne WD, Dunn DL, et al. Renal transplant function after ten years of cyclosporine. Transplantation 1992;53(2):316–23.

155. Burke JF Jr, Pirsch JD, Ramos EL, Salomon DR, Stablein DM, Van Buren DH, West JC. Long-term efficacy and safety of cyclosporine in renal-transplant recipients. N Engl J Med 1994;331(6):358–63.

156. Ruggenenti P, Perico N, Amuchastegui CS, Ferrazzi P, Mamprin F, Remuzzi G. Following an initial decline, glomerular filtration rate stabilizes in heart transplant patients on chronic cyclosporine. Am J Kidney Dis 1994;24(4):549–53.

157. Parving HH, Tarnow L, Nielsen FS, Rossing P, Mandrup-Poulsen T, Osterby R, Nerup J. Cyclosporine nephrotoxicity in type 1 diabetic patients. A 7-year follow-up study. Diabetes Care 1999;22(3):478–83.

158. Lipkowitz GS, Madden RL, Mulhern J, Braden G, O'Shea M, O'Shaughnessy J, Nash S, Kurbanov A, Freeman J, Rennke H, Germain M. Long-term maintenance of therapeutic cyclosporine levels leads to optimal graft survival without evidence of chronic nephrotoxicity. Transpl Int 1999;12(3):202–7.

159. Vercauteren SB, Bosmans JL, Elseviers MM, Verpooten GA, De Broe ME. A meta-analysis and morphological review of cyclosporine-induced nephrotoxicity in auto-immune diseases. Kidney Int 1998;54(2):536–45.

160. Feutren G, Mihatsch MJ. Risk factors for cyclosporine-induced nephropathy in patients with autoimmune diseases. International Kidney Biopsy Registry of Cyclosporine in Autoimmune Diseases. N Engl J Med 1992;326(25):1654–60.

161. Pei Y, Scholey JW, Katz A, Schachter R, Murphy GF, Cattran D. Chronic nephrotoxicity in psoriatic patients treated with low-dose cyclosporine. Am J Kidney Dis 1994;23(4):528–36.

162. Korstanje MJ, Bilo HJ, Stoof TJ. Sustained renal function loss in psoriasis patients after withdrawal of low-dose cyclosporin therapy. Br J Dermatol 1992;127(5):501–4.

163. Young EW, Ellis CN, Messana JM, Johnson KJ, Leichtman AB, Mihatsch MJ, Hamilton TA, Groisser DS, Fradin MS, Voorhees JJ. A prospective study of renal structure and function in psoriasis patients treated with cyclosporin. Kidney Int 1994;46(4):1216–22.

164. Shupack J, Abel E, Bauer E, Brown M, Drake L, Freinkel R, Guzzo C, Koo J, Levine N, Lowe N, McDonald C, Margolis D, Stiller M, Wintroub B, Bainbridge C, Evans S, Hilss S, Mietlowski W, Winslow C, Birnbaum JE. Cyclosporine as maintenance therapy in patients with severe psoriasis. J Am Acad Dermatol 1997;36(3 Pt 1):423–32.

165. van den Borne BE, Landewe RB, The HS, Breedveld FC, Dijkmans BA. Low dose cyclosporine in early rheumatoid arthritis: effective and safe after two years of therapy when compared with chloroquine. Scand J Rheumatol 1996;25(5):307–16.

166. Zachariae H, Kragballe K, Hansen HE, Marcussen N, Olsen S. Renal biopsy findings in long-term cyclosporin treatment of psoriasis. Br J Dermatol 1997;136(4):531–5.

167. Lowe NJ, Wieder JM, Rosenbach A, Johnson K, Kunkel R, Bainbridge C, Bourget T, Dimov I, Simpson K, Glass E, Grabie MT. Long-term low-dose cyclosporine therapy for severe psoriasis: effects on renal function and structure. J Am Acad Dermatol 1996;35(5 Pt 1):710–9.

168. Rodriguez F, Krayenbuhl JC, Harrison WB, Forre O, Dijkmans BA, Tugwell P, Miescher PA, Mihatsch MJ. Renal biopsy findings and followup of renal function in rheumatoid arthritis patients treated with cyclosporin A. An update from the International Kidney Biopsy Registry. Arthritis Rheum 1996;39(9):1491–8.

169. Landewe RB, Dijkmans BA, van der Woude FJ, Breedveld FC, Mihatsch MJ, Bruijn JA. Longterm low dose cyclosporine in patients with rheumatoid arthritis: renal function loss without structural nephropathy. J Rheumatol 1996;23(1):61–4.

170. Feehally J, Walls J, Mistry N, Horsburgh T, Taylor J, Veitch PS, Bell PR. Does nifedipine ameliorate cyclosporin A nephrotoxicity? BMJ (Clin Res Ed) 1987;295(6593):310.

171. Tindall RS, Rollins JA, Phillips JT, Greenlee RG, Wells L, Belendiuk G. Preliminary results of a double-blind, randomized, placebo-controlled trial of cyclosporine in myasthenia gravis. N Engl J Med 1987;316(12):719–24.

172. Hadj-Aissa A, Labeeuw M, Lareal MC, et al. Effets de la cyclosporine (CyA) sur le rein isole: comparaison avec l'excipient (Exc). Nephrologie 1987;8:73.

173. Hoyer PF, Krohn HP, Offner G, Byrd DJ, Brodehl J, Wonigeit K, Pichlmayr R. Renal function after kidney transplantation in children. A comparison of conventional immunosuppression with cyclosporine. Transplantation 1987;43(4):489–93.

174. Wheatley HC, Datzman M, Williams JW, Miles DE, Hatch FE. Long-term effects of cyclosporine on renal function in liver transplant recipients. Transplantation 1987;43(5):641–7.

175. Albengres E, Le Louet H, d'Athis P, Tillement JP. S15176 and S16950 interaction with cyclosporin A antiproliferative effect on cultured human lymphocytes. Fundam Clin Pharmacol 2001;15(1):41–6.

176. Mihatsch MJ, Thiel G, Ryffel B. Brief review of the morphology of cyclosporin A nephropathy. Nephrologie 1987;8(3):143–5.

177. Palestine AG, Austin HA 3rd, Balow JE, Antonovych TT, Sabnis SG, Preuss HG, Nussenblatt RB. Renal histopathologic alterations in patients treated with cyclosporine for uveitis. N Engl J Med 1986;314(20):1293–8.

178. Serkova N, Christians U. Transplantation: toxicokinetics and mechanisms of toxicity of cyclosporine and macrolides. Curr Opin Investig Drugs 2003;4:1287–96.

179. Parra Cid T, Conejo Garcia JR, Carballo Alvarez F, de Arriba G. Antioxidant nutrients protect against cyclosporine A nephrotoxicity. Toxicology 2003;189:99–111.

180. Raphael L, Fish JC. An in vitro model for analyzing the nephrotoxicity of cyclosporine and preservation injury. Transplantation 1987;43(5):703–8.

181. Anaise D, Waltzer WC, Arnold AN, Rapaport FT. Adverse effects of cyclosporine A on the microcirculation of the cold preserved kidney. NY State J Med 1987;87(3):141–2.

182. Nankivell BJ, Chapman JR, Bonovas G, Gruenewald SM. Oral cyclosporine but not tacrolimus reduces renal transplant blood flow. Transplantation 2004;77(9):1457–9.

183. Nankivell BJ, Borrows RJ, Fung CL, O'Connell PJ, Chapman JR, Allen RD. Calcineurin inhibitor nephrotoxicity: longitudinal assessment by protocol histology. Transplantation 2004;78(4):557–65.

184. Nankivell BJ, Borrows RJ, Fung CL, O'Connell PJ, Chapman JR, Allen RD. Delta analysis of posttransplantation tubulointerstitial damage. Transplantation 2004;78(3):434–41.

185. Lewis RM. Long-term use of cyclosporine A does not adversely impact on clinical outcomes following renal transplantation. Kidney Int Suppl 1995;52:S75–8.

186. Sehgal V, Radhakrishnan J, Appel GB, Valeri A, Cohen DJ. Progressive renal insufficiency following cardiac transplantation: cyclosporine, lipids, and hypertension. Am J Kidney Dis 1995;26(1):193–201.

187. Camara NO, Matos AC, Rodrigues DA, Pereira AB, Pacheco-Silva A. Early detection of heart transplant patients with increased risk of ciclosporin nephrotoxicity. Lancet 2001;357(9259):856–7.

188. Iijima K, Hamahira K, Tanaka R, Kobayashi A, Nozu K, Nakamura H, Yoshikawa N. Risk factors for cyclosporine-induced tubulointerstitial lesions in children with minimal change nephrotic syndrome. Kidney Int 2002;61(5):1801–5.

189. Hauser IA, Schaeffeler E, Gauer S, Scheuermann EH, Wegner B, Gossmann J, Ackermann H. ABCB1 genotype of the donor but not of the recipient is a major risk factor for cyclosporine-related nephrotoxicity after renal transplantation. J Am Soc Nephrol 2005;16(5):1501–11.

190. Murphy GJ, Waller JR, Sandford RS, Furness PN, Nicholson ML. Randomized clinical trial of the effect of microemulsion cyclosporin and tacrolimus on renal allograft fibrosis. Br J Surg 2003;90:680–6.

191. Stallone G, Di Paolo S, Schena A, Infante B, Grandaliano G, Battaglia M, Gesualdo L, Schena FP. Early withdrawal of cyclosporine A improves 1-year kidney graft structure and function in sirolimus-treated patients. Transplantation 2003;75:998–1003.

192. Saunders RN, Bicknell GR, Nicholson ML. The impact of cyclosporine dose reduction with or without the addition of rapamycin on functional, molecular, and histological markers of chronic allograft nephropathy. Transplantation 2003;75:772–80.

193. Hollander AAMJ, Van der Woude FJ. Efficacy and tolerability of conversion from cyclosporin to azathioprine after kidney transplantation. A review of the evidence. BioDrugs 1998;9:197–210.

194. Kasiske BL, Heim-Duthoy K, Ma JZ. Elective cyclosporine withdrawal after renal transplantation. A meta-analysis. JAMA 1993;269(3):395–400.

195. Heim-Duthoy KL, Chitwood KK, Tortorice KL, Massy ZA, Kasiske BL. Elective cyclosporine withdrawal 1 year after renal transplantation. Am J Kidney Dis 1994;24(5):846–53.

196. Smith SR, Minda SA, Samsa GP, Harrell FE Jr, Gunnells JC, Coffman TM, Butterly DW. Late withdrawal of cyclosporine in stable renal transplant recipients. Am J Kidney Dis 1995;26(3):487–94.

197. Mourad G, Vela C, Ribstein J, Mimran A. Long-term improvement in renal function after cyclosporine reduction in renal transplant recipients with histologically proven chronic cyclosporine nephropathy. Transplantation 1998;65(5):661–7.

198. Bunke M, Sloan R, Brier M, Ganzel B. An improved glomerular filtration rate in cardiac transplant recipients with once-a-day cyclosporine dosing. Transplantation 1995;59(4):537–40.

199. Thervet E, Martinez F, Legendre C. Benefit-risk assessment of ciclosporin withdrawal in renal transplant recipients. Drug Saf 2004;27(7):457–76.

200. Ramsay HM, Harden PN. Cyclosporin-induced flushing in a renal transplant recipient resolving after substitution with tacrolimus. Br J Dermatol 2000;142(4):832–3.

201. Azurdia RM, Graham RM, Weismann K, Guerin DM, Parslew R. Acne keloidalis in caucasian patients on cyclosporin following organ transplantation. Br J Dermatol 2000;143(2):465–7.

202. Carnero L, Silvestre JF, Guijarro J, Albares MP, Botella R. Nuchal acne keloidalis associated with cyclosporin. Br J Dermatol 2001;144(2):429–30.

203. Gupta S, Radotra BD, Kumar B, Pandhi R, Rai R. Multiple, large, polypoid infundibular (epidermoid) cysts in a cyclosporin-treated renal transplant recipient. Dermatology 2000;201(1):78.

204. Mahendran R, Grech C. Generalized pustular psoriasis following a short course of cyclosporin (Neoral). Br J Dermatol 1998;139(5):934.

205. Halpert E, Tunnessen WW Jr, Fivush B, Case B. Cutaneous lesions associated with cyclosporine therapy in pediatric renal transplant recipients. J Pediatr 1991;119(3):489–91.

206. Reznik VM, Jones KL, Durham BL, Mendoza SA. Changes in facial appearance during cyclosporin treatment. Lancet 1987;1(8547):1405–7.

207. Hivnor C, Nosauri C, James W, Poh-Fitzpatrick M. Cyclosporine-induced pseudoporphyria. Arch Dermatol 2003;139:1373–4.

208. Heaphy MR, Jr., Shamma HN, Hickmann M, White MJ. Cyclosporine-induced folliculodystrophy. J Am Acad Dermatol 2004;50(2):310–5.

209. Flicinski J, Brzosko M, Olewniczak S. Multiple haemangiomas in a psoriatic arthritis patient treated with cyclosporine. Acta Derm Venereol 2006;86(3):271–2.

210. Boschnakow A, May T, Assaf C, Tebbe B, Zouboulis ChC. Ciclosporin A-induced sebaceous gland hyperplasia. Br J Dermatol 2003;149:198–200.

211. Harman KE, Higgins EM. Case 4: eruption on the face of a diabetic man suffering from retinopathy, hypertension, and nephropathy. Diagnosis: ciclosporin-associated hyperplastic folliculitis. Clin Exp Dermatol 2003;28:341–2.

212. Lee MO, Park SK, Choi JH, Sung KJ, Moon KC, Koh JK. Juxta-clavicular beaded lines in a kidney transplant patient receiving immunosuppressants. J Dermatol 2002;29(4):235–7.

213. Lear J, Bourke JF, Burns DA. Hyperplastic pseudofolliculitis barbae associated with cyclosporin. Br J Dermatol 1997;136(1):132–3.

214. Rebora A, Delmonte S, Parodi A. Cyclosporin A-induced hair darkening. Int J Dermatol 1999;38(3):229–30.

215. Siragusa M, Alberti A, Schepis C. Mees' lines due to cyclosporin. Br J Dermatol 1999;140(6):1198–9.

216. Arellano F, Krupp P. Muscular disorders associated with cyclosporin. Lancet 1991;337(8746):915.

217. Breil M, Chariot P. Muscle disorders associated with cyclosporine treatment. Muscle Nerve 1999;22(12):1631–6.

218. Fujii Y, Arimura Y, Takahashi N, Toki T, Marumo T, Yoshihara K, Nakabayashi K, Yamada A. A case of Behçet's disease associated with neuromyopathy induced by combination therapy with colchicine and cyclosporin. Ryumachi 2003;43:44–50.

219. Courtney AE, Doherty C, Herron B, McCarron MO, Connolly JK, Jefferson JA. Acute polymyositis following renal transplantation. Am J Transplant 2004;4(7):1204–7.

220. Khan S, El Dars L, Holt PJ. Musculoskeletal and myotoxic side-effects in a patient treated for psoriasis. Br J Dermatol 2006;155(2):481.

221. Stevens JM, Hilson AJ, Sweny P. Post-renal transplant distal limb bone pain. An under-recognized complication of transplantation distinct from avascular necrosis of bone? Transplantation 1995;60(3):305–7.

222. Barbosa LM, Gauthier VJ, Davis CL. Bone pain that responds to calcium channel blockers. A retrospective and prospective study of transplant recipients. Transplantation 1995;59(4):541–4.

223. Kart-Koseoglu H, Yucel AE, Isiklar I, Turker I, Akcali Z, Haberal M. Joint pain and arthritis in renal transplant recipients and correlation with cyclosporine therapy. Rheumatol Int 2003;23:159–62.

224. Hokken-Koelega AC, Van Zaal MA, de Ridder MA, Wolff ED, De Jong MC, Donckerwolcke RA, De Muinck Keizer-Schrama SM, Drop SL. Growth after renal transplantation in prepubertal children: impact of various treatment modalities. Pediatr Res 1994;35(3):367–71.

225. Monegal A, Navasa M, Guanabens N, Peris P, Pons F, Martinez de Osaba MJ, Rimola A, Rodes J, Munoz-Gomez J. Bone mass and mineral metabolism in liver transplant patients treated with FK506 or cyclosporine A. Calcif Tissue Int 2001;68(2):83–6.

226. Wada C, Kataoka M, Seto H, Hayashi N, Kido J, Shinohara Y, Nagata T. High-turnover osteoporosis is induced by cyclosporin A in rats. J Bone Miner Metab 2006;24(3):199–205.

227. Baildam AD, Higgins RM, Hurley E, Furlong A, Walls J, Venning MC, Ackrill P, Mansel RE. Cyclosporin A and multiple fibroadenomas of the breast. Br J Surg 1996;83(12):1755–7.

228. Foxwell BM, Woerly G, Husi H, Mackie A, Quesniaux VF, Hiestand PC, Wenger RM, Ryffel B. Identification of several cyclosporine binding proteins in lymphoid and non-lymphoid cells in vivo. Biochim Biophys Acta 1992;1138(2):115–21.

229. Lopez-Calderon A, Soto L, Villanua MA, Vidarte L, Martin AI. The effect of cyclosporine administration on growth hormone release and serum concentrations of insulin-like growth factor-I in male rats. Life Sci 1999;64(17):1473–83.

230. Russell DH, Kibler R, Matrisian L, Larson DF, Poulos B, Magun BE. Prolactin receptors on human T and B lymphocytes: antagonism of prolactin binding by cyclosporine. J Immunol 1985;134(5):3027–31.

231. Larson DF. Cyclosporin. Mechanism of action: antagonism of the prolactin receptor. Prog Allergy 1986;38:222–38.

232. Alkhunaizi AM, Ismail A, Yousif BM. Breast fibroadenomas in renal transplant recipients. Transplant Proc 2004;36(6):1839–40.

233. Kanaan N, Goffin E. Multiple bilateral fibroadenomas of the breasts requiring mastectomy in a renal transplant patient. Clin Nephrol 2004;61(2):151–4..

234. Son EJ, Oh KK, Kim EK, Cho N, Lee JD, Kim SH, Jung WH. Characteristic imaging features of breast fibroadenomas in women given cyclosporin A after renal transplantation. J Clin Ultrasound 2004;32(2):69–77.

235. Weinstein SP, Orel SG, Collazzo L, Conant EF, Lawton TJ, Czerniecki B. Cyclosporin A-induced fibroadenomas of the breast: report of five cases. Radiology 2001;220(2):465–8.

236. Volcheck GW, Van Dellen RG. Anaphylaxis to intravenous cyclosporine and tolerance to oral cyclosporine: case report and review. Ann Allergy Asthma Immunol 1998;80(2):159–63.

237. Liau-Chu M, Theis JG, Koren G. Mechanism of anaphylactoid reactions: improper preparation of high-dose intravenous cyclosporine leads to bolus infusion of Cremophor EL and cyclosporine. Ann Pharmacother 1997;31(11):1287–91.

238. Garcia VD, Keitel E, Almeida P, Santos AF, Becker M, Goldani JC. Morbidity after renal transplantation: role of bacterial infection. Transplant Proc 1995;27(2):1825–6.

239. Wade JJ, Rolando N, Hayllar K, Philpott-Howard J, Casewell MW, Williams R. Bacterial and fungal infections after liver transplantation: an analysis of 284 patients. Hepatology 1995;21(5):1328–36.

240. Singh N, Yu VL. Infections in organ transplant recipients. Curr Opin Infect Dis 1996;9:223–9.

241. Reis MA, Costa RS, Ferraz AS. Causes of death in renal transplant recipients: a study of 102 autopsies from 1968 to 1991. J R Soc Med 1995;88(1):24–7.

242. Dai MS, Kao WY, Shyu RY, Chao TY. Restoration of immunity and reactivation of hepatitis B virus after immunosuppressive therapy in a patient with severe aplastic anaemia. J Viral Hepat 2004;11(3):283–5.

243. Lee YA, Kim HJ, Lee TW, Kim MJ, Lee MH, Lee JH, Ihm CG. First report of Cryptococcus albidus-induced disseminated cryptococcosis in a renal transplant recipient. Korean J Intern Med 2004;19(1):53–7.

244. Fukuda M, Ohmori Y, Aikawa I, Yoshimura N, Oka T. Mutagenicity of cyclosporine in vivo. Transplant Proc 1988;20(3 Suppl 3):929–30.

245. Penn I. Tumors after renal and cardiac transplantation. Hematol Oncol Clin North Am 1993;7(2):431–45.

246. Qunibi WY, Akhtar M, Ginn E, Smith P. Kaposi's sarcoma in cyclosporine-induced gingival hyperplasia. Am J Kidney Dis 1988;11(4):349–52.

247. Penn I. Cancers after cyclosporine therapy. Transplant Proc 1988;20(1 Suppl 1):276–9.

248. Penn I. Posttransplant malignancies. World J Urol 1988;6:125.

249. Penn I, Brunson ME. Cancers after cyclosporine therapy. Transplant Proc 1988;20(3 Suppl 3):885–92.

250. Pilgrim M. Spontane Manifestation und Regression eines Kaposi-Sarkoms unter Cyclosporin A. [Spontaneous manifestation and regression of a Kaposi's sarcoma under cyclosporin A therapy.] Hautarzt 1988;39(6):368–70.

251. Gaya SB, Rees AJ, Lechler RI, Williams G, Mason PD. Malignant disease in patients with long-term renal transplants. Transplantation 1995;59(12):1705–9.

252. London NJ, Farmery SM, Will EJ, Davison AM, Lodge JP. Risk of neoplasia in renal transplant patients. Lancet 1995;346(8972):403–6.

253. Corazza M, Zampino MR, Montanari A, Altieri E, Virgili A. Primary cutaneous CD30+ large T-cell lymphoma in a patient with psoriasis treated with cyclosporine. Dermatology 2003;206:330–3.

254. Ogata M, Kikuchi H, Ono K, Ohtsuka E, Gamachi A, Kashima K, Nasu M. Spontaneous remission of Epstein–Barr virus-negative non-Hodgkin's lymphoma after withdrawal of cyclosporine in a patient with refractory anemia. Int J Hematol 2004;79(2):161–4.

255. Kirby B, Owen CM, Blewitt RW, Yates VM. Cutaneous T cell lymphoma developing in a patient on cyclosporin therapy. J Am Acad Dermatol 2002;47(Suppl 2):S165–7.

256. Kehinde EO, Petermann A, Morgan JD, Butt ZA, Donnelly PK, Veitch PS, Bell PR. Triple therapy and incidence of de novo cancer in renal transplant recipients. Br J Surg 1994;81(7):985–6.

257. Opelz G, Henderson R. Incidence of non-Hodgkin lymphoma in kidney and heart transplant recipients. Lancet 1993;342(8886–8887):1514–6.

258. Gruber SA, Gillingham K, Sothern RB, Stephanian E, Matas AJ, Dunn DL. De novo cancer in cyclosporine-treated and non-cyclosporine-treated adult primary renal allograft recipients. Clin Transplant 1994;8(4):388–95.

259. Hiesse C, Kriaa F, Rieu P, Larue JR, Benoit G, Bellamy J, Blanchet P, Charpentier B. Incidence and type of malignancies occurring after renal transplantation in conventionally and cyclosporine-treated recipients: analysis of a 20-year period in 1600 patients. Transplant Proc 1995;27(1):972–4.

260. Andre N, Roquelaure B, Conrath J. Molecular effects of cyclosporine and oncogenesis: a new model. Med Hypotheses 2004;63(4):647–52.

261. Hojo M, Morimoto T, Maluccio M, Asano T, Morimoto K, Lagman M, Shimbo T, Suthanthiran M. Cyclosporine induces cancer progression by a cell-autonomous mechanism. Nature 1999;397(6719):530–4.

262. Jensen P, Hansen S, Moller B, Leivestad T, Pfeffer P, Geiran O, Fauchald P, Simonsen S. Skin cancer in kidney and heart transplant recipients and different long-term immunosuppressive therapy regimens. J Am Acad Dermatol 1999;40(2 Pt 1):177–86.

263. De Felipe I, Redondo P. Eruptive angiomas after treatment with cyclosporine in a patient with psoriasis. Arch Dermatol 1998;134(11):1487–8.

264. Zavos G, Papaconstantinou I, Chrisostomidis C, Kostakis A. Metastatic melanoma within a transplanted kidney: a case report. Transplant Proc 2004;36(5):1411–2.

265. Ho VC. The use of ciclosporin in psoriasis: a clinical review. Br J Dermatol 2004;150 Suppl 67:1–10.

266. Lain EL, Markus RF. Early and explosive development of nodular basal cell carcinoma and multiple keratoacanthomas in psoriasis patients treated with cyclosporine. J Drugs Dermatol 2004;3(6):680–2.

267. Armenti VT, Ahlswede KM, Ahlswede BA, Cater JR, Jarrell BE, Mortiz MJ, Burke JF Jr. Variables affecting birthweight and graft survival in 197 pregnancies in cyclosporine-treated female kidney transplant recipients. Transplantation 1995;59(4):476–9.

268. Cararach V, Carmona F, Monleon FJ, Andreu J. Pregnancy after renal transplantation: 25 years experience in Spain. Br J Obstet Gynaecol 1993;100(2):122–5.

269. Dor R, Blanshard C. Caution with the use of cyclosporin in pregnancy. Gut 2003;52:1070.

270. Day C, Hewins P, Sheikh L, Kilby M, McPake D, Lipkin G. Cholestasis in pregnancy associated with ciclosporin therapy in renal transplant recipients. Transpl Int 2006;19(12):1026-9.

271. Ramsey-Goldman R, Schilling E. Immunosuppressive drug use during pregnancy. Rheum Dis Clin North Am 1997;23(1):149–67.

272. Armenti VT, Moritz MJ, Davison JM. Drug safety issues in pregnancy following transplantation and immunosuppression: effects and outcomes. Drug Saf 1998;19(3):219–32.

273. Armenti VT, Ahlswede KM, Ahlswede BA, Jarrell BE, Moritz MJ, Burke JF. National Transplantation Pregnancy Registry—outcomes of 154 pregnancies in cyclosporine-treated female kidney transplant recipients. Transplantation 1994;57(4):502–6.

274. Armenti VT, Ahlswede BA, Moritz MJ, Jarrell BE. National Transplantation Pregnancy Registry: analysis of pregnancy outcomes of female kidney recipients with relation to time interval from transplant to conception. Transplant Proc 1993;25(1 Pt 2):1036–7.

275. Pilarski LM, Yacyshyn BR, Lazarovits AI. Analysis of peripheral blood lymphocyte populations and immune function from children exposed to cyclosporine or to azathioprine in utero. Transplantation 1994;57(1):133–44.

276. Baarsma R, Kamps WA. Immunological responses in an infant after cyclosporine A exposure during pregnancy. Eur J Pediatr 1993;152(6):476–7.

277. Giudice PL, Dubourg L, Hadj-Aissa A, Said MH, Claris O, Audra P, Martin X, Cochat P. Renal function of children exposed to cyclosporin in utero. Nephrol Dial Transplant 2000;15(10):1575–9.

278. Shaheen FA, al-Sulaiman MH, al-Khader AA. Long-term nephrotoxicity after exposure to cyclosporine in utero. Transplantation 1993;56(1):224–5.

279. Bar Oz B, Hackman R, Einarson T, Koren G. Pregnancy outcome after cyclosporine therapy during pregnancy: a meta-analysis. Transplantation 2001;71(8):1051–5.

280. Nyberg G, Haljamae U, Frisenette-Fich C, Wennergren M, Kjellmer I. Breast-feeding during treatment with cyclosporine. Transplantation 1998;65(2):253–5.

281. Dirks NL, Huth B, Yates CR, Meibohm B. Pharmacokinetics of immunosuppressants: a perspective on ethnic differences. Int J Clin Pharmacol Ther 2004;42(12):701-18.

282. Rayhill SC, Barbeito R, Katz D, Voigt M, Labrecque D, Kirby P, Miller R, Stolpen A, Wu Y, Schmidt W. A cyclosporine-based immunosuppressive regimen may be better than tacrolimus for long-term liver allograft survival in recipients transplanted for hepatitis C. Transplant Proc 2006;38(10):3625-8.

283. Villamil F, Levy G, Grazi GL, Mies S, Samuel D, Sanjuan F, Rossi M, Lake J, Munn S, Mühlbacher F, Leonardi L, Cillo U. Long-term outcomes in liver transplant patients with hepatic C infection receiving tacrolimus or cyclosporine. Transplant Proc 2006;38(9):2964-7.

284. O'Grady JG, Hardy P, Burroughs AK, Elbourne D. Randomized controlled trial of tacrolimus versus microemulsified cyclosporin (TMC) in liver transplantation: post-study surveillance to 3 years. Am J Transplant 2007;7(1):137-41.

285. Olyaei AJ, deMattos AM, Bennett WM. Switching between cyclosporin formulations. What are the risks? Drug Saf 1997;16(6):366–73.

286. Wijdicks EF, Dahlke LJ, Wiesner RH. Oral cyclosporine decreases severity of neurotoxicity in liver transplant recipients. Neurology 1999;52(8):1708–10.

287. Keown P, Landsberg D, Halloran P, Shoker A, Rush D, Jeffery J, Russell D, Stiller C, Muirhead N, Cole E, Paul L, Zaltzman J, Loertscher R, Daloze P, Dandavino R, Boucher A, Handa P, Lawen J, Belitsky P, Parfrey P. A randomized, prospective multicenter pharmacoepidemiologic study of cyclosporine microemulsion in stable renal graft recipients. Report of the Canadian Neoral Renal Transplantation Study Group. Transplantation 1996;62(12):1744–52.

288. Shah MB, Martin JE, Schroeder TJ, First MR. Evaluation of the safety and tolerability of Neoral and Sandimmune: a meta-analysis. Transplant Proc 1998;30(5):1697–700.

289. Freise CE, Galbraith CA, Nikolai BJ, Ascher NL, Lake JR, Stock PG, Roberts JP. Risks associated with conversion of stable patients after liver transplantation to the microemulsion formulation of cyclosporine. Transplantation 1998;65(7):995–7.

290. Shah MB, Martin JE, Schroeder TJ, First MR. Validity of open labeled versus blinded trials: a meta-analysis comparing Neoral and Sandimmune. Transplant Proc 1999;31(1–2):217–9.

291. Sheil AG, Disney AP, Mathew TH, Amiss N, Excell L. Cancer development in cadaveric donor renal allograft recipients treated with azathioprine (AZA) or cyclosporine (CyA) or AZA/CyA. Transplant Proc 1991;23(1 Pt 2): 1111–2.

292. Hiesse C, Rieu P, Kriaa F, Larue JR, Goupy C, Neyrat N, Charpentier B. Malignancy after renal transplantation: analysis of incidence and risk factors in 1700 patients followed during a 25-year period. Transplant Proc 1997; 29(1–2):831–3.

293. Hoshida Y, Tsukuma H, Yasunaga Y, Xu N, Fujita MQ, Satoh T, Ichikawa Y, Kurihara K, Imanishi M, Matsuno T, Aozasa K. Cancer risk after renal transplantation in Japan. Int J Cancer 1997;71(4):517–20.

294. Dantal J, Hourmant M, Cantarovich D, Giral M, Blancho G, Dreno B, Soulillou JP. Effect of long-term immunosuppression in kidney-graft recipients on cancer incidence: randomised comparison of two cyclosporin regimens. Lancet 1998;351(9103):623–8.

295. Feutren G. The optimal use of cyclosporin A in autoimmune diseases. J Autoimmun 1992;5(Suppl A):183–95.

296. Arellano F, Krupp P. Malignancies in rheumatoid arthritis patients treated with cyclosporin A. Br J Rheumatol 1993;32(Suppl 1):72–5.

297. van den Borne BE, Landewe RB, Houkes I, Schild F, van der Heyden PC, Hazes JM, Vandenbroucke JP, Zwinderman AH, Goei The HS, Breedveld FC, Bernelot Moens HJ, Kluin PM, Dijkmans BA. No increased risk of malignancies and mortality in cyclosporin A-treated patients with rheumatoid arthritis. Arthritis Rheum 1998;41(11):1930–7.

298. Arellano F. Risk of cancer with cyclosporine in psoriasis. Int J Dermatol 1997;36(Suppl 1):15–7.

299. Tarantino A, Passerini P, Campise M, Bonizzoni E, Ceccarini F, Montagnino G, Aroldi A, Ponticelli C. Is cyclosporine in renal-transplant recipients more effective when given twice a day than in a single daily dose? Transplantation 2004;78(5):675-80.

300. Arellano F, Monka C, Krupp PF. Acute cyclosporin overdose. A review of present clinical experience. Drug Saf 1991;6(4):266–76.

301. Sketris IS, Onorato L, Yatscoff RW, Givner M, Nicol D, Abraham I. Eight days of cyclosporine overdose: a case report. Pharmacotherapy 1993;13(6):658–60.

302. Dussol B, Reynaud-Gaubert M, Saingra Y, Daniel L, Berland Y. Acute tubular necrosis induced by high level of cyclosporine A in a lung transplant. Transplantation 2000;70(8):1234–6.

303. de Perrot M, Spiliopoulos A, Cottini S, Nicod L, Ricou B. Massive cerebral edema after I.V. cyclosporin overdose Transplantation 2000;70(8):1259–60.

304. Tabbara KF, Al-Faisal Z, Al-Rashed W. Interaction between acetazolamine and cyclosporine. Arch Ophthalmol 1998;116(6):832–3.

305. Lill J, Bauer LA, Horn JR, Hansten PD. Cyclosporine-drug interactions and the influence of patient age. Am J Health Syst Pharm 2000;57(17):1579–84.

306. Ahmed T, Fenton T, McGraw M. Reversible renal failure in renal transplant patients receiving acyclovir. Pediatr Nephrol 1993;7:C58.

307. Dugandzic RM, Sketris IS, Belitsky P, Schlech WF 3rd, Givner ML. Effect of coadministration of acyclovir and cyclosporine on kidney function and cyclosporine concentrations in renal transplant patients. DICP 1991;25(3): 316–7.

308. Termeer A, Hoitsma AJ, Koene RA. Severe nephrotoxicity caused by the combined use of gentamicin and cyclosporine in renal allograft recipients. Transplantation 1986;42(2):220–1.

309. Schmitt U, Abou El-Ela A, Guo LJ, Glavinas H, Krajcsi P, Baron JM, Tillmann C, Hiemke C, Langguth P, Härtter S. Cyclosporine A (CsA) affects the pharmacodynamics and pharmacokinetics of the atypical antipsychotic amisulpride probably via inhibition of P-glycoprotein (P-gp). J Neural Transm 2006;113(7):787-801.

310. Guaraldi G, Cocchi S, Codeluppi M, Di Benedetto F, Bonora S, Motta A, Luzi K, Pecorari M, Gennari W, Masetti M, Gerunda GE, Esposito R. Pharmacokinetic interaction between amprenavir/ritonavir and fosamprenavir on cyclosporine in two patients with human immunodeficiency virus infection undergoing orthotopic liver transplantation. Transplant Proc 2006;38(4):1138-40.

311. Vogel M, Voigt E, Michaelis HC, Sudhop T, Wolff M, Turler A, Sauerbruch T, Rockstroh JK, Spengler U. Management of drug-to-drug interactions between cyclosporine A and the protease-inhibitor lopinavir/ritonavir in liver-transplanted HIV-infected patients. Liver Transpl 2004;10(7):939-44.

312. Sketris IS, Methot ME, Nicol D, Belitsky P, Knox MG. Effect of calcium-channel blockers on cyclosporine clearance and use in renal transplant patients. Ann Pharmacother 1994;28(11):1227–31.

313. Smith CL, Hampton EM, Pederson JA, Pennington LR, Bourne DW. Clinical and medicoeconomic impact of the cyclosporine–diltiazem interaction in renal transplant recipients. Pharmacotherapy 1994;14(4):471–81.

314. Jones TE, Morris RG, Mathew TH. Formulation of diltiazem affects cyclosporin-sparing activity. Eur J Clin Pharmacol 1997;52(1):55–8.

315. Kuypers DR, Neumayer HH, Fritsche L, Budde K, Rodicio JL, Vanrenterghem Y. Lacidipine Study Group. Calcium channel blockade and preservation of renal graft function in cyclosporine-treated recipients: a prospective randomized placebo-controlled 2-year study. Transplantation 2004;78(8):1204–11.

316. Bui L, Huang DD. Possible interaction between cyclosporine and chloramphenicol. Ann Pharmacother 1999; 33(2):252–3.

317. Thurnheer R, Laube I, Speich R. Possible interaction between clindamycin and cyclosporin. BMJ 1999; 319(7203):163.

318. Ducloux D, Schuller V, Bresson-Vautrin C, Chalopin JM. Colchicine myopathy in renal transplant recipients on cyclosporin. Nephrol Dial Transplant 1997;12(11):2389–92.

319. Minetti EE, Minetti L. Multiple organ failure in a kidney transplant patient receiving both colchicine and cyclosporine. J Nephrol 2003;16:421–5.

320. Tweddle DA, Windebank KP, Hewson QC, Yule SM. Cyclosporin neurotoxicity after chemotherapy. BMJ 1999;318(7191):1113.

321. Pea F, Damiani D, Michieli M, Ermacora A, Baraldo M, Russo D, Fanin R, Baccarani M, Furlanut M. Multidrug resistance modulation in vivo: the effect of cyclosporin A alone or with dexverapamil on idarubicin pharmacokinetics in acute leukemia. Eur J Clin Pharmacol 1999;55(5):361–8.

322. Meerum Terwogt JM, Beijnen JH, ten Bokkel Huinink WW, Rosing H, Schellens JH. Co-administration of cyclosporin enables oral therapy with paclitaxel. Lancet 1998;352(9124):285.

323. Malingre MM, Beijnen JH, Rosing H, Koopman FJ, van Tellingen O, Duchin K, Ten Bokkel Huinink WW, Swart M, Lieverst J, Schellens JH. A phase I and pharmacokinetic study of bi-daily dosing of oral paclitaxel in combination with cyclosporin A. Cancer Chemother Pharmacol 2001;47(4):347–54.

324. Bisogno G, Cowie F, Boddy A, Thomas HD, Dick G, Pinkerton CR. High-dose cyclosporin with etoposide—toxicity and pharmacokinetic interaction in children with solid tumours. Br J Cancer 1998;77(12):2304–9.

325. Rushing DA, Raber SR, Rodvold KA, Piscitelli SC, Plank GS, Tewksbury DA. The effects of cyclosporine on the pharmacokinetics of doxorubicin in patients with small cell lung cancer. Cancer 1994;74(3):834–41.

326. Carcel-Trullols J, Torres-Molina F, Araico A, Saadeddin A, Peris JE. Effect of cyclosporine A on the tissue distribution and pharmacokinetics of etoposide. Cancer Chemother Pharmacol 2004;54(2):153–60.

327. Hoey LL, Lake KD. Does ciprofloxacin interact with cyclosporine? Ann Pharmacother 1994;28(1):93–6.

328. McLellan RA, Drobitch RK, McLellan H, Acott PD, Crocker JF, Renton KW. Norfloxacin interferes with cyclosporine disposition in pediatric patients undergoing renal transplantation. Clin Pharmacol Ther 1995;58(3):322–7.

329. Wynckel A, Toupance O, Melin JP, David C, Lavaud S, Wong T, Lamiable D, Chanard J. Traitement des légionelloses par ofloxacine chez le transplanté rénal. Absence d'interférence avec la ciclosporine A. [Treatment of legionellosis with ofloxacin in kidney transplanted patients. Lack of interaction with cyclosporin A.] Presse Méd 1991;20(7):291–3.

330. Morales JM, Munoz MA, Fernandez Zatarain G, Garcia Canton C, Garcia Rubiales MA, Andres A, Aguado JM, Gonzalez Pinto I. Reversible acute renal failure caused by the combined use of foscarnet and cyclosporin in organ transplanted patients. Nephrol Dial Transplant 1995;10(6):882–3.

331. Cantarovich M, Latter D. Effect of prophylactic ganciclovir on renal function and cyclosporine levels after heart transplantation. Transplant Proc 1994;26(5):2747–8.

332. Johnston A, Holt DW. Effect of grapefruit juice on blood cyclosporin concentration. Lancet 1995;346(8967):122–3.

333. Lewis SM, McCloskey WW. Potentiation of nephrotoxicity by H2-antagonists in patients receiving cyclosporine. Ann Pharmacother 1997;31(3):363–5.

334. Rodriguez JA, Crespo-Leiro MG, Paniagua MJ, Cuenca JJ, Hermida LF, Juffe A, Castro-Beiras A. Rhabdomyolysis in heart transplant patients on HMG-CoA reductase inhibitors and cyclosporine. Transplant Proc 1999;31(6):2522–3.

335. Gullestad L, Nordal KP, Berg KJ, Cheng H, Schwartz MS, Simonsen S. Interaction between lovastatin and cyclosporine A after heart and kidney transplantation. Transplant Proc 1999;31(5):2163–5.

336. Maltz HC, Balog DL, Cheigh JS. Rhabdomyolysis associated with concomitant use of atorvastatin and cyclosporine. Ann Pharmacother 1999;33(11):1176–9.

337. East C, Alivizatos PA, Grundy SM, Jones PH, Farmer JA. Rhabdomyolysis in patients receiving lovastatin after cardiac transplantation. N Engl J Med 1988;318(1):47–8.

338. Campana C, Iacona I, Regazzi MB, Gavazzi A, Perani G, Raddato V, Montemartini C, Vigano M. Efficacy and pharmacokinetics of simvastatin in heart transplant recipients. Ann Pharmacother 1995;29(3):235–9.

339. Cheung AK, DeVault GA Jr, Gregory MC. A prospective study on treatment of hypercholesterolemia with lovastatin in renal transplant patients receiving cyclosporine. J Am Soc Nephrol 1993;3(12):1884–91.

340. Wanner C, Kramer-Guth A, Galle J. Use of HMG-CoA reductase inhibitors after kidney and heart transplantation. BioDrugs 1997;8:387–93.

341. Olbricht C, Wanner C, Eisenhauer T, Kliem V, Doll R, Boddaert M, O'Grady P, Krekler M, Mangold B, Christians U. Accumulation of lovastatin, but not pravastatin, in the blood of cyclosporine-treated kidney graft patients after multiple doses. Clin Pharmacol Ther 1997;62(3):311–21.

342. Ichimaru N, Takahara S, Kokado Y, Wang JD, Hatori M, Kameoka H, Inoue T, Okuyama A. Changes in lipid metabolism and effect of simvastatin in renal transplant recipients induced by cyclosporine or tacrolimus. Atherosclerosis 2001;158(2):417–23.

343. Muck W, Mai I, Fritsche L, Ochmann K, Rohde G, Unger S, Johne A, Bauer S, Budde K, Roots I, Neumayer HH, Kuhlmann J. Increase in cerivastatin systemic exposure after single and multiple dosing in cyclosporine-treated kidney transplant recipients. Clin Pharmacol Ther 1999;65(3):251–61.

344. Taylor PJ, Kubler PA, Lynch SV, Allen J, Butler M, Pillans PI. Effect of atorvastatin on cyclosporine pharmacokinetics in liver transplant recipients. Ann Pharmacother 2004;38(2):205–8.

345. Gumprecht J, Zychma M, Grzeszczak W, Kuzniewicz R, Burak W, Zywiec J, Karasek D, Otulski I, Mosur M. Simvastatin-induced rhabdomyolysis in a CsA-treated renal transplant recipient. Med Sci Monit 2003;9:CS89–91.

346. Shitara Y, Itoh T, Sato H, Li AP, Sugiyama Y. Inhibition of transporter-mediated hepatic uptake as a mechanism for drug–drug interaction between cerivastatin and cyclosporin A. J Pharmacol Exp Ther 2003;304:610–6.

347. Neuvonen PJ, Niemi M, Backman JT. Drug interactions with lipid-lowering drugs: mechanisms and clinical relevance. Clin Pharmacol Ther 2006;80(6):565–81.

348. Ruschitzka F, Meier PJ, Turina M, Luscher TF, Noll G. Acute heart transplant rejection due to Saint John's wort. Lancet 2000;355(9203):548–9.

349. Breidenbach T, Hoffmann MW, Becker T, Schlitt H, Klempnauer J. Drug interaction of St. John's wort with cyclosporin. Lancet 2000;355(9218):1912.

350. Barone GW, Gurley BJ, Ketel BL, Lightfoot ML, Abul-Ezz SR. Drug interaction between St. John's wort and cyclosporine. Ann Pharmacother 2000;34(9):1013–6.

351. Karliova M, Treichel U, Malago M, Frilling A, Gerken G, Broelsch CE. Interaction of *Hypericum perforatum* (St. John's wort) with cyclosporin A metabolism in a patient after liver transplantation. J Hepatol 2000;33(5):853–5.

352. Mai I, Kruger H, Budde K, Johne A, Brockmoller J, Neumayer HH, Roots I. Hazardous pharmacokinetic interaction of Saint John's wort (*Hypericum perforatum*) with the immunosuppressant cyclosporin. Int J Clin Pharmacol Ther 2000;38(10):500–2.

353. Bauer S, Stormer E, Johne A, Kruger H, Budde K, Neumayer HH, Roots I, Mai I. Alterations in cyclosporin A pharmacokinetics and metabolism during treatment

with St John's wort in renal transplant patients. Br J Clin Pharmacol 2003;55:203–11.

354. Izzo AA. Drug interactions with St. John's wort (Hypericum perforatum): a review of the clinical evidence. Int J Clin Pharmacol Ther 2004;42(3):139–48.

355. Mai I, Bauer S, Perloff ES, Johne A, Uehleke B, Frank B, Budde K, Roots I. Hyperforin content determines the magnitude of the St John's wort–cyclosporine drug interaction. Clin Pharmacol Ther 2004;76(4):330–40.

356. Knuppel L, Linde K. Adverse effects of St. John's wort: a systematic review. J Clin Psychiatry 2004;65(11):1470–9.

357. Alscher DM, Klotz U. Drug interaction of herbal tea containing St. John's wort with cyclosporine. Transplant Int 2003;16:543–4.

358. Schroeder TJ, Melvin DB, Clardy CW, Wadhwa NK, Myre SA, Reising JM, Wolf RK, Collins JA, Pesce AJ, First MR. Use of cyclosporine and ketoconazole without nephrotoxicity in two heart transplant recipients. J Heart Transplant 1987;6(2):84–9.

359. Florea NR, Capitano B, Nightingale CH, Hull D, Leitz GJ, Nicolau DP. Beneficial pharmacokinetic interaction between cyclosporine and itraconazole in renal transplant recipients. Transplant Proc 2003;35:2873–7.

360. First MR, Schroeder TJ, Michael A, Hariharan S, Weiskittel P, Alexander JW. Cyclosporine–ketoconazole interaction. Long-term follow-up and preliminary results of a randomized trial. Transplantation 1993;55(5):1000–4.

361. Keogh A, Spratt P, McCosker C, Macdonald P, Mundy J, Kaan A. Ketoconazole to reduce the need for cyclosporine after cardiac transplantation. N Engl J Med 1995;333(10):628–33.

362. Sobh M, el-Agroudy A, Moustafa F, Harras F, el-Bedewy M, Ghoneim M. Coadministration of ketoconazole to cyclosporin-treated kidney transplant recipients: a prospective randomized study. Am J Nephrol 1995;15(6):493–9.

363. Groll AH, Kolve H, Ehlert K, Paulussen M, Vormoor J. Pharmacokinetic interaction between voriconazole and ciclosporin A following allogeneic bone marrow transplantation. J Antimicrob Chemother 2004;53(1):113–4.

364. Romero AJ, Pogamp PL, Nilsson LG, Wood N. Effect of voriconazole on the pharmacokinetics of cyclosporine in renal transplant patients. Clin Pharmacol Ther 2002;71(4):226–34.

365. Turhal NS. Cyclosporin A and imipenem associated seizure activity in allogeneic bone marrow transplantation patients. J Chemother 1999;11(5):410–3.

366. Jones TE. The use of other drugs to allow a lower dosage of cyclosporin to be used. Therapeutic and pharmacoeconomic considerations. Clin Pharmacokinet 1997;32(5):357–67.

367. Chester JD, Joel SP, Cheeseman SL, Hall GD, Braun MS, Perry J, Davis T, Button CJ, Seymour MT. Phase I and pharmacokinetic study of intravenous irinotecan plus oral ciclosporin in patients with fluorouracil-refractory metastatic colon cancer. J Clin Oncol 2003;21:1125–32.

368. Innocenti F, Undevia SD, Ramirez J, Mani S, Schilsky RL, Vogelzang NJ, Prado M, Ratain MJ. A phase I trial of pharmacologic modulation of irinotecan with cyclosporine and phenobarbital. Clin Pharmacol Ther 2004;76(5):490–502.

369. Agarwal A, Raza M, Dhiraaj S, Saxena R, Singh PK, Pandey R. Is ketamine a safe anesthetic for percutaneous liver biopsy in a liver transplant recipient immunosuppressed with cyclosporine? Anesth Analg 2005;100(1):85–6.

370. Amsden GW. Macrolides versus azalides: a drug interaction update. Ann Pharmacother 1995;29(9):906–17.

371. Rheeders M, Bouwer M, Goosen TC. Drug-drug interaction after single oral doses of the furanocoumarin methoxsalen and cyclosporine. J Clin Pharmacol 2006;46(7):768–75.

372. Gregoor PJ, de Sevaux RG, Hene RJ, Hesse CJ, Hilbrands LB, Vos P, van Gelder T, Hoitsma AJ, Weimar W. Effect of cyclosporine on mycophenolic acid trough levels in kidney transplant recipients. Transplantation 1999;68(10):1603–6.

373. Helms-Smith KM, Curtis SL, Hatton RC. Apparent interaction between nefazodone and cyclosporine. Ann Intern Med 1996;125(5):424.

374. Garton T. Nefazodone and CYP450 3A4 interactions with cyclosporine and tacrolimus1. Transplantation 2002;74(5):745.

375. Wright DH, Lake KD, Bruhn PS, Emery RW Jr. Nefazodone and cyclosporine drug–drug interaction. J Heart Lung Transplant 1999;18(9):913–5.

376. Constantopoulos A. Colitis induced by interaction of cyclosporine A and non-steroidal anti-inflammatory drugs. Pediatr Int 1999;41(2):184–6.

377. Kovarik JM, Mueller EA, Gerbeau C, Tarral A, Francheteau P, Guerret M. Cyclosporine and nonsteroidal antiinflammatory drugs: exploring potential drug interactions and their implications for the treatment of rheumatoid arthritis. J Clin Pharmacol 1997;37(4):336–43.

378. Kovarik JM, Kurki P, Mueller E, Guerret M, Markert E, Alten R, Zeidler H, Genth-Stolzenburg S. Diclofenac combined with cyclosporine in treatment refractory rheumatoid arthritis: longitudinal safety assessment and evidence of a pharmacokinetic/dynamic interaction. J Rheumatol 1996;23(12):2033–8.

379. Tugwell P, Ludwin D, Gent M, Roberts R, Bensen W, Grace E, Baker P. Interaction between cyclosporin A and nonsteroidal antiinflammatory drugs. J Rheumatol 1997;24(6):1122–5.

380. Barbaro D, Orsini P, Pallini S, Piazza F, Pasquini C. Obesity in transplant patients: case report showing interference of orlistat with absorption of cyclosporine and review of literature. Endocr Pract 2002;8(2):124–6.

381. Nagele H, Petersen B, Bonacker U, Rodiger W. Effect of orlistat on blood cyclosporin concentration in an obese heart transplant patient. Eur J Clin Pharmacol 1999;55(9):667–9.

382. Evans S, Michael R, Wells H, Maclean D, Gordon I, Taylor J, Goldsmith D. Drug interaction in a renal transplant patient: cyclosporin-Neoral and orlistat. Am J Kidney Dis 2003;41:493–6.

383. Nagele H, Petersen B, Bonacker U, Rodiger W. Effect of orlistat on blood cyclosporin concentration in an obese heart transplant patient. Eur J Clin Pharmacol 1999;55:667–9.

384. Barbaro D, Orsini P, Pallini S, Piazza F, Pasquini C. Obesity in transplant patients: case report showing interference of orlistat with absorption of cyclosporine and review of literature. Endocr Pract 2002;8:124–6.

385. Colman E, Fossler M. Reduction in blood cyclosporine concentrations by orlistat. N Engl J Med 2000;342(15):1141–2.

386. Le Beller C, Bezie Y, Chabatte C, Guillemain R, Amrein C, Billaud EM. Co-administration of orlistat and cyclosporine in a heart transplant recipient. Transplantation 2000;70(10):1541–2.

387. Schnetzler B, Kondo-Oestreicher M, Vala D, Khachatourian G, Faidutti B. Orlistat decreases the

plasma level of cyclosporine and may be responsible for the development of acute rejection episodes. Transplantation 2000;70(10):1540–1.

388. Asberg A. Interactions between cyclosporin and lipid-lowering drugs: implications for organ transplant recipients. Drugs 2003;63:367–78.

389. Actis GC, Debernardi-Venon W, Lagget M, Marzano A, Ottobrelli A, Ponzetto A, Rocca G, Boggio-Bertinet D, Balzola F, Bonino F, et al. Hepatotoxicity of intravenous cyclosporin A in patients with acute ulcerative colitis on total parenteral nutrition. Liver 1995;15(6):320–3.

390. Gregoor PJ, van Gelder T, van der Ende ME, Ijzermans JN, Weimar W. Cyclosporine and triple-drug treatment with human immunodeficiency virus protease inhibitors. Transplantation 1999;68(8):1210.

391. Brinkman K, Huysmans F, Burger DM. Pharmacokinetic interaction between saquinavir and cyclosporine. Ann Intern Med 1998;129(11):914–5.

392. Schouler L, Dumas F, Couzigou P, Janvier G, Winnock S, Saric J. Omeprazole–cyclosporin interaction. Am J Gastroenterol 1991;86(8):1097.

393. Arranz R, Yanez E, Franceschi JL, Fernandez-Ranada JM. More about omeprazole–cyclosporine interaction. Am J Gastroenterol 1993;88(1):154–5.

394. Blohme I, Idstrom JP, Andersson T. A study of the interaction between omeprazole and cyclosporine in renal transplant patients. Br J Clin Pharmacol 1993;35(2):156–60.

395. Wauters JP, Uehlinger D, Marti HP. Drug interaction between sevelamer and cyclosporin. Nephrol Dial Transplant 2004;19(7):1939–40.

396. Guillen-Anaya MA, Jadoul M. Drug interaction between sevelamer and cyclosporin. Nephrol Dial Transplant 2004;19(2):515.

397. Pieper AK, Buhle F, Bauer S, Mai I, Budde K, Haffner D, Neumayer HH, Querfeld U. The effect of sevelamer on the pharmacokinetics of cyclosporin A and mycophenolate mofetil after renal transplantation. Nephrol Dial Transplant 2004;19(10):2630–3.

398. Clerbaux G, Goffin E, Pirson Y. Interaction between sibutramine and cyclosporine. Am J Transplant 2003;3:906.

399. Zimmerman JJ, Harper D, Getsy J, Jusko WJ. Pharmacokinetic interactions between sirolimus and microemulsion cyclosporine when orally administered jointly and 4 hours apart in healthy volunteers. J Clin Pharmacol 2003;43:1168–76.

400. Du Cheyron D, Debruyne D, Lobbedez T, Richer C, Ryckelynck JP, Hurault de Ligny B. Effect of sulfasalazine on cyclosporin blood concentration. Eur J Clin Pharmacol 1999;55(3):227–8.

401. Caforio AL, Gambino A, Tona F, Feltrin G, Marchini F, Pompei E, Testolin L, Angelini A, Dalla Volta S, Casarotto D. Sulfinpyrazone reduces cyclosporine levels: a new drug interaction in heart transplant recipients. J Heart Lung Transplant 2000;19(12):1205–8.

402. Pichard L, Fabre I, Fabre G, Domergue J, Saint Aubert B, Mourad G, Maurel P. Cyclosporin A drug interactions. Screening for inducers and inhibitors of cytochrome P-450 (cyclosporin A oxidase) in primary cultures of human hepatocytes and in liver microsomes. Drug Metab Dispos 1990;18(5):595–606.

403. Islam SI, Masuda QN, Bolaji OO, Shaheen FM, Sheikh IA. Possible interaction between cyclosporine and glibenclamide in posttransplant diabetic patients. Ther Drug Monit 1996;18(5):624–6.

404. Verdejo A, de Cos MA, Zubimendi JA, Lopez-Lazaro L. Drug points. Probable interaction between cyclosporin A and low dose ticlopidine. BMJ 2000;320(7241):1037.

405. Kaplan B, Friedman G, Jacobs M, Viscuso R, Lyman N, DeFranco P, Bonomini L, Mulgaonkar SP. Potential interaction of troglitazone and cyclosporine. Transplantation 1998;65(10):1399–400.

406. Park MH, Pelegrin D, Haug MT 3rd, Young JB. Troglitazone, a new antidiabetic agent, decreases cyclosporine level. J Heart Lung Transplant 1998;17(11):1139–40.

407. Blackhall MR, Fassett RG, Sharman JE, Geraghty DP, Coombes JS. Effects of antioxidant supplementation on blood cyclosporin A and glomerular filtration rate in renal transplant recipients. Nephrol Dial Transplant 2005;20(9):1970–5.

408. de Vries AP, Oterdoom LH, Gans RO, Bakker SJ. Supplementation with anti-oxidants vitamin C and E decreases cyclosporine A trough-levels in renal transplant recipients. Nephrol Dial Transplant 2006;21(1):231–2.

409. Cantarovich D, Renou M, Megnigbeto A, Giral-Classe M, Hourmant M, Dantal J, Blancho G, Karam G, Soulillou JP. Switching from cyclosporine to tacrolimus in patients with chronic transplant dysfunction or cyclosporine-induced adverse events. Transplantation 2005;79(1):72–8.

410. Le Bigot JF, Lavene D, Kiechel JR. Pharmacocinétique et métabolisme di la cyclosporine: interaction médicamenteuse. [Pharmacokinetics and metabolism of cyclosporin; drug interactions.] Nephrologie 1987;8(3): 135–41.

411. Keown PA. New concepts in cyclosporine monitoring. Curr Opin Nephrol Hypertens 2002;11(6):619–26.

412. Levy G, Burra P, Cavallari A, Duvoux C, Lake J, Mayer AD, Mies S, Pollard SG, Varo E, Villamil F, Johnston A. Improved clinical outcomes for liver transplant recipients using cyclosporine monitoring based on 2-hr post-dose levels (C2). Transplantation 2002; 73(6):953–9.

413. Lindholm A, Ringden O, Lonnqvist B. The role of cyclosporine dosage and plasma levels in efficacy and toxicity in bone marrow transplant recipients. Transplantation 1987; 43(5):680–4.

414. Azoulay D, Lemoine A, Dennison A, Gries JM, Dolizy I, Castaing D, Beaune P, Bismuth H. Incidence of adverse reactions to cyclosporine after liver transplantation is predicted by the first blood level. Hepatology 1993; 17(6):1123–6.

415. Caforio AL, Tona F, Piaserico S, Gambino A, Feltrin G, Fortina AB, Angelini A, Alaibac M, Bontorin M, Calzolari D, Peserico A, Thiene G, Iliceto S, Gerosa G. C2 is superior to C0 as predictor of renal toxicity and rejection risk profile in stable heart transplant recipients. Transpl Int 2005;18(1):116–24.

416. Meiser BM, Groetzner J, Kaczmarek I, Landwehr P, Muller M, Jung S, Uberfuhr P, Fraunberger P, Stempfle HU, Weis M, Reichart B. Tacrolimus or cyclosporine: which is the better partner for mycophenolate mofetil in heart transplant recipients? Transplantation 2004;78(4):591–8.

417. Wang CH, Chou NK, Wu FL, Ko WJ, Tsao CI, Chi NH, Hsu RB, Wang SS. Therapeutic drug monitoring of cyclosporine Neoral in de novo Chinese cardiac transplant recipients treated with an everolimus–cyclosporine immunosuppressive regimen. Transplant Proc 2006;38(7):2132–4.

Corticosteroids—glucocorticoids

General Information

Nomenclature

The two main classes of adrenal corticosteroids are properly known as glucocorticoids and mineralocorticosteroids. The former are often known by shorter names and are commonly referred to as "glucocorticoids", "corticosteroids", "corticoids", or even simply "steroids"; the latter are often referred to as "mineralocorticoids". Here we shall use the terms "glucocorticoids" and "mineralocorticoids". When referring to both we shall use the term "corticosteroids".

Relative potencies

The main human anti-inflammatory corticosteroid, the glucocorticoid cortisol (hydrocortisone), as secreted by the adrenal gland, has generally been replaced by related glucocorticoids of synthetic origin for therapeutic purposes. These Δ^1-dehydrated glucocorticoids are designed to imitate the physiological hormone. They have marked glucocorticoid potency but only minor effects on sodium retention and potassium excretion; the relative glucocorticoid and mineralocorticoid potencies of the best-known compounds, insofar as these potencies are agreed, are compared in Table 1.

Over many years, a great deal of research has been devoted to producing better glucocorticoids for therapeutic use. Those endeavors have succeeded only in part; from the start the mineralocorticoid effects were sufficiently minor to be nonproblematic; the fact that successive synthetic glucocorticoids had an increasing potency in terms of weight was not of direct therapeutic significance; and the most hoped-for aim, that of dissociating wanted from unwanted glucocorticoid effects has not been achieved (1). Most untoward effects, such as those due to the catabolic and gluconeogenic activities of the glucocorticoid family, probably cannot be dissociated entirely from the anti-inflammatory activity (2) it is possible that myopathy and muscle wasting are actually more common when triamcinolone or dexamethasone are used, but this may merely reflect overdosage of these potent drugs. However, some progress in achieving a dissociation of effects has been made. Beclomethasone does have a relatively greater local than systemic effect. Deflazacort, one of the few new glucocorticoids to have been developed in recent years, originally promised reduced intensity of adverse effects, for example on bone mineral density, but the early promise has not held up (SEDA-18, 389). Cloprednol seems to affect the hypothalamic–pituitary–adrenal axis much less than other glucocorticoids, and to cause less excretion of nitrogen and calcium (3).

Uses

Most patients who are treated therapeutically with glucocorticoids do not have glucocorticoid deficiency. Adverse reactions to glucocorticoids depend very largely on the ways in which, and the purposes for which, they are used. There are four groups of uses.

(1) Substitution therapy is used in cases of primary and secondary adrenocortical insufficiency; the aim is to provide glucocorticoids and mineralocorticoids in physiological amounts, and the better the dosage regimen is adapted to the individual's needs, the less the chance of adverse effects (1).

(2) Anti-inflammatory and immunosuppressive therapy exploits the immunosuppressive, anti-allergic, anti-inflammatory, anti-exudative, and anti-proliferative effects of the glucocorticoids (2). The desired pharmacodynamic effects reflect a general influence of these substances on the mesenchyme, where they suppress reactions that result in the symptoms of inflammation, exudation, and proliferation; the non-specific effects of glucocorticoids on the mesenchyme are part of their physiological actions, but they can only be obtained to a clinically useful extent by using dosages at which the more specific (and unwanted) physiological effects also occur. High doses sufficient to suppress immune reactions are used in patients who have undergone organ transplantation.

(3) Hormone suppression therapy can be used, for example, to inhibit the adrenogenital syndrome (3). Higher doses are used. The treatment of the adrenogenital syndrome is only partly substitutive and has to be adapted to the individual case, but doses are needed at which various hormonal effects of the glucocorticoids and mineralocorticoids are likely to become troublesome.

Table 1 Relative potencies of glucocorticoids

Compound	Glucocorticoid potency relative to hydrocortisone	Mineralocorticoid potency	Equivalent doses (mg)
Cortisone	0.8	++	25
Hydrocortisone	1.0	++	20
Prednisone	4	+	5
Prednisolone	4	+	5
Methylprednisolone	5	0	4
Triamcinolone	5	0	4
Paramethasone	10	0	2
Fluprednisolone	10	0	1.5
Dexamethasone	30	0	0.75

(4) Massive doses of glucocorticoids, far exceeding physiological amounts, are given in the immediate management of anaphylaxis, although their beneficial effects are delayed for several hours. This is because, in severely ill patients, early administration of hydrocortisone 100–300 mg as the sodium succinate salt can gradually enhance the actions of adrenaline (4). Glucocorticoids have been used as an adjunct to the use of inotropic and vasopressor drugs for septic shock. Their efficacy, as well as their proposed mechanisms of action, is controversial; inhibition of complement-mediated aggregation and resultant endothelial injury, and inhibition of the release of beta-endorphin are current theories of their mechanism of action. However, controlled studies have not indicated a beneficial effect of high-dose glucocorticoid therapy in treating septic shock (5,6). Hence, there is no established role for glucocorticoids in the treatment of shock, except shock caused by adrenal insufficiency.

Routes of administration

Glucocorticoids can be given by the following routes:

- oral
- rectal
- intravenous
- intramuscular
- inhalation
- nasal
- topical (skin, eyes, ears)
- intradermal
- intra-articular and periarticular
- intraspinal (epidural, intrathecal)
- intracapsular (breast)

All of these routes are covered in this monograph, except the inhalation route, which is the subject of a separate monograph.

Observational studies

A study has been undertaken to clarify whether glucocorticoid excess affects endothelium-dependent vascular relaxation in glucocorticoid treated patients and whether dexamethasone alters the production of hydrogen peroxide and the formation of peroxynitrite, a reactive molecule between nitric oxide and superoxide, in cultured human umbilical endothelial cells (7). Glucocorticoid excess impaired endothelium-dependent vascular relaxation in vivo and enhanced the production of reactive oxygen species to cause increased production of peroxynitrite in vitro. Glucocorticoid-induced reduction in nitric oxide availability may cause vascular endothelial dysfunction, leading to hypertension and atherosclerosis.

Comparative studies

In another randomized trial, the effects and adverse effects of early dexamethasone on the incidence of chronic lung disease have been evaluated in 50 high-risk preterm infants (8). The treated infants received dexamethasone intravenously from the fourth day of life for 7 days (0.5 mg/kg/day for the first 3 days, 0.25 mg/kg/day for the next 3 days, and 0.125 mg/kg/day on the seventh day). The incidence of chronic lung disease at 28 days of life and at 36 weeks of postconceptional age was significantly lower in the infants who were given dexamethasone, who also remained intubated and required oxygen therapy for a shorter period. Hyperglycemia, hypertension, growth failure, and left ventricular hypertrophy were the transient adverse effects associated with early glucocorticoid administration. Early dexamethasone administration may be useful in preventing chronic lung disease, but its use should be restricted to preterm high-risk infants.

Placebo-controlled studies

Patients taking glucocorticoids have an increased risk of infections, including those produced by opportunistic and rare pathogens. However, it has been suggested that glucocorticoid administration in severe community-acquired pneumonia could attenuate systemic inflammation and lead to earlier resolution of pneumonia and a reduction in sepsis-related complications. In a placebo-controlled study in 46 patients with severe community-acquired pneumonia who received protocol-guided antibiotic treatment hydrocortisone (intravenous 200 mg bolus followed by infusion at a rate of 10 mg/hour) for 7 days produced significant clinical improvement (9). Adverse effects were not described.

Although there have been several trials of early dexamethasone to determine whether it would reduce mortality and chronic lung disease in infants with respiratory distress, the optimal duration and adverse effects of such therapy are unknown. The purpose of one study was: (a) to determine if a 3-day course of early dexamethasone therapy would reduce chronic lung disease and increase survival without chronic lung disease in neonates who received surfactant therapy for respiratory distress syndrome and (b) to determine the associated adverse effects (10). This was a prospective, placebo-controlled, multicenter, randomized study of a 3-day course of early dexamethasone therapy, beginning at 24–48 hours of life in 241 neonates, who weighed 500–1500 g, had received surfactant therapy, and were at significant risk of chronic lung disease or death. Infants randomized to dexamethasone received a 3-day tapering course (total dose 1.35 mg/kg) given in six doses at 12-hour intervals. Chronic lung disease was defined by the need for supplementary oxygen at a gestational age of 36 weeks. Neonates randomized to early dexamethasone were more likely to survive without chronic lung disease (RR = 1.3; CI = 1.0, 1.7) and were less likely to develop chronic lung disease (RR = 0.6; CI = 0.3, 0.98). Mortality rates were not significantly different. Subsequent dexamethasone therapy was less in early dexamethasone-treated neonates (RR = 0.8; CI = 0.70, 0.96). Very early (before 7 days of life) intestinal perforations were more common among dexamethasone-treated neonates (8 versus 1%). The authors concluded that an early 3-day course of dexamethasone increases survival without chronic lung disease, reduces chronic lung disease, and reduces late dexamethasone therapy in high-risk, low birthweight infants who receive surfactant therapy for respiratory distress syndrome. The potential benefits of early dexamethasone therapy in the regimen used in this trial need to be weighed against the risk of early intestinal perforation.

Although dexamethasone is commonly associated with transient adverse effects, several randomized trials have shown that it rapidly reduces oxygen requirements and shortens the duration of ventilation. A randomized study was designed to evaluate the effects of two different dexamethasone courses on growth in preterm infants (11). The first phase included 30 preterm infants at high risk of chronic lung disease, of whom 15 (8 boys) were given dexamethasone for 14 days, from the tenth day of life; they received a total dose of 4.75 mg/kg; 15 babies were assigned to the control group (8 boys). The second phase included 30 preterm infants at high risk of chronic lung disease, of whom 15 babies (7 boys) were treated with dexamethasone for 7 days, from the fourth day of life; they received a total dose of 2.38 mg/kg; 15 babies were assigned to the control group (9 boys). Infants given dexamethasone had significantly less weight gain than controls, but they caught up soon after the end of treatment. At 30 days of life, the gains in weight and length in each group were similar to those in control infants, but those given dexamethasone had significantly less head growth. There were no differences between the groups at discharge. The longer-term impact of postnatal dexamethasone on mortality and morbidity is less clear. Better data, from larger clinical trials with longer follow-up, will determine whether this kind of treatment enhances lives, makes little difference, causes significant harm, or does several of these things (12).

Systematic reviews

A systematic review of glucocorticoid adjunctive therapy in adults with acute bacterial meningitis has been published (13). Five trials involving 623 patients were included (pneumococcal meningitis = 234, meningococcal meningitis = 232, others = 127, unknown = 30). Treatment with glucocorticoids was associated with a significant reduction in mortality (RR = 0.6; 95% CI = 0.4, 0.8) and in neurological sequelae (RR = 0.6; 95% CI = 0.4, 1), and with a reduction in case-fatality in pneumococcal meningitis of 21% (RR = 0.5; 95% CI = 0.3, 0.8). In meningococcal meningitis, mortality (RR = 0.9; 95% CI = 0.3, 2.1) and neurological sequelae (RR = 0.5; 95% CI = 0.1, 1.7) were both reduced, but not significantly. Adverse events were similar in the treatment and placebo groups (RR = 1; CI = 0.5, 2), with gastrointestinal bleeding in 1% of glucocorticoid-treated patients and 4% of the rest. The authors recommended the early use of glucocorticoid therapy in adults in whom acute community-acquired bacterial meningitis is suspected.

A systematic review of randomized controlled trials has been performed to determine whether dexamethasone therapy in the first 15 days of life prevents chronic lung disease in premature infants (14). Studies were identified by a literature search using Medline (1970–97)

supplemented by a search of the Cochrane Library (1998, Issue 4). Inclusion criteria were: (a) prospective randomized design with initiation of dexamethasone therapy within the first 15 days of life; (b) report of the outcome of interest; and (c) less than 20% crossover between the treatment and control groups during the study period. The primary outcomes were mortality at hospital discharge and the development of chronic lung disease at 28 days of life and 36 weeks postconceptional age. The secondary outcomes were the presence of a patent ductus arteriosus and treatment adverse effects. Dexamethasone reduced the incidence of chronic lung disease by 26% at 28 days (RR = 0.74; CI = 0.57, 0.96) and 48% at 36 weeks postconceptional age (RR = 0.52; CI = 0.33, 0.81). These reductions were more significant when dexamethasone was started in the first 72 hours of life. The 24% relative risk reduction of deaths was marginally significant (RR = 0.76; CI = 0.56, 1.04). The 27% reduction in patent ductus arteriosus and the 11% increase in infections were not statistically significant, nor were any other changes. The conclusion from this meta-analysis was that systemic dexamethasone given to at-risk infants soon after birth may reduce the incidence of chronic lung disease. There was no evidence of significant short-term adverse effects.

General adverse effects

The incidence and severity of adverse reactions to glucocorticoids depend on the dose and duration of treatment. Even the very high single doses of glucocorticoids, such as methylprednisolone, which are sometimes used, do not cause serious adverse effects, whereas an equivalent dose given over a long period of time can cause many long-term effects.

The two major risks of long-term glucocorticoid therapy are adrenal suppression and Cushingoid changes. During prolonged treatment with anti-inflammatory doses, glucose intolerance, osteoporosis, acne vulgaris, and a greater or lesser degree of mineralocorticoid-induced changes can occur. In children, growth can be retarded, and adults who take high doses can have mental changes. There may be a risk of gastroduodenal ulceration, although this is much less certain than was once thought. Infections and abdominal crises can be masked. Some of these effects reflect the catabolic properties of the glucocorticoids, that is their ability to accelerate tissue breakdown and impair healing. Allergic reactions can occur.

Anyone who prescribes long-term glucocorticoids should have a checklist in mind of the undesired effects that they can exert, both during treatment and on withdrawal, so that any harm that occurs can be promptly detected and countered. The main groups of risks arising from long-term treatment with glucocorticoids are summarized in Table 2.

The adverse reactions that were reported in a study of 213 children are listed in Table 3 (15).

Drug interactions that affect the efficacy of glucocorticoids have been reviewed (16).

Table 2 Risks of long-term glucocorticoid therapy

1. Exogenous hypercorticalism with Cushing's syndrome
Moon face (facial rounding)
Central obesity
Striae
Hirsutism
Acne vulgaris
Ecchymoses
Hypertension
Osteoporosis
Proximal myopathy
Disorders of sexual function
Diabetes mellitus
Hyperlipidemia
Disorders of mineral and fluid balance (depending on the type of glucocorticoid)
2. Adrenal insufficiency
Insufficient or absent stress reaction
Withdrawal effects
3. Unwanted results accompanying desired effects
Increased risk of infection
Impaired wound healing
Peptic ulceration, bleeding, and perforation
Growth retardation
4. Other adverse effects
Mental disturbances
Encephalopathy
Increased risk of thrombosis
Posterior cataract
Increased intraocular pressure and glaucoma
Aseptic necrosis of bone

Table 3 Adverse reactions in 213 children given intravenous methylprednisolone

Adverse effect	Number
Behavioral changes	21
Abdominal disorders	11
Pruritus	9
Urticaria	5
Hypertension	5
Bone pain	3
Dizziness	3
Fatigue	2
Fractures	2
Hypotension	2
Lethargy	2
Tachycardia	2
Anaphylactoid reaction	1
"Grey appearance"	1

Organs and Systems

Cardiovascular

The considerable body of evidence that glucocorticoids can cause increased rates of vascular mortality and the underlying mechanisms (increased blood pressure, impaired glucose tolerance, dyslipidemia, hypercoagulability, and increased fibrinogen production) have been reviewed (17). In view of their adverse cardiovascular effects, the therapeutic options should be carefully considered before long-term glucocorticoids are begun; although they can be life-saving, dosages should be regularly reviewed during long-term therapy, in order to minimize complications.

The benefit of glucocorticoid therapy is often limited by several adverse reactions, including cardiovascular disorders such as hypertension and atherosclerosis. Plasma volume expansion due to sodium retention plays a minor role, but increased peripheral vascular resistance, due in part to an increased pressor response to catecholamines and angiotensin II, plays a major role in the pathogenesis of hypertension induced by glucocorticoid excess. However, the molecular mechanism remains unclear.

Long-term systemic administration of glucocorticoids might be expected, because of their effects on vascular fragility and wound healing, to increase the risk of vascular complications during percutaneous coronary intervention. To assess the potential risk of long-term glucocorticoid use in the setting of coronary angioplasty, 114 of 12 883 consecutively treated patients who were taking long-term glucocorticoids were compared with those who were not. Glucocorticoid use was not associated with an increased risk of composite events of major ischemia but was associated with a threefold risk of major vascular complications and a three- to fourfold risk of coronary perforation (18).

Hypertension

The secondary mineralocorticoid activity of glucocorticoids can lead to salt and water retention, which can cause hypertension. Although the detailed mechanisms are as yet uncertain, glucocorticoid-induced hypertension often occurs in elderly patients and is more common in patients with total serum calcium concentrations below the reference range and/or in those with a family history of essential hypertension (SEDA-20, 368) (19).

Hemangioma is the most common tumor of infancy, with a natural history of spontaneous involution. Some hemangiomas, however, as a result of their proximity to vital structures, destruction of facial anatomy, or excessive bleeding, can be successfully treated with systemic glucocorticoids between other therapies. The risk of hypertension is poorly documented in this setting. In one prospective study of 37 infants (7 boys, 17 girls; mean age 3.5 months, range 1.5–10) with rapidly growing complicated hemangiomas treated with oral prednisone 1–5 mg/kg/day, blood pressure increased in seven cases (20). Cardiac ultrasound examination in five showed two cases of myocardial hypertrophy, which was unrelated to the hypertension and which regressed after withdrawal of the prednisone.

Myocardial ischemia

Cortisone-induced cardiac lesions are sometimes reported and electrocardiographic changes have been seen in patients taking glucocorticoids (21). Whereas abnormal myocardial hypertrophy in children has perhaps been associated more readily with corticotropin, it has been seen on occasion during treatment with high dosages of glucocorticoids, with normalization after dosage reduction and withdrawal.

Fatal myocardial infarction occurred after intravenous methylprednisolone for an episode of ulcerative colitis (22).

- A day after a dose of intravenous methylprednisolone 60 mg a 79-year-old woman developed acute thoracic pain and collapsed. An electrocardiogram showed signs of a myocardial infarction and her cardiac enzyme activities were raised. She died within several hours. Autopsy showed an anterior transmural myocardial infarction and mild atheromatous lesions in the coronary arteries.

This report highlights the risk of cardiovascular adverse effects with short courses of glucocorticoid therapy in elderly patients with inflammatory bowel disease, even with rather low-dosage regimens. Acute myocardial infarction occurred in an old man with coronary insufficiency and giant cell arteritis after treatment with prednisolone (SEDA-10, 343) but could well have been coincidental.

Myocardial ischemia has been reportedly precipitated by intramuscular administration of betamethasone (SEDA-21, 413; 23). It has been suggested that long-term glucocorticoid therapy accelerates atherosclerosis and the formation of aortic aneurysms, with a high risk of rupture (SEDA-20, 369; 24).

Patients with seropositive rheumatoid arthritis taking long-term systemic glucocorticoids are at risk of accelerated cardiac rupture in the setting of transmural acute myocardial infarction treated with thrombolytic drugs (25).

- Two women and one man, aged 53–74 years, died after they received thrombolytic therapy for acute myocardial infarction. All three had a long history of seropositive rheumatoid arthritis treated with prednisone 5–20 mg/day for many years.

Cardiomyopathy

Postnatal exposure to glucocorticoids has been associated with hypertrophic cardiomyopathy in neonates. Such an effect has not previously been described in infants born to mothers who received antenatal glucocorticoids. Three neonates (gestational ages 36, 29, and 34 weeks), whose mothers had been treated with betamethasone prenatally in doses of 12 mg twice weekly for 16 doses, 8 doses, and 5 doses respectively, developed various degrees of hypertrophic cardiomyopathy diagnosed by echocardiography (26). There was no maternal evidence of diabetes, except for one infant whose mother had a normal fasting and postprandial blood glucose before glucocorticoid therapy, but an abnormal 1-hour postprandial glucose after 8 weeks of betamethasone therapy, with a normal HbA_{1C} concentration. There was no family history of hypertrophic cardiomyopathy, no history of maternal intake of other relevant medications, no hypertension, and none of the infants received glucocorticoids postnatally. Follow-up echocardiography showed complete resolution in all infants. The authors suggested that repeated antenatal maternal glucocorticoids might cause hypertrophic cardiomyopathy in neonates. These changes appear to be dose- and duration-related and are mostly reversible.

Transient hypertrophic cardiomyopathy is a rare sequel of the concurrent administration of glucocorticoid and insulin excess (SEDA-21, 412; 27). The heart is also almost certainly a site for myopathic changes analogous to those that affect other muscles.

Transient hypertrophic cardiomyopathy has been attributed to systemic glucocorticoid administration for a craniofacial hemangioma (28).

- A 69-day-old white child presented with a rapidly growing 2.5 × 1.5 cm hemangioma of the external left nasal side wall. He was normotensive and there was no family history of cardiomyopathy or maternal gestational diabetes. Because of nasal obstruction and possible visual obstruction, he was given prednisolone 3 mg/kg/day. After 10 weeks his weight had fallen from 7.6 to 7.1 kg and 2 weeks later he became tachypneic with a respiratory rate of 40/minutes. A chest X-ray showed cardiomegaly and pulmonary venous congestion. An echocardiogram showed hypertrophic cardiomyopathy. The left ventricular posterior wall thickness was 10 mm (normal under 4 mm), and the peak left ventricular outflow gradient was 64 mmHg. He was given a beta-blocker and a diuretic and the glucocorticoid dose was tapered. The cardiomyopathy eventually resolved.

Dilated cardiomyopathy caused by occult pheochromocytoma has been described infrequently.

- A 34-year-old woman had acute congestive heart failure 12 hours after administration of dexamethasone 16 mg for an atypical migraine (29). The authors postulated that the acute episode had been induced by the dexamethasone, which increased the production of adrenaline, causing beta$_2$-adrenoceptor stimulation, peripheral vasodilatation, and congestive heart failure.

In an addendum the authors reported another similar case. Obstructive cardiomyopathy has been attributed to a glucocorticoid in a child with subglottal stenosis (30).

- A 4-month-old boy (weight 4 kg) developed fever, nasal secretions, and stridor due to a subglottal granuloma. Dexamethasone 1 mg/kg/day was started and tapered over 1 week. The mass shrank to 25% of its original size but the symptoms recurred 2 weeks later. The granuloma was excised and dexamethasone 1 mg/kg/day was restarted. After 5 days he developed a tachycardia (140/minute) and a new systolic murmur. Echocardiography showed severe ventricular hypertrophy with dynamic left ventricular outflow tract obstruction. The dexamethasone was weaned over several days. Over the next 3 weeks several echocardiograms showed rapid resolution of the outflow tract obstruction and gradual improvement of the cardiac hypertrophy. After 8 months there was no further problem.

Cardiac dysrhythmias

Serious cardiac dysrhythmias and sudden death have been reported with pulsed methylprednisolone. Oral methylprednisolone has been implicated in a case of sinus bradycardia (31).

- A 14-year-old boy received an intravenous dose of methylprednisolone 30 mg/kg for progressive glomerulonephritis. After 5 hours, his heart rate had fallen to 50/minute and an electrocardiogram showed sinus bradycardia. His heart rate then fell to 40/minutes and a temporary transvenous pacemaker was inserted and methylprednisolone was withdrawn. His heart rate increased to 80/minutes over 3 days. After a further 3 days, he was treated with oral methylprednisolone 60 mg/m^2/day and his heart rate fell to 40/minutes in 5 days. Oral methylprednisolone was stopped on day 8 of treatment and his heart rate normalized.

Hypokalemia, secondary to mineralocorticoid effects, can cause cardiac dysrhythmias and cardiac arrest. Recurrent cardiocirculatory arrest has been reported (32).

- A 60-year-old white man was admitted for kidney transplantation. Immediately after reperfusion and intravenous methylprednisolone 500 mg, he developed severe bradycardia with hypotension and then cardiac arrest. After resuscitation, his clinical state improved quickly, but on the morning of the first postoperative day directly after the intravenous administration of methylprednisolone 250 mg, he had another episode of severe

bradycardia, hypotension, and successful cardiopulmonary resuscitation. A third episode occurred 24 hours later after intravenous methylprednisolone 100 mg, again followed by rapid recovery after resuscitation. Two weeks later, during a bout of acute rejection, he was given intravenous methylprednisolone 500 mg, after which he collapsed and no heartbeat or breathing was detectable; after cardiopulmonary resuscitation he was transferred to the intensive care unit, where he died a few hours later.

If patients at risk are identified, glucocorticoid bolus therapy should be avoided or, if that is not possible, should only be done under close monitoring.

Pericarditis

- Disseminated *Varicella* and staphylococcal pericarditis developed in a previously healthy girl after a single application of triamcinolone cream 0.1% to relieve pruritus associated with *Varicella* skin lesions (SEDA-22, 443) (33).

Vasculitis

Long-term treatment with glucocorticoids can cause arteritis, but patients with rheumatoid arthritis have a special susceptibility to vascular reactions, and cases of periarteritis nodosa after withdrawal of long-term glucocorticoids have been reported (34).

Respiratory

Local adverse effects are common in patients with asthma who use inhaled glucocorticoids, as suggested by a survey of the prevalence of throat and voice symptoms in patients with asthma using glucocorticoids by metered-dose pressurized aerosol (SEDA-20, 369; 35).

There have been no reports of an increased frequency of lower respiratory tract infections. However, patients with aspiration of gastric material who were treated with glucocorticoids did not have improved survival but had a higher incidence of pneumonia (SED-12, 982).

In cases of pneumothorax with closed thoracotomy tube drainage, chronic glucocorticoid treatment has been reported to delay and impede re-expansion of the lung (SED-8, 820).

Hiccup is a rare complication of glucocorticoid therapy; five cases have been published at various times (36).

- A 59-year-old man had intractable hiccups during treatment with dexamethasone for multiple myeloma (37).
- Persistent hiccupping has been described in a 30-year-old man after the administration of a single intravenous dose of dexamethasone (16 mg) (38). The symptom was resistant to metoclopramide and resolved spontaneously after 4 days. On rechallenge, the hiccups recurred within 2 hours and disappeared after 36 hours.

Low-dose metoclopramide can be effective and may allow a patient to continue beneficial therapy without the discomfort and exhaustion that can accompany intractable hiccups.

Ear, nose, throat

Atrophic changes and fungal and other infections can alter the nasal mucosa after aerosol treatment (39), and since most systematic published documentation on these intranasal products is limited to 1–2 years of experience (although they have been in use for a far longer period), some reserve is warranted with respect to their long-term safety and the wisdom of continual use.

Nervous system

Cerebral venous thrombosis associated with glucocorticoid treatment has rarely been reported. A relation between glucocorticoids and venous thrombosis has already been suggested but has never been clearly understood. Three young patients, two women (aged 28 and 45) and one man (aged 38 years), developed cerebral venous thrombosis after intravenous high-dose glucocorticoids (40). All presented with probable multiple sclerosis according to clinical, CSF, and MRI criteria. All had a lumbar puncture and were then treated with methylprednisolone 1 g/day for 5 days. All the usual causes of cerebral venous thrombosis were systematically excluded. The authors proposed that glucocorticoids interfere with blood coagulation and suggested that the administration of glucocorticoids after a lumbar puncture carries a particular risk of complications.

Dexamethasone is widely used for the prevention and treatment of chronic lung disease in premature infants, in whom follow-up studies have raised the possibility of an association with alterations in neuromotor function and somatic growth. In 159 survivors (mean age 53 months) of a previous placebo-controlled study, the children who had received dexamethasone had a significantly higher incidence of cerebral palsy (39/80 versus 12/79; OR = 4.62; 95% CI = 2.38, 8.98) (41). The most common form of cerebral palsy was spastic diplegia. Developmental delay was more frequent in the dexamethasone group (44/80 versus 23/79; OR = 2.9; CI = 1.5, 5.4).

In a systematic review the authors concluded that postnatal dexamethasone at currently recommended doses should be avoided because of long-term neurological adverse effects (42). Lower doses of dexamethasone or inhaled glucocorticoids might be indicated for ill ventilator-dependent infants with chronic lung disease after the age of 2 weeks.

In 146 children who participated in a placebo-controlled trial of early postnatal dexamethasone therapy for the prevention of the chronic lung disease of prematurity, follow-up at school age (mean age 8 years old) showed that the children who had received dexamethasone were significantly shorter than the controls (mean height 122.8 cm versus 126.4 cm for boys and 121.3 cm versus 124.7 cm for girls) and had a significantly smaller head circumference (49.8 cm versus 50.6 cm) (43). They also had significantly poorer motor skills, motor coordination, and visuomotor integration. Compared with the controls, the children who had received dexamethasone had significantly lower IQ scores, including full scores (mean 78.2 versus 84.4), verbal scores (84.1 versus 88.4), and performance scores (76.5 versus 84.5). The frequency of clinically significant disabilities was higher among the children who had received dexamethasone than among the controls (39% versus 22%). The authors did not recommend the routine use of dexamethasone therapy for the prevention or treatment of chronic lung disease.

Long-term treatment with glucocorticoids can cause cerebral atrophy (44).

Severe organic brain syndrome has been seen in six patients taking long-term glucocorticoids (SEDA-3, 304). The manifestations included confusion, disorientation, apathy, confabulation, irrelevant speech, and slow thinking; the symptoms occurred abruptly.

Latent epilepsy can be made manifest by glucocorticoid treatment. Seizures in patients with lung transplants were related to glucocorticoids, which had been used in high dosages to prevent organ rejection. There was an increased risk of seizures in younger patients (under 25 years) and with intravenous methylprednisolone (SEDA-21, 413) (45).

Long-term glucocorticoid treatment can result in papilledema and increased intracranial pressure (the syndrome of pseudotumor cerebri or so-called "benign intracranial hypertension"), particularly in children.

- Benign intracranial hypertension occurred in a 7-month-old child after withdrawal of topical betamethasone ointment and in a 7-year-old boy treated with a 1% cortisol ointment in large amounts.
- A 6-year-old girl, who had taken prednisone for 2.5 years for nephrotic syndrome with seven relapses in 3 years, developed symptoms of benign intracranial hypertension after oral glucocorticoid dosage reduction over 10 months from 30 mg/day to 2.5 mg/every other day (46). Laboratory studies and head CT scan were normal, but there was bilateral papilledema and the cerebrospinal fluid pressure was increased. She was given prednisone 1 mg/kg/day initially, with acetazolamide, and 25 ml of cerebrospinal fluid was removed. All her symptoms resolved and treatment was gradually withdrawn. She developed no further visual failure.

The symptoms can simulate those of an intracranial tumor. All patients taking large doses of glucocorticoids who complain of headache or blurred vision, particularly after a reduction in dosage, should have an ophthalmoscopic examination to exclude this complication. Paradoxically, cerebral edema occurring during a surgical procedure can be partly prevented by glucocorticoids (47).

An encephalopathy can occur at any age (SEDA-18, 387), not necessarily in association with intracranial hypertension.

There have been repeated reports of epidural lipomatosis, which can lead to spinal cord compression (48,49) or spinal fracture (50); in one instance, the excised lipomata contained brown fat, a phenomenon that may prove to be not unusual in glucocorticoid-induced lipomata (SEDA-16, 451).

- A 40-year-old woman with ulcerative colitis took cortisone 20 mg/day and developed progressive paraplegia (50). There was kyphosis of the thoracic spine from T7 to T9, with pathological fractures. An MRI scan showed massive epidural fat extending from T1 to T9. She recovered 3 months after surgical removal of the epidural fat.

- A 78-year-old man was given methylprednisolone (60 mg/day reducing to 8 mg/day) for temporal arteritis (51). After 4 months, he developed numbness and paresis of the legs and hyperalgesia at dermatomes T3 and T4. After 10 months he had marked disturbance of proprioception combined with spinal ataxia and an increasing loss of motor bladder control. There was an intraspinal epidural lipoma in the dorsal part of the spine from T1-10. The fat was removed surgically and within 4 weeks his gait disturbance and proprioception improved, the sensory deficit abated, and the bladder disorder disappeared completely.

- A 57-year-old man took prednisone 20–30 mg/day for 13 years for rheumatoid arthritis (52). He had been treated unsuccessfully with gold, azathioprine, hydroxychloroquine, and sulfasalazine; tapering his glucocorticoid dosage had been unsuccessful. He developed worsening back pain in his thoracic spine and lateral leg weakness. He was unable to walk. He was Cushingoid and had marked thoracic kyphosis associated with multiple vertebral body fractures in T5-8. An MRI scan at T5-6 showed displacement and compression of the spinal cord by high-signal epidural fat, which had caused anterior thecal displacement and total effacement of cerebrospinal fluid.

The authors of the last report commented on the high dose of prednisone used.

Glucocorticoid-induced spinal epidural lipomatosis is not very common in children. Spinal magnetic resonance imaging was performed in 125 children with renal diseases (68 boys); they either had back pain or numbness, were obese, or had taken a cumulative dose of prednisone of more than 500 mg/kg; there was lipomatosis in five patients (53).

In the past there was reason to think that glucocorticoids might precipitate multiple sclerosis. However, this has not been confirmed, and there is evidence that a special glucocorticoid regimen can actually be capable of retarding deterioration in multiple sclerosis (SEDA-18, 387).

A Guillain–Barré-like syndrome occurred in a patient receiving high-dose intravenous glucocorticoid therapy (SEDA-16, 449). Although glucocorticoids have been used successfully to treat weakness due to chronic inflammatory demyelinating sensorimotor neuropathy, other types of acquired chronic demyelinating neuropathies can be impaired by these drugs.

- In four patients with a pure motor demyelinating neuropathy treated with oral prednisolone (60 mg/day) motor function rapidly deteriorated within 4 weeks of starting prednisolone (SEDA-19, 375; 54). Intravenous immunoglobulin some months later in two of them produced clear improvement in strength and motor nerve conduction.

Sensory systems

The eye can be involved in generalized adverse reactions to systemically administered glucocorticoids. For example, conjunctivitis can occur as part of an allergic reaction and infections of the eye can be masked as a result of anti-inflammatory and analgesic effects. Ophthalmoplegia can occur as one of the consequences of glucocorticoid myopathy (SEDA-16, 450). Two complications that require special discussion are cataract and glaucoma.

The ocular adverse effects of glucocorticoids are well documented. However, patients are now able to browse the internet and purchase medications freely and are often not aware of their adverse effects.

- A 64-year-old woman developed bilateral decreased vision and had evidence of steroid-induced glaucoma and cataract (55). She had been purchasing oral steroids via the internet for 4 years for a self-diagnosis of myalgic encephalomyelitis and had taken prednisolone 10–40 mg/day without medical advice.

Cataract

Oral glucocorticoid treatment is a risk factor for the development of posterior subcapsular cataract. A review of nine studies including 343 asthmatics treated with oral glucocorticoids showed a prevalence of posterior subcapsular cataracts of 0–54% with a mean value of 9% (56). In a 1993 study in children taking low-dose prednisone there were cataracts in seven of 23 cases (57). Some studies have shown a clear correlation with the duration of treatment and total dosage, others have not (SEDA-17, 449). The use of inhaled glucocorticoids was associated with a dose-dependent increased risk of posterior subcapsular and nuclear cataracts in 3654 patients aged 49–97 years (SEDA-22, 446; 58). Data on glucocorticoid use were available for 3313 of these patients; glucocorticoid use was classified as none in 2784 patients, inhaled only in 241, systemic only in 177, and both inhaled and systemic in 111. Compared with nonuse, current or prior use of inhaled glucocorticoids was associated with a significant increase in the prevalence of nuclear cataracts (adjusted relative prevalence = 1.5; 95% CI = 1.2, 1.9) and posterior subcapsular cataracts (1.9; 1.3, 2.8), but not cortical cataracts. The increased prevalence of posterior subcapsular cataracts was significantly associated with current use of inhaled glucocorticoids (2.6; 1.7, 4.0); there was no association with past use. Current use of inhaled glucocorticoids was also associated with an increased prevalence of cortical cataracts (1.4; 1.1, 1.7). The highest prevalences of posterior subcapsular and grade 4 or 5 nuclear cataracts were found in patients who had taken a cumulative dose of beclomethasone over 2000 mg.

It has been suggested that the risk of cataract is higher in patients with rheumatoid arthritis than in patients with bronchial asthma, and it is also higher in children. The reversibility of the lenticular changes has often been discussed (59,60), but even without glucocorticoid withdrawal regression has been found in children taking long-term treatment (61). Nevertheless, some 7% of the patients who develop cataract caused by glucocorticoid treatment have to be operated on. A change in permeability of the lens capsule, followed by altered electrolyte concentrations in the lens and a change in the mucopolysaccharides in the lens have been advanced as reasons for the development of cataract.

Increased intraocular pressure and glaucoma

Ocular hypertension and open-angle glaucoma are well-known adverse effects of ophthalmic administration of glucocorticoids (SEDA-17, 449).

Frequency

A total of 113 patients with angiographically proven subretinal neovascularization were enrolled into a prospective study of the effects of intravitreal triamcinolone (62). About 30% developed a significant rise in intraocular pressure (at least 5 mmHg) above baseline during the first 3 months.

A large case-control study, in which 9793 elderly patients with ocular hypertension or open-angle glaucoma were compared with 38 325 controls, has shown an increased risk of these complications with oral glucocorticoids (SEDA-22, 446; 63). The risk of ocular hypertension or open-angle glaucoma increased with increasing dose and duration of use of the oral glucocorticoid. There was no significant increase in the risk of ocular hypertension or open-angle glaucoma in patients who had stopped taking oral glucocorticoids 15–45 days before. The authors estimated that the excess risk of ocular hypertension or open-angle glaucoma with current oral glucocorticoid use is 43 additional cases per 10 000 patients per year. However, in patients taking over 80 mg/day of hydrocortisone equivalents, the excess risk is 93 additional cases per 10 000 patients per year. Monitoring of intraocular pressure may be justified in long-term users of oral glucocorticoids, as it is in long-term users of topical glucocorticoids.

Prolonged use of high doses of inhaled glucocorticoids also increases the risk of ocular hypertension and open-angle glaucoma (SEDA-22, 446; 64). In a case-control study of the records of 9793 elderly patients with ocular hypertension or open-angle glaucoma over a 6-year period, there was a significantly increased risk of ocular hypertension and open-angle glaucoma in patients who had taken high doses of inhaled glucocorticoids (1500–1600 micrograms) for 3 months or longer (OR = 1.44; 95% CI = 1.01, 2.06). Both a high dosage of inhaled glucocorticoid and prolonged continuous duration of therapy had to be present to increase the risk.

Glaucoma and ocular hypertension have been reported after dermal application of glucocorticoids for facial atopic eczema (SEDA-19, 376; 65), and after treatment with beclomethasone by nasal spray and inhalation (SEDA-20, 373; 66).

The effects of topical dexamethasone on intraocular pressure have been compared with those of fluorometholone (SEDA-22, 446; 67). The ocular hypertensive response to topical dexamethasone in children occurs more often, more severely, and more rapidly than that reported in adults. It should be avoided in children if possible and it is desirable to monitor the intraocular pressure when it is being used. Fluorometholone may be more acceptable.

Pathogenesis

The pathogenesis of glucocorticoid-induced glaucoma is still unknown, but there is reduced outflow, and excessive accumulation of mucopolysaccharides may be a major factor. An association with cataract and papilledema has often been observed. The rise in intraocular pressure is variable: in the pediatric study of low dose cited above there was a reversible effect in only two of 23 subjects compared with controls, but in other studies serious increases in pressure have occurred, with a risk of blindness.

There is almost certainly a genetic predisposition to glucocorticoid-induced glaucoma, as there is to glaucoma in general.

Susceptibility factors

Children have more frequent, more severe, and more rapid ocular hypertensive responses to topical dexamethasone than adults. In one case a systemic glucocorticoid caused significant but asymptomatic ocular hypertension in a child (68).

• A 9-year-old girl with acute lymphoblastic leukemia received a 5-week course of oral prednisolone 60 mg/day (2.3 mg/kg/day). She did not receive any other systemic medications that have a known effect on intraocular pressure. Her baseline pressures in the right and left eyes were 16 and 17 mmHg with visual acuities of 20/20 and 20/15 respectively. The cup-to-disk ratio was 0.5 in both eyes, with normal visual fields. She was not myopic and had no family history of glaucoma or glucocorticoid responsiveness. After 8 days of systemic glucocorticoid therapy, her intraocular pressures increased to 39 mmHg and 38 mmHg in the right and left eyes respectively. Gonioscopy confirmed an open drainage angle in both eyes. She was given topical betaxolol 0.25% and dorzolamide 2% bd. However, her intraocular pressure continued to increase to 52 mm Hg in the right eye and 47 mm Hg in the left eye on day 10. Topical latanoprost 0.001% od and brimonidine 0.2% bd were added, and the intraocular pressures fell to 38 mmHg and 36 mmHg. Two days after withdrawal of the prednisolone, the intraocular pressure returned rapidly to 17 mm Hg in both eyes. Over the next 6 weeks, this was maintained despite stepwise withdrawal of all glaucoma medications. Four months later, she was given a 4-week course of oral dexamethasone 10 mg/day and had similar patterns of changes in intraocular pressure. Oral acetazolamide was prescribed. She remained largely asymptomatic throughout, except for one episode of reduced visual acuity from 20/20 to 20/40 in the right eye when the intraocular pressure reached 52 mmHg.

Chorioretinopathy

Systemic glucocorticoid treatment can cause severe exacerbation of bullous exudative retinal detachment and lasting visual loss in some patients with idiopathic central serous chorioretinopathy (SEDA-20, 374; 69). The atypical presentation of this condition can include peripheral retinal capillary nonperfusion and retinal neovascularization. The treatment of choice in patients with idiopathic central serous chorioretinopathy is laser photocoagulation.

In a prospective, case-control study 38 consecutive patients (28 men and 10 women), aged 28–63 years with central serous chorioretinopathy, were compared with 38 age- and sex-matched controls (28 men and 10 women) aged 27–65 years (70). Eleven patients (29%; eight men and three women) with central serous chorioretinopathy were taking glucocorticoids, compared with two patients (5.2%; one man and one woman) in the control group (OR = 7.33, 95% CI = 1.49, 36).

Subtenon local injection of a glucocorticoid is effective in the treatment of certain forms of uveitis. Central serous chorioretinopathy, confirmed by optical coherence tomography, developed after a single local subtenon glucocorticoid injection to treat HLA-B27-associated iritis (71).

- A healthy 37-year-old man developed progressive blurred vision, photophobia, and floaters in the left eye. Best-corrected visual acuity was 20/20 in the right eye and 20/50 in the left eye. The intraocular pressures were 21 mmHg in the right eye and 16 mmHg in the left eye. The anterior and posterior segments of the right eye were normal, but the anterior segment of the left eye showed 2+ conjunctival injection and mild keratitic precipitates. There was a 2+ anterior chamber cellular reaction with a 1 mm hypopyon, engorged iris vessels, and fibrinous iris posterior synechiae that were released after pupillary dilatation. Binocular and indirect ophthalmoscopy of the left eye showed a normal optic nerve, macula, retinal vasculature, and periphery. There was no evidence of retinal or vitreous inflammation, vasculitis, or cystoid macular edema. The fovea was well visualized after pupillary dilatation, with a normal and distinct foveal reflex. HLA-B27 iritis was suspected and subsequently confirmed with positive serotyping. He was given prednisolone acetate 1% every hour, cycloplegic eye drops, and a 1.0 ml periocular injection of triamcinolone acetonide (40 mg/ml) into the subtenon space of the left eye. Within 1 week, there was a marked therapeutic response, with complete resolution of the hypopyon and fibrin deposition and partial improvement in acuity to 20/40 in the left eye. There were only occasional residual anterior chamber inflammatory cells. Macular biomicroscopy showed the new development of subretinal fluid and serous pigment epithelial detachment at the fovea. Fluorescein angiography confirmed an enlarging pinpoint spot of hyperfluorescence. Optical coherence tomography confirmed the subretinal location of this fluid collection, consistent with a diagnosis of central serous chorioretinopathy. The topical glucocorticoid drops were rapidly tapered and withdrawn over 5 days. There was progressive reduction in subretinal fluid and gradual improvement in visual acuity. By 12 weeks the fluid had resolved and visual acuity recovered to 20/20 in the left eye.

Endophthalmitis

Intravitreal triamcinolone injection is safe and effective for cystoid macular edema caused by uveitis, diabetic maculopathy, and central retinal vein occlusion, and for pseudophakic cystoid macular edema. Potential risks include glaucoma, cataract, retinal detachment, and endophthalmitis. Infectious endophthalmitis is extremely rare when appropriate sterile technique is practised. Seven patients developed a clinical picture simulating endophthalmitis after intravitreal injection of triamcinolone (72). The authors believed that this effect was a toxic reaction to the injected material and explained that the differential diagnosis of infectious endophthalmitis in eyes that have been injected with triamcinolone under sterile conditions includes a sterile toxic endophthalmitis that requires careful monitoring, perhaps every 8-12 hours, in order to determine whether the inflammation is worsening or improving. Resolution occurs spontaneously, and in the absence of eye pain unnecessary intervention can be avoided.

Hypopyon associated with non-infectious endophthalmitis after intravitreal injection of triamcinolone has been described previously (73). Pseudohypopyon and sterile endophthalmitis after intravitreal injection of triamcinolone for pseudophakic cystoid macular edema has been reported (74).

- An 88-year-old woman underwent phacoemulsification surgery, which was complicated by posterior capsule rupture. Anterior vitrectomy was performed, with implantation of a silicone intraocular lens into the sulcus. Postoperatively, she developed cystoid macular edema, which failed to respond to topical dexamethasone, topical ketorolac, and posterior subtenon injection of triamcinolone, limiting visual acuity to 6/24 at 7 months after the surgery. An intravitreal injection of triamcinolone acetonide (4 mg in 0.1 ml) (Kenalog®, Bristol-Myers Squibb, Middlesex, UK) was administered through the pars plana with a 30-gauge needle using a sterile technique. Three days later she reported painless loss of vision, which had developed immediately after the injection. Visual acuity was reduced to perception of hand movements. There was minimal conjunctival injection and the cornea was clear. A 3 mm pseudohypopyon, consisting of refractile crystalline particles, was visible in the anterior chamber, associated with 3+ anterior chamber cells (or particles). Severe vitreous haze prevented visualization of the retina. Because infectious endophthalmitis could not be excluded, she was treated with intravitreal injections of ceftazidime and vancomycin. Vitreous and aqueous taps were performed and the pseudohypopyon was completely aspirated from the anterior chamber. The next day a 2 mm pseudohypopyon had reformed. The position of the pseudohypopyon depended on gravity and shifted with changes in head position. Aqueous and vitreous cultures were negative. Microscopy of the aspirated pseudohypopyon showed triamcinolone particles with no cells. The pseudohypopyon, vitreous haze, and cystoid macular edema (as demonstrated on optical coherence tomography) resolved spontaneously over 6 weeks and visual acuity recovered to 6/12.

The pseudohypopyon was a unique feature of this case and was due to the presence of a posterior capsule defect enabling the passage of triamcinolone from the vitreous cavity into the anterior chamber. The authors commented that presumably the triamcinolone crystals had been carried into the anterior chamber by currents generated by saccadic eye movements in the partially vitrectomized vitreous cavity. In this case the pseudohypopyon was distinguishable from an infective or inflammatory hypopyon by its ground glass appearance, the presence of refractile particles, and its shifting position, which depended on the patient's head position. The absence of ocular pain, photophobia, ciliary injection, or iris vessel dilatation suggested a non-inflammatory response and perhaps it would be appropriate to monitor such patients closely rather than administering intravitreal antibiotics.

Keratopathy and keratitis

Band-shaped keratopathy is caused by the deposition of calcium salts in the basement membrane of the corneal epithelium and superficial stroma. It is typically a chronic process that develops over a period of months and years, and is associated with chronic corneal or intraocular inflammation.

- Infectious crystalline keratopathy developed in a 73-year-old woman with noninsulin-dependent diabetes mellitus after the use of topical prednisolone 1% eye-drops, for conjunctival injection over 12 months (SEDA-20, 372; 75).
- Acute-onset calcific band keratopathy has been reported in a woman using topical prednisolone (SEDA-20, 372; 76).

Patients with severe keratoconjunctivitis sicca are at definite risk of this complication, and the addition of phosphate-containing eye-drops tilted the precariously balanced situation toward precipitation of calcium in the cornea and bandage contact lens. Acetate-containing rather than phosphate-containing glucocorticoid eye drops may be a safer alternative in patients with such predisposing factors.

Bacterial keratitis is one of the most frequent ophthalmic infections. In a meta-analysis of publications from 1950 to 2000, the use of a topical glucocorticoid before the diagnosis of bacterial keratitis significantly predisposed to ulcerative keratitis in eyes with pre-existing corneal disease (OR = 2.63; 95% CI = 1.41, 4.91). Previous glucocorticoid use significantly increased the risk of antibiotic failure or other infectious complications (OR = 3.75; 95% CI = 2.52, 5.58). The use of glucocorticoids with an antibiotic for the treatment of bacterial keratitis did not increase the risk of complications, but neither did it improve the outcome of treatment.

Retinal damage

An apparent association between severe retinopathy of prematurity and dexamethasone therapy has been shown in a retrospective study (SEDA-20, 372; 77). Infants treated with dexamethasone required longer periods of mechanical ventilation (44 versus 26 days), had a longer duration of supplemental oxygen (57 versus 29 days), had a higher incidence of patent ductus arteriosus (28/38 versus 18/52), and required surfactant therapy more often for respiratory distress syndrome (17/38 versus 11/52). Prospective, randomized, controlled studies are needed to correct for differences in severity of cardiorespiratory disease. Until such studies are available, careful consideration must be given to indications, dosage, time of initiation, and duration of treatment with dexamethasone in infants of extremely low birthweight.

Retinal hemorrhage occurred in four women after they had received epidural methylprednisolone for chronic back and hip pain (SEDA-20, 373; 78). Retinal and choroidal vascular occlusions are a serious and sometimes lasting complication of periocular and facial injections of glucocorticoids (SEDA-21, 416).

Toxic optic neuropathy

Toxic optic neuropathy can occur and may underlie various reports of sudden blindness in patients taking glucocorticoids. In one case, transient visual loss occurred on several occasions, each time after administration of a glucocorticoid (SEDA-17, 447). In another case, blindness occurred suddenly and paradoxically after glucocorticoid injections into the nasal turbinates (79). Although glucocorticoids are sometimes used successfully to relieve pre-existing optic neuritis, a number of such patients react adversely with increased episodes of visual loss.

Exophthalmos

Exophthalmos has been described incidentally as a complication of long-term glucocorticoid therapy and there has been a series of 21 cases (80).

Psychological

The psychostimulant effects of the glucocorticoids are well known (81), and their dose dependency is recognized (SED-11, 817); they may amount to little more than euphoria or comprise severe mental derangement, for example mania in an adult with no previous psychiatric history (SEDA-17, 446) or catatonic stupor demanding electroconvulsive therapy (82). In their mildest form, and especially in children, the mental changes may be detectable only by specific tests of mental function (83). Mental effects can occur in patients treated with fairly low doses; they can also occur after withdrawal or omission of treatment, apparently because of adrenal suppression (84,85).

- A 32-year-old woman developed irritability, anger, and insomnia after taking oral prednisone (60 mg/day) for a relapse of ileal Crohn's disease (86). The prednisone was withdrawn and replaced by budesonide (9 mg/day), and the psychiatric adverse effects were relieved after 3 days. A good clinical response was maintained, with no relapse after 2 months of budesonide therapy.

Seventeen patients taking long-term glucocorticoid therapy (16 women, mean age 47 years, mean prednisone dose 16 mg, mean length of current treatment 92 months) and 15 matched controls were assessed with magnetic resonance imaging and proton magnetic resonance spectroscopy, neurocognitive tests (including the Rey Auditory Verbal Learning Test, Stroop Colour Word Test, Trail Making Test, and estimated overall intelligent quotient), and psychiatric scales (including the Hamilton Rating Scale for Depression, Young Mania Rating Scale, and Brief Psychiatric Rating Scale) (87). Glucocorticoid-treated patients had smaller hippocampal volumes and lower N-acetylaspartate ratios than controls. They had lower scores on the Rey Auditory Verbal Learning Test and Stroop Colour Word Test (declarative memory deficit) and higher scores on the Hamilton Rating Scale for Depression and the Brief Psychiatric Rating Scale (depression). These findings support the idea that chronic glucocorticoid exposure is associated with changes in hippocampal structure and function.

Development
Dexamethasone has been used in ventilator-dependent preterm infants to reduce the risk and severity of chronic lung disease. Usually it is given in a tapering course over a long period (42 days). The effects of dexamethasone on developmental outcome at 1 year of age has been evaluated in 118 infants of very low birthweights (47 boys and 71 girls, aged 15–25 days), who were not weaning from assisted ventilation (88). They were randomly assigned double-blind to receive placebo or dexamethasone (initial dose 0.25 mg/kg) tapered over 42 days. A neurological examination, including ultrasonography, was done at 1 year of age. Survival was 88% with dexamethasone and 74% with placebo. Both groups obtained similar scores in mental and psychomotor developmental indexes. More dexamethasone-treated infants had major intracranial abnormalities (21 versus 11%), cerebral palsy (25 versus 7%; OR = 5.3; CI = 1.3, 21), and unspecified neurological abnormalities (45 versus 16%; OR = 3.6; CI = 1.2, 11). Although the authors suggested an adverse effect, they added other possible explanations for these increased risks (improved survival in those with neurological injuries or at increased risk of such injuries).

Behavioral disorders
Children have marked increases in behavioral problems during treatment with high-dose prednisone for relapse of nephrotic syndrome, according to the results of a study conducted in the USA (89). Ten children aged 2.9–15 years (mean 8.2 years) received prednisone 2 mg/kg/day, tapering at the time of remission, which was at week 2 in seven patients. At baseline, eight children had normal behavioral patterns and two had anxious/depressed and aggressive behavior using the Child Behaviour Checklist (CBCL). During high-dose prednisone therapy, five of the eight children with normal baseline scores had CBCL scores for anxiety, depression, and aggressive behavior above the 95th percentile for age. The two children with high baseline CBCL scores had worsening behavioral problems during high-dose prednisone. Behavioral problems occurred almost exclusively in the children who received over 1 mg/kg every 48 hours.

Regression analysis showed that prednisone dosage was a strong predictor of increased aggressive behaviour.

Intravenous methylprednisolone was associated with a spectrum of adverse reactions, most frequently behavioral disorders, in 213 children with rheumatic disease, according to the results of a US study (15). However, intravenous methylprednisolone was generally well tolerated. The children received their first dose of intravenous methylprednisolone 30 mg/kg over at least 60 minutes, and if the first dose was well tolerated they were given further infusions at home under the supervision of a nurse. There was at least one adverse reaction in 46 children (22%) of whom 18 had an adverse reaction within the first three doses. The most commonly reported adverse reactions were behavioral disorders (21 children), including mood changes, hyperactivity, hallucinations, disorientation, and sleep disorders. Several children had serious acute reactions, which were readily controlled. Most of them were able to continue methylprednisolone therapy with premedication or were given an alternative glucocorticoid. The researchers emphasized the need to monitor treatment closely and to have appropriate drugs readily available to treat adverse reactions.

Large doses are most likely to cause the more serious behavioral and personality changes, ranging from extreme nervousness, severe insomnia, or mood swings to psychotic episodes, which can include both manic and depressive states, paranoid states, and acute toxic psychoses. A history of emotional disorders does not necessarily preclude glucocorticoid treatment, but existing emotional instability or psychotic tendencies can be aggravated by glucocorticoids. Such patients as these should be carefully and continuously observed for signs of mental changes, including alterations in the sleep pattern. Aggravation of psychiatric symptoms can occur not only during high-dose oral treatment, but also after any increase in dosage during long-term maintenance therapy; it can also occur with inhalation therapy (90). The psychomotor stimulant effect is said to be most pronounced with dexamethasone and to be much less with methylprednisolone, but this concept of a differential psychotropic effect still has to be confirmed.

Memory
The effects of prednisone on memory have been assessed (SEDA-21, 413) (91). Glucocorticoid-treated patients performed worse than controls in tests of explicit memory. Pulsed intravenous methylprednisolone (2.5 g over 5 days, 5 g over 7 days, or 10 g over 5 days) caused impaired memory in patients with relapsing-remitting multiple sclerosis, but this effect is reversible, according to the results of an Italian study (92). Compared with ten control patients, there was marked selective impairment of explicit memory in 14 patients with relapsing-remitting multiple sclerosis treated with pulsed intravenous methylprednisolone. However, this memory impairment completely resolved 60 days after methylprednisolone treatment.

Glucocorticoids can regulate hippocampal metabolism, physiological functions, and memory. Despite evidence of memory loss during glucocorticoid treatment (SEDA-23,

428), and correlations between memory and cortisol concentrations in certain diseases, it is unclear whether exposure to the endogenous glucocorticoid cortisol in amounts seen during physical and psychological stress in humans can inhibit memory performance in otherwise healthy individuals. In an elegant experiment on the effect of cortisol on memory, 51 young healthy volunteers (24 men and 27 women) participated in a double-blind, randomized, crossover, placebo-controlled trial of cortisol 40 mg/day or 160 mg/day for 4 days (93). The lower dose of cortisol was equivalent to the cortisol delivered during a mild stress and the higher dose to major stress. Cognitive performance and plasma cortisol were evaluated before and until 10 days after drug administration. Cortisol produced a dose-related reversible reduction in verbal declarative memory without effects on nonverbal memory, sustained or selective attention, or executive function. Exposure to cortisol at doses and plasma concentrations associated with physical and psychological stress in humans can reversibly reduce some elements of memory performance.

Prednisone, 10 mg/day for 1 year, has been evaluated in 136 patients with probable Alzheimer's disease in a double-blind, randomized, placebo-controlled trial (94). There were no differences in the primary measures of efficacy (cognitive subscale of the Alzheimer Disease Assessment Scale), but those treated with prednisone had significantly greater memory impairment (Clinical Dementia sum of boxes), and agitation and hostility/suspicion (Brief Psychiatric Rating Scale). Other adverse effects in those who took prednisone were reduced bone density and a small rise in intraocular pressure.

In healthy individuals undergoing acute stress, there was specifically impaired retrieval of declarative long-term memory for a word list, suggesting that cortisol-induced impairment of retrieval may add significantly to the memory deficits caused by prolonged treatment (95).

In 52 renal transplant recipients (mean age 45 years, 34 men and 18 women) taking prednisone (100 mg/day for 3 days followed by 10 mg/day for as long as needed; mean dose 11 mg/day) there was a major reduction in immediate recall but not delayed recall (96). However, there was a significant correlation between mean prednisone dose and delayed recall. In animals, phenytoin pretreatment blocks the effects of stress on memory and hippocampal histology.

In a double blind, randomized, placebo-controlled trial 39 patients (mean age 44 years, 8 men) with allergies or pulmonary or rheumatological illnesses who were taking prednisone (mean dose 40 mg/day) were randomized to either phenytoin (300 mg/day) or placebo for 7 days (97). Those who took phenytoin had significantly smaller increases in a mania self-report scale. There was no effect on memory. Thus, phenytoin blocked the hypomanic effects of prednisone, but not the effects on declarative memory.

Sleep

The effects of acute systemic dexamethasone administration on sleep structure have been investigated.

Dexamethasone caused significant increases in REM latency, the percentage time spent awake, and the percentage time spent in slow-wave sleep. There were also significant reductions in the percentage time spent in REM sleep and the number of REM periods (SEDA-21, 413) (98).

Psychiatric

Use of glucocorticoids is associated with adverse psychiatric effects, including mild euphoria, emotional lability, panic attacks, psychosis, and delirium. Although high doses increase the risks, psychiatric effects can occur after low doses and different routes of administration. Of 92 patients with systemic lupus erythematosus (78 women, mean age 34 years) followed between 1999 and 2000, psychiatric events occurred in six of those who were treated with glucocorticoids for the first time or who received an augmented dose, an overall 4.8% incidence (99). The psychiatric events were mood disorders with manic features (delusions of grandiosity) (n = 3) and psychosis (auditory hallucinations, paranoid delusions, and persecutory ideas) (n = 3). Three patients were first time users (daily prednisone dose 30–45 mg/day) and three had had mean increases in daily prednisone dose from baseline of 26 (range 15–33) mg. All were hypoalbuminemic and none had neuropsychiatric symptoms before glucocorticoid treatment. All the events occurred within 3 weeks of glucocorticoid administration. In five of the six episodes, the symptoms resolved completely after dosage reduction (from 40 mg to 18 mg) but in one patient an additional 8-week course of a phenothiazine was given. In a multivariate regression analysis, only hypoalbuminemia was an independent predictor of psychiatric events (HR = 0.8, 95% CI = 0.60, 0.97).

Although mood changes are common during short-term, high-dose, glucocorticoid therapy, there are virtually no data on the mood effects of long-term glucocorticoid therapy. Mood has been evaluated in 20 outpatients (2 men, 18 women), aged 18–65 years taking at least 7.5 mg/day of prednisone for 6 months (mean current dose 19 mg/day; mean duration of current prednisone treatment 129 months) and 14 age-matched controls (1 man, 13 women), using standard clinician-rated measures of mania (Young Mania Rating Scale, YMRS), depression (Hamilton Rating Scale for Depression, HRSD), and global psychiatric symptoms (Brief Psychiatric Rating Scale, BPRS, and the patient-rated Internal State Scale, ISS) (100). Syndromal diagnoses were evaluated using a structured clinical interview. The results showed that symptoms and disorders are common in glucocorticoid-dependent patients. Unlike short-term prednisone therapy, long-term therapy is more associated with depressive than manic symptoms, based on the clinician-rated assessments. The Internal State Scale may be more sensitive to mood symptoms than clinician-rated scales.

Psychoses
Mania has been attributed to glucocorticoids (101).

- A 46-year-old man, with an 8-year history of cluster headaches and some episodes of endogenous depression, took glucocorticoids 120 mg/day for a week and then a tapering dosage at the start of his latest cluster episode. His headaches stopped but then recurred after 10 days. He was treated prophylactically with verapamil, but a few days later, while the dose of glucocorticoid was being tapered, he developed symptoms of mania. The glucocorticoids were withdrawn, he was given valproic acid, and his mania resolved after 10 days. Verapamil prophylaxis was restarted and he had no more cluster headaches.

The authors commented that the manic symptoms had probably been caused by glucocorticoids or glucocorticoid withdrawal. They concluded that patients with cluster headache and a history of affective disorder should not be treated with glucocorticoids, but with valproate or lithium, which are effective in both conditions. Lamotrigine, an anticonvulsive drug with mood-stabilizing effects, may prevent glucocorticoid-induced mania in patients for whom valproate or lithium are not possible (102).

Glucocorticoids can cause neuropsychiatric adverse effects that dictate a reduction in dose and sometimes withdrawal of treatment. Of 32 patients with asthma (mean age 47 years) who took prednisone in a mean dosage of 42 mg/day for a mean duration of 5 days, those with past or current symptoms of depression had a significant reduction in depressive symptoms during prednisone therapy compared with those without depression (103). After 3–7 days of therapy there was a significant increase in the risk of mania, with return to baseline after withdrawal.

The management of a psychotic reaction in an Addisonian patient taking a glucocorticoid needs special care (SED-8, 820). Psychotic reactions that do not abate promptly when the glucocorticoid dosage is reduced to the lowest effective value (or withdrawn) may need to be treated with neuroleptic drugs; occasionally these fail and antidepressants are needed (SEDA-18, 387). However, in other cases, antidepressants appear to aggravate the symptoms.

- Two patients with prednisolone-induced psychosis improved on giving the drug in three divided daily doses. Recurrence was avoided by switching to enteric-coated tablets.

This suggests that in susceptible patients the margin of safety may be quite narrow (SED-12, 982). It is possible that reduced absorption accounted for the improvement in this case, but attention should perhaps be focused on peak plasma concentrations rather than average steady-state concentrations.

Two women developed secondary bipolar disorder associated with glucocorticoid treatment and deteriorated to depressive–catatonic states without overt hallucinations and delusions (104).

- A 21-year-old woman, who had taken prednisolone 60 mg/day for dermatomyositis for 1 year developed a depressed mood, pessimistic thought, irritability, poor concentration, diminished interest, and insomnia. Although the dose of prednisolone was tapered and she

was treated with sulpiride, a benzamide with mild antidepressant action, she never completely recovered. After 5 months she had an exacerbation of her dermatomyositis and received two courses of methylprednisolone pulse therapy. Two weeks after the second course, while taking prednisolone 50 mg/day, she became hypomanic and euphoric. She improved substantially with neuroleptic medication and continued to take prednisolone 5 mg/day. About 9 months later she developed depressive stupor without any significant psychological stressor or changes in prednisolone dosage. She had mutism, reduction in contact and reactivity, immobility, and depressed mood. Manic or mixed state and psychotic symptoms were not observed. She was initially treated with intravenous clomipramine 25 mg/day followed by oral clomipramine and lithium carbonate. She improved markedly within 2 weeks with a combination of clomipramine 100 mg/day and lithium carbonate 300 mg/day. Prednisolone was maintained at 5 mg/day.

- A 23-year-old woman with ulcerative colitis and no previous psychiatric disorders developed emotional lability, euphoria, persecutory delusions, irritability, and increased motor and verbal activity 3 weeks after starting to take betamethasone 4 mg/day. She improved within a few weeks with bromperidol 3 mg/day. After 10 months she became unable to speak and eat, was mute, depressive, and sorrowful, and responded poorly to questions. There were no neurological signs and betamethasone had been withdrawn 10 months before. She was treated with intravenous clomipramine 25 mg/day and became able to speak. Intravenous clomipramine caused dizziness due to hypotension, and amoxapine 150 mg/day was substituted after 6 days. All of her symptoms improved within 10 days. Risperidone was added for mood lability and mild persecutory ideation.

In one case, glucocorticoid-induced catatonic psychosis unexpectedly responded to etomidate (105).

- A 27-year-old woman with myasthenia gravis taking prednisolone 100 mg/day became unresponsive and had respiratory difficulties. She was given etomidate 20 mg intravenously to facilitate endotracheal intubation. One minute later she became alert and oriented, with normal muscle strength, and became very emotional. Eight hours later she again became catatonic and had a similar response to etomidate 10 mg. Glucocorticoid-induced catatonia was diagnosed, her glucocorticoid dosage was reduced, and she left hospital uneventfully 4 days later.

The effect of etomidate on catatonia, similar to that of amobarbital, was thought to be due to enhanced GABA receptor function in patients with an overactive reticular system.

A case report has suggested that risperidone, an atypical neuroleptic drug, can be useful in treating adolescents with glucocorticoid-induced psychosis and may hasten its resolution (106).

- A 14-year-old African-American girl with acute lymphocytic leukemia was treated with dexamethasone

24 mg/day for 25 days. Four days after starting to taper the dose she had a psychotic reaction with visual hallucinations, disorientation, agitation, and attempts to leave the floor. Her mother refused treatment with haloperidol. Steroids were withdrawn and lorazepam was given as needed. Nine days later the symptoms had not improved. She was given risperidone 1 mg/day; within 3 days the psychotic reaction began to improve and by 3 weeks the symptoms had completely resolved.

Obsessive-compulsive disorder

Obsessive-compulsive behavior after oral cortisone has been described (107).

- A 75-year-old white man, without a history of psychiatric disorders, took cortisone 50 mg/day for 6 weeks for pulmonary fibrosis and developed severe obsessive-compulsive behavior without affective or psychotic symptoms. He was given risperidone without any beneficial effect. The dose of cortisone was tapered over 18 days. An MRI scan showed no signs of organic brain disease and an electroencephalogram was normal. His symptoms improved 16 days after withdrawal and resolved completely after 24 days. Risperidone was withdrawn without recurrence.

Endocrine

The endocrine effects of the glucocorticoids variously involve the pituitary–adrenal axis, the ovaries and testes, the parathyroid glands, and the thyroid gland.

Pituitary gland

Empty sella syndrome occurred in a boy who developed hypopituitarism after long-term pulse therapy with prednisone for nephrotic syndrome (108).

- A 16-year-old Japanese boy's growth and development was normal until the age of 2 years. He then developed nephrotic syndrome and was treated with pulsed glucocorticoid therapy nine times over the next 14 years. After the age of 3 years, his rate of growth had fallen. At 16 years, when he was taking prednisone 60 mg/m²/day he was given prednisone on alternate days and the dose was gradually tapered. The secretion of pituitary hormones, except antidiuretic hormone, was impaired and an MRI scan of his brain showed an empty sella and atrophy of the pituitary gland.

When markedly impaired growth is noted in patients treated with glucocorticoids long-term or in pulses, it is necessary to assess pituitary function and the anatomy of the pituitary gland. Children who receive glucocorticoid pulse therapy may develop an empty sella more frequently than is usually recognized.

Pituitary–adrenal axis

Raised glucocorticoid plasma concentrations usually result, after 2 weeks, in the first signs of iatrogenic Cushing's syndrome. The characteristic symptoms can occur individually or in combination. Whereas in Cushing's

disease or corticotropin–induced Cushing's syndrome, the predominant symptoms are in part determined by hyperandrogenicity and tend to comprise hypertension, acne, impaired sight, disorders of sexual function, hirsutism or virilism, striae of the skin, and plethora, Cushing's syndrome due to glucocorticoid therapy is likely to cause benign intracranial hypertension, glaucoma, subcapsular cataract, pancreatitis, aseptic necrosis of the bones, and panniculitis. Obesity, facial rounding, psychiatric symptoms, edema, and delayed wound healing are common to these different forms of Cushing's syndrome.

It has been said that Cushing-like effects are to be expected if the function of the adrenal cortex is suppressed by daily doses of more than 50 mg hydrocortisone or its equivalent. However, pituitary–adrenal suppression has been described at lower dosage equivalents, for example during prolonged intermittent therapy with dexamethasone (109). The secondary adrenal insufficiency caused by therapeutically effective doses can be observed even after giving prednisone 5 mg tds for only 1 week; after withdrawal, adrenal suppression lasts for some days. If one continues this treatment for about 20 weeks, maximal atrophy of the adrenal cortex results, and lasts for some months. This effect begins with inhibition of the hypothalamus, and culminates in true atrophy of the adrenal cortex. It can occur even with glucocorticoids given by inhalation (110). Inhaled fluticasone is associated with at least a twofold greater suppression of adrenal function than inhaled budesonide microgram for microgram, according to the results of a crossover study (SEDA-21, 415) (111). Patients with liver disease may experience adrenal suppression with lower doses of glucocorticoids (112). It is advisable to use alternate-day therapy to avoid suppression of corticotropin secretion in patients who will need long-term therapy; it will produce the same therapeutic effect as daily dosage. It can be helpful to measure the degree of suppression of corticotropin secretion during long-term glucocorticoid treatment of asthmatic children, as a means of optimizing therapy and avoiding excessive dosage (113). The period of time during which the patient should be considered at risk of adrenal insufficiency after withdrawal of oral prednisolone treatment in childhood nephrotic syndrome is still controversial. A study in such patients has suggested that adrenal insufficiency may occur up to 9 months after treatment has ended (SEDA-19, 376; 114).

Many protocols for treating children with early B cell acute lymphoblastic leukemia involve 28 consecutive days of high-dose glucocorticoids during induction. The effect of this therapy on adrenal function has been prospectively evaluated (115) in 10 children by tetracosactide stimulation before the start of dexamethasone therapy and every 4 weeks thereafter until adrenal function returned to normal. All had normal adrenal function before dexamethasone treatment and impaired adrenal responses 24 hours after completing therapy. Each child felt ill for 2–4 weeks after completing therapy. Seven patients recovered normal adrenal function after 4 weeks, but three did not have normal adrenal function until 8 weeks after withdrawal. Thus, high-dose dexamethasone therapy can cause adrenal insufficiency lasting more than 4 weeks after the end of treatment. This problem might be avoided by tapering doses of glucocorticoids and providing supplementary glucocorticoids during periods of increased stress.

Tolerance to glucocorticoids in this, as in some other respects, varies from individual to individual; some patients tolerate 30 mg of prednisone for a long time without developing Cushing's syndrome, while others develop symptoms at 7.5 mg; the doses recommended today to avoid Cushing's syndrome in most patients are usually equivalent to hydrocortisone 20 mg. Cushing's syndrome and other systemic adverse effects can occur not only from oral and injected glucocorticoids, but also from topical and intranasal treatment (116) and intrapulmonary or epidural administration (SEDA-19, 376; SEDA-20, 370; 117,118).

- Two patients developed hypopituitarism and empty sella syndrome during glucocorticoid pulse therapy for nephrotic syndrome (SEDA-22, 444; 119).

Glucocorticoid-treated patients with inadequate adrenal function who have an intercurrent illness or are due to undergo surgery will have an inadequate reaction to the resulting stress and need to be temporarily protected by additional glucocorticoid (120).

Iatrogenic Cushing's syndrome after a single low dose is exceptional (121).

- A 45-year-old woman was given a single-dose of intramuscular triamcinolone acetonide 40 mg for acute laryngitis and 1 month later was noted to have a cushingoid appearance. Endocrinological tests confirmed hypothalamic–pituitary–adrenal (HPA) axis suppression. Eight months later, the cushingoid appearance had completely disappeared and HPA function had spontaneously recovered.

Pseudohyperaldosteronism has been reported even after intranasal application of 9-alpha-fluoroprednisolone (SEDA-11, 340).

Parathyroid function

There is antagonism between the parathyroid hormone and glucocorticoids (122). Latent hyperparathyroidism can be unmasked by glucocorticoids (123).

Thyroid function

Even a single dose of corticotropin briefly inhibits the secretion of thyrotrophic hormone. The uptake of radioactive iodine is also suppressed by corticotropin and by glucocorticoids, but this has no clinical relevance. Pathological changes in thyroid function induced by glucocorticoid treatment are reportedly rare.

Metabolism

Glucose metabolism

All glucocorticoids increase gluconeogenesis. The turnover of glucose is increased, more being metabolized to fat, and blood glucose concentration is increased by 10–20%. Glucose tolerance and sensitivity to insulin are reduced, but provided pancreatic islet function is normal, carbohydrate metabolism will not be noticeably altered. So-called "steroid diabetes," a benign diabetes without a tendency to ketosis, but with a low sensitivity to insulin and a low renal threshold to glucose, only develops in one-fifth of patients treated with high glucocorticoid dosages. Even in patients with diabetes, ketosis is not to be expected, since glucocorticoids have antiketotic activity, presumably through suppression of growth hormone secretion.

Glucocorticoid treatment of known diabetics normally leads to deregulation, but this can be compensated for by adjusting the dose of insulin. The increased gluconeogenesis induced by glucocorticoids mainly takes place in the liver, but glucocorticoid treatment is especially likely to disturb carbohydrate metabolism in liver disease.

When hyperglycemic coma occurs it is almost always of the hyperosmolar nonketotic type. After termination of glucocorticoid treatment, steroid diabetes normally disappears. An apparent exception to these findings is provided by the case of a patient in whom glucocorticoid treatment was followed by severe diabetes with diabetic nephropathy, but this was a seriously ill individual who had already undergone renal transplantation (SEDA-17, 449). Gestational diabetes mellitus was more common in women who had received glucocorticoids with or without beta-adrenoceptor agonists for threatened preterm delivery compared with controls (SEDA-22, 445; 124).

Glucocorticoids probably have more than one effect on carbohydrate metabolism. An increase in fasting glucagon concentration has been observed in volunteers given prednisolone 40 mg/day for 4 days, and this effect may be involved, alongside gluconeogenesis, in glucocorticoid-induced hyperglycemia. Some newer glucocorticoids have been claimed to have smaller effects on blood glucose (as well as less salt and water retention), but further studies are needed to confirm whether this interesting therapeutic approach has been successful (SEDA-13, 353).

Deflazacort, an oxazoline derivative of prednisolone, was introduced as a potential substitute for conventional glucocorticoids in order to ameliorate glucose intolerance. In a randomized study in kidney transplant recipients with pre- or post-transplantation diabetes mellitus, 42 patients who switched from prednisone to deflazacort (in the ratio 5:6 mg) were prospectively compared with 40 patients who continued to take prednisone (SEDA-22, 445; 125). During the mean follow-up period of 13 months, neither graft dysfunction nor acute rejection developed in the conversion group, and there was improvement in blood glucose control. When the conversion group was stratified into those with pre- or post-transplantation diabetes, there were promising effects in the patients with post-transplantation diabetes. More than a 50% dosage reduction of hypoglycemic drugs was possible in 42% of those with post-transplantation diabetes.

The risk of hyperglycemia requiring treatment in patients receiving oral glucocorticoids has been quantified in a case-control study of 11 855 patients, 35 years of age or older, with newly initiated treatment with a hypoglycemic drug (SEDA-19, 375; 126). The risk for initiating hypoglycemic therapy increased with the recent use of a glucocorticoid. The risk grew with increasing average daily glucocorticoid dosage (in mg of hydrocortisone equivalents): 1.77 for 1–39 mg/day, 3.02 for 40–79 mg/day, 5.82 for 80–119 mg/day, and 10.34 for 120 mg/day or more.

Lipid metabolism

High-dose glucocorticoid therapy can cause marked hypertriglyceridemia, with milky plasma (SEDA-15, 421; SEDA-16, 450). It has been suggested that this is caused by abnormal accumulation of dietary fat, reduced post-heparin lipolytic activity, and glucose intolerance (127). An association between glucocorticoid exposure and hypercholesterolemia has been found in several studies (128) and can contribute to an increased risk of athero-sclerotic vascular disease.

Most premature neonates need intravenous lipids during the first few weeks of life to acquire adequate energy intake and prevent essential fatty acid deficiency before they can tolerate all nutrition via enteral feeds. Dexamethasone is associated with multiple adverse effects in neonates, including poor weight gain and impairment of glucose and protein metabolism. In ten neonates (four boys, mean age 17.3 days) taking dexamethasone for bronchopulmonary dysplasia, intravenous lipids (3 g/kg/day) caused hypertriglyceridemia in the presence of hyperinsulinemia and increased free fatty acid concentrations (129). Because of concomitant hyperinsulinemia, the authors speculated that dexamethasone reduced fatty acid oxidation, explaining poor weight gain.

Altered fat deposition has been repeatedly reported. Fat can be deposited epidurally and at other sites. Adiposis dolora, which involves the symmetrical appearance of multiple painful fat deposits in the subcutaneous tissues, has on one occasion been attributed to glucocorticoids (SEDA-16, 451).

Tumor lysis syndrome

Acute tumor lysis syndrome is a life-threatening metabolic emergency that results from rapid massive necrosis of tumor cells. There have been repeated reports of an acute tumor lysis syndrome when glucocorticoids are administered in patients with pre-existing lymphoid tumors (130).

- A 60-year-old woman took dexamethasone 4 mg 8-hourly for dyspnea due to a precursor T lymphoblastic lymphoma-leukemia with bilateral pleural effusions and a large mass in the anterior mediastinum (131). She developed acute renal insufficiency and laboratory evidence of the metabolic effects of massive cytolysis. She received vigorous hydration, a diuretic, allopurinol, and hemodialysis. She recovered within 2 weeks and then underwent six courses of CHOP chemotherapy. The mediastinal mass regressed completely. She remained asymptomatic until she developed full-blown acute lymphoblastic leukemia, which was resistant to treatment.

Electrolyte balance

The severity of potassium loss due to glucocorticoids depends partly on the amount of sodium in the diet; the most widely used synthetic glucocorticoids cause less potassium excretion than natural hydrocortisone does. Prednisone and prednisolone have a glucocorticoid activity 4–5 times that of hydrocortisone, but their mineralocorticoid activity is less (see Table 1); even at high dosages they do not cause noteworthy sodium and water retention. Of the major synthetic glucocorticoids, dexamethasone has the strongest anti-inflammatory, hyperglycemic, and corticotropin-inhibitory activity; sodium retention is completely absent; the degree of glucocorticoid-induced metabolic alkalosis may also be less with dexamethasone than with hydrocortisone or methylprednisolone (SEDA-10, 343).

Mineral balance

There can be increases in calcium and phosphorus loss because of effects on both the kidney and the bowel, with increased excretion and reduced resorption (132). Tetany, which has been seen in patients receiving high-dose long-term intravenous glucocorticoids, has been explained as being due to hypocalcemia, and there are also effects on bone. Tetany has also been reported in a patient with latent hyperparathyroidism after the administration of a glucocorticoid (123).

Hypocalcemic encephalopathy occurred in a 35-year-old woman with hypoparathyroidism. It was believed that the administration of methylprednisolone intramuscularly had precipitated severe hypocalcemia, which had led to a metabolic encephalopathy (SEDA-20, 371; 133).

The administration of large doses of glucocorticoids to patients with major burns presenting with low cardiac output has been reported to produce a reversible drop in serum zinc, which might lead to impaired tissue repair (SED-8, 824), but it is not clear whether this has clinical effects.

Metal metabolism

Glucocorticoids increase chromium losses and glucocorticoid-induced diabetes can be reversed by chromium supplementation (134). Doses of hypoglycemic drugs were also reduced by 50% in all patients when they were given supplementary chromium.

Hematologic

Erythrocytes

Polycythemia is a symptom of Cushing's syndrome, and conversely anemia correlates with Addison's disease, but polycythemia is not generally encountered as a consequence of treatment with glucocorticoids, perhaps because there is no increased secretion of androgens; an increase in hemoglobin was nevertheless the most frequent adverse effect observed in a study over 8 years of 77 patients treated for hyperergic-allergic reactions. At the beginning of treatment more than 40% (and during continuous therapy more than 70%) of patients showed this change in erythrocytes (135). There was leukocytosis in more than 60% in the early phases and in more than 40% later (135). Thrombocytosis occurred in 5–10% during continuous treatment. This report agrees fairly well with some older publications, but it has been noted in the past that in the long run very high-dose glucocorticoid treatment can result in suppression of the activity of the bone marrow with fatty infiltration replacing hemopoietic tissue.

Leukocytes

Not all classes of leukocytes are affected by glucocorticoids in the same way. The total leukocyte count is increased, but the number of eosinophilic leukocytes falls, as does the lymphocyte count. The number of monocytes is reduced, as is their capacity to perform phagocytosis.

In children, a leukemoid reaction has been induced by betamethasone treatment (136); this possibility must always be borne in mind, since glucocorticoids can actually be used to treat leukemia or its complications. A case of very high white blood cell count with neutrophilia in a preterm infant whose mother had received two doses of betamethasone prenatally to enhance fetal lung maturation is one of a short list of leukemoid reactions possibly attributable to antenatal glucocorticoid treatment (137).

It is possible that in children with acute lymphoblastic leukemia, glucocorticoid therapy adversely affects the duration of remissions, and it has therefore been suggested that leukemia should be ruled out in children before starting long-term therapy with glucocorticoids (SEDA-11, 340). Depression of the lymphocyte count seems to be a general and direct action of the glucocorticoids (138), but the mechanism is still incompletely understood; certainly, lymphocytolysis seems to be increased by glucocorticoids. Studies of lymphocyte subpopulations show a preferential reduction in T cells, while B cells are constant or slightly reduced. B lymphocyte function (measured as immunoglobulin synthesis) falls, suppressor T lymphocyte activity is suppressed, and helper T lymphocyte function is unaffected by glucocorticoids (SEDA-3, 308) (139).

- Fever and leukopenia with methylprednisolone and prednisolone has been reported in a 29-year-old woman with systemic lupus erythematosus (140).

The authors commented that fever associated with glucocorticoids occurs frequently, whereas leukopenia is rare. Fever and leukopenia are important signs of an exacerbation of systemic lupus erythematosus, and it would be difficult to distinguish between an exacerbation of the disease and an adverse effect of glucocorticoids.

Platelets and coagulation

In heart transplant recipients, intramuscular glucocorticoids can impair fibrinolysis, producing susceptibility to thrombotic disease (SEDA-22, 443) (141). They can also increase the platelet count. In one patient the blue toe syndrome occurred repeatedly when glucocorticoids were used to increase the platelet count (SEDA-16, 451).

Mouth

Oral candidiasis is seen in some 5–10% of patients who use inhaled glucocorticoids, particularly when oral hygiene is poor, but is rarely symptomatic. The risk can be reduced by the use of a large-volume spacer (142,143).

Hypertrophy of the tongue has been attributed to inhaled beclomethasone and may have been related to edema of the buccal mucosa and tongue from direct contact with the glucocorticoid, infection, glossitis caused by glucocorticoid therapy, a direct effect of glucocorticoids on the tongue muscle, or excess localized deposition of fat, as is seen in patients given systemic glucocorticoids (SEDA-20, 371; 144).

Geographic tongue is a common condition, with a prevalence in adults of 0.28–2.4%. It is characteristically asymptomatic. There are multiple, well-demarcated, erythematous areas, of variable sizes, usually surrounded by a slightly elevated circinate linear border, usually on the anterior two-thirds of the dorsum of the tongue. In a population-based case-control study, data from 16 833 US adults who were examined during The Third National Health and Nutrition Examination Survey 1988–1994 (NHANES III) were included (145). There was an overall prevalence of geographic tongue of 1.8%. Individuals who were taking glucocorticoids had a higher prevalence (5.7%; OR = 3.3; 95% CI = 1.3, 8.2) than those who were not (1.8%). There was no relation to the use of inhaled glucocorticoids. Multivariate logistic regression showed significant effects of current glucocorticoid therapy (adjusted OR = 3.7; 95% CI = 1.54, 8.6) and race (Whites and Afro–Americans versus Mexican–Americans) but not with age, sex, oral contraceptive use, diabetes mellitus, allergy or atopy, or psychological or dermatological conditions

Gastrointestinal

Peptic ulceration

It is no longer seriously believed that glucocorticoid treatment in adults markedly increases the risk of peptic ulceration (146,147). However, the symptoms of an existing peptic ulcer can certainly be masked. There may also be a genuine risk of ulcerative disorders in premature children. The issue has often been complicated by the simultaneous (sometimes unrecorded) use of ulcerogenic non-steroidal anti-inflammatory agents. A meta-analysis of whether glucocorticoid therapy caused peptic ulcer and other putative complications of glucocorticoid therapy was negative: peptic ulcers occurred in nine of 3267 patients in the placebo group (0.03%) and 13 of 3335 patients in the glucocorticoid group (0.04%).

Peptic ulcer should not be considered a contraindication when glucocorticoid therapy is indicated (SEDA-19, 376; 148). However, the risk of a fatal outcome due to ulcer complications was increased about fourfold in a previous case-control study. Gastrointestinal hemorrhage occurred more often in glucocorticoid-treated patients (2.25%) than in controls (1.6%) (149). The frequency of gastrointestinal bleeding in these studies compares well with earlier observations in the Boston Collaborative Surveillance Program's 1978 report, according to which

0.5% of a large series of medical inpatients taking gluco-corticoids had gastrointestinal bleeding sufficiently severe to require transfusions and 28% had minor bleeding (SED-12, 986).

- A 47-year-old woman developed a gastrocolic fistula during treatment with aspirin (dosage and duration of therapy not stated) and prednisone for chronic rheuma-toid arthritis (150).

The author commented that 50–75% of gastrocolic fistu-las are related to benign gastric ulcers secondary to the use of NSAIDs. The use of aspirin plus prednisone, as in this patient, increases the risk of complication of peptic ulcer disease two- to fourfold.

In a study of 2061 patients with a first-time hospital discharge diagnosis of perforated peptic ulcer, using population-based discharge registries in three Danish counties, 228 patients (11%) were exposed to glucocorti-coids within 60 days of admission (151). Overall 30-day mortality rate was 25%, the corresponding rate among current glucocorticoid users being 39%. Compared with "never users", the adjusted mortality ratio among current users of oral glucocorticoids alone was 2.1 (95% CI = 1.5, 3.1). Among current users of oral glucocorticoids in com-bination with other ulcer-related drugs the mortality ratio was 1.5 (95% CI = 1.1, 2.1). Thus, pre-admission use of oral glucocorticoids was associated with up to a twofold increase in 30-day mortality among patients hospitalized with perforated peptic ulcer.

The mechanism of whatever harm glucocorticoids may do to the stomach is not clear; cortisol neither consistently increases acid or pepsinogen secretion, nor reduces the protective production of mucin by the gastric mucosa. Serum gastrin concentrations are raised in Cushing's syn-drome and in patients taking prolonged glucocorticoid treatment. On the other hand, the secretion of prostaglan-din E_2 in gastric juice in response to pentagastrin was impaired during glucocorticoid therapy in children. Since PGE_2 has a cytoprotective effect on the gastric mucosa, impaired secretion in response to increased acid secretion during glucocorticoid therapy may be related to the development of peptic ulcer (SEDA-19, 376; 152).

Some reports suggest that people with hepatic cirrhosis or nephrotic syndrome are particularly at risk. Whatever the degree of risk, patients taking long-term glucocorti-coids should be regularly checked to detect peptic ulcers, which can bleed and even perforate without producing pain. There do not seem to be differences in gastric tolerance between the various synthetic glucocorticoids.

Regional ileitis

While glucocorticoids may have a beneficial effect on regional ileitis, perforation of the ileum, lymphatic dilata-tion, and microscopic fistulae have been observed after treatment.

Ischemic colitis

Glucocorticoids should be used with caution in progres-sive systemic sclerosis, and concomitant administration of anticoagulants to prevent ischemic colitis is recommended when administering glucocorticoids in high doses, especially by pulse therapy (SEDA-21, 415; 153).

Ulcerative colitis

A possible risk of glucocorticoid treatment of ulcerative colitis is the development of toxic megacolon or colonic perforation. A change from ulcerative colitis to Crohn's disease may have been induced by prolonged treatment with glucocorticoids (SEDA-19, 376; 154). This case pro-vides further evidence for the view that ulcerative colitis and Crohn's disease may represent a continuous spectrum of inflammatory bowel disease and raises the possibility that reduced polymorphonuclear leukocyte function caused by glucocorticoids may have provoked the devel-opment of granulomata.

Diverticular disease

Existing diverticula can perforate during glucocorticoid therapy (SEDA-18, 387). Abdominal tenderness is the most common and often the only early sign of perforated diverticula in patients taking glucocorticoids. However, in some cases, even abdominal tenderness is absent (SEDA-22, 445; 155).

- Perforation of the sigmoid colon occurred in a 61-year-old Caucasian man with colonic diverticular disease and rheumatoid arthritis treated with pulses of methylpred-nisolone 1 g (156).

The authors suggested that methylprednisolone pulses should be used carefully in patients over 50 years of age and/or people with demonstrated or suspected diverticu-lar disease.

The importance of treatment with glucocorticoids and NSAIDs in the development of sigmoid diverticular abscess perforation has been the subject of a case-control study in 64 patients (38 women), median age 70 years (range 39–91) and 320 age- and sex-matched controls (157). Independently of rheumatic diagnosis glucocorti-coid treatment was strongly associated with sigmoid diverticular abscess perforation (OR = 32; 95% CI = 6.4, 159).

Liver

The process of gluconeogenesis, which is promoted by glucocorticoids, takes place mainly in the liver. The gly-colytic enzymes of the liver are also activated by these glucocorticoids. The synthesis of ribonucleic acid and of enzymes involved in protein catabolism is increased, but the process of protein catabolism takes place outside the liver as well, for example in the muscles. There is experi-mental evidence for glucocorticoid-induced enhancement of hepatic lipid synthesis (SEDA-3, 308), but the main effect of glucocorticoids in this connection is lipid mobi-lization from adipose tissue. The influence of long-term glucocorticoid treatment on liver function is still unknown. If pathological changes are diagnosed, the pos-sible influence of the disease which is being treated has to be borne in mind.

Liver damage from glucocorticoids is rarely severe, but fatal liver failure has been reported.

- A 71-year-old white woman with a compressive optic neuropathy was given five cycles of intravenous methyl-prednisolone 1 g/day for 3 days followed by tapering oral cortisone for 10–14 days (158). The intervals between cycles were 14 days to 6 weeks. She was other-wise healthy and had no history of liver disease. Her liver function tests were normal or only slightly raised during the first five cycles. She then developed raised liver enzymes, a prolonged prothrombin time, and fatal liver failure. Postmortem examination showed necrosis of the liver parenchyma. Hepatitis serology (A, B, and C) was negative as was in situ hybridization for immu-nohistochemical proof of hepatitis Bs and Bc or delta virus antibodies in the liver.
- A 53-year-old woman who took prednisolone 20 mg/day for systemic lupus erythematosus for 38 days devel-oped increased aspartate transaminase and alanine transaminase activities (175 and 144 IU/l respectively on day 38 and 871 and 658 IU/l on day 69) (159). She denied taking hepatotoxic drugs. Serological tests for hepatitis viruses were all negative. Autoantibodies against mitochondria and smooth muscle were not detected. Ultrasound and CT scan were consistent with fatty infiltration. Histology showed macrovesicular fat infiltration, periportal cell infiltration with fibrosis, and a few Mallory bodies. The glucocorticoid was gra-dually tapered and the transaminases gradually fell.
- A 67-year-old teetotaler was given intravenous predni-solone 25 mg tds for primary dermatomyositis and 8 days later developed painless icteric hepatitis, with daily pro-gressive marked deterioration of liver biochemistry (160). She had not taken any other hepatotoxic drugs, and serological tests for hepatitis and hepatotropic viruses were all negative. Antinuclear, antimitochon-drial, and smooth muscle autoantibodies were negative. Ultrasound and CT scan of the upper abdomen showed liver fatty infiltration. Prednisolone was tapered gradu-ally, and she gradually improved. However, on day 26 she developed pneumonia and died 6 days later.

Glucocorticoid treatment in the early phase of acute viral hepatitis carries the risk of transition to chronic active hepatitis (SEDA-3, 308).

Three children developed hepatomegaly and raised liver enzymes after receiving high-dose dexamethasone therapy (0.66–1.09 mg/kg/day) (161).

There has been a report of seven cases of acute severe liver damage associated with intravenous glucocorticoid pulse therapy in patients with Grave's ophthalmopathy (162).

Methylprednisolone-associated toxic hepatitis has been reported (163).

- A 47-year-old woman developed weakness, fatigue, pruritus, and scleral icterus. She had been taking topir-amate (dose not stated) for 1 year for chronic isolated central nervous system vasculitis. One week before her symptoms developed, she had completed a self-prescribed 7-day course of oral methylprednisolone

(32 mg/day) for left arm weakness. She believed that methylprednisolone was appropriate, since it had been used previously for acute episodes of vasculitis. Her liver function tests were: alanine transaminase 2478 U/l (reference range 0–50), aspartate transaminase 1600 U/l (0– 40), total bilirubin 10 mg/dl (0.2–1.2), direct bilirubin 8 mg/dl (0–0.4), alkaline phosphatase 138 U/l (40–150), and gamma-glutamyl transferase 242 U/l (5–64). Topiramate was withdrawn, and the liver func-tion tests normalized within 45 days without treatment.

Based on the history and laboratory findings, the authors suggested that the hepatocellular and cholestatic liver injury had been caused by methylprednisolone, a rare adverse effect.

Pancreas

Pancreatitis and altered pancreatic secretion can occur at any time during long-term glucocorticoid treatment (SED-12, 986; SEDA-14, 339; 164). Necrosis of the pan-creas during glucocorticoid treatment has been described and can be lethal. Impairment of pancreatic function can predispose to glucocorticoid-induced pancreatitis. Two other cases of glucocorticoid-induced pancreatitis have been reported (165).

- A 74-year-old woman with seronegative rheumatoid arthritis was given sulfasalazine followed by methotrex-ate, both of which were withdrawn because of adverse effects. She also took prednisone 10 mg/day. She devel-oped acute abdominal pain and fever (38.7°C) with no chills. Her serum amylase was 269 IU/l, serum lipase 300 IU/l, and urinary amylase 2895 IU/l. There was no evidence of tumor, hypertriglyceridemia, or lithiasis. In addition to prednisone, she was taking amlodipine, bro-mazepam, and omeprazole, none of which have been reported to cause pancreatitis. A marked improvement was noted after prednisone withdrawal.
- A 68-year-old woman who had taken prednisone 30 mg/day for polymyalgia rheumatica for 6 months developed sharp stabbing abdominal pain, fever (39°C), and vomiting. Her serum amylase was 310 IU/l, serum lipase 340 IU/l, and urinary amylase 1560 IU/l. Other causes of pancreatitis were ruled out. She had been taking a thiazide diuretic therapy for the past 10 years. Her symptoms improved noticeably after predni-sone withdrawal.

Although the literature suggests a causal relation between glucocorticoid therapy and these various pancreatic com-plications there is still no certainty; glucocorticoid treat-ment is, after all, often given simultaneously with other forms of therapy which can cause pancreatitis (SED-11, 82). The strongest evidence that there is a causal relation is provided by a Japanese report on 52 autopsies, which showed marked changes in pancreatic histology in gluco-corticoid-treated patients compared with controls (SEDA-17, 449).

Acute pancreatitis after rechallenge provides direct evidence that hydrocortisone can cause acute pancreatitis in a patient with ulcerative colitis (166).

- An 18-year old youth was admitted with a history of large bowel diarrhea off and on for 6 months before admission. There was a history of passage of blood mixed with stools for the same duration. There was no history of fever, arthralgias, jaundice, or red eyes. At the time of admission he was passing 10-12 stools in 24 hours, and 6-7 of them contained blood. His pulse rate was 100/minute and there was pallor and minimal pedal edema. He was tender in the flanks with exaggerated bowel sounds. Sigmoidoscopy showed ulceration, erythema, friability, and loss of vascular pattern in the rectum and sigmoid colon, suggestive of ulcerative colitis. A rectal biopsy showed crypt atrophy, crypt abscesses, a mixed cellular infiltrate, goblet cell depletion, and submucosal edema. He was given intravenous fluids and injectable hydrocortisone 100 mg six times an hour. Injections of ofloxacin and metronidazole were added later, because his leukocyte count was 15.6 x 10^9/l. On the second day of treatment he developed epigastric pain radiating to the back. The pain was continuous, associated with vomiting, and relieved by sitting in the knee-chest position. Acute pancreatitis was corroborated by a serum lipase activity of 650 units/l and high serum amylase activity (550 units/l). Ultrasonography showed a bulky, heterogeneous pancreas with ill defined margins, suggestive of pancreatitis. There were no gallstones. Hydrocortisone was withdrawn and the rest of the treatment continued. Mesalazine was added after 1 day. The pancreatitis resolved in 48 hours, as did the diarrhea. After 1 month the patient was readmitted with a relapse of ulcerative colitis. This time his stool frequency was 4–5 stools in 24 hours, and most contained some blood. There was no fever and his total leukocyte count was normal. He was given mesalazine enemas and injectable hydrocortisone. On the second day after admission, he had a similar bout of acute pancreatitis. Hydrocortisone was withdrawn and he recovered.

Urinary tract

Urinary calculi are more likely during glucocorticoid treatment because of increased excretion of calcium and phosphate (132).

Prednisolone can cause an abrupt rise in proteinuria in patients with nephrotic syndrome. A placebo-controlled study in 26 patients aged 18–68 years with nephrotic syndrome has clarified the mechanisms responsible for this (167). Systemic and renal hemodynamics and urinary protein excretion were measured after prednisolone (125 mg or 150 mg when body weight exceeded 75 kg) and after placebo. Prednisolone increased proteinuria by changing the size–selective barrier of the glomerular capillaries. Neither the renin–angiotensin axis nor prostaglandins were involved in these effects of prednisolone on proteinuria.

Changes resembling diabetic nodular glomerular sclerosis have been seen in glucocorticoid-treated nephrosis.

Treatment with glucocorticoids can result in minor increases in the urinary content of leukocytes and erythrocytes without clear renal injury (168).

The use of high doses of glucocorticoids to counter rejection of renal transplants is still a matter of intensive study; the optimal dose to ensure an effect without undue risk of complications has yet to be agreed on (169).

Vasopressin-resistant polyuria induced by intravenous administration of a therapeutic dose of dexamethasone has been reported (SEDA-20, 370; 170) and nocturia is fairly common during glucocorticoid treatment (171).

The administration of glucocorticoids should be undertaken with caution in progressive systemic sclerosis and the concomitant administration of anticoagulants to prevent scleroderma renal crisis is recommended when administering glucocorticoids in high doses, especially by pulse therapy (SEDA-21, 415; 153).

Skin

Acne is common during treatment, particularly after topical application, and is said to be correlated with the use of compounds that have a particularly strong local effect (172), although this is not proven.

Leukoderma can occur, accompanied by normal melanocyte function but reduced phagocytic activity of the keratinocytes to eliminate the melanosomes (173). Depigmentation can occur at the site of injection of glucocorticoids.

Three cases of severe lipoatrophy, one also with leukoderma, occurring within the same family after intramuscular injection of triamcinolone, suggested genetic susceptibility to this adverse effect (SEDA-3, 303).

Inhibition of the function of the sebaceous glands in the skin is caused by glucocorticoids whilst androgens stimulate their function (174).

A delayed hypersensitivity reaction, characterized by a skin rash, due to dexamethasone has been reported (175). These kinds of reactions to systemic glucocorticoids are rarely reported.

- A 59-year-old woman, who had not used glucocorticoids before, developed an exfoliative rash on her face, upper chest, and skin folds after 3 days treatment with oral dexamethasone (dosage not stated) for an acute episode of encephalomyelitis disseminata. Dexamethasone was immediately withdrawn and her skin lesions resolved over several days. Patch tests were positive to dexamethasone, betamethasone, and clobetasol, but negative to other glucocorticoids, including prednisolone, hydrocortisone butyrate, methylprednisolone, and triamcinolone. Prick tests with all of these glucocorticoids were negative. She tolerated oral methylprednisolone without adverse effects.

Linear hypopigmentation after intralesional or intra-articular injection of triamcinolone acetonide has been reported as a very rare adverse effect. The hypopigmentation is oriented linearly, spreads proximally, and may or may not be associated with skin atrophy. Another case has been reported (176)

- An 11-year-old girl had an elevated scar on the back of her wrist, which had remained erythematous, gradually increasing in size. The scar had recurred after excision, and a silicon sheet was applied and triamcinolone injected intralesionally (20 mg in 0.5 ml) three times at intervals of 8 weeks. Hypopigmentation developed around the scar in the form of a halo about 2 weeks after the last injection and a linear hypopigmented streak progressed proximally over the forearm. At 4 weeks after the last injection, the hypopigmented streak stopped progressing and the lesion on the wrist started to repigment. At 6 months the perilesional halo of hypopigmentation and the linear streak were only very faintly discernible.

The authors commented that the hypopigmentation could have been due to lymphatic spread after inadvertent intradermal injection in the peripheral part of the keloid.

Acute generalized exanthematous pustulosis (AGEP) due to a glucocorticoid has been reported (SEDA-21, 416; 271).

Reduced skin thickness and bruising

The glucocorticoids reduce subcutaneous collagen and cause atrophic changes in the skin (177). Subcutaneous atrophy after intramuscular and intra-articular injection has often been reported. Ecchymosis and paper-thin skin folds recall those seen in old people. An increased incidence of subcutaneous ecchymosis in older women has been observed during treatment with triamcinolone acetate (178). Purpura has been observed during glucocorticoid treatment and an increased fragility of the capillaries is thought to occur in about 60% of these patients. There have been reports of cutaneous bruising after the use of high doses of inhaled glucocorticoids (budesonide and beclomethasone), suggesting systemic absorption (SEDA-21, 416; 179).

Prednicarbate is a topical glucocorticoid that seems to have an improved benefit–harm balance, as has been shown in 24 healthy volunteers (7 men, 17 women, aged 25–49 years) in a double-blind, randomized, placebo-controlled study of the effects of prednicarbate, mometasone furoate, and betamethasone 17-valerate on total skin thickness over 6 weeks (180). On day 36, total skin thickness was reduced by a mean of 1% in test fields treated with vehicle; the relative reductions were 13, 17, and 24% for prednicarbate, mometasone furoate, and betamethasone 17-valerate respectively. There were visible signs of atrophy or telangiectasia in two subjects each with betamethasone 17-valerate and mometasone furoate, but not with prednicarbate or its vehicle.

Contact allergy

Topical glucocorticoids are well-known contact sensitizers. Immediate allergic or allergic-like reactions to systemic glucocorticoids also occur, but less often. Two atopic patients developed urticaria, possibly IgE-mediated, from a hydrocortisone injection or infusion (181) and other reactions have been reported.

- A 50-year-old woman developed contact dermatitis on her legs after she applied hydrocortisone aceponate cream (Efficort) to psoriatic lesions on her lower back (182). Similar lesions also occurred on her legs after she used topical betamethasone cream (Diprosone). However, no eczema developed on or around the site of application. Patch tests were negative to a range of glucocorticoids, including Efficort and Diprosone creams. However, a repeated open application test was positive with Efficort cream, hydrocortisone aceponate 0.127% in petroleum, and tixocortol pivalate 1% in petroleum.

- A 42-year-old woman developed a nonpigmented fixed drug eruption after skin testing and an intra-articular injection of triamcinolone acetonide, which has not been previously reported (183).

Contact allergy to glucocorticoids was evaluated in 7238 patients in a multicenter multinational study of five drugs: budesonide, betamethasone-17-valerate, clobetasol-17-propionate, hydrocortisone-17-butyrate, and tixocortol-21-pivalate. There was a positive patch-test reaction to at least one of the glucocorticoids in 189 patients (2.6%). The incidence ranged from 0.4% in Spain to 6.4% in Belgium. Positive reactions were more frequent with budesonide (100 results) and tixocortol (98 reactions) (SEDA-21, 415; 184). Contact allergic reactions to intranasal budesonide and fluticasone propionate have been described. Many of these cases were characterized by perinasal eczema, often with vesicles, and edema as the initial symptoms. Lesions sometimes spread to the upper lip, cheeks, and eyelids. For fluticasone propionate, analysis of data on adverse events from the Spontaneous Reporting System of the US FDA Division of Epidemiology and Surveillance showed that, in the first 5 months after its introduction into the USA in 1995, 46 patients reported 89 adverse events suspected to be caused by fluticasone propionate intranasal spray. Central nervous system symptoms occurred in 46%, cardiac symptoms in 28%, dermatological symptoms in 39%, and epistaxis in 6.5%. These numbers may underestimate the problem, since no cases reported by the drug manufacturer were included. These results suggest that safety issues may differentiate budesonide and fluticasone propionate from other intranasal glucocorticoids, such as beclomethasone dipropionate (SEDA-21, 415; 185).

Budesonide is advocated as a marker molecule for glucocorticoid contact allergy. When patch testing glucocorticoids, one must consider both their sensitizing potential and their anti-inflammatory properties, as well as the possibility of different time courses of such properties. The dose–response relation for budesonide has therefore been investigated with regard to dose, occlusion time, and reading time in 10 patients (ages not stated) who were patch tested with budesonide in ethanol in serial dilutions from 2.0% down to 0.0002%, with occlusion times of 48, 24, and 5 hours (186). Readings were on days 2, 4, and 7. The 48-hour occlusion detected most positive reactors (8/10) at a reading time of 4 days and 0.002% detected most contact allergies. The "edge effect" (reactions with a peripheral ring due to suppression of the allergic reaction under the patch because of the intrinsic anti-inflammatory effect of the glucocorticoid itself) was noted with several concentrations at early readings. That lower concentrations can detect budesonide allergy better at early readings and that patients with an "edge reaction" can have positive reactions to lower concentrations can be explained by individual glucocorticoid reactivity, the dose–response relation, and the time-courses of the elicitation and the anti-inflammatory capacity.

- A 36-year-old man, who had a long history of atopic dermatitis of the neck, chest, and arms, developed allergic contact dermatitis after topical administration of clobetasone ointment 0.05% (Kindavate) and prednisolone ointment 0.3% (Lidomex) (187). Patch tests with both ointments showed a positive reaction only to Kindavate. Further testing with the separate ingredients of Kindavate showed positive reactions to 0.05, 0.01, and 0.005% clobetasone on day 7.
- A 40-year-old woman had a flare-up of her eczema (188). She had had previous negative patch tests 10 years before. She had taken topical glucocorticoids and emollients for a few months, but had not used budesonide. Patch testing with the European standard series showed a positive reaction to budesonide 0.1% at 3 days. All other allergens were negative. The only antecedent exposure was that she had three children with asthma, all of whom regularly used inhaled budesonide and occasionally nebulizers. She had not used the inhaler but had helped her children to manage the devices. A subsequent patch test with powdered budesonide from the inhaler was positive.
- A 14-year-old girl with newly diagnosed systemic lupus erythematosus developed a pruritic bullous eruption while taking prednisone 20 mg/day (189). She was given a single daily dose of intravenous methylprednisolone 60 mg with rapid improvement. In preparation for discharge, the glucocorticoid was changed to oral prednisone 60 mg/day, to which she developed a pruritic bullous eruption consistent with erythema multiforme. She underwent immediate and delayed hypersensitivity tests. Intradermal and patch tests to liquid prednisone were positive. She was given oral methylprednisolone 48 mg/day and has not had recurrence of the skin lesions.
- A 27-year-old woman, a pharmacist, had dermatitis on three separate occasions a few hours after she started to take oral deflazacort 6 mg for vesicular hand eczema (190). On each occasion, her symptoms included a widespread macular rash mainly on the inner aspects of her arms and legs and buttocks. She also had severe scaling, fever, nausea, vomiting, malaise, and hypotension. A skin biopsy was consistent with erythema multiforme, and direct immunofluorescence showed granular deposits at the dermoepidermal junction. Patch tests to the commercial formulation of deflazacort 6 mg (1% aqueous solution) and to pure deflazacort (1% aqueous solution) were positive, but there were no cross-reactions to other glucocorticoids.

The author of the last report commented that the patient probably developed hypersensitivity to deflazacort as a result of occupational exposure.

Other cases of erythema multiforme-like contact dermatitis after topical budesonide have been reported (SEDA-21, 415) (191). In a large case-control study,

potential cases of severe forms of erythema multiforme, toxic epidermal necrolysis and Stevens–Johnson syndrome, were collected in four European countries (France, Portugal, Italy, and Germany) (SEDA-20, 371; 192). There was a significant relation with glucocorticoid use in the preceding week (multivariate analysis relative risk = 4.4; 95% CI = 1.9, 10), or when prescribed for long-term therapy (crude relative risk for use less than 2 months = 54; 95% CI = 23, 124). The estimates of excess risks associated with glucocorticoids or sulfonamides (which are well-known to cause these syndromes), expressed as the number of cases attributable to the drug per million users in 1 week, were 1.5 and 4.5 respectively.

Cross-reactivity between glucocorticoids and progestogens has been described (193).

- A 68-year-old woman, with a prolonged history of pityriasis lichenoides chronica treated with topical glucocorticoids, including hydrocortisone, took a formulation containing conjugated estrogens 0.625 mg and hydroxyprogesterone acetate 5 mg (frequency of administration not stated) for late menopausal syndrome. Years later she started to have pruritus, a maculopapular rash, and flu-like symptoms for several days before menstruation. On this occasion, she presented with a severe, pruritic, papulovesicular eruption on her chest, back, abdomen, and legs. The eruption had developed after treatment for 7 days with the estrogen–progestogen formulation; she had developed similar symptoms on several previous occasions after taking the same medication. She was treated with antihistamines and her skin eruption resolved within a few days. Patch tests were positive to 17-OH-progesterone, tixocortol pivalate, and budesonide.

The authors hypothesized that this patient, who had taken topical glucocorticoids for several years, had become sensitive and that the recurrent episodes of autoimmune progestogen dermatitis were related to endogenous progestogen sensitivity following cross-sensitivity to glucocorticoids. This hypothesis was supported by the development of recurrent eczema several times after she took an estrogen–progestogen preparation.

Musculoskeletal

Osteoporosis

The use of glucocorticoids is associated with reduced bone mineral density, bone loss, osteoporosis, and fractures. This has been described during the long-term use of glucocorticoid by any route of administration (SEDA-19, 377; SEDA-20, 374). The effects of glucocorticoids on bone have been reviewed (SEDA-21, 417; 194)195,196. Biochemical markers of bone mineral density are listed in Table 4. In patients with secondary hypoadrenalism, hydrocortisone 30 mg/day for replacement produced a significant fall in osteocalcin, indicating bone loss. Lower doses of hydrocortisone (10 mg and 20 mg) produced similar efficacy in terms of quality of life but smaller effects on osteocalcin concentrations and therefore a reduction in bone loss (197). Three studies add evidence

Table 4   Biochemical markers of bone mineral density

Bone formation
Blood
Alkaline phosphatase (bone-specific)
Osteocalcin
Procollagen type I carboxy-terminal propeptide (PICP)
Procollagen type I amino-terminal propeptide (PINP)
Procollagen type III amino-terminal propeptide (PIIINP)
Bone resorption
Blood
Acid phosphatase (acid-resistant)
Type I collagen carboxy-terminal telopeptide (ICTP)

Urine
Calcium
Hydroxyproline
Cross-linked peptides (pyridinium and deoxypyridinoline)

of the deleterious effects of oral glucocorticoids and high doses of inhaled glucocorticoids on bone mineral density (198) and the risk of fractures (199,200).

The fluorinated glucocorticoids are said to have relatively more catabolic activity than others and might have a greater effect on the skeleton but such impressions may merely reflect the general potency of some newer glucocorticoids and a tendency to use them in inappropriate doses. A relatively new glucocorticoid, deflazacort, has been proposed to have less effect on bone metabolism, but a double-blind study has failed to show an advantage compared with prednisolone (SEDA-21, 417; 201).

Osteoporosis induced by chronic glucocorticoid therapy has been reviewed in patients with obstructive lung diseases (202) and patients with skin diseases (203).

Presentation
Of the effects of glucocorticoids on the skeleton, osteoporosis is the most important clinically; manifestations can include vertebral compression fractures, scoliosis resulting in respiratory embarrassment, and fractures of the long bones. The risk of vertebral fractures is not different in patients taking or not taking glucocorticoids in whom bone mineral density is similar (204).

Glucocorticoids can even cause osteoporosis when they are used for long-term replacement therapy in the Addison's disease, as has been shown by a study of 91 patients who had taken glucocorticoids for a mean of 10.6 years, in whom bone mineral density was reduced by 32% compared with age-matched controls (SEDA-19, 377; 205). However, these results contrasted with the results of a Spanish study in patients with Addison's disease, in which no direct relation was found between replacement therapy and either bone density or biochemical markers of bone turnover of calcium metabolism (alkaline phosphatase, osteocalcin, procollagen I type, parathormone, and 1,25-dihydroxycolecalciferol) (SEDA-19, 377; 206).

Atraumatic posterior pelvic ring fractures that simulate the form of presentation of metastatic diseases can be produced by glucocorticoid administration (SEDA-19, 377; 207).

Accelerated bone loss, with an increased risk of first hip fracture, occurred in elderly women taking oral glucocorticoids (208). At baseline, 122 (1.5%) women were taking inhaled glucocorticoids only (median dose equivalent to inhaled beclomethasone 168 micrograms/day), 228 (2.8%) were taking oral glucocorticoids (median dose equivalent to prednisone 5 mg/day) with or without inhaled glucocorticoids, and 7718 were not taking any glucocorticoids. The women who were taking oral glucocorticoids had lower mean bone mineral density at 3.6 years than nonusers, with an interim fall that was twice as fast. First hip fracture occurred in 4.8% of the women who were taking oral glucocorticoids and in 2.8% of the women who were not (RR = 2.1; CI = 1.0, 4.4). The researchers said that the power of the study was not sufficient to determine the relative risk of hip fracture in women taking inhaled glucocorticoids.

A reduction in bone mineral density has been described in 23 patients (19 men) with chronic fatigue syndrome taking low-dose glucocorticoids in a double-blind, randomized, placebo-controlled study (209). The patients took hydrocortisone 25–35 mg/day or matched placebo for 3 months. Mean bone mineral density in the spine fell by 2% with hydrocortisone and increased by 1% with placebo.

A group of 367 patients with lung disease taking oral glucocorticoids (177 women, mean age 68 years, 190 men, mean age 70 years) and 734 matched controls completed a questionnaire about lifestyle, fractures, and other possible adverse effects of glucocorticoids (210). The cumulative incidence of fractures from the time of diagnosis was 23% in patients taking oral glucocorticoids and 15% in the controls (OR = 1.8; 95% CI = 1.3, 2.6). Fractures of the vertebrae were more likely (OR = 10; 95% CI = 2.9, 35). The adverse effects were dose-related, with a higher risk of all fractures (OR = 2.22; 95% CI = 1.04, 4.8) and vertebral fractures (OR = 9.2; 95% CI = 2.4, 36) in those who took the highest compared with the lowest cumulative doses (61 versus 5 g).

Systemic glucocorticoids are often prescribed for rheumatoid arthritis. Even in low doses they can have clinical benefits and can inhibit joint damage, but they can cause osteoporotic fractures. In a 2-year double-blind, randomized, placebo-controlled trial in 81 patients (29 men, mean age 62 years) with early active rheumatoid arthritis who had not been treated with disease-modifying antirheumatic drugs, 41 were assigned to oral prednisone 10 mg/day and 40 to placebo. NSAIDs were allowed in both groups and after 6 months, sulfasalazine (2 g/day) could be prescribed as rescue medication. Those who took prednisone had more clinical improvement with less use of concomitant drugs. After month 6, radiological scores had progressed significantly less in those who took prednisone. After 24 months, seven patients had new vertebral fractures, five in the prednisone group and two in the placebo group (211).

Mechanisms
There have been reviews of the mechanisms and adverse effects of glucocorticoids in rheumatoid arthritis (212)

and the pathogenesis, diagnosis, and treatment of glucocorticoid-induced osteoporosis in patients with pulmonary diseases (213). Several mechanisms underlie the effect of glucocorticoids on bone, both biochemical and cellular. Effects on calcium are:

(a) increased excretion of calcium into the bowel and inhibition of its absorption;
(b) inhibition of the tubular re-absorption of calcium in the kidney;
(c) increased mobilization of calcium from the skeleton.

When calcium homeostasis cannot be maintained, the resulting hypocalcemia can have serious consequences (SEDA-18, 388; 214,215). This so-called "glucocorticoid hyperparathyroidism" was the explanation traditionally most prominently advanced for glucocorticoid osteoporosis, but it is not the only one and may not be the most central. Other biochemical effects include:

(a) a catabolic effect on protein metabolism, causing a reduction in the bone matrix;
(b) altered vitamin D metabolism, with reduced concentrations of vitamin D metabolites (216);
(c) a dose-dependent reduction of serum osteocalcin, a bone matrix protein that appears to correlate with bone formation.

Measurement of serum osteocalcin is a useful marker for glucocorticoid-induced osteoporosis, and can be used alongside other measures noted below.

Various cellular mechanisms are involved in the production of glucocorticoid-induced osteoporosis (SEDA-20, 375; 217). The major change is a reduction in osteoblast activity that results in a reduced working rate (mean appositional rate), and a reduced active life-span of osteoblasts. The cellular mechanism seems to be related to diminished production of cytokines and other locally acting factors. Increased bone resorption and reduced calcium absorption have also been described. A sophisticated mathematical model has been used to describe changes in calcium kinetics in patients treated with glucocorticoids (SEDA-20, 375; 218). Plasma calcium concentrations were higher than in controls, with a marked reduction in calcium flow into the irreversible stable bone compartment in glucocorticoid-treated patients. The authors concluded that prednisone has direct effects on osteoblast function.

Osteoprotegerin (osteoclastogenesis inhibitory factor, OCIF) has been identified as a novelly secreted cytokine receptor that plays an important role in the negative regulation of osteoclastic bone resorption. There are reports that suggest that glucocorticoids promote osteoclastogenesis by inhibiting osteoprotegerin production in vitro, thereby enhancing bone resorption. However, there are only a few clinical reports in which the regulatory functions of osteoprotegerin have been explored. In order to clarify the potential role of osteoprotegerin in the pathogenesis of glucocorticoid-induced osteoporosis, Japanese investigators have measured serum osteoprotegerin and other markers of bone metabolism before and after glucocorticoid therapy in patients with various renal diseases (219). The findings suggested that short-term administration of glucocorticoids significantly suppresses serum osteoprotegerin and osteocalcin. This might be relevant to the development of glucocorticoid-induced osteoporosis via enhancement of bone resorption and suppression of bone formation. Further long-term studies are needed to elucidate the mechanism of the glucocorticoid-induced reduction in circulating osteoprotegerin and its participation in the pathogenesis of osteoporosis.

Although glucocorticoids can cause changes in trabecular microarchitecture, loss of bone (reduced bone density) seems to be the major determinant of osteoporosis (220). Bone resorption seems to involve the receptor of the activator of the nucleus factor KB ligand (RANK-L) and osteoprotegerin. RANK-L binds to a specific receptor in osteoclasts, and in the presence of the macrophage colony stimulating factor (M-CSF) it induces osteoclastogenesis (the development of mature osteoclasts) and suppression of normal osteoclast apoptosis. Osteoprotegerin is a soluble decoy receptor that binds to and neutralizes RANK-L and so reduces osteoclastogenesis. Glucocorticoids increase the expression of RANK-L and M-CSF and reduce osteoprotegerin production by osteoblasts. The net result is enhanced osteoclastic activity. Other inflammatory mediators, such as tumor necrosis factor-alfa and interleukin-6, have similar biological actions to glucocorticoids. Glucocorticoids reduce osteoblast numbers and function by reducing the replication and differentiation of osteoblasts and by increasing apoptosis in mature osteoblasts. Glucocorticoids inhibit osteoblastic synthesis of type I collagen, the major component of bone extracellular matrix. They can induce apoptosis of osteocytes, and this could be the mechanism of osteonecrosis. Two other factors are involved in bone loss: firstly, glucocorticoids increase renal calcium elimination and reduce intestinal calcium absorption, leading to a negative calcium balance, which can lead to secondary hyperparathyroidism; secondly, glucocorticoids reduce the production of gonadal hormones. The histological effects of glucocorticoids are a reduced rate of bone formation, reduced trabecular wall thickness, and apoptosis of bone cells. These effects lead to osteoporosis and fractures.

Although glucocorticoid use seems to be an important factor for low mineral density, sex hormones have also been suggested as an important determinant of bone mineral content. Bone mineral density and sex hormone status have been studied in 99 men with rheumatoid arthritis and 68 age-matched controls (SEDA-20, 375; 221). There were significant reductions in lumbar and femoral density, and salivary testosterone, androstenedione, and dehydroepiandrosterone in the patients. Salivary testosterone correlated with femoral density. By multiple regression analysis, weight, serum testosterone concentrations, and cumulative dose of glucocorticoid were significant predictors of lumbar bone density. Weight, age, androstenedione concentrations, and cumulative dose of glucocorticoids were significant predictors of femoral bone density.

Dose relation

Dose is an important factor, but these adverse effects have been described after low doses. The risk of hip fracture associated with glucocorticoid use has been studied in Denmark in a population-based case-control study in 6660 subjects with hip fractures and 33 272 age-matched population controls (222). Data on prescriptions for glucocorticoid within the last 5 years before the index date were retrieved from a population-based prescription database. Doses were recalculated to prednisolone equivalents. Cases and controls were grouped according to cumulative glucocorticoid dose:

1. not used;
2. under 130 mg (equivalent to prednisolone 30 mg/day for 4 days given for an acute exacerbation of asthma);
3. 130-499 mg (equivalent to a short course of prednisolone of 450 mg) for acute asthma;
4. 500-1499 mg (equivalent to prednisolone 7.5 mg/day for 6 months or 800 micrograms/day of inhaled budesonide for 1 year);
5. 1500 mg or more (equivalent to more than 4.1 mg day for 1 year, a long-term high dose).

A conditional logistic regression was used and adjusted for potential confounders including sex, redeemed prescriptions for hormone replacement therapy, antiosteoporotic, anxiolytic, antipsychotic, and antidepressant drugs. Compared with never users, there was an increased risk of hip fracture in glucocorticoid users, with increasing cumulative doses of any type of drug used during the preceding 5 years. For doses of prednisolone under 130 mg, the adjusted risk (OR) was 0.96 (95% CI = 0.89, 1.04); for 130-499 mg the OR was 1.17 (1.01, 1.35); for 500-1499 mg the OR was 1.36 (1.19, 1.56); and for 1500 mg or more the OR was 1.65 (1.43, 1.92). There was an also increased risk when the study population was stratified according to sex, age, and type of glucocorticoid (systemic or topical). This study showed that even a limited daily dose of glucocorticoids (more than an average dose of prednisolone of about 71 micrograms/day) was associated with an increased risk of hip fracture.

Doses of prednisone of 7.5 mg/day can cause premature or exaggerated osteoporosis. However, it is unclear whether a dose of 5 mg/day has the same effect. In a double-blind, randomized, placebo-controlled, 8-week trial 50 healthy postmenopausal women (mean age 57 years) were randomly assigned to prednisone 5 mg/day or matching placebo for 6 weeks, followed by a 2-week recovery phase (223). Prednisone rapidly and significantly decreased serum concentrations of propeptide of type I N-terminal procollagen, propeptide of type I C-terminal procollagen, and osteocalcin, and free urinary deoxypyridinoline compared with placebo. These changes were largely reversed during the recovery period. In conclusion, low-dose prednisone significantly reduced indices of bone formation and bone resorption in postmenopausal women.

Lumbar spine bone mineral density has been assessed in 76 prepubertal asthmatics (mean age 7.7 years, 26 girls) using glucocorticoids (224). After stratification for dose and route of administration, the children who used over 800 micrograms/day of inhaled glucocorticoids, with or without intermittent oral glucocorticoids, had a significant lower weight-adjusted bone density than children who used

400–800 micrograms/day of inhaled glucocorticoids (mean difference -0.05 g/cm^2; 95% CI = -0.02, -0.09). Bone mass was similar in children who did not use inhaled glucocorticoids and those who used 400–800 micrograms/day.

In kidney transplant recipients, lumbar bone loss was significantly higher in 20 patients who took daily prednisone (5.9%, mean dosage 0.19 mg/kg/day) than in 27 patients who used alternate-day prednisone (1.1%, mean dosage 0.15 mg/kg/day) (225).

Time course

The loss of bone mineral after organ and tissue transplant associated with immunosuppressive therapy follows a delayed time course. The long-term effects of immunosuppressive therapy on bone density have been determined in 25 cardiac transplant patients (SEDA-20, 375; 226). As expected, there was bone loss in the spine during the first year, but this was not maintained during the second and third years after transplantation, despite continuing maintenance immunosuppression with prednisolone. Only four patients, all of whom were hypogonadal, continued to lose bone.

Susceptibility factors

The overall effect of glucocorticoids on bone mineral content differs between patients on comparable treatments, which suggests that some patients are more predisposed than others (SEDA-3, 306), and probably also that the standards of evaluation used in different clinics are not comparable. This variability and the wide range of products and dosage schemes used mean that one does not have a clear impression of what constitutes a safe regimen as far as the skeleton is concerned (SEDA-20, 374), or whether any regimen is safe in this respect. Certainly, in a series of men with rheumatoid arthritis, even a very low dose of glucocorticoids (for example 10 mg or less of prednisolone daily) has proved to have a significant effect on bone mineral density (227); other work has provided similar results (SEDA-20, 374; 228). In another published study, patients who took 1–4 mg/day had the same density as those who were not taking glucocorticoids. Patients who took 5–9 mg/day and those who took more than 10 mg/day had significantly lower bone density (84 and 81% of control values respectively) (SEDA-20, 374; 229).

Glucocorticoid-related complications have been described in 748 adult kidney transplant recipients, followed for at least 1 year. For bone/joint complications, the multivariate analysis showed that the only significant variable was the cumulative duration of glucocorticoid therapy. For avascular necrosis, no variables were significant (SEDA-19, 377; 230).

In a similar study of 65 renal transplant patients treated with immunosuppressive drugs for at least 6 months, multivariate analysis showed that cumulative glucocorticoid dose and female sex were the major predictors of low vertebral bone density (SEDA-19, 377; 231).

In another study, the loss of bone density correlated with the cumulative dose of prednisolone (21 g total dose at 11.4 mg/day) and renal function (SEDA-21, 417; 232).

In a review of renal transplantation during 1974–94, 166 patients were classified into those with osteonecrosis of the femoral head (22 patients) and those without (47 patients) (SEDA-21, 417; 233). The total dose of methyl-prednisolone was higher in those with osteonecrosis. All five patients who had received intravenous pulse doses over 2000 mg had osteonecrosis.

The risk of vertebral deformity is increased by the combination of an oral glucocorticoid and advanced age, according to the findings in 229 patients (69% women) taking long-term oral glucocorticoids (prednisone equivalents of 5 mg/day or more) and 286 untreated controls (234). The duration of treatment was 0.5–37 (median 4.8) years. More than 60% of the treatment group were aged over 60 years, and most (62%) had been treated for rheumatoid arthritis. Bone mineral density data were analysed in 194 patients. The researchers identified at least one vertebral deformity (defined as a more than 20% reduction in anterior, middle, or posterior vertebral height) in 65 (28%) of the patients in the treatment group, and two or more fractures were identified in 25 (11%). In the treatment group, vertebral deformities were significantly more common in men than in women, and the prevalence of deformities increased with age. Compared with patients aged under 60 years, glucocorticoid-treated patients aged 70–79 years had a five-fold increased risk of vertebral deformity (OR = 5.1; 95% CI = 2.0, 13). The prevalence of vertebral deformities increased significantly with age in the glucocorticoid group. While the mean spine and femoral bone mineral density scores were lower in the glucocorticoid group, logistic regression analysis showed that bone mineral density was only a modest predictor of deformity. Age is an important independent risk factor, with very high prevalence rates in those over 70 years. Increasing duration of glucocorticoid use may increase the risk of fracture.

Osteoporosis is common in Crohn's disease, often because of glucocorticoids. Budesonide as controlled-release capsules is a locally acting glucocorticoid with low systemic availability. In a randomized study in 272 patients with Crohn's disease involving the ileum and/or ascending colon, budesonide and prednisolone were compared for 2 years in doses adapted to disease activity (235). There was active disease in 181, of whom 98 were glucocorticoid-naive; 90 had quiescent disease and were corticosteroid-dependent. Efficacy was similar in the two groups, but treatment-related adverse effects were less frequent with budesonide. The glucocorticoid-naive patients who took budesonide had smaller reductions in bone mineral density than those who took prednisolone (mean –1.04% versus –3.84%).

The risk of fractures is increased in patients with rheumatoid arthritis. In a database study of 30 262 patients with rheumatoid arthritis (older than 40 years) and 30 783 controls with similar characteristics, followed for a mean of 7.6 years, there were 2460 fractures in the case group (236). Compared with controls, the cases had an increased risk of hip fracture (RR = 2.0; 95% CI = 1.8, 2.3) and spine (RR = 2.4; 95% CI = 2.0, 2.8). Factors related to an increased risk of hip fracture included more than 10 years' duration of rheumatoid arthritis (RR = 3.4; 95% CI = 3.0, 3.9), a low body mass index (RR = 3.9; 95%

CI = 3.1, 4.9), and use of oral glucocorticoids (RR = 3.4; 95% CI = 3.0, 4.0).

Comparisons of glucocorticoids

Bone loss induced by glucocorticoids has been assessed in three different populations. A group of 374 subjects (mean age 35 years, 55% women) with mild asthma taking beta-adrenoceptor agonists only, were randomized to inhaled glucocorticoids (budesonide or beclomethasone) or non-glucocorticoid treatment for 2 years (237). Bone mineral density was measured blind after 6, 12, and 24 months. Mean doses of budesonide and beclomethasone were 389 micrograms/day and 499 micrograms/day, respectively. At the end of follow-up, the subjects who had used glucocorticoids had better asthma control. The mean changes in bone density over 2 years in the budesonide, beclomethasone, and control groups were 0.1%, –0.4%, and 0.4% for the lumbar spine and –0.9%, –0.9%, and –0.4% for the neck of the femur. The daily dose of inhaled glucocorticoid was related to the reduction in bone mineral density only at the lumbar spine. Low to moderate doses of inhaled glucocorticoids caused little change in bone mineral density over 2 years and provided better asthma control.

Diagnosis

Several techniques are used to measure bone density. Cortical bone can be assessed in peripheral sites by single-photon absorptiometry and a combination of cortical and trabecular bone in central sites by dual X-ray absorptiometry. Trabecular bone can be assessed by quantitative computer tomography scanning of the lumbar spine. Since single-photon absorptiometry and dual X-ray absorptiometry give a negligible dose of radiation, they are useful for population screening. However, these two techniques are not sensitive enough to show subtle changes in bone density over short periods of time. Quantitative computed tomography gives a significant dose of radiation (of the order of one-tenth of a lateral X-ray of the spine) but can focus on trabecular bone, which has a tenfold greater turnover, compared with cortical bone. Quantitative computed tomography is more sensitive to changing bone density over time.

Other methods, such as the fasting urinary hydroxyproline/creatinine ratio, alkaline phosphatase activity, dual-absorption photometry of the hip, and serum osteocalcin measurements, can also be used, depending on an individual clinic's equipment and experience (SEDA-17, 447).

Management

The prevention and treatment of glucocorticoid bone loss in patients with skin diseases have been reviewed (203). Strategies for the management of this problem have been discussed (SEDA-22, 184) and the clinical implications of trials in the management of glucocorticoid-induced osteoporosis have been reviewed (238). Provided no fractures have occurred, loss of bone mineral density seems to be reversible when treatment is withdrawn (SEDA-18, 389). The management of glucocorticoid-induced osteoporosis has been revised by the UK Consensus Group Meeting on

Osteoporosis (SEDA-20, 376; 219) and by the American College of Rheumatology (SEDA-21, 417; 239).

Guidelines for the prevention and treatment of glucocorticoid-induced osteoporosis have been published (240). Although there are several consensus statements and recommendations for prophylactic measures against glucocorticoid-induced osteoporosis in patients with rheumatoid arthritis, prophylaxis is commonly underprescribed. In two recent studies of 191 and 92 patients taking long-term glucocorticoids, relatively few were taking primary prevention, although some were taking vitamin D and calcium tablets. Around 65–68% of all those who qualified for prophylaxis for glucocorticoid-induced osteoporosis did not receive therapy, and only 9% of those in one study and 21% in the other were taking bisphosphonates (241,242).

Low availability compounds
Bone loss in patients taking oral budesonide has been evaluated in a longitudinal study in which bone mineral density was measured annually for 2 years in 138 patients (67 men, mean age 36 years old) with quiescent Crohn's disease (243). They took budesonide (8.5 mg/day; $n = 48$), prednisone (10.5 mg/day, $n = 45$), or non-steroidal drugs ($n = 45$). After 1 year, the bone mineral density in the lumbar spine fell by 2.36% in those who took budesonide, by 0.61% in those who took prednisone, and by 0.09% in those who took non-steroidal drugs. In the second year, the largest fall occurred in those who took budesonide (1.97%), but the differences between the groups were not significant. After 2 years, bone mineral density in the femoral neck fell by 2.94% with budesonide, 0.36% with prednisone, and 1.05% with the non-steroidal drugs. These results suggest that budesonide can cause bone loss, but the non-randomized design of the study limits conclusions about the comparison between budesonide and prednisone.

Pulse administration
The administration of glucocorticoids in sporadic pulses has been shown not to reduce bone density in patients with multiple sclerosis. In a prospective study, 30 patients were given 1000 mg/day of methylprednisolone intravenously for 3 days, followed by oral prednisone in tapering dosage for 2 weeks. Bone density was determined in the lumbar spine and femoral neck before and at 2, 4, and 6 months after therapy. At baseline, the patients had a reduced bone mass compared with controls; this reduction did not correlate with previous exposure to glucocorticoids. Ambulant patients during follow-up after glucocorticoid pulse therapy had an increase in lumbar bone density (+1.7% at 6 months). Average femoral density did not change; however, in patients who required a walking stick or other aid, femoral density fell (–1.6%), while in those with better ambulation it increased (+2.9%). These results suggest that inactivity is the main factor causing bone loss in patients treated with sporadic pulses of glucocorticoids (SEDA-21, 417; 244).

Calcium and vitamin D
Infusion of ionic calcium has sometimes been used to counteract the malabsorption of calcium in patients taking long-term glucocorticoids, particularly in patients who develop secondary hypoparathyroidism (SEDA-3, 306). There is also evidence that in amenorrheic or menopausal women requiring glucocorticoids, the adverse effects on the vertebrae can be countered by hormonal replacement therapy with estrogen and progesterone (245); progestogens similarly seem to have a promising effect in men, and while they cause a fall in serum testosterone they apparently do not undermine the desired effects of glucocorticoids (SEDA-16, 449).

Vitamin D or calcitriol plus calcium did not prevent the bone loss associated with glucocorticoids in two studies, one in patients with asthma taking glucocorticoid therapy in a double-blind placebo-controlled trial (246), and another in which a group of steroid-treated children with nephrotic syndrome were compared with a similar group without treatment (247). However, calcium and vitamin D3 can prevent bone loss induced by glucocorticoids, and trials have confirmed its efficacy when given for 2 years. Patients taking prednisone and placebo lost bone density in the lumbar spine at a rate of 2% per year. Those taking prednisone and calcium plus vitamin D3 gained bone mineral density at a rate of 0.72% per year. Calcium plus vitamin D3 did not improve bone mineral density in patients who were not taking prednisone (SEDA-21, 417; 248).

In a similar randomized double-blind study, the effects of vitamin D (50 000 units/week) and calcium (1000 mg/day) were evaluated in 62 patients with different rheumatic diseases treated with prednisone (10–100 mg/day) (SEDA-21, 418; 249). The primary outcome was bone mineral density in the lumbar spine at 36 months. Patients taking placebo had reductions of 4.1, 3.8, and 1.5% at 12, 24, and 36 months respectively. Patients taking calcium and vitamin D had reductions of 2.6, 3.7, and 2.2% respectively. The results suggested that preventive therapy could be beneficial early in the prevention of glucocorticoid-induced bone loss, but there was no evidence of long-term beneficial effects. In kidney transplant patients, the preventive administration of 25-hydroxycolecalciferol and calcium reduced bone loss in the spine and femoral neck and the number of new vertebral crush fractures (SEDA-21, 418) (250). In children with rheumatic diseases taking glucocorticoids, calcium and vitamin D supplementation improved spinal bone density, although osteocalcin concentrations remained low (SEDA-19, 378; 251).

A meta-analysis has shown that alfacalcidol and calcitriol prevent bone loss induced by glucocorticoid (effect size = 0.43) but not fractures (252).

Alfacalcidol and vitamin D3 have been compared in patients with established glucocorticoid-induced osteoporosis with or without vertebral fractures (253). Patients taking long-term glucocorticoids were included as matched pairs to receive randomly either alfacalcidol 1 microgram/day plus calcium 500 mg/day (n = 103) or vitamin D3 1000 IU/day plus calcium 500 mg/day (n = 101). The two groups were well matched in terms of mean age, sex ratio, mean height and weight, daily dosage and duration of glucocorticoid therapy, and the percentages of the three underlying diseases (chronic obstructive pulmonary disease, rheumatoid arthritis, and polymyalgia rheumatica). The baseline mean bone mineral density values (expressed as T scores, the number of standard deviations from the mean of the healthy population) at the lumbar spine were –3.26 (alfacalcidol) and –3.25 (vitamin D_3) and at the femoral neck –2.81 and –2.84 respectively. The prevalence rates of vertebral and non-vertebral fractures did not differ. During the 3-year study, the median percentage bone mineral density increased at the lumbar spine by 2.4% with alfacalcidol and decreased by 0.8% with vitamin D_3. There also was a significantly larger median increase at the femoral neck with alfacalcidol (1.2%) than with vitamin D_3 (0.8%). The 3-year rates of patients with at least one new vertebral fracture were 9.7% with alfacalcidol and 25% with vitamin D_3 (RR = 0.61; 95% CI = 0.24, 0.81). The 3-year rates of patients with at least one new non-vertebral fracture were 15% with alfacalcidol and 25% with vitamin D_3 (RR = 0.41; 95% CI = 0.06, 0.68). The 3-year rates of patients with at least one new fracture of any kind were 19% with alfacalcidol and 41% with vitamin D3 (RR = 0.52; 95% CI = 0.25, 0.71). Those who took alfacalcidol had a substantially larger reduction in back pain than those who took vitamin D_3. Generally, adverse effects in both groups were mild, and only three patients taking alfacalcidol and two taking vitamin D_3 had moderate hypercalcemia. The authors concluded that alfacalcidol plus calcium is greatly superior to vitamin D_3 plus calcium in the treatment of established glucocorticoid-induced osteoporosis.

Calcitonin

Less clear are the results observed after the administration of salmon calcitonin. The usefulness of intranasally administered salmon calcitonin for 2 years has been evaluated in 44 glucocorticoid-dependent asthmatics (SEDA-19, 378; 254). All were taking calcium supplements (1000 mg/day), but one group also took calcitonin (100 IU every other day). Calcitonin increased spinal bone mass during first year of treatment, and maintained bone mass in a steady state during the second year. However, the rate of vertebral fractures was similar in the two groups. The addition of salmon calcitonin did not increase the efficacy of calcium plus vitamin D in the prevention of bone loss in 48 newly diagnosed patients taking glucocorticoids for temporal arteritis and polymyalgia rheumatica in a double-blind, randomized, placebo-controlled trial (SEDA-21, 418; 255). However, salmon calcitonin nasal spray prevented bone loss in the lumbar spine of 31 patients treated with prednisone for polymyalgia rheumatica (SEDA-22, 448; 256). They were randomized to salmon calcitonin nasal spray (200 IU/day) or matched placebo for 1 year. Both groups were treated with calcium supplements if their dietary intake was below 800 mg/day. With calcitonin, the mean bone mineral density in the lumbar spine fell by 1.3% and with placebo by 5% after 1 year. There were no differences in the hip, including the femoral neck and trochanter, or in total body bone density.

Bisphosphonates

There have been several studies of the use of bisphosphonates in preventing glucocorticoid-induced osteoporosis.

Intermittent cyclical etidronate prevented bone loss induced by prednisone in 10 postmenopausal women with temporal arteritis (SEDA-19, 378; 257). Cyclical etidronate (400 mg/day for 2 weeks every 3 months) plus ergocalciferol (0.5 mg/week) was given to 15 postmenopausal women (mean age 63 years) starting glucocorticoid therapy (prednisone 5–20 mg/day). A control group of 11 postmenopausal women (mean age 60 years) with glucocorticoid-induced osteoporosis were treated with calcium supplements only (1 g/day). During the first year, the cyclical regimen significantly increased lumbar and femoral neck bone density compared with placebo (7 and 2.5% for spine and femur respectively). After the second year of cyclical therapy, femoral neck bone density continued to increase while lumbar spine density remained stable (SEDA-20, 376; 258). The effect of intermittent cyclical therapy with etidronate has been investigated in the prevention of bone loss in 117 patients taking high-dose glucocorticoid therapy (a mean daily dose of at least 7.5 mg for 90 days followed by at least 2.5 mg/day for at least 12 months) (259). The patients were randomized to oral etidronate 400 mg/day or placebo for 14 days, followed by 76 days of oral calcium carbonate (500 mg elemental calcium), cycled over 12 months. The mean lumbar spine bone density changed 0.30% and –2.79% in the etidronate and placebo groups respectively. The mean difference between the groups after 1 year (3.0%) was significant. The changes in the femoral neck and greater trochanter were not different between the groups. There was a reduction in pyridinium cross-links, significant from baseline at both 6 and 12 months, in the etidronate group. Osteocalcin increased in the placebo group, and the differences between the groups at 6 and 12 months were –25% and –35% respectively. There was no significant difference between the groups in the number of adverse events, including gastrointestinal disorders. In a placebo-controlled study of the effects of 104 weeks of intermittent cyclical etidronate therapy in 49 patients, the same dose and cycles were used as in the previous study, but calcium (97 mg/day) was given with vitamin D (400 IU) (260). Intermittent cyclical etidronate therapy with vitamin D supplementation significantly increased lumbar spine bone mineral density by 4.5 in patients with osteoporosis resulting from long-term treatment with glucocorticoids.

Intermittent etidronate has been evaluated in a randomized controlled trial in 102 Japanese patients who had taken over 7.5 mg/day of prednisolone for at least 90 days (261). They were randomized to etidronate disodium 200 mg/day for 2 weeks plus calcium lactate 3.0 g/day and alfacalcidol 0.75 micrograms/day) or control (calcium lactate 3.0 g and alfacalcidol 0.75 micrograms/day). Bone mineral density in the lumbar spine and the rate of new vertebral fractures at 48 and 144 weeks were evaluated. With etidronate the mean lumbar spine bone mineral density increased by 3.7% and 4.8% at 48 and 144 weeks respectively. In the control group, the mean lumbar spine bone mineral density increased by 1.5% and 0.4% at 48 and 144 weeks respectively. Of three subgroups, men, premenopausal women, and postmenopausal women, the postmenopausal women had the greatest benefit. Two control patients had new vertebral fractures, whereas there were no fractures with etidronate.

Clodronate 100 mg by intramuscular route once a week was effective in the prevention of glucocorticoid-induced bone loss and fractures in patients with arthritis compared with calcium 1000 mg/day and vitamin D 800 mg/day (262).

Ibandronate can be given intravenously every 3 months. Its efficacy has been demonstrated in men and women with established glucocorticoid-induced osteoporosis in 115 subjects who were randomly assigned to daily calcium supplements (500 mg) plus either ibandronate injections 2 mg every 3 months or daily oral alfacalcidol 1 microgram for up to 3 years (263,264). After 3 years, intermittent intravenous ibandronate produced significantly greater increases than daily oral alfacalcidol in mean bone mineral density in the lumbar spine (13% versus 2.6%), and femoral neck (5.2% versus 1.9%). However, there were no differences between the groups with respect to fractures.

Contradictory results have been published about the prophylactic use of two other bisphosphonates in patients treated with glucocorticoids. There were no bone losses after therapy, and no differences in bone density or biochemical bone markers between placebo and clodronate (SEDA-22, 447; 265).

Pamidronate disodium has been compared with calcium supplementation in an open trial of primary prevention of glucocorticoid-induced osteoporosis in 27 patients with different rheumatic conditions, randomly assigned to pamidronate (90 mg intravenously every 3 months) plus calcium (800 mg calcium carbonate) or calcium only for 1 year (SEDA-22, 448; 266). The glucocorticoids were given in a starting dosage of 10–80 mg/day. With pamidronate there was a significant increase in bone density (3.6% lumbar, 2.2% femoral neck), but there was a significant reduction with calcium (–5.3% in both spine and femoral neck).

The effects of risedronate on bone density and vertebral fracture have been studied in 518 patients (mean age 59 years, 40% with rheumatoid arthritis, 56% men, 64% of the women postmenopausal) taking moderate to high doses of oral glucocorticoids (equivalent to prednisone 7.5 mg/day or more) (267). The patients were randomized double-blind to placebo, or risedronate 2.5 or 5 mg/day for 1 year. All took elemental calcium 1000 mg/day and vitamin D 400 IU/day. The mean density of the lumbar spine fell by 1% in the placebo group and increased by 1.3% and 1.9% with risedronate 2.5 and 5 mg respectively. There was a significant reduction of 70% in the risk of vertebral fracture with risedronate 5 mg compared with placebo. There were similar incidences of adverse effects in all the groups.

Similar results have been reported in a clinical trial in 290 patients (38% men, 55% of the women postmenopausal) taking high-dose glucocorticoid therapy (prednisone over 7.5 mg/day or equivalent) (268). The subjects were randomized to receive placebo or risedronate 2.5 or 5 mg/day for 1 year. All took elemental calcium 1000 mg/day and vitamin D 400 IU/day. Risedronate 5 mg increased bone mineral density at 1 year by a mean of 2.9% in the lumbar spine, 1.8% in the femoral neck, and 2.4% in the trochanter. The values for placebo were 0.4%, –0.3%, and 1.0% respectively. The results for risedronate 2.5 mg were positive but not significant compared with placebo. The incidence of spinal fractures was reduced by 70% in the combined risedronate treatment groups compared with placebo. Risedronate and placebo caused similar adverse effects.

In a 1-year extension of a previous double-blind, randomized, placebo-controlled study, two doses of alendronate (5 and 10 mg/day) were compared in 66 men and 142 women taking glucocorticoids (at least 7.5 mg/day of prednisone or equivalent) (269). The extension was also double-blind, but those who had taken alendronate 2.5 mg/day in the previous study were given 10 mg/day. All the patients took supplementary calcium and vitamin D. The primary end-point was the mean percentage change in lumbar spine bone mineral density from baseline to 2 years. In those who took alendronate 5, 10, and 2.5/10 mg/day, bone mineral density increased significantly by 2.8, 3.9, and 3.7% respectively, and fell by – 0.8% with placebo. There were significantly fewer patients with new vertebral fractures in the alendronate group compared with placebo (0.7 versus 6.8%). Adverse events were similar across the groups.

Calcitriol was less effective than alendronate in a randomized, double-blind, placebo-controlled trial that included patients with a rheumatic disease who took glucocorticoids in a daily dose that was equivalent to at least 7.5 mg of prednisone (mean dose equivalent 23 mg) (270). The 201 patients (mean age 61 years, 66% women) were randomized to alendronate (10 mg/day) or alfacalcidol (1 micrograms/day) for 18 months. The bone mineral density of the lumbar spine increased by 2.1% in the alendronate group (95 CI = 1.1, 3.1) and fell by 1.9% in the alfacalcidol group (95 CI = –3.1, –0.7). Three patients in the alendronate group had a new vertebral deformity, compared with eight patients in the alfacalcidol group (of whom three had symptomatic vertebral fractures).

No data are available about the effects on bone mineral density of withdrawing bisphosphonates. Of 183 patients who participated in a randomized, placebo-controlled trial of the efficacy of alendronate 5 and 10 mg/day on the prevention and treatment of glucocorticoid-induced osteoporosis during 1 year 90 participated in a follow-up study for 3.3-4.6 years (271). In the subgroup that continued to take a glucocorticoid (more than 6 mg/day of prednisone or equivalent for more than 1 year) and took alendronate for less than 90 days (n = 11), there was bone loss after the end of the trial (–5.1% at the lumbar spine to –9.2% at the femoral neck). In the subgroup that continued to take glucocorticoids and alendronate for more than 300 days (n = 31), there was a small gain in the lumbar spine (+0.1%) and no significant loss in the femoral neck (−0.1%). Although the study had limitations, particularly loss to follow-up of a considerable number of patients, the results suggested that sustained treatment with alendronate maintains bone mineral density, and that patients who discontinue alendronate and continue to take glucocorticoids lose bone mass in the femoral neck and lumbar spine.

Parathyroid hormone

Parathyroid hormone (parathormone) is an anabolic osteotrophic agent. Randomized controlled trials have shown the efficacy of human parathormone, hPTH (1-34), in improving bone mass and reducing the risk of fractures in postmenopausal osteoporosis. In 51 women who had been postmenopausal for at least 3 years and who had taken both glucocorticoids (mean dose of prednisone 5-20 mg/day or equivalent for at least 1 year) and hormone replacement therapy (HRT; Premarin 0.625 mg/day or equivalent) were randomized to either HRT + parathormone 40 micrograms/day for 1 year or HRT only (272). Vertebral cross-sectional area increased by 4.8%, and 1 year after treatment was withdrawn it was still 2.6% higher than at baseline. In the control group there was no change. In addition, estimated vertebral compressive strength increased by more than 200% over baseline with parathormone and there was no change in the control group.

Fluoride

Fluoride is a potent stimulator of trabecular bone formation. Sodium monofluorophosphate was given to 48 patients with osteoporosis due to glucocorticoids (more than 10 mg of prednisone equivalents/day). Patients were randomly allocated to 1 g of calcium carbonate (control) or 200 mg of sodium monofluorophosphate plus 1 g of calcium carbonate for 18 months. At the end of the study lumbar spine bone density had increased by 7.8% in the fluoride group versus 3.3% in the controls. There were no changes in femoral neck density (SEDA-20, 376; 273).

Growth hormone

Growth hormone is a potent anabolic agent that stimulates protein synthesis, cell growth, and osteoblast activity. Recombinant human growth hormone has been used in patients taking long-term glucocorticoid treatment with suppressed endogenous growth hormone responses to GH-releasing hormone (SEDA-20, 376; 274). A single daily dose of 0.1 IU/kg of human growth hormone was given subcutaneously to nine nonobese patients. There was a significant increase in nitrogen balance, osteocalcin, carboxy-terminal propeptide of type I procollagen, and carboxy-terminal telopeptide of type I collagen. Growth hormone also lowered total high density lipoprotein, and low density lipoprotein cholesterol. These preliminary data suggest that growth hormone could ameliorate some adverse effects induced by long-term glucocorticoids.

Others

Other agents are effective in special populations. Vitamin K prevented bone loss in 20 patients with chronic glomerulonephritis treated with prednisolone (275) and ciclosporin 4.8 mg/kg/day prevented glucocorticoid-induced osteopenia in 52 patients taking prednisone 10 mg/day after kidney transplantation (276).

Avascular necrosis

Avascular aseptic necrosis of bone (SEDA-19, 377; 277,278) is a well-recognized adverse effect related to high-dose glucocorticoid therapy (equivalent to more than 4000 mg of prednisone) for extended periods (3 months or longer) but can occur after short-term glucocorticoid therapy. It occurs in a wide range of patients with many different disorders and is particularly likely to involve the femoral and humeral heads. The first lesions are often localized small osteolytic areas in the subchondral bone, where they can be diagnosed early by X-radiography. Magnetic resonance imaging (MRI) is one of the more sensitive techniques to diagnose avascular necrosis of the femoral head. The development and changes in avascular necrosis of the femoral head had been studied by MRI in patients with systemic lupus erythematosus treated with long-term prednisolone administration (SEDA-19, 377; SEDA-19, 193). MRI abnormalities could be detected soon after the start of glucocorticoid therapy or were associated with increased dosages for treating exacerbation of the disease. Normal hips are rarely involved in avascular osteonecrosis. However, aseptic osteonecrosis of the femoral head is often seen in young patients; the lunate, capitate, and patella are their locations. Usually only one joint is involved, although lesions can be multiple. Whether intra-articular injections of glucocorticoids can cause necrosis of bone is still uncertain.

Femoral head necrosis in kidney transplant recipients who receive postoperative immunosuppression with prednisone can be prevented, at least to some extent, by minimizing the dosage of prednisone whenever feasible (279). Of 750 patients (445 men and 305 women) who had undergone kidney transplantation in 1968–95, 374 had received an average of 12.5 g of prednisone during the first year after surgery (high-dose prednisone group) and 276 had received an average of 6.5 g during this time (low-dose prednisone group) plus ciclosporin. Femoral head necrosis occurred in 42/374 patients (11%) in the high-dose prednisone group, an average of 26 months after transplantation. In contrast, femoral head necrosis occurred in only 19/376 patients (5.1%) in the low-dose group an average of 21 months after transplantation. The difference between the high- and low-dose groups was highly significant.

The risk of avascular necrosis has been assessed in a nested case-control study using computer records (280). There were 31 cases during 720 000 person-years Avascular necrosis was strongly associated with glucocorticoid exposure (RR = 16). When total prednisone exposure over 35 months was stratified into three levels (under 440 mg, 440–1290 mg, and over 1290 mg), there was no excess risk for cumulative doses of up to 440 mg (RR = 0; 95% CI = 0, 5). The relative risk was increased for doses between 440 and 1290 mg (RR = 6; CI = 1, 43) and indeterminately increased at doses over 1290 mg (CI = 26, infinity).

In 15 men with osteonecrosis of the femoral head after short-term therapy the mean duration of therapy was 21 (range 7–39) days and the mean dose in milligram equivalents of prednisone was 850 (range 290–3300) mg (281). The time from administration of glucocorticoids to hip pain was 17 (range 6–33) months. A new case of bilateral avascular necrosis of the femoral heads after high-dose short-term dexamethasone therapy as an antiemetic in cancer chemotherapy has been reported (282).

Avascular necrosis of the bilateral femoral head resulting from long-term steroid administration for radiation pneumonitis has been reported (283).

- A 50-year-old postmenopausal woman with breast cancer and radiation pneumonitis was given oral glucocorticoids followed by steroid pulse administration and more oral therapy. She improved immediately, but the radiation pneumonitis relapsed when the steroid medication was stopped. The period of medication was 423 days and the cumulative dose of steroids was 7365 mg before complete resolution occurred. In the 19 months after therapy she developed bilateral avascular necrosis of the femoral heads.

Patients treated with long-term or high-dose glucocorticoids have been suggested to be at great risk of avascular necrosis, but this hypothesis is controversial. The probability of avascular necrosis may be very small, but it should be considered as one of the complications of glucocorticoids.

Myopathy

The presence of physiological amounts of glucocorticoids is necessary for the normal functioning of muscle. Excessive glucocorticoid concentrations, in contrast, result in protein catabolism and a reduced rate of muscle protein synthesis (284), and hence in muscle atrophy and fibrosis. The molecular and biochemical basis of myopathy has been widely studied, and the mechanism has been attributed to impairment of glycogen synthesis. Muscle glycogen synthase protein content and activity was measured in samples from 14 patients taking glucocorticoids after kidney transplantation and from 20 healthy subjects (SEDA-21, 418; 285). The patients had impaired activation of glycogen synthase and reduced enzyme activity. Muscular weakness can of course also result from glucocorticoid-induced hypokalemia. In spontaneous Cushing's syndrome, there is muscle involvement in some 50% of cases (286).

Among reports of myopathy in patients taking glucocorticoids, involvement of the respiratory muscles is often mentioned (287,288), possibly because this is particularly likely to have clinical consequences. Patients on mechanically assisted ventilation may be particularly at risk of myopathy (SEDA-18, 390). However, any muscle can be affected; one often sees weakness and atrophy of the hip muscles and (in about half the cases) the shoulder muscles and the proximal muscles of the limbs.

The myopathy usually develops gradually, without pain, and symmetrically. However, a single epidural injection of a glucocorticoid for lumbar radicular pain has caused Cushing's syndrome and myopathy (SEDA-20, 370; 118).

There is a suggestion that the incidence of myopathy is greatest during treatment with compounds that are fluorinated at the 9-alpha position, such as triamcinolone, but this may simply reflect its general potency. In children, the risk of effects on muscles is relatively high.

Biopsy is not justified as a routine, but it is useful as a diagnostic tool in distinguishing suspected corticoid myopathy from diseases of the muscles or vascular system with inflammation that may have been the indication for giving glucocorticoids in the first place; electromyographic measurements cannot confirm the diagnosis.

After termination of treatment the myopathy normally improves over a period of several months.

Damage to tendons and fascia

Tendons can be injured by glucocorticoids and can rupture (289). Ten cases of Achilles tendon rupture were seen in a single clinic over a 10-year period (SEDA-17, 448). The risk seems to be greater if local (for example intra-articular) injections are used.

Rupture of the plantar fascia induced by glucocorticoids has usually been reported in athletes. However, a case of spontaneous degenerative rupture has been reported in a 72-year-old man who had received four glucocorticoid injections over 1 year for plantar fasciitis (SEDA-21, 418; 290).

- A 69-year-old man with newly diagnosed giant cell arteritis was given prednisone 30 mg bd, and 2 weeks later developed severe pain along his Achilles tendons bilaterally; 1 week later the left tendon ruptured (291). Despite immobilization his pain worsened. The prednisone was gradually tapered and the symptoms abated, with complete recovery.

In the previous literature this adverse reaction was described in patients taking glucocorticoids for from 4 months to several years.

Joints

Among the adverse effects of pulse glucocorticoid therapy, joint manifestations are rare. A woman with systemic lupus erythematosus and nephritis developed transient bilateral knee effusions during pulse therapy with high doses of glucocorticoids (292).

- A 62-year old woman was admitted to hospital with lupus nephritis. A kidney biopsy showed a mesangio-proliferative glomerulonephritis (WHO class III). After 4 months of inadequate response to traditional treatment, she started monthly pulse glucocorticoid therapy (methylprednisolone 1 g for 3 days) before immunosuppressive drugs. After 2 days of pulse glucocorticoid therapy she complained of pain and flexion discomfort in both knees, which were swollen. At arthrocentesis synovial fluid was aspirated (5 ml from the right knee and 6 ml from the left). The fluid was colorless, with a high viscosity and excellent mucin clot formation.

There was only 1 mononuclear cell/mm^3 in the right knee synovial fluid and no cells in the left. There were no crystals. Inflammatory laboratory measurements carried out simultaneously were unchanged. X-rays of the affected joints were normal. The effusion resolved with arthrocentesis and did not recur.

The author proposed that raised arterial pressure, which is an adverse effect of high dose glucocorticoid treatment, and low oncotic pressure due to a low protein plasma concentration in a patient with nephrotic syndrome, could have increased trans-synovial fluid flow at a lower arterial pressure than normal.

Growth in children
The possibility that inhaled glucocorticoids may impair growth in children is of concern, but difficult to assess, as severe chronic asthma can impair growth. If not adequately controlled, asthma modifies the prepubertal growth spurt, the pubertal growth spurt, and the catch-up phase, which allows the child to attain adult height. There is a wide range of individual responses and some children have adverse effects with relatively small doses of glucocorticoids. It is still not clear whether this is a transient phenomenon, causing a slowing of growth and maturational delay with no adverse effect on adult height, or whether growth can be permanently impaired. Ideally studies should establish the effect of asthma treatments on final adult height (compared with predicted values for sex and parental height). Such studies pose considerable logistic problems. For this reason most studies have measured growth over shorter time spans. Outcome measures have been expressed as the height velocity or growth rate, that is changes in height over a defined time. Alternatively height is measured and compared with that of age- and sex-matched controls. Such relatively short-term studies do not necessarily predict the effects of treatment on eventual adult height.

The growth-inhibiting effects of glucocorticoids in children are related not only to inhibition of growth hormone secretion, but also to the sensitivity of the peripheral tissues to the effects of growth hormone. By means of overnight profile analysis it was shown that glucocorticoid treatment reduces the amplitude but not the number of pulses of the physiological growth hormone secretion (SEDA-14, 335; 293).

Effects on growth occur early in treatment: with sensitive testing methods they can be detected in growing children within a few weeks of starting therapy. The effects can be produced by any route of administration, including even inhalation therapy (at least with dexamethasone) (SEDA-18, 391). Comparisons of attained heights with expected heights in children who have used inhaled or oral glucocorticoids have been summarized in a meta-analysis (SEDA-19, 375; 294). There was a significant but small tendency for glucocorticoid therapy in general to be associated with reduced final height. However, this effect varied according to the route of administration. As expected, there was significant impairment of growth with prednisone and other oral glucocorticoids. On the other hand, inhaled

beclomethasone dipropionate was associated with normal stature, even when it was used in higher dosages, for longer durations, or in patients with more severe asthma. In another study in 94 children aged 7–9 years, beclomethasone in a dosage taken by many children with mild asthma (400 micrograms/day) significantly reduced growth (SEDA-20, 369; 295). In children with growth suppression during therapy with inhaled beclomethasone or budesonide (200–400 micrograms/day) there was catch-up growth when they switched to equipotent dosages of inhaled fluticasone (100–200 micrograms/day) (SEDA-21, 414; 296). However, in six children with severe asthma, treatment with inhaled high-dosage fluticasone 1000 micrograms/day was associated with growth retardation and adrenal insufficiency (SEDA-21, 414; 297). In one child, growth rate and adrenal function normalized 9 months after the fluticasone dosage was reduced to 500 micrograms/day.

It is generally agreed that the use of single doses of prednisone on alternate mornings minimizes growth retardation but does not avoid it; in children it has been shown that biochemical markers of growth are lower in patients receiving daily glucocorticoid therapy than in patients treated with an alternate-day regimen or not receiving glucocorticoids (SED-12, 988; 298).

It has long been thought by some physicians that the impairment of growth caused by glucocorticoids can be lessened by switching to corticotropin, but this is uncertain. Compensatory treatment with anabolic hormones is definitely not recommended today, since they do not stimulate growth but actually impede it by promoting closure of the epiphyses. Recombinant growth hormone (rGH) treatment of poorly growing children with glucocorticoid-dependent renal disease has often been observed to improve linear growth. However, the dosage of prednisone has been reported to be a critical factor in determining the efficacy of rGH therapy in glucocorticoid-dependent children (SEDA-19, 375; 299). When the dose of prednisone was greater than 0.35 mg/kg/day, rGH did not increase the linear growth rate. At lower doses, the response was inversely related to the amount of prednisone.

Provided glucocorticoid treatment is terminated before the end of puberty, total growth may catch up with the physiological norm (SEDA-17, 448). Concern has been expressed that fear of growth retardation can result in unjustifiable denial of glucocorticoid therapy. It does, however, seem highly advisable to keep doses as low as possible and to switch to a therapeutic regimen that excludes glucocorticoids as children approach the expected onset of puberty (SEDA-14, 335).

Serum osteocalcin determinations appear to be a helpful marker to evaluate the effects of glucocorticoids on growth in children.

One unanswered question is whether the growth suppression that occurs in children during glucocorticoid treatment persists after treatment is withdrawn and affects final adult height. In an attempt to answer this question, growth 6–7 years after withdrawal of alternate-day prednisone has been evaluated in children (aged 6–14 years) with cystic fibrosis who had participated in a multicenter trial from 1986 to 1991 (300). Of 224 children, 161 had been randomized to prednisone (1 or 2 mg/kg) and 73 to placebo. At the time of the study, 68% were aged 18 years or more. Height fell during prednisone therapy, but catch-up growth began 2 years after withdrawal. However, the heights of the boys treated with prednisone remained significantly lower by 4 cm than those who took placebo. In contrast, in the girls there were no differences in height at 2–3 years after prednisone withdrawal.

In a retrospective study of 13 infants with hemangiomas treated with systemic glucocorticoids there was slowed linear growth but "catch-up" growth after the end of treatment (301). Glucocorticoids did not affect bone mineralization adversely. Only one of 10 infants who had been treated with dexamethasone had clear evidence of adrenal insufficiency after therapy was stopped.

Reproductive system

Reduced sperm count and motility and inhibition of the secretory function of the testicles during glucocorticoid treatment have been reported and discussed in relation to the suppression of adrenal androgen production. These reports still await confirmation.

Since amenorrhea is a symptom of Cushing's syndrome, disorders of menstruation are common in fertile women taking higher doses of glucocorticoids (SEDA-3, 305). On the other hand, plasma cortisol concentrations in normally menstruating women have marked circadian variation, the extent of which can reach 200% or more (302), with the peak of the cortisol plasma concentrations at mid-cycle and near its end. Inhibition of ovulation by triamcinolone 25 mg has been reported when the drug is given on day 1 or 2 of the cycle. How glucocorticoids interfere with the hormonal control of the menstrual cycle is still unknown (303).

Women should be warned about the possibility of menstrual disorders after local triamcinolone injections (304). When premenopausal women received their first injection of triamcinolone intra-articularly ($n = 46$), injected into soft tissue ($n = 24$), or epidurally ($n = 7$) they were specifically asked to report flushing or menstrual irregularities during a mean follow-up period of 6 weeks. Of the 77 women in the study, 39 reported menstrual disorders. The onset of menstruation was later than expected in ten women and earlier in 16 women. There was reduced loss of blood and/or a shorter duration of menstruation in four women and increased loss of blood and/or a longer duration of menstruation in 18. Also, 22 women had flushing. Menstrual disorders occurred significantly less often in women who were taking oral contraceptives.

Immunologic

Since the glucocorticoids have immunosuppressive and anti-inflammatory properties, one would not expect allergic reactions to be a problem, except when excipients act as allergens. Nevertheless, allergic reactions to glucocorticoids themselves have been reported (SEDA-21, 419) (305). Immunological reactions to glucocorticoids have been reviewed (306). Reactions can be of types I, III, or

IV. Immediate reactions usually occur in patients with asthma and in those who have to use glucocorticoids repeatedly. Other susceptibility factors include female sex and hypersensitivity to acetylsalicylic acid. Often excipients are implicated (succinates, sulfites, and carboxymethylcellulose). Cross-reactivity does not necessarily occur; patients with immediate reactions to hydrocortisone and methylprednisolone can often tolerate prednisone and prednisolone and second-generation compounds, such as dexamethasone and betamethasone. Urticaria after glucocorticoid treatment has been explained as a reaction of the mesenchyme. Also, an increase in eosinophilic leukocytes (which normally are diminished by glucocorticoids) has been reported as a first reaction to treatment with glucocorticoids.

Class I reactions

To date, there have been about 100 published reports of immediate hypersensitivity reactions after oral and parenteral administration of glucocorticoids. Although there is evidence that glucocorticoids themselves can cause these reactions, there is debate about the mechanism. Anaphylactic shock has been described after intranasal hydrocortisone acetate, intramuscular methylprednisolone (SEDA-21, 419; 307), intravenous methylprednisolone (SEDA-22, 448; 308), intramuscular dexamethasone (SEDA-22, 448; 309), and intra-articular methylprednisolone (SEDA-22, 449; 310). A life-threatening anaphylactic-like reaction to intravenous hydrocortisone has been described in patients with asthma (311). Acute laryngeal obstruction has been described for the first time after the intravenous administration of hydrocortisone (SEDA-22, 449; 312). There is some reason to believe that sodium succinate esters are more likely to cause hypersensitivity reactions (SEDA-17, 449), but unconjugated glucocorticoids can definitely produce allergy in some cases (SEDA-16, 452).

- A 64-year-old woman with a history of bronchial asthma developed increasing shortness of breath after an upper respiratory tract infection (313). Her medication included inhaled salbutamol as necessary, theophylline 300 mg bd, and aspirin 325 mg/day. She was given nebulized salbutamol and ipratropium and hydrocortisone 200 mg intravenously. Within 30 minutes, she developed a generalized rash, fever (38.3°C), and respiratory distress. She was promptly intubated and mechanical ventilation was started. No further doses of glucocorticoid were given. Skin testing with various parenteral formulations of glucocorticoids produced a 5 mm wheal at the site of hydrocortisone and methylprednisolone injections. She was subsequently given a challenge dose of triamcinolone using a metered-dose inhaler with no reaction, and was therefore continued on this medication.
- An anaphylactoid reaction (angioedema, generalized urticaria, worsening bronchospasm, and marked hypotension) occurred in a 35-year-old man with multiple sclerosis who became allergic to methylprednisolone (dose not stated) after starting treatment with interferon beta-1b (314). He had previously been treated

with different courses of methylprednisolone. Clinicians should be aware that the complexity of the effects of interferon beta-1b on the immune system can lead to unexpected outcomes. It is uncertain whether the sequence of events here was due to an effect of interferon beta-1b or to coincidence.

- A 17-year-old boy, with an 11-year history of asthma, had anaphylaxis with respiratory distress shortly after he received intravenous methylprednisolone for an exacerbation of asthma while taking a tapering course of oral prednisone 15 mg/day (315). He had been glucocorticoid-dependent for at least 1 year. He reported having received intravenous glucocorticoids previously. He was treated with inhaled salbutamol and then intravenous methylprednisolone 125 mg over 15–30 seconds, and 3–4 minutes later became flushed and dyspneic, and developed diffuse urticarial lesions on his trunk and face and an undetectable blood pressure. He was treated with adrenaline, but required intubation. Sinus bradycardia developed and then asystole. He was successfully resuscitated and a 10–15 seconds period of generalized tonic-clonic activity was treated with diazepam. He remained unresponsive to stimulation for 30 minutes. However, he awoke 1 hour after his respiratory arrest and was extubated and discharged the following day taking a tapering dosage of prednisone.

- An anaphylactoid reaction occurred in a 68-year-old woman after treatment with intravenous methylprednisolone for asthma. She had developed urticaria with methylprednisolone 1 year earlier, but the reaction had been thought to be related to the solvent in the formulation (316).

- Forty minutes after a first dose of prednisone 25 mg, a 17-year-old girl with a history of aspirin intolerance had generalized flushing, hives, hypogastric pain, and abdominal cramps, followed by vomiting and diarrhea (317). She lost consciousness and developed arterial hypotension. She responded to intravenous diphenhydramine and hydrocortisone. Intradermal skin tests were positive for prednisone and negative for methylprednisolone and hydrocortisone. An oral challenge test with prednisone led to flushing, nausea, dizziness, tachycardia, and hypotension and responded to intravenous diphenhydramine and hydrocortisone. Challenge tests with intravenous methylprednisolone and hydrocortisone were negative.

- A 75-year-old man developed triamcinolone-induced anaphylaxis and dose-related positive prick skin tests to triamcinolone, suggesting that an IgE-mediated hypersensitivity mechanism may have played a part (318).

- A 30-year-old man with recurrent atopic eczema of the head and neck, generalized xerosis, keratosis pilaris of the arms, and a history of dyshidrosis was initially treated with prednisolone-21-acetate ointment (319). His skin eruption became worse. He was given oral prednisolone 25 mg, and 5 hours after the first dose developed intense generalized pruritus with erythema and swelling of the face. After 24 hours there was generalized erythema with disseminated partly follicular papules. There was an eosinophilia (1.1×10^9/l). Total IgE was not raised.

Patch tests showed delayed reactions to hydrocortisone 1%, prednisolone 1%, prednisolone-21-acetate ointment, and prednisolone 2.5%. Prick and intradermal tests with methylprednisolone succinate, hydrocortisone succinate, betamethasone, and triamcinolone acetonide in concentrations up to 1 : 10 were negative at 15 minutes. However, 4 hours after intradermal testing, generalized pruritus developed and 24 hours later there was a disseminated partly follicular eczematous reaction with involvement of the flexural areas. Biopsy of the eruptions caused by prednisolone and of the positive skin reaction to methylprednisolone succinate showed superficial dermatitis with a perivascular infiltration consisting predominantly of CD4+ cells and some eosinophils. Immunofluorescence showed increased expression of HLA-DR molecules on the CD4+ and CD8+ cells. During the exanthema caused by prednisolone, interleukin-5 (14 pg/ml), interleukin-6 (38 pg/ml), and interleukin-10 (26 pg/ml) were detected in the blood; 2 months after recovery these cytokines were not detectable.

The authors of the last report commented that generalized delayed type hypersensitivity to systemic administration of a glucocorticoid is rare. Despite the potent immunosuppressive effect of glucocorticoids on immunocompetent cells, the clinical features, the skin biopsy specimen, and the positive delayed skin test reactions strongly suggested an immunological mechanism: T cells were clearly involved and the high concentrations of interleukins 5, 6, and 10 were consistent with a T helper type 2 reaction. The raised concentrations of interleukin-5 were probably responsible for the blood and tissue eosinophilia.

Skin prick tests and intradermal tests to hydrocortisone and methylprednisolone, intradermal tests to betamethasone and dexamethasone, and oral challenge tests to betamethasone and deflazacort were performed in 10 patients with adverse reactions to systemic hemisuccinate esters of hydrocortisone and methylprednisolone (320). The skin prick tests and intradermal tests results suggested the possibility of an IgE-mediated mechanism for allergic reactions to hydrocortisone and methylprednisolone. The authors hypothesized that this mechanism is probably due, at least in part, to a glucocorticoid-glyoxal compound, a degradation product of cortisol, which in aqueous solution may be responsible for presenting steroid carbon rings to the immune system. They suggested that betamethasone and deflazacort could be reserved for emergency use in patients with adverse reactions to other glucocorticoids. Budesonide has been marketed in oral form for intestinal inflammatory disease. An non-IgE-mediated anaphylactic reaction has been associated with oral budesonide (321).

- A 32-year-old woman with Crohn's disease, who had taken prednisone 20 mg/day and azathioprine 150 mg/day, switched to budesonide 9 mg/day because of weight gain, and 5 minutes after the first capsule her tongue and throat swelled, accompanied by wheeziness and diarrhea. She was given clemastine and recovered after 4 ays. Intracutaneous tests with diluted budesonide suggested a non-IgE-mediated reaction. She had a previous history of a similar reaction to mesalazine.

One year later her tongue and throat swelled after intravenous dexamethasone.

Urticaria with angioedema has been described in a patient taking deflazacort (322).

- A 64-year-old woman with allergic alveolitis caused by parakeet feathers improved with intravenous methylprednisolone, and was given oral deflazacort 60 mg/day, to be reduced progressively. After 30 days she developed generalized itchy blotches and lip edema. At that time she was mistakenly taking deflazacort in a dose of 120 mg/day. She was given an antihistamine, without any improvement. Deflazacort was then replaced by prednisolone and her symptoms disappeared immediately. Skin tests (a prick test and an epicutaneous test) were positive with deflazacort. Oral provocation with deflazacort 30 mg was positive, with the immediate appearance of the same symptoms as in the initial episode.

Class III reactions

Allergy to topical glucocorticoids in inflammatory bowel disease has been reported (323).

- A 57-year old Caucasian man with inflammatory bowel disease was given prednisolone metasulfobenzoate sodium enemas twice daily and oral mesalazine 800 mg tds for about 5 months, without improvement. He stopped using the prednisolone enemas but continued to take mesalazine. Within 48 hours of stopping prednisolone his symptoms resolved completely. The theoretical possibility of contact allergy was entertained. Patch tests with a standard battery of contact allergens, including tixocortol pivalate and budesonide, were ++ positive with budesonide. At follow up 3 months later he was symptom free.

The authors advised that allergy to topical glucocorticoids should be considered in patients using rectal steroids whose condition unexpectedly fails to improve or in whom there is unexpected deterioration.

Vasculitis

Exacerbation of giant cell arteritis, with clinical signs of an evolving vertebrobasilar stroke, has been attributed to prednisolone (324).

- A 64-year-old man with giant cell arteritis was given prednisolone 60 mg/day. Within 5 days he developed double vision and agitation and became drowsy and confused. A cranial MRI scan showed recent cerebral lesions and a Doppler scan showed high-resistant blood flow in both vertebral arteries. He had an episode of complete loss of vision and was given dexamethasone and intravenous heparin followed by warfarin. He gradually improved over the next few weeks but was left with cognitive and memory deficits.

Immunosuppression

Glucocorticoids inhibit the formation of antibodies. Of 111 consecutive heart transplant recipients taking oral prednisone (mean 13.8 months), 57% developed hypogammaglobulinemia (IgG below 7 g/l) (325). Those with severe hypogammaglobulinemia (IgG below 3.5 g/l) were at increased risk of opportunistic infections compared with those with IgG concentrations over 3.5 g/l (55 versus 5%, OR = 23). Parenteral glucocorticoid pulse therapy was associated with a significantly increased risk of severe hypogammaglobulinemia (OR = 15).

With long-term treatment, IgG subclass deficiencies can become marked (326). There is suppression of the antigen–antibody reaction, and since this reaction itself normally results in liberation of kinins, the latter is also suppressed. Failure of kinin liberation leads in turn to inhibition of invasion of sensitized leukocytes and reduced production and maturation of phagocytes. Undoubtedly, it is true that using minimal effective doses will avoid the most serious consequences, but the problem cannot be fully circumvented, since the anti-inflammatory effects themselves involve some inhibition of the migration of leukocytes and phagocytosis.

Dexamethasone significantly affected the antibody response of preterm infants with chronic lung disease to immunization against *Haemophilus influenzae* (327). Serum samples were obtained before and after immunization from an unselected cohort of 59 preterm infants (30 boys; gestational age 175–208 days). *Haemophilus influenzae* antibodies were measured using ELISA. IgG antibody concentrations in 16 infants who received no dexamethasone were 0.16 and 4.63 microgram/ml before and after immunization respectively. The corresponding values for those who received dexamethasone were 0.10 and 0.51 microgram/ml.

Infection risk

The consequence of this interference with immune responses can be multiplication of bacteria and an increased risk of bacterial intoxication when infection does occur; hence, the frequency and severity of clinical infections tend to increase during glucocorticoid therapy. Aggravation of existing tuberculosis and reactivation of completely quiescent cases of this infection are classic consequences demanding prophylactic measures; atypical mycobacteria have also caused tissue infections (SEDA-17, 449). Other bacterial infections, some severe and proceeding to sepsis, have followed glucocorticoid treatment. There is little evidence that glucocorticoids, even in high dosages and early in the course of infection, significantly alter the ultimate outcome (328). Use of glucocorticoids in the treatment of septic shock is not recommended in the absence of adrenal suppression.

It has been suggested that there are some differences between drugs. The use of fluticasone nasal spray to control polyp recurrence after functional endoscopic sphenoethmoidectomy should be viewed with caution, as it has been said to be associated with a high incidence of severe postoperative infection compared with beclomethasone (SEDA-21, 375; 329).

In a retrospective study, postoperative infectious complications were evaluated in 159 patients with inflammatory bowel disease undergoing elective surgery (330,33). Immunosuppression consisted of glucocorticoid monotherapy (n = 56), a glucocorticoid + azathioprine or mercaptopurine (n = 52), and neither a glucocorticoid nor azathioprine or mercaptopurine (n = 51). The adjusted odds ratios for any infection and major infections in patients who took glucocorticoid were 3.69 and 5.54 respectively, and in patients who took azathioprine or mercaptopurine 1.68 and 1.20. Thus, preoperative use of glucocorticoid in patients with inflammatory bowel disease increased the risk of postoperative infectious complications.

The risk of hospitalization for pneumonia in relation to drugs has been evaluated in 16 788 patients with rheumatoid arthritis from the US National Data Bank for Rheumatic Diseases followed semiannually for 3.5 years (332). In 644 patients hospitalization for pneumonia was required on 749 occasions. The use of prednisone increased the risk of pneumonia by 70% (HR = 1.7; 95% CI = 1.5, 2.1); leflunomide increased the risk by 30% (HR = 1.3; 95% CI = 1.0,1.5). There was a dose-related increase in the risk with prednisone: under 5 mg/day (HR = 1.4, 95% CI = 1.1, 1.6), 5–10 mg/day (HR = 2.1; 95% CI = 1.7, 2.7), and over 10 mg/day (HR = 2.3; 95% CI = 1.6, 3.2). There was no increased risk with anti-TNF therapy or methotrexate.

In a case-control study of the effects of glucocorticoids in a trauma Intensive Care Unit in 2002–3, 100 patients were compared with 100 controls with similar APACHE II scores and medical histories (333). Steroid use was associated in the multivariate analysis with an increased rate of pneumonia (OR = 2.64; 95% CI = 1.21, 5.75) and bloodstream infections (OR = 3.25; 95% CI = 1.26, 8.37). There was a trend towards increased urinary tract infections (OR = 2.31; 95% CI = 0.94, 5.69), other infections (OR = 2.57; 95% CI = 0.87, 7.67), and deaths (OR + 1.89; 95% CI = 0.81, 4.40).

Bacterial infections

Infections with *Clostridium difficile*, *Pseudomonas aeruginosa*, and *Listeria monocytogenes* (SEDA-22, 450; 334) have occasionally been precipitated or aggravated by glucocorticoids, as has tuberculous peritonitis (SEDA-20, 377; 335).

The cumulative and mean daily dosages of glucocorticoids in patients with systemic lupus erythematosus, inflammatory myopathy, overlap syndrome, or mixed connective tissue disease were the most important risk factors for the development of tuberculosis, according to a study conducted in Korea (336). Records were analysed from 269 patients who had been hospitalized during a 5-year period. In 21 patients active tuberculosis developed after a mean duration of 27 months from diagnosis of their rheumatic disease, an incidence rate of 20 cases per 1000 patient-years. The mean cumulative and daily dosages of prednisolone during the follow-up period were 31 594 and 25 mg respectively in patients who developed tuberculosis, compared with 17 043 and 18 mg in patients who did not. Glucocorticoid pulse therapy was a risk factor for the development of tuberculosis.

- A 43-year-old woman developed cavitary lung tuberculosis after she received methotrexate and glucocorticoid pulse therapy for rheumatoid arthritis (337).

The authors commented that the onset of the lung infection appeared to be closely related to methotrexate and glucocorticoid pulse therapy, because of the interval between drug administration and the onset of tuberculosis, and the lack of other risk factors for opportunistic infections.

In a retrospective study, the use of glucocorticoids during *Pneumocystis jiroveci* pneumonia (mean total dose methylprednisolone 420 mg, mean treatment duration 12 days) did not increase the risk of development or relapse of tuberculosis or other AIDS-related diseases (SEDA-20, 377; 338). The study included 129 patients (72 who took glucocorticoids and 57 who did not) who were followed up at 6, 12, 18, and 24 months of glucocorticoid therapy. The rates of infections were similar in both groups, and the cumulative rate of tuberculosis at 2 years was 12–13%.

Mycobacterium avium septic arthritis has been reported in two patients with pre-existing rheumatic disease (scleroderma and polymyositis) who were taking prednisolone and azathioprine; the infection was in the left shoulder in one patient and in the knee in the other (339).

The use of glucocorticoids in patients with hematological diseases is a factor that facilitates the occurrence of *Legionella pneumophila* pneumonia, and 10 episodes of this infection were possibly related to glucocorticoids in a series of 67 cases of Legionnaires' disease diagnosed in a single institution during 2.5 years (340).

Viral infections

Infections such as chickenpox can have serious consequences, including death, in patients taking systemic glucocorticoids (SEDA-19, 378; SEDA-20, 377; 341,342). It has been suggested that *Varicella zoster* immunoglobulin should be given to patients in contact with chickenpox if they have taken glucocorticoids in dosages over 0.5 mg/kg/day during the preceding 3 months, in the context of near-fatal chickenpox in a child receiving prednisolone (SEDA-20, 377; 343). Smallpox vaccination has in the past resulted in vaccinia gangrenosum in patients taking glucocorticoids, and the current type of *Varicella* vaccine is much more likely to produce rashes in children who are already taking glucocorticoids than in controls (SEDA-16, 452).

Herpes simplex virus encephalitis after myxedema coma has been described in an 81-year-old man treated with hydrocortisone (100 mg 8-hourly) and levothyroxine (344). In renal transplantation, two cases of death from *Herpes simplex* as a result of glucocorticoid treatment are on record (SED-8, 827; SEDA-17, 449).

Fungal and yeast infections

Fungal and yeast infections (including cases of fulminant fungal pericarditis, mucormycosis, *Aspergillus fumigatus* infection, and cutaneous alternariosis) can be precipitated or aggravated by glucocorticoid treatment (SEDA-17, 449; SEDA-18, 390; SEDA-20, 377; SEDA-21, 418; SEDA-22, 449; 345–348).

Primary esophageal histoplasmosis must be considered in patients who have a history of gastroesophageal reflux disease and are immunosuppressed by long-term glucocorticoids (SEDA-22, 450; 349). Oropharyngeal candidiasis is a well-described adverse effect of inhaled glucocorticoids. However, few cases of esophageal candidiasis have been reported (SEDA-22, 179).

Invasive pulmonary aspergillosis with cerebromeningeal involvement has been described after short-term intravenous administration of methylprednisolone (SEDA-22, 449; 350). Of 473 HIV-infected children, 7 (1.5%) developed invasive aspergillosis during the study period (1987–95; SEDA-22, 449; 335). Sustained neutropenia or glucocorticoid therapy as predisposing factors for invasive aspergillosis were found in only two patients.

- Fatal pulmonary infection with *Aspergillus fumigatus* and *Nocardia asteroides* has been described in a patient who took prednisone 1 mg/kg/day for 1 month for bronchiolitis obliterans (352).
- Fatal *Aspergillus* myocarditis, probably related to short-term administration of glucocorticoids, has been described in a 58-year-old man, who had an acute exacerbation of his chronic obstructive pulmonary disease and received oxygen, bronchodilators, omeprazole, co-amoxiclav, and intravenous methylprednisolone 40 mg 8-hourly; he died 5 days later and postmortem examination showed a fungal myocarditis (353).
- Fatal aspergillosis with a thyroid gland abscess occurred in a 74-year-old man after treatment with prednisolone for polymyalgia rheumatica (354).
- *Cryptoccocus neoformans* meningitis occurred in a 15-year old child with acute lymphoblastic leukemia (355). The clinical signs, headache, and a sixth nerve palsy on the right side, occurred at the end of the maintenance therapy when complete remission had been obtained (after 100 weeks of maintenance therapy, including multiple intermittent doses of dexamethasone). Culture of the cerebrospinal fluid confirmed cryptoccocal meningitis, and antifungal therapy produced a complete clinical response.
- *Scedosporium apiospermum* infection occurred in the left forearm of an 81-year-old man who was taking chronic oral prednisone (increased to 40 mg/day 1 month before presentation) for lung fibrosis (356).

Cutaneous alternariosis (infection with *Alternaria alternata*) has been described in a 78-year-old farmer with idiopathic pulmonary fibrosis taking oral prednisone 20 mg/day (357).

The effect of dexamethasone has been assessed in a retrospective chart review study in neonates weighing less than 1200 g, both with ($n = 65$) and without ($n = 269$) *Candida* sepsis; dexamethasone therapy and prolonged antibiotic therapy were associated with *Candida* infection (358).

In a retrospective study that included 163 consecutive recipients of allogenic hemopoietic stem cell transplants with invasive fungal infections, the possible role of glucocorticoid therapy was evaluated. The administration of high-dose glucocorticoids (2 mg/kg/day or more) was associated with an increased risk of mold infection (HR = 4.0, 95% CI = 1.7, 9.6) and an increased risk of mold infection-related death (1 year survival 11% compared with 44% when patients took doses less than 2 mg/kg/day) (359).

Fatal cerebral involvement in systemic aspergillosis has been described in a 25–year old woman with severe thrombocytopenia (platelet count 10 x 10^9/l) and mild intermittent leukopenia (granulocytes 0.375–3 x 10^9/l) who was taking prednisone 1–1.5 mg/kg/day and azathioprine 100–200 mg/day (360).

Helminth infections
Strongyloidiasis (SEDA-20, 377; SEDA-21, 419; SEDA-22, 449; 361–363) has been precipitated or aggravated by glucocorticoids.

Protozoal infections
Toxoplasmosis has been precipitated by glucocorticoids (364,365).

Pneumocystis jiroveci pneumonia has been precipitated or aggravated by glucocorticoids (SEDA-20, 377; SEDA-22, 450; 334,366,367). There is some concern about the use of glucocorticoids as adjunctive therapy in patients with AIDS who develop *Pneumocystis jiroveci* pneumonia. The immunosuppressant properties of glucocorticoids have been reported to enhance the risk of tuberculosis and other AIDS-related diseases (for example Kaposi's sarcoma or cytomegalovirus infection).

Amebic dysentery has been precipitated by glucocorticoids (368).

Death

Mortality associated with glucocorticoid has been retrospectively studied in 556 patients with chronic obstructive pulmonary disease admitted to a rehabilitation center (369). Median survival was 38 months and 280 patients died during follow-up. On multivariate analysis, oral glucocorticoid use at a prednisone equivalent of 10 mg/day without inhaled glucocorticoid was associated with an increased risk of death (RR = 2.34; 95% CI = 1.24, 4.44), and 15 mg/day increased the risk further (RR = 4.03; 95% CI = 1.99, 8.15). The risk of death was not increased in those using 5 mg/day or when patients used any oral dose in combination with inhaled glucocorticoids.

Long-Term Effects

Drug withdrawal

Suppression of adrenocortical function is one of the consequences of repeated administration of glucocorticoids; after termination of treatment a withdrawal syndrome can occur. In many cases this is unpleasant rather than acutely dangerous; in such instances the patients may have headache, nausea, dizziness, anorexia, weakness, emotional changes, lethargy, and perhaps fever; in some cases severe mental disorders occur and there are repeated reports of benign intracranial hypertension (370). The glucocorticoid withdrawal syndrome also seems to underlie the "glucocorticoid pseudorheumatism" that can occur when the drugs are withdrawn in rheumatic patients.

Withdrawal symptoms disappear if the glucocorticoid is resumed, but as a rule they will in any case vanish spontaneously within a few days. More serious consequences can ensue, however, in certain types of cases and if adrenal cortical atrophy is severe. In patients treated with corticoids for the nephrotic syndrome and apparently cured, the syndrome is particularly likely to relapse on withdrawal of therapy if the adrenal cortex is atrophic (SEDA-3, 305). In some cases, acute adrenocortical insufficiency after glucocorticoid treatment has actually proved fatal. It is advisable to withdraw long-term glucocorticoid therapy gradually so that the cortex has sufficient opportunity to recover. Table 5 lists methods of withdrawing prednisolone after long-term therapy in different circumstances (371).

Anorexia nervosa has been precipitated by withdrawal of oral prednisolone for asthma (SEDA-21, 414; 372).

A case of papilledema as a manifestation of raised intracranial pressure has been reported following withdrawal of topical glucocorticoids (SEDA-3, 305).

Panniculitis, which causes erythematous, firm, warm subcutaneous nodules, can occur within 2 weeks of withdrawal of large doses of glucocorticoids, but case reports confirm that resolution without scarring is the rule and that reintroduction of glucocorticoids is not necessary for improvement (373).

Churg–Strauss syndrome has come into prominence with the introduction of the leukotriene receptor antagonists, because they allow glucocorticoid-dependent asthmatics to discontinue their oral prednisolone. Five patients developed Churg–Strauss syndrome when their oral glucocorticoids were withdrawn (374). The duration of oral glucocorticoid therapy was 3–216 months and the dosage of prednisolone was 2.5–25.5 mg/day. The diagnosis of Churg–Strauss syndrome was made from 6 to 83 months after withdrawal of the oral glucocorticoids. These case reports support the hypothesis that it is the withdrawal of glucocorticoids that unmasks the underlying systemic vasculitis in these patients with asthma, rather than an effect of the new therapeutic agents that permits the reduction (and withdrawal) of prednisolone. Case-control studies are needed to determine the respective roles of the new therapeutic agents, prednisolone withdrawal, or other factors in the emergence of Churg–Strauss syndrome in these asthmatic patients

Tumorigenicity

Direct tumor-inducing effects of the glucocorticoids are not known, but the particular risk that malignancies in patients undergoing immunosuppression with these or other drugs will spread more rapidly is a well-recognized problem.

- Progressive endometrial carcinoma associated with azathioprine and prednisone therapy has been reported (375).
- Rapid progression of Kaposi's sarcoma 10 weeks after combined treatment with glucocorticoids and cyclophosphamide has been described; marked improvement of the skin lesions was noted after discontinuation of prednisone therapy (376).

Patients (mean age 39 years, $n = 1862$) who underwent 1924 renal transplantations from March 1995 to May 1997 were followed for 3–150 months. They received one of the following regimens: prednisolone plus azathioprine (group 1; $n = 100$); prednisolone plus azathioprine plus ciclosporin (group 2; $n = 1464$); and the same therapy as group 2 plus either muromonab-CD3 or antithymocyte globulin as induction or antirejection therapy (group 3; $n = 298$). The mean time to appearance of neoplasia after renal transplantation was 48 months. Malignancies developed earlier in group 3 patients (mean time to appearance 31 months) than in group 2 (39 months) and in group 1 (90 months). Seven of the patients who developed malignancies had also received pulse methylprednisolone for acute rejection. The authors concluded that the treatment of acute rejection with pulsed methylprednisolone and the use of muromonab-CD3 and antithymocyte globulin may lead to an increased incidence of malignancies after renal transplantation. They recommended that strategies be implemented for the early detection of malignancy (377)

Table 5 Suggested methods of withdrawing prednisolone

Circumstances	Change in daily dose
The problem has resolved and treatment has been given for only a few weeks	Reduce by 2.5 mg every 3 or 4 days down to 7.5 mg/day; then reduce more slowly, for example by 2.5 mg every week, fortnight, or month
There is uncertainty about disease resolution and/or therapy has been given for many weeks	Reduce by 2.5 mg every fortnight or month down to 7.5 mg/day then reduce by 1 mg every month
Symptoms of the disease are likely to recur on withdrawal (for example rheumatoid arthritis)	Reduce by 1 mg every month

In seven patients, accelerated growth of Kaposi's sarcoma lesions during glucocorticoid therapy suggested that glucocorticoids can alter the biological behavior of this malignant disease (378). Hydrocortisone accelerates the growth of cell lines derived from Kaposi's sarcoma cells cultured in vitro and this may partially explain these findings. Reports continue to point to the reversibility of the condition when glucocorticoids are withdrawn (379).

Kaposi's sarcoma has been associated with prednisolone therapy in two elderly women (380).

- An 84-year-old woman with polymyalgia rheumatica and a 79-year-old woman with undifferentiated connective tissue disease and leukocytoclastic vasculitis were given prednisolone 20 mg/day with subsequent dosage reductions. The first patient developed a raised purpuric rash and lymphedema of the left leg within 5 months and the second developed large purple nodules on the soles of her feet and the backs of her hands accompanied by periorbital and peripheral edema. Skin biopsies showed Kaposi's sarcoma, and both patients had raised IgG antibody titers to human herpesvirus-8.

Prior infection with herpesvirus-8 is a requisite for the development of Kaposi's sarcoma. The question arises as to how glucocorticoid treatment alone can lead to the emergence of this malignancy. In vitro evidence supports the hypothesis that glucocorticoids have a direct role in stimulating tumor development and the activation of herpesvirus-8.

A possible relation between systemic glucocorticoid use and a risk of esophageal cancer has been described in a population-based study in Denmark, in which the prescriptions database and the Danish cancer registry were linked (381). There was an increase in the number of cases observed (n = 36) compared with the number expected (n = 19), with a standardized incidence ratio of 1.92 (95% CI = 1.34, 2.65).

Second-Generation Effects

Pregnancy

A single course of a glucocorticoid given to women at risk of preterm delivery promotes fetal lung maturation, reduces the incidence of respiratory distress syndrome, and reduces neonatal morbidity and mortality. In a retrospective analysis of 306 infants of gestational age under 34 weeks, there was an association between glucocorticoid use and gastroesophageal reflux (382). In this series, 71% of the neonates (216/306) received antenatal glucocorticoids. More babies who received antenatal glucocorticoids had clinical evidence of gastroesophageal reflux (27% versus 12%). There was a significant increase in the incidence of gastroesophageal reflux with increasing courses of antenatal steroids: no course 12%, one course 25%, and two or more courses 32%.

However, there is still controversy about the use of single or repeat courses. It seems that betamethasone is more active in reducing neonatal deaths and produces fewer adverse effects than dexamethasone (383).

In a statement, the American Academy of Pediatrics and the Canadian Paediatric Society did not recommend the routine use of systemic dexamethasone for the prevention or treatment of chronic lung disease in infants with very low birthweights, because it does not reduce overall mortality and is associated with impaired growth and neurodevelopment delay (384,385).

In an analysis of 595 preterm infants born at 26–32 weeks gestation during a randomized controlled trial for the prevention of lung disease, glucocorticoids given to women at risk of preterm delivery promoted fetal lung maturation, reduced the incidence of respiratory distress syndrome, and reduced neonatal morbidity and mortality (386). Dexamethasone was given as either two doses of 12 mg 24 hours apart or four doses of 6 mg every 6 hours. Mortality was 9.2% after three or more courses, compared with 4.8% after one or two courses. This association was not explained by other factors (maternal or other common preterm morbidities).

The effects of glucocorticoids on uterine activity and preterm labor in high-order multiple gestations have been retrospectively reviewed (SEDA-20, 377; 387). In 15 women with triplet or quadruplet pregnancies, 17 out of 57 courses of betamethasone were associated with episodes of significant contractions requiring tocolytic intervention; 11 of these episodes were associated with cervical change and four resulted in premature delivery. The authors did not recommend the use of glucocorticoids if patients have more than 3.5 contractions per hour.

Prenatal glucocorticoid therapy to enhance fetal lung maturation reduces neonatal morbidity and mortality. However, adverse effects of serial courses of betamethasone on mother and fetus can occur.

For example, single versus multiple courses of antenatal glucocorticoids have been compared retrospectively in 704 pregnancies that resulted in pre-term births at 24–32 weeks. There three groups: 294 neonates whose mothers had not received glucocorticoids, 257 who had received a single dose, and 153 who had received multiple doses. Multiple doses compared with a single dose was associated with increased positive maternal cultures (44% versus 31%), small for gestational age infants (35% versus 21%), and intraventricular haemorrhage (45% versus 34%) (388).

In a retrospective study of the use of betamethasone every 12 hours versus 24 hours for anticipated preterm delivery in 909 pregnancies, three groups were identified: those who had not received antenatal glucocorticoids, those who had received betamethasone 12 hours apart, and those who received 24-hour dosing (389). There was significantly more maternal antibiotic use (90% versus 84%) and more neonatal surfactant use (40% versus 26%) in the 12-hour group compared with the 24-hour group. For all other outcomes there was no clinically significant difference.

Endocrine

Maternal hyperadrenalism occurred after five courses of betamethasone to enhance fetal lung maturation (390).

• A 26-year-old woman was given intravenous salbutamol 0.3 mg/hour for preterm labor, and intramuscular betamethasone 12 mg/day for 2 days. Daily oral tocolysis (salbutamol 2 mg every 6 hours plus nicardipine 50 mg every 12 hours) and betamethasone every week were continued at home for 3 weeks. The mother developed amyotrophy, acne on the face and trunk, moon face, hirsutism with whiskers, and thin skin. Free urinary cortisol was less than 5 micrograms/day (reference range 25–90), plasma cortisol was less than 10 ng/ml (100–200), and the salivary cortisol was less than 0.6 ng/ml (2.3–4.7). One hour after intramuscular tetracosactide 250 micrograms, her plasma cortisol was 102 ng/ml (reference range over 210) and the salivary cortisol was 3.1 ng/ml (13–25), indicating no adrenocortical response. She was given hydrocortisone 20 mg/day, and 2 months later adrenocortical insufficiency persisted, with a plasma cortisol of 152 ng/ml after corticotropin stimulation. One year later, she still required hydrocortisone 10 mg/day.

Hyperadrenalism has never otherwise been reported after the sequential use of glucocorticoids for fetal lung maturation.

A study in 10 women has been conducted to determine whether betamethasone administered at risk of preterm delivery causes adrenal suppression (391). After adrenal stimulation with corticotropin 1 microgram at 24–25 weeks, each woman received two intramuscular doses of betamethasone 12 mg 24 hours apart; 1 week later, another corticotropin test was followed by another two doses of betamethasone; a third corticotropin stimulation test was carried out 1 week later. All the women had normal baseline and stimulated cortisol concentrations during the first corticotropin stimulation test. Mean baseline serum cortisol concentrations fell with each corticotropin stimulation test (from 700 nmol/l (254 micrograms/l) before betamethasone to 120 nmol/l (43 micrograms/l) 1 week after the second course of betamethasone). The mean stimulated cortisol concentrations also fell significantly, from 910 nmol/l (330 micrograms/l) to 326 nmol/l (118 micrograms/l). There was evidence of adrenal suppression in four patients after the first course of betamethasone and in seven patients after the second course. There was no evidence of Addisonian crisis antepartum or intrapartum.

Musculoskeletal

Osteonecrosis of the femoral head can occur with glucocorticoids in nonpregnant individuals, but has not previously been reported in pregnancy (392).

• A 37-year-old white woman was given betamethasone, two doses of 12 mg over a day, at 24 weeks of a twin pregnancy, because of a history of growth restriction in her first pregnancy. At 25 weeks Doppler of the umbilical vessels suggested a reduction in end-diastolic flow in one twin. Betamethasone was prescribed again and was repeated weekly to a total of six courses because of the high risk of preterm delivery. At 30 weeks she complained of pain in the right hip exacerbated by weight bearing, which increased over the following 7 days until standing was impossible. An MRI scan showed avascular necrosis of the femoral head.

Infection risk

The use of betamethasone for the treatment of premature rupture of membranes during pregnancy is associated with an increased prevalence of maternal and neonatal infections. Two reports have described the risk of infections associated with the use of glucocorticoids during pregnancy. Of 374 patients with preterm premature rupture of membranes, 99 received a single course of glucocorticoids, 72 received multiple courses, and 203 were not treated with glucocorticoids (393). Only multiple courses of betamethasone increased the incidence of early-onset neonatal sepsis, chorioamnionitis, and endometritis in mothers. A single course of glucocorticoid was not significantly associated with any maternal or neonatal infectious complications. The incidence of maternal infections in 37 patients who received three or more courses of betamethasone (median 6, range 3–10) because of the risk of preterm delivery has been evaluated, with 70 healthy pregnant women as controls (394). Of those treated with betamethasone, 65% developed infectious diseases compared with 18% of controls. Symptomatic lower urinary tract infections (35 versus 2.7%) and serious bacterial infections (24 versus 0%) were more frequent in treated mothers. Eight of nine serious infections occurred in patients exposed to five or more courses of glucocorticoids.

Singleton pregnancies delivered at 24–34 weeks after antenatal betamethasone exposure have been prospectively analysed, in order to study the incidence of perinatal infection (395). There were 453 patients, 267 of whom took a single course of betamethasone (two doses of 12 mg in 24 hours), and 186 of whom took a multiple course (more than two doses in the 24 hours after the initial course). Multiple courses were significantly associated with early-onset neonatal sepsis (OR = 5.0; 95% CI = 1.0, 23), neonatal death (OR = 2.9; CI = 1.3, 6.9), chorioamnionitis (OR = 10; CI = 2.1, 65), and endometritis (OR = 3.6; CI = 1.7, 8.1). Respiratory distress and intraventricular hemorrhage were similar in the two groups. Although the study was non-randomized the results suggest an increased risk of neonatal infection and death after multiple courses of dexamethasone during pregnancy.

In a retrospective study in 609 mothers and their 713 infants who were treated with 1–12 courses of antenatal glucocorticoids, data from 369 singleton preterm infants born at 34 weeks or later, 210 multiple gestations, and 134 infants delivered at 35 weeks or later were analysed (396). The incidence of respiratory distress syndrome was 45% for single courses and 35% for multiple courses of glucocorticoids (OR = 0.44; 95% CI = 0.25, 0.79). The multiple-course group also had significantly less cases of patent ductus arteriosus (20 versus 13%). The incidences of death before discharge and other neonatal morbidities were similar. The multiple-course group had a significant reduction of 0.46 cm in head circumference at birth when adjusted for gestational age and pre-eclampsia. The two groups had similar birthweights. Infants born at more than 35 weeks, multiple-gestation infants, and infants who were born more than 7 days after the last dose of glucocorticoid had similar outcomes, regardless of the number of courses they had received. Mothers treated with multiple courses compared with a single course had a significantly higher incidence of postpartum endometritis, even though they had a lower incidence of prolonged rupture of membranes (24 versus 33%) and similar cesarean delivery rates. In conclusion, antenatal exposure to multiple courses of glucocorticoids compared with a single course resulted in a significant reduction in the incidence of respiratory distress syndrome in singleton preterm infants delivered within a week of the last glucocorticoid dose. This was associated with a reduction in head circumference at birth and an increased incidence of maternal endometritis. Whether the potential benefits of repeated therapy outweigh the risks will ultimately be determined in randomized controlled trials.

In a retrospective study of the benefits and risks of multiple courses of glucocorticoids in patients with preterm premature rupture of membranes, 170 preterm singleton infants were evaluated (397). They were divided into three groups: non-use (n = 50), single courses (n = 76), and multiple courses (n = 44). There was a higher incidence of chorioamnionitis those who had received multiple courses.

Teratogenicity

Teratogenic effects of glucocorticoids, which have been demonstrated in animal experiments since 1950, have not generally been confirmed in man. The question whether a disease that has had to be treated with glucocorticoids in pregnancy or the glucocorticoid treatment itself may have caused congenital anomalies reported anecdotally usually cannot be answered in any individual case. Dexamethasone, for instance, given in a suppressive dosage, seems to have been therapeutically effective in endocrine abnormal pregnancy with congenital adrenogenital syndrome (398); how is one to distinguish cause and effect here? Cleft lip and palate, seen in animal studies, have not been encountered more often in the offspring of glucocorticoid-treated women than in those of untreated women. In several small series of patients in whom glucocorticoids were used before and during pregnancy, no congenital abnormalities were seen on follow-up, but material on which to base a firm judgement is lacking. Certainly, the evidence to date does not suggest that on teratological grounds one should hesitate to administer glucocorticoids for therapeutic reasons during pregnancy (SEDA-3, 306).

However, first trimester in utero exposure to a glucocorticoid was associated with a small risk of major neonatal malformations, according to the results of a Canadian meta-analysis (399). Six cohort studies and one case-control study were analysed, and the results showed that women who had taken long-term glucocorticoid therapy during pregnancy were more likely to have a baby with a major malformation than women who had not (OR = 2.46; 95% CI = 1.41, 4.29).

Glucocorticoids have been used in cases of hyperemesis gravidarum when standard antiemetics are ineffective. In an observational comparison of women with complicated hyperemesis gravidarum and weight loss, over 5% of prepregnant weight treated with (n = 30) or without (n = 25) glucocorticoids, gestational evolution and singleton birthweights were not different in the two groups (400).

A hydatidiform mole during pregnancy may have been due to the glucocorticoids used in an immunosuppressive regimen (401).

- A 33-year-old woman took immunosuppressive therapy after renal transplantation: ciclosporin (dosage adjusted to achieve blood concentrations of 120–160 ng/ml), azathioprine 1 mg/kg (frequency of administration not stated), and methylprednisolone 40 mg/day from day 1 after transplantation, tapered weekly by 4–8 mg/day. Because of rejection symptoms at weeks 1, 4, and 7, she received three cycles of intravenous methylprednisolone 250 mg/day, each cycle lasting 5–7 days; she also received a bolus dose of methylprednisolone 500 mg on day 0. Pregnancy was diagnosed on day 12 after transplantation (9 weeks after conception). At week 6 after transplantation she had a missed abortion. Curettage was performed and a partial hydatidiform mole was detected. She was discharged at week 10 and immunosuppressive therapy was tapered.

The teratogenic effects of prednisone have been evaluated in a placebo-controlled study in 372 women and a meta-analysis (402). There was no statistical difference in the rate of major anomalies between the glucocorticoid-exposed women and the controls. The meta-analysis included 10 studies (six cohort and four case-control studies), with data from 535 exposed and 50 845 nonexposed women. The odds ratios for major malformations were 1.5 (95% CI = 0.8, 2.6) for the cohort studies and 3.4 (CI = 2.0, 5.7) for the case-control studies. The results suggest that although prednisone does not represent a major teratogenic risk in humans in therapeutic doses, it does increase the risk of oral cleft defects by an order of 3.4-fold.

Fetotoxicity

The effect of prolonged antenatal betamethasone (three or more weekly administrations) has been studied in 414 fetuses (403). Multidose betamethasone was not associated with higher risks of antenatal maternal fever, chorioamnionitis, reduced birthweight, neonatal adrenal suppression, neonatal sepsis, or neonatal death.

The effects of antenatal dexamethasone on birthweight have been studied in 961 infants and matched controls (404). Dexamethasone-treated infants had significantly lower birthweights (after adjustment for week of gestation). The average differences from controls were 12 g at 24–26 weeks, 63 g at 27–29 weeks, 161 g at 30–32 weeks, and 80 g at 33–34 weeks. In the case of preterm rupture of membranes, the data were not conclusive.

Betamethasone, two doses of 12 mg a day apart, in 40 pregnant women (27–34 weeks) caused important changes in fetal physiology (405). Fetal breathing (the number of breathing episodes and the total breathing time in 30 minutes) fell by 83% and fetal limb and trunk movements fell by 53% and 49% respectively. These changes were transient and returned to the range of normality 96 hours after administration. There were no changes in Doppler velocimetry of the umbilical and middle cerebral arteries. Awareness of these effects may prevent unnecessary iatrogenic delivery of preterm infants who present abnormal biophysical profile scores 2 days after glucocorticoid exposure.

Prenatal glucocorticoids given weekly to women at risk of preterm birth have been studied in 982 women who were randomly assigned to repeated intramuscular doses of either 11.4 mg betamethasone (as Celestone Chronodose) or saline (7 or more days after receiving a first course of prenatal glucocorticoids) (406). The primary outcomes were the occurrence and severity of neonatal respiratory distress syndrome, the use and duration of oxygen and mechanical ventilation, and weight, length, and head circumference at birth and hospital discharge. Fewer babies exposed to repeated doses of corticosteroids had respiratory distress syndrome (33% versus 41%; RR = 0.82; 95% CI = 0.71, 0.95) and fewer had severe lung disease (12% versus 20%; RR = 0.60; 95% CI = 0.46, 0.79). Mean weight, length, and head circumference at birth and hospital discharge did not differ. There were no differences in adverse effects (chorioamnionitis, postpartum pyrexia, postnatal hypertension, and cesarean sections). Pending long-term outcomes, the short-term benefits support the use of repeat doses of glucocorticoids in women who are at risk of very preterm birth 7 or more days after an initial course.

The adverse neonatal outcomes associated with antenatal dexamethasone or betamethasone have been studied retrospectively in 3600 infants (407). Compared with betamethasone, dexamethasone was associated with a statistically significant increase in the risk of neonatal death (OR = 1.66; 95% CI = 1.07, 2.57). There were trends for greater risks associated with dexamethasone compared with betamethasone for intraventricular haemorrhage (OR = 1.21; 95% CI = 0.93, 1.59) and severe retinopathy of prematurity (OR = 1.50; 95% CI = 0.93, 2.42). Betamethasone seemed preferable to dexamethasone, but this must be confirmed in a comparative randomized trial.

Retardation of intrauterine growth by glucocorticoids has been reported not only in animals but also in man. In a 1990 case from France, dwarfism (as well as Cushing's syndrome) was recorded in a child whose mother had received high-dose glucocorticoids during pregnancy.

It has been suggested that the risk of stillbirth may be increased by glucocorticoid treatment; the figures are suggestive, but the possibility that the disorder that led to the use of the glucocorticoid was itself responsible for the less favorable outcome cannot be excluded (408).

Prevention of the respiratory distress syndrome in anticipated prematurity has become a widely accepted (though not uncontroversial) indication for glucocorticoids in late pregnancy, the compound most often used being dexamethasone. The timing of such treatment in late pregnancy seems to be of crucial importance (SEDA-3, 306); the possible adverse effects on the mother and child are still being discussed. The issue has been extensively reviewed (SEDA-17, 445). A meta-analysis of 15 trials, involving 1780 patients treated with glucocorticoids and 1780 controls, has shown a lower risk of the syndrome, and a substantial reduction in neonatal mortality (OR = 0.60; 95% CI = 0.48, 0.76), without a higher risk of infection in the mother or maternal pulmonary edema (SEDA-20, 377; 409). In the mother, labor can be delayed by such glucocorticoid therapy (SEDA-3, 306); the combination of this treatment with sympathomimetic drugs may put the mother at risk of fluid retention with pulmonary edema (SED-12, 990), although it is not clear whether this problem only occurs when both drugs are used.

As far as the child is concerned, there may be only moderate adrenal suppression (410), although in some cases substitution treatment with glucocorticoids can be necessary in such babies; short-term treatment with betamethasone shortly before birth generally does not inhibit the infant's adrenal capacity to react to corticotropin (411). A single case of a leukemoid reaction in a preterm infant has been observed, after the mother was given betamethasone shortly before delivery (SEDA-3, 306).

On the other hand, there are many reports of hypertension (412), and electrocardiographic and other studies have often confirmed the presence of a disproportionately serious and bilateral hypertrophic obstructive cardiomyopathy, which unless it proves fatal is, in general, reversible once the glucocorticoids are withdrawn (SEDA-18, 386). Although the issue is confounded by the possibility that infants with bronchopulmonary dysplasia may be innately hypertensive, there seems no doubt as to the effect.

Most babies treated with glucocorticoids for lung dysplasia also show an appreciable rise in blood urea nitrogen, due almost entirely to an increase in structural protein catabolism (413). Serious gastrointestinal complications can occur. In one typical series of premature neonates treated in this way there were three such instances (perforated duodenal ulcer, perforated gastric ulcer, and upper gastrointestinal hemorrhage, the last two proving fatal; 413); the symptoms are apparently not masked by the glucocorticoid, as one would expect in adults. Treated infants also tend to have a low pH, which is unusual in premature babies (SEDA-18, 445).

In 534 individuals aged 30 years, whose mothers had participated in a double-blind, randomized, placebo-controlled trial of antenatal betamethasone (two intramuscular doses 24 hours apart) for the prevention of neonatal respiratory distress syndrome, there were no differences between those exposed to betamethasone and placebo in body size, blood lipids, blood pressure, plasma cortisol, prevalence of diabetes, or history of cardiovascular disease (415). After the oral glucose tolerance test, those who had been exposed to betamethasone had higher plasma insulin concentrations at 30 minutes (61 versus 52 mIU/l) and lower glucose concentrations at 120 minutes (4.8 versus 5.1 mmol/l) than did those exposed to placebo. Antenatal exposure to betamethasone might result in insulin resistance in adult offspring, but has no effect on cardiovascular risk factors at 30 years of age.

In an Italian prospective study, 201 preterm singleton infants received one or more antenatal courses of a glucocorticoid (416). Neurodevelopment was evaluated at 2 years; 138 subjects received at least one complete course of betamethasone (37 multiple) and 63 patients received dexamethasone (33 multiple). The prevalence of infant leukomalacia was 26% after a complete course of glucocorticoid, 40% after one additional course, 42% after two additional courses, and 44% after more than two additional courses. The corresponding prevalences of 2-year infant neurodevelopmental abnormalities, considering the same categories of glucocorticoid exposure, were 18%, 21%, 29%, and 35% respectively. However, most of the risk was related to dexamethasone administration. Compared with betamethasone, exposure to multiple doses of dexamethasone was associated with an increased risk of leukomalacia (OR = 3.21; 95% CI = 1.07, 9.77) and overall 2-year infant neurodevelopmental abnormalities (OR = 3.63; 95% CI = 1.03, 14).

In an Australian cohort study, 541 very preterm infants were followed for physical, cognitive, and psychological assessment up to 6 years after administration of glucocorticoids during pregnancy (417). Although increasing numbers of antenatal glucocorticoid courses (two intramuscular doses of betamethasone 11.4 mg) were associated with a reduction in the rate of cerebral palsy, three or more courses were also associated with increased rates of aggressive/destructive, distractible, and hyperkinetic behavior, and these effects were present at ages 3 and 6 years. Intelligence quotients were unaffected by antenatal use of a glucocorticoid.

In 192 adult offspring (mean age 31 years) of mothers who had taken part in a randomized controlled trial of antenatal betamethasone for the prevention of neonatal respiratory distress syndrome (87 exposed to betamethasone two doses 24 hours apart, and 105 exposed to placebo) there were no alterations in cognitive functioning, working memory and attention, psychiatric morbidity, handedness, or health-related quality-of-life in adulthood (418).

The effects of a single antenatal dose of a glucocorticoid on prostanoids have been evaluated in 43 singleton pregnancies in women who were taking betamethasone or not (419). Betamethasone (dose not described) reduced maternal PGE_2 concentrations, with concomitant increases in the fetoplacental compartment. Umbilical cord thromboxane B_2 concentrations in the treated group were significantly lower than the non-treated group, resulting in a higher ratio of 6-keto$PGF_{1\alpha}$ to thromboxane B2. Considering the regulatory role of PGE_2 and PGI_2 in fetal lung development and neonatal transition homeostasis, these results suggest a mechanism, at least in part, for the beneficial effects of antenatal glucocorticoids on fetal lung maturation and neonatal cardiopulmonary homeostasis at birth.

Clearly, the duration of such treatment after delivery should be as brief as possible, but there is no reason for such concern as would lead to withholding therapy; one

Dutch study with a 10-year follow-up detected no problems with exposed children's intellectual, motor, or social functioning compared with controls (136).

A meta-analysis, including 15 controlled trials and involving more than 1400 women, has shown that antenatal glucocorticoids in women with ruptured membranes may be beneficial in reducing the risks of neonatal death (RR = 0.68; 95% CI = 0.43, 1.07) and respiratory distress syndrome (RR = 0.56; CI = 0.46, 0.70), with no increase in the risk of infection in either the mother (RR = 0.88; CI = 0.61, 1.20) or baby (RR = 1.05; CI = 0.66, 1.68; 420).

A reduction in fetal response to vibroacoustic stimulation (vibroacoustic startle reflex) has been reported during 48 hours after the administration to pregnant women of two doses of betamethasone (12 mg 2 days apart; 421). The authors recommended that this test should not be used to evaluate well-being in fetuses exposed to glucocorticoids.

Susceptibility Factors

Genetic factors

Significant differences in the pharmacokinetics of methylprednisolone have been described in black and white renal transplant patients. Black patients had a slower clearance rate and a lower apparent volume of distribution. They had higher cortisol concentrations throughout the day, with higher nadir concentrations. Some of them had glucocorticoid-associated diabetes, and no white patients did. Further studies are needed to define the differences between the races (SEDA-20, 377; 422).

Age

Children

Inhaled glucocorticoids are recommended as first-line therapy for persistent asthma in children, to reduce both asthma symptoms and inflammatory markers. Treatment should be begun early in the course of the disease, because inhaled glucocorticoids can preserve airway function and prevent airway remodelling and subsequent irreversible airway obstruction (423). Because asthma is a chronic disease requiring long-term treatment, it is very important to balance the safety and efficacy of inhaled glucocorticoids to achieve optimal long-term results. Major safety concerns in children are the potential adverse effects on growth, adrenal function, and bone mass. Overall, the benefits of inhaled glucocorticoids clearly outweigh their potential adverse effects and the risks of poor asthma control. However, high doses of inhaled glucocorticoids in children are still of concern (424). It is of utmost importance to use the lowest effective dose, to limit systemic availability by selecting drugs with high first-pass hepatic inactivation, and to instruct patients on proper inhalation technique. Moreover, the use of adjuvant asthma medications acting by different mechanisms can help to reduce inhaled glucocorticoid dosages (423,424). These add-on therapies include leukotriene modifiers, long-acting beta$_2$-agonists, cromoglicate and nedocromil, and in selected cases theophylline. These agents should be added to, but should not in any case replace, inhaled glucocorticoid therapy (423,424).

The use of postnatal glucocorticoids in very premature infants is controversial; although dexamethasone reduces bronchopulmonary dysplasia, it has been associated with severe adverse effects (425). In 220 infants with a birth-weight of 501–1000 g randomized to placebo or dexamethasone (0.15 mg/kg/day for 3 days and tapering over a period of 7 days) the relative risk of death or chronic lung disease compared with controls was 0.9 (95% CI = 0.8–1.1) at 36 weeks of gestational age (426). Infants treated with dexamethasone were less likely to need supplementary oxygen. Dexamethasone was associated with increased risks of hypertension (RR = 7.4; 95% CI = 2.7, 20.2), hyperglycemia (RR = 2.0; 95% CI = 1.1, 3.6), spontaneous gastrointestinal perforation (13 versus 4%), lower weight, and a smaller head circumference.

Elderly people

Prolonged use of glucocorticoids in elderly people can exacerbate diabetes, hypertension, congestive heart failure, and osteoporosis, or cause depression. In a retrospective, controlled study, the risks of high-dose intravenous or oral glucocorticoid therapy were assessed in 55 patients with Crohn's disease who were over the age of 50 years (427). They had a higher risk of developing hypertension, hypokalemia, and changes in mental state.

Hepatic disease

In patients with acute hepatitis and active hepatitis, protein binding of the glucocorticoids will be reduced and peak concentrations of administered glucocorticoids increased. Conversion of prednisone to prednisolone has been reported to be impaired in chronic active liver disease (427). However, although plasma prednisolone concentrations were more predictable after the administration of prednisolone than of prednisone to a group of healthy subjects (429), there was no difference in patients with chronic active hepatitis. There was also impaired elimination of prednisolone in these patients. In a review of the pharmacokinetics of prednisone and prednisolone it was concluded that fear of inadequate conversion of prednisone into prednisolone was not justified (430). Patients with hepatic disease suffer adrenal suppression more readily (112).

Other features of the patient

Menopause

Significant differences in the pharmacokinetics of prednisolone amongst menopausal women have been described (SEDA-21, 419; 431). The postmenopausal women had reduced unbound clearance (30%), reduced total clearance, and an increased half-life. Similar results are seen in the postmenopausal women who took estrogen or estrogen–progestogen therapy.

Protein binding

The association between low serum albumin concentrations and complications of prednisone has been long recognized, and it is an elementary pharmacokinetic principle that concentrations of unbound drug in plasma (the fraction that can reach the tissues) will be increased when binding of a drug to serum albumin is reduced (432).

Systemic lupus erythematosus

In 539 patients with systemic lupus erythematosus, organ damage was associated with glucocorticoid therapy compared with controls (433). Oral prednisone 10 mg/day for 10 years (cumulative dose 36.6 g) was significantly associated with osteoporotic fractures (RR = 2.5; 95% CI = 1.7, 3.7), symptomatic coronary artery disease (RR = 1.7; CI = 1.1, 2.5), and cataracts (RR = 1.7; CI = 1.4, 2.5). Avascular necrosis was associated with high-dose prednisone (at least 60 mg/day for at least 2 months; RR = 1.2; CI = 1.1, 1.4). Intravenous pulses of methylprednisolone (1000 mg for 1–3 days) were associated with a small increase in the risk of osteoporotic fractures (RR = 1.3; CI = 1.0, 1.8).

Drug Administration

Drug formulations

The development of adverse effects has been evaluated after switching from conventional glucocorticoids to a pH-modified release formulation, Eudragit L-coated budesonide, in 178 patients with Crohn's disease who had taken 5–30 mg/day of prednisolone equivalents for at least 2 weeks (434). The percentage of patients with glucocorticoid-related adverse effects fell from 65% at entry to 43% at the end of the study. The total number of glucocorticoid-related adverse effects fell significantly from 269 to 90. In conclusion, switching from conventional glucocorticoids to budesonide leads to a significant reduction in glucocorticoid-related adverse effects in patients with Crohn's disease without causing rapid deterioration of the disease.

Drug contamination

Unregulated Chinese herbal products adulterated with glucocorticoids have been detected (435). Dexamethasone was present in eight of 11 Chinese herbal creams analysed by UK dermatologists. The creams contained dexamethasone in concentrations inappropriate for use on the face or in children (64–1500 micrograms/g). The cream with the highest concentration of dexamethasone was prescribed to treat facial eczema in a 4-month-old baby. In all cases, it had been assumed that the creams did not contain glucocorticoids. The authors were concerned that these patients received both unlabelled and unlicensed topical glucocorticoids. They wrote that "greater regulation and restriction needs to be imposed on herbalists, and continuous monitoring of side effects of these medications is necessary."

Drug dosage regimens

Daily or alternate-day administration

The unwanted effects of the glucocorticoids can be reduced to some extent by altering the dosage routine, for example by giving them on alternate days or giving the total daily dose every morning.

Because of circadian variation in endogenous glucocorticoid secretion, the pituitary–adrenal axis is suppressed more easily in the night than during the day (436). Thus, administration of the total dose as a single dose in the morning is preferable to twice daily dosing or administration in the evening alone.

Alternate-day therapy (giving twice the daily dose on alternate days) can in some cases maintain the therapeutic efficacy of oral glucocorticoids, while reducing their adverse effects (437–439).

Use in fixed combinations

Fixed combinations of oral glucocorticoids with nonsteroidal anti-inflammatory analgesics or broncholytic drugs that have to be given repeatedly during the day are undesirable, since their pattern of administration is determined in part by the demands of the other components; the glucocorticoid is thus likely to be given in such a way that it alters the circadian rhythm of endogenous glucocorticoids.

Pulse or megadose therapy

Extremely large intravenous doses of glucocorticoids given at longer intervals can sometimes be effective when a patient does not respond to conventional high doses. Systemic lupus erythematosus, various rheumatic diseases, and the treatment of renal graft rejection are indications for this type of use (SEDA-6, 331). High doses of glucocorticoids also have an antiemetic effect in patients with cancers.

No adverse effects are to be expected after a single injection of a high dose of a glucocorticoid, but some serious complications have been observed with repeated use, including both infections and the known direct adverse effects of glucocorticoids. Cases of ventricular dysrhythmias and atrial fibrillation have been reported (SEDA-18, 391). With pulse therapy, the nature of the injected glucocorticoid seems to be important; for example, hydrocortisone, which is more rapidly metabolized, seems to be better tolerated than dexamethasone (SEDA-6, 331).

Pulsed glucocorticoid therapy for moderately severe ulcerative colitis, given on an out-patient basis, can induce remission more quickly than conventional oral glucocorticoid therapy (440). There were no serious adverse effects in 11 patients given pulsed glucocorticoids or in eight treated conventionally. The two regimens were equally efficacious.

Drug administration route

Most knowledge of the adverse effects of glucocorticoids has been acquired in connection with their use as oral products. However, various other routes of administration have been developed, sometimes specifically in the hope of securing a local therapeutic effect while avoiding systemic adverse reactions. Although experience has shown that the latter cannot be eliminated in this way,

they can be diminished in some cases. In other cases, new problems arise.

Topical administration to the skin

The percutaneous absorption of high-potency topical glucocorticoids has been documented, but hypothalamic–pituitary–adrenal axis suppression, leading to clinically significant adrenal insufficiency or Cushing's syndrome, is infrequent. Two patients developed adrenal suppression after the unregulated use of betamethasone dipropionate 0.05% ointment (about 80 g/week) or clobetasol 0.05% ointment (up to 100 g/week), obtained without prescription to treat psoriasis (441).

Although glucocorticoids are used to treat eczema, they can sometimes exacerbate it (442).

- A 74-year-old man developed worsening eczema 24 hours after he applied clobetasol (Decloban) to treat chronic eczema of his external ear. Twelve years earlier he had noted exacerbation of a cutaneous lesion after he had applied a topical glucocorticoid. He had also had generalized erythema after an intra-articular injection of paramethasone. Patch tests to a series of glucocorticoids were positive for all drugs except flupametasone, fluocortine, and tixocortol. In addition, intradermal tests were positive to hydrocortisone and prednisolone, despite negative patch tests.

The authors commented that most glucocorticoid-sensitized patients react to several of the same group and less frequently of different groups. No case of hypersensitivity to glucocorticoids of all four classes has previously been reported.

- Chronic lichenified eczema has been attributed to prolonged use of topical methylprednisolone aceponate and budesonide (strength and duration of therapy not stated) in a 26-year-old woman (443). Patch tests were positive for methylprednisolone aceponate and budesonide cream, but negative for all other topical glucocorticoids.
- A 4-month old boy developed iatrogenic Cushing's syndrome, which occurred when his mother used excessive amounts of clobetasol 17-propionate and hydrocortisone 17-butyrate cream for 2 months to treat a diaper rash (444).
- An 18-year-old woman presented with a pruritic eczematous eruption that developed after topically applying an ointment containing hydrocortisone acetate, neomycin sulfate, and Centella asiatica (445). She was positive to all three ingredients of the ointment.

Two patients developed central serous chorioretinopathy after prolonged treatment with glucocorticoids applied locally to the skin (446).

- A 32-year-old man complained of reduced vision and metamorphopsia in the right eye. Best-corrected visual acuity was 20/25 in right eye and 20/20 in left eye. The left fundus was normal but in the right eye there was a well-circumscribed, shallow, serous detachment of the sensory retina. The clinical appearance was consistent with central serous chorioretinopathy, and the diagnosis was confirmed by fluorescein angiography, which showed a leakage point at the superior macula, spreading slowly in an inkblot configuration into the subretinal space. He had had seborrheic dermatitis involving the central face, eyebrows, eyelids, and scalp for 2 years treated with topical hydrocortisone acetate cream 1%. After the initial prescription, he used the cream without further medical consultation when his symptoms got worse and used it for 4 weeks, 3–4 times a day before developing central serous chorioretinopathy.

- A 37-year-old man developed blurred vision in the left eye. He had had central serous chorioretinopathy in the contralateral eye 5 years before, for which he had been treated with laser photocoagulation. Best-corrected visual acuity was 20/20 in each eye. There were scars from previous laser photocoagulation at the superior macula in the right eye. In the left eye there was a well-delineated area of serous detachment temporal to the fovea and small yellowish precipitates at the posterior aspect of the detached retina. Fluorescein angiography showed a leakage point at the upper pole of the detachment. He had had pityriasis versicolor, for which he had used local diflucortolone valerate cream 0.1% in combination with isoconazole nitrate 1%. He had used the cream occasionally but had used it for 3 weeks before the onset of symptoms. He also used diflucortolone valerate cream 0.1% during the first episode of central serous chorioretinopathy.

The effects of exposure to topical glucocorticoids during pregnancy have been evaluated in a population-based follow-up study in 363 primigravida exposed to topical glucocorticoids during pregnancy and 9263 controls who received no prescriptions at all (445). The prevalence of malformations was 2.9% among 170 infants exposed to glucocorticoids during the first trimester and 3.6% among the controls. There were no increases in the risks of low birthweight, malformations, or preterm delivery in the offspring of women who were exposed to topical glucocorticoids during pregnancy.

Topical administration to the eye

Glucocorticoids that have been used for local ophthalmic treatment include medrysone, fluorometholone, tetrahydroxytriamcinolone, and clobetasone. Loteprednol etabonate 0.5% increases intraocular pressure less than dexamethasone. Studies on animal models of uveitis and two randomized double-masked trials showed that loteprednol etabonate 0.5% was less potent than dexamethasone, prednisolone acetate 1%, or fluorometholone, which may partly explain the improved toxicity profile of loteprednol etabonate (448).

Clinicians should not prescribe glucocorticoid-containing eye-drops unless they have performed a slit-lamp examination with tonometry, have assurance of appropriate follow-up, and understand the differential diagnosis, evaluation, and treatment. Unless clearly indicated, prescribing volumes larger than 5 ml or providing refillable prescriptions should be avoided. It should be stressed that excessive use of glucocorticoids can result in corneal Herpes infection and mycosis.

Since glucocorticoids reduce the immunological defences of the body to most types of infection, their use in the eyes should be monitored carefully. When long-term use is necessary, even with oral or inhalation therapy, eye examination should be performed every 6 months. The ophthalmological follow-up of patients using topical glucocorticoids should include tonometry at least twice a year, careful slit-lamp examination for early signs of herpetic or fungal keratitis and for changes in the equatorial and posterior subcapsular portions of the lens, examination of pupillary size and lid position, and staining of the cornea to detect possible punctate keratitis. Blood glucose concentrations should be checked if there are symptoms that suggest hyperglycemia.

Sensory systems

Ocular adverse effects of local or systemic administration of glucocorticoids include cataracts, glaucoma, papilledema, pseudotumor cerebri, activation of corneal infections, superficial keratitis, ptosis, pupillary dilatation, conjunctival palpebral petechiae, uveitis, and scleromalacia. Topical ocular application and facial application can cause high glucocorticoid concentrations in the anterior compartment of the eye. Serious visual loss can occur owing to the development of cataract in patients using glucocorticoid creams.

Glucocorticoid creams applied topically to the skin are routinely used in the treatment of many skin disorders, and their use on the face in severe atopic eczema is relatively common. Three patients developed advanced glaucoma while using topical facial glucocorticoids. Two other patients developed ocular hypertension secondary to topical facial glucocorticoids (449).

The use of a combination of a glucocorticoid with an antimicrobial drug is illogical and should generally be avoided because of the possibility of the emergence of resistant bacterial strains. It would be highly preferable if prescriptions for these drugs were issued by ophthalmologists only, at least in those parts of the world where adequate medical services are available.

Three vision-threatening complications have been described due to the indiscriminate use of glucocorticoid-containing eyedrops (450).

- A 31-year-old man noted a blind spot in his right eye. He had worn contact lenses for 10 years to correct his myopia. He had applied Tobradex ointment (tobramycin 0.3% and dexamethasone 0.1%) to each eye every evening for the past 4 years because of irritation due to contact lenses, and continuous refills of this prescription were obtained through an acquaintance who was employed in a pharmacy. With spectacle correction his visual acuity was 20/25 in each eye. The intraocular pressure was 52 mmHg in his right eye and 37 mmHg in his left eye. The optic discs showed glaucomatous cupping in each eye. Automated visual field testing showed superior and inferior arcuate defects typical of glaucoma in both eyes. Slit-lamp biomicroscopy showed mild papillary conjunctivitis bilaterally due to contact lenses. The antibiotic + glucocorticoid ointment was withdrawn and his bilateral glucocorticoid-induced open-angle glaucoma was treated with antiglaucomatous drugs.

- A 15-year-old boy felt a foreign body sensation in his right eye after he had been raking hay. His local physician prescribed a suspension of tobramycin 0.3% + dexamethasone 0.1% tds, but 6 days later referred him for evaluation of a suspected fungal keratitis. He had a corneal epithelial defect with an underlying dense inflammatory infiltrate. Corneal scrapings contained fungal hyphae and *Fusarium* species was identified. Natamycin 5% was administered topically every hour, the infection resolved, and his visual acuity returned to 20/20 despite a dense corneal scar.

- A 56-year-old woman had bilateral primary open-angle glaucoma without visual field loss, which was well controlled with a long-term topical beta-blocker in each eye. She underwent a left dacryocystorhinostomy for nasolacrimal duct obstruction, but developed persistent tearing and irritation of the left eye several months postoperatively. A suspension of tobramycin 0.3% + dexamethasone 0.1% was prescribed, which she continued to use as needed for 6 months. Pain and reduced vision persisted in her left eye. Corrected visual acuity was 20/20 in her right eye and 20/60 in her left eye. The intraocular pressures were 18 mmHg in her right eye and 68 mmHg in her left eye. Automated visual field testing showed a normal field in her right eye, but only a central island and a crescent of temporal visual field in her left eye. External examination showed persistent nasolacrimal duct obstruction on the left side with mild conjunctival injection. The diagnosis was primary open-angle glaucoma in both eyes, which was exacerbated by topically applied glucocorticoids in her left eye. The antibiotic + glucocorticoid suspension was withdrawn, and a topical ocular hypotensive therapeutic regimen was initiated in her left eye.

Susceptibility factors

Local and systemic adverse effects of ophthalmic glucocorticoids occur in children more often, more severely, and more rapidly than in adults, for unknown reasons. It could be that children have relatively immature chamber angles, giving rise to a rapidly increasing intraocular pressure (445).

Glaucoma has been reported after the use of a glucocorticoid ointment in a young boy (445).

- A 6-year-old boy underwent a resection of levator palpebrae superioris for congenital blepharoptosis. Postoperatively, an ointment containing 0.1% dexamethasone and neomycin (Maxitrol) was applied to the operated eyelid three times a day to reduce lid edema. Four days later the surgical correction was satisfactory and there were no symptoms, but the intraocular pressure was raised to 44 mmHg in the operated eye, although normal in the other eye. The glucocorticoid was withdrawn and topical ocular hypotensive agents were prescribed. The intraocular pressure returned to normal the next day, and the antiglaucoma treatments were maintained for 1 week and tapered over the next 2

weeks. Subsequent follow-up confirmed normal intraocular pressure and no glaucomatous damage.

The ocular hypertensive response in this case could have been due to systemic absorption of glucocorticoid through the skin of the eyelid, especially when there was a surgical wound. Alternatively, a sufficient amount of ointment could have seeped over the eyelid margins, causing the rise in intraocular pressure, similar to the application of eye-drops, as has been reported in another child, who also had Cushing's syndrome, a rare result of ophthalmic glucocorticoids (452).

- An 11-year-old boy with iridocyclitis developed Cushing's syndrome, a posterior subcapsular cataract, and increased intraocular pressure in both eyes after the topical administration of prednisolone acetate 1% eye-drops bilaterally for 6 months. The Cushing's syndrome was aggravated when periocular methylprednisolone acetate was started while bilateral posterior subtenon injections of 80 mg of suspension were continued every 6 weeks for 6 months. He had not used systemic glucocorticoids before.

Topical administration to the nose

The safety of nasal glucocorticoids in the treatment of allergic rhinitis has been reviewed (453,454). The local application of glucocorticoids for seasonal or perennial rhinitis often results in systemic adverse effects. The use of nasal sprays containing a glucocorticoid that has specific topical activity (such as beclomethasone dipropionate or flunisolide) seems to reduce the systemic adverse effects, but they can nevertheless occur, even to the extent of suppression of basal adrenal function in children (455). Local adverse effects include *Candida* infection, nasal stinging, epistaxis, throat irritation (456), and, exceptionally, anosmia (457).

Nervous system

Benign intracranial hypertension with nasal glucocorticoids has been reported (458).

- A 13-year-old boy with Crohn's disease in remission, who had taken fluticasone aqueous nasal spray 50 micrograms to each nostril od regularly for 5 days, gave a 10-day history of head and back pain. He had a right sixth nerve palsy with bilateral swelling of his optic discs. An unenhanced computer tomogram was normal and magnetic resonance imaging excluded cavernous sinus thrombosis. The cerebrospinal fluid was clear with no cells, and protein and glucose concentrations were normal.

Although there was no clear temporal relation between the onset of the symptoms and the regular use of fluticasone, the authors proposed that the fluticasone was responsible, because the symptoms resolved after drug withdrawal. The association remains unproven but it does highlight the possibility of an association.

Sensory systems

Nasal budesonide or beclomethasone 100 micrograms bd for 3–9 months had no effect on the eyes in 26 patients who had undergone endoscopic sinus surgery (458). Ophthalmologic examination, tonometry, visual field testing, and biomicroscopic studies showed no evidence of ocular hypertension or posterior subcapsular cataract.

Ear, nose, and throat

The use of intranasal glucocorticoids in the treatment of allergic and vasomotor rhinitis in Sweden has doubled over a period of 5 years, and the number of reported cases of nasal septum perforation increased over the same time (460). The most common risk factor in 32 patients with nasal septum perforation (21 women, 11 men) was glucocorticoid treatment. Information from the Swedish Drug Agency showed that 38 cases of glucocorticoid-induced perforation had been reported over 10 years. The number of adverse effects per million Defined Daily Doses averaged 0.21. The risk of perforation was greatest during the first 12 months of treatment and most cases were in young women.

Endocrine

Aqueous nasal triamcinolone spray 220 or 440 micrograms od for the treatment of allergic rhinitis reportedly had no measurable adverse effects on adrenocortical function in 80 children (aged 6–12 years) in a placebo-controlled, double-blind study (446). Plasma triamcinolone concentrations measured over 6 hours fell rapidly and there was little or no accumulation during 6 weeks.

There have been reports of Cushing's syndrome after prolonged use of intranasal betamethasone 0.1% for chronic catarrh in two boys (462) and from an interaction of nasal fluticasone with ritonavir (463).

- A 30-year-old man who was using an intranasal formulation of fluticasone (therapeutic indication not stated), developed Cushing's syndrome about 5 months after starting ritonavir 600 mg bd, zidovudine, and lamivudine for HIV infection. His plasma cortisol concentrations were undetectable, his corticotrophin was low (under 2 pmol/l), and his 24-hours urinary cortisol excretion was under 30 nmol/l. Further investigations were consistent with secondary adrenal failure or with glucocorticoid use. He admitted to having used a topical glucocorticoid cream for 2 months. However, 6 weeks after he stopped using this cream, his plasma cortisol concentrations were still undetectable. It was then established that he had used nasal fluticasone propionate 200 micrograms/day for about 1 year before starting ritonavir. Ritonavir was replaced by nevirapine, and he continued to use fluticasone nasal spray. Three weeks later, his plasma cortisol concentration had increased to 290 nmol/l. Ritonavir was then added and his plasma cortisol concentration fell rapidly. Ritonavir was stopped again and his cortisol concentration normalized and his Cushingoid facies improved.

The authors thought it likely that inhibition of cytochrome P-450 by ritonavir increased the systemic availability of fluticasone and thus caused Cushing's syndrome in this patient.

Musculoskeletal

Osteonecrosis of the femoral head after the use of a glucocorticoid nasal spray has been reported (464).

- A 48-year-old man taking losartan, low-dose amitriptyline, and triamcinolone acetonide nasal spray developed pain in the abdomen and hips. Radiography and magnetic resonance imaging showed rapidly progressive bilateral osteonecrosis of the femoral heads. He had used excessive amounts of nasal glucocorticoids, and during the previous 12 months had used triamcinolone acetonide 110 micrograms qds in each nostril.

Intralesional injection

Intralesional triamcinolone acetonide has been used extensively for the treatment of hypertrophic and keloid scars. Complications are few, usually being local skin color changes, prominent vascular markings, or subcutaneous atrophy. Cushing's syndrome after intralesional administration of triamcinolone acetate has been described in two adults and two children (aged 10 years and 21 months) after treatment of hypertrophic burn scars with intralesional triamcinolone acetonide (SEDA-21, 419; 350). These two children may have had a form of hypersensitivity to triamcinolone acetonide, as Cushing's syndrome was not the result of overdosage.

- Acute anaphylaxis occurred in an 18-year-old man after the third course of intradermal injections of triamcinolone suspension ("Kenalog" 10 mg per treatment) for alopecia areata (465). Subsequent rechallenge with intradermal triamcinolone 1 ml resulted in the same anaphylactic reaction as before and his serum IgE concentration was increased.

Immediate hypersensitivity reactions to paramethasone acetate, causing widespread eruptions, have been described in at least four cases. Delayed allergic reactions are less common.

- A woman had received intralesional paramethasone and other topical glucocorticoids several times for alopecia between the ages of 7 and 18 years (466). When she was 30 she was again treated with intralesional paramethasone for a relapse of alopecia. She developed pruritus after the first intralesional injection and erythema, edema, and vesicles 6–8 hours later. A biopsy showed spongiform lymphocytic folliculitis with spongiosis and exocytosis in the sweat gland ducts and in the pilosebaceous unit. She was treated with triamcinolone cream and her skin lesions resolved. Patch tests were positive for paramethasone, with cross-reactivity to tixocortol pivalate, hydrocortisone, and hydrocortisone butyrate.

Intraspinal injection
Intrathecal

The effects of intrathecal administration, both wanted and unwanted, are still much debated (467). The question as to whether oral glucocorticoid therapy should be preferred to intrathecal injections is raised by the harmful effects that have sometimes occurred after the latter, although some of these may have been caused by irritative substances in the injection fluid (SEDA-6, 331). The same local glucocorticoid concentrations can probably be attained with fewer problems with oral administration. Epidural injection of glucocorticoids seems to be safer than intrathecal injection, but injection of high doses can cause the same systemic adverse effects as seen with oral treatment. Facial flushing and erythema after lumbar epidural glucocorticoid administration have been reported (SEDA-20, 378; 468).

Glucocorticoids given intrathecally can cause a rise in cerebrospinal fluid protein and carry the risk of arachnoiditis (SED-8, 820). Chemical meningitis has been reported after two intrathecal injections of methylprednisolone acetate (469) and after lumbar facet joint block (SEDA-17, 450). Intraspinal injections of hydrocortisone for multiple sclerosis apparently led in one case to a cauda equina syndrome, with subsequent ulceromutilating acropathy (SEDA-17, 450). Intra-discal injections of triamcinolone acetonide in a number of French cases led to disk or epidural calcification, sometimes symptomless (SEDA-17, 450).

Postlumbar puncture syndrome with abducent nerve palsy followed the use of intrathecal prednisolone for the treatment of low back pain and sciatica (470).

- A 38-year-old woman received intrathecal prednisolone 3 ml (strength not stated) and 1 day later developed a postural headache, nausea, and dizziness. She was treated with intravenous fluids and analgesics. Eight days later she suddenly developed a complete palsy of the right abducent nerve. An MRI brain scan showed contrast meningeal enhancement typical of postlumbar puncture syndrome. She was treated with oral glucocorticoids and blood patching was performed. Her headache began to resolve a week later. Four months later she had almost completely recovered function of her abducent nerve and a repeat MRI scan was normal.

Epidural

The indications, rationale, techniques, alternatives, contraindications, complications, and efficacy of lumbar and caudal epidural glucocorticoid injections have been reviewed (SEDA-21, 420; 471).

Bilateral posterior subcapsular cataracts have been reported after treatment with epidural methylprednisolone for low back pain secondary to degenerative joint disease and disk protrusion (472).

- A 42-year-old man had received 15 epidural injections of methylprednisolone 80 mg over 10 years. About 6 weeks after his last injection, he developed progressively worsening cloudy vision. He had bilateral posterior subcapsular cataracts and subsequently underwent bilateral cataract removal.

The authors commented that it is possible that multiple epidural glucocorticoid injections had contributed to cataract formation. The patient also had several other risk factors for cataracts (cigarette smoking, alcohol consumption, exposure to ultraviolet radiation, low socioeconomic class, and low intake of antioxidant vitamins). However, the role of these other risk factors was speculative.

Symptoms consistent with complex regional pain syndrome have been reported after a cervical epidural glucocorticoid injection (SEDA-22, 451; 473).

Spinal epidural lipomatosis secondary to exogenous administration of glucocorticoids is a rare condition that has been reported almost exclusively in association with systemic treatment. However, local epidural administration has also been implicated (474).

One case of *Staphylococcus aureus* meningitis, a rare complication of epidural analgesia, has been published. The same patient developed a cauda equina syndrome of uncertain etiology, although neural ischemia as a result of meningitis secondary to immunosuppression was possible (SEDA-21, 420; 475). A unique case of transient profound paralysis after epidural glucocorticoid injection (acute paraplegia) has now been reported (SEDA-22, 451; 476). Diplopia associated with the peridural or intrathecal infiltration of prednisolone have not been previously reported (SEDA-22, 451; 477).

Of 31 patients who received 1 ml (40 mg) of methylprednisolone epidurally at the end of microdiscectomy, three developed epidural abscesses (478). These results were compared with a historical series of 400 patients not taking glucocorticoids, who had no deep infection. Although the data were limited, epidural glucocorticoids after discectomy should not be recommended.

Cervical epidural glucocorticoid injection is often used for the treatment of cervical radiculopathy. Subjective patient satisfaction has been reported, but controlled trials have not yet delineated the effectiveness of this procedure. Three cases of severe pain consistent with nerve injury have been reported immediately after cervical epidural glucocorticoid injection, bringing into question the benefit–harm balance of this technique (479).

Intra-articular and periarticular administration

Local injections of glucocorticoids into and around the joints can have a dramatic therapeutic effect, but the catabolic effect can have serious consequences, including adverse effects on joint structure (480) and on local tendons, subcutaneous atrophy, and possibly osteonecrosis. Provided the state of the joint is carefully inspected before any new injection is given, and the interval between the injections is not less than 4 weeks, the risk seems to be small enough to justify treatment in invalidating cases (SEDA-3, 307).

Respiratory

Hiccups have been reported after intra-articular administration (481).

- A 38-year-old man had an intra-articular injection of betamethasone dipropionate (dose not stated) into his right ankle, and the day after had hiccups that lasted for 24 hours and then resolved without treatment. Some months later, because of persistent arthritis, he received a further injection of betamethasone dipropionate into his right ankle. Once again, he had hiccups the following day. On this occasion, the hiccups resolved after 2 weeks, following treatment with levomepromazine.

Psychiatric

Neuropsychiatric effects of glucocorticoids, like hallucinations, can result from intra-articular administration (SEDA-22, 444; 482).

Endocrine

An acute adrenal crisis occurred in a woman who received an intra-articular glucocorticoid for pseudogout of the knee (483).

- An 87-year-old woman received intra-articular betamethasone (Diprophos) 7 mg on three occasions for painful knee joints over 6 months. Six weeks after the last injection she developed diffuse pain and contractures in the legs, fatigue, nausea, abdominal pain, and weight loss of 6 kg. Both knee joints were tender but there was no effusion. Her serum sodium concentration was 123 mmol/l, serum osmolality 254 mosmol/kg, urine sodium 136 mmol/l, and urinary osmolality 373 mosmol/kg. The syndrome of inappropriate antidiuretic hormone secretion was diagnosed, but despite treatment she remained drowsy and hyponatremic. About a week later, she developed hypotension and symptoms of an acute abdomen. Further investigations showed that her basal cortisol concentration was low (36 nmol/l) but it increased to 481 nmol/l after a short tetracosactide test, consistent with acute adrenal crisis. She recovered rapidly after treatment with oral hydrocortisone, but still required glucocorticoid substitution several months later.

skin

An erythema multiforme-like eruption has been reported after intra-articular triamcinolone in the right knee, with cross-sensitivity to budesonide (484).

- A 70-year-old man had received three intra-articular injections of triamcinolone (dose not stated) into the same knee over 3 months without any allergic reactions. However, 12–24 hours after the last injection he developed pruritus and erythema at the injection site. This eruption was treated with topical budesonide, but within the next few hours, acute eczema developed. The lesions spread to his legs and abdomen, and were erythematous, edematous, and resembled erythema multiforme. He was treated with boric acid solution dressings, emollients, and oral antihistamines. His lesions gradually resolved and did not recur during 8 months of follow-up. A month after the lesions had resolved, he underwent patch testing, which was positive to triamcinolone 1% and budesonide 1% in petrolatum, but negative to other glucocorticoids.

Musculoskeletal

An arthropathy induced by glucocorticoid crystals has been reported (485).

- A 65-year-old man with bilateral osteoarthritis of the knees developed an effusion in the left knee. The swollen joint was treated with an intra-articular injection of triamcinolone hexacetonide 40 mg. The next day, he developed acute arthritis in the injected knee; the joint was swollen and tender and he was unable to walk. Examination of the joint fluid showed 35 ml of a thick, turbid, yellowish synovial fluid with a leukocyte count of 13 x 10^6/l (95% neutrophils). Gram and acridine orange stains were negative. Wet preparations of the specimen with polarizing compensated microscopy showed numerous birefringent, pleomorphic intra- and extracellular crystals of glucocorticoid. He underwent joint lavage with 1 l of isotonic saline and recovered completely within one day.

The conclusive diagnosis in this case was triamcinolone hexacetonide crystal-induced arthropathy.

Osteomyelitis after three glucocorticoid injections for tennis elbow has been reported; the second injection was given 3 months after the first and the third 2 days later (486). This case illustrates the need for vigilance, even after common procedures, and that exacerbation of symptoms after local glucocorticoid injections should prompt the doctor to review the diagnosis and consider the need for further investigation.

Immunologic

Anaphylaxis occurred in two women after intra-articular administration of paramethasone plus mepivacaine 2% (487).

- A 44-year-old woman developed generalized pruritus 10 minutes after intra-articular paramethasone and mepivacaine and 30 minutes later developed generalized urticaria, tachycardia, and dyspnea. She received emergency treatment and her condition initially improved. However, her symptoms recurred after 6 hours and she was treated again and then discharged taking oral dexchlorpheniramine. She had a history of allergic contact dermatitis due to nickel sulfate sensitization, and 7 years before had had generalized urticaria and dyspnea after intra-articular administration of a glucocorticoid.
- A 31-year-old woman developed generalized pruritus and urticaria, facial edema, and dyspnea 2 hours after the intra-articular administration of paramethasone and mepivacaine. She was treated with an intramuscular glucocorticoid and antihistamines, with worsening of her symptoms. She received intravenous fluids and dexchlorpheniramine, but her symptoms recurred after 1 hour, when she was given subcutaneous adrenaline, intravenous fluids and dexchlorpheniramine. She was later discharged taking oral diphenhydramine. She had a history of a systemic reaction after the administration of a glucocorticoid and a local anesthetic.

Skin prick tests were positive for isolated paramethasone in both patients, but negative for mepivacaine. There has only been one previous report of anaphylaxis in association with paramethasone.

Inadvertent intra-arterial injection

Particularly when injecting glucocorticoids locally, for example to relieve arthritis of the wrist, accidental injection into an artery is possible. Severe local ischemia can result (SEDA-17, 450).

Intracapsular injection

The use of implants for augmentation of the breast can lead to capsular contracture. Patients with intractable capsular contracture are treated with intracapsular injection of triamcinolone. Major complications included three cases of major atrophy requiring surgical correction. This problem appeared to have been eliminated by reduction of the dose of triamcinolone from 50 to 25 mg. There was one implant puncture (SEDA-19, 379; 488).

Rectal administration

Systemic absorption of glucocorticoids can occur after rectal administration.

- A 48-year-old woman developed avascular necrosis 9 months after she had completed a 3-month course of hydrocortisone 100 mg retention enemas once or twice daily for ulcerative proctitis (489). An MRI scan showed multiple bony infarcts in her distal femora, proximal tibiae, and posterior proximal right fibular head, extending from the diaphysis to the epiphysis, consistent with avascular necrosis.
- Cushing's syndrome occurred in a 65-year-old woman with ulcerative colitis who received a daily betamethasone enema (490).

The authors of the second report reported the pharmacokinetics of betamethasone after rectal dosing, with plasma concentrations of betamethasone high enough to cause Cushing's syndrome. Suppression of the hypothalamic–pituitary–adrenal axis disappeared after the dosage schedule was changed from daily to three times a week. These findings suggest that a considerable amount of betamethasone is absorbed after rectal dosing.

Occupational exposure

Occupational exposure to glucocorticoids can cause adverse effects. Facial plethora has been found in workers manufacturing synthetic glucocorticoids, some of them having grossly abnormal responses to tetracosactide.

- A 58-year-old woman, who had been involved in the manufacturing of glucocorticoid creams and ointments for over 10 years, developed occupational contact sensitization to topical glucocorticoids (491). Patch tests were positive to hydrocortisone, hydrocortisone butyrate, and tixocortol pivalate. Intradermal tests were positive to hydrocortisone succinate, methylprednisolone, and prednisolone. An oral challenge with betamethasone 0.75 mg, 2.5 mg, and 8 mg on three consecutive days resulted in no adverse reactions.

It has been recommended that all workers manufacturing potent glucocorticoids should be screened regularly for glucocorticoid overdosage and should be moved regularly to units processing other drugs (492).

Drug overdose

High doses of glucocorticoids in patients with cancers can increase the risk of metastases, for example in breast cancer; this has been attributed in some cases to immunosuppression (493). These hormones should therefore only be used in patients with those types of tumors for which they are known to improve the efficacy of the cancer treatment.

A curious reaction to intravenous high-dose dexamethasone, used as an antiemetic agent in cancer chemotherapy or for other purposes, is sudden severe itching, burning, and constrictive pain in the perineal region, which has been described in several published reports (SEDA-11, 336; 494).

Drug–Drug Interactions

Albendazole

Dexamethasone reduced the clearance of albendazole and increased its half-life; plasma concentrations almost doubled (SEDA-22, 450; 495).

Amiodarone

Budesonide for collagenous colitis caused Cushing's syndrome in a patient with chronic renal insufficiency taking amiodarone for paroxysmal atrial fibrillation (496).

- An 81-year-old man with persistent diarrhea was given oral budesonide 9 mg/day, following unsuccessful treatment with mesalazine and prednisone. He was also taking amiodarone 100 mg/day. His diarrhea resolved within 6 weeks, and attempts to reduce the dosage of bzudesonide resulted in recurrent diarrhea. After 11 months he developed Cushing's syndrome, which persisted despite a reduction in dosage to 3 mg/day. His mild diarrhea recurred and the dosage of budesonide was increased to 6 mg/day with worsening of Cushing's syndrome; the dosage was reduced to 3 mg/day. Four weeks later amiodarone was withdrawn. The symptoms of Cushing's syndrome resolved within 4 weeks.

The authors suggested that the development of Cushing's syndrome and its persistence at a low dosage of budesonide was caused by inhibition of the metabolism of budesonide by amiodarone.

Anticoagulants

Intravenous methylprednisolone (1 g/day for 3 days) has been reported to inhibit the metabolism of oral anticoagulants (acenocoumarol and fluindione) in 10 patients, increasing the INR by 8 (range 5–20; 497).

Glucocorticoids can also alter the response to anticoagulants. A raised tolerance to heparin has been reported and a fall in fibrinolytic activity has been seen during glucocorticoid treatment (SED-8, 816). The entire clotting mechanism and particularly the prothrombin time should therefore be checked periodically in patients taking glucocorticoids concomitantly with anticoagulants, particularly if the glucocorticoid dose is changed. In addition there is an increased risk of gastric bleeding in patients taking both glucocorticoids and anticoagulants.

Antifungal azoles

Itraconazole 200 mg/day markedly increased plasma methylprednisolone concentrations and reduced morning plasma cortisol concentrations by over 80% in 10 healthy volunteers (498). The C_{max}, AUC, and half-life of methylprednisolone were increased 1.9, 3.9, and 2.4 times respectively.

Itraconazole 200 mg/day orally for 4 days markedly reduced the clearance and increased the half-life of intravenous methylprednisolone from 2.1 to 4.8 hours in a double-blind, randomized, two-phase, crossover study in nine healthy volunteers (SEDA-23, 430; 499). The volume of distribution was not affected. The mean morning plasma cortisol concentration during the itraconazole phase, measured 24 hours after methylprednisolone, was only 9% of that during the placebo phase (11 versus 117 ng/ml).

The authors of these two reports recommended that care be taken when methylprednisolone is prescribed in combination with itraconazole or other potent inhibitors of CYP3A4.

- Cushing's syndrome developed rapidly in a 55-year-old man who took itraconazole for 6 weeks in addition to inhaled fluticasone and resolved after withdrawal of itraconazole (500). Cushing's syndrome was attributed to increased systemic concentrations of fluticasone associated with adrenal insufficiency due to suppression of pituitary corticotropin secretion.

Although itraconazole can also directly inhibit adrenal steroidogenesis, this usually happens at a much higher dose and there was no concomitant rise in corticotropin.

Itraconazole, given orally increased oral prednisolone concentrations by only 24% (501) but increased intravenous dexamethasone concentrations 3.3-fold and oral dexamethasone 3.7-fold (502).

In another study, ketoconazole was given orally as 200 mg od for 4 days, following a single oral dose of budesonide 3 mg either at the same time as ketoconazole or 12 hours before (501). Ketoconazole increased budesonide concentrations (C_{max} and AUC) 6.8- to 7.6-fold when the two drugs were co-administered; with a 12-hour separation, budesonide concentrations increased only 1.7- to 2.1-fold.

Aprepitant

Aprepitant is a neurokinin-1 receptor antagonist that, in combination with a glucocorticoid and a $5HT_3$ receptor antagonist, is very effective in preventing chemotherapy-induced nausea and vomiting. At therapeutic doses it is also a moderate inhibitor of CYP3A4. Coadministration of aprepitant with dexamethasone or methylprednisolone resulted in increased plasma glucocorticoid concentrations (504). These findings suggest that the dose of these glucocorticoids should be adjusted when aprepitant is given.

Calcium channel blockers

Methylprednisolone concentrations increased with the co-administration of diltiazem (2.6-fold) and mibefradil (3.8-fold; 505).

Ciclosporin

Glucocorticoids cause additive immunosuppression when they are given with other immunosuppressants, such as ciclosporin (SEDA-22, 451; 506).

The AUC of plasma prednisolone has been studied in patients with stable renal transplants (507). The prednisolone AUC was significantly higher in women and in those who took ciclosporin. The highest AUC was in women taking estrogen supplements and ciclosporin. A significantly higher proportion of patients taking ciclosporin + azathioprine + prednisolone had glucocorticoid adverse effects compared with those taking azathioprine + prednisolone. Furthermore, more women than men had adverse effects and the prednisone AUC was greater in those with adverse effects than without. Ciclosporin was thought to have increased the systemic availability of prednisolone, most probably by inhibiting P glycoprotein. Because the major contributor to AUC is the maximum post-dose concentration, it may be possible to use single-point monitoring (2 hours after the dose) for routine clinical studies.

Clarithromycin

Clarithromycin inhibits CYP3A4, which is responsible for the metabolic clearance of prednisolone, the biologically active metabolite of prednisone. Clarithromycin (500 mg bd for 2 days) reduced the clearance of methylprednisolone by 65% and significantly increased its plasma concentrations; clarithromycin did not influence the clearance or plasma concentrations of prednisone (508). Acute mania has been reported to be related to inhibition of the metabolic clearance of prednisone by clarithromycin (SEDA-22, 444; 509).

Cyclophosphamide

The effect of prednisone 1 mg/kg on the pharmacokinetics of cyclophosphamide and its initial metabolites 4-hydroxycyclophosphamide and aldophosphamide (the acyclic tautomer of 4-hydroxycyclophosphamide) has been studied between the first and sixth cycles in seven patients (two men) with systemic vasculitis receiving intravenous cyclophosphamide 0.6 g/m² as a 1-hour intravenous infusion every 3 weeks for six cycles (510). Prednisone reduced the clearance of cyclophosphamide from 5.8 to 4.0 l/hour, reducing the amount of initial metabolites formed. Although the clinical significance of this interaction is unclear, 4-hydroxycyclophosphamide and aldophosphamide are probably responsible for the cytotoxic activity of cyclophosphamide, and increased cyclophosphamide dosages should be considered in patients taking prednisone.

Diuretics

Glucocorticoids with mineralocorticoid activity potentiate potassium loss when they are given with potassium-wasting diuretics (511).

Globulin

A case report with a review of 27 cases of thromboembolic events after the administration of intravenous globulin with or without glucocorticoids has been published (512). The authors suggested that this combined therapy should be administered with caution because of its potential synergistic thrombotic risk.

Grapefruit juice

Methylprednisolone concentrations increased with the co-administration of grapefruit juice (1.75-fold; 513).

Leukotriene receptor antagonists

In a probable pharmacodynamic interaction, severe peripheral edema followed treatment with montelukast and prednisone for asthma (514).

- A 23-year-old man, with a history of asthma, house dust mite allergy, and rhinoconjunctivitis, presented with acute respiratory symptoms. He was given oral cetirizine, inhaled salmeterol, and fluticasone propionate, and oral prednisone 40 mg/day for 1 week and 20 mg/day for 1 week. His asthma recurred when prednisone was withdrawn and he took oral prednisone 60 mg/day for 1 week and 40 mg/day for 1 week. He also took montelukast 10 mg/day. He then developed severe peripheral edema with a gain in weight of 13 kg. Prednisone was withdrawn and his edema resolved. Montelukast was continued.

The author commented that the patient had tolerated prednisone without montelukast and montelukast without prednisone. However, he had severe edema when both drugs were used together. Montelukast may have potentiated glucocorticoid-induced renal tubular sodium and fluid retention. Both have been associated with edema.

Oral contraceptives

Oral contraceptives increased budesonide concentrations by only 22%, but prednisolone concentrations increased by 131%, suggesting a clinically important interaction (515).

Phenobarbital

Phenobarbital increases the metabolism of glucocorticoids, reducing the half-life by some 50% (516).

Phenytoin

Phenytoin increases the metabolism of glucocorticoids, reducing the half-life by some 50% (516).

Rifampicin

Rifampicin and other drugs that induce liver enzymes increase the metabolism of glucocorticoids (517), sufficient to reduce their therapeutic effects, for example in asthma (518).

Ritonavir

Iatrogenic Cushing's syndrome with secondary adrenal insufficiency has been described in two children (12 and 15 year-old girls) with HIV infection taking oral ritonavir and inhaled fluticasone (519). The combination of these drugs can cause Cushing syndrome and adrenal suppression in children, potentially leading to misdiagnosis of lipodystrophy syndrome and to an increased risk of adrenal crisis during acute illnesses (520).

Salicylates

Glucocorticoids reduce the plasma concentrations of salicylates (521). If they are given with aspirin or other anti-inflammatory drugs, there may be an additive effect on the gastric wall, leading to an increased risk of bleeding and ulceration (522–524).

Warfarin

In a retrospective study using the medical records of 387 patients to evaluate a possible interaction between corticoids and warfarin; 32 fulfilled the inclusion criteria of stable anticoagulation therapy, short-term oral glucocorticoid therapy, an INR recorded within 30 days before the start of glucocorticoid therapy, and an INR recorded during corticosteroid therapy or within 14 days of withdrawal (525). Most of the patients had a raised INR after concomitant use of warfarin and glucocorticoids. The mean difference between pre- and post-INR values was 1.24 (95% CI = 0.86, 1.62). The change in INR occurred at a mean of 7 days after the first dose of glucocorticoid. Only one adverse event, minor epistaxis, was reported, and no visits or hospitalizations occurred as a consequence of the interaction. Thus, the use of oral glucocorticoids in patients taking long-term warfarin therapy may result in a clinically important interaction, which requires INR monitoring and possible warfarin dosage reduction.

Diagnosis of Adverse Drug Reactions

The short Synacthen (tetracosactide) test is the most commonly used test for assessing adrenal suppression. The potential of a simpler and more cost-effective procedure, the morning salivary cortisol concentration, as an out-patient screening tool to detect adrenal suppression in patients using topical intranasal glucocorticoids for rhinosinusitis has been investigated in 48 patients who were using topical glucocorticoids (526). The morning salivary cortisol measurement was a useful screening tool for adrenal suppression in this setting.

Osteoporosis and osteopenia are usually evaluated by measuring bone density using dual-energy X-ray absorptiometry (DXA). However, there is increased interest in measuring not only bone density but also some structural properties of the bone, such as elasticity and trabecular stiffness and connectivity, which are more closely related to bone strength. Quantitative ultrasound could theoretically provide information on bone structure, as has been suggested by a prospective study in patients with glucocorticoid-induced osteoporosis (527), but further studies are needed to define the role of quantitative ultrasonography in the prediction of fracture and in the clinical management of glucocorticoid-induced osteoporosis.

Management of Adverse Drug Reactions

Mood stabilizers, such as lithium, lamotrigine, and carbamazepine, may be effective in treating glucocorticoid-induced mood symptoms. In an open trial, 12 patients with glucocorticoid-induced manic or mixed symptoms were treated with olanzapine 2.5 mg/day initially, increasing to a maximum of 20 mg/day; 11 of the 12 patients had significant improvement (528).

References

1. Kaiser H. Cortisone derivate in Klinik und PraxisStuttgart-New York: Thieme;. 1987.
2. Labhart A. Adrenal cortex. In: Labhart A, editor. Clinical Endocrinology. Berlin-Heidelberg-New York: Springer, 1985:373.
3. Medici TC, Ruegsegger P. Does alternate-day cloprednol therapy prevent bone loss? A longitudinal double-blind, controlled clinical study. Clin Pharmacol Ther 1990;48(4):455–66.
4. Iwasaki E, Baba M. [Pharmacokinetics and pharmacodynamics of hydrocortisone in asthmatic children.]Arerugi 1993;42(10):1555–62.
5. Bone RC, Fisher CJ Jr, Clemmer TP, Slotman GJ, Metz CA, Balk RA. A controlled clinical trial of high-dose methylprednisolone in the treatment of severe sepsis and septic shock. N Engl J Med 1987;317(11):653–8.
6. The Veterans Administration Systemic Sepsis Cooperative Study Group. Effect of high-dose glucocorticoid therapy on mortality in patients with clinical signs of systemic sepsis. N Engl J Med 1987;317(11):659–65.
7. Iuchi T, Akaike M, Mitsui T, Ohshima Y, Shintani Y, Azuma H, Matsumoto T. Glucocorticoid excess induces superoxide production in vascular endothelial cells and elicits vascular endothelial dysfunction. Circ Res 2003; 92:81–7.
8. Romagnoli C, Zecca E, Vento G, De Carolis MP, Papacci P, Tortorolo G. Early postnatal dexamethasone for the prevention of chronic lung disease in high-risk preterm infants. Intensive Care Med 1999;25(7):717–21.
9. Confalonieri M, Urbino R, Potena A, Piattella M, Parigi P, Puccio G, Della Porta R, Giorgio C, Blasi F, Umberger R, Meduri GU. Hydrocortisone infusion for severe community-acquired pneumonia: a preliminary randomized study. Am J Respir Crit Care Med 2005; 171(3): 242-8.
10. Garland JS, Alex CP, Pauly TH, Whitehead VL, Brand J, Winston JF, Samuels DP, McAuliffe TL. A three-day course of dexamethasone therapy to prevent chronic lung disease in ventilated neonates: a randomized trial. Pediatrics 1999;104(1 Part 1):91–9.
11. Romagnoli C, Zecca E, Vento G, Maggio L, Papacci P, Tortorolo G. Effect on growth of two different dexamethasone courses for preterm infants at risk of chronic lung disease. A randomized trial. Pharmacology 1999;59(5):266–74.
12. Tarnow-Mordi W, Mitra A. Postnatal dexamethasone in preterm infants is potentially lifesaving, but follow up studies are urgently needed. BMJ 1999;319(7222):1385–6.
13. van de Beek D, de Gans J, McIntyre P, Prasad K. Steroids in adults with acute bacterial meningitis: a systematic review. Lancet Infect Dis 2004; 4: 139-43.
14. Arias-Camison JM, Lau J, Cole CH, Frantz ID 3rd. Meta-analysis of dexamethasone therapy started in the first 15 days of life for prevention of chronic lung disease in premature infants. Pediatr Pulmonol 1999;28(3):167–74.
15. Klein-Gitelman MS, Pachman LM. Intravenous corticosteroids: adverse reactions are more variable than expected in children. J Rheumatol 1998;25(10):1995–2002.
16. Feldweg AM, Leddy JP. Drug interactions affecting the efficacy of corticosteroid therapy. A brief review with an illustrative case. J Clin Rheumatol 1999;5:143–50.
17. Maxwell SR, Moots RJ, Kendall MJ. Corticosteroids: do they damage the cardiovascular system? Postgrad Med J 1994;70(830):863–70.
18. Ellis SG, Semenec T, Lander K, Franco I, Raymond R, Whitlow PL. Effects of long-term prednisone (> = 5 mg) use on outcomes and complications of percutaneous coronary intervention. Am J Cardiol 2004; 93: 1389-90.
19. Sato A, Funder JW, Okubo M, Kubota E, Saruta T. Glucocorticoid-induced hypertension in the elderly. Relation to serum calcium and family history of essential hypertension. Am J Hypertens 1995;8(8):823–8.
20. Thedenat B, Leaute-Labreze C, Boralevi F, Roul S, Labbe L, Marliere V, Taieb A. Surveillance tensionnelle des nourrissons traites par corticotherapie generale pour un hemangiome. [Blood pressure monitoring in infants with hemangiomas treated with corticosteroids.] Ann Dermatol Venereol 2002;129(2):183–5.
21. Stewart IM, Marks JSECG. Abnormalities in steroid-treated rheumatoid patients. Lancet 1977;2(8050):1237–8.
22. Baty V, Blain H, Saadi L, Jeandel C, Canton P. Fatal myocardial infarction in an elderly woman with severe ulcerative colitis. what is the role of steroids? Am J Gastroenterol 1998;93(10):2000–1.
23. Machiels JP, Jacques JM, de Meester A. Coronary artery spasm during anaphylaxis. Ann Emerg Med 1996;27(5):674–5.
24. Sato O, Takagi A, Miyata T, Takayama Y. Aortic aneurysms in patients with autoimmune disorders treated with corticosteroids. Eur J Vasc Endovasc Surg 1995;10(3):366–9.
25. Kotha P, McGreevy MJ, Kotha A, Look M, Weisman MH. Early deaths with thrombolytic therapy for acute myocardial infarction in corticosteroid-dependent rheumatoid arthritis. Clin Cardiol 1998;21(11):853–6.
26. Yunis KA, Bitar FF, Hayek P, Mroueh SM, Mikati M. Transient hypertrophic cardiomyopathy in the newborn following multiple doses of antenatal corticosteroids. Am J Perinatol 1999;16(1):17–21.
27. Gill AW, Warner G, Bull L. Iatrogenic neonatal hypertrophic cardiomyopathy. Pediatr Cardiol 1996;17(5):335–9.
28. Pokorny JJ, Roth F, Balfour I, Rinehart G. An unusual complication of the treatment of a hemangioma. Ann Plast Surg 2002;48(1):83–7.
29. Kothari SN, Kisken WA. Dexamethasone-induced congestive heart failure in a patient with dilated cardiomyopathy caused by occult pheochromocytoma. Surgery 1998;123(1):102–5.
30. Balys R, Manoukian J, Zalai C. Left ventricular hypertrophy with outflow tract obstruction-a complication of dexamethasone treatment for subglottic stenosis. Int J Pediatr Otorhinolaryngol 2005; 69(2): 271–3.

31. Kucukosmanoglu O, Karabay A, Ozbarlas N, Noyan A, Anarat A. Marked bradycardia due to pulsed and oral methylprednisolone therapy in a patient with rapidly progressive glomerulonephritis. Nephron 1998;80(4):484.

32. Schult M, Lohmann D, Knitsch W, Kuse ER, Nashan B. Recurrent cardiocirculatory arrest after kidney transplantation related to intravenous methylprednisolone bolus therapy. Transplantation 1999;67(11):1497–8.

33. Brumund MR, Truemper EJ, Lutin WA, Pearson-Shaver AL. Disseminated varicella and staphylococcal pericarditis after topical steroids. J Pediatr 1997;131(1 Part 1):162–3.

34. Kaiser H. Cortisonderivate in Klink und Praxis. 7th edn.. Stuttgart: G.Thieme;. 1977.

35. Williamson IJ, Matusiewicz SP, Brown PH, Greening AP, Crompton GK. Frequency of voice problems and cough in patients using pressurized aerosol inhaled steroid preparations. Eur Respir J 1995;8(4):590–2.

36. Lim BS, Choi WY, Choi JW. A case of steroid-induced intractable hiccup. Tuberc Respir Dis 1991;38:304–7.

37. Cersosimo RJ, Brophy MT. Hiccups with high dose dexamethasone administration: a case report. Cancer 1998;82(2):412–4.

38. Ross J, Eledrisi M, Casner P. Persistent hiccups induced by dexamethasone. West J Med 1999;170(1):51–2.

39. Poynter D. Beclomethasone dipropionate aerosol and nasal mucosa. Br J Clin Pharmacol 1977;4(Suppl 3):S295–301.

40. Albucher JF, Vuillemin-Azais C, Manelfe C, Clanet M, Guiraud-Chaumeil B, Chollet F. Cerebral thrombophlebitis in three patients with probable multiple sclerosis. Role of lumbar puncture or intravenous corticosteroid treatment. Cerebrovasc Dis 1999;9(5):298–303.

41. Shinwell ES, Karplus M, Reich D, Weintraub Z, Blazer S, Bader D, Yurman S, Dolfin T, Kogan A, Dollberg S, Arbel E, Goldberg M, Gur I, Naor N, Sirota L, Mogilner S, Zaritsky A, Barak M, Gottfried E. Early postnatal dexamethasone treatment and increased incidence of cerebral palsy. Arch Dis Child Fetal Neonatal Ed 2000;83(3):F177–81.

42. Halliday HL. Postnatal steroids and chronic lung disease in the newborn. Paediatr Respir Rev 2004; 5 Suppl A: S245-8.

43. Yeh TF, Lin YJ, Lin HC, Huang CC, Hsieh WS, Lin CH, Tsai CH. Outcomes at school age after postnatal dexamethasone therapy for lung disease of prematurity. N Engl J Med 2004; 350: 1304-13.

44. Bentson J, Reza M, Winter J, Wilson G. Steroids and apparent cerebral atrophy on computed tomography scans. J Comput Assist Tomogr 1978;2(1):16–23.

45. Vaughn BV, Ali II, Olivier KN, Lackner RP, Robertson KR, Messenheimer JA, Paradowski LJ, Egan TM. Seizures in lung transplant recipients. Epilepsia 1996;37(12):1175–9.

46. Lorrot M, Bader-Meunier B, Sebire G, Dommergues JP. Hypertension intracranienne benigne: une complication meconnue de la corticotherapie. [Benign intracranial hypertension: an unrecognized complication of corticosteroid therapy.] Arch Pediatr 1999;6(1):40–2.

47. Kalapurakal JA, Silverman CL, Akhtar N, Laske DW, Braitman LE, Boyko OB, Thomas PR. Intracranial meningiomas: factors that influence the development of cerebral edema after stereotactic radiosurgery and radiation therapy. Radiology 1997;204(2):461–5.

48. Laroche F, Chemouilli R, Carlier P. Efficacy of conservative treatment in a patient with spinal cord compression due to corticosteroid-induced epidural lipomatosis. Rev Rheum (English Edn) 1993;30:729–31.

49. Roy-Camille R, Mazel C, Husson JL, Saillant G. Symptomatic spinal epidural lipomatosis induced by a long-term steroid treatment. Review of the literature and report of two additional cases. Spine 1991;16(12):1365–71.

50. Andress HJ, Schurmann M, Heuck A, Schmand J, Lob G. A rare case of osteoporotic spine fracture associated with epidural lipomatosis causing paraplegia following long-term cortisone therapy. Arch Orthop Trauma Surg 2000;120(7–8):484–6.

51. Pinsker MO, Kinzel D, Lumenta CB. Epidural thoracic lipomatosis induced by long-term steroid treatment case illustration. Acta Neurochir (Wien) 1998;140(9):991–2.

52. Parker CT, Jarek MJ, Finger DR. Corticosteroid-associated epidural lipomatosis. J Clin Rheumatol 1999;5:141–2.

53. Kano K, Kyo K, Ito S, Nishikura K, Ando T, Yamada Y, Arisaka O. Spinal epidural lipomatosis in children with renal diseases receiving steroid therapy. Pediatr Nephrol 2005; 20(2): 184-9.

54. Donaghy M, Mills KR, Boniface SJ, Simmons J, Wright I, Gregson N, Jacobs J. Pure motor demyelinating neuropathy: deterioration after steroid treatment and improvement with intravenous immunoglobulin. J Neurol Neurosurg Psychiatry 1994;57(7):778–83.

55. Sevem PS, Fraser SG. Bilateral cataracts and glaucoma induced by long-term use of oral prednisolone bought over the internet. Lancet 2006; 386: 618.

56. Urban RC Jr, Cotlier E. Corticosteroid-induced cataracts. Surv Ophthalmol 1986;31(2):102–10.

57. Kaye LD, Kalenak JW, Price RL, Cunningham R. Ocular implications of long-term prednisone therapy in children. J Pediatr Ophthalmol Strabismus 1993;30(3):142–4.

58. Cumming RG, Mitchell P, Leeder SR. Use of inhaled corticosteroids and the risk of cataracts. N Engl J Med 1997;337(1):8–14.

59. Abramson HA. May corticosteroid cataracts be reversible. J Asthma Res 1977;14(3):vii–viii.

60. Lubkin VL. Steroid cataract – a review and a conclusion. J Asthma Res 1977;14(2):55–9.

61. Forman AR, Loreto JA, Tina LU. Reversibility of corticosteroid-associated cataracts in children with the nephrotic syndrome. Am J Ophthalmol 1977;84(1):75–8.

62. Wingate RJ, Beaumont PE. Intravitreal triamcinolone and elevated intraocular pressure. Aust NZ J Ophthalmol 1999;27(6):431–2.

63. Garbe E, LeLorier J, Boivin JF, Suissa S. Risk of ocular hypertension or open-angle glaucoma in elderly patients on oral glucocorticoids. Lancet 1997;350(9083):979–82.

64. Garbe E, LeLorier J, Boivin JF, Suissa S. Inhaled and nasal glucocorticoids and the risks of ocular hypertension or open-angle glaucoma. JAMA 1997;277(9):722–7.

65. Novack GD. Ocular toxicology. Curr Opin Ophthalmol 1994;5(6):110–4.

66. Opatowsky I, Feldman RM, Gross R, Feldman ST. Intraocular pressure elevation associated with inhalation and nasal corticosteroids. Ophthalmology 1995;102(2):177–9.

67. Kwok AK, Lam DS, Ng JS, Fan DS, Chew SJ, Tso MO. Ocular-hypertensive response to topical steroids in children. Ophthalmology 1997;104(12):2112–6.

68. Tham CCY, Ng JSK, Li RTH, Chik KW, Lam DSC. Intraocular pressure profile of a child on a systemic corticosteroid. Am J Ophthalmol 2004; 137: 198–201.

69. Gass JD, Little H. Bilateral bullous exudative retinal detachment complicating idiopathic central serous chorioretinopathy during systemic corticosteroid therapy. Ophthalmology 1995;102(5):737–47.

70. Karadimas P, Bouzas EA. Glucocorticoid use represents a risk factor for central serous chorioretinopathy: a prospective, case-control study. Graefe's Arch Clin Exp Ophthalmol 2004; 242: 800–2.

71. Baumal CR, Martidis A, Truong SN. Central serous chorioretinopathy associated with periocular corticosteroid injection treatment for HLA-B27-associated iritis. Arch Ophthalmol 2004; 122: 926-8.

72. Roth DB, Chieh J, Spirn MJ, Green SN, Yarian DL, Chaudhry NA. Noninfectious endophthalmitis associated with intravitreal triamcinolone injection. Arch Ophthalmol 2003; 121: 1279-82.

73. Roth DB, Chieh J, Spirn MJ, Green SN, Yarian DL, Chaudhry NA. Noninfectious endophthalmitis associated with intravitreal triamcinolone injection. Arch Ophthalmol 2003; 121: 1279-82.

74. Chen SDM, Lochhead J, McDonald B, Patel CK. Pseudohypopyon after intravitreal triamcinolone injection for the treatment of pseudophakic cystoid macular oedema. Br J Ophthalmol 2004; 88: 843-4.

75. Apel A, Campbell I, Rootman DS. Infectious crystalline keratopathy following trabeculectomy and low-dose topical steroids. Cornea 1995;14(3):321–3.

76. Rao GP, O'Brien C, Hicky-Dwyer M, Patterson A. Rapid onset bilateral calcific band keratopathy associated with phosphate-containing steroid eye drops. Eur J Implant Refractive Surg 1995;7:251–2.

77. Ramanathan R, Siassi B, deLemos RA. Severe retinopathy of prematurity in extremely low birth weight infants after short-term dexamethasone therapy. J Perinatol 1995;15(3):178–82.

78. Kushner FH, Olson JC. Retinal hemorrhage as a consequence of epidural steroid injection. Arch Ophthalmol 1995;113(3):309–13.

79. Byers B. Blindness secondary to steroid injections into the nasal turbinates. Arch Ophthalmol 1979;97(1):79–80.

80. Van Dalen JT, Sherman MD. Corticosteroid-induced exophthalmos. Doc Ophthalmol 1989;72(3–4):273–7.

81. Klein JF. Adverse psychiatric effects of systemic glucocorticoid therapy. Am Fam Physician 1992;46(5):1469–74.

82. Doherty M, Garstin I, McClelland RJ, Rowlands BJ, Collins BJ. A steroid stupor in a surgical ward. Br J Psychiatry 1991;158:125–7.

83. Satel SL. Mental status changes in children receiving glucocorticoids. Review of the literature. Clin Pediatr (Phila) 1990;29(7):383–8.

84. Alpert E, Seigerman C. Steroid withdrawal psychosis in a patient with closed head injury. Arch Phys Med Rehabil 1986;67(10):766–9.

85. Hassanyeh F, Murray RB, Rodgers H. Adrenocortical suppression presenting with agitated depression, morbid jealousy, and a dementia-like state. Br J Psychiatry 1991;159:870–2.

86. Nahon S, Pisanté L, Delas N. A successful switch from prednisone to budesonide for neuropsychiatric adverse effects in a patient with ileal Crohn's disease. Am J Gastroenterol 2001;96(1):1953–4.

87. Brown ES, J Woolston D, Frol A, Bobadilla L, Khan DA, Hanczyc M, Rush AJ, Fleckenstein J, Babcock E, Cullum CM. Hippocampal volume, spectroscopy, cognition, and mood in patients receiving corticosteroid therapy. Biol Psychiatry 2004; 55: 538-45.

88. O'Shea TM, Kothadia JM, Klinepeter KL, Goldstein DJ, Jackson BG, Weaver RG III, Dillard RG. Randomized placebo-controlled trial of a 42-day tapering course of dexamethasone to reduce the duration of ventilator dependency in very low birth weight infants: outcome of study participants at 1-year adjusted age. Pediatrics 1999;104(1 Part 1):15–21.

89. Soliday E, Grey S, Lande MB. Behavioral effects of corticosteroids in steroid–sensitive nephrotic syndrome. Pediatrics 1999;104(4):e51.

90. Kaiser H. Psychische Storungen nach Beclomethasondipropionat-Inhalation?. [Mental disorders following beclomethasone dipropionate inhalation?.] Med Klin 1978;73(38):1334.

91. Keenan PA, Jacobson MW, Soleymani RM, Mayes MD, Stress ME, Yaldoo DT. The effect on memory of chronic prednisone treatment in patients with systemic disease. Neurology 1996;47(6):1396–402.

92. Oliveri RL, Sibilia G, Valentino P, Russo C, Romeo N, Quattrone A. Pulsed methylprednisolone induces a reversible impairment of memory in patients with relapsing-remitting multiple sclerosis. Acta Neurol Scand 1998;97(6):366–9.

93. Newcomer JW, Selke G, Melson AK, Hershey I, Craft S, Richards K, Alderson AL. Decreased memory performance in healthy humans induced by stress-level cortisol treatment. Arch Gen Psychiatry 1999;56(6):527–33.

94. Aisen PS, Davis KL, Berg JD, Schafer K, Campbell K, Thomas RG, Weiner MF, Farlow MR, Sano M, Grundman M, Thal LJ. A randomized controlled trial of prednisone in Alzheimer's disease. Alzheimer's Dis Cooperative Study. Neurology 2000;54(3):588–93.

95. de Quervain DJ, Roozendaal B, Nitsch RM, McGaugh JL, Hock C. Acute cortisone administration impairs retrieval of long-term declarative memory in humans. Nat Neurosci 2000;3(4):313–4.

96. Bermond B, Surachno S, Lok A, ten Berge IJ, Plasmans B, Kox C, Schuller E, Schellekens PT, Hamel R. Memory functions in prednisone-treated kidney transplant patients. Clin Transplant 2005; 19(4): 512-7.

97. Brown ES, Stuard G, Liggin JD, Hukovic N, Frol A, Dhanani N, Khan DA, Jeffress J, Larkin GL, McEwen BS, Rosenblatt R, Mageto Y, Hanczyc M, Cullum CM. Effect of phenytoin on mood and declarative memory during prescription corticosteroid therapy. Biol Psychiatry 2005; 57(5): 543-8.

98. Moser NJ, Phillips BA, Guthrie G, Barnett G. Effects of dexamethasone on sleep. Pharmacol Toxicol 1996;79(2):100–2.

99. Chau SY, Mok CC. Factors predictive of corticosteroid psychosis in patients with systemic lupus erythematosus. Neurology 2003; 61: 104-7.

100. Bolanos SH, Khan DA, Hanczyc M, Bauer MS, Dhanani N, Brown ES. Assessment of mood states in patients receiving long-term corticosteroid therapy and in controls with patient-rated and clinician-rated scales. Ann Allergy Asthma Immunol 2004; 92: 500-5.

101. Preda A, Fazeli A, McKay BG, Bowers MB Jr, Mazure CM. Lamotrigine as prophylaxis against steroid-induced mania. J Clin Psychiatry 1999;60(10):708–9.

102. Preda A, Fazeli A, McKay BG, Bowers MB Jr, Mazure CM. Lamotrigine of prophylaxis against steroid-induced mania. J. Clin Psychiatry 1999;60(10):708–9.

103. Brown ES, Suppes T, Khan DA, Carmody TJ 3rd. Mood changes during prednisone bursts in outpatients with asthma. J Clin Psychopharmacol 2002;22(1):55–61.

104. Wada K, Suzuki H, Taira T, Akiyama K, Kuroda S. Successful use of intravenous clomipramine in depressive–catatonic state associated with corticosteroid treatment. Int J Psych Clin Pract 2004; 8: 131-3.

105. Ilbeigi MS, Davidson ML, Yarmush JM. An unexpected arousal effect of etomidate in a patient on high-dose steroids. Anesthesiology 1998;89(6):1587–9.

106. Kramer TM, Cottingham EM. Risperidone in the treatment of steroid-induced psychosis. J Child Adolesc Psychopharmacol 1999;9(4):315–6.

107. Scheschonka A, Bleich S, Buchwald AB, Ruther E, Wiltfang J. Development of obsessive-compulsive behaviour following cortisone treatment. Pharmacopsychiatry 2002;35(2):72–4.

108. Kamoda T, Nakahara C, Matsui A. A case of empty sella after steroid pulse therapy for nephrotic syndrome. J Rheumatol 1998;25(4):822–3.

109. Rabhan NB. Pituitary-adrenal suppression and Cushing's syndrome after intermittent dexamethasone therapy. Ann Intern Med 1968;69(6):1141–8.

110. Zwaan CM, Odink RJ, Delemarre-van de Waal HA, Dankert-Roelse JE, Bokma JA. Acute adrenal insufficiency after discontinuation of inhaled corticosteroid therapy. Lancet 1992;340(8830):1289–90.

111. Clark DJ, Grove A, Cargill RI, Lipworth BJ. Comparative adrenal suppression with inhaled budesonide and fluticasone propionate in adult asthmatic patients. Thorax 1996;51(3):262–6.

112. Marazzi MG, Agnese G, Gremmo M, Cotellessa M, Garibaldi L. Problemi relativi alla funzionalita surrenalica in corso di terapia cortisonica protratta in soggetti con epatite cronica: nota preliminare. [Problems concerning adrenal function during prolonged corticoid treatment in patients with chronic hepatitis. Preliminary note.] Minerva Pediatr 1978;30(11):937–44.

113. Dutau G, Rochiccioli P. Exploration corticotrope au cours des traitements prolongés par le dipropionate de béclométhasone chez l'enfant. [Corticotropic testing during long-term beclomethasone dipropionate treatment asthmatic children.] Poumon Coeur 1978;34(4):247–53.

114. Sumboonnanonda A, Vongjirad A, Suntornpoch V, Petrarat S. Adrenal function after prednisolone treatment in childhood nephrotic syndrome. J Med Assoc Thai 1994;77(3):126–9.

115. Felner EI, Thompson MT, Ratliff AF, White PC, Dickson BA. Time course of recovery of adrenal function in children treated for leukemia. J Pediatr 2000;137(1):21–4.

116. Reiner M, Galeazzi RL, Studer H. Cushing-Syndrom und Nebennierenrinden-Suppression durch intranasale Anwendung von Dexamethasonpraparaten. [Cushing's syndrome and adrenal suppression by means of intranasal use of dexamethasone preparations.] Schweiz Med Wochenschr 1977;107(49):1836–7.

117. Kay J, Findling JW, Raff H. Epidural triamcinolone suppresses the pituitary–adrenal axis in human subjects. Anesth Analg 1994;79(3):501–5.

118. Boonen S, Van Distel G, Westhovens R, Dequeker J. Steroid myopathy induced by epidural triamcinolone injection. Br J Rheumatol 1995;34(4):385–6.

119. Kobayashi S, Warabi H, Hashimoto H. Hypopituitarism with empty sella after steroid pulse therapy. J Rheumatol 1997;24(1):236–8.

120. Grabner W. Zur induzierten NNR-Insuffizienz bei chirurgischen Eingriffen. [Problems of corticosteroid-induced adrenal insufficiency in surgery.] Fortschr Med 1977;95(30):1866–8.

121. Iglesias P, González J, Díez JJ. Acute and persistent iatrogenic Cushing's syndrome after a single dose of triamcinolone acetonide. J Endocrinol Invest 2005; 28(11): 1019-23.

122. Mukai T. [Antagonism between parathyroid hormone and glucocorticoids in calcium and phosphorus metabolism.]Nippon Naibunpi Gakkai Zasshi 1965;41(8):950–9.

123. Kahn A, Snapper I, Drucker A. Corticosteroid-induced tetany in latent hypoparathyroidism. Arch Intern Med 1964;114:434–8.

124. Fisher JE, Smith RS, Lagrandeur R, Lorenz RP. Gestational diabetes mellitus in women receiving beta-adrenergics and corticosteroids for threatened preterm delivery. Obstet Gynecol 1997;90(6):880–3.

125. Kim YS, Kim MS, Kim SI, Lim SK, Lee HY, Han DS, Park K. Post-transplantation diabetes is better controlled after conversion from prednisone to deflazacort: a prospective trial in renal transplants. Transpl Int 1997;10(3):197–201.

126. Gurwitz JH, Bohn RL, Glynn RJ, Monane M, Mogun H, Avorn J. Glucocorticoids and the risk for initiation of hypoglycemic therapy. Arch Intern Med 1994;154(1): 97–101.

127. Bagdade JD, Porte D Jr, Bierman EL. Steroid-induced lipemia. A complication of high-dosage corticosteroid therapy. Arch Intern Med 1970;125(1):129–34.

128. Ettinger WH Jr, Hazzard WR. Elevated apolipoprotein-B levels in corticosteroid-treated patients with systemic lupus erythematosus. J Clin Endocrinol Metab 1988;67(3):425–8.

129. Amin SB, Sinkin RA, McDermott MP, Kendig JW. Lipid intolerance in neonates receiving dexamethasone for bronchopulmonary dysplasia. Arch Pediatr Adolesc Med 1999;153(8):795–800.

130. Tiley C, Grimwade D, Findlay M, Treleaven J, Height S, Catalano J, Powles R. Tumour lysis following hydrocortisone prior to a blood product transfusion in T-cell acute lymphoblastic leukaemia. Leuk Lymphoma 1992;8(1–2):143–6.

131. Lerza R, Botta M, Barsotti B, Schenone E, Menconi M, Bogliolo G, Pannacciulli I, Arboscello E. Dexamethazone-induced acute tumor lysis syndrome in a T-cell malignant lymphoma. Leuk Lymphoma 2002;43(5):1129–32.

132. Balli F, Benatti C. Terapia corticosteroidea protratta e metabolismo fosfo-calcico. II. Modificazioni del metabolismo fosfo-calcico in soggetti nefrosici sattoposti a terapia carticosteroidea protratta. [Prolonged corticosteroid therapy and phospho-calcic metabolism. II. Changes of phospho-calcic metabolism in nephrotic subjects subjected to prolonged corticoid therapy.] Minerva Pediatr 1968;20(45):2315–25.

133. Handa R, Wali JP, Singh RI, Aggarwal P. Corticosteroids precipitating hypocalcemic encephalopathy in hypoparathyroidism. Ann Emerg Med 1995;26(2):241–2.

134. Ravina A, Slezak L, Mirsky N, Bryden NA, Anderson RA. Reversal of corticosteroid-induced diabetes mellitus with supplemental chromium. Diabet Med 1999;16(2):164–7.

135. Schneider J, Burmeister H, Ruiz-Torres A. Langzeitstudien uber die Wirksamkeit der Dauertherapie bei hyperergisch-allergischen Erkrankungen mit Prednisolon. [Longitudinal study about the efficacy of long term prednisolone therapy in hyperergic-allergic diseases.] Verh Dtsch Ges Inn Med 1977;83:1785–8.

136. Schmand B, Neuvel J, Smolders-de Haas H, Hoeks J, Treffers PE, Koppe JG. Psychological development of children who were treated antenatally with corticosteroids to prevent respiratory distress syndrome. Pediatrics 1990;86(1):58–64.

137. Bielawski D, Hiatt IM, Hegyi T. Betamethasone-induced leukaemoid reaction in pre-term infant. Lancet 1978;1(8057):218–9.

138. Craddock CG. Corticosteroid-induced lymphopenia, immunosuppression, and body defense. Ann Intern Med 1978;88(4):564–6.

139. Saxon A, Stevens RH, Ramer SJ, Clements PJ, Yu DT. Glucocorticoids administered in vivo inhibit human suppressor T lymphocyte function and diminish B lymphocyte responsiveness in in vitro immunoglobulin synthesis. J Clin Invest 1978;61(4):922–30.

140. Maeshima E, Yamada Y, Yukawa S. Fever and leucopenia with steroids. Lancet 2000;355(9199):198.

141. Patrassi GM, Sartori MT, Livi U, Casonato A, Danesin C, Vettore S, Girolami A. Impairment of fibrinolytic potential in long-term steroid treatment after heart transplantation. Transplantation 1997;64(11):1610–4.

142. The British Thoracic and Tuberculosis Association. Inhaled corticosteroids compared with oral prednisone in patients starting long-term corticosteroid therapy for asthma. Lancet 1975;2(7933):469–73.

143. Salzman GA, Pyszczynski DR. Oropharyngeal candidiasis in patients treated with beclomethasone dipropionate delivered by metered-dose inhaler alone and with Aerochamber. J Allergy Clin Immunol 1988;81(2):424–8.

144. Linder N, Kuint J, German B, Lubin D, Loewenthal R. Hypertrophy of the tongue associated with inhaled corticosteroid therapy in premature infants. J Pediatr 1995;127(4):651–3.

145. Shulman JD, Carpenter WM. Prevalence and risk factors associated with geographic tongue among US adults. Oral Dis 2006; 12(4): 381-6.

146. Spiro HM. Is the steroid ulcer a myth? N Engl J Med 1983;309(1):45–7.

147. Messer J, Reitman D, Sacks HS, Smith H Jr, Chalmers TC. Association of adrenocorticosteroid therapy and peptic-ulcer disease. N Engl J Med 1983;309(1):21–4.

148. Conn HO, Poynard T. Corticosteroids and peptic ulcer: meta-analysis of adverse events during steroid therapy. J Intern Med 1994;236(6):619–32.

149. Henry DA, Johnston N, Dobson A, Duggan J. Fatal peptic ulcer complications and the use of non-steroidal antiinflammatory drugs, aspirin, and corticosteroids. BMJ (Clin Res Ed) 1987;295:1227.

150. Suazo-Barahona J, Gallegos J, Carmona-Sanchez R, Martinez R, Robles-Diaz G. Nonsteroidal anti-inflammatory drugs and gastrocolic fistula. J Clin Gastroenterol 1998;26(4):343–5.

151. Christensen S, Riis A, Nørgaard M, Thomsen RW, Tønnesen EM, Larsson A, Sorensen HT. Perforated peptic ulcer: use of pre-admission oral glucocorticoids and 30-day mortality. Aliment Pharmacol Ther 2006; 23(1): 45-52.

152. Shimizu T, Yamashiro Y, Yabuta K. Impaired increase of prostaglandin E2 in gastric juice during steroid therapy in children. J Paediatr Child Health 1994;30(2):169–72.

153. Yamanishi Y, Yamana S, Ishioka S, Yamakido M. Development of ischemic colitis and scleroderma renal crisis following methylprednisolone pulse therapy for progressive systemic sclerosis. Intern Med 1996;35(7):583–6.

154. Dwarakanath AD, Nash J, Rhodes JM. "Conversion" from ulcerative colitis to Crohn's disease associated with corticosteroid treatment. Gut 1994;35(8):1141–4.

155. Sharma R, Gupta KL, Ammon RH, Gambert SR. Atypical presentation of colon perforation related to corticosteroid use. Geriatrics 1997;52(5):88–90.

156. Candelas G, Jover JA, Fernandez B, Rodriguez-Olaverri JC, Calatayud J. Perforation of the sigmoid colon in a rheumatoid arthritis patient treated with methylprednisolone pulses. Scand J Rheumatol 1998;27(2):152–3.

157. Mpofu S, Mpofu CMA, Hutchinson D, Maier AE, Dodd SR, Moots RJ. Steroids, non-steroidal anti-inflammatory drugs, and sigmoid diverticular abscess perforation in rheumatic conditions. Ann Rheum Dis 2004; 63: 588–90.

158. Weissel M, Hauff W. Fatal liver failure after high-dose glucocorticoid pulse therapy in a patient with severe thyroid eye disease. Thyroid 2000;10(6):521.

159. Nanki T, Koike R, Miyasaka N. Subacute severe steatohepatitis during prednisolone therapy for systemic lupus erythematosis. Am J Gastroenterol 1999;94(11):3379.

160. Dourakis SP, Sevastianos VA, Kaliopi P. Acute severe steatohepatitis related to prednisolone therapy. Am J Gastroenterol 2002;97(4):1074–5.

161. Verrips A, Rotteveel JJ, Lippens R. Dexamethasone-induced hepatomegaly in three children. Pediatr Neurol 1998;19(5):388–91.

162. Marinò M, Morabito E, Brunetto MR, Bartalena L, Pinchera A, Marocci C. Acute and severe liver damage associated with intravenous glucocorticoid pulse therapy in patients with Graves' ophthalmopathy. Thyroid 2004; 14: 403–6.

163. Topal F, Özaslan E, Akbulut S, Küçükazman M, Yuksel O, Altiparmak E. Methylprednisolone-induced toxic hepatitis. Ann Pharmacother 2006; 40(10): 1868-71.

164. Hamed I, Lindeman RD, Czerwinski AW. Case report: acute pancreatitis following corticosteroid and azathioprine therapy. Am J Med Sci 1978;276(2):211–9.

165. Di Fazano CS, Messica O, Quennesson S, Quennesson ER, Inaoui R, Vergne P, Bonnet C, Bertin P, Treves R. Two new cases of glucocorticoid-induced pancreatitis. Rev Rhum Engl Ed 1999;66(4):235.

166. Khanna S, Kumar A. Acute pancreatitis due to hydrocortisone in a patient with ulcerative colitis. J Gastroenterol Hepatol 2003; 18: 1010–1.

167. Reichert LJ, Koene RA, Wetzels JF. Acute haemodynamic and proteinuric effects of prednisolone in patients with a nephrotic syndrome. Nephrol Dial Transplant 1999;14(1):91–7.

168. Charpin J, Arnaud A, Boutin C, Aubert J, Murisasco A, Gotte G. Long-term corticosteroid therapy and its effect on the kidney. Acta Allergol 1969;24(1):49–56.

169. Gray D, Shepherd H, Daar A, Oliver DO, Morris PJ. Oral versus intravenous high-dose steroid treatment of renal allograft rejection. The big shot or not? Lancet 1978;1(8056):117–8.

170. Toftegaard M, Knudsen F. Massive vasopressin-resistant polyuria induced by dexamethasone. Intensive Care Med 1995;21(3):238–40.

171. Editorial. Nocturia during steroid therapy. BMJ 1970;4(729):193–4.

172. Wendt H. Klinisch-pharmakologische Untersuchungen zur akneinduzierenden Wirkung von Fluorcortinbutylester. [Clinico-pharmacological studies on the acne-inducing action of fluocortin butylester.] Arzneimittelforschung 1977;27(11a):2245–6.

173. Bioulac P, Beylot C. Etude ultrastructurale d'une leucodermie secondaire à une injection intraarticulaire de corticoides. [Ultrastructural study of a leukoderma secondary to an intra-articular injection of corticoides.] Ann Dermatol Venereol 1977;104(12):883–5.

174. Bondy PhK. Disorders of the adrenal cortex. In: Wilson JD, Foster DW, editors. Williams' Textbook of Endocrinology. 7th edn.. Philadelphia: Saunders, 1985:816.

175. Reinhold K, Schneider L, Hunzelmann N, Krieg T, Scharffetter-Kochanek K. Delayed-type allergy to systemic corticosteroids. Allergy 2000;55(11):1095–6.

176. Nanda V, Parwaz MA, Handa S. Linear hypopigmentation after triamcinolone injection: a rare complication of a common procedure. Aesthetic Plast Surg 2006; 30(1): 118–9.

177. Shuster S, Raffle EJ, Bottoms E. Skin collagen in rheumatoid arthritis and the effect of corticosteroids. Lancet 1967;2:525.

178. Mathov E, Grad P, Scaglia H. Provocación de hemorragias uterinas anormales y hematomas subcutáneos por el uso de la acetonida de la triamcinoona en pacientes alérgicas. [Provocation of uterine hemorrhages and subcutaneous hematomas by the use of triamcinolone acetonide in allergic patients.] Prensa Med Argent 1971;58(16): 826–9.

179. Roy A, Leblanc C, Paquette L, Ghezzo H, Cote J, Cartier A, Malo JL. Skin bruising in asthmatic subjects treated with high doses of inhaled steroids: frequency and association with adrenal function. Eur Respir J 1996;9(2):226–31.

180. Korting HC, Unholzer A, Schafer-Korting M, Tausch I, Gassmueller J, Nietsch KH. Different skin thinning potential of equipotent medium-strength glucocorticoids. Skin Pharmacol Appl Skin Physiol 2002;15(2):85–91.

181. Sener O, Caliskaner Z, Yazicioglu K, Karaayvaz M, Ozanguc N. Nonpigmenting solitary fixed drug eruption after skin testing and intra-articular injection of triamcinolone acetonide. Ann Allergy Asthma Immunol 2001;86(3):335–6.

182. Weber F, Barbaud A, Reichert-Penetrat S, Danchin A, Schmutz JL. Unusual clinical presentation in a case of contact dermatitis due to corticosteroids diagnosed by ROAT. Contact Dermatitis 2001;44(2):105–6.

183. Sener O, Caliskaner Z, Yazicioglu K, Karaayvaz M, Ozanguc N. Nonpigmenting solitary fixed drug eruption after skin testing and intra-articular injection of triamcinolone acetonide. Ann Allergy Asthma Immunol 2001;86(3):335–6.

184. Dooms-Goossens A, Andersen KE, Brandao FM, Bruynzeel D, Burrows D, Camarasa J, Ducombs G, Frosch P, Hannuksela M, Lachapelle JM, Lahti A, Menne T, Wahlberg JE, Wilkinson JD. Corticosteroid contact allergy: an EECDRG multicentre study. Contact Dermatitis 1996;35(1):40–4.

185. Quintiliani R. Hypersensitivity and adverse reactions associated with the use of newer intranasal corticosteroids for allergic rhinitis. Curr Ther Res Clin Exp 1996;57:478–88.

186. Isaksson M, Bruze M, Goossens A, Lepoittevin JP. Patch testing with budesonide in serial dilutions. the significance of dose, occlusion time and reading time. Contact Dermatitis 1999;40(1):24–31.

187. Murata T, Tanaka M, Dekio I, Tanikawa A, Nishikawa T. Allergic contact dermatitis due to clobetasone butyrate. Contact Dermatitis 2000;42(5):305.

188. O'Hagan AH, Corbett JR. Contact allergy to budesonide in a breath-actuated inhaler. Contact Dermatitis 1999;41(1):53.

189. Lew DB, Higgins GC, Skinner RB, Snider MD, Myers LK. Adverse reaction to prednisone in a patient with systemic lupus erythematosus. Pediatr Dermatol 1999;16(2):146–50.

190. Garcia-Bravo B, Repiso JB, Camacho F. Systemic contact dermatitis due to deflazacort. Contact Dermatitis 2000;43(6):359–60.

191. Stingeni L, Caraffini S, Assalve D, Lapomarda V, Lisi P. Erythema-multiforme-like contact dermatitis from budesonide. Contact Dermatitis 1996;34(2):154–5.

192. Roujeau JC, Kelly JP, Naldi L, Rzany B, Stern RS, Anderson T, Auquier A, Bastuji-Garin S, Correia O, Locati F, Mockenhaupt M, Paoletti C, Shapiro S, Shear N, Schüpf E, Kaufman DW. Medication use and the risk of Stevens–Johnson syndrome or toxic epidermal necrolysis. N Engl J Med 1995;333(24):1600–7.

193. Ingber A, Trattner A, David M. Hypersensitivity to an oestrogen–progesterone preparation and possible relationship to autoimmune progesterone dermatitis and corticosteroid hypersensitivity. J Dermatol Treat 1999;10:139–40.

194. Picado C, Luengo M. Corticosteroid-induced bone loss. Prevention and management. Drug Saf 1996;15(5):347–59.

195. van Staa TP. The pathogenesis, epidemiology and management of glucocorticoid-induced osteoporosis. Calcif Tissue Int 2006; 79(3): 129-37.

196. Summey BT, Yosipovitch G. Glucocorticoid-induced bone loss in dermatologic patients: an update. Arch Dermatol 2006; 142(1): 82-90.

197. Wichers M, Springer W, Bidlingmaier F, Klingmuller D. The influence of hydrocortisone substitution on the quality of life and parameters of bone metabolism in patients with secondary hypocortisolism. Clin Endocrinol (Oxf) 1999;50(6):759–65.

198. Langhammer A, Norjavaara E, de Verdier MG, Johnsen R, Bjermer L. Use of inhaled corticosteroids and bone mineral density in a population based study: the Nord–Trondelag Health Study (the HUNT Study). Pharmacoepidemiol Drug Saf 2004; 13: 569-79.

199. Suissa S, Baltzan M, Kremer R, Ernst P. Inhaled and nasal corticosteroid use and the risk of fracture. Am J Respir Crit Care Med 2004; 169: 83-8.

200. Steinbuch M, Youket TE, Cohen S. Oral glucocorticoid use is associated with an increased risk of fracture. Osteoporos Int 2004; 15: 323-8.

201. Krogsgaard MR, Thamsborg G, Lund B. Changes in bone mass during low dose corticosteroid treatment in patients with polymyalgia rheumatica. a double blind, prospective comparison between prednisolone and deflazacort. Ann Rheum Dis 1996;55(2):143–6.

202. Goldstein MF, Fallon JJ Jr, Harning R. Chronic glucocorticoid therapy-induced osteoporosis in patients with obstructive lung disease. Chest 1999;116(6):1733–49.

203. Yosipovitch G, Hoon TS, Leok GC. Suggested rationale for prevention and treatment of glucocorticoid-induced bone loss in dermatologic patients. Arch Dermatol 2001;137(4):477–81.

204. Selby PL, Halsey JP, Adams KR, Klimiuk P, Knight SM, Pal B, Stewart IM, Swinson DR. Corticosteroids do not alter the threshold for vertebral fracture. J Bone Miner Res 2000;15(5):952–6.

205. Zelissen PM, Croughs RJ, van Rijk PP, Raymakers JA. Effect of glucocorticoid replacement therapy on bone mineral density in patients with Addison disease. Ann Intern Med 1994;120(3):207–10.

206. Valero MA, Leon M, Ruiz Valdepenas MP, Larrodera L, Lopez MB, Papapietro K, Jara A, Hawkins F. Bone density and turnover in Addison's disease: effect of glucocorticoid treatment. Bone Miner 1994;26(1):9–17.

207. Heiner JP, Joyce MJ, Carter JR, Makley JT. Atraumatic posterior pelvic ring fractures simulating metastatic disease in patients with metabolic bone disease. Orthopedics 1994;17(3):285–9.

208. Baltzan MA, Suissa S, Bauer DC, Cummings SR. Hip fractures attributable to·corticosteroid use. Study Osteoporotic Fractures Group. Lancet 1999;353(9161):1327.

209. McKenzie R, Reynolds JC, O'Fallon A, Dale J, Deloria M, Blackwelder W, Straus SE. Decreased bone mineral density during low dose glucocorticoid administration in a randomized, placebo controlled trial. J Rheumatol 2000;27(9):2222–6.

210. Walsh LJ, Wong CA, Oborne J, Cooper S, Lewis SA, Pringle M, Hubbard R, Tattersfield AE. Adverse effects of oral corticosteroids in relation to dose in patients with lung disease. Thorax 2001;56(4):279–84.

211. van Everdingen AA, Jacobs JW, Siewertsz Van Reesema DR, Bijlsma JW. Low-dose prednisone therapy for patients with early active rheumatoid arthritis: clinical efficacy, disease-modifying properties, and side effects: a randomized, double-blind, placebo-controlled clinical trial. Ann Intern Med 2002;136(1):1–12.

212. Townsend HB, Saag KG. Glucocorticoid use in rheumatoid arthritis: benefits, mechanisms, and risks. Clin Exp Rheumatol 2004; 22 (Suppl 35): S77-82.

213. Gluck O, Colice G. Recognizing and treating glucocorticoid-induced osteoporosis in patients with pulmonary diseases. Chest 2004; 125: 1859-76.

214. Lukert BP, Adams JS. Calcium and phosphorus homeostasis in man. Effect Corticosteroids. Arch Intern Med 1976;136(11):1249–53.

215. Hahn TJ. Corticosteroid-induced osteopenia. Arch Intern Med 1978;138(Spec No):882–5.

216. Chesney RW, Mazess RB, Hamstra AJ, DeLuca HF, O'Reagan S. Reduction of serum-1, 25-dihydroxyvitamin-D3 in children receiving glucocorticoids. Lancet 1978;2(8100):1123–5.

217. Eastell R. Management of corticosteroid-induced osteoporosis. UK Consensus Group Meeting on Osteoporosis. J Intern Med 1995;237(5):439–47.

218. Goans RE, Weiss GH, Abrams SA, Perez MD, Yergey AL. Calcium tracer kinetics show decreased irreversible flow to bone in glucocorticoid treated patients. Calcif Tissue Int 1995;56(6):533–5.

219. Sasaki N, Kusano E, Ando Y, Yano K, Tsuda E, Asano Y. Glucocorticoid decreases circulating osteoprotegerin (OPG): possible mechanism for glucocorticoid induced osteoporosis. Nephrol Dial Transplant 2001;16(3):479–82.

220. Lespessailles E, Siroux V, Poupon S, Andriambelosoa N, Pothuaud L, Harba R, Benhamou CL. Long-term corticosteroid therapy induces mild changes in trabecular bone texture. J Bone Miner Res 2000;15(4):747–53.

221. Mateo L, Nolla JM, Bonnin MR, Navarro MA, Roig-Escofet D. Sex hormone status and bone mineral density in men with rheumatoid arthritis. J Rheumatol 1995;22(8):1455–60.

222. Vestergaard P, Olsen ML, Paaske Johnsen S, Rejnmark L, Sorensen HT, Mosekilde L. Corticosteroid use and risk of hip fracture: a population-based case-control study in Denmark. J Intern Med 2003; 254: 486-93.

223. Ton FN, Gunawardene SC, Lee H, Neer RM. J. Effects of low-dose prednisone on bone metabolism. Bone Miner Res 2005; 20(3): 464-70.

224. Harris M, Hauser S, Nguyen TV, Kelly PJ, Rodda C, Morton J, Freezer N, Strauss BJ, Eisman JA, Walker JL. Bone mineral density in prepubertal asthmatics receiving corticosteroid treatment. J Paediatr Child Health 2001;37(1):67–71.

225. Lane NE. An update on glucocorticoid-induced osteoporosis. Rheum Dis Clin North Am 2001;27(1):235–53.

226. Henderson NK, Sambrook PN, Kelly PJ, Macdonald P, Keogh AM, Spratt P, Eisman JA. Bone mineral loss and recovery after cardiac transplantation. Lancet 1995;346(8979):905.

227. Garton MJ, Reid DM. Bone mineral density of the hip and of the anteroposterior and lateral dimensions of the spine in men with rheumatoid arthritis. Effects of low-dose corticosteroids. Arthritis Rheum 1993;36(2):222–8.

228. Saito JK, Davis JW, Wasnich RD, Ross PD. Users of low-dose glucocorticoids have increased bone loss rates: a longitudinal study. Calcif Tissue Int 1995;57(2):115–9.

229. Buckley LM, Leib ES, Cartularo KS, Vacek PM, Cooper SM. Effects of low dose corticosteroids on the bone mineral density of patients with rheumatoid arthritis. J Rheumatol 1995;22(6):1055–9.

230. Fryer JP, Granger DK, Leventhal JR, Gillingham K, Najarian JS, Matas AJ. Steroid-related complications in the cyclosporine era. Clin Transplant 1994;8(3 Part 1):224–9.

231. Wolpaw T, Deal CL, Fleming-Brooks S, Bartucci MR, Schulak JA, Hricik DE. Factors influencing vertebral bone density after renal transplantation. Transplantation 1994;58(11):1186–9.

232. Yun YS, Kim BJ, Hong SP, Lee TW, Lim CG, Kim MJ. Changes of bone metabolism indices in patients receiving immunosuppressive therapy including low doses of steroids after renal transplantation. Transplant Proc 1996;28(3):1561–4.

233. Saisu T, Sakamoto K, Yamada K, Kashiwabara H, Yokoyama T, Iida S, Harada Y, Ikenoue S, Sakamoto M, Moriya H. High incidence of osteonecrosis of femoral head in patients receiving more than 2 g of intravenous methylprednisolone after renal transplantation Transplant Proc 1996;28(3):1559–60.

234. Naganathan V, Jones G, Nash P, Nicholson G, Eisman J, Sambrook PN. Vertebral fracture risk with long-term corticosteroid therapy: prevalence and relation to age, bone density, and corticosteroid use. Arch Intern Med 2000;160(19):2917–22.

235. Schoon EJ, Bollani S, Mills PR, Israeli E, Felsenberg D, Ljunghall S, Persson T, Haptén-White L, Graffner H, Bianchi Porro G, Vatn M, Stockbrügger RW; Matrix Study Group. Bone mineral density in relation to efficacy and side effects of budesonide and prednisolone in Crohn's disease. Clin Gastroenterol Hepatol 2005; 3(2): 113-21.

236. van Staa TP, Geusens P, Bijlsma JW, Leufkens HG, Cooper C. Clinical assessment of the long-term risk of fracture in patients with rheumatoid arthritis. Arthritis Rheum 2006; 54(10): 3104-12.

237. Tattersfield AE, Town GI, Johnell O, Picado C, Aubier M, Braillon P, Karlstrom R. Bone mineral density in subjects with mild asthma randomized to treatment with inhaled corticosteroids or non-corticosteroid treatment for two years. Thorax 2001;56(4):272–8.

238. Sambrook PN. Corticosteroid osteoporosis: practical implications of recent trials. J Bone Miner Res 2000;15(9):1645–9.

239. American College of Rheumatology Task Force on Osteoporosis Guidelines. Recommendations for the prevention and treatment of glucocorticoid-induced osteoporosis. Arthritis Rheum 1996;39(11):1791–801.

240. Bone and Tooth Society. National Osteoporosis Society, Royal College of Physicians. Glucocorticoid-induced Osteoporosis. Guidelines for Prevention and TreatmentLondon: Royal College of Physicians;. 2002.

241. Hart SR, Green B. Osteoporosis prophylaxis during corticosteroid treatment: failure to prescribe. Postgrad Med J 2002;78(918):242–3.

242. Gudbjornsson B, Juliusson UI, Gudjonsson FV. Prevalence of long term steroid treatment and the frequency of decision making to prevent steroid induced

osteoporosis in daily clinical practice. Ann Rheum Dis 2002;61(1):32–6.

243. Cino M, Greenberg GR. Bone mineral density in Crohn's disease: a longitudinal study of budesonide, prednisone, and nonsteroid therapy. Am J Gastroenterol 2002;97(4):915–21.

244. Schwid SR, Goodman AD, Puzas JE, McDermott MP, Mattson DH. Sporadic corticosteroid pulses and osteoporosis in multiple sclerosis. Arch Neurol 1996;53(8):753–7.

245. Lukert BP, Johnson BE, Robinson RG. Estrogen and progesterone replacement therapy reduces glucocorticoid-induced bone loss. J Bone Miner Res 1992;7(9):1063–9.

246. McDonald CF, Zebaze RM, Seeman E. Calcitriol does not prevent bone loss in patients with asthma receiving corticosteroid therapy: a double-blind placebo-controlled trial. Osteoporos Int 2006; 17(10): 1546-51.

247. Bak M, Serdaroglu E, Guclu R. Prophylactic calcium and vitamin D treatments in steroid-treated children with nephrotic syndrome. Pediatr Nephrol 2006; 21(3): 350-4.

248. Buckley LM, Leib ES, Cartularo KS, Vacek PM, Cooper SM. Calcium and vitamin D3 supplementation prevents bone loss in the spine secondary to low-dose corticosteroids in patients with rheumatoid arthritis. A randomized, double-blind, placebo-controlled trial. Ann Intern Med 1996;125(12):961–8.

249. Adachi JD, Bensen WG, Bianchi F, Cividino A, Pillersdorf S, Sebaldt RJ, Tugwell P, Gordon M, Steele M, Webber C, Goldsmith CH. Vitamin D and calcium in the prevention of corticosteroid induced osteoporosis: a 3 year followup. J Rheumatol 1996;23(6):995–1000.

250. Talalaj M, Gradowska L, Marcinowska-Suchowierska E, Durlik M, Gaciong Z, Lao M. Efficiency of preventive treatment of glucocorticoid-induced osteoporosis with 25-hydroxyvitamin D3 and calcium in kidney transplant patients. Transplant Proc 1996;28(6):3485–7.

251. Warady BD, Lindsley CB, Robinson FG, Lukert BP. Effects of nutritional supplementation on bone mineral status of children with rheumatic diseases receiving corticosteroid therapy. J Rheumatol 1994;21(3):530–5.

252. Richy F, Ethgen O, Bruyere O, Reginster JY. Efficacy of alphacalcidol and calcitriol in primary and corticosteroid-induced osteoporosis: a meta-analysis of their effects on bone mineral density and fracture rate. Osteoporos Int 2004; 15: 301-10.

253. Ringe JD, Dorst A, Faber H, Schacht E, Rahlfs VW. Superiority of alfacalcidol over plain vitamin D in the treatment of glucocorticoid-induced osteoporosis. Rheumatol Int 2004; 24: 63-70.

254. Luengo M, Pons F, Martinez de Osaba MJ, Picado C. Prevention of further bone mass loss by nasal calcitonin in patients on long term glucocorticoid therapy for asthma: a two year follow up study. Thorax 1994;49(11):1099–102.

255. Healey JH, Paget SA, Williams-Russo P, Szatrowski TP, Schneider R, Spiera H, Mitnick H, Ales K, Schwartzberg P. A randomized controlled trial of salmon calcitonin to prevent bone loss in corticosteroid-treated temporal arteritis and polymyalgia rheumatica. Calcif Tissue Int 1996;58(2):73–80.

256. Adachi JD, Bensen WG, Bell MJ, Bianchi FA, Cividino AA, Craig GL, Sturtridge WC, Sebaldt RJ, Steele M, Gordon M, Themeles E, Tugwell P, Roberts R, Gent M. Salmon

257. calcitonin nasal spray in the prevention of corticosteroid-induced osteoporosis. Br J Rheumatol 1997;36(2):255–9.

257. Mulder H, Struys A. Intermittent cyclical etidronate in the prevention of corticosteroid-induced bone loss. Br J Rheumatol 1994;33(4):348–50.

258. Diamond T, McGuigan L, Barbagallo S, Bryant C. Cyclical etidronate plus ergocalciferol prevents glucocorticoid-induced bone loss in postmenopausal women. Am J Med 1995;98(5):459–63.

259. Roux C, Oriente P, Laan R, Hughes RA, Ittner J, Goemaere S, Di Munno O, Pouilles JM, Horlait S, Cortet B. Randomized trial of effect of cyclical etidronate in the prevention of corticosteroid-induced bone loss. Ciblos Study Group. J Clin Endocrinol Metab 1998;83(4):1128–33.

260. Pitt P, Li F, Todd P, Webber D, Pack S, Moniz C. A double blind placebo controlled study to determine the effects of intermittent cyclical etidronate on bone mineral density in patients on long-term oral corticosteroid treatment. Thorax 1998;53(5):351–6.

261. Sato S, Ohosone Y, Suwa A, Yasuoka H, Nojima T, Fujii T, Kuwana M, Nakamura K, Mimori T, Hirakata M. Effect of intermittent cyclical etidronate therapy on corticosteroid induced osteoporosis in Japanese patients with connective tissue disease: 3 year follow up. J Rheumatol 2003; 30: 2673-9.

262. Frediani B, Falsetti P, Baldi F, Acciai C, Filippou G, Marcolongo R. Effects of 4-year treatment with once-weekly clodronate on prevention of corticosteroid-induced bone loss and fractures in patients with arthritis: evaluation with dual-energy X-ray absorptiometry and quantitative ultrasound. Bone 2003; 33: 575-81.

263. Ringe JD, Dorst A, Faber H, Ibach K, Preuss J. Three-monthly ibandronate bolus injection offers favorable tolerability and sustained efficacy advantage over two years in established corticosteroid-induced osteoporosis. Rheumatol (Oxf) 2003; 42: 743-9.

264. Ringe JD, Dorst A, Faber H, Ibach K, Sorenson F. Intermittent intravenous ibandronate injections reduce vertebral fracture risk in corticosteroid-induced osteoporosis: results from a long-term comparative study. Osteoporos Int 2003; 14: 801-7.

265. Nordborg E, Schaufelberger C, Andersson R, Bosaeus I, Bengtsson BA. The ineffectiveness of cyclical oral clodronate on bone mineral density in glucocorticoid-treated patients with giant-cell arteritis. J Intern Med 1997;242(5):367–71.

266. Boutsen Y, Jamart J, Esselinckx W, Stoffel M, Devogelaer JP. Primary prevention of glucocorticoid-induced osteoporosis with intermittent intravenous pamidronate: a randomized trial. Calcif Tissue Int 1997;61(4):266–71.

267. Wallach S, Cohen S, Reid DM, Hughes RA, Hosking DJ, Laan RF, Doherty SM, Maricic M, Rosen C, Brown J, Barton I, Chines AA. Effects of risedronate treatment on bone density and vertebral fracture in patients on corticosteroid therapy. Calcif Tissue Int 2000;67(4):277–85.

268. Reid DM, Hughes RA, Laan RF, Sacco-Gibson NA, Wenderoth DH, Adami S, Eusebio RA, Devogelaer JP. Efficacy and safety of daily risedronate in the treatment of corticosteroid-induced osteoporosis in men and women: a randomized trial. European Corticosteroid-Induced

Osteoporosis Treatment Study. J Bone Miner Res 2000;15(6):1006–13.

269. Adachi JD, Saag KG, Delmas PD, Liberman UA, Emkey RD, Seeman E, Lane NE, Kaufman JM, Poubelle PE, Hawkins F, Correa-Rotter R, Menkes CJ, Rodriguez-Portales JA, Schnitzer TJ, Block JA, Wing J, McIlwain HH, Westhovens R, Brown J, Melo-Gomes JA, Gruber BL, Yanover MJ, Leite MO, Siminoski KG, Nevitt MC, Sharp JT, Malice MP, Dumortier T, Czachur M, Carofano W, Daifotis A. Two-year effects of alendronate on bone mineral density and vertebral fracture in patients receiving glucocorticoids: a randomized, double-blind, placebo-controlled extension trial. Arthritis Rheum 2001;44(1):202–11.

270. de Nijs RN, Jacobs JW, Lems WF, Laan RF, Algra A, Huisman AM, Buskens E, de Laet CE, Oostveen AC, Geusens PP, Bruyn GA, Dijkmans BA, Bijlsma JW; STOP Investigators. Alendronate or alfacalcidol in glucocorticoid-induced osteoporosis. N Engl J Med 2006; 355(7): 675-84.

271. Emkey R, Delmas PD, Goemaere S, Liberman UA, Poubelle PE, Daifotis AG, Verbruggen N, Lombardi A, Czachur M. Changes in bone mineral density following discontinuation or continuation of alendronate therapy in glucocorticoid-treated patients: a retrospective, observational study. Arthritis Rheum 2003; 48: 1102-8.

272. Rehman Q, Lang TF, Arnaud CD, Modin GW, Lane NE. Daily treatment with parathyroid hormone is associated with an increase in vertebral cross-sectional area in postmenopausal women with glucocorticoid-induced osteoporosis. Osteoporos Int 2003; 14: 77-81.

273. Rizzoli R, Chevalley T, Slosman DO, Bonjour JP. Sodium monofluorophosphate increases vertebral bone mineral density in patients with corticosteroid-induced osteoporosis. Osteoporos Int 1995;5(1):39–46.

274. Giustina A, Bussi AR, Jacobello C, Wehrenberg WB. Effects of recombinant human growth hormone (GH) on bone and intermediary metabolism in patients receiving chronic glucocorticoid treatment with suppressed endogenous GH response to GH-releasing hormone. J Clin Endocrinol Metab 1995;80(1):122–9.

275. Yonemura K, Kimura M, Miyaji T, Hishida A. Short-term effect of vitamin K administration on prednisolone-induced loss of bone mineral density in patients with chronic glomerulonephritis. Calcif Tissue Int 2000;66(2): 123–8.

276. Westeel FP, Mazouz H, Ezaitouni F, Hottelart C, Ivan C, Fardellone P, Brazier M, El Esper I, Petit J, Achard JM, Pruna A, Fournier A. Cyclosporine bone remodeling effect prevents steroid osteopenia after kidney transplantation. Kidney Int 2000;58(4):1788–96.

277. Abe H, Sako H, Okino K, Nakane Y, Kodama M, Park KI, Inoue H, Kim CJ, Tomoyoshi T. Clinical study of aseptic necrosis of bone after renal transplantation. Transplant Proc 1994;26(4):1987.

278. Alarcon GS, Mikhail I, Jaffe KA, Bradley LA, Bailey WC. Hip osteonecrosis secondary to the administration of corticosteroids for feigned bronchial asthma. The clinical spectrum of the factitious disorders. Arthritis Rheum 1994;37(1):139–41.

279. Lausten GS, Lemser T, Jensen PK, Egfjord M. Necrosis of the femoral head after kidney transplantation. Clin Transplant 1998;12(6):572–4.

280. Bauer M, Thabault P, Estok D, Chrinstiansen C, Platt R. Low-dose corticosteroids and avascular necrosis of the hip and knee. Pharmacoepidemiol Drug Saf 2000;9:187–91.

281. McKee MD, Waddell JP, Kudo PA, Schemitsch EH, Richards RR. Osteonecrosis of the femoral head in men following short-course corticosteroid therapy: a report of 15 cases. CMAJ 2001;164(2):205–6.

282. Virik K, Karapetis C, Droufakou S, Harper P. Avascular necrosis of bone: the hidden risk of glucocorticoids used as antiemetics in cancer chemotherapy. Int J Clin Pract 2001;55(5):344–5.

283. Kosaka Y, Mitsumori M, Araki N, Yamauchi C, Nagata Y, Hiraoka M, Kodama H. Avascular necrosis of bilateral femoral head as a result of long-term steroid administration for radiation pneumonitis after tangential irradiation of the breast. Int J Clin Oncol 2006; 11(6): 482-6.

284. Gibson JN, Poyser NL, Morrison WL, Scrimgeour CM, Rennie MJ. Muscle protein synthesis in patients with rheumatoid arthritis: effect of chronic corticosteroid therapy on prostaglandin F2 alpha availability. Eur J Clin Invest 1991;21(4):406–12.

285. Ekstrand A, Schalin-Jantti C, Lofman M, Parkkonen M, Widen E, Franssila-Kallunki A, Saloranta C, Koivisto V, Groop L. The effect of (steroid) immunosuppression on skeletal muscle glycogen metabolism in patients after kidney transplantation. Transplantation 1996;61(6):889–93.

286. Anonymous. Corticosteroid myopathy. Lancet 1970;2:1118.

287. Janssens S, Decramer M. Corticosteroid-induced myopathy and the respiratory muscles. Report of two cases. Chest 1989;95(5):1160–2.

288. Weiner P, Azgad Y, Weiner M. The effect of corticosteroids on inspiratory muscle performance in humans. Chest 1993;104(6):1788–91.

289. Halpern AA, Horowitz BG, Nagel DA. Tendon ruptures associated with corticosteroid therapy. West J Med 1977;127(5):378–82.

290. Pai VS. Rupture of the plantar fascia. J Foot Ankle Surg 1996;35(1):39–40.

291. Bunch TJ, Welsh GA, Miller DV, Swaroop VS. Acute spontaneous Achilles tendon rupture in a patient with giant cell arteritis. Ann Clin Lab Sci 2003; 33: 326-8.

292. Schiavon F. Transient joint effusion: a forgotten side effect of high dose corticosteroid treatment. Ann Rheum Dis 2003; 62: 491-2.

293. Motson RW, Glass DN, Smith DA, Daly JR. The effect of short- and long-term corticosteroid treatment on sleep-associated growth hormone secretion. Clin Endocrinol (Oxf) 1978;8(4):315–26.

294. Allen DB, Mullen M, Mullen B. A meta-analysis of the effect of oral and inhaled corticosteroids on growth. J Allergy Clin Immunol 1994;93(6):967–76.

295. Doull IJ, Freezer NJ, Holgate ST. Growth of prepubertal children with mild asthma treated with inhaled beclomethasone dipropionate. Am J Respir Crit Care Med 1995;151(6):1715–9.

296. Whitaker K, Webb J, Barnes J, Barnes ND. Effect of fluticasone on growth in children with asthma. Lancet 1996;348(9019):63–4.

297. Todd G, Dunlop K, McNaboe J, Ryan MF, Carson D, Shields MD. Growth and adrenal suppression in asthmatic children treated with high-dose fluticasone propionate. Lancet 1996;348(9019):27–9.

298. Travis LB, Chesney R, McEnery P, Moel D, Pennisi A, Potter D, Talwalkar YB, Wolff E. Growth and glucocorticoids in children with kidney disease. Kidney Int 1978;14(4):365–8.

299. Rivkees SA, Danon M, Herrin J. Prednisone dose limitation of growth hormone treatment of steroid-induced growth failure. J Pediatr 1994;125(2):322–5.

300. Lai HC, FitzSimmons SC, Allen DB, Kosorok MR, Rosenstein BJ, Campbell PW, Farrell PM. Risk of persistent growth impairment after alternate-day prednisone

treatment in children with cystic fibrosis. N Engl J Med 2000;342(12):851–9.

301. Lomenick, JP, Backeljauw, PF, Lucky, AW. Growth, bone mineral accretion, and adrenal function in glucocorticoid-treated infants with hemangiomas—a retrospective study. Pediatr Dermatol 2006; 23 (2): 169-74.

302. Diczfalusy E, Landgren BM. Hormonal changes in the menstrual cycle. In: Diczfalusy D, editor. Regulation of Human Fertility. Copenhagen: Scriptor, 1977:21.

303. Cunningham GR, Goldzieher JW, de la Pena A, Oliver M. The mechanism of ovulation inhibition by triamcinolone acetonide. J Clin Endocrinol Metab 1978;46(1):8–14.

304. Mens JM, Nico de Wolf A, Berkhout BJ, Stam HJ. Disturbance of the menstrual pattern after local injection with triamcinolone acetonide. Ann Rheum Dis 1998;57(11):700.

305. Lopez-Serrano MC, Moreno-Ancillo A, Contreras J, Ortega N, Cabanas R, Barranco P, Munoz-Pereira M. Two cases of specific adverse reactions to systemic corticosteroids. J Invest Allergol Clin Immunol 1996;6(5):324–7.

306. Ventura MT, Muratore L, Calogiuri GF, Dagnello M, Buquicchio R, Nicoletti A, Altamura M, Sabba C, Tursi A. Allergic and pseudoallergic reactions induced by glucocorticosteroids: a review. Curr Pharm Des 2003; 9: 1956-64.

307. Moreno-Ancillo A, Martin-Munoz F, Martin-Barroso JA, Diaz-Pena JM, Ojeda JA. Anaphylaxis to 6-alpha-methylprednisolone in an eight-year-old child. J Allergy Clin Immunol 1996;97(5):1169–71.

308. van den Berg JS, van Eikema Hommes OR, Wuis EW, Stapel S, van der Valk PG. Anaphylactoid reaction to intravenous methylprednisolone in a patient with multiple sclerosis. J Neurol Neurosurg Psychiatry 1997;63(6):813–4.

309. Figueredo E, Cuesta-Herranz JI, De Las Heras M, Lluch-Bernal M, Umpierrez A, Sastre J. Anaphylaxis to dexamethasone. Allergy 1997;52(8):877.

310. Mace S, Vadas P, Pruzanski W. Anaphylactic shock induced by intraarticular injection of methylprednisolone acetate. J Rheumatol 1997;24(6):1191–4.

311. Hayhurst M, Braude A, Benatar SR. Anaphylactic-like reaction to hydrocortisone. S Afr Med J 1978;53(7):259–60.

312. Srinivasan V, Lanham PR. Acute laryngeal obstruction – reaction to intravenous hydrocortisone? Eur J Anaesthesiol 1997;14(3):342.

313. Vaghjimal A, Rosenstreich D, Hudes G. Fever, rash and worsening of asthma in response to intravenous hydrocortisone. Int J Clin Pract 1999;53(7):567–8.

314. Clear D. Anaphylactoid reaction to methyl prednisolone developing after starting treatment with interferon beta-1b. J Neurol Neurosurg Psychiatry 1999;66(5):690.

315. Schonwald S. Methylprednisolone anaphylaxis. Am J Emerg Med 1999;17(6):583–5.

316. Vanpee D, Gillet JB. Allergic reaction to intravenous methylprednisolone in a woman with asthma. Ann Emerg Med 1998;32(6):754.

317. Polosa R, Prosperini G, Pintaldi L, Rey JP, Colombrita R. Anaphylaxis after prednisone. Allergy 1998;53(3):330–1.

318. Karsh J, Yang WH. An anaphylactic reaction to intra-articular triamcinolone: a case report and review of the literature. Ann Allergy Asthma Immunol 2003; 90: 254-8.

319. Yawalkar N, Hari Y, Helbing A, von Greyerz S, Kappeler A, Baathen LR, Pichler WJ. Elevated serum levels of interleukins 5, 6, and 10 in a patient with drug-induced exanthem caused by systemic corticosteroids. J Am Acad Dermatol 1998;39(5 Part 1):790–3.

320. Ventura MT, Calogiuri GF, Matino MG, Dagnello M, Buquicchio R, Foti C, Di Corato R. Alternative glucocorticoids for use in cases of adverse reaction to systemic glucocorticoids: a study on 10 patients. Br J Dematol 2003; 148: 139-41.

321. Heeringa M, Zweers P, de Man RA, de Groot H. Drug Points: Anaphylactic-like reaction associated with oral budesonide. BMJ 2000;321(7266):927.

322. Gomez CM, Higuero NC, Moral de Gregorio A, Quiles MH, Nunez Aceves AB, Lara MJ, Sanchez CS. Urticaria–angioedema by deflazacort. Allergy 2002;57(4):370–1.

323. Monk BE, Skipper D. Allergy to topical corticosteroids in inflammatory bowel disease. Gut 2003; 52: 597.

324. Staunton H, Stafford F, Leader M, O'Riordain D. Deterioration of giant cell arteritis with corticosteroid therapy. Arch Neurol 2000;57(4):581–4.

325. Schols AM, Wesseling G, Kester AD, de Vries G, Mostert R, Slangen J, Wouters EF. Dose dependent increased mortality risk in COPD patients treated with oral glucocorticoids. Eur Respir J 2001;17(3):337–42.

326. Klaustermeyer WB, Gianos ME, Kurohara ML, Dao HT, Heiner DC. IgG subclass deficiency associated with corticosteroids in obstructive lung disease. Chest 1992;102(4):1137–42.

327. Robinson MJ, Campbell F, Powell P, Sims D, Thornton C. Antibody response to accelerated Hib immunisation in preterm infants receiving dexamethasone for chronic lung disease. Arch Dis Child Fetal Neonatal Ed 1999;80(1):F69–71.

328. Sprung CL, Caralis PV, Marcial EH, Pierce M, Gelbard MA, Long WM, Duncan RC, Tendler MD, Karpf M. The effects of high-dose corticosteroids in patients with septic shock. A prospective, controlled study. N Engl J Med 1984;311(18):1137–43.

329. Mostafa BE. Fluticasone propionate is associated with severe infection after endoscopic polypectomy. Arch Otolaryngol Head Neck Surg 1996;122(7):729–31.

330. Demitsu T, Kosuge A, Yamada T, Usui K, Katayama H, Yaoita H. Acute generalized exanthematous pustulosis induced by dexamethasone injection. Dermatology 1996;193(1):56–8.

331. Aberra FN, Lewis JD, Hass D, Rombeau JL, Osborne B, Lichtenstein GR. Corticosteroids and immunomodulators: postoperative infectious complication risk in inflammatory bowel disease patients. Gastroenterology 2003; 125: 320-7.

332. Wolfe F, Caplan L, Michaud K. Treatment for rheumatoid arthritis and the risk of hospitalization for pneumonia: associations with prednisone, disease-modifying antirheumatic drugs, and anti-tumor necrosis factor therapy. Arthritis Rheum 2006; 54(2): 628-34.

333. Britt RC, Devine A, Swallen KC, Weireter LJ, Collins JN, Cole FJ, Britt LD. Corticosteroid use in the intensive care unit: at what cost? Arch Surg 2006; 141(2): 145-9.

334. Hedderwick SA, Bonilla HF, Bradley SF, Kauffman CA. Opportunistic infections in patients with temporal arteritis treated with corticosteroids. J Am Geriatr Soc 1997;45(3):334–7.

335. Korula J. Tuberculous peritonitis complicating corticosteroid therapy for acute alcoholic hepatitis. Dig Dis Sci 1995;40(10):2119–20.

336. Kim HA, Yoo CD, Baek HJ, Lee EB, Ahn C, Han JS, Kim S, Lee JS, Choe KW, Song YW. *Mycobacterium tuberculosis* infection in a corticosteroid-treated rheumatic disease patient population. Clin Exp Rheumatol 1998;16(1):9–13.

337. di Girolamo C, Pappone N, Melillo E, Rengo C, Giuliano F, Melillo G. Cavitary lung tuberculosis in a rheumatoid arthritis patient treated with low-dose

methotrexate and steroid pulse therapy. Br J Rheumatol 1998;37(10):1136–7.

338. Martos A, Podzamczer D, Martinez-Lacasa J, Rufi G, Santin M, Gudiol F. Steroids do not enhance the risk of developing tuberculosis or other AIDS-related diseases in HIV-infected patients treated for *Pneumocystis carinii* pneumonia. AIDS 1995;9(9):1037–41.

339. Bridges MJ, McGarry F. Two cases of *Mycobacterium avium* septic arthritis. Ann Rheum Dis 2002;61(2):186–7.

340. Fernandez-Aviles F, Batlle M, Ribera JM, Matas L, Sabria M, Feliu E. *Legionella* sp pneumonia in patients with hematologic diseases. A study of 10 episodes from a series of 67 cases of pneumonia. Haematologica 1999;84(5):474–5.

341. Rice P, Simmons K, Carr R, Banatvala J. Near fatal chickenpox during prednisolone treatment. BMJ 1994;309(6961):1069–70.

342. Choong K, Zwaigenbaum L, Onyett H. Severe varicella after low dose inhaled corticosteroids. Pediatr Infect Dis J 1995;14(9):809–11.

343. Burnett I. Severe chickenpox during treatment with corticosteroids. Immunoglobulin should be given if steroid dosage was > or = 0.5 mg/kg/day in preceding three months BMJ 1995;310(6975):327Erratum in BMJ 1995; 310(6978):534.

344. Doherty MJ, Baxter AB, Longstreth WT Jr. Herpes simplex virus encephalitis complicating myxedema coma treated with corticosteroids. Neurology 2001;56(8):1114–5.

345. Pingleton WW, Bone RC, Kerby GR, Ruth WE. Oropharyngeal candidiasis in patients treated with triamcinolone acetonide aerosol. J Allergy Clin Immunol 1977;60(4):254–8.

346. Nenoff P, Horn LC, Mierzwa M, Leonhardt R, Weidenbach H, Lehmann I, Haustein UF. Peracute disseminated fatal *Aspergillus fumigatus* sepsis as a complication of corticoid-treated systemic lupus erythematosus. Mycoses 1995;38(11–12):467–71.

347. Wald A, Leisenring W, van Burik JA, Bowden RA. Epidemiology of *Aspergillus infections* in a large cohort of patients undergoing bone marrow transplantation. J Infect Dis 1997;175(6):1459–66.

348. Machet L, Jan V, Machet MC, Vaillant L, Lorette G. Cutaneous alternariosis: role of corticosteroid-induced cutaneous fragility. Dermatology 1996;193(4):342–4.

349. Fucci JC, Nightengale ML. Primary esophageal histoplasmosis. Am J Gastroenterol 1997;92(3):530–1.

350. Monlun E, de Blay F, Berton C, Gasser B, Jaeger A, Pauli G. Invasive pulmonary aspergillosis with cerebromeningeal involvement after short-term intravenous corticosteroid therapy in a patient with asthma. Respir Med 1997;91(7):435–7.

351. Shetty D, Giri N, Gonzalez CE, Pizzo PA, Walsh TJ. Invasive aspergillosis in human immunodeficiency virus-infected children. Pediatr Infect Dis J 1997;16(2):216–21.

352. Fernandez JM, Sanchez E, Polo FJ, Saez L. Infección pulmonar por *Aspergillus fumigatus* y *Nocardia asteroides* como complicación del tratamiento con glucocorticoides. Med Clin (Barc) 2000;114:358.

353. Carrascosa Porras M, Herreras Martinez R, Corral Mones J, Ares Ares M, Zabaleta Murguiondo M, Ruchel R. Fatal *Aspergillus* myocarditis following short-term corticosteroid therapy for chronic obstructive pulmonary disease. Scand J Infect Dis 2002;34(3):224–7.

354. Vogeser M, Haas A, Ruckdeschel G, von Scheidt W. Steroid-induced invasive aspergillosis with thyroid gland abscess and positive blood cultures. Eur J Clin Microbiol Infect Dis 1998;17(3):215–6.

355. Mavinkurve-Groothuis AMC, Bokkerink JPM, Verweij PE, Veerman AJP, Hoogerbrugge PM. Cryptococcal meningitis in a child with acute lymphoblastic leukemia. Pediatr Infect Dis J 2003; 22: 576.

356. Bower CP, Oxley JD, Campbell CK, Archer CB. Cutaneous *Scedosporium apiospermum* infection in an immunocompromised patient. J Clin Pathol 1999;52(11):846–8.

357. Ioannidou DJ, Stefanidou MP, Maraki SG, Panayiotides JG, Tosca AD. Cutaneous alternariosis in a patient with idiopathic pulmonary fibrosis. Int J Dermatol 2000;39(4):293–5.

358. Pera A, Byun A, Gribar S, Schwartz R, Kumar D, Parimi P. Dexamethasone therapy and *Candida* sepsis in neonates less than 1250 grams. J Perinatol 2002;22(3):204–8.

359. Fukuda T, Boeckh M, Carter RA, Sandmaier BM, Maris MB, Maloney DG, Martin PJ, Storb RF, Marr KA. Risks and outcomes of invasive fungal infections in recipients of allogenic hematopoietic stem cell transplants after nonmyeloablative conditioning. Blood 2003; 102: 827-33.

360. Buchheidt D, Hummel M, Diehl S, Hehlmann R. Fatal cerebral involvement in systemic aspergillosis: a rare complication of steroid-treated autoimmune bicytopenia. Eur J Haematol 2004; 72: 375-6.

361. Sen P, Gil C, Estrellas B, Middleton JR. Corticosteroid-induced asthma: a manifestation of limited hyperinfection syndrome due to *Strongyloides stercoralis*. South Med J 1995;88(9):923–7.

362. Mariotta S, Pallone G, Li Bianchi E, Gilardi G, Bisetti A. *Strongyloides stercoralis* hyperinfection in a case of idiopathic pulmonary fibrosis. Panminerva Med 1996;38(1):45–7.

363. Leung VK, Liew CT, Sung JJ. Fatal strongyloidiasis in a patient with ulcerative colitis after corticosteroid therapy. Am J Gastroenterol 1997;92(8):1383–4.

364. Schipperijn AJM. Flare-up of toxoplasmosis due to corticosteroid therapy in pulmonary sarcoidosis. Ned T Geneesk 1970;114:1710.

365. Cohen SN. Toxoplasmosis in patients receiving immunosuppressive therapy. JAMA 1970;211(4):657–60.

366. Sy ML, Chin TW, Nussbaum E. *Pneumocystis carinii* pneumonia associated with inhaled corticosteroids in an immunocompetent child with asthma. J Pediatr 1995;127(6):1000–2.

367. Bachelez H, Schremmer B, Cadranel J, Mouly F, Sarfati C, Agbalika F, Schlemmer B, Mayaud CM, Dubertret L. Fulminant *Pneumocystis carinii* pneumonia in 4 patients with dermatomyositis. Arch Intern Med 1997;157(13):1501–3.

368. Kanani SR, Knight R. Amoebic dysentery precipitated by corticosteroids. BMJ 1969;3(662):114.

369. Stark AR, Carlo WA, Tyson JE, Papile LA, Wright LL, Shankaran S, Donovan EF, Oh W, Bauer CR, Saha S, Poole WK, Stoll BJ. National Institute of Child Health and Human Development Neonatal Research Network. Adverse effects of early dexamethasone in extremely-low-birth-weight infants. National Institute of Child Health and Human Development Neonatal Research Network. N Engl J Med 2001;344(2):95–101.

370. Lucas A, Coll J, Salinas I, Sanmarti A. Hipertensión intracraneal benigna tras suspensión de corticoterapia en una paciente previaments intervenida por enfermedad de Cushing. [Benign intracranial hypertension following the suspension of corticotherapy in a female patient previously operated on for Cushing's disease.] Med Clin (Barc) 1991;97(12):473.

371. Richards D, Aronson J. The Oxford Handbook of Practical Drug TherapyOxford: Oxford University Press;. 2004.

372. Morgan J, Lacey JH. Anorexia nervosa and steroid withdrawal. Int J Eat Disord 1996;19(2):213–5.

373. Silverman RA, Newman AJ, LeVine MJ, Kaplan B. Poststeroid panniculitis: a case report. Pediatr Dermatol 1988;5(2):92–3.

374. Le Gall C, Pham S, Vignes S, Garcia G, Nunes H, Fichet D, Simonneau G, Duroux P, Humbert M. Inhaled corticosteroids and Churg–Strauss syndrome: a report of five cases. Eur Respir J 2000;15(5):978–81.

375. Hodgkinson DJ, Williams TJ. Endometrial carcinoma associated with azathioprine and cortisone therapy. A case report. Gynecol Oncol 1977;5(3):308–12.

376. Erban SB, Sokas RK. Kaposi's sarcoma in an elderly man with Wegener's granulomatosis treated with cyclophosphamide and corticosteroids. Arch Intern Med 1988;148(5):1201–3.

377. Thiagarajan CM, Divakar D, Thomas SJ. Malignancies in renal transplant recipients. Transplant Proc 1998;30(7):3154–5.

378. Gill PS, Loureiro C, Bernstein-Singer M, Rarick MU, Sattler F, Levine AM. Clinical effect of glucocorticoids on Kaposi sarcoma related to the acquired immunodeficiency syndrome (AIDS). Ann Intern Med 1989;110(11):937–40.

379. Tebbe B, Mayer-da-Silva A, Garbe C, von Keyserlingk HJ, Orfanos CE. Genetically determined coincidence of Kaposi sarcoma and psoriasis in an HIV-negative patient after prednisolone treatment. Spontaneous regression 8 months after discontinuing therapy. Int J Dermatol 1991;30(2):114–20.

380. Vincent T, Moss K, Colaco B, Venables PJ. Kaposi's sarcoma in two patients following low-dose corticosteroid treatment for rheumatological disease. Rheumatology (Oxford) 2000;39(11):1294–6.

381. Sorensen HT, Mellemkjaer L, Friis S, Olsen JH. Use of systemic corticosteroids and risk of esophageal cancer. Epidemiology 2002;13(2):240–1.

382. Chin S-OS, Brodsky NL, Bhandari V. Antenatal steroid use is associated with increased gastroesophageal reflux in neonates. Am J Perinatol 2003; 20: 205-13.

383. Jobe AH, Soll RF. Choice and dose of corticosteroid for antenatal treatments. Am J Obstet Gynecol 2004; 190: 878–81.

384. Committee on Fetus and Newborn. Postnatal corticosteroids to treat or prevent chronic lung disease in preterm infants. Pediatrics 2002;109(2):330–8.

385. Canadian Paediatric Society and American Academy of Pediatrics. Postnatal corticosteroids to treat or prevent chronic lung disease in preterm infants. Pediatr Child Health 2002;7:20–8.

386. Banks BA, Macones G, Cnaan A, Merrill JD, Ballard PL, Ballard RA. North American TRH Study Group. Multiple courses of antenatal corticosteroids are associated with early severe lung disease in preterm neonates. J Perinatol 2002;22(2):101–7.

387. Elliott JP, Radin TG. The effect of corticosteroid administration on uterine activity and preterm labor in high-order multiple gestations. Obstet Gynecol 1995;85(2):250–4.

388. Ogunyemi D. A comparison of the effectiveness of single-dose vs multi-dose antenatal corticosteroids in pre-term neonates. Obstet Gynaecol 2005; 25(8): 756-60.

389. Haas DM, McCullough W, Olsen CH, Shiau DT, Richard J, Fry EA, McNamara MF. Neonatal outcomes with different betamethasone dosing regimens: a comparison. J Reprod Med 2005; 50(12): 915-22.

390. Schmitz T, Goffinet F, Barrande G, Cabrol D. Maternal hypercorticism from serial courses of betamethasone. Obstet Gynecol 1999;94(5 Part 2):849.

391. Helal KJ, Gordon MC, Lightner CR, Barth WH Jr. Adrenal suppression induced by betamethasone in women at risk for premature delivery. Obstet Gynecol 2000;96(2):287–90.

392. Spencer C, Smith P, Rafla N, Weatherell R. Corticosteroids in pregnancy and osteonecrosis of the femoral head. Obstet Gynecol 1999;94(5 Part 2):848.

393. Vermillion ST, Soper DE, Chasedunn-Roark J. Neonatal sepsis after betamethasone administration to patients with preterm premature rupture of membranes. Am J Obstet Gynecol 1999;181(2):320–7.

394. Rotmensch S, Vishne TH, Celentano C, Dan M, Ben-Rafael Z. Maternal infectious morbidity following multiple courses of betamethasone. J Infect 1999;39(1):49–54.

395. Vermillion ST, Soper DE, Newman RB. Neonatal sepsis and death after multiple courses of antenatal betamethasone therapy. Am J Obstet Gynecol 2000;183(4):810–4.

396. Abbasi S, Hirsch D, Davis J, Tolosa J, Stouffer N, Debbs R, Gerdes JS. Effect of single versus multiple courses of antenatal corticosteroids on maternal and neonatal outcome. Am J Obstet Gynecol 2000;182(5):1243–9.

397. Yang SH, Choi SJ, Roh CR, Kim JH. Multiple courses of antenatal corticosteroid therapy in patients with preterm premature rupture of membranes. J Perinat Med 2004; 32: 42–8.

398. Stockli A, Keller M. Kongenitales adrenogenitales Syndrom und Schwangerschaft. [Congenital adrenogenital syndrome and pregnancy.] Schweiz Med Wochenschr 1969;99(4):126–8.

399. Beique LC, Friesen MH, Park LY, Diaz-Citrin O, Koren G, Einarson TR. Major malformations associated with corticosteroid exposure during the first trimester: a meta-analysis. Can J Hosp Pharm 1998;51:83.

400. Moran P, Taylor R. Management of hyperemesis gravidarum: the importance of weight loss as a criterion for steroid therapy. QJM 2002;95(3):153–8.

401. Markert UR, Klemm A, Flossmann E, Werner W, Sperschneider H, Funfstuck R. Renal transplantation in early pregnancy with acute graft rejection and development of a hydatidiform mole. Clin Nephrol 1998;49(6):391–2.

402. Park-Wyllie L, Mazzotta P, Pastuszak A, Moretti ME, Beique L, Hunnisett L, Friesen MH, Jacobson S, Kasapinovic S, Chang D, Diav-Citrin O, Chitayat D, Nulman I, Einarson TR, Koren G. Birth defects after maternal exposure to corticosteroids: prospective cohort study and meta-analysis of epidemiological studies. Teratology 2000;62(6):385–92.

403. Harding JE, Pang J, Knight DB, Liggins GC. Do antenatal corticosteroids help in the setting of preterm rupture of membranes? Am J Obstet Gynecol 2001;184(2):131–9.

404. Bloom SL, Sheffield JS, McIntire DD, Leveno KJ. Antenatal dexamethasone and decreased birth weight. Obstet Gynecol 2001;97(4):485–90.

405. Rotmensch S, Liberati M, Celentano C, Efrat Z, Bar-Hava I, Kovo M, Golan A, Moravski G, Ben-Rafael Z. The effect of betamethasone on fetal biophysical activities and Doppler velocimetry of umbilical and middle cerebral arteries. Acta Obstet Gynecol Scand 1999;78(9):768–73.

406. Crowther CA, Haslam RR, Hiller JE, Doyle LW, Robinson JS; Australasian Collaborative Trial of Repeat Doses of Steroids (ACTORDS) Study Group. Neonatal respiratory distress syndrome after repeat exposure to

antenatal corticosteroids: a randomised controlled trial. Lancet 2006; 367(9526): 1913–9.

407. Lee BH, Stoll BJ, McDonald SA, Higgins RD; National Institute of Child Health and Human Development Neonatal Research Network. Adverse neonatal outcomes associated with antenatal dexamethasone versus antenatal betamethasone. Pediatrics 2006; 117(5): 1503-10.

408. Warrell DW, Taylor R. Outcome for the foetus of mothers receiving prednisolone during pregnancy. Lancet 1968;1(7534):117–8.

409. Crowley PA. Antenatal corticosteroid therapy: a meta-analysis of the randomized trials, 1972–94. Am J Obstet Gynecol 1995;173(1):322–35.

410. Kairalla AB. Hypothalamic–pituitary–adrenal axis function in premature neonates after extensive prenatal treatment with betamethasone: a case history. Am J Perinatol 1992;9(5–6):428–30.

411. Ohrlander S, Gennser G, Nilsson KO, Eneroth P. ACTH test to neonates after administration of corticosteroids during gestation. Obstet Gynecol 1977;49(6):691–4.

412. Ohlsson A, Calvert SA, Hosking M, Shennan AT. Randomized controlled trial of dexamethasone treatment in very-low-birth-weight infants with ventilator-dependent chronic lung disease. Acta Paediatr 1992;81(10):751–6.

413. Brownlee KG, Ng PC, Henderson MJ, Smith M, Green JH, Dear PR. Catabolic effect of dexamethasone in the preterm baby. Arch Dis Child 1992;67(1 Spec No):1–4.

414. O'Neil EA, Chwals WJ, O'Shea MD, Turner CS. Dexamethasone treatment during ventilator dependency: possible life threatening gastrointestinal complications. Arch Dis Child 1992;67(1 Spec No):10–1.

415. Dalziel SR, Walker NK, Parag V, Mantell C, Rea HH, Rodgers A, Harding JE. Cardiovascular risk factors after antenatal exposure to betamethasone: 30-year follow-up of a randomised controlled trial. Lancet 2005; 365(9474): 1856-62.

416. Spinillo A, Viazzo F, Colleoni R, Chiara A, Maria Cerbo R, Fazzi E. Two-year infant neurodevelopmental outcome after single or multiple antenatal courses of corticosteroids to prevent complications of prematurity. Am J Obstet Gynecol 2004; 191: 217-24.

417. French NP, Hagan R, Evans SF, Mullan A, Newnham JP. Repeated antenatal corticosteroids: effects on cerebral palsy and childhood behavior. Am J Obstet Gynecol 2004; 190: 588-95.

418. Dalziel SR, Lim VK, Lambert A, McCarthy D, Parag V, Rodgers A, Harding JE. Antenatal exposure to betamethasone: psychological functioning and health related quality of life 31 years after inclusion in randomised controlled trial. BMJ 2005; 331(7518): 665.

419. Cho S, Beharry KD, Valencia AM, Guajardo L, Nageotte MP, Modanlou HD. Maternal and feto-placental prostanoid responses to a single course of antenatal betamethasone. Prostaglandins Other Lipid Mediat 2005; 78(1-4): 139-59.

420. Harding JE, Pang J, Knight DB, Liggins GC. Do antenatal corticosteroids help in the setting of preterm rupture of membranes? Am J Obstet Gynecol 2001;184(2):131–9.

421. Rotmensch S, Celentano C, Liberati M, Sadan O, Glezerman M. The effect of antenatal steroid administration on the fetal response to vibroacoustic stimulation. Acta Obstet Gynecol Scand 1999;78(10):847–51.

422. Tornatore KM, Biocevich DM, Reed K, Tousley K, Singh JP, Venuto RC. Methylprednisolone pharmacokinetics, cortisol response, and adverse effects in black and white renal transplant recipients. Transplantation 1995;59(5):729–36.

423. Skoner DP. Balancing safety and efficacy in pediatric asthma management. Pediatrics 2002;109(Suppl 2):381–92.

424. Allen DB. Safety of inhaled corticosteroids in children. Pediatr Pulmonol 2002;33(3):208–20.

425. Thebaud B, Lacaze-Masmonteil T, Watterberg K. Postnatal glucocorticoids in very preterm infants: "the good, the bad, and the ugly"? Pediatrics 2001;107(2):413–5.

426. O'Callaghan JW, Brooks PM. Disease-modifying agents and immunosuppressive drugs in the elderly. Clin Rheum Dis 1986;2(1):275–89.

427. Akerkar GA, Peppercorn MA, Hamel MB, Parker RA. Corticosteroid-associated complications in elderly Crohn's disease patients. Am J Gastroenterol 1997;92(3):461–4.

429. Powell LW, Axelsen E. Corticosteroids in liver disease: studies on the biological conversion of prednisone to prednisolone and plasma protein binding. Gut 1972;13(9):690–6.

429. Davis M, Williams R, Chakraborty J, English J, Marks V, Ideo G, Tempini S. Prednisone or prednisolone for the treatment of chronic active hepatitis? A comparison of plasma availability. Br J Clin Pharmacol 1978;5(6):501–5.

430. Frey BM, Frey FJ. Clinical pharmacokinetics of prednisone and prednisolone. Clin Pharmacokinet 1990;19(2): 126–46.

431. Harris RZ, Tsunoda SM, Mroczkowski P, Wong H, Benet LZ. The effects of menopause and hormone replacement therapies on prednisolone and erythromycin pharmacokinetics. Clin Pharmacol Ther 1996;59(4):429–35.

432. Lewis GP, Jusko WJ, Graves L, Burke CW. Prednisone side-effects and serum-protein levels. A collaborative study. Lancet 1971;2(7728):778–80.

433. Zonana-Nacach A, Barr SG, Magder LS, Petri M. Damage in systemic lupus erythematosus and its association with corticosteroids. Arthritis Rheum 2000;43(8):1801–8.

434. Andus T, Gross V, Caesar I, Schulz HJ, Lochs H, Strohm WD, Gierend M, Weber A, Ewe K, Scholmerich J; German/Austrian Budesonide Study Group. Replacement of conventional glucocorticoids by oral pH-modified release budesonide in active and inactive Crohn's disease: results of an open, prospective, multicenter trial. Dig Dis Sci 2003; 48: 373-8.

435. Keane FM, Munn SE, du Vivier AW, Taylor NF, Higgins EM. Analysis of Chinese herbal creams prescribed for dermatological conditions. BMJ 1999;318(7183):563–4.

436. Reinberg AE. Chronopharmacology of corticosteroids and ACTH. In: Lammer B, editor. Chronopharmacology. Cellular and Biochemical Interactions. New York and Basel: Marcel Dekker Inc, 1989:137–67.

437. Kimura Y, Fieldston E, Devries-Vandervlugt B, Li S, Imundo L. High dose, alternate day corticosteroids for systemic onset juvenile rheumatoid arthritis. J Rheumatol 2000;27(8):2018–24.

438. Kaiser BA, Polinsky MS, Palmer JA, Dunn S, Mochon M, Flynn JT, Baluarte HJ. Growth after conversion to alternate-day corticosteroids in children with renal transplants: a single-center study. Pediatr Nephrol 1994;8(3):320–5.

439. Blair GP, Light RW. Treatment of chronic obstructive pulmonary disease with corticosteroids. Comparison of daily vs alternate-day therapy. Chest 1984;86(4):524–8.

440. Oshitani N, Kamata N, Ooiso R, Kawashima D, Inagawa M, Sogawa M, Iimuro M, Jinno Y, Watanabe K, Higuchi K, Matsumoto T, Arakawa T. Outpatient treatment of moderately severe active ulcerative colitis with pulsed steroid therapy and conventional steroid therapy. Dig Dis Sci 2003; 4: 1002–5.

441. Gilbertson EO, Spellman MC, Piacquadio DJ, Mulford MI. Super potent topical corticosteroid use associated with adrenal suppression: clinical considerations. J Am Acad Dermatol 1998;38(2 Part 2):318–21.

442. Marcos C, Allegue F, Luna I, Gonzalez R. An unusual case of allergic contact dermatitis from corticosteroids. Contact Dermatitis 1999;41(4):237–8.

443. Corazza M, Virgili A. Allergic contact dermatitis from 6alpha-methylprednisolone aceponate and budesonide. Contact Dermatitis 1998;38(6):356–7.

444. Ermis B, Ors R, Tastekin A, Ozkan B. Cushing's syndrome secondary to topical corticosteroids abuse. Clin Endocrinol 2003;58:795-7.

445. Oh C, Lee J. Contact allergy to various ingredients of topical medicaments. Contact Dermatitis 2003;49:49–5.

446. Karadimas P, Kapetanios A, Bouzas EA. Central serous chorioretinopathy after local application of glucocorticoids for skin disorders. Arch Ophthalmol 2004; 122: 784-6.

447. Mygind H, Thulstrup AM, Pedersen L, Larsen H. Risk of intrauterine growth retardation, malformations and other birth outcomes in children after topical use of corticosteroid in pregnancy. Acta Obstet Gynecol Scand 2002;81(3):234–9.

448. Whitcup SM, Ferris FL 3rd. New corticosteroids for the treatment of ocular inflammation. Am J Ophthalmol 1999;127(5):597–9.

449. Aggarwal RK, Potamitis T, Chong NH, Guarro M, Shah P, Kheterpal S. Extensive visual loss with topical facial steroids. Eye 1993;7(5):664–6.

450. Baratz KH, Hattenhauer MG. Indiscriminate use of corticosteroid-containing eyedrops. Mayo Clin Proc 1999;74(4):362–6.

451. Chua JK, Fan DS, Leung AT, Lam DS. Accelerated ocular hypertensive response after application of corticosteroid ointment to a child's eyelid. Mayo Clin Proc 2000;75(5):539.

452. Ozerdem U, Levi L, Cheng L, Song MK, Scher C, Freeman WR. Systemic toxicity of topical and periocular corticosteroid therapy in an 11-year-old male with posterior uveitis. Am J Ophthalmol 2000;130(2):240–1.

453. Mehle ME. Are nasal steroids safe? Curr Opin Otolaryngol Head Neck Surg 2003; 11: 201-5.

454. Salib RJ, Howarth PH. Safety and tolerability profiles of intranasal antihistamines and intranasal corticosteroids in the treatment of allergic rhinitis. Drug Saf 2003; 26: 863-93.

455. Priftis K, Everard ML, Milner AD. Unexpected side-effects of inhaled steroids: a case report. Eur J Pediatr 1991;150(6):448–9.

456. Stead RJ, Cooke NJ. Adverse effects of inhaled corticosteroids. BMJ 1989;298(6671):403–4.

457. Whittet HB, Shinkwin C, Freeland AP. Anosmia due to nasal administration of corticosteroid. BMJ 1991;303(6803):651.

455. Bond DW, Charlton CP, Gregson RM. Benign intracranial hypertension secondary to nasal fluticasone propionate. BMJ 2001;322(7291):897.

459. Ozturk F, Yuceturk AV, Kurt E, Unlu HH, Ilker SS. Evaluation of intraocular pressure and cataract formation following the long-term use of nasal corticosteroids. Ear Nose Throat J 1998;77(10):846–51.

460. Cervin A, Andersson M. Intranasal steroids and septum perforation – an overlooked complication? A description of the course of events and a discussion of the causes. Rhinology 1998;36(3):128–32.

461. Nayak AS, Ellis MH, Gross GN, Mendelson LM, Schenkel EJ, Lanier BQ, Simpson B, Mullin ME, Smith JA. The effects of triamcinolone acetonide aqueous nasal spray on adrenocortical function in children with allergic rhinitis. J Allergy Clin Immunol 1998;101(2 Part 1):157–62.

462. Findlay CA, Macdonald JF, Wallace AM, Geddes N, Donaldson MD. Childhood Cushing's syndrome induced by betamethasone nose drops, and repeat prescriptions. BMJ 1998;317(7160):739–40.

463. Hillebrand-Haverkort ME, Prummel MF, ten Veen JH. Ritonavir-induced Cushing's syndrome in a patient treated with nasal fluticasone. AIDS 1999;13(13):1803.

464. Downs AM, Lear JT, Kennedy CT. Anaphylaxis to intradermal triamcinolone acetonide. Arch Dermatol 1998;134(9):1163–4.

465. Mistlin A, Gibson T. Osteonecrosis of the femoral head resulting from excessive corticosteroid nasal spray use. J Clin Rheumatol 2004; 10: 45-6.

466. Miranda-Romero A, Bajo-del Pozo C, Sanchez-Sambucety P, Martinez-Fernandez M, Garcia-Munoz M. Delayed local allergic reaction to intralesional parametasone acetate. Contact Dermatitis 1998;39(1):31–2.

467. Wilkinson HA. Intrathecal Depo-Medrol: a literature review. Clin J Pain 1992;8(1):49–56.

468. DeSio JM, Kahn CH, Warfield CA. Facial flushing and/or generalized erythema after epidural steroid injection. Anesth Analg 1995;80(3):617–9.

469. Plumb VJ, Dismukes WE. Chemical meningitis related to intrathecal corticosteroid therapy. South Med J 1977;70(10):1241–3.

470. Dumont D, Hariz H, Meynieu P, Salama J, Dreyfus P, Boissier MC. Abducens palsy after an intrathecal glucocorticoid injection. Evidence for a role of intracranial hypotension. Rev Rhum Engl Ed 1998;65(5):352–4.

471. Spaccarelli KC. Lumbar and caudal epidural corticosteroid injections. Mayo Clin Proc 1996;71(2):169–78.

472. Chen YC, Gajraj NM, Clavo A, Joshi GP. Posterior subcapsular cataract formation associated with multiple lumbar epidural corticosteroid injections. Anesth Analg 1998;86(5):1054–5.

473. Siegfried RN. Development of complex regional pain syndrome after a cervical epidural steroid injection. Anesthesiology 1997;86(6):1394–6.

474. Sandberg DI, Lavyne MH. Symptomatic spinal epidural lipomatosis after local epidural corticosteroid injections: case report. Neurosurgery 1999;45(1):162–5.

475. Cooper AB, Sharpe MD. Bacterial meningitis and cauda equina syndrome after epidural steroid injections. Can J Anaesth 1996;43(5 Part 1):471–4.

476. McLain RF, Fry M, Hecht ST. Transient paralysis associated with epidural steroid injection. J Spinal Disord 1997;10(5):441–4.

477. Brocq O, Breuil V, Grisot C, Flory P, Ziegler G, Euller-Ziegler L. Diplopie après infiltrations peridurale et intradurale de prédnisolone. Deux observations. [Diplopia after peridural and intradural infiltrations of prednisolone. 2 cases.] Presse Méd 1997;26(6):271.

478. Lowell TD, Errico TJ, Eskenazi MS. Use of epidural steroids after discectomy may predispose to infection. Spine 2000;25(4):516–9.

479. Field J, Rathmell JP, Stephenson JH, Katz NP. Neuropathic pain following cervical epidural steroid injection. Anesthesiology 2000;93(3):885–8.

480. Sparling M, Malleson P, Wood B, Petty R. Radiographic followup of joints injected with triamcinolone hexacetonide for the management of childhood arthritis. Arthritis Rheum 1990;33(6):821–6.

481. Gutierrez-Urena S, Ramos-Remus C. Persistent hiccups associated with intraarticular corticosteroid injection. J Rheumatol 1999;26(3):760.

482. Daragon A, Vittecoq O, Le Loet X. Visual hallucinations induced by intraarticular injection of steroids. J Rheumatol 1997;24(2):411.

483. Wicki J, Droz M, Cirafici L, Vallotton MB. Acute adrenal crisis in a patient treated with intraarticular steroid therapy. J Rheumatol 2000;27(2):510–1.

484. Valsecchi R, Reseghetti A, Leghissa P, Cologni L, Cortinovis R. Erythema-multiforme-like lesions from triamcinolone acetonide. Contact Dermatitis 1998;38(6):362–3.

485. Selvi E, De Stefano R, Lorenzini S, Marcolongo R. Arthritis induced by corticosteroid crystals. J Rheumatol 2004; 31: 622.

486. Jawed S, Allard SA. Osteomyelitis of the humerus following steroid injections for tennis elbow. Rheumatology (Oxford) 2000;39(8):923–4.

487. Montoro J, Valero A, Serra-Baldrich E, Amat P, Lluch M, Malet A. Anaphylaxis to paramethasone with tolerance to other corticosteroids. Allergy 2000;55(2):197–8.

488. Caffee HH. Intracapsular injection of triamcinolone for intractable capsule contracture. Plast Reconstr Surg 1994;94(6):824–8.

489. Braverman DL, Lachmann EA, Nagler W. Avascular necrosis of bilateral knees secondary to corticosteroid enemas. Arch Phys Med Rehabil 1998;79(4):449–52.

490. Tsuruoka S, Sugimoto K, Fujimura A. Drug-induced Cushing syndrome in a patient with ulcerative colitis after betamethasone enema: evaluation of plasma drug concentration. Ther Drug Monit 1998;20(4):387–9.

491. Lauerma AI. Occupational contact sensitization to corticosteroids. Contact Dermatitis 1998;39(6):328–9.

492. Newton RW, Browning MC, Iqbal J, Piercy N, Adamson DG. Adrenocortical suppression in workers manufacturing synthetic glucocorticoids. BMJ 1978;1(6105):73–4.

493. Nixon DW, Shlaer SM. Fulminant lung metastases from cancer of the breast. Med Pediatr Oncol 1981;9(4):381–5.

494. Klygis LM. Dexamethasone-induced perineal irritation in head injury. Am J Emerg Med 1992;10(3):268.

495. Takayanagui OM, Lanchote VL, Marques MP, Bonato PS. Therapy for neurocysticercosis: pharmacokinetic interaction of albendazole sulfoxide with dexamethasone. Ther Drug Monit 1997;19(1):51–5.

496. Ahle GB, Blum AL, Martinek J, Oneta CM, Dorta G. Cushing's syndrome in an 81-year-old patient treated with budesonide and amiodarone. Eur J Gastroenterol Hepatol 2000;12(9):1041–2.

497. Costedoat-Chalumeau N, Amoura Z, Aymard G, Sevin O, Wechsler B, Du Cacoub PLT, Diquet B, Ankri A, Piette JC. Potentiation of vitamin K antagonists by high-dose intravenous methylprednisolone. Ann Intern Med 2000;132(8):631–5.

498. Varis T, Kaukonen KM, Kivisto KT, Neuvonen PJ. Plasma concentrations and effects of oral methylprednisolone are considerably increased by itraconazole. Clin Pharmacol Ther 1998;64(4):363–8.

499. Varis T, Kivisto KT, Backman JT, Neuvonen PJ. Itraconazole decreases the clearance and enhances the effects of intravenously administered methylprednisolone in healthy volunteers. Pharmacol Toxicol 1999;85(1):29–32.

500. Woods DR, Arun CS, Corris PA, Perros P. Cushing's syndrome without excess cortisol. BMJ 2006; 332: 469-70.

501. Varis T, Kivisto KT, Neuvonen PJ. The effect of itraconazole on the pharmacokinetics and pharmacodynamics of oral prednisolone. Eur J Clin Pharmacol 2000;56(1):57–60.

502. Varis T, Kivisto KT, Backman JT, Neuvonen PJ. The cytochrome P450 3A4 inhibitor itraconazole markedly increases the plasma concentrations of dexamethasone and enhances its adrenal-suppressant effect. Clin Pharmacol Ther 2000;68(5):487–94.

503. Seidegard J. Reduction of the inhibitory effect of ketoconazole on budesonide pharmacokinetics by separation of their time of administration. Clin Pharmacol Ther 2000;68(1):13–7.

504. McCrea JB, Majumdar AK, Goldberg MR, Iwamoto M, Gargano C, Panebianco DL, Hesney M, Lines CR, Petty KJ, Deutsch PJ, Murphy MG, Gottesdiener KM, Goldwater DR, Blum RA. Effects of the neurokinin1 receptor antagonist aprepitant on the pharmacokinetics of dexamethasone and methylprednisolone. Clin Pharmacol Ther 2003; 74: 17-24.

505. Varis T, Backman JT, Kivisto KT, Neuvonen PJ. Diltiazem and mibefradil increase the plasma concentrations and greatly enhance the adrenal-suppressant effect of oral methylprednisolone. Clin Pharmacol Ther 2000;67(3):215–21.

506. Quan VA, Saunders BP, Hicks BH, Sladen GE. Cyclosporin treatment for ulcerative colitis complicated by fatal *Pneumocystis carinii* pneumonia. BMJ 1997;314(7077):363–4.

507. Potter JM, McWhinney BC, Sampson L, Hickman PE. Area-under-the-curve monitoring of prednisolone for dose optimization in a stable renal transplant population. Ther Drug Monit 2004; 26: 408–14.

508. Fost DA, Leung DY, Martin RJ, Brown EE, Szefler SJ, Spahn JD. Inhibition of methylprednisolone elimination in the presence of clarithromycin therapy. J Allergy Clin Immunol 1999;103(6):1031–5.

509. Finkenbine R, Gill HS. Case of mania due to prednisone–clarithromycin interaction. Can J Psychiatry 1997;42(7):778.

510. Belfayol-Pisante L, Guillevin L, Tod M, Fauvelle F. Possible influence of prednisone on the pharmacokinetics of cyclophosphamide in systemic vasculitis. Clin Drug Invest 1999;18:225–31.

511. Manchon ND, Bercoff E, Lemarchand P, Chassagne P, Senant J, Bourreille J. Frequence et gravité des interactions médicamenteuses dans une population agée: étude prospective concernant 639 malades. [Incidence and severity of drug interactions in the elderly. a prospective study of 639 patients.] Rev Med Interne 1989;10(6):521–525.

512. Feuillet L, Guedj E, Laksiri N, Philip E, Habib G, Pelletier J, Cherif AA. Deep vein thrombosis after intravenous immunoglobulins associated with methylprednisolone. Thromb Haemost 2004; 92: 662-5.

513. Varis T, Kivisto KT, Neuvonen PJ. Grapefruit juice can increase the plasma concentrations of oral methylprednisolone. Eur J Clin Pharmacol 2000;56(6–7):489–93.

514. Geller M. Marked peripheral edema associated with montelukast and prednisone. Ann Intern Med 2000;132(11):924.

515. Seidegard J, Simonsson M, Edsbacker S. Effect of an oral contraceptive on the plasma levels of budesonide and prednisolone and the influence on plasma cortisol. Clin Pharmacol Ther 2000;67(4):373–81.

516. Schönhofer PS. Interaktionen antirheumatisch wirksamer Substanzen. [Interactions of antirheumatic agents.] Internist (Berl) 1979;20(9):433–8.

517. Strayhorn VA, Baciewicz AM, Self TH. Update on rifampin drug interactions III. Arch Intern Med 1997;157(21):2453–8.

518. Dhanoa J, Natu M, Massey S. Worsening of steroid depending bronchial asthma following rifampicin administration. J Assoc Physicians India 1998;46(2):242.

519. Johnson SR, Marion AA, Vrchoticky T, Emmanuel PJ, Lujan-Zilbermann J. Cushing syndrome with secondary adrenal insufficiency from concomitant therapy with ritonavir and fluticasone. J Pediatr 2006; 148(3): 386–8.

520. Arrington-Sanders R, Hutton N, Siberry GK. Ritonavir–fluticasone interaction causing Cushing syndrome in HIV-infected children and adolescents. Pediatr Infect Dis J 2006; 25(11): 1044-8.

521. Edelman J, Potter JM, Hackett LP. The effect of intra-articular steroids on plasma salicylate concentrations. Br J Clin Pharmacol 1986;21(3):301–7.

522. Nielsen GL, Sorensen HT, Mellemkjoer L, Blot WJ, McLaughlin JK, Tage-Jensen U, Olsen JH. Risk of hospitalization resulting from upper gastrointestinal bleeding among patients taking corticosteroids: a register-based cohort study. Am J Med 2001;111(7):541–5.

523. Garcia Rodriguez LA, Hernandez-Diaz S. The risk of upper gastrointestinal complications associated with nonsteroidal anti-inflammatory drugs, glucocorticoids, acetaminophen, and combinations of these agents. Arthritis Res 2001;3(2):98–101.

524. Weil J, Langman MJ, Wainwright P, Lawson DH, Rawlins M, Logan RF, Brown TP, Vessey MP, Murphy M, Colin-Jones DG. Peptic ulcer bleeding: accessory risk factors and interactions with nonsteroidal anti-inflammatory drugs. Gut 2000;46(1):27–31.

525. Hazlewood KA, Fugate SE, Harrison DL. Effect of oral corticosteroids on chronic warfarin therapy. Ann Pharmacother 2006; 40(12): 2101-6.

526. Patel RS, Shaw SR, McIntyre HE, McGarry GW, Wallace AM. Morning salivary cortisol versus short Synacthen test as a test of adrenal suppression. Ann Clin Biochem 2004; 41: 408-10.

527. Cepollaro C, Gonnelli S, Rottoli P, Montagnani A, Caffarelli C, Bruni D, Nikiforakis N, Fossi A, Rossi S, Nuti R. Bone ultrasonography in glucocorticoid-induced osteoporosis. Osteoporos Int 2005; 16(8): 743-8.

528. Brown ES, Chamberlain W, Dhanani N, Paranjpe P, Carmody TJ, Sargeant M. An open-label trial of olanzapine for corticosteroid-induced mood symptoms. J Affect Disord 2004; 83(2-3): 277-81.

Cyclophosphamide

General Information

Cyclophosphamide is an alkylating nitrogen mustard derivative mainly used in oncology patients (1) or in conditioning regimens for bone marrow transplantation. Its immunosuppressant properties have been used in organ transplantation and more often in chronic inflammatory disorders or autoimmune diseases.

Observational studies

Cyclophosphamide has been investigated in a wide range of diseases, but results in aplastic anemia and idiopathic pulmonary fibrosis have been disappointing. In a low dose (2 mg/kg/day), it produced minimal efficacy in 19 patients with idiopathic pulmonary fibrosis who had failed to respond to a glucocorticoid or who had had adverse effects (2). Moreover, 13 patients had cyclophosphamide-induced adverse effects, which required drug withdrawal in nine. The most frequent were severe gastrointestinal effects, leukopenia, and skin rashes. In another study, high-dose cyclophosphamide plus ciclosporin (50 mg/kg/day for 4 days) was compared with antithymocyte globulin plus ciclosporin in patients with severe aplastic anemia, but the trial was prematurely stopped after only 31 patients had been enrolled because of three early deaths in patients taking cyclophosphamide (3). Subsequent analysis showed excess morbidity and mortality in patients taking cyclophosphamide, with six proven or suspected cases of systemic fungal infection (including the three deaths) compared with no cases in the other group, but no significant difference in the hematological response rates between the groups. In addition, the durations of hospital stay, neutropenia, and antibacterial treatment were longer with cyclophosphamide. Based on these results, the authors concluded that cyclophosphamide should not be used in aplastic anemia.

Comparative studies

The beneficial effects of cyclophosphamide must be weighed against its considerable toxicity during long-term therapy in patients with proliferative lupus nephritis. Patients with lupus nephritis (n = 59; 12 of WHO class III, 46 of class IV, and one of class Vb) received induction therapy with up to seven monthly intravenous boluses of cyclophosphamide 0.5–1.0 g/m^2 plus glucocorticoids (4). They were subsequently randomized to quarterly intravenous cyclophosphamide, oral azathioprine 1–3 mg/kg/day, or oral mycophenolate mofetil 0.5–3 g/day for 1–3 years. During maintenance therapy, five patients died (four taking cyclophosphamide and one taking mycophenolate mofetil), and five developed chronic renal insufficiency (three taking cyclophosphamide, one taking azathioprine, and one taking mycophenolate mofetil). The 72-month event-free survival rate for the composite end-point of death or chronic renal insufficiency was significantly higher in the mycophenolate mofetil and azathioprine groups than in the cyclophosphamide group. The rate of relapse-free survival was significantly higher in the mycophenolate mofetil group than in the cyclophosphamide group. The incidences of hospitalization, amenorrhea, infections, nausea, and vomiting were significantly lower in the mycophenolate mofetil and azathioprine groups than in the cyclophosphamide group. Therefore, short-term therapy with intravenous cyclophosphamide followed by maintenance therapy with mycophenolate mofetil or azathioprine appears to be more efficacious and safer than long-term therapy with intravenous cyclophosphamide.

General adverse effects

Common adverse effects observed at low doses of cyclophosphamide are similar to, but less frequent than, those observed in oncology patients. They include gastrointestinal disturbances (mostly nausea), hematological toxicity (mostly leukopenia), alopecia, and infectious complications (5,6).

Organs and Systems

Cardiovascular

Cardiac toxicity can be observed at high doses of cyclophosphamide (usually over 1.5 g/m^2/day), and acute myocardial necrosis or severe cardiac failure have been anecdotally reported after smaller dosages (SEDA-21, 386).

High-dose cyclophosphamide (120–200 mg/kg) can cause lethal cardiotoxicity, and severe congestive heart failure can develop 1–10 days after the first dose. Severe congestive heart failure is accompanied by electrocardiographic findings of diffuse voltage loss, cardiomegaly, pulmonary vascular congestion, and pleural and pericardial effusions. Pathological findings include hemorrhagic myocardial necrosis, thickening of the left ventricular wall, and fibrinous pericarditis.

Of 80 patients who received cyclophosphamide 50 mg/kg/day for 4 days in preparation for bone marrow grafting 17% had symptoms consistent with cyclophosphamide cardiotoxicity (7). Six died from congestive heart failure. Older patients were at greatest risk of developing cardiotoxicity.

In six patients who developed heart failure after high-dose conditioning therapy before stem cell transplantation, cyclophosphamide was suspected, despite the possible involvement of four drugs (8). The authors suggested monitoring high-risk patients.

Corrected QT dispersion was a predictor of acute heart failure after high-dose cyclophosphamide chemotherapy (5.6 g/m^2 over 4 days) in 19 patients (9).

Respiratory

Cyclophosphamide-induced pneumonitis has been described in 29 cases (10). Considering the widespread use of this drug over many years, this is a rare adverse effect. It does not clearly correlate with dosage (SED-8, 1112; SED-13, 1122). From a review of 12 case reports and a retrospective analysis of six other patients (including four with Wegener's granulomatosis), in whom cyclophosphamide was thought to be the only causative factor, two distinct clinical patterns of pneumonitis with different prognoses were identified (11). Early-onset pneumonitis ($n = 8$) occurred acutely within 1–8 months of treatment, and complete recovery was noted after cyclophosphamide withdrawal and prednisone treatment. In contrast, late-onset pneumonitis ($n = 10$) developed insidiously over several months (eventually after cyclophosphamide withdrawal) in patients maintained taking low daily doses for months to years. These patients had progressive pulmonary fibrosis unresponsive to glucocorticoid therapy, and six died of respiratory failure. Radiological pleural thickening may be an early sign of late-onset lung toxicity.

Nervous system

Progressive multifocal leukoencephalopathy is sometimes associated with Wegener's granulomatosis, but one case occurred in a patient who was taking low-dose cyclophosphamide, with subsequent significant improvement on withdrawal of the drug (SEDA-19, 347).

Sensory systems

Blurred vision is sometimes reported after high intravenous doses of cyclophosphamide, and there has been one report of transient myopia that recurred after each monthly intravenous pulse (12).

Endocrine

Even low-dose intravenous cyclophosphamide can cause a syndrome that resembles inappropriate secretion of antidiuretic hormone, with severe hyponatremia and symptoms of water intoxication (SEDA-19, 347; SEDA-21, 386). A direct effect on the renal tubules is likely, but no other nephrotoxic effects have been documented.

Hematologic

Leukopenia, and less commonly thrombocytopenia or anemia, due to cyclophosphamide are typically dose-related in the therapeutic range. Cyclophosphamide-induced anemia has led to retinopathy presenting as striated hemorrhage of the retina (13).

Relative eosinophilia and increased interleukin-4 secretion were found in one study, suggesting that an immune deviation toward a type-2 T helper cell (Th2) response can occur (14). The clinical relevance of these findings as regards hypersensitivity reactions is unknown.

The idea that the degree of leukocyte suppression can be used to predict the success of adjuvant chemotherapy has been applied to combined treatment with cyclophosphamide, methotrexate, and 5-fluorouracil for breast cancer; the lower the nadir leukocyte count, the greater the incidence of metastatic disease-free survival (15).

Mouth

Unilateral necrosis of the tongue has been attributed to cyclophosphamide (16).

- A 62-year-old woman with invasive ductal carcinoma of the breast was treated with epirubicin and cyclophosphamide. She rapidly developed swelling and necrosis of the tongue and consequent airway obstruction necessitating tracheostomy. After excision of the necrosis, the swelling of the tongue and the airway obstruction resolved.

Because of the temporal connection between the necrosis and the chemotherapy, the authors suspected an adverse effect, although they could not exclude a paraneoplastic pathogenesis.

Gastrointestinal

Nausea and vomiting are infrequent with daily low-dose cyclophosphamide (5).

Two-thirds of patients treated with cyclophosphamide orally for 4 months plus intravenous 5-fluorouracil and methotrexate for breast cancer developed Barrett's epithelium (17), perhaps as a result of esophagitis, rather than through mucosal re-epithelialization by undifferentiated stem cells (18).

Toxic megacolon occurred after five cycles of epirubicin 70 mg/m^2, 5-fluorouracil 500 mg/m^2, and oral cyclophosphamide 75 mg/m^2 for 14 days (19). The clinical presentation included a raised erythrocyte sedimentation rate and a colonic diameter of greater than 9 cm; the outcome can be fatal.

Liver

Cyclophosphamide-induced, dose-related liver damage is probably caused as a result of impaired clearance of its metabolite acrolein (20). This causes raised serum transaminases (21) and can be aggravated by prior exposure to azathioprine.

Acute reversible cytolytic or cholestatic jaundice can also occur after low-dose cyclophosphamide in adults and children (SED-13, 1122; SEDA-19, 347; SEDA-20, 342; SEDA-21, 386). Acute liver failure required liver transplantation in one patient (22). Although glucocorticoids were given concomitantly in most of these patients, no data are available to indicate a possibly increased hepatotoxic potential of this drug combination.

Hepatic veno-occlusive disease was attributed to low-dose cyclophosphamide in a 2-year-old child, and in repeated episodes of serum transaminase fluctuations in a patient with hepatitis C virus infection (SEDA-19, 347).

Late hepatotoxicity has also been reported with low-dose cyclophosphamide (23).

- A 67-year-old man with Sjögren's syndrome took cyclophosphamide for 2 years, a cumulative dose of 40.5 g. He then developed severe progressive jaundice due to acute hepatocellular injury. Gallstones and acute viral hepatitis were excluded, and only anti-smooth muscle antibodies were weakly positive. Liver histology showed marked ballooning of the hepatocytes and cell loss, cytoplasmic and canalicular cholestasis, and infiltration of the portal tract with inflammatory cells. Complete resolution occurred 6 weeks after cyclophosphamide withdrawal.

The authors emphasized this was the first case suggesting a cumulative hepatotoxic effect of low-dose cyclophosphamide. Previous rare cases of low-dose cyclophosphamide-induced acute hepatitis have usually occurred within the first 2 months.

Cyclophosphamide 60 mg/kg was infused over 1-2 hours on each of 2 consecutive days, followed by total body irradiation in 147 patients (24). Hepatotoxicity was scored by the development of sinusoidal obstruction syndrome (veno-occlusive disease) and by total serum bilirubin concentrations. The hazards of liver toxicity, non-relapse mortality, tumor relapse, and survival were calculated using regression analysis that included exposure to cyclophosphamide metabolites (as AUC). Of 147 patients, 23 (16%) developed moderate or severe veno-occlusive disease. The median peak serum bilirubin concentration to day 20 was 44 (range 9–700) µmol/l. Metabolism of cyclophosphamide was highly variable, particularly for the metabolite O-carboxyethylphosphoramide mustard, whose AUC varied 16-fold. Exposure to this metabolite was significantly related to veno-occlusive disease, a raised bilirubin, non-relapse mortality, and survival, after adjusting for age and irradiation dose. Patients in the highest quartile of O-carboxyethylphosphoramide mustard exposure had a 5.9-fold higher risk of non-relapse mortality than patients in the lowest quartile. Engraftment and tumor relapse were not significantly related to cyclophosphamide metabolite exposure.

Urinary tract

Hemorrhagic cystitis and bladder cancer are well-known complications of cyclophosphamide. The damage to the urinary bladder epithelium is caused by acrolein, a metabolite of cyclophosphamide that is excreted in the urine. In bone marrow transplant recipients, prior administration of busulfan, which itself causes hemorrhagic cystitis, can increase this risk (25). Mesna (2-mercaptoethane sodium sulfonate) is used to prevent this adverse effect. It is excreted by the kidney, and it binds and detoxifies acrolein in the urine; mesna also prevents the breakdown of acrolein precursors. Intravesical prostaglandin E$_2$ has been suggested as an alternative treatment (25).

The incidence of cystitis and/or dysuria was only 8% in 531 women with breast cancer who were given oral cyclophosphamide 60 mg/m^2/day for 1 year; the majority of cases were only grade 1 (26).

Upper renal tract disorders with ureteric reflux and bilateral hydronephrosis has been briefly reported in a patient with a history of cyclophosphamide-induced cystitis (SEDA-22, 410–411).

In 155 patients with Wegener's granulomatosis, of whom 142 took daily oral cyclophosphamide, the most frequent long-term cyclophosphamide-related adverse effects were cystitis despite mesna therapy (12%) and myelodysplasia (8%; 27). Patients who took a cumulative dose of over 100 g had a two-fold greater risk of cystitis and/or myelodysplasia than patients who took under 100 g. The authors emphasized that cyclophosphamide therapy should be as short as possible, with mesna and close surveillance in order to reduce treatment-associated morbidity.

Cyclophosphamide was thought to have favored the development of emphysematous cystitis in a 73-year-old man (28).

Skin

High doses of cyclophosphamide can cause the erythro-dysesthesia syndrome, that is erythema of the hands and feet (29).

Stevens–Johnson syndrome developed in two patients, including one with positive rechallenge (SEDA-20, 342).

Five of thirty-two patients treated with the alternating drug regimen CAMBO-VIP (cyclophosphamide, doxorubicin, methotrexate, bleomycin, vincristine, etoposide, ifosfamide, and prednisolone) for non-Hodgkin's lymphoma developed blisters under the thickened skin of the palms and/or soles, followed by desquamation (30).

Discrete cutaneous hyperpigmentation occurred in two patients after high-dose chemotherapy with cyclophosphamide, etoposide, and carboplatin (31).

Hair

Alopecia occurs in patients taking cyclophosphamide, but it is less common and less severe in patients taking low doses. Mild to moderate alopecia was observed in 17% of patients with Wegener's granulomatosis (5).

Nails

Beau's lines (transverse ridging of the nails) developed after multiple drug therapy for Hodgkin's disease, including cyclophosphamide (32).

Reproductive system

In autoimmune diseases cyclophosphamide can cause menstrual disorders (oligomenorrhea or sustained amenorrhea) and ultimately sterility or premature menopause. This has been particularly exemplified in lupus erythematosus, and several studies have shown a high prevalence of menstrual disorders or premature ovarian failure in cyclophosphamide-treated patients, or a significantly higher incidence of both complications compared with other immunosuppressive regimens or healthy controls (32–35).

Of 17 adult men who had been treated before puberty for sarcoma with high-dose pulse cyclophosphamide (median dose 20.5 m/m^2) as part of regimens containing vincristine, dactinomycin, and cyclophosphamide, with or without doxorubicin, 10 had azoospermia, five had oligospermia, and only two had normal sperm counts (36). The authors concluded that a previous suggestion that puberty acts as a protection to infertility was not borne out and that the risk of infertility was proportional to the cumulative dose of cyclophosphamide.

Susceptibility factors have been investigated in a large retrospective study of 274 patients aged under 45 years, of whom 70 had received cyclophosphamide, 84 azathioprine but not cyclophosphamide, and 88 either no drug or hydroxychloroquine alone (37). The overall incidence of ovarian failure, defined as sustained amenorrhea for at least 12 months and documented by reduced estradiol concentrations, was 26, 1, and 0% respectively. The mean delay to onset of the first missed menses was 4.4 months. A higher age at the start of treatment and cumulative dose were independent risk factors for cyclophosphamide-induced ovarian failure. The incidences were 14, 28, and 50% in patients aged under 30 years, 30–39 years, and over 40 years respectively, and 4, 26, 31, 70% for cumulative doses of under 10, 10–20, 20–30, and over 40 g, respectively.

Immunologic

Type I hypersensitivity

Anaphylactic reactions have very rarely occurred after intravenous cyclophosphamide (SED-8, 1126; SEDA-17, 522; 38), and positive skin tests to the parent drug and/or 4-hydroxycyclophosphamide were found in several well-documented case reports (SEDA-19, 347). Although other mechanisms could be considered, a possible IgE antibody-mediated reaction was substantiated by the positivity of immediate skin tests to cyclophosphamide metabolites in five patients, and the recurrence of symptoms following intravenous or oral rechallenge in several of them (39).

Cyclophosphamide reportedly caused a type I hypersensitivity reaction in a patient with systemic lupus erythematosus (40).

- A 17-year-old Chinese girl with systemic lupus erythematosus developed acute angioedema over the neck, chest, and larynx, and required mechanical ventilation. She had received two previous courses of cyclophosphamide without incident. She developed urticaria 30 minutes after an infusion of cyclophosphamide, without angioedema, stridor, wheezing, or hypotension. Skin prick testing with cyclophosphamide was negative. Four weeks later, 15 minutes after the start of an infusion of cyclophosphamide, she developed generalized urticaria. Further infusions were given with diphenhydramine premedication.

In the absence of drug-induced angioedema or anaphylaxis, monthly therapy with cyclophosphamide can be continued with antihistamine premedication in patients who have allergic reactions.

Infection risk

Owing to its effects on cellular and humoral immune responses, and independently of leukopenia, cyclophosphamide can induce more frequent and more severe infectious complications (SED-13, 1123; SEDA-20, 343). Older age and total cumulative dose are possible susceptibility factors for severe infectious episodes. More specifically, an increased risk of severe, life-threatening *Pneumocystis jiroveci* pneumonia has been identified, particularly in patients with lymphopenia (41,42). There was also a 10- to 20-fold increase in *Herpes zoster* infections (43,44). Fatal aspergillosis and disseminated cryptococcosis have been sometimes reported (SEDA-20, 343; 45). Infections were mostly reported in patients who were also taking glucocorticoids, and a synergistic effect with glucocorticoids is likely to be relevant in causation (43,46); all the same, there is direct evidence that cyclophosphamide itself is involved. Its role was investigated in a retrospective study of 100 patients with systemic lupus erythematosus: 45% developed serious bacterial infections (58%), opportunistic infections (24%), or *H. zoster* infections (18%), compared with 12% in 43 patients taking high-dose glucocorticoids alone (47). Infections were more frequent with sequential intravenous and oral cyclophosphamide (68%) than with intravenous cyclophosphamide (39%) or oral cyclophosphamide (40%), and leukopenia was an additional risk factor. Other investigators have similarly adduced evidence of more frequent infections, particularly *P. jiroveci* pneumonia, in patients receiving cyclophosphamide plus glucocorticoids daily rather than alternate-day glucocorticoids (43).

- A 72-year-old man with autoimmune thrombocytopenia had taken prednisone (30 mg/day) for 1 year, when he was found to have systemic lupus erythematosus (48). Prednisone was continued and he started to take chloroquine (250 mg/day) and monthly cyclophosphamide (0.75 g/m^2). Three weeks after the first bolus of cyclophosphamide, he complained of fever and dyspnea, and chest X-rays showed bilateral pulmonary infiltrates. Despite prompt medical management, he died 5 days after admission with cytomegalovirus-induced interstitial pneumonia.

In addition to cyclophosphamide, this patient had several susceptibility factors for fatal infection, namely age (older than 50 years) and a low leukocyte nadir (2900 × 10^6/l) after treatment with cyclophosphamide and prednisone.

Long-Term Effects

Tumorigenicity

Although tumor induction has mostly been documented in patients treated for cancer, long-term cyclophosphamide treatment for non-neoplastic conditions can also increase the incidence of certain neoplasms. Whether this oncogenic effect is a consequence of drug-induced chromosomal aberrations rather than immunosuppression is unclear. An increased incidence of bladder cancers, skin cancers, and myeloproliferative disorders was found in a 20-year follow-up study of 119 patients with rheumatoid arthritis, and a high dose of cyclophosphamide (mean total dose of 80 g) was the main susceptibility factor (49).

In another study in patients with Wegener's granulomatosis there was an 11-fold increase in the incidence of lymphomas compared with the general population (43). In contrast, previous exposure to cyclophosphamide did not appear to be associated with a significantly higher risk of cancer in patients with systemic lupus erythematosus, but the number of cases was very low (50).

Myelodysplastic syndromes

Cyclophosphamide can cause myelodysplastic syndromes, particularly after prolonged treatment. The type of myelodysplastic syndromes and cytogenetic abnormalities that developed after treatment with alkylating agents for rheumatic diseases have been described in eight patients (mean age 57 years), of whom seven had taken oral cyclophosphamide and one chlorambucil (51). The mean cumulative dose of cyclophosphamide was 118 g for a mean cumulative duration of 4.4 years, and the myelodysplastic syndrome was diagnosed 0–4 years (mean 2.4 years) after the end of treatment. Concomitant immunosuppressive drugs were given in four of seven cyclophosphamide-treated patients. Cytogenetic abnormalities of chromosome 5 and/or 7, which are characteristic of treatment-related myelodysplastic syndromes, were found in all patients. Only two patients were still alive at the time of the report, and the outcome was remarkably poor in patients with chromosome 5 deletion. This study suggested that a high cumulative dose of cyclophosphamide is a risk factor for hematological malignancies, and that patients require long-term surveillance.

Urinary tract tumors

Squamous cell carcinoma of the bladder has been reported 4 years after pulsed cyclophosphamide therapy (52). However, the authors noted that other susceptibility factors, such as bladder diverticula and human papilloma virus infection, occurred in the intervening period and they speculated on the cumulative risk.

- A 72-year old woman who received 1400 mg cyclophosphamide over 2 weeks for Wegener's granulomatosis had gross hematuria and dysuria (53). Cystoscopy was normal, but there was marked irregularity of the mucosa of the upper ureteric mucosa, the renal pelvis, and the renal calyces on retrograde ureteropyelography. Nephroscopy showed a gray necrotic uroepithelium with dystrophic calcification.

The risk of bladder cancer persists for as long as 20 years after cyclophosphamide withdrawal. In a retrospective analysis, half of the 145 patients on long-term treatment for Wegener's granulomatosis had microscopic or gross hematuria, among whom 70% had cystoscopic features compatible with cyclophosphamide-induced bladder injury (54). Seven patients (5%) developed bladder cancer, a 31-fold higher incidence than in the general population. As previous episodes of hematuria were found in all seven patients and the drug was the only significant risk factor for bladder cancer, prompt cystoscopy should be done in any patient who develops gross hematuria, even after treatment withdrawal. Another study showed an excess in the incidence of bladder cancer in patients with multiple sclerosis who received cyclophosphamide and who also had an indwelling catheter (55).

Renal adenocarcinoma has been reported in a 50-year-old man after 3 years of cyclophosphamide treatment for hepatic sarcoidosis (56).

Other tumors

It has been suggested that cyclophosphamide can contribute to the risk of cervical dysplasia. In a retrospective study of 110 patients with systemic lupus erythematosus, cervical dysplasia was significantly more frequent in patients who had received intravenous cyclophosphamide (10 of 61) than in a control group who did not receive cyclophosphamide (two of 49; 57). In addition, cervical pathology worsened during cyclophosphamide therapy in all four patients with pre-existing cervical dysplasia, and one patient developed in situ cervical carcinoma.

- A 54-year-old man with polyarteritis nodosa developed hepatic angiosarcoma after taking cyclophosphamide for 13 years (58). Although this may have been coincidental, the authors found two other published reports of this very rare tumor in patients taking long-term cyclophosphamide.

To determine the frequency and types of malignancies that occur in children with end-stage renal insufficiency who required renal replacement therapy, data from 249 patients were analysed retrospectively (59). There were 22 malignancies in 21 patients; skin cancers accounted for 59% and non-Hodgkin's lymphomas for 23%. At 25 years after first renal replacement therapy, the probability of developing a malignancy was 17%. The incidence of cancers overall was 10-fold higher than in the general population. For cancers other than melanoma and non-Hodgkin's lymphoma, the standardized risks were 222 and 46 respectively. The use of more than 20 mg/kg cyclophosphamide was associated with an increased risk of malignancy. Six patients died as a result of their malignancy, accounting for 9.5% of overall mortality. The long-term risk of certain malignancies is significantly increased in children who have undergone renal replacement therapy, especially after treatment with cyclophosphamide.

Second-Generation Effects

Fertility

Cyclophosphamide, or testicular and cranial irradiation, in the treatment of childhood malignancies can lead to small testicular size and decreased sperm production in adulthood (60). Of 17 adult male survivors of childhood sarcomas treated before puberty with high-dose cyclophosphamide, only two had normal sperm counts, 10 had azoospermia, and five had oligospermia (36). The two patients with normal sperm counts had taken the lowest doses of cyclophosphamide.

Gonadal toxicity has been documented in both men and women receiving cyclophosphamide (5). In men, the incidence of transient or permanent oligospermia/azoospermia is 50–90%, and in prepubertal patients spermatogenesis will more readily return to normal than adults. In one study, testosterone prophylaxis given at the same time as cyclophosphamide reduced the incidence of disorders of spermatogenesis and accelerated spermatogenesis recovery after cyclophosphamide discontinuation, but few patients were evaluable (61).

Of 23 men treated with either cyclophosphamide or non-alkylating agent combinations, there was a dose-related disturbance of gonadotrophin secretion in the cyclophosphamide group (62). The chances of maintaining normal gonadal function after combined treatment of Hodgkin's disease are significantly greater among girls than boys at 9-year follow-up (63). Pre- and post-pubescent boys were affected by six cycles of MOPP, whether or not pelvic radiation was administered; on the other hand, in girls similarly treated, ovarian function was directly affected by the number of courses of chemotherapy and the ovarian radiation dose (64). In a study of male gonadal function at 9 years follow-up after regimens containing cyclophosphamide, mechlorethamine, vincristine, or procarbazine, there was azoospermia, whereas regimens containing dactinomycin and vinblastine did not have a toxic effect on spermatogenesis (65). Testicular volume and sperm count in 18 patients, 1–3 years after chemotherapy, showed that all those who had received chemotherapy that did not include cisplatin had normal testicular size and sperm counts, whereas of seven who had received cisplatin, six had small testes and azoospermia and one was oligozoospermic with normal-sized testes (66).

The risk of ovarian failure and infertility has been studied in 84 women with an underlying inflammatory disease receiving intravenous cyclophosphamide (67). The incidence of sustained amenorrhea was 22% and was independent of the underlying inflammatory disease. After treatment with cyclophosphamide following bone marrow transplantation, ovarian function can occasionally recover, resulting in a successful pregnancy up to 7 years after treatment (68). No specific factors correlated with recovery of normal ovarian function. However, recovery was rare if the patient had undergone concurrent total body irradiation (69).

Table 1 The FDA's classification of teratogenic drug risk

Category	Description of Risk
A	No fetal risk shown in controlled human studies
B	No human data available and animal studies show no fetal risk or Animal studies show a risk but human studies do not show fetal risk
C	No controlled studies on fetal risk available for humans or animals or Fetal risk shown in controlled animal studies but no human data available (the benefit of drug use must clearly justify the potential fetal risk in this category)
D	Studies show fetal risk in humans (use of the drug may be acceptable even with risks such as in life-threatening illness or when safer drugs are ineffective)
X	Risk to fetus clearly outweighs any benefits from the drug

Pregnancy

Cyclophosphamide crosses the placenta and reaches an amniotic fluid concentration of 25%. Cyclophosphamide is a pregnancy category D agent (see Table 1).

- A 37-year-old Caucasian woman with an infiltrating ductal breast carcinoma in situ was given doxorubicin and cyclophosphamide in the second and third trimesters and delivered a premature baby boy at 31 weeks (70). The neonate had respiratory distress and failure. There were no physical anomalies, but the baby had neutropenia and anemia probably because of the chemotherapy. The infant grew and developed normally during his first year of life and remained in good health.

Six pregnancies occurred in women taking cyclophosphamide; three had induced abortions, one had a spontaneous abortion, and two had normal pregnancies. After withdrawal of cyclophosphamide, 16 women became pregnant; three had induced abortions for severe morphological anomalies, three had spontaneous miscarriages, and 10 delivered healthy infants. Contraception during intravenous cyclophosphamide therapy is recommended, and after withdrawal, pregnancy is possible, with a favourable outcome in two-thirds of cases.

Teratogenicity

The FDA has classified cyclophosphamide as a pregnancy risk factor D drug: it is teratogenic in animals, but population studies have not conclusively shown teratogenicity in humans. However, in a study of in utero first-trimester exposure to four doses of cyclophosphamide 20 mg/kg it was concluded that cyclophosphamide is a human teratogen, that there is a distinct embryopathic phenotype, and that there are serious doubts about the safety of cyclophosphamide in pregnancy (71). The congenital malformation rate has been estimated at 10–44% (72).

Reported congenital abnormalities are many and include facial and palate defects, skin and skeletal anomalies, and visceral malformations. Based on one case and a review of six previous reports of malformations after in utero exposure to cyclophosphamide in the first trimester, a distinct embryopathy due to

cyclophosphamide has been suggested (71). The proposed phenotype included growth deficiency, developmental delay, craniosynostosis, blepharophimosis, flat nasal bridge, abnormal ears, and distal limb defects; chromosomes were normal.

In one case of first-trimester exposure to cyclophosphamide in a woman pregnant with twins, the male twin was born with multiple congenital abnormalities and developed papillary thyroid cancer at 11 years of age and stage III neuroblastoma at 14 years of age; the female twin was unaffected (73).

Most cases have been reported in patients with cancer who were also exposed to other antineoplastic drugs or to irradiation. The potential for congenital abnormalities in the offspring of men treated with cyclophosphamide is yet unknown.

Fetotoxicity

The effects of second- or third-trimester exposure to cyclophosphamide are poorly documented, although normal children have been described (74). However, in other cases growth retardation and neutropenia have been reported (75).

Drug Administration

Drug dosage regimens

In inflammatory or autoimmune diseases, both daily oral and cyclic pulse intravenous cyclophosphamide regimens are used, but it is unclear whether one route of administration should be preferred to another. The cumulative dose obtained in those given an intravenous pulse regimen is consistently lower than in those given daily oral administration, and the incidence of bladder cancer or infection is expected to be lower in the former. However, the choice of the maintenance regimen remains a dilemma as regards efficacy and toxicity (76). For example, in one study in 50 patients with Wegener's granulomatosis there was a similar overall incidence of adverse effects in patients treated with prednisone plus oral cyclophosphamide compared with those who received prednisone plus intravenous pulse cyclophosphamide (77). Patients in the oral group had a higher incidence of severe or fatal infectious complications, but a lower incidence of cumulative relapse rates at 4.5 years.

In 47 patients intravenous pulsed cyclophosphamide was as effective as daily oral cyclophosphamide, but caused fewer adverse effects (78). The patients were randomized to receive monthly intravenous pulses of cyclophosphamide (0.75 g/m^2, $n = 22$) or daily oral cyclophosphamide (2 mg/kg/day, $n = 25$) for at least 1 year. Both groups received glucocorticoids. Whereas efficacy end-points did not show significant differences between the two groups, leukopenia (18 versus 60%) and severe infections (14% with no deaths versus 40% with three deaths) were significantly less frequent with intravenous pulsed cyclophosphamide. As a result, the probability of freedom from adverse effects (no deaths, severe infections, leukopenia, or thrombocytopenia) over a 12-month period was only about 25% in the oral group, compared with 70% in the intravenous group. In addition, and based on the findings of a significantly lower serum follicle-stimulating hormone concentration at 3 and 6 months and a 57% reduction in the total dose in the intravenous pulse group, the intravenous pulse regimen was expected to produce fewer adverse gonadal effects and a reduced risk of malignancies.

Drug–Drug Interactions

Cisplatin

A 4-year follow-up of comparison of a combination of cyclophosphamide with either 50 mg/m^2 or 100 mg/m^2 of cisplatin in ovarian cancer has been reported (79). Peripheral neuropathy was dose-limiting and persistent. Ten of thirty-one patients had significant toxicity in the high-dose group compared with one of 24 in the low-dose group.

Fluconazole

Cyclophosphamide is a prodrug that requires cytochrome P$_{450}$-dependent hepatic activation to produce alkylating species and several inactive by-products. However, very few metabolic interactions involving cyclophosphamide have been reported. In a retrospective study of 22 children treated with cyclophosphamide for cancer or bone marrow transplantation, cyclophosphamide clearance was significantly lower in nine patients taking fluconazole compared with 13 patients not taking it (80). In vitro studies in human liver microsomes confirmed that the rate of 4-hydroxylation of cyclophosphamide was inhibited by fluconazole.

Prednisolone

Daily prednisolone significantly reduced the total clearance of cyclophosphamide and the peak concentration and AUC of 4-hydroxycyclophosphamide (81). It is not known whether this interaction has clinical consequences.

References

1. Fraiser LH, Kanekal S, Kehrer JP. Cyclophosphamide toxicity. Characterising and avoiding the problem. Drugs 1991;42(5):781–95.
2. Zisman DA, Lynch JP 3rd, Toews GB, Kazerooni EA, Flint A, Martinez FJ. Cyclophosphamide in the treatment of idiopathic pulmonary fibrosis: a prospective study in patients who failed to respond to corticosteroids. Chest 2000;117(6):1619–26.
3. Tisdale JF, Dunn DE, Geller N, Plante M, Nunez O, Dunbar CE, Barrett AJ, Walsh TJ, Rosenfeld SJ, Young NS. High-dose cyclophosphamide in severe aplastic anaemia: a randomised trial. Lancet 2000;356(9241):1554–1559.
4. Contreras G, Pardo V, Leclercq B, Lenz O, Tozman E, O'Nan P, Roth D. Sequential therapies for proliferative lupus nephritis. N Engl J Med 2004;350(10):971–8.
5. Langford CA. Complications of cyclophosphamide therapy. Eur Arch Otorhinolaryngol 1997;254(2):65–72.
6. Omdal R, Husby G, Koldingsnes W. Intravenous and oral cyclophosphamide pulse therapy in rheumatic diseases: side effects and complications. Clin Exp Rheumatol 1993;11(3):283–8.
7. Goldberg MA, Antin JH, Guinan EC, Rappeport JM. Cyclophosphamide cardiotoxicity: an analysis of dosing as a risk factor. Blood 1986;68(5):1114–8.
8. Mugitani A, Yamane T, Park K, Im T, Tatsumi N, Tatsumi Y. Cardiac complications after high-dose chemotherapy with peripheral blood stem cell transplantation. J Jpn Soc Cancer Ther 1996;31:255–62.
9. Nakamae H, Tsumura K, Hino M, Hayashi T, Tatsumi N. QT dispersion as a predictor of acute heart failure after high-dose cyclophosphamide. Lancet 2000;355(9206):805–806.
10. Glatt E, Henke M, Sigmund G, Costabel U. Cyclophosphamid-induzierte Pneumonitis. [Cyclophosphamide-induced pneumonitis.] Rofo 1988;148(5):545–9.
11. Malik SW, Myers JL, DeRemee RA, Specks U. Lung toxicity associated with cyclophosphamide use. Two distinct patterns. Am J Respir Crit Care Med 1996;154(6 Pt 1):1851–6.
12. Arranz JA, Jimenez R, Alvarez-Mon M. Cyclophosphamide-induced myopia. Ann Intern Med 1992;116(1):92–3.
13. Kadoya K, Suda Y, Tonaki M, et al. Two cases of anemic retinopathy. Folia Ophthalmol Jpn 1989;40:148.
14. Smith DR, Balashov KE, Hafler DA, Khoury SJ, Weiner HL. Immune deviation following pulse cyclophosphamide/methylprednisolone treatment of multiple sclerosis: increased interleukin-4 production and associated eosinophilia. Ann Neurol 1997;42(3):313–8.
15. Poikonen P, Saarto T, Lundin J, Joensuu H, Blomqvist C. Leucocyte nadir as a marker for chemotherapy efficacy in node-positive breast cancer treated with adjuvant CMF. Br J Cancer 1999;80(11):1763–6.
16. Buch RS, Schmidt M, Reichert TE. Akute Nekrose der Zunge unter Epirubicin-Cyclophosphamid-Therapie bei einem invasiv duktalen Mammakarzinom. [Acute tongue necrosis provoked by epirubicin–cyclophosphamide treatment for invasive ductal breast cancer.] Mund Kiefer Gesichtschir 2003;7(3):175–9.
17. Spechler S. Columnar-lined (Barrett's) esophagus. Curr Opin Gastroenterol 1991;7:557–61.
18. Mullai N, Sivarajan KM, Shiomoto G. Barrett esophagus. Ann Intern Med 1991;114(10):913.

19. De Gara CJ, Gagic N, Arnold A, Seaton T. Toxic mega-colon associated with anticancer chemotherapy. Can J Surg 1991;34(4):339–41.

20. Honjo I, Suou T, Hirayama C. Hepatotoxicity of cyclophosphamide in man: pharmacokinetic analysis. Res Commun Chem Pathol Pharmacol 1988;61(2):149–65.

21. Shaunak S, Munro JM, Weinbren K, Walport MJ, Cox TM. Cyclophosphamide-induced liver necrosis: a possible interaction with azathioprine. Q J Med 1988;67(252):309–17.

22. Gustafsson LL, Eriksson LS, Dahl ML, Eleborg L, Ericzon BG, Nyberg A. Cyclophosphamide-induced acute liver failure requiring transplantation in a patient with genetically deficient debrisoquine metabolism: a causal relationship? J Intern Med 1996;240(5):311–4.

23. Mok CC, Wong WM, Shek TW, Ho CT, Lau CS, Lai CL. Cumulative hepatotoxicity induced by continuous low-dose cyclophosphamide therapy. Am J Gastroenterol 2000;95(3):845–6.

24. McDonald GB, Slattery JT, Bouvier ME, Ren S, Batchelder AL, Kalhorn TF, Schoch HG, Anasetti C, Gooley T. Cyclophosphamide metabolism, liver toxicity, and mortality following hematopoietic stem cell transplantation. Blood 2003;101:2043–8.

25. Thomas AE, Patterson J, Prentice HG, Brenner MK, Ganczakowski M, Hancock JF, Pattinson JK, Blacklock HA, Hopewell JP. Haemorrhagic cystitis in bone marrow transplantation patients: possible increased risk associated with prior busulphan therapy. Bone Marrow Transplant 1987;1(4):347–55.

26. Budd GT, Green S, O'Bryan RM, Martino S, Abeloff MD, Rinehart JJ, Hahn R, Harris J, Tormey D, O'Sullivan J, et al. Short-course FAC-M versus 1 year of CMFVP in node-positive, hormone receptor-negative breast cancer: an inter-group study. J Clin Oncol 1995;13(4):831–9.

27. Reinhold-Keller E, Beuge N, Latza U, de Groot K, Rudert H, Nolle B, Heller M, Gross WL. An interdisciplinary approach to the care of patients with Wegener's granulomatosis: long-term outcome in 155 patients. Arthritis Rheum 2000;43(5):1021–32.

28. Abuzarad H, Gadallah MF, Rabb H, Vermess M, Ramirez G. Emphysematous cystitis: possible side-effect of cyclophosphamide therapy. Clin Nephrol 1998;50(6):394–6.

29. Matsuyama JR, Kwok KK. A variant of the chemotherapy-associated erythrodysesthesia syndrome related to high-dose cyclophosphamide. DICP 1989;23(10):776778–9.

30. Hirano M, Okamoto M, Maruyama F, Ezaki K, Shimizu K, Ino T, Matsui T, Sobue R, Shinkai K, Miyazaki H, et al. Alternating non-cross-resistant chemotherapy for non-Hodgkin's lymphoma of intermediate-grade and high-grade malignancy. A pilot study. Cancer 1992;69(3):772–7.

31. Singal R, Tunnessen WW Jr, Wiley JM, Hood AF. Discrete pigmentation after chemotherapy. Pediatr Dermatol 1991;8(3):231–5.

32. Requena L. Chemotherapy-induced transverse ridging of the nails. Cutis 1991;48(2):129–30.

33. Wang CL, Wang F, Bosco JJ. Ovarian failure in oral cyclophosphamide treatment for systemic lupus erythematosus. Lupus 1995;4(1):11–4.

34. Gonzalez-Crespo MR, Gomez-Reino JJ, Merino R, Ciruelo E, Gomez-Reino FJ, Muley R, Garcia-Consuegra J, Pinillos V, Rodriguez-Valverde V. Menstrual disorders in girls with systemic lupus erythematosus treated with cyclophosphamide. Br J Rheumatol 1995;34(8):737–41.

35. McDermott EM, Powell RJ. Incidence of ovarian failure in systemic lupus erythematosus after treatment with pulse cyclophosphamide. Ann Rheum Dis 1996;55(4):224–9.

36. Kenney LB, Laufer MR, Grant FD, Grier H, Diller L. High risk of infertility and long term gonadal damage in males treated with high dose cyclophosphamide for sarcoma during childhood. Cancer 2001;91(3):613–21.

37. Mok CC, Lau CS, Wong RW. Risk factors for ovarian failure in patients with systemic lupus erythematosus receiving cyclophosphamide therapy. Arthritis Rheum 1998;41(5):831–7.

38. Salles G, Vial T, Archimbaud E. Anaphylactoid reaction with bronchospasm following intravenous cyclophosphamide administration. Ann Hematol 1991;62(2–3):74–5.

39. Popescu N, Sheehan M, Kouides P, Loughner JE, Condemi JJ, Looney RJ, Leddy JP. Allergic reactions to cyclophosphamide: delayed clinical expression associated with positive immediate skin tests to drug metabolites in five patients. J Allerg Clin Immunol 1995;95:288.

40. Thong BY, Leong KP, Thumboo J, Koh ET, Tang CY. Cyclophosphamide type I hypersensitivity in systemic lupus erythematosus. Lupus 2002;11(2):127–9.

41. Jarrousse B, Guillevin L, Bindi P, Hachulla E, Leclerc P, Gilson B, Remy P, Rossert J, Jacquot C, Gilson B. Increased risk of *Pneumocystis carinii* pneumonia in patients with Wegener's granulomatosis. Clin Exp Rheumatol 1993;11(6):615–21.

42. Porges AJ, Beattie SL, Ritchlin C, Kimberly RP, Christian CL. Patients with systemic lupus erythematosus at risk for *Pneumocystis carinii* pneumonia. J Rheumatol 1992;19(8):1191–4.

43. Hoffman GS, Kerr GS, Leavitt RY, Hallahan CW, Lebovics RS, Travis WD, Rottem M, Fauci AS. Wegener granulomatosis: an analysis of 158 patients. Ann Intern Med 1992;116(6):488–98.

44. Kahl LE. *Herpes zoster* infections in systemic lupus erythematosus: risk factors and outcome. J Rheumatol 1994;21(1):84–6.

45. Kattwinkel N, Cook L, Agnello V. Overwhelming fatal infection in a young woman after intravenous cyclophosphamide therapy for lupus nephritis. J Rheumatol 1991;18(1):79–81.

46. Bradley JD, Brandt KD, Katz BP. Infectious complications of cyclophosphamide treatment for vasculitis. Arthritis Rheum 1989;32(1):45–53.

47. Pryor BD, Bologna SG, Kahl LE. Risk factors for serious infection during treatment with cyclophosphamide and high-dose corticosteroids for systemic lupus erythematosus. Arthritis Rheum 1996;39(9):1475–82.

48. Garcia-Porrua C, Gonzalez-Gay MA, Perez de Llano LA, Alvarez-Ferreira J. Fatal interstitial pneumonia due to cytomegalovirus following cyclophosphamide treatment in a patient with systemic lupus erythematosus. Scand J Rheumatol 1998;27(6):465–6.

49. Radis C, Kwoh C, Morgan M, et al. Risk of malignancy in cyclophosphamide treated patients with rheumatoid arthritis: a 20-year follow-up study. Arthr Rheum 1993;36(Suppl):R19.

50. Pettersson T, Pukkala E, Teppo L, Friman C. Increased risk of cancer in patients with systemic lupus erythematosus. Ann Rheum Dis 1992;51(4):437–9.

51. McCarthy CJ, Sheldon S, Ross CW, McCune WJ. Cytogenetic abnormalities and therapy-related myelodysplastic syndromes in rheumatic disease. Arthritis Rheum 1998;41(8):1493–6.

52. Wang JS, Hsieh SP, Jiaan BP, Tseng HH. Human papillomavirus in cyclophosphamide and diverticulum-associated

squamous cell carcinoma of urinary bladder: a case report. Zhonghua Yi Xue Za Zhi (Taipei) 1996;57(4):305–9.

53. Aviles RJ, Vlahakis SA, Elkin PL. Cyclophosphamide-associated uroepithelial toxicity. Ann Intern Med 1999;131(7):549.

54. Talar-Williams C, Hijazi YM, Walther MM, Linehan WM, Hallahan CW, Lubensky I, Kerr GS, Hoffman GS, Fauci AS, Sneller MC. Cyclophosphamide-induced cystitis and bladder cancer in patients with Wegener granulomatosis. Ann Intern Med 1996;124(5):477–84.

55. De Ridder D, van Poppel H, Demonty L, D'Hooghe B, Gonsette R, Carton H, Baert L. Bladder cancer in patients with multiple sclerosis treated with cyclophosphamide. J Urol 1998;159(6):1881–4.

56. Das D, Smith A, Warnes TW. Hepatic sarcoidosis and renal carcinoma. J Clin Gastroenterol 1999;28(1):61–3.

57. Bateman H, Yazici Y, Leff L, Peterson M, Paget SA. Increased cervical dysplasia in intravenous cyclophosphamide-treated patients with SLE: a preliminary study. Lupus 2000;9(7):542–4.

58. Rosenthal AK, Klausmeier M, Cronin ME, McLaughlin JK. Hepatic angiosarcoma occurring after cyclophosphamide therapy: case report and review of the literature. Am J Clin Oncol 2000;23(6):581–3.

59. Coutinho HM, Groothoff JW, Offringa M, Gruppen MP, Heymans HS. De novo malignancy after paediatric renal replacement therapy. Arch Dis Child 2001;85(6):478–83.

60. Siimes MA, Rautonen J. Small testicles with impaired production of sperm in adult male survivors of childhood malignancies. Cancer 1990;65(6):1303–6.

61. Masala A, Faedda R, Alagna S, Satta A, Chiarelli G, Rovasio PP, Ivaldi R, Taras MS, Lai E, Bartoli E. Use of testosterone to prevent cyclophosphamide-induced azoospermia. Ann Intern Med 1997;126(4):292–5.

62. Hoorweg-Nijman JJ, Delemarre-van de Waal HA, de Waal FC, Behrendt H. Cyclophosphamide-induced disturbance of gonadotropin secretion manifesting testicular damage. Acta Endocrinol (Copenh) 1992;126(2):143–8.

63. Jackson DV Jr, Craig JB, Spurr CL, White DR, Muss HB, Cruz JM, Richards F, Powell BL. Vincristine infusion with CHOP-CCNU in diffuse large-cell lymphoma. Cancer Invest 1990;8(1):7–12.

64. Ortin TT, Shostak CA, Donaldson SS. Gonadal status and reproductive function following treatment for Hodgkin's disease in childhood: the Stanford experience. Int J Radiat Oncol Biol Phys 1990;19(4):873–80.

65. Aubier F, Flamant F, Brauner R, Caillaud JM, Chaussain JM, Lemerle J. Male gonadal function after chemotherapy for solid tumors in childhood. J Clin Oncol 1989;7(3):304–9.

66. Siimes MA, Elomaa I, Koskimies A. Testicular function after chemotherapy for osteosarcoma. Eur J Cancer 1990;26(9):973–5.

67. Huong du L, Amoura Z, Duhaut P, Sbai A, Costedoat N, Wechsler B, Piette JC. Risk of ovarian failure and fertility after intravenous cyclophosphamide. A study in 84 patients. J Rheumatol 2002;29(12):2571–6.

68. Sanders JE, Buckner CD, Amos D, Levy W, Appelbaum FR, Doney K, Storb R, Sullivan KM, Witherspoon RP, Thomas ED. Ovarian function following marrow transplantation for aplastic anemia or leukemia. J Clin Oncol 1988;6(5):813–8.

69. Gradishar WJ, Schilsky RL. Effects of cancer treatment on the reproductive system. Crit Rev Oncol Hematol 1988;8(2):153–71.

70. Kerr JR. Neonatal effects of breast cancer chemotherapy administered during pregnancy. Pharmacotherapy 2005;25(3):438–4.

71. Enns GM, Roeder E, Chan RT, Ali-Khan Catts Z, Cox VA, Golabi M. Apparent cyclophosphamide (Cytoxan) embryopathy: a distinct phenotype? Am J Med Genet 1999;86(3):237–41.

72. Roubenoff R, Hoyt J, Petri M, Hochberg MC, Hellmann DB. Effects of antiinflammatory and immunosuppressive drugs on pregnancy and fertility. Semin Arthritis Rheum 1988;18(2):88–110.

73. Zemlickis D, Lishner M, Erlich R, Koren G. Teratogenicity and carcinogenicity in a twin exposed in utero to cyclophosphamide. Teratog Carcinog Mutagen 1993;13(3):139–43.

74. Peretz B, Peretz T. The effect of chemotherapy in pregnant women on the teeth of offspring. Pediatr Dent 2003;25(6):601–4.

75. Kerr JR. Neonatal effects of breast cancer chemotherapy administered during pregnancy. Pharmacotherapy 2005;25(3):438–41.

76. Werth VP. Pulse intravenous cyclophosphamide for treatment of autoimmune blistering disease. Is there an advantage over oral routes? Arch Dermatol 1997;133(2):229–30.

77. Guillevin L, Cordier JF, Lhote F, Cohen P, Jarrousse B, Royer I, Lesavre P, Jacquot C, Bindi P, Bielefeld P, Desson JF, Detree F, Dubois A, Hachulla E, Hoen B, Jacomy D, Seigneuric C, Lauque D, Stern M, Longy-Boursier M. A prospective, multicenter, randomized trial comparing steroids and pulse cyclophosphamide versus steroids and oral cyclophosphamide in the treatment of generalized Wegener's granulomatosis. Arthritis Rheum 1997; 40(12):2187–98.

78. Haubitz M, Schellong S, Gobel U, Schurek HJ, Schaumann D, Koch KM, Brunkhorst R. Intravenous pulse administration of cyclophosphamide versus daily oral treatment in patients with antineutrophil cytoplasmic antibody-associated vasculitis and renal involvement: a prospective, randomized study. Arthritis Rheum 1998;41(10):1835–1844.

79. Kaye SB, Paul J, Cassidy J, Lewis CR, Duncan ID, Gordon HK, Kitchener HC, Cruickshank DJ, Atkinson RJ, Soukop M, Rankin EM, Davis JA, Reed NS, Crawford SM, MacLean A, Parkin D, Sarkar TK, Kennedy J, Symonds RP. Mature results of a randomized trial of two doses of cisplatin for the treatment of ovarian cancer. Scottish Gynecology Cancer Trials Group. J Clin Oncol 1996;14(7):2113–9.

80. Yule SM, Walker D, Cole M, McSorley L, Cholerton S, Daly AK, Pearson AD, Boddy AV. The effect of fluconazole on cyclophosphamide metabolism in children. Drug Metab Dispos 1999;27(3):417–21.

81. Belfayol-Pisante L, Guillevin L, Tod M, Fauvelle F. Possible influence of prednisone on the pharmacokinetics of cyclophosphamide in systemic vasculitis. Clin Drug Invest 1999;18:225–31.

Etanercept

General Information

Etanercept is a dimeric fusion protein consisting of two recombinant p75 tumor necrosis factor receptors fused with the Fc portion of human IgG1. It inhibits the binding of tumor necrosis factor alfa to its receptor and thereby neutralizes its biological activity. It has been used in the treatment of moderate to severe active rheumatoid arthritis, ankylosing spondylitis, psoriatic arthropathy, and juvenile rheumatoid arthritis in patients who have failed to respond to previous disease-modifying antirheumatic drugs. The clinical pharmacology and adverse effects of etanercept in patients with rheumatoid disorders have been reviewed (1).

Comparative studies

In a study of weekly oral methotrexate in two different doses (10 or 25 mg) or twice-weekly etanercept in 632 patients, etanercept produced fewer systemic adverse effects than methotrexate, but a higher incidence of injection site reactions (2). Despite theoretical concerns about the development of autoimmune reactions in patients taking etanercept, no evidence of clinical autoimmune disease emerged from this large trial.

In a double-blind study of 682 patients with rheumatoid arthritis randomized to etanercept alone, methotrexate alone, or a combination of the two, the rate of adverse events or study discontinuation related to an adverse event was similar in the three groups (3). In particular, there were no differences in the rates of infection and severe infections. There were no cases of tuberculosis, opportunistic infections, demyelinating diseases, or severe blood dyscrasias among the 454 patients who received etanercept, but only 363 completed the 1-year study. One etanercept-treated patient died from heart failure and suspected sepsis.

Placebo-controlled studies

In a double-blind study in 672 patients randomized to either placebo or etanercept subcutaneously at a low dose (25 mg once weekly), a medium dose (25 mg twice weekly), or a high dose (50 mg twice weekly) significantly more patients had improved psoriasis area-and-severity indices with etanercept compared with placebo at weeks 12 and 24 (4). Adverse events and infections occurred in similar proportions in each group. There were no cases of tuberculosis or opportunistic infections. Laboratory abnormalities were of mild to moderate intensity and did not necessitate withdrawal. Eight patients who received etanercept had serum samples positive for anti-etanercept antibodies. There were no differences in efficacy or adverse event profiles between these patients and those without antibodies.

In a double-blind, placebo-controlled study, 112 patients were randomized to placebo or etanercept 25 mg subcutaneously twice a week for 24 weeks (5).

Etanercept resulted in significant improvements in psoriasis area-and-severity indices. Similar numbers of patients had adverse events in the two groups. Injection site reactions occurred more often with etanercept than placebo (9% versus 0% respectively). One patient who received etanercept developed guttate psoriasis, which was considered to be possibly related to the drug and another had worsening psoriasis after 4 days. Both withdrew from the study.

Favorable safety data have been observed in a phase III randomized controlled study (24-week studies) of etanercept in patients with chronic plaque psoriasis (6).

Systematic reviews

In a systematic review of double-blind, randomized, controlled trials of alefacept (n = 3), efalizumab (n = 5), etanercept (n = 4), and infliximab (n = 4); in patients with psoriasis the relative risks of one or more adverse events in were significantly increased compared with placebo:

- alefacept: $RR = 1.09$; $NNT_H = 15$;
- efalizumab: $RR = 1.15$; $NNT_H = 9$;
- infliximab: $RR = 1.18$; $NNT_H = 9$

Serious adverse events were increased in a sensitivity analysis of four efalizumab trials (n = 2443; $RR = 1.92$; $NNT_H = 60$) (7).

General adverse effects

The therapeutic use and safety of etanercept have been reviewed (8). Mild-to-moderate injection site reactions were the most common adverse effects (42–49%), with a frequency 3.8 to 6 times greater than with placebo. Non-neutralizing antibodies to etanercept were rarely detected. Etanercept-treated patients more often developed new antinuclear antibodies or anti-double-stranded DNA antibodies, but no patient developed symptoms suggestive of an autoimmune disease during clinical trials.

Organs and Systems

Respiratory

The typical histological morphology of pulmonary rheumatoid nodules that developed during etanercept treatment has been reported (9,10). Pulmonary granulomas during etanercept treatment can be coincidental and difficult to distinguish from other pulmonary complications, such as relapse of tuberculosis. In two patients with rheumatoid arthritis who underwent lung biopsy for etanercept-associated pulmonary granulomas, there were non-caseating granulomas containing birefringent particulate in one (11) and caseating necrosis in the other (12). Infectious causes were ruled out. After etanercept withdrawal, the lesions resolved completely with steroid treatment in the first patient but persisted over 1 year despite antituberculosis treatment in the other.

Two patients receiving etanercept developed severe diffuse alveolar infiltrates culminating in ground-glass changes on high-resolution CT scans of the lung (13).

- A 59-year-old woman with a 5-year history of seropositive erosive rheumatoid arthritis developed a demyelinating syndrome during etanercept therapy (14).

Nervous system

Postmarketing warnings about etanercept that have been issued by regulatory agencies and the manufacturers relate to a possible increased risk of demyelinating disorders, such as multiple sclerosis, myelitis, and optic neuritis, in patients with pre-existing or a recent history of demyelinating disorders (SEDA-26, 399). This was in keeping with the results obtained in a placebo-controlled trial of lenercept, another recombinant tumor necrosis factor alfa receptor immunoglobulin fusion protein, in 168 patients with multiple sclerosis; compared with placebo, significantly more patients randomized to lenercept had exacerbation of multiple sclerosis, and exacerbation also occurred earlier (15).

Transverse myelitis of abrupt onset has also been reported (16).

- A 45-year-old woman with resistant rheumatoid arthritis was given etanercept 25 mg twice weekly. Nine days later she developed total acute sensory loss, with flaccid paraplegia, fecal incontinence, and urinary retention. MRI imaging and cerebrospinal fluid analysis were consistent with a diagnosis of transverse myelitis. She also had positive antinuclear and anticardiolipin antibodies. After etanercept withdrawal and treatment with dexamethasone and cyclophosphamide, her motor function improved with no change in sensory function.

Neurological events suggestive of demyelinating disorders in patients treated with tumor necrosis factor alfa antagonists and reported to the FDA's Adverse Events Reporting System have been reviewed (17). These included 17 cases temporarily associated with etanercept and two with infliximab, but complete information was lacking in a number of cases. One additional case with etanercept was more extensively detailed. The first symptoms occurred after a large range of delay after first drug administration (1 week to 15 months; mean 5 months) and mostly included paresthesia, optic neuritis, and confusion. MRI scans in 19 patients showed demyelination in various brain areas in 16. Although a causal relation was not proven, it is noteworthy that most patients improved after withdrawal and one patient had recurrent neurological symptoms after etanercept readministration. The various hypothetical mechanisms by which tumor necrosis factor alfa antagonists might produce demyelinating events have been discussed elsewhere (18). Briefly, they cause increased peripheral T cell autoreactivity, and their inability to cross the blood–brain barrier may account for exacerbation of central demyelinating disorders.

Sensory systems

There have been two reports of anterior uveitis associated with etanercept in a 44-year-old woman with ankylosing spondylitis and a 31-year-old woman with juvenile rheumatic disease, both of whom had responded well to etanercept (19,20). Both had a long-standing rheumatic disease with no previous episodes of uveitis before etanercept and one patient had severe relapse of uveitis on etanercept rechallenge. By contrast, two other patients who responded to etanercept, but also developed scleritis or uveitis, fully recovered with local and systemic treatment despite etanercept continuation (21). Although it was difficult to establish whether this condition was related to the underlying disease or to etanercept, these reports at least suggest that etanercept may fail to prevent ocular involvement in rheumatic disease.

- A 59-year-old woman developed symptomatic bilateral peripheral visual field loss shortly after starting to take etanercept (22).

Four cases of optic neuritis associated with etanercept were revealed by a retrospective chart review between January 2003 and January 2005 in two Israeli medical centers (the Assaf Harofeh Medical Center and the Kaplan Medical Center) (23).

Endocrine

- Transient hyperthyroidism occurred after 6 months of etanercept treatment in a 37-year-old woman with rheumatoid arthritis (24).

However, a direct causal relation with etanercept was debatable, because there was complete resolution with propranolol and despite continuation of etanercept.

Metabolism

Type 1 diabetes mellitus occurred after 5 months treatment with etanercept for juvenile rheumatoid arthritis in a 7-year-old girl (25). Antiglutamic acid decarboxylase antibodies were positive both before and during treatment, suggesting that etanercept may have prematurely triggered an underlying disease.

Hematologic

Postmarketing warnings about etanercept that have been issued by regulatory agencies and the manufacturers relate to a possible risk of aplastic anemia and pancytopenia (10 reported cases, of which 5 ended in fatal sepsis; 8).

- Reversible aplastic anemia occurred in a 78-year-old man who had taken etanercept during the previous 16 weeks (26). Although he had taken methotrexate uneventfully for 3 years, the potential role of methotrexate or a synergistic effect of the drug combination could not be ruled out.

Etanercept has reportedly caused abrupt exacerbation of the macrophage activation syndrome (27).

- A 22-year-old woman with adult-onset Still's disease developed symptoms suggestive of the macrophage activation syndrome. After initial glucocorticoid treatment, she received two doses of etanercept, and within 6 days her white blood cell count fell from $6.4 \times 10^9/l$ to $2.5 \times 10^9/l$ and the neutrophil count from $0.8 \times 10^9/l$ to $0.2 \times 10^9/l$. There was also thrombocytopenia and impaired coagulation and her liver enzymes were raised. A bone marrow aspirate showed delayed myelopoiesis. She received multiple transfusions, intravenous immunoglobulin, and granulocyte-macrophage colony-stimulating factor. The macrophage activation syndrome was diagnosed at that time and she was successfully treated with pulse methylprednisolone and ciclosporin. Epstein–Barr virus infection was subsequently confirmed.

Because soluble tumor necrosis factor alfa receptors are supposedly involved in the macrophage activation syndrome, the authors speculated that the administration of additional soluble receptors may have been the cause of a prolonged and exacerbated syndrome.

- Etanercept was a probable triggering factor of the macrophage activation syndrome in a 4-year-old girl with juvenile rheumatoid arthritis (28). Her symptoms abated after etanercept withdrawal and glucocorticoid treatment.

Gastrointestinal

Previous clinical trials have shown that etanercept is not effective in Crohn's disease. This has been indirectly illustrated in a 7-year-old boy with juvenile idiopathic arthritis had developed an exacerbation of severe Crohn's disease after each administration of etanercept (29). Infliximab was later successfully used for both diseases.

Urinary tract

Glomerulonephritis has been discussed as a possible consequence of etanercept treatment in two patients, with biopsy-proven mesangial deposits of IgA in one (30).

Henoch–Schönlein purpura with acute renal failure has been associated with an increase in the dose of etanercept after 11 months of use for psoriasis (31). Withdrawal of the drug and treatment with a course of systemic glucocorticoids produced complete resolution of the vasculitis and improved renal function.

Skin

The dermatological adverse effects of etanercept have been reviewed (32). Injection site reactions are common and usually self-limiting. Some patients have recall site reactions, in which rotated injection sites simultaneously develop a hypersensitivity reaction. In all cases, the rash has responded to antihistamines and etanercept therapy has been continued. Other injection site reactions have included discoid lupus and cutaneous vasculitis, which respond to withdrawal of treatment and appropriate therapy. Skin reactions more distant from the injection site include erythema nodosum, widespread lupus rashes, infections, and skin tumors. One patient developed a purpuric rash at the site of the last injection associated with thrombocytopenia.

Histological findings in one patient showed a mild transient inflammatory response that did not suggest sensitization (33). The clinical and histological characteristics of these lesions have been analysed in a retrospective review of 103 etanercept-treated patients and in three other patients assessed prospectively (34). Of 103 patients, 21 had injection site reactions (erythema, pain, pruritus, or edema) within the first 2 months of treatment, and typically within 1–2 days after the last injection. In addition, eight patients developed recall reactions while continuing to take etanercept. Skin biopsies and immunohistological analysis of reaction sites in three patients showed an inflammatory infiltrate consistent with a T cell-mediated delayed hypersensitivity reaction.

Exacerbation of atopic dermatitis has been attributed to etanercept (35).

- Atopic dermatitis worsened soon after etanercept was started in a 10-year-old girl. Although initial concomitant withdrawal of ciclosporin made interpretation difficult, the dermatitis persisted during the whole 6 months of etanercept treatment and resolved only after withdrawal. Etanercept-induced abnormalities of Th2 cytokines were suggested as the most likely mechanism.

A 55-year-old woman with no previous personal or family history of skin lesions developed clinical and histological features of psoriasis after taking etanercept for 3 months for seronegative rheumatoid arthritis (36). Etanercept was continued, but the lesions were poorly controlled by topical steroids and phototherapy. Two other patients aged 25 and 34 years had acute exacerbations of palmar and plantar psoriasis 4 and 7 months after starting to take etanercept for ankylosing spondylitis (37).

Paradoxical new-onset psoriasis has been attributed to etanercept, as has paradoxical worsening of pre-existing psoriasis.

- A 13-year-old girl developed new-onset psoriasis after starting to take etanercept for extending oligo-articular juvenile idiopathic arthritis (38).
- A 35-year-old man with severe plaque psoriasis and disabling psoriatic arthropathy, poorly controlled with conventional therapies, and recurrent episodes of erythroderma or pustular exanthematous psoriasis after intercurrent infections, was given subcutaneous. etanercept 25 mg twice a week (39). After about 7 weeks of treatment he had flu-like symptoms with upper respiratory tract involvement, followed 10 days later by sudden aggravation of his skin lesions, despite resolution of joint pain and stiffness. There were diffuse skin lesions and some pustules, submandibular lymphadenopathy, a mild pyrexia, a neutrophil leukocytosis, and a slight increase in erythrocyte sedimentation rate. No specific infection was identified. Etanercept was withdrawn and he was given topical therapy and oral paracetamol for 1 week, when the fever abated. Methotrexate 10 mg weekly and ciclosporin 2.5 mg/kg then caused regression of the pustular lesions and erythema after 2

months, but the articular symptoms reappeared and etanercept was restarted with a good clinical response and no complications.

In the second case the authors proposed that exacerbation of psoriasis had resulted from an interaction between etanercept and an infection, an unproven association.

A rash has been attributed to etanercept (40).

- A 70-year-old woman long-standing erosive seropositive rheumatoid arthritis was given etanercept 25 mg subcutaneously twice a week. After the fourth injection, she developed erythematous macular lesions, which were diagnosed as discoid eczema. Histopathology was consistent with a drug-induced dermatitis.

There have been several descriptions of new cutaneous or pulmonary nodulosis in patients with rheumatoid arthritis treated with etanercept (9,41); concomitant cutaneous vasculitis was also reported in two patients (41). Although this may have been due to the natural history of rheumatoid arthritis or a lack of response to treatment, the short time to the occurrence of cutaneous nodulosis after the start of therapy in some patients implicated the etanercept.

Cutaneous vasculitis can also be the sole cutaneous manifestation of etanercept treatment (42). Purpuric lesions with histological features of leukocytoclastic vasculitis have been reported in a 58-year-old man (43) and a necrotizing vasculitis with eosinophils in a skin biopsy in a woman with rheumatoid arthritis (44). However, it is not known whether this resulted from the deposition of specific immune complexes.

- A 13-year-old girl developed a slowly reversible purpuric rash after 6 weeks of etanercept treatment, and the lesions recurred on re-administration (45). However, further administration of a gradually increasing dose of etanercept, with concomitant high-dose glucocorticoids, and antihistamines, was well tolerated, suggesting that tolerance can be obtained.

One patient who had separate episodes of vascular purpura during each of three sequences of treatment with etanercept, with leukocytoclastic vasculitis during the third episode, later developed similar cutaneous lesions after a third injection of infliximab (42).

Other types of skin reactions that have been described in isolated reports include urticaria-like eruptions with prurigo in two patients with juvenile arthritis (46) and discoid lupus erythematosus in a woman with rheumatoid arthritis (44). Erythema multiforme in three patients and a lichenoid eruption in one were attributed to infliximab; however, one patient had similar lesions after etanercept (47).

Musculoskeletal

Painless orbital myositis has been reported in a 42-year-old woman taking etanercept, but a causal relation was not established (48).

Direct injection of etanercept into arthritic joints has been used in some patients with mono- or oligoarticular arthritis. This was presumably the cause of an acute intra-articular injection site reaction with painful local effusion in a 35-year-old man (49).

Immunologic

Although patients treated with etanercept commonly develop new antinuclear antibodies or anti-double-stranded DNA antibodies, there were no reports of cutaneous or systemic lupus erythematosus in early clinical trials. However, since then, at least eight cases have been reported, including five patients with a lupus-like syndrome, two with acute discoid lupus, and one with subacute cutaneous lupus erythematosus (50–53). All were women and they developed their first symptoms 6 weeks to 14 months after the first injection of etanercept. Antinuclear and/or anti-DNA antibodies were positive in most of them. Etanercept was withdrawn in all patients with features of systemic lupus erythematosus, and the symptoms resolved within 2–8 weeks. The skin lesions also improved with local glucocorticoids, despite continued etanercept treatment in two patients with discoid lupus or subacute cutaneous lupus erythematosus. This suggests that etanercept-induced autoantibodies are sometimes associated with clinical autoimmune disease.

There were no major changes in global immune functions, assessed by cell surface antigen expression of peripheral leucocytes, delayed-type hypersensitivity, T cell proliferation, serum immunoglobulin concentrations, and neutrophil function, in 33 patients taking etanercept compared with 16 patients taking placebo (54). The incidence of infections was also similar in the two groups. Although these results may account for a lower number of reports of infection with etanercept than with infliximab, etanercept also contributed to the occurrence of severe infectious complications.

Giant cell arteritis of the left temporal artery has been attributed to etanercept in a 79-year-old woman with rheumatoid arthritis (55). However, the patient had tolerated etanercept for 2 years before the onset of the symptoms and was also taking methotrexate. As the outcome was also unknown, any causal relationship is purely speculative.

Severe glomerulonephritis and cutaneous vasculitis have been reported (56).

- A 28-year-old woman with rheumatoid arthritis and positive antinuclear autoantibodies was given 18 infusions of infliximab because she did not continue to respond to hydroxychloroquine and methotrexate after 10 years of treatment, during which renal function had been normal. When infliximab became ineffective she was given etanercept 35 mg twice a week. Six months later she developed a dot-like eruption, an increase in serum creatinine concentration, and proteinuria. Etanercept was withdrawn. Skin and renal biopsies showed a non-specific lymphocytic vasculitis with a lupus band in the skin and glomerulonephritis. The cutaneous vasculitis resolved within a few days, but she developed status epilepticus and aggravation of renal function and required short-term dialysis. Persistent albuminuria was later noted.

Although anti-double-stranded DNA and antihistone antibodies were negative, a lupus-like syndrome was not completely excluded in this patient.

In a case of necrotizing crescentic glomerulonephritis with positive pANCA and progressive renal insufficiency in a 32-year-old woman with rheumatoid arthritis, the authors thought that etanercept given for the previous 11 months had failed to control the development of pANCA-associated vasculitis rather than precipitating or causing the adverse event (57).

The adverse events reporting system of the US Food and Drug Administration has recorded 35 cases of leukocytoclastic vasculitis, 20 after etanercept and 15 after infliximab (58). In most cases the symptoms developed within 3 months. In only one case was direct immunofluorescence performed on tissues and no specific immunoreactivity was found.

Infection risk

See also Adalimumab and Infliximab

Severe or uncommon infectious complications (severe viral pneumonia, fatal pneumococcal sepsis due to necrotizing fasciitis, osteoarticular tuberculosis) have been described in patients taking etanercept and long-term glucocorticoids (59–62).

The risk of infectious complications associated with TNF-alfa antagonists and current recommendations to be used before and during treatment have been reviewed (63,64,65,66).

Immunological and clinical studies have suggested that there is a higher risk of infection in patients with rheumatoid arthritis or ankylosing spondylitis who receive TNF-α antagonists, because they have active and more severe disease. They should therefore be closely monitored for serious infections, and rapid and adequate treatment of infections that are not mild and transient is recommended. Atypical signs and symptoms can occur and atypical pathogens can be involved. Patients should be educated about how to avoid infectious complications

Tumor necrosis factor inhibitor therapy may increase the risk of serious postoperative orthopedic infections in patients with rheumatoid arthritis (67). The risk of infection was studied in 546 patients who underwent at least one orthopedic surgical procedure during January 1999 to March 2004. Seven of 21 patients were receiving TNF-α antagonists at the time of procedure and one developed an infection. All together 10 of 91 patients who underwent an orthopedic surgical procedure developed a serious postoperative orthopedic infection. The authors concluded that the prescription of TNF-α inhibitor therapy was significantly associated with the development of serious postoperative infections. This association persisted after adjusting for other susceptibility factors for infection, such as age, use of prednisone, diabetes mellitus, disease duration, and rheumatoid factor seropositivity.

Patients with psoriatic arthropathy who were being treated with etanercept were able to produce antibodies in response to pneumococcal immunization, whereas patients receiving methotrexate had lower mean antibody titers in response to the vaccine (68). This suggests that patients treated with etanercept will have normal humoral responses to a T cell-independent antigen.

Detailed reports in patients with for rheumatoid arthritis have included:

- late recurrence of *Mycobacterium xenopi* infection manifesting as Pott's disease and severe spinal infection in a 49-year-old man taking methotrexate, prednisone, and sulfasalazine about 2 years after etanercept was begun (69).
- pulmonary aspergillosis in a 55-year-old woman who had received etanercept alone for 10 months (70).
- *Listeria monocytogenes* meningitis in a 45-year-old patient treated with etanercept monotherapy for 20 months (71).
- septic arthritis due to *Actinobacillus ureae*, which necessitated synovectomy and debridement in a 59-year-old woman also taking methotrexate (72).

All these patients developed their infection after a long course of etanercept and fully recovered from the infectious episode.

Incidence

TNF plays a key role in granuloma formation, which is an essential component for host control of several infections. Although infliximab and etanercept share the same therapeutic target, differences in their mode of action may account for a differential infection risk (73).

The general infection rate with etanercept over an entire course of therapy has been estimated to be 35% in placebo-controlled trials (74).

The data on spontaneous reports received by the FDA's Adverse Event Reporting System have been analysed to compare the reporting incidence and characteristics of granulomatous infectious diseases associated with etanercept or infliximab (75,76). A large number of granulomatous infections were selected for this purpose, but tuberculosis, histoplasmosis, candidiasis, and listeriosis accounted for more than 80% of the reported cases. Among 639 episodes of granulomatous infections, 556 were associated with infliximab and 83 with etanercept. According to the estimated number of patients treated in the USA during the reporting period and taking into account only those cases that occurred in there, the calculated reporting rate of granulomatous infections was 130 per 100 000 patients treated with infliximab and 60 per 100 000 patients treated with etanercept. The rates of tuberculosis were 54 per 100 000 and 28 per 100 000 respectively. Overall, there was a significantly higher rate of reporting with infliximab than with etanercept for coccidioidomycosis, histoplasmosis, listeriosis, and tuberculosis. From an analysis of the whole database, extrapulmonary presentation of tuberculosis was more frequent with infliximab (26%) than etanercept (10%), as was meningeal disease (17% versus 7%). In addition,

44% of tuberculosis cases attributed to infliximab were observed within the first 90 days of treatment compared with only 10% in those associated with etanercept. For all types of granulomatous infections, the median time to onset was 40 days for infliximab and 236 days for etanercept. The authors correctly argued that these differences can be explained by the different mechanisms of action of these drugs, with a higher risk of reactivation of latent tuberculosis infection with infliximab than with etanercept. The same conclusion probably applies in other granulomatous infections.

In a retrospective study of 180 patients taking etanercept for various systemic rheumatic diseases, there was no difference in the frequency of serious infections between the periods that preceded or followed etanercept use, but two of the five patients who developed serious infections while taking etanercept died as a result of complicated sepsis (77). The possible role of etanercept in the development of multifocal septic arthritis (78,79), tonsil or peritoneal tuberculosis (80,81), and cerebral toxoplasmosis (82) has also been discussed in recent isolated case reports.

All serious infections were analysed in a national prospective observational study in 7664 patients with severe rheumatoid arthritis who were given TNF-α antagonists and 1354 who were given DMARDs (83). There were 525 serious infections in those who received TNF-α antagonists and 56 in the comparison cohort (9868 and 1352 person-years of follow-up respectively). The incidence rate ratio (IRR), adjusted for baseline risk, in those who received TNF-α antagonists compared with those who did not was 1.03 (95% CI = 0.68, 1.57). However, the frequency of serious skin and soft tissue infections was increased in those who received TNF-α antagonists, with an adjusted IRR of 4.28 (95% CI = 1.06, 17). There was no difference in infection risk between the three main TNF-α antagonists. There were 19 cases of serious bacterial intracellular infections, exclusively in patients who received TNF-α antagonists. In patients with active rheumatoid arthritis, TNF-α antagonists were not associated with an increased overall risk of serious infections compared with DMARDs, after adjustment for baseline risk. In contrast, the rates of serious skin and soft tissue infections were increased, suggesting an important physiological role of TNF in host defences in the skin and soft tissues beyond that in other tissues.

The extent to which anti-TNF-α antibodies increase the risk of serious infections and malignancies has been assessed in patients with rheumatoid arthritis by performing a meta-analysis to derive estimates of sparse harmful events occurring in randomized trials of TNF-α antagonists (84). From a systematic literature search (EMBASE, MEDLINE, Cochrane Library, and electronic abstract databases, annual scientific meetings of both the European League Against Rheumatism and the American College of Rheumatology, interviews of the manufacturers of the two licensed anti-TNF-α antibodies, and randomized placebo-controlled trials of infliximab and adalimumab), nine trials met the inclusion criteria; 3493 patients received TNF-α antagonists and 1512 patients received placebo. The pooled odds ratio for serious infections was 2.0 (95% CI = 1.3, 3.1). For serious infections the number needed to treat for harm (NNT_H) was 59 (95% CI = 39, 125) during 3–12 months.

Bacterial infections

In a prospective study of 50 consecutive patients with rheumatoid arthritis who were given etanercept, there were serious infections, defined as requiring hospitalization and parenteral antibiotics, in six, including one patient with *Streptococcus G* septicemia, diverticular disease, and diabetic gangrene, two with streptococcal pneumonia, two with *Staphylococcus aureus* soft tissue infections and ulceration, and one with *Campylobacter jejuni* diarrhea (85).

Mycobacterium tuberculosis

Following a 2001 report that the voluntary Adverse Event Reporting System of the US Food and Drug Administration had received reports of nine cases of tuberculosis in patients taking etanercept (30) 25 cases were reviewed; the number of cases of tuberculosis reported to the FDA for each person-year of treatment with etanercept among patients with rheumatoid arthritis was estimated at about 10 per 100 000 patient-years of exposure (86). It is unclear from these data whether etanercept increases the risk of tuberculosis beyond the increased rates already documented among patients with rheumatoid arthritis.

Tuberculosis in patients taking the monoclonal TNF-α inhibitor frequently presents as extrapulmonary or disseminated disease, and clinicians should be vigilant for tuberculosis in any patient taking a TNF-α inhibitor who develops fever, weight loss, or cough. To prevent reactivation of latent tuberculosis infection during TNF-α inhibitor therapy, clinicians should screen all patients for tuberculosis and begin treatment if latent infection is found, before therapy is started. Specific tuberculosis screening and treatment strategies vary between geographical regions. The screening strategies used in Europe and North America have reduced the occurrence of TNF-α inhibitor-associated tuberculosis and are to be recommended. However, the role of screening in preventing other opportunistic (e.g. fungal) infections is far less certain (87).

Staphylococcus aureus

Etanercept has been used in two children with severe atopic dermatitis: it was minimally effective and was associated with complications. One patient developed a superinfection with methicillin-resistant *Staphylococcus aureus* (MRSA) and the other had viral-like symptoms followed by a generalized urticarial eruption (88). This was a limited study, which the authors suggested should not rule out the use of biologicals for severe atopic dermatitis, but should encourage a larger controlled study.

Viral infections

Preliminary data suggest that TNF-α inhibitor therapy may be safe in chronic hepatitis C. However, TNF antagonists have resulted in re-activation of chronic hepatitis B if not given concurrently with antiviral therapy.

Fungal infections
Coccidioidomycosis

To explore the risk of coccidioidomycosis associated with TNF-alfa antagonists, cases collected from five practices in an endemic area were retrospectively examined (89). There were 12 cases associated with infliximab (four with documented dissemination, including two deaths) and one case of resolved pneumonia with etanercept. Two patients had a prior history of coccidioidomycosis, but all of them were also taking other immunosuppressive agents, methotrexate being the most frequent. The disease occurred after a median time of 12.5 weeks (1–48 weeks) after starting infliximab, whereas the time to onset was 96 weeks in the only case involving etanercept. From a cohort of patients with inflammatory arthritis identified in one of these centers, there were seven cases of coccidioidomycosis among 247 patients treated with infliximab and four among 738 patients taking other antirheumatic drugs. The relative risk for infection with infliximab compared with other drugs was 5.2 (CI = 1.5, 18) and remained significant after adjusting for age and use of methotrexate or prednisone.

Histoplasmosis

Pulmonary fungal infections have been reported with TNF-α antagonists (66). The risk of histoplasmosis, which can be fatal, was reported as 27 per million with etanercept and 1990 per million with infliximab. Other pulmonary fungal infections include cryptococcal infection, invasive pulmonary aspergillosis, and coccidioidomycosis. The incidence of aspergillus was reported as 86 per million with infliximab and 62 per million with etanercept.

Pneumocystis jiroveci

Pneumocystis jiroveci pneumonia as a complication from treatment with infliximab for rheumatoid arthritis has been reported in a 63-year-old woman (90). There was no dyspnea and no typical observations on chest X-ray.

Long-Term Effects

Tumorigenicity

There is great concern about the potential development of malignancy after blockade of tumor necrosis factor alfa, and it is biologically plausible. The FDA received reports of 26 cases of lymphoproliferative disorders in patients treated with etanercept ($n = 18$) or infliximab ($n = 8$) over 20 months (91). Although this reporting rate does not exceed the age-adjusted incidence of lymphomas in the USA, spontaneous reporting underestimates the true incidence. In addition, several findings were similar to those reported in patients taking immunosuppressive drugs after transplantation. For example, 81% of the reported cases were non-Hodgkin's lymphomas. Also, the median time to occurrence after the start of anti-TNF-alfa treatment was only 8 weeks. Finally, lymphoma regressed in two patients after withdrawal and without specific cytotoxic therapy. Although the actual incidence of neoplasia was low, additional long-term data that take into account concomitant or previous immunosuppressive treatment are needed before firm conclusions can be reached.

According to the Australian Adverse Drug Reactions Advisory Committee (ADRAC), TNF-α antagonists may predispose patients to an increased risk of malignancy or accelerate its development (92). Since 2000, ADRAC has received 319 reports involving infliximab, etanercept, and adalimumab. The more serious reports were as follows: malignant melanoma (3 reports), tuberculosis ($n = 4$), lymphoma ($n = 5$), anaphylaxis ($n = 9$), sepsis ($n = 10$), lupus or lupus-like syndrome ($n = 22$), and pneumonia/lower respiratory tract infections ($n = 23$). The Australian Product Information has advised caution when considering these drugs in patients with a history of malignancy, or when considering continued treatment in those who develop a malignancy.

The potential risk of lymphoma in patients treated with TNF-alfa antagonists has been discussed (93). Whether these agents are independently associated with an increased risk of lymphoma continues to be debated (94). This issue was analysed in two large cohorts of rheumatoid arthritis patients. From the data registered in the South Swedish Arthritis Treatment Group, which covered over 90% of arthritic patients treated with anti-TNF-alfa drugs in this area of Sweden, there were 11 cases of tumors and five of lymphomas among 757 patients treated with etanercept or infliximab (1603 person-years of risk) (95). Although there was no increase in the overall risk of total tumors, the relative risk of lymphoma was 11 times higher than that expected in the background population. More importantly, a direct comparison showed that the relative risk of lymphoma was five times higher in patients treated with anti-TNF-alfa drugs than in a community-based control group of 800 patients treated with conventional antirheumatic drugs and never exposed to biological agents. This difference persisted after adjustment with the Health Assessment Questionnaire, used as a marker of disease severity. The other cohort consisted of 18 572 patients and included 29 cases of lymphoma, with a standardized incidence ratio of 2.6 for infliximab, 3.8 for etanercept, 1.7 for methotrexate, and 1.0 for patients not receiving methotrexate or anti-TNF-alfa agents (96). Although both studies suggested an increased rate of lymphoma in patients treated with infliximab or etanercept, these results should be interpreted with caution, because of the very small number of cases and a possible role of higher disease activity in these patients.

In 180 patients with active Wegener's granulomatosis enrolled in the Wegener's Granulomatosis Etanercept Trial (WGET) there were more solid malignancies in the etanercept group than in those treated with standard therapy alone (97). All six solid malignancies were associated with etanercept treatment; they included two cases of mucinous adenocarcinoma of the colon, one each of metastatic cholangiocarcinoma, renal cell carcinoma, and breast carcinoma, and one recurrent liposarcoma. Those who received etanercept were older at baseline and those who developed solid tumors were older than those who did not. In addition, all etanercept-treated patients who developed solid tumors had also received cyclophosphamide. This suggests that this combination may increase the risk of cancer beyond that observed with cyclophosphamide alone.

Second-Generation Effects

Lactation

Etanercept was secreted in breast milk in small amounts in one patient (98). The milk to plasma ratio was 0.04 and the calculated amount of etanercept orally ingested by a breast-fed newborn was 50–90 micrograms/day. Based on these findings, and since the systemic availability of etanercept by the oral route is assumed to be very low, breast-feeding during treatment is probably safe.

Susceptibility Factors

Age

In eight children with juvenile rheumatoid arthritis, who had failed to respond to disease-modifying anti-rheumatic drugs, high-dose etanercept was well tolerated (99). None withdrew because of etanercept-related adverse events. One child reported transient erythema at the injection site after the first injection. Three had mild transient upper respiratory tract infections. There were no laboratory abnormalities.

Special attention has been paid to the safety of infliximab and etanercept in children with juvenile idiopathic arthritis, in particular as regards to the possible risk of autoimmune disease and severe infectious disease, such as varicella zoster virus infection or tuberculosis (100). Whereas there were no cases of demyelination or lupus in these children, there were two cases of type I diabetes mellitus after etanercept treatment. A genetic predisposition was likely, but accelerated development of diabetes should be also considered, as suggested by experimental data that suggest an important role of TNF suppression in the progression of diabetes.

The risks of infections in elderly people taking TNF-α antagonists have been reviewed (101). Compared with younger people, elderly patients have more co-morbidities and are likely to be taking more medications. Moreover, the aging process causes an increase in the rate of infections. In analyses of the databases of etanercept trials, the normalized incidence of adverse events, serious adverse events, medically important infections, and deaths was not increased in patients aged 65 years and over. However, these trials included patients who might have been healthier than elderly patients with rheumatoid arthritis and therefore not truly representative. Conflicting results have been reported in several observational studies. Taken together, the available data are reassuring for carefully selected populations, at least for etanercept, but it is not possible to claim that TNF-α antagonists do or do not pose a particular risk for the general population of older patients.

Drug Administration

Drug dosage regimens

Two etanercept dosing regimens have been compared—50 mg twice weekly and 100 mg once weekly, each for 12 weeks in 108 patients with moderate-to-severe recalcitrant psoriasis (102). The two regimens caused comparable improvements after 4 weeks and 12 weeks. Treatment was well tolerated and adverse events ware of similar type and frequency in the two groups.

Etanercept and sulfasalazine, alone and in combination, have been compared in 254 adults with active rheumatoid arthritis, despite sulfasalazine treatment, in a double-blind, randomized study (103). Lack of efficacy was the primary reason for withdrawal (sulfasalazine, n = 12/50; etanercept, n = 1/103; etanercept and sulfasalazine, n = 4/101). Several common adverse events (headache, nausea, weakness) were less common with etanercept alone than with the combination, but infections and injection site reactions were more common.

In a prospective open study of added etanercept in 119 patients with active rheumatoid arthritis despite stable therapy with sulfasalazine (n = 50), hydroxychloroquine (n = 50), or intramuscular gold (n = 19), withdrawals because of adverse effects by 48 weeks included proteinuria (etanercept + gold, n = 1); septic wrist and bilateral pneumonia, rash, optic neuritis, breast cancer, and squamous cancer of the tongue (etanercept + hydroxychloroquine, n = 5); and otitis media, abnormal liver function tests, pericarditis, rash, and gastroenteritis (etanercept + sulfasalazine, n = 5) (104). The most common adverse events not requiring withdrawal were injection site reactions (43%) and upper respiratory infections (34%).

In 714 patients with rheumatoid arthritis refractory to disease modifying antirheumatic drugs (DMARD) who received etanercept for 8 years in one of seven initial trials or a long-term extension, the overall rate of serious adverse events was 15 events/100 patient-years. Other rates were: serious infections 4.2, cancers 1.0, and deaths 0.7 (105).

Interference with Diagnostic Tests

Troponin concentration

Non-neutralizing antibodies to etanercept have been identified in clinical trials. Although there was no correlation between these antibodies and the development of adverse effects (2), their presence was suggested as a likely explanation of false-positive rises in troponin concentrations in an assay that used mouse antihuman troponin (106).

References

1. Culy CR, Keating GM. Etanercept: an updated review of its use in rheumatoid arthritis, psoriatic arthritis and juvenile rheumatoid arthritis. Drugs 2002;62(17):2493–537.
2. Bathon JM, Martin RW, Fleischmann RM, Tesser JR, Schiff MH, Keystone EC, Genovese MC, Wasko MC,

Moreland LW, Weaver AL, Markenson J, Finck BK. A comparison of etanercept and methotrexate in patients with early rheumatoid arthritis. N Engl J Med 2000;343(22):1586–93.

3. Klareskog L, van der Heijde D, de Jager JP, Gough A, Kalden J, Malaise M, Martin Mola E, Pavelka K, Sany J, Settas L, Wajdula J, Pedersen R, Fatenejad S, Sanda M; TEMPO (Trial of Etanercept and Methotrexate with Radiographic Patient Outcomes) study investigators. Therapeutic effect of the combination of etanercept and methotrexate compared with each treatment alone in patients with rheumatoid arthritis: double-blind randomised controlled trial. Lancet 2004;363:675–81.

4. Leonardi C, Powers J, RT, Goffe B, Zitnik R, Wang A, Gottlieb A. Etanercept as monotherapy in patients with psoriasis. New Engl J Med 2003;349:2014–22.

5. Gottlieb AB, Matheson RT, Lowe N, Krueger GG, Kang S, Goffe BS, Gaspari AA, Ling M, Weinstein GD, Nayak A, Gordon KB, Zitnik R. A randomized trial of etanercept as monotherapy for psoriasis. Arch Dermatol 2003;139:1627–32.

6. Papp KA, Tyring S, Lahfa M, Prinz J, Griffiths CEM, Nakanishi AM, Zitnik R, van de Kerkhof PCM. A global phase III randomized controlled trial of etanercept in psoriasis: safety, efficacy, and effect of dose reduction. Br J Dermatol 2005;152:1304–12.

7. Brimhall AK, King LN, Licciardone JC, Jacobe H, Menter A. Safety and efficacy of alefacept, efalizumab, etanercept and infliximab in treating moderate to severe plaque psoriasis: a meta-analysis of randomized controlled trials. Br J Dermatol 2008;159(2):274–85.

8. Jarvis B, Faulds D. Etanercept: a review of its use in rheumatoid arthritis. Drugs 1999;57(6):945–66.

9. Kekow J, Welte T, Kellner U, Pap T. Development of rheumatoid nodules during anti-tumor necrosis factor alpha therapy with etanercept. Arthritis Rheum 2002; 46(3):843–4.

10. Hubscher O, Re R, Iotti R. Pulmonary rheumatoid nodules in an etanercept-treated patient. Arthritis Rheum 2003; 48(7):2077–8.

11. Peno-Green L, Lluberas G, Kingsley T, Brantley S. Lung injury linked to etanercept therapy. Chest 2002; 122(5):1858–60.

12. Vavricka SR, Wettstein T, Speich R, Gaspert A, Bachli EB. Pulmonary granulomas after tumour necrosis factor alpha antagonist therapy. Thorax 2003;58(3):278–9.

13. Lindsay K, Melsom R, Jacob BK, Mestry N. Acute progression of interstitial lung disease: acomplication of etanercept particularly in the presence of rheumatoid lung and methotrexate treatment. Rheumatology 2006;45(8):1048–9.

14. Mart nez-Taboada VM, Val-Bernal JF, Pesquera LC, Fern ndez-Llanio NE, Esteban JMP, Blanco R, Alonso-Bartolome P, Gonzalez-Vela C, Rodr guez-Valverde V. Demyelinating disease and cutaneous lymphocitic vasculitis after etanercept therapy in a patient with rheumatoid arthritis. Scand J Rheumatol 2006;35(4):322–3.

15. Arnason BGWThe Lenercept Multiple Sclerosis Study GroupThe University of British Columbia MS/MRI Analysis Group. TNF neutralization in MS: results of a randomized, placebo-controlled multicenter study. Neurology 1999;53(3):457–65.

16. van der Laken CJ, Lems WF, van Soesbergen RM, van der Sande JJ, Dijkmans BA. Paraplegia in a patient receiving anti-tumor necrosis factor therapy for rheumatoid arthritis: comment on the article by Mohan et al. Arthritis Rheum 2003;48(1):269–70.

17. Mohan N, Edwards ET, Cupps TR, Oliverio PJ, Sandberg G, Crayton H, Richert JR, Siegel JN. Demyelination occurring during anti-tumor necrosis factor alpha therapy for inflammatory arthritides. Arthritis Rheum 2001;44(12):2862–9.

18. Robinson WH, Genovese MC, Moreland LW. Demyelinating and neurologic events reported in association with tumor necrosis factor alpha antagonism: by what mechanisms could tumor necrosis factor alpha antagonists improve rheumatoid arthritis but exacerbate multiple sclerosis? Arthritis Rheum 2001;44(9):1977–83.

19. Kaipiainen-Seppanen O, Leino M. Recurrent uveitis in a patient with juvenile spondyloarthropathy associated with tumour necrosis factor alfa inhibitors. Ann Rheum Dis 2003;62:88–9.

20. Reddy AR, Backhouse OC. Does etanercept induce uveitis? Br J Ophthalmol 2003;87:925.

21. Tiliakos AN, Tiliakos NA. Ocular inflammatory disease in patients with RA taking etanercept: is discontinuation of etanercept necessary? J Rheumatol 2003;30:2727.

22. Clifford L, Rossiter J. Peripheral visual field loss following treatment with etanercept. Br J Ophthalmol 2004;88:842.

23. Tauber T, Turetz J, Barash J, Avni I, Morad Y. Optic neuritis associated with etanercept therapy for juvenile arthritis. J Am Assoc Pediatr Ophthalmol Strabismus 2006;10(1):26–9.

24. Allanore Y, Bremont C, Kahan A, Menkes CJ. Transient hyperthyroidism in a patient with rheumatoid arthritis treated by etanercept. Clin Exp Rheumatol 2001;19(3):356–7.

25. Bloom BJ. Development of diabetes mellitus during etanercept therapy in a child with systemic-onset juvenile rheumatoid arthritis. Arthritis Rheum 2000;43(11):2606–8.

26. Kuruvilla J, Leitch HA, Vickars LM, Galbraith PF, Li CH, Al-Saab S, Naiman SC. Aplastic anemia following administration of a tumor necrosis factor-alfa inhibitor. Eur J Haematol 2003;71:396–8.

27. Stern A, Buckley L. Worsening of macrophage activation syndrome in a patient with adult onset Still's disease after initiation of etanercept therapy. J Clin Rheumatol 2001; 7:252–6.

28. Ramanan AV, Schneider R. Macrophage activation syndrome following initiation of etanercept in a child with systemic onset juvenile rheumatoid arthritis. J Rheumatol 2003;30:401–3.

29. Ruemmele FM, Prieur AM, Talbotec C, Goulet O, Schmitz J. Development of Crohn disease during anti-TNF-alpha therapy in a child with juvenile idiopathic arthritis. J Pediatr Gastroenterol Nutr 2004;39:203–6.

30. Kemp E, Nielsen H, Petersen LJ, Gam AN, Dahlager J, Horn T, Larsen S, Olsen S. Newer immunomodulating drugs in rheumatoid arthritis may precipitate glomerulonephritis. Clin Nephrol 2001;55(1):87–8.

31. Lee A, Kasama R, Evangelisto A, Elfenbein B, Falasca G. Henoch–Schönlein purpura after etanercept therapy for psoriasis. J Clin Rheumatol 2006;12(5):249–51.

32. Rajakulendran S, Deighton C. Adverse dermatological reactions in rheumatoid arthritis patients treated with etanercept, an anti-TNFalpha drug. Curr Drug Saf 2006;1(3):259–64.

33. Murphy FT, Enzenauer RJ, Battafarano DF, David-Bajar K. Etanercept-associated injection-site reactions. Arch Dermatol 2000;136(4):556–7.

34. Zeltser R, Valle L, Tanck C, Holyst MM, Ritchlin C, Gaspari AA. Clinical, histological, and immunophenotypic characteristics of injection site reactions associated with etanercept: a recombinant tumor necrosis factor alpha

receptor: Fc fusion protein. Arch Dermatol 2001; 137(7):893–9.

35. Mangge H, Gindl S, Kenzian H, Schauenstein K. Atopic dermatitis as a side effect of anti-tumor necrosis factor-alfa therapy. J Rheumatol 2003;30:2506–7.

36. Dereure O, Guillot B, Jorgensen C, Cohen JD, Combes B, Guilhou JJ. Psoriatic lesions induced by antitumour necrosis factor-alpha treatment: two cases. Br J Dermatol 2004;151:506–7.

37. Haibel H, Spiller I, Strasser C, Rudwaleit M, Dorner T, et al. Unexpected new onset or exacerbation of psoriasis in treatment of active ankylosing spondylitis with TNF-alpha blocking agents: four case reports. Ann Rheum Dis 2004;63(Suppl 1):405.

38. Peek R, Scott-Jupp R, Strike H, Clinch J, Ramanan AV. Psoriasis after treatment of juvenile idiopathic arthritis with etanercept. Ann Rheum Dis 2006;65:1259.

39. Cassano N, Coviello C, Loconsole F, Miracapillo A, Vena GA. Psoriasis exacerbation after a flu-like syndrome during anti-TNF-alpha therapy. Eur J Dermatol 2006;16(3):316–7.

40. Lai-Cheong J, Warren R, Bucknall R, Parslew R. Etanercept-induced dermatitis in a patient with rheumatoid arthritis. J Eur Acad Dermatol Venereol 2006;20(5):614–5.

41. Cunnane G, Warnock M, Fye KH, Daikh DI. Accelerated nodulosis and vasculitis following etanercept therapy for rheumatoid arthritis. Arthritis Rheum 2002;47(4):445–9.

42. McCain ME, Quinet RJ, Davis WE. Etanercept and infliximab associated with cutaneous vasculitis. Rheumatology (Oxford) 2002;41(1):116–7.

43. Galaria NA, Werth VP, Schumacher HR. Leukocytoclastic vasculitis due to etanercept. J Rheumatol 2000;27(8):2041–4.

44. Brion PH, Mittal-Henkle A, Kalunian KC. Autoimmune skin rashes associated with etanercept for rheumatoid arthritis. Ann Intern Med 1999;131(8):634.

45. Livermore PA, Murray KJ. Anti-tumour necrosis factor therapy associated with cutaneous vasculitis. Rheumatology (Oxford) 2002;41(12):1450–2.

46. Skytta E, Pohjankoski H, Savolainen A. Etanercept and urticaria in patients with juvenile idiopathic arthritis. Clin Exp Rheumatol 2000;18(4):533–4.

47. Vergara G, Silvestre JF, Betlloch I, Vela P, Albares MP, Pascual JC. Cutaneous drug eruption to infliximab: report of 4 cases with an interface dermatitis pattern. Arch Dermatol 2002;138(9):1258–9.

48. Caramaschi P, Biasi D, Carletto A, Bambara LM. Orbital myositis in a rheumatoid arthritis patient during etanercept treatment. Clin Exp Rheumatol 2003;21(1):136–7.

49. Arnold EL, Khanna D, Paulus H, Goodman MP. Acute injection site reaction to intraarticular etanercept administration. Arthritis Rheum 2003;48:2078–9.

50. Bleumink GS, ter Borg EJ, Ramselaar CG, Ch Stricker BH. Etanercept-induced subacute cutaneous lupus erythematosus. Rheumatology (Oxford) 2001;40(11):1317–9.

51. De Bandt MJ, Descamps V, Meyer O. Two cases of etanercept-induced systemic lupus erythematosus in patients with rheumatoid arthritis. Ann Rheum Dis 2001;60:175.

52. Misery L, Perrot JL, Gentil-Perret A, Pallot-Prades B, Cambazard F, Alexandre C. Dermatological complications of etanercept therapy for rheumatoid arthritis. Br J Dermatol 2002;146(2):334–5.

53. Shakoor N, Michalska M, Harris CA, Block JA. Drug-induced systemic lupus erythematosus associated with etanercept therapy. Lancet 2002;359(9306):579–80.

54. Moreland LW, Bucy RP, Weinblatt ME, Mohler KM, Spencer-Green GT, Chatham WW. Immune function in patients with rheumatoid arthritis treated with etanercept. Clin Immunol 2002;103:13–21.

55. Seton M. Giant cell arteritis in a patient taking etanercept and methotrexate. J Rheumatol 2004;31:1467.

56. Roux CH, Brocq O, Albert C Breuil V, Euller-Ziegler L. Cutaneous vasculitis and glomerulonephritis in a patient taking the anti-TNF alpha agent etanercept for rheumatoid arthritis. Joint Bone Spine 2004;71:444–5.

57. Doulton TWR, Tucker B, Reardon J, Velasco N. Antineutrophil cytoplasmic antibody-associated necrotizing crescentic glomerulonephritis in a patient receiving treatment with etanercept for severe rheumatoid arthritis. Clin Nephrol 2004;62:234–8.

58. Mohan N, Edwards ET, Cupps TR, Slifman N, Lee JH, Siegel JN, Braun MM. Leukocytoclastic vasculitis associated with tumor necrosis factor-alpha blocking agents. J Rheumatol 2004;31(10):1955–8.

59. Keane J, Gershon S, Wise RP, Mirabile-Levens E, Kasznica J, Schwieterman WD, Siegel JN, Braun MM. Tuberculosis associated with infliximab, a tumor necrosis factor alpha-neutralizing agent. N Engl J Med 2001;345(15):1098–104.

60. Baghai M, Osmon DR, Wolk DM, Wold LE, Haidukewych GJ, Matteson EL. Fatal sepsis in a patient with rheumatoid arthritis treated with etanercept. Mayo Clin Proc 2001;76(6):653–6.

61. Myers A, Clark J, Foster H. Tuberculosis and treatment with infliximab. N Engl J Med 2002;346(8):623–6.

62. Smith D, Letendre S. Viral pneumonia as a serious complication of etanercept therapy. Ann Intern Med 2002;136(2):174.

63. Bakleh M, Tleyjeh I, Matteson EL, Osmon DR, Berbari EF. Infectious complications of tumor necrosis factor-alpha antagonists. Int J Dermatol 2005;44:443–8.

64. Bieber J, Kavanaugh A. Tuberculosis and opportunistic infections: relevance to biologic agents. Clin Exp Rheumatol 2004;22(Suppl 35):S126-33.

65. Desai SB, Furst DE. Problems encountered during anti-tumour necrosis factor therapy. Best Pract Res Clin Rheumatol 2006;20(4):757–90.

66. Strangfeld A, Listing J. Infection and musculoskeletal conditions: bacterial and opportunistic infections during anti-TNF therapy. Best Pract Res Clin Rheumatol 2006;20(6):1181–95.

67. Giles JT, Bartlett SJ, Gelber AC, Nanda S, Fontaine K, Ruffing V, Bathon JM. Tumor necrosis factor inhibitor therapy and risk of serious postoperative orthopedic infection in rheumatoid arthritis. Arthritis Rheum 2006;55(2):333–7.

68. Mease PJ, Ritchlin CT, Martin RW, Gottlieb AB, Baumgartner SW, Burge DJ, Whitmore JB. Pneumococcal vaccine response in psoriatic arthritis patients during treatment with etanercept. J Rheumatol 2004;31(7):1356–61.

69. Yim K, Nazeer SH, Kiska D, Rose FB, Brown D, Cynamon MH. Recurrent Mycobacterium xenopi infection in a patient with rheumatoid arthritis receiving etanercept. Scand J Infect Dis 2004;36:150–4.

70. Lassoued S, Sire S, Farny M, Billey T, Lassoued K. Pulmonary aspergillosis in a patient with rheumatoid arthritis treated by etanercept. Clin Exp Rheumatol 2004;22:267–8.

71. Pagliano P, Attanasio V, Fusco U, Mohamed DA, Rossi M, Faella FS. Does etanercept monotherapy enhance the

risk of *Listeria monocytogenes meningitis? Ann Rheum Dis* 2004;63:462–3.

72. Kaur PP, Derk CT, Chatterji M, Dehoratius RJ. Septic arthritis caused by *Actinobacillus ureae* in a patient with rheumatoid arthritis receiving anti-tumor necrosis factor-alpha therapy. J Rheumatol 2004;31:1663–5.

73. Ehlers S. Why does tumor necrosis factor targeted therapy reactivate tuberculosis? J Rheumatol 2005;74(Suppl):35–9.

74. Scheinfeld N. A comprehensive review and evaluation of the side effects of the tumor necrosis factor alpha blockers etanercept, infliximab and adalimumab. J Dermatol Treat 2004;15:280–94.

75. Wallis RS, Broder MS, Wong JY, Hanson ME, Beenhouwer DO. Granulomatous infectious diseases associated with tumor necrosis factor antagonists. Clin Infect Dis 2004;38:1261–5.

76. Wallis RS, Broder M, Wong J, Beenhouwer D. Granulomatous infections due to tumor necrosis factor blockade: correction. Clin Infect Dis 2004;39:1254–5.

77. Phillips K, Husni ME, Karlson EW, Coblyn JS. Experience with etanercept in an academic medical center: are infection rates increased? Arthritis Rheum 2002;47:17–21.

78. Amital H, Aamar S, Rubinow A. Bilateral septic arthritis of the hip: does etanercept play a role? A case report. J Bone Joint Surg Am 2003;85:2205–6.

79. Elwood RL, Pelszynski MM, Corman LI. Multifocal septic arthritis and osteomyelitis caused by group A streptococcus in a patient receiving immunomodulating therapy with etanercept. Pediatr Infect Dis J 2003;22:286–8.

80. Derk CT, DeHoratius RJ. Tuberculous tonsillitis in a patient receiving etanercept treatment. Ann Rheum Dis 2003;62:372.

81. Manadan AM, Block JA, Sequeira W. Mycobacteria tuberculosis peritonitis associated with etanercept therapy. Clin Exp Rheumatol 2003;21:526.

82. Gonzalez-Vicent M, Diaz MA, Sevilla J, Madero L. Cerebral toxoplasmosis following etanercept treatment for idiophatic pneumonia syndrome after autologous peripheral blood progenitor cell transplantation (PBPCT). Ann Hematol 2003;82:649–53.

83. Dixon WG, Watson K, Lunt M, Hyrich KL, Silman AJ, Symmons DP; British Society for Rheumatology Biologics Register. Rates of serious infection, including site-specific and bacterial intracellular infection, in rheumatoid arthritis patients receiving anti-tumor necrosis factor therapy: results from the British Society for Rheumatology Biologics Register. Arthritis Rheum 2006;54(2):2368–76.

84. Bongartz T, Sutton AJ, Sweeting MJ, Buchan I, Matteson EL, Montori V. Anti-TNF antibody therapy in rheumatoid arthritis and the risk of serious infections and malignancies: systematic review and meta-analysis of rare harmful effects in randomized controlled trials. JAMA 2006;295(19):2275-85. Erratum: 2006;295(21):2482.

85. Perera LC, Tymms KE, Wilson BJ, Shadbolt B, Brook AS, Dorai Raj AK, Khoo KBK. Etanercept in severe active rheumatoid arthritis: first Australian experience. Intern Med J 2006;36(10):625–31.

86. Mohan A, Cote T, Block J, Manadan A, Siegel J, Braun M. Tuberculosis following the use of etanercept, a tumor necrosis factor inhibitor. Clin Infect Diseases 2004;39:295–9.

87. Winthrop KL. Risk and prevention of tuberculosis and other serious opportunistic infections associated with the inhibition of tumor necrosis factor. Nat Clin Pract Rheumatol 2006;2(11):602–10.

88. Buka RL, Resh B, Roberts B, Cunningham B, Friedlander S. Etanercept is minimally effective in 2 children with atopic dermatitis. J Am Acad Dermatol 2005;53:358–9.

89. Bergstrom L, Yocum DE, Ampel NM, Villanueva I, Lisse J, Gluck O, Tesser J, Posever J, Miller M, Araujo J, Kageyama DM, Berry M, Karl L, Yung CM. Increased risk of coccidioidomycosis in patients treated with tumor necrosis factor alpha antagonists. Arthritis Rheum 2004;50:1959–66.

90. Mori S, Imamura F, Kiyofuji C, Ito K, Koga Y, Honda I, Sugimoto M. *Pneumocystis jiroveci* pneumonia in a patient with rheumatoid arthritis as a complication of treatment with infliximab, anti-tumor necrosis factor alpha neutralizing antibody. Modern Rheumatol 2006;16(1):58–62.

91. Brown SL, Greene MH, Gershon SK, Edwards ET, Braun MM. Tumor necrosis factor antagonist therapy and lymphoma development: twenty-six cases reported to the Food and Drug Administration. Arthritis Rheum 2002;46(12):3151–8.

92. Anonymous. Tumor necrosis factor (TNF)-α inhibitors. Increased risk of malignancy. WHO Pharm Newslett 2007;1:5.

93. van Vollenhoven RF. Benefits and risks of biological agents: lymphomas. Clin Exp Rheumatol 2004;22(Suppl 35):S122-5.

94. Symmons DP, Silman AJ. Anti-tumor necrosis factor alpha therapy and the risk of lymphoma in rheumatoid arthritis: no clear answer. Arthritis Rheum 2004;50:1703–6.

95. Geborek P, Bladstrom A, Turesson C, Gulfe A, Petersson IF, Saxne T, Olsson H, Jacobsson LT. Tumour necrosis factor blockers do not increase overall tumour risk in patients with rheumatoid arthritis, but may be associated with an increased risk of lymphomas. Ann Rheum Dis 2005;64:699–703.

96. Wolfe F, Michaud K. Lymphoma in rheumatoid arthritis: the effect of methotrexate and anti-tumor necrosis factor therapy in 18,572 patients. Arthritis Rheum 2004;50:1740–51.

97. Stone JH, Holbrook JT, Marriott MA, Tibbs AK, Sejismundo LP, Min YI, Specks U, Merkel PA, Spiera R, Davis JC, St Clair EW, McCune WJ, Ytterberg SR, Allen NB, Hoffman GS; Wegener's Granulomatosis Etanercept Trial Research Group. Solid malignancies among patients in the Wegener's Granulomatosis Etanercept Trial. Arthritis Rheum 2006;54(5):1608–18.

98. Ostensen M, Eigenmann GO. Etanercept in breast milk. J Rheumatol 2004;31:1017–8.

99. Takei S, Groh D, Bernstein B, Shaham B, Gallagher K, Reiff A. Safety and efficacy of high dose etanercept in treatment of juvenile rheumatoid arthritis. J Rheumatol 2001;28(7):1677–80.

100. Dekker L, Armbrust W, Rademaker CM, Prakken B, Kuis W, Wulffraat NM. Safety of anti-TNFalpha therapy in children with juvenile idiopathic arthritis. Clin Exp Rheumatol 2004;22:252–8.

101. Ornetti P, Chevillotte H, Zerrak A, Maillefert JF. Anti-tumour necrosis factor-alpha therapy for rheumatoid and other inflammatory arthropathies: update on safety in older patients. Drugs Aging 2006;23(11):855–60.

102. Cassano N, Loconsole F, Galluccio A, Miracapillo A, Pezza M, Vena GA. Once-weekly administration of high-dosage etanercept in patients with plaque psoriasis: results of a pilot experience (power study). Int J Immunopathol Pharmacol 2006;19(1):225–9.

103. Combe B, Codreanu C, Fiocco U, Gaubitz M, Geusens PP, Kvien TK, Pavelka K, Sambrook PN, Smolen JS, Wajdula J, Fatenejad S; Etanercept European Investigators Network (Etanercept Study 309 Investigators). Etanercept and sulfasalazine, alone and combined, in patients with active rheumatoid arthritis despite receiving sulfasalazine: a double-blind comparison. Ann Rheum Dis 2006;65(10):1357–62.

104. O'Dell JR, Petersen K, Leff R, Palmer W, Schned E, Blakely K, Haire C, Fernandez A. Etanercept in combination with sulfasalazine, hydroxychloroquine, or gold in the treatment of rheumatoid arthritis. J Rheumatol 2006;33(2):213–8.

105. Moreland LW, Weinblatt ME, Keystone EC, Kremer JM, Martin RW, Schiff MH, Whitmore JB, White BW. Etanercept treatment in adults with established rheumatoid arthritis: 7 years of clinical experience. J Rheumatol 2006;33(5):854–61.

106. Russell E, Zeihen M, Wergin S, Litton T. Patients receiving etanercept may develop antibodies that interfere with monoclonal antibody laboratory assays. Arthritis Rheum 2000;43(4):944.

Gold and gold salts

General Information

Gold is a heavy yellow-colored element (symbol Au; atomic no. 79). Its symbol derives from the Latin word aurum. It is usually found as the metallic element but can occur as salts such gold telluride (sylvanite).

Metallic gold is used in dentistry, and gold salts still form one of the mainstays of treatment for rheumatoid arthritis. The radioactive isotope ^{198}Au is used therapeutically in the treatment of certain malignancies. In Japan, chrysotherapy has a reputation for efficacy in bronchial asthma. The antitumor activity of novel gold compounds is being pursued (1,2). The molecular mechanisms of action of gold have been reviewed (3,4).

Gold salts

Sodium aurothiomalate is water-soluble and is given intramuscularly as an aqueous solution. Aurothioglucose is water-soluble and is given intramuscularly in either an aqueous solution or an oily suspension. Sodium aurothiopropanol sulfonate, aurotioprol, and aurothiosulfate have similar actions and uses to those of sodium aurothiomalate. They are given by intramuscular injection.

Auranofin

Auranofin is a triethylphosphine gold derivative for oral administration. It is in some respects strikingly different from the rest. Some 25% of an oral dose is absorbed through the intestinal wall and blood concentrations are some 15–25% of those reached with parenteral therapy. Auranofin is bound to cellular elements of the blood, is excreted mainly in the feces, and exhibits less tissue retention and total body gold accumulation than parenteral

forms. It is more effective in acute inflammatory models and is a potent inhibitor of lysosomal enzyme release, antibody-dependent cellular toxicity, and superoxide production. Auranofin also affects humoral and cellular immune reactions. However, some have found auranofin to be rather less effective than parenteral gold. Auranofin is used in doses of 2–9 mg/day (generally 6 mg/day), which is less than the dose originally recommended.

In view of all this it is not surprising that auranofin has a distinct profile of therapeutic and adverse effects, the differences being so great that one actually suspects differences in the mechanism of action between oral and parenteral forms. Like the latter, however, auranofin shows no clear correlation between whole blood gold concentrations and either efficacy or adverse effects.

Use in rheumatoid arthritis

In rheumatoid arthritis the most commonly used gold salts are sodium aurothiomalate and aurothioglucose (5). There is some reason to believe that adverse effects are less frequent with the suspensions (of aurothioglucose or aurothiosulfate) than with the more rapidly absorbed solution (of sodium gold thiomalate; SEDA-16, 233; 6).

Whereas gold was previously regarded as one of the most toxic drugs in the pharmacopeia, many authors now share the view that its adverse effects can to an important extent be contained by individually adapted dosage regimens and careful monitoring. However, it is not strictly possible to predict the nature or timing of the complications that an individual may experience, and it has to be borne in mind that some reactions are immunological (SEDA-21, 236). The prevalence of adverse gold reactions seems to be similar in patients given 25 or 50 mg of gold weekly (SED-12, 520; 7). Some studies have suggested that the frequency of mucocutaneous and renal adverse reactions may be higher in the initial months of treatment. In one series of patients receiving gold sodium thiomalate, a plateau in the cumulative incidence of withdrawals due to rash was reached only after 40 months (45% of all patients), while withdrawals due to proteinuria reached a plateau after 18 months (15%; 8). Hematological complications can occur at any stage.

It is widely considered that the patients who are most likely to develop adverse reactions to gold salts are those who react most favorably. In the past, many rheumatologists intensified treatment with high doses of gold salts until a skin eruption occurred, only then seeking to reduce to a maintenance dosage.

After withdrawal due to adverse reactions, treatment with gold compounds can be cautiously reintroduced without the previous adverse effects necessarily reappearing. However, clearly one will not take this course if life-threatening reactions have occurred. It should always be borne in mind that many adverse reactions allegedly due to chrysotherapy may have other causes, particularly in the case of skin reactions. Most patients have been or are using other drugs at the same time. The concomitant use of penicillamine can be particularly confusing, since its pattern of adverse effects closely resembles that produced by gold.

Use in dentistry

Dental gold alloys continue to be used and remain a source of contact hypersensitivity (9), including contact stomatitis and skin eruptions at sites not usually associated with dentistry. Contact dermatitis to metallic gold, for example in jewellery, has also repeatedly been observed (SED-8, 510; SEDA-22, 245). A gold surgical clip has also caused an apparently allergic reaction, characterized by sterile abscess formation (10). However, such reactions are rare and may in part be due to other metals contained in the alloy.

General adverse effects

Intravenous gold salts

Adverse effects of gold salts occur in about one-third of systemically treated patients, the incidence varying from 25 to 40%. The dropout rate due to adverse reactions has been assessed as 22–26% (11). Children are considered to show the same pattern of adverse reactions as adults.

Cutaneous lesions are the most frequent adverse effects of gold salts, followed by involvement of the mucous membranes and kidneys. Pruritus and a wide range of skin reactions can occur. In the gastrointestinal system inflammation can occur at all levels, from the buccal cavity to the colon. Glossitis, cheilitis, and stomatitis are less common than dermatitis. Enterocolitis is a rare but very serious complication. Mild proteinuria is often seen in patients receiving chrysotherapy, while severe nephrotic syndrome is much less common. Blood dyscrasias of any type can occur either during therapy or after withdrawal. Leukopenia and thrombocytopenia are the most common hematological complications, although both are clearly less common than the mucocutaneous and renal adverse effects. Unusual reactions include pulmonary infiltration, intrahepatic cholestasis, and peripheral neuropathy. By and large, undesirable effects are transient and mild, but occasional deaths continue to be reported, usually because of hematological complications.

Apart from the "nitritoid" cardiovascular reaction, which is unique to sodium aurothiomalate, and possible differences between slowly and rapidly absorbed gold salts in the relative frequency of adverse effects, the general pattern of adverse reactions is similar for all parenteral gold salts.

Although most adverse effects of gold have traditionally been characterized as toxic, various factors show that some of the complications due to chrysotherapy are, at least in part, manifestations of hypersensitivity. Eosinophilia, raised IgE concentrations, immune complexes, and a positive reaction to gold in the lymphocyte transformation test have been observed in association with many adverse reactions to chrysotherapy and point to immunological mechanisms (12). With aurothiomalate both pemphigus and erythroderma have been described (SEDA-22, 246). It may be that gold facilitates the development of autoimmunity in patients with rheumatoid arthritis. Gold-induced membranous glomerulonephritis is believed to be an immune complex (type III) reaction, although the role of gold in the development of

proteinuria has not yet been clarified. Gold-induced antibody deficiency may be more common than is usually recognized. In 22 patients with rheumatoid arthritis subnormal serum immunoglobulin concentrations developed as a consequence of gold treatment (13). There were mild deficiencies of single immunoglobulin isotypes or severe deficiencies affecting two or three isotypes. There may be transient exacerbation of rheumatoid symptoms before a therapeutic response to gold occurs. In one series of 43 patients with rheumatoid arthritis serious exacerbation of the disease occurred in 17% (14). Tumor-inducing effects have not been observed.

Auranofin

Auranofin is well tolerated by most patients; its adverse effects resemble those of parenteral gold salts, but the pattern differs, with gastrointestinal reactions predominating. Adverse reactions to auranofin are also generally less severe. Where serious adverse effects have been attributed to auranofin, cause and effect has usually remained in doubt. Adverse effects on the lower gastrointestinal tract are the most common; early studies showed a change in bowel habit in some 40% of cases, but this does not often amount to frank diarrhea (15). The same authors noted proteinuria (4%) and hematological reactions (2%). Mucocutaneous reactions (pruritus, conjunctivitis, stomatitis) often occur but are rarely severe and are less problematic than with sodium aurothiomalate. Most adverse effects occur during the first few months; age, sex, and duration of disease do not influence the risk of developing an adverse effect. The adverse effect-related withdrawal rates for injectable gold, auranofin, and placebo were 40, 14, and 6% respectively. Rashes occur in some 20% of cases but rarely require withdrawal. Tumor-inducing effects have not been observed.

Aurothiomalate

Of 120 patients with rheumatoid arthritis who switched from aurothioglucose to aurothiomalate after the former was withdrawn from the Dutch market because of insufficient quality of the raw material at the end of 2001, 19 reported an adverse drug reaction with aurothiomalate that they had not previously experienced with aurothioglucose (16). The most common adverse effects were pruritus, dermatitis/stomatitis, and chrysiasis/hyperpigmentation. There were 29 withdrawals within 12 months because of lack of efficacy (n = 17), adverse drug reactions (n = 8), or remission (n = 3). Kaplan–Meier plots showed a survival rate with aurothiomalate of 79% after 12 months. There were no statistically significant differences in disease activity indicators during follow-up visits compared with baseline.

Metallic gold

Dental gold alloys can cause contact hypersensitivity (9). Contact dermatitis to metallic gold, for example in jewellery, has also repeatedly been observed (SED-8, 510; SEDA-22, 245). A gold surgical clip has also caused an apparently allergic reaction, characterized by sterile abscess formation (10). However, such reactions are rare and may in part be due to other metals contained in the alloy.

Organs and Systems

Cardiovascular

Acute vasodilatory (nitritoid) reactions occur in a minority of patients receiving parenteral gold, especially sodium aurothiomalate (SEDA-22, 245). A few minutes after injection the patient experiences weakness, flushing, hypotension, tachycardia, palpitation, sweating, and sometimes syncope (17). Very rarely myocardial infarction and stroke follow (17,18). The mechanism is unknown, but it has been suggested that the vehicle might be responsible, and that aurothioglucose might therefore be preferable to sodium aurothiomalate in elderly patients or in those with a history of cardiovascular disease.

Respiratory

Gold-induced lung toxicity is an infrequent adverse effect in patients with rheumatoid arthritis and psoriatic arthritis. There are three types: interstitial pneumonitis, bronchiolitis obliterans with organizing pneumonia, and bronchiolitis obliterans; the first is the most frequent.

'Fatal interstitial pneumonitis has been attributed to gold (19).

- A 65-year-old woman with seronegative rheumatoid arthritis was treated for 6 weeks with intramuscular sodium aurothiomalate 50 mg/week and prednisone 5 mg/day. Her joint symptoms improved but later she developed a rash, a dry cough, oppressive chest pain, dyspnea on exertion, weakness, and low-grade fever. An X-ray showed reduced lung volumes and a diffuse bilateral interstitial infiltrate, most marked in the lower zones. Infectious causes for the lung disorder were excluded; gold was withdrawn. She required progressively higher concentrations of oxygen to avoid hypoxemia. A chest CT scan showed a small left pleural effusion and multiple alveolar infiltrates and ground-glass opacities, which were most marked in the middle and lower zones of both lungs. Her condition deteriorated and she died of respiratory failure 18 days after admission.

There have been two reports of gold-induced lung toxicity in psoriatic arthritis (20).

- A 54-year-old woman with psoriatic polyarthritis was treated with aurothiomalate 50 mg/week. When the cumulative dose reached 250 mg she developed weakness, dyspnea, fever, nausea, vomiting and erythematous skin lesions. Chest X-ray and CT scan showed diffuse interstitial pneumonitis. Gold was withdrawn and she was given prednisone 60 mg/day. She recovered in 6 months.
- A 62-year old woman with psoriatic arthritis was given aurothiomalate 50 mg/week. After a cumulative dose of 135 mg she developed an itchy rash, dyspnea, and fever. Chest X-ray and CT scan suggested pneumonitis and she

was given prednisone 40 mg/day. She recovered in 6 months.

More than 60 cases of "gold lung" have been reported and there must be many more unpublished cases. Beginning as a rule some weeks or months after starting treatment, the patient develops dyspnea on exertion, weakness, a dry cough, and malaise. Chest X-rays show bilateral pulmonary infiltrates of varying extent, but cases have been described in which the radiography is entirely normal (21). If chrysotherapy is continued, pulmonary insufficiency can follow. In fact two types of process need to be distinguished; fibrosing alveolitis and obliterative bronchiolitis occur and can co-exist (22); some patients develop proliferative and immunoallergic changes, perhaps even mimicking malignant processes. In treating rheumatism, it can be difficult to distinguish "gold lung" from rheumatoid lung disease (SEDA-21, 236).

Bronchoalveolar lavage in "gold lung" tends to show an increase in the total cell count and predominance of the percentage of lymphocytes with an inverse helper/suppressor ratio. The prognosis is generally good; if gold is immediately withdrawn, the pulmonary lesions as a rule subside, although incomplete regression or even persistence of dyspnea and impaired lung function have been described, despite glucocorticoid therapy (23).

The pulmonary toxicity of gold salts uncommonly causes life-threatening respiratory failure. Patients who suffer from this do not usually need mechanical ventilation, and the toxicity can be difficult to diagnose when it occurs in patients with an illness with pulmonary involvement. However, severe respiratory failure requiring mechanical ventilation has been attributed to gold salt toxicity in a patient with rheumatoid arthritis (24). Glucocorticoid therapy was life-saving and induced complete resolution of the lung damage.

Pneumonitis associated with gold has been reported in a woman with rheumatoid arthritis.

- A 77-year-old woman with rheumatoid arthritis was given sodium aurothiomalate 50 mg intramuscularly weekly, following a test dose of 10 mg (25). Her rheumatoid arthritis responded well, but after a cumulative dose of 560 mg she became progressively short of breath on exertion and generally felt unwell. She had bilateral basal inspiratory crackles and widespread ill-defined shadowing on the chest X-ray, predominantly in the middle and lower zones of both lungs. A high-resolution CT scan showed ground glass opacities, particularly in the upper zones, and thickening of the peribronchovascular interstitium and interlobular septa in the middle and lower zones. Pulmonary function tests showed a restrictive lung defect. The gold injections were discontinued and she responded well to methylprednisolone. A CT scan 10 months later showed almost complete resolution, with some heterogeneity of lung density posteriorly in the lower lobes.

Interstitial pneumonia has been described in an adult who had taken auranofin for only 6 days; glucocorticoids were required (SEDA-17, 276).

Nervous system

Gold can damage nervous tissue. Peripheral neuropathy due to gold is possibly not as rare as was previously assumed and can co-exist with a neuroencephalopathy or other symptoms, such as dizziness and nausea (26). Nervous damage can take other forms: peripheral pain, general malaise, psychiatric disorders, and insomnia can be the first uncharacteristic symptoms and can easily be overlooked as adverse effects. Acute polyneuropathy of the Guillain-Barré type (SED-12, 521; 27), myokymia (Morvan-type fibrillating chorea; SEDA-6, 216; 28), and gold encephalopathy (29) are rare neurological complications of chrysotherapy that have, however, all been well documented from different sources (28).

- A woman in whom gold had been withdrawn because of a rash developed a severe parkinsonian tremor of the hands a week later (26).

An axonal polyneuropathy has been attributed to gold (30).

- A 63-year-old man with a 4-month history of rheumatoid arthritis developed progressive malaise, anorexia, and weight loss, and had a 2-day history of diarrhea, fever, and chills. He had epigastric and periumbilical pain radiating to the back, associated with nausea, abdominal distension, and jaundice. He was taking prednisone 5 mg bd and diclofenac sodium 100 mg bd. He had recently started weekly gold injections (total dose of gold 150 mg). He received two test doses before starting induction therapy, with no adverse effects. Both gold and diclofenac sodium were withdrawn and 2 weeks later he complained of symmetrical distal paresthesia in a glove and stocking distribution. There was no weakness, parallel reflexes were diminished, and the ankle reflexes were both absent. Nerve conduction studies showed a reduction in sensory nerve action potential amplitude in the sural and median nerves, with normal motor conduction. There was a slightly increased threshold for warm and cold sensations in the foot, with normal results in the hand. A liver needle biopsy showed preserved liver architecture with marked cholestasis mainly in the central and mid zones. A positive lymphocyte transformation test to gold suggested a cell-mediated hypersensitivity reaction.

Intrathecal colloidal gold has been used as an adjunct in the treatment of childhood neoplasms, including medulloblastoma and leukemia. Long-term follow-up of patients treated with intrathecal colloidal gold has been described and the high incidence of delayed cerebrovascular complications and their management has been emphasized (31).

Between 1967 and 1970, 14 children with a posterior fossa medulloblastoma underwent treatment consisting of surgical resection, external beam radiotherapy, and intrathecal colloidal gold. All had persistent or recurrent disease and six died within 2 years of treatment. The eight surviving patients developed significant neurovascular complications 5–20 years after treatment. Three patients died as a result of aneurysmal subarachnoid hemorrhage

and five developed cerebral ischemic symptoms from a severe vasculopathy that resembled moyamoya disease. Although therapy with colloidal gold results in long-term survival in a number of cases of childhood medulloblastoma, this study suggests that its severe cerebrovascular adverse effects fail to justify its use. The authors recommended routine screening of any long-term survivors after colloidal gold therapy, to exclude the presence of an intracranial aneurysm and to document the possibility of moyamoya disease.

Sensory systems

Chrysiasis corneae (deposition of gold crystals in the cornea) occurs rarely in patients treated with a cumulative dose of up to 500 mg of gold, but they occur in nearly all patients who have received 1500 mg or more (32). Deposition of gold as such has no clinical consequences. Gold can occasionally cause a keratitis or keratoconjunctivitis, but these are usually associated with skin involvement and are not a consequence of gold deposits in the cornea.

- A 50-year-old white man who had received colloidal gold 50 mg intramuscularly on alternate weeks since 1980 had a slate-grey complexion and fine scattered yellow brown deposits on the central corneal epithelium. In the deep central corneal stroma the deposits were confluent (33). The lens was clear. Ophthalmoscopy was normal. The ocular chrysiasis was not sufficiently severe to warrant withdrawal of the gold therapy.

Gold keratopathy has been reported in a woman with rheumatoid arthritis (34).

- A-60-year-old woman with rheumatoid arthritis who was taking prednisone, azathioprine, sulindac, plaquenil, and receiving intramuscular injections of gold sodium thiomalate (50 mg once weekly) developed intense, bilateral ocular irritation and photophobia. She had received a total of 7.4 g of gold over the past 3 years. Her conjunctivae were mildly injected, with bilateral perilimbal chemosis. The peripheral corneae showed 360° stromal edema. Mid-stromal vessels were seen entering the edematous stroma from the limbus. She was given topical prednisolone acetate hourly for rheumatoid marginal keratitis. Over the next 2 months her symptoms gradually resolved, but granular, golden-brown, pigmented deposits appeared in the corneal stroma in the same peripheral ring-like distribution as the resolved stromal keratitis. Gold was discontinued. Over the next 6 months, the stromal deposits partially cleared. She then had a milder episode of photophobia and irritation, with stromal edema in the same distribution. This was controlled by topical prednisolone. One year later, she continued to use topical prednisolone once a day and was asymptomatic, with no stromal inflammation, but persistent fine golden granules.

Conjunctivitis has occurred in some 10% of patients treated with auranofin, either early or late in treatment, and has led to withdrawal in about in 1% (35).

Metabolism

In one case, diabetes was destabilized after 3 weeks of auranofin treatment (36).

Hematologic

Because of the hematological effects of gold salts, full blood counts should be monitored regularly at least during the first 2 years of treatment (37).

Pure red cell aplasia occurred in a patient with cholestatic jaundice taking sodium aurothiomalate (SEDA-17, 275). Anemia has been reported occasionally with auranofin (0.1%) either as a direct effect or secondary to hematuria.

Eosinophilia in the peripheral blood is the most frequent hematological effect of parenteral gold salts, affecting up to 40% of patients. It is no longer believed that it is a reliable advance marker of more serious reactions of any type (38). Among the latter are severe blood dyscrasias, which sometimes appear unexpectedly, despite regular blood counts.

Auranofin has been associated with eosinophilia (range of incidence in various reports 0.1–13%). In a retrospective study of 82 patients with rheumatoid arthritis there was eosinophilia in 21% taking sodium aurothiomalate and 13% taking auranofin (38). However, early eosinophilia is not a reliable indicator of potential toxicity.

Leukopenia is rare, sometimes very mild, and not always related to gold (SED-12, 522). Granulocytopenia can evolve slowly or suddenly, and its course can be transient or prolonged. Some workers have found gold-associated granulocytopenias to be brief and self-limiting; indeed, if other marrow elements are unimpaired, full recovery can occur even from severe agranulocytosis. Full-fledged aplastic anemia and pancytopenia are the most serious and feared conditions, and although they are today uncommon, deaths continue to occur (SEDA-13, 192), particularly because of superimposed infections or hemorrhage. Auranofin has been associated with leukopenia (0.1%), lymphopenia, and neutropenia (SEDA-10, 207).

Leukopenia with liver damage has been reported (39).

- A 62-year-old woman with rheumatoid arthritis developed swelling and pain of both knees. Aurothiomalate was given in a test dose of 12.5 mg, followed the next day by a dose of 25 mg, and then 50 mg twice weekly (total cumulative dose 137.5 mg). She had a leukocyte count of $2.2 \times 10^9/l$, a normochromic anemia, and a normal platelet count. Her liver enzyme activities were raised. Aurothiomalate was withdrawn and about 6 weeks later her liver function tests returned to normal and her white cell count rose to $6.9 \times 10^9/l$.

Thrombocytopenia occurs in 0.7–3% of cases and can be severe (40). It presents with petechiae, hematuria, oral mucosal bleeding, and other hemorrhagic phenomena. Some cases are due to immune reactions, others to a direct toxic effect of gold on the megakaryocytes, and it is important to distinguish the two types. For an immunologically mediated thrombocytopenia, high-dose steroid therapy should be used if necessary, followed or accompanied by immunosuppressive drugs, infusions of fresh frozen plasma or high-dose immunoglobulin, and even splenectomy. Toxic thrombocytopenia probably demands gold chelator therapy. There is no correlation between the appearance of thrombocytopenia and effects on the skin or kidney (41). Thrombocytopenia is known with auranofin but rare (0.5%). Three patients developed serious thrombocytopenia after taking auranofin for 3 months (40). Auranofin was withdrawn and two of the patients were given oral glucocorticoids; platelet counts normalized within 8 weeks.

Thrombocytopenia has been attributed to aurothioglucose (42).

- A 51-year-old woman with rheumatoid arthritis was treated with intramuscular aurothioglucose 100 mg/week to a cumulative dose of 1000 mg then 50 mg aurothioglucose once every 2 weeks. When the cumulative dose was 1350 mg she developed petechiae and hematomas and the platelet count had fallen from $238 \times 10^9/l$ to $6 \times 10^9/l$.
- A 47-year old woman with rheumatoid arthritis was given intramuscular aurothioglucose 50 mg weekly to a cumulative dose of 1000 mg and then 25 mg every third week. After a cumulative dose of 2700 mg she mentioned that hematomas had started tot develop. Three days after the previous injection she had petechiae and hematomas and the platelet count had fallen from $280 \times 10^9/l$ to $18 \times 10^9/l$.

Both patients made an uneventful recovery and the platelet count returned to normal within several weeks without further treatment. As a cause for the thrombocytopenia a rapid autoantibody induction was considered.

It has been postulated that early treatment with very high doses of intravenous *N*-acetylcysteine and the use of immunomodulatory drugs, such as antithymocyte globulin and ciclosporin, can improve the recovery of hematological parameters, even in the case of pancytopenia (43). One case of gold-induced aplastic anemia, unresponsive to various treatments, recovered after therapy with antithymocyte globulin (SED-12, 522).

Lymphadenopathy is a rare complication of gold injections (SEDA-12, 188). In one case lymphadenopathy in association with a patient with rheumatoid arthritis; biopsy of the lymph nodes showed crystalline material containing gold (SEDA-16, 234).

- A 34-year-old woman was given intramuscular sodium aurothiomalate for rheumatoid arthritis after little response to anti-inflammatory drugs (44). After the sixth injection she developed enlarged neck and axillary lymph nodes. Biopsy showed subtotal infarction of a reactive node, confirmed by histochemical, immunohistochemical, and molecular techniques. Gold was withdrawn and the lymphadenopathy gradually resolved over the next 2 months. She continued to suffer from rheumatoid arthritis with no evidence of malignant lymphoma after 3 years.

This case provides strong evidence that gold salts can cause malignant lymphoma.

Although there is no direct evidence of potentiation of hematological toxicity, the concomitant use of drugs that are known to carry a risk of blood dyscrasias is unwise. Simultaneous use of glucocorticoids in small doses is not thought to detract from the beneficial effects of gold and can delay the onset of adverse reactions (45)

Mouth

Stomatitis, sometimes preceded by a metallic taste, is a frequent complication of gold. It can take the form of superficial buccal erosions, which produce mild symptoms but tend to run a protracted course (46).

There has been one unusual report of obstructive sialadenitis caused by local compression of the excretory ducts of the parotid glands due to deposits of gold in the intraparotid lymphoid tissues; there was swelling of both parotid glands on eating (47).

Gastrointestinal

Fulminant enterocolitis or panenteritis are rare manifestations of gold intolerance; more than 30 cases have been published since 1945 (48) and one-third of them have been fatal. The presenting symptoms are diarrhea, rectal bleeding, and vomiting. Bowel dilatation can develop. The course of the disease is occasionally complicated by overwhelming infection. The X-ray picture sometimes simulates regional or ischemic enteritis. Pathological findings include intense mucosal edema, ulceration, hemorrhage, and infiltration of lymphocytes and plasma cells. No treatment is known. However, there is a milder eosinophilic type of enterocolitis due to gold, which, it has been suggested, responds to treatment with cromoglicate. Two cases of ischemic colitis have also been described, presenting as abdominal pain and rectal bleeding (SEDA-21, 236; 49).

The most common adverse effects of auranofin are gastrointestinal. About half of all users have loose stools at some time during treatment; this effect can be transient, can occur at any time, and is rarely severe. No infective cause or signs of malabsorption has been found in any case and neither was gold absorption adversely affected. In a long-term study, diarrhea was mainly observed in the first 6 months of therapy with auranofin 6 mg/day; in 8% of the cases this was a reason for withdrawal (50). There is experimental evidence in animals of a direct effect of auranofin on ion and water absorption from the intestine with inhibition of enterocyte Na^+/K^+-ATPase activity (SED-12, 525).

Stomatitis occurs in about 10% of patients taking auranofin, generally early in treatment, demanding withdrawal in up to 1% (SEDA-9, 217; (51).

Two patients developed fulminant colitis with toxic megacolon during treatment with auranofin (52,53). Both recovered completely within 4–6 weeks with supportive treatment, including high doses of prednisone.

Liver

Liver injury is an extremely rare complication of gold therapy (SEDA-14, 189; 54). The underlying mechanisms are probably complex and certainly variable. Overdosage can cause centrilobular necrosis and bile stasis. With normal doses intrahepatic cholestasis with an absence of necrosis is more likely, although there can be both bile duct damage and canalicular damage (55); an immunological mechanism for this disorder has been suggested. Several cases of a severe form of idiosyncratic hepatic necrosis soon after starting chrysotherapy have been described (13,56). However, most hepatic lesions as a rule resolve rapidly after withdrawal of chrysotherapy, and mild or moderate liver injury of any type is not necessarily a contraindication to gold treatment.

- A 62-year-old man with rheumatoid factor positive rheumatoid arthritis developed painless icterus, nausea and vomiting, and discolored stools (57). He had previously been given methotrexate without effect, and was instead given aurothioglucose 50 mg/week (cumulative dose 160 mg). He reported sweating, fatigue, and myalgia shortly after each gold injection. The liver was tender but not enlarged, and there were no signs of splenomegaly. Liver function tests showed a cholestatic pattern and predominantly conjugated hyperbilirubinemia. All potentially hepatotoxic drugs (aurothioglucose, naproxen, and aspirin) were withdrawn and his dose of prednisone was increased to 15 mg/day. His liver function tests normalized 4 weeks later.

Mild and transient abnormalities in serum transaminase and alkaline phosphatase activities have been reported during therapy with auranofin (0.4%). This is noteworthy, since almost all patients were taking acetylsalicylic acid or other non-steroidal anti-inflammatory drugs, which also can cause increases in transaminases. There has been a report of two cases of toxic hepatosis in patients taking auranofin (58).

Urinary tract

Mild proteinuria develops in 2–3% of patients receiving chrysotherapy; it is usually benign and reversible within a few weeks after discontinuation of therapy (59). No deterioration in creatinine clearance has been found at periodic follow-up. It is not always necessary to stop gold treatment if a patient develops proteinuria, provided there is no marked loss of renal function and proteinuria is not in the nephrotic range. Gold therapy can be continued under close monitoring for at least 10 months without causing permanent renal damage (60).

Proteinuria has been observed in many trials of auranofin, but in contrast to cases associated with parenteral gold it has only rarely progressed to nephrotic syndrome. Of 1283 auranofin-treated patients, 38 had a raised urinary protein concentration, but only in nine it was heavy, and in most patients who continued treatment the proteinuria did not persist beyond the first 12 months of treatment; seven of eight who were rechallenged, after auranofin had been withdrawn and the protein had cleared, were able to continue treatment without relapse. Biopsy showed membranous glomerulonephritis, suggesting an underlying immunopathological mechanism (61).

Microhematuria has long been considered a manifestation of nephrotoxicity from chrysotherapy, but one multicenter study showed no higher an incidence than in patients receiving placebo (SED-12, 522). Hematuria associated with auranofin has been reported in a few patients, generally after at least 2–3 months of treatment (62).

Serious nephrotoxicity is uncommon, but nephrotic syndrome can develop in about 0.3% of patients, generally among those who have experienced mild proteinuria earlier in treatment. Very exceptionally, acute renal insufficiency can occur; peritoneal dialysis has been reported to promote recovery.

The histological findings in cases of gold nephropathy range from essentially normal glomeruli to a focal increase in mesangium, glomerular basement membrane thickening or splitting, membranous glomerulonephritis (63,64), periglomerular fibrosis with proliferation of Bowman's capsule, and even hyalinization of glomeruli. Chronic interstitial nephritis can also occur (65). Fortunately, many cases of renal complications run a benign course if gold is withdrawn (64).

Gold nephropathy is often considered to be an immunological disorder, and IgG and C3 are usually present in fine granular immune complex deposits along the capillary walls of the glomeruli. Oddly, however, X-ray microanalysis fails to detect gold as a component of the deposited immune complexes, throwing doubt on the concept that gold itself acts as an antigen or a hapten. Gold might however alter the proximal tubular cells in such a way that tubular autoantigens are released, resulting in the development of antigen–antibody complexes; these would then become attached to the glomerular basement membrane, inducing membranous glomerulopathy and proteinuria. That gold does damage the tubular cells is well known, although there appears to be no correlation with dosage and duration of therapy. Gold-containing, electron-dense, filamentous, cytoplasmic inclusions have been found in proximal tubular cells. The urinary excretion of beta-glucosaminidase, leucine aminopeptidase, beta$_2$-microglobulin, and other tubular proteins has often been found to be increased in patients treated with gold compounds (SEDA-15, 229). Tubular dysfunction can persist for up to 2 years after the end of chrysotherapy.

Skin

Skin reactions are the most frequent of all adverse effects of gold; they develop in about 25% of patients, sometimes in association with other forms of gold intolerance. Up to 30% of patients taking auranofin develop mucocutaneous adverse effects and 18–24% develop a rash or pruritus, meriting withdrawal in some 4% of cases (SEDA-10, 208).

Skin reactions to gold salts can be toxic or immunological, and patch-testing is often positive (57). No increase in gold concentration in the skin has been found, nor is there any correlation with blood concentrations of gold. Skin biopsies show that both macrophages and Langerhans cells are actively involved in the pathogenesis of gold dermatitis (66).

Pruritus is the commonest and earliest manifestation of such reactions and can precede an eruption by some

weeks. Lesions are of every conceivable type, ranging from transient, non-specific, localized, or generalized dermatitis (eczema) and erythematous, maculopapular rash to lichen planus-like eruptions, discoid eczema, pityriasis rosacea, erythema multiforme, erythema nodosum, scaling eruptions, urticaria, photosensitivity, hyperkeratosis, seborrheic dermatitis, toxic epidermal necrolysis, and granuloma annulare. Exacerbation of pre-existing psoriasis has been reported (67). Patients receiving aurothioglucose have sometimes developed a dermatitis closely resembling contact dermatitis (SED-12, 523). More than one of these effects can occur in the same patient.

Gold can also cause pemphigus (68).

- A 53-year-old woman with rheumatoid arthritis who had reacted to D-penicillamine treatment by developing myasthenia gravis was given gold instead and 12 months later developed pemphigus vulgaris (69).

Not every gold-induced skin disorder is necessarily wholly disfiguring; in one curious case, the patient was seen to "glitter" with tiny specks of a gold-coloured (and gold-containing) material covering the skin of the neck, upper arms, and back (70).

Chrysiasis, a gray, blue, or purple pigmentation on light-exposed skin areas, is a complication that tends to be permanent (SEDA-20, 210). In one series of 40 patients receiving sodium aurothiomalate it appeared in 31 (71).

Laser therapy of lentigines in patients with a history of gold therapy can lead to localized chrysiasis (72).

- A 49-year-old woman developed persistent multiple 6-mm, well circumscribed, blue-gray circular macules on the backs of her hands, forehead, and thighs 7 months after several of her solar lentigines had been treated with a Q-switched ruby laser. The lesions, which had been stable over the previous 7 months and were otherwise asymptomatic, corresponded exactly to the treated areas. She had rheumatoid arthritis, previously controlled with aurothioglucose 50 mg intramuscularly every 1–3 weeks for 10 years.

The authors diagnosed chrysiasis related to laser therapy for solar lentigines and recommended that all patients treated with lasers should be routinely screened for previous gold therapy, even gold therapy that may have been withdrawn many years before.

Inadvertent gold administration has reportedly caused an allergic skin rash (73).

- A 31-year-old woman developed a rash, similar to the rash she had experienced after wearing gold jewellery. The evening before she had taken about 90–120 ml of Goldschlager liquor, a cinnamon schnapps that can contain as much as 8–17 mg of gold in 750 ml. The rash was isolated to her neck, upper chest, and hands and was erythematous and pruritic with no borders or margins. Her rash resolved over 2 weeks without desquamation.

Of 49 respondents to a questionnaire that was sent to 102 gold-allergic patients, all but one were women (74). Most of them reported that their dermatitis had improved after patch testing, but most had avoided other allergens as well as gold. The authors concluded that avoidance of gold earrings did not appear to benefit patients with ear-lobe dermatitis, but that total avoidance of gold jewelry on the hands and wrists did seem to benefit a subgroup of patients with facial and eyelid dermatitis who wore powder, eye shadow, or foundation on affected areas.

There is increasing documentation of allergic contact dermatitis and other effects from gold jewelry, gold dental restorations, and gold implants (75). These effects are especially pronounced among women who wear body-piercing gold objects. Eczema of the head and neck is the most common response in individuals who are hypersensitive to gold, and sensitivity can last for several years. Ingestion of beverages containing flake gold can result in allergic-type reactions similar to those seen in gold-allergic individuals exposed to gold through dermal contact and other routes.

In patients with a history of localized hypersensitivity to metallic gold, allergic skin reactions can develop in the sensitized region after gold injections (SEDA-13, 193).

Worldwide experience with auranofin points to a 2% incidence of alopecia, but this included older experience at high doses; at current doses, alopecia is rather less common (35).

If skin reactions are not serious, withdrawal of gold is not essential, and some physicians deliberately increase the dosage to the point where some skin reaction occurs, as a means of securing the best possible therapeutic effect. Once troublesome reactions have appeared they can often be relieved simply by reducing the dosage or the frequency of administration. More troublesome reactions will demand withdrawal of gold, and in that case most skin lesions will begin to subside within a few days or a week, and disappear within several weeks more; it may then be possible to resume gold at a reduced dosage (76). On the other hand, some gold-induced skin lesions can run a protracted course, in certain cases necessitating topical or systemic glucocorticoid treatment. A patchy brown discoloration can persist after the disorders have resolved. When gold has been withdrawn it can often be restarted later without recurrence of the lesion.

Nails

Gold rarely causes yellow thickening of the nails and onycholysis, followed by irreversible nail dystrophy (SED-9, 373).

- A 34-year-old woman with severe rheumatoid arthritis developed yellow thickening of all 20 nails 2 years after starting gold therapy (77). She had received 50 mg of gold salts intramuscularly at intervals of 2–4 weeks after an initial course of weekly injections (total cumulative dose 90 mg/kg) over 4 years. There was associated thickening of the nail plate, increased transverse curvature, and mild subungual hyperkeratosis. There was onycholysis of both thumbnails and the right little fingernail. There was no associated chrysiasis. Gold was withdrawn. The yellow discoloration began to grow out and fingernail growth increased in the next 3 months. Six months later there was further improvement, although light yellow discoloration of all nails persisted

and there was markedly increased longitudinal growth. Both thumbnails showed transverse depressions of the nail plate (Beau's lines) where the change in growth rate had presumably occurred.

Immunologic

Several patients with selective IgA deficiency and even a panhypogammaglobulinemia during intramuscular gold treatment have been described (SEDA-14, 190; SEDA-15, 230; SEDA-21, 237).

Polyarteritis (78) and systemic lupus erythematosus (79) have been reported after the administration of gold compounds.

- After taking sodium aurothiomalate for 10 months (cumulative dose 550 mg) a 12-year-old girl with severe exudative polyarthritis developed pericarditis, high titers of antinuclear antibodies, and antibodies to native double-stranded DNA (79). After withdrawal her symptoms rapidly disappeared and did not recur after a follow-up period of 5 years. The titers of autoantibodies fell to normal within 1 year.

In one series of some 5500 patients with juvenile rheumatoid arthritis, 105 were found to have developed secondary amyloidosis; 37 of the latter had been receiving sodium aurothiomalate. In 12 of these children the time between withdrawal of gold (because of adverse effects) and the finding of amyloid A was less than six months (SEDA-21, 237).

- A 63-year-old woman with rheumatoid arthritis was given intramuscular gold sodium thiomalate and began to have nausea, vomiting, anorexia, and watery diarrhea (80). A year later the watery diarrhea became more frequent (more than 10 times within a day) and she developed proteinuria. Biopsies from the stomach, duodenum, and kidney showed systemic amyloidosis. This was a rare case of secondary systemic amyloidosis associated with rheumatoid arthritis. It is not clear from the report what the role of gold was in this case.

Infection risk

An increased incidence of *Herpes zoster* was found in a series of patients receiving sodium aurothiomalate; the mechanism is unknown, but herpesvirus infection can also occur in association with some other heavy metals, for example in environmental poisoning.

The incidence of *H. zoster* infection in auranofin-treated patients was slightly higher (0.9%) than in patients with rheumatoid arthritis not receiving gold therapy (0.4%), but less frequent than in patients given parenteral gold compounds (3.1%).

Body temperature

There may be transient exacerbation of rheumatoid symptoms before a therapeutic response to gold occurs. In one series of 43 patients with rheumatoid arthritis serious exacerbation of the disease occurred in 17% (14).

Second-Generation Effects

Teratogenicity

In 1980, alarm was caused by a report of a seriously malformed child born to a mother who had been treated with sodium aurothiomalate during pregnancy (81), particularly since a partially congruent pattern of neural abnormalities had earlier been described in rats and rabbits, and given the fact that gold crosses the placenta. On the other hand, a Danish team in 1983 studied eight children born after exposure to gold in utero from weeks 2–9 or longer; no abnormalities were found, and the children appeared to develop normally during a follow-up period averaging 8.6 years (82). In view of the lack of further incriminating evidence some physicians today adopt the view that chrysotherapy can be continued in selected pregnant women whose rheumatoid arthritis is of such severity as to warrant treatment.

Lactation

Breastfeeding is not recommended since gold salts are excreted in the milk (SEDA-12, 188; SEDA-13, 193).

Susceptibility Factors

Genetic factors

There is good evidence that patients with rheumatoid arthritis who carry the DR3 antigen run a greater risk of proteinuria (83), mucocutaneous reactions (84), and hematological actions (85) to parenteral gold compounds as well as to penicillamine, although such patients also tend to react rather better than others to aurothioglucose (86). The same applies to the B8, DR3 haplotype (87). The prevalence of the HLA antigens DR2 and DR7 is lower among rheumatoid arthritis patients with toxic reactions than among patients without toxic reactions or among controls (88). Because of conflicting results and the low relative risk, HLA typing has not been of much practical help as a guide to forecasting the risk of therapy.

Patients with rheumatoid arthritis and poor sulfoxidation state are six times more susceptible than others to the adverse effects of sodium aurothiomalate (89). This parallels an earlier similar finding with penicillamine, which has the same sulfhydryl group in its structure.

Age

Several studies have shown that in juvenile chronic arthritis auranofin gives rise to fewer adverse reactions than in adults, but the therapeutic effect is dubious and variable (SEDA-17, 277).

Elderly patients were once thought to be more likely than younger individuals to develop severe reactions (90) but this seems not to be so (91).

Rheumatoid arthritis

The question of whether features associated with severe rheumatoid arthritis are predictive of adverse drug reactions to gold salts, independent of HLA-DR3 status, has been studied in 41 patients with rheumatoid arthritis who developed thrombocytopenia (platelet count below $100 \times 10^9/l$) or proteinuria (over 1.0 g/24 hours) whole receiving gold sodium thiomalate, 41 patients treated with gold without adverse reactions and 161 patients who had received gold for at least as long without adverse reactions (92). All were typed for HLA-DRB1, and the presence of rheumatoid factor, antinuclear antibodies, and nodules before the start of therapy. Patients with adverse reactions were more likely to have nodular disease than their matched controls (51% versus 26%; OR = 3.0) and were more likely to be HLA-DR3 positive (41% versus 18%; OR = 3.0). There were no differences between the groups I rheumatoid factor or antinuclear antibodies. Nodular disease was associated with development of adverse reactions independent of HLA-DR3 status, although a combination of the two factors significantly increased the likelihood of an adverse reaction. The data suggested that nodular disease may be a predictor of adverse reactions to gold independent of HLA-DR3.

Other features of the patient

There are various contraindications to gold therapy (93): active hepatic disease, impaired renal function, colitis, patients with a history of hematological disorders, and patients who have recently had radiotherapy (because of the depressant action of radiotherapy on hemopoietic tissue).

Drug Administration

Drug overdose

- Severe overdosage of sodium aurothiopropanol sulfonate (1.1 g daily for 13 days) caused jaundice and skin eruptions. Liver biopsies showed modest centrilobular necrosis and significant bile stasis. Serum hepatic enzyme activities were increased. The patient was treated with dimercaprol and recovered after 2 months, although alkaline phosphatase and gamma-glutamyltransferase activities remained high for 6 months.

It seems advisable in cases of acute gold intoxication to adopt a conservative strategy. Should severe complications occur, supportive therapy can be given in combination with such treatments as chelation, glucocorticoids, or gamma-globulin.

Drug–Drug Interactions

Glucocorticoids

In a placebo-controlled study auranofin reduced the doses of glucocorticoids needed in asthma (94). This is perhaps a parallel effect rather than an interaction since, as noted above, gold itself may have an effect in asthma.

References

1. Tiekink ER. Gold derivatives for the treatment of cancer. Crit Rev Oncol Hematol 2002;42(3):225–48.

2. Kostova I. Gold coordination complexes as anticancer agents. Anticancer Agents Med Chem 2006;6(1):19–32.

3. Burmester GR. Molekulare Wirkungsmechanismen von Gold bei der Behandlung der Rheumatoiden Arthritis—ein Update. [Molecular mechanisms of action of gold in treatment of rheumatoid arthritis—an update.] Z Rheumatol 2001;60(3):167–73.

4. Youn HS, Lee JY, Saitoh SI, Miyake K, Hwang DH. Auranofin, as an anti-rheumatic gold compound, suppresses LPS-induced homodimerization of TLR4. Biochem Biophys Res Commun 2006;350(4):866–71.

5. Gabriel SE, Coyle D, Moreland LW. A clinical and economic review of disease-modifying antirheumatic drugs. Pharmacoeconomics 2001;19(7):715–28.

6. Rothermich NO, Philips VK, Bergen W, Thomas MH. Chrysotherapy. A prospective study. Arthritis Rheum 1976;19(6):1321–7.

7. Griffin AJ, Gibson T, Huston G. A comparison of conventional and low dose sodium aurothiomalate treatment in rheumatoid arthritis. Br J Rheumatol 1983;22(2):82–8.

8. Sambrook PN, Browne CD, Champion GD, Day RO, Vallance JB, Warwick N. Terminations of treatment with gold sodium thiomalate in rheumatoid arthritios. J Rheumatol 1982;9(6):932–4.

9. Vamnes JS, Morken T, Helland S, Gjerdet NR. Dental gold alloys and contact hypersensitivity. Contact Dermatitis 2000;42(3):128–33.

10. Trathen WT, Stanley RJ. Allergic reaction to Hulka clips. Obstet Gynecol 1985;66(5):743–4.

11. Arrigoni-Martelli E. Antirheumatic drugs. Med Actual 1982;18:461.

12. Rau R. Hepatotoxicity of gold compounds. In: Schattenkirchner M, Muller W, editors. Modern Aspects of Gold Therapy. Rheumatology, an Annual Review 8. Basel-New York: Karger, 1983:188.

13. Watkins PB, Schade R, Mills AS, Carithers RL Jr, Van Thiel DH. Fatal hepatic necrosis associated with parenteral gold therapy. Dig Dis Sci 1988;33(8):1025–9.

14. Vlak T, Jajic I. Nepozeljni ucinci lijecenja solima zlata u bolesnika s reumatoidnim artritisom. [Side effects of gold salt therapy in patients with rheumatoid arthritis.] Reumatizam 1992;39(2):25–8.

15. Heuer MA, Pietrusko RG, Morris RW, Scheffler BJ. An analysis of worldwide safety experience with auranofin. J Rheumatol 1985;12(4):695–9.

16. van Roon EN, van de Laar MA, Janssen M, Kruijsen MW, Jansen TL, Brouwers JR. Parenteral gold preparations. Efficacy and safety of therapy after switching from aurothioglucose to aurothiomalate. J Rheumatol 2005;32:1026–30.

17. Hill C, Pile K, Henderson D, Kirkham B. Neurological side effects in two patients receiving gold injections for rheumatoid arthritis. Br J Rheumatol 1995;34(10):989–90.

18. Gottlieb NL, Gray RG. Diagnosis and management of adverse reactions from gold compounds. J Anal Toxicol 1978;2:173.

19. Soler MJ, Barroso E, Aranda FI, Alonso S, Romero S. Fatal, gold-induced pneumonitis. Rheumatol Int 2003;23:207–10.

20. Manero Ruiz FJ, Larraga Palacio R, Herrero Labarga I, Ferrer Peralta M. Neumonitis por sales de oro en la artritis psoriasica: a proposito de dos casos. [Pneumonitis caused by gold salts in psoriatic arthritis: report of 2 cases.] An Med Interna 2002;19(5):237–40.

21. Blackwell TS, Gossage JR. Gold pulmonary toxicity in a patient with a normal chest radiograph. South Med J 1995;88(6):644–6.

22. Evans RB, Ettensohn DB, Fawaz-Estrup F, Lally EV, Kaplan SR. Gold lung: recent developments in pathogenesis, diagnosis, and therapy. Semin Arthritis Rheum 1987;16(3):196–205.

23. Liebetrau G. Alveolitis-eine seltene Nebenwirkung der Goldtherapie. [Alveolitis—a rare side effect of gold therapy.] Z Erkr Atmungsorgane 1984;163(2):200–4.

24. Blancas R, Moreno JL, Martin F, de la Casa R, Onoro JJ, Gomez V, Prados J. Alveolar-interstitial pneumopathy after gold-salts compounds administration, requiring mechanical ventilation. Intensive Care Med 1998;24(10):1110–2.

25. Sinha A, Silverstone EJ, O'Sullivan MM. Gold-induced pneumonitis: computed tomography findings in a patient with rheumatoid arthritis. Rheumatology (Oxford) 2001;40(6):712–4.

26. Machtey I. Neurological signs in RA patients receiving gold. Br J Rheumatol 1996;35(8):804.

27. Dick DJ, Raman D. The Guillain–Barré syndrome following gold therapy. Scand J Rheumatol 1982;11(2):119–20.

28. Fam AG, Gordon DA, Sarkozi J, Blair GR, Cooper PW, Harth M, Lewis AJ. Neurologic complications associated with gold therapy for rheumatoid arthritis. J Rheumatol 1984;11(5):700–6.

29. Perry RP, Jacobsen ES. Gold induced encephalopathy: case report. J Rheumatol 1984;11(2):233–4.

30. Ben-Ami H, Pollack S, Nagachandran P, Lashevsky I, Yarnitsky D, Edoute Y. Reversible pancreatitis, hepatitis, and peripheral polyneuropathy associated with parenteral gold therapy. J Rheumatol 1999;26(9):2049–50.

31. Nussbaum ES, Sebring LA, Neglia JP, Chu R, Mattsen ND, Erickson DL. Delayed cerebrovascular complications of intrathecal colloidal gold. Neurosurgery 2001;49(6):1308–12.

32. Rodenhauser JH, Behrend T. Art und Häufigkeit der Augenbeteiligung nach parenteraler Goldtherapie. [Nature and frequency of ocular involvement after parenteral gold therapy.] Dtsch Med Wochenschr 1969;94(46):2389–92.

33. Singh AD, Puri P, Amos RS. Deposition of gold in ocular structures, although known, is rare. A case of ocular chrysiasis in a patient of rheumatoid arthritis on gold treatment is presented. Eye. 2004;18:443–4.

34. Zamir E, Read RW, Affeldt JC, Ramaswamy D, Rao NA. Gold induced interstitial keratitis. Br J Ophthalmol 2001;85(11):1386–7.

35. Rau R, Kaik B, Muller-Fassbender H, et al. Auranofin (SK&F 39 162) and sodium aurothiomalate in the treatment of rheumatoid arthritis. Rheumatology 1983;8:162.

36. Anonymous. Auranofin–Diabetes situation impaired/hypoglycemia. Bull SADRAC, June/October (English version), 3.

37. Cervi PL, Wright P, Casey EB. Audit of full blood count monitoring in patients on longterm gold therapy for rheumatoid arthritis. Ir J Med Sci 1992;161(3):73–4.

38. Edelman J, Davis P, Owen ET. Prevalence of eosinophilia during gold therapy for rheumatoid arthritis. J Rheumatol 1983;10(1):121–3.

39. Uhm WS, Yoo DH, Lee JH, Kim TH, Jun JB, Lee IH, Bae SC, Kim SY. Injectable gold-induced hepatitis and neutropenia in rheumatoid arthritis. Korean J Intern Med 2000;15(2):156–9.

40. Bakke E, Myklebust G, Gran JT. Trombocytopeni utlost ved auranofinbehandling. [Thrombocytopenia induced by auranofin treatment.] Tidsskr Nor Laegeforen 1997;117(28):4081–2.

41. Davis P. Undesirable effects of gold salts. J Rheumatol Suppl 1979;5:18–24.
42. Levin M-D, Van 't Veer MB, De Veld JC, Markusse HM. Two patients with acute thrombocytopenia following gold administration and five-year follow-up. Neth J Med 2003;61:223–5.
43. Yan A, Davis P. Gold induced marrow suppression: a review of 10 cases. J Rheumatol 1990;17(1):47–51.
44. Roberts C, Batstone PJ, Goodlad JR. Lymphadenopathy and lymph node infarction as a result of gold injections. J Clin Pathol 2001;54(7):562–4.
45. Corkill MM, Kirkham BW, Chikanza IC, Gibson T, Panayi GS. Intramuscular depot methylprednisolone induction of chrysotherapy in rheumatoid arthritis: a 24-week randomized controlled trial. Br J Rheumatol 1990; 29(4):274–9.
46. Glenert U. Drug stomatitis due to gold therapy. Oral Surg Oral Med Oral Pathol 1984;58(1):52–6.
47. Zuazua JS, de la Fuente AM, Rodriguez JC, Garcia GB, Rodriguez AP. Obstructive sialadenitis caused by intraparotid deposits of gold salts: a case report. Oral Surg Oral Med Oral Pathol Oral Radiol Endod 1996;81(6):649–51.
48. Jackson CW, Haboubi NY, Whorwell PJ, Schofield PF. Gold induced enterocolitis. Gut 1986;27(4):452–6.
49. Cobeta Garcia JC, Ruiz Jimeno MT. Ischemic colitis associated with gold salts treatment. Rev Esp Reumatol 1996;23:105–7.
50. Wallin BA, McCafferty JP, Fox MJ, Cooper DR, Goldschmidt MS. Incidence and management of diarrhea during longterm auranofin therapy. J Rheumatol 1988; 15(12):1755–8.
51. Furst DE. Mechanism of action, pharmacology, clinical efficacy and side effects of auranofin. An orally administered organic gold compound for the treatment of rheumatoid arthritis. Pharmacotherapy 1983;3(5):284–98.
52. Horing E. Goldinduzierte kolitis. Med Welt 1989;40:876.
53. Jarner D, Nielsen AM. Auranofin (SK + F 39162) induced enterocolitis in rheumatoid arthritis. A case report Scand J Rheumatol 1983;12(3):254–6.
54. Harats N, Ehrenfeld M, Shalit M, Lijovetzky G. Gold-induced granulomatous hepatitis. Isr J Med Sci 1985; 21(9):753–6.
55. Murphy M, Hunt S, McDonald GSA, et al. Intrahepatic cholestasis secondary to gold therapy. Eur J Gastroenterol Hepatol 1991;3:855–9.
56. Van Linthoudt D, Buss W, Beyner F, Ott H. Nécrose hépatique fatale au cours d'un traitement aux sels d'or d'une polyarthrite rhumatoide. [Fatal hepatic necrosis due to a treatment course of rheumatoid arthritis with gold salts.] Schweiz Med Wochenschr 1991;121(30):1099–102.
57. te Boekhorst PA, Barrera P, Laan RF, van de Putte LB. Hepatotoxicity of parenteral gold therapy in rheumatoid arthritis: a case report and review of the literature. Clin Exp Rheumatol 1999;17(3):359–62.
58. Goebel KM, Storck U, Kohl FV, et al. Klinischer Effekt und unerwünschte Arzneimittelwirkungen von Auranofin bei rheumatoider Arthritis. Inn Med 1985;12:39.
59. Hall CL, Fothergill NJ, Blackwell MM, Harrison PR, MacKenzie JC, MacIver AG. The natural course of gold nephropathy: long term study of 21 patients. BMJ (Clin Res Ed) 1987;295(6601):745–8.
60. Hall CL, Tighe R. The effect of continuing penicillamine and gold treatment on the course of penicillamine and gold nephropathy. Br J Rheumatol 1989;28(1):53–7.
61. Katz WA, Blodgett RC Jr, Pietrusko RG. Proteinuria in gold-treated rheumatoid arthritis. Ann Intern Med 1984;101(2):176–9.
62. Smith PR, Brown GM, Meyers OL. An open comparative study of auranofin vs. gold sodium thiomalate. J Rheumatol Suppl 1982;8:190–6.
63. Davenport A, Maciver AG, Hall CL, MacKenzie JC. Do mesangial immune complex deposits affect the renal prognosis in membranous glomerulonephritis? Clin Nephrol 1994;41(5):271–6.
64. Pospishil' IuA. Patogistologicheskie i ul'trastrukturnye osobennosti medikamentoznogo membranoznogo glomerulonefrita. [Pathohistologic and ultrastructural features of drug-induced membranous glomerulonephritis.] Arkh Patol 1996;58(5):52–6.
65. Cramer CR, Hagler HK, Silva FG, Eigenbrodt EH, Meltzer JI, Pirani CL. Chronic interstitial nephritis associated with gold therapy. Arch Pathol Lab Med 1983;107(5):258–63.
66. Ranki A, Niemi KM, Kanerva L. Clinical, immunohistochemical, and electron-microscopic findings in gold dermatitis. Am J Dermatopathol 1989;11(1):22–8.
67. Smith DL, Wernick R. Exacerbation of psoriasis by chrysotherapy. Arch Dermatol 1991;127(2):268–70.
68. Papacharalambous VG, Pramatarov KD, Tsankov NK. Development of pemphigus in a patient with rheumatoid arthritis during a course of gold therapy. Eur J Dermatol 1997;7(1):65–6.
69. Ciompi ML, Marchetti G, Bazzichi L, Puccetti L, Agelli M. D-penicillamine and gold salt treatments were complicated by myasthenia and pemphigus, respectively, in the same patient with rheumatoid arthritis. Rheumatol Int 1995;15(3):95–7.
70. Michalski JP, Isphording W, Parker S, Hardin JG. All that glitters may be gold. Arthritis Rheum 1991;34(8):1069.
71. Smith RW, Leppard B, Barnett NL, Millward-Sadler GH, McCrae F, Cawley MI. Chrysiasis revisited: a clinical and pathological study. Br J Dermatol 1995;133(5):671–8.
72. Geist DE, Phillips TJ. Development of chrysiasis after Q-switched ruby laser treatment of solar lentigines. J Am Acad Dermatol 2006;55(2 Suppl):S59-60.
73. Guenthner T, Stork CM, Cantor RM. Goldschlager allergy in a gold allergic patient. Vet Hum Toxicol 1999;41(4):246.
74. Nedorost S, Wagman A. Positive patch-test reactions to gold: patients' perception of relevance and the role of titanium dioxide in cosmetics. Dermatitis 2005;16(2):67–70.
75. Eisler R. Mammalian sensitivity to elemental gold (Au degrees). Biol Trace Elem Res 2004;100:1–18.
76. Klinkhoff AV, Teufel A. How low can you go? Use of very low dosage of gold in patients with mucocutaneous reactions. J Rheumatol 1995;22(9):1657–9.
77. Roest MA, Ratnavel R. Yellow nails associated with gold therapy for rheumatoid arthritis. Br J Dermatol 2001;145(5):855–6.
78. Oochi N, Kbayashi K, Nanishi F, Tsuruda H, Onoyama K, Fujishima M, Omae T. [A case of gold nephropathy associated with polyarteritis nodosa.] Nippon Jinzo Gakkai Shi 1986;28(1):87–94.
79. Korholz D, Nurnberger W, Göbel U, Wahn V. Gold-induzierter systemischer Lupus erythematodes. [Gold-induced systemic lupus erythematosus.] Monatsschr Kinderheilkd 1988;136(9):644–6.
80. Tahara K, Nishiya K, Yoshida T, Matsubara Y, Matsumori A, Ito H, Kumon Y, Hashimoto K, Moriki T, Ookubo S. [A case of secondary systemic amyloidosis associated with rheumatoid arthritis after 3-year disease duration.] Ryumachi 1999;39(1):27–32.
81. Rogers JG, Anderson RM, Chow CW, Gillam GL, Markman L. Possible teratogenic effects of gold. Aust Paediatr J 1980;16(3):194–5.

82. Tarp U, Graudal H, Muller-Madsen B, et al. In: A follow-up study of children exposed to gold salts in utero. Abstracts, X European Congress of Rheumatology, Abstract No. 646. Moscow 1983:188.

83. Hakala M, van Assendelft AH, Ilonen J, Jalava S, Tiilikainen A. Association of different HLA antigens with various toxic effects of gold salts in rheumatoid arthritis. Ann Rheum Dis 1986;45(3):177–82.

84. Speerstra F, van Riel PL, Reekers P, van de Putte LB, Vandenbroucke JP. The influence of HLA phenotypes on the response to parenteral gold in rheumatoid arthritis. Tissue Antigens 1986;28(1):1–7.

85. Speerstra F, Reekers P, van de Putte LB, Vandenbroucke JP. HLA associations in aurothioglucose- and D-penicillamine-induced haematotoxic reactions in rheumatoid arthritis. Tissue Antigens 1985;26(1):35–40.

86. van Riel PL, Reekers P, van de Putte LB, Gribnau FW. Association of HLA antigens, toxic reactions and therapeutic response to auranofin and aurothioglucose in patients with rheumatoid arthritis. Tissue Antigens 1983; 22(3):194–9.

87. Singal DP, Green D, Reid B, Gladman DD, Buchanan WW. HLA-D region genes and rheumatoid arthritis (RA): importance of DR and DQ genes in conferring susceptibility to RA. Ann Rheum Dis 1992;51(1):23–8.

88. Rodriguez Perez M, Gonzalez Dominguez J, Mataran Perez L, Salvatierra Rios D. HLA DR7 como factor de proteccion frente a la toxicidad por sales de oro en la artritis reumatoide. [HLA DR7 as a protective factor against gold salt toxicity in rheumatoid arthritis.] An Med Interna 1993;10(10):484–6.

89. Madhok R, Capell HA, Waring R. Does sulphoxidation state predict gold toxicity in rheumatoid arthritis? BMJ (Clin Res Ed) 1987;294(6570):483.

90. Prupas HM. Stroke-like syndrome after gold sodium thiomalate induced vasomotor reaction. J Rheumatol 1984; 11(2):235–6.

91. Kean WF, Bellamy N, Brooks PM. Gold therapy in the elderly rheumatoid arthritis patient. Arthritis Rheum 1983; 26(6):705–11.

92. Shah P, Griffith SM, Shadforth MF, Fisher J. Dawes PT, Poulton KV, Thomson W, Ollier WE, Mattey DL. Can gold therapy be used more safely in rheumatoid arthritis? Adverse drug reactions are more likely in patients with nodular disease, independent of HLA-DR3 status. J Rheumatol 2004;31:1903–5.

93. Wijnands MJ, van Riel PL, Gribnau FW, van de Putte LB. Risk factors of second-line antirheumatic drugs in rheumatoid arthritis. Semin Arthritis Rheum 1990;19(6):337–52.

94. Nierop G, Gijzel WP, Bel EH, Zwinderman AH, Dijkman JH. Auranofin in the treatment of steroid dependent asthma: a double blind study. Thorax 1992; 47(5):349–54.

Infliximab

See also Monoclonal antibodies

General Information

Infliximab is a chimeric, human-murine anti-TNF monoclonal antibody. It was initially approved by the Food and Drug and Administration in August 1998 for the treatment of moderately to severely active Crohn's disease (1,2) in patients with an inadequate response to conventional therapies and those with enterocutaneous fistulae. The indications were expanded in June 2002 and April 2003 to include maintenance of clinical remission, treatment of enterocutaneous and rectovaginal fistulae, and maintaining fistula closure. It is also used to treat rheumatoid arthritis (3) and ankylosing spondylitis (4,5).

From the available data submitted for Crohn's disease to the US and European regulatory agencies, the most significant acute adverse reactions were infusion reactions, defined as symptoms within 2 hours after intravenous infusion. The symptoms consisted of fever, chills, urticaria, dyspnea, chest pain, or hypotension, and occurred in 16% of infliximab-treated patients versus 6–7% of placebo-treated patients. They can cause flushing, palpitation, sweating, chest pain, hypotension/hypertension, or dyspnea (6).

Several adverse effects, such as upper respiratory tract infections, headaches, rash, or cough, were more common than with placebo, but severe adverse effects were only slightly more frequent (3.6 versus 2.6%). Clinical trials also showed an increase in the prevalence of antinuclear antibodies or the development of double-stranded DNA antibodies (9% of patients). Although there were clinical features suggestive of the lupus-like syndrome in only very few patients, this issue needs to be further investigated. Also of great concern is the report in several patients of lymphoma (7) or severe opportunistic infections (8). Patients taking concomitant immunosuppressive drugs should be carefully observed for such complications.

Other reports have highlighted several potential serious adverse effects associated with infliximab, including congestive heart failure, drug-induced lupus-like syndrome, and demyelination. In addition, reactivation of mycobacterial and fungal infections can occur in patients taking infliximab, mandating appropriate tuberculosis screening before drug therapy (9).

Centocor has issued a "Dear Healthcare Professional" letter advising of changes to the USA infliximab (Remicade) label, following post-marketing reports of hematological and neurological events (10). "A Warning on Hematological Events" has been added to the label to advise of reports of neutropenia, leukopenia, thrombocytopenia, and pancytopenia, some of which were fatal. The "Warning on Neurological Events" has also been updated to detail cases of nervous system manifestations of systemic vasculitis. In addition, pericardial effusion, neutropenia, and cutaneous and systemic vasculitis have been added to the "Adverse Reactions" sections of infliximab prescribing information. Physicians are advised that they should consider withdrawal of infliximab in patients who develop significant adverse nervous system reactions or hematological abnormalities.

Observational studies

A total of 33 patients with plaque psoriasis were treated with infliximab 5 or 10 mg/kg by intravenous infusion (11). One patient treated with 10 mg/kg infliximab complained of severe itching of the feet, which resolved on withdrawal. Three of 33 patients had infusion reactions, which were generally mild and transient. There were infections (for example cellulitis, tooth abscess, ear infection, infected wisdom tooth, bronchitis, pneumonia) in seven patients.

Seven patients with various inflammatory disorders were treated with infliximab 5 mg/kg by intravenous infusion; three had pityriasis rubra pilaris, one had panniculitis, one had eosinophilic fasciitis, one had discoid lupus erythematosus, and one had necrobiosis lipoidica diabeticorum (12). One patient with discoid lupus erythematosus did not respond to treatment and reported insomnia and mild confusion, which resolved after 1 month.

Five patients with hidradenitis suppurativa were treated with infliximab 5 mg/kg by intravenous infusion (13). All improved. One developed a tender submandibular swelling; a fine needle aspirate of the enlarged lymph node showed acid-fast bacteria, but culture was negative. This patient was treated for presumed Mycobacterium tuberculosis, with reduction of the size of the node. The number of patients in this series was small, but the authors commented that tuberculosis in infliximab-treated patients has previously been reported to be more common than expected.

Infliximab-related adverse drug reactions have been studied in 32 patients with rheumatoid arthritis (14). In all, there were 43 reactions in 21 patients, four patients had serious reactions, and in five patients infliximab was withdrawn. Adverse reactions consisted of infections (n=21), allergies (n=3) and cardiovascular complications (n=3). The incidence of reactions was as follows: respiratory 28%; urinary 22%; cutaneous 16%; allergic 9.4%; cardiovascular 9.4%.

TNF-alfa has been suggested to be an important mediator of circulatory disturbances in alcoholic hepatitis. The effects of infliximab on portal and systemic hemodynamics have been studied in 10 patients with severe biopsy proven alcoholic hepatitis (15). After treatment, serum bilirubin, C-reactive protein, white cell count, and plasma concentrations of interleukin-6 and interleukin-8 were significantly reduced. Nine of 10 patients were alive at 28 days. Mean hepatic venous pressure gradient fell significantly at 24 hours. Mean arterial pressure and systemic vascular resistance increased significantly, mirrored by a reduction in cardiac index. Hepatic and renal blood flow also increased significantly. There was also a reduction in hepatic inflammation and improved organ blood flow, suggesting an important role for TNF-alfa in mediating circulatory disturbances in alcoholic hepatitis. The authors concluded that infliximab produces a highly significant, early, and sustained reduction in hepatic venous pressure gradient in patients with alcoholic hepatitis, possibly by a combination of reduced cardiac output and intrahepatic resistance.

In 23 patients with refractory autoimmune uveitis, who were given three infusions of inflixiamb at weeks 0, 2, and 6, 78% had clinical success, but only 50% continued infliximab therapy for at least 1 year (16). There was an unexpectedly high rate of adverse events. Seven patients had serious adverse events, including three cases of serious thrombosis, two vitreous hemorrhages, one malignancy, one new-onset congestive heart failure, and two possible cases of drug-induced lupus-like syndrome.

Data from 5000 patients with active rheumatoid arthritis treated with infliximab have been collected by Tanabe Seiyaku Co, Ltd (17). The overall risk of adverse reactions was 28% and of serious adverse reactions 6.2%, including bacterial pneumonia 2.2%, tuberculosis (n = 14), *Pneumocystis* pneumonia (n = 22), interstitial pneumonitis (n = 25), and serious infusion reactions (n = 24); other adverse reactions included transient liver damage, gastroenteritis, and local skin infections. Most recovered after intensive treatment, but three patients (one with bacterial pneumonia and two with interstitial pneumonitis) died. There were 14 cases of tuberculosis in the early stages of treatment and half were extra-pulmonary. Serious infusion reactions included anaphylactic reactions (n = 8) and hypotension (n = 9); all recovered completely.

Adverse effects possibly related to infliximab have been retrospectively examined in 500 consecutive patients with Crohn's disease who had received a median of three infusions (18). The median duration of follow-up was 17 months. Serious adverse effects were attributed to infliximab in 30 patients (6%). The most frequent adverse effects were infections (41 patients, of whom 15 had a serious infection), acute infusion reactions (19 patients, of whom two had life-threatening reactions), serum sickness-like diseases (14 patients, of whom five had severe disease), lupus-like syndrome (three patients, including one with positive rechallenge after a subsequent infusion), malignant disorders (two solid tumors and one case of non-Hodgkin's lymphoma), worsening of heart failure (one patient with a previously diagnosed cardiomyopathy), and demyelination syndrome (one patient). Among 10 deaths, five were considered to be possibly related to the treatment (four severe infections and one case of lung cancer).

Of 217 patients who received infliximab (mean number of infusions 2.6) for inflammatory bowel diseases, 41 had 42 severe adverse events (19). Most of these consisted of hypersensitivity reactions (n = 13), infections (n = 11), postoperative complications (n = 7), thromboembolic events (n = 5), or lymphomas (n = 3). There was also one case each of lupus-like syndrome, depression, and vestibular neuronitis. Six patients died, and the cause of death was lymphoma in two patients, infections in three, and pulmonary embolism in one. However, it was not stated how the causal relation to infliximab treatment was assessed. The authors noted that the annual incidence of lymphoma in their patients was 1.5%, which is considerably higher than the 0.015% expected from the background population data in their country. They also commented on the unexpectedly 2.8% mortality rate during the 2-year follow-up period.

In 100 patients treated with infliximab for inflammatory bowel disease there were adverse events in 10 patients after a median follow-up of 26 months (20). There were acute infusion reactions in two patients, a serum sickness-like reaction in one, bacterial or viral infections in four, pancytopenia in one, and surgical complications in two. There were no malignancies, autoimmune diseases, or neurological or cardiovascular adverse events.

Comparative studies

In a retrospective study, 122 patients with Crohn's disease who received infliximab infusions were also given azathioprine (n=47), mercaptopurine (n=11), methotrexate (n=23), prednisone (n=64), mesalazine (n=51), and antibiotics (n=16) (21). Mean follow-up was 52 weeks (14–864 days). The overall response rate to infliximab was similar between patients who received immunomodulators and patients who received infliximab alone. There were more frequent adverse drug reactions in those who took infliximab alone (22%) than in those who took methotrexate (13%) and azathioprine/mercaptopurine (14%), but this was not statistically significant. Concomitant use of immunomodulators with infliximab in patients with Crohn's disease did not improve clinical response rates, dosage reduction of prednisone, fistula response, and mean intervals between infliximab infusions.

Organs and Systems

Cardiovascular

The preliminary results of a phase II trial in patients with moderate to severe congestive heart failure showed a higher incidence of worsening congestive heart failure and death in patients treated with infliximab compared with placebo (22). This led to warnings from regulatory agencies and to the limited use of infliximab in patients with congestive heart failure.

Venous thrombosis has been associated with infliximab in two patients.

- A 55-year-old woman with psoriatic arthritis and possible systemic lupus erythematosus developed inspiratory pain, slight dyspnea, and left leg pain 1 week after receiving a second infusion of infliximab 3 mg/kg (23). A respiratory infection was suspected and she

recovered. Similar pulmonary symptoms with right leg pain recurred 6 days after her third infusion of infliximab, and a pulmonary embolism was suggested on spiral CT. She also had raised anti-DNA antibodies and slightly raised cardiolipin antibodies.

- A 45-year-old woman with no history of hypertension, hypercholesterolemia, or diabetes received infliximab for Crohn's disease (24). She had visual changes after her third dose of infliximab and ophthalmoscopy showed retinal vein thrombosis. There was no underlying coagulation disorder.

Although vascular complications have been associated with Crohn's disease or rheumatoid arthritis, there was a close temporal relation with infliximab treatment in both cases. In addition, the second patient had no evidence of susceptibility factors.

There are reports that suggest that infliximab can precipitate thrombotic events in patients with various underlying diseases (Table 1).

It is not yet known whether infliximab has a negative procoagulant effect, but experimental data suggest that TNF-alpha has a strong antithrombotic activity in mice (30). In contrast, prolonged use of infliximab in seven patients with rheumatoid arthritis improved endothelial function assessed by brachial ultrasonography, at least during the first 7 days after infusion (31).

Respiratory

Allergic granulomatosis of the lung has been described after a second infusion of infliximab in one of 35 patients with active ankylosing spondylitis (32). The clinical and radiological symptoms resolved 8 weeks after withdrawal, but no other details were given.

- A 32-year-old man with Crohn's disease developed an eosinophilic pleural effusion soon after a second infusion of infliximab (33). He recovered within 8 weeks, but the effusion recurred after infliximab re-treatment 1 year later.

Table 1 Reports of thrombotic disorders associated with infliximab

Age Sex	Disease and susceptibility factors	Time to onset	Adverse reaction	Outcome	Ref.
31 M	Ankylosing spondylitis	Headache rapidly after 1st infusion	Cerebral thrombophlebitis on day 3	Recovery	(25)
31 F	Crohn's disease	1 day after 3rd infusion	Extensive deep venous thrombosis in the infusion arm	Recovery	(26)
63 M	Rheumatoid arthritis, diabetes mellitus, hypertension, hypercholesterolemia	3 days after 1st infusion	Myocardial infarction	Infliximab continued; 2nd infarction after 8th infusion	(27)
63 F	Non-insulin- dependent diabetes	Within 30 min of 1st infusion	Myocardial infarction	Recovery	(28)
41 M	Ankylosing spondylitis, paroxysmal nocturnal hemoglobinuria	2 months after 6th infusion	Hepatic vein thrombosis (Budd–Chiari syndrome)	Recovery	(29)

Severe interstitial pneumonitis has been attributed to infliximab.

- A 22-year-old woman with colonic and perianal Crohn's disease developed a cough within hours of her first dose of infliximab (34). It became worse after the second dose and 5 weeks after the first infusion she was hospitalized with progressive breathlessness. A high-resolution CT scan of the thorax showed extensive ground glass shadowing with right apical peribronchial consolidation. Pulmonary function tests showed a marked restrictive pattern. Bronchoscopy showed normal endobronchial appearances and bronchial washings were negative for *Pneumocystis jiroveci*, fungi, acid-fast bacilli, and viruses.
- A 66-year-old woman developed non-infectious interstitial pneumonitis after a second infusion of infliximab (35).

Four patients developed severe features of methotrexate pneumonitis shortly after they received their third infusion of infliximab, raising the possibility that infliximab could potentiate the pulmonary toxicity of methotrexate (36,37). Three patients with rheumatoid arthritis and asymptomatic fibrosing alveolitis had acute fatal exacerbations of their lung disease after having received two or three doses of infliximab (38).

Pulmonary damage in patients without prior pulmonary disease has also been attributed to infliximab.

- Two men aged 21 and 71 years developed hypersensitivity pneumonitis after infliximab treatment for Crohn's disease (39). The first developed pulmonary symptoms after a single dose of infliximab, whereas the second had previously tolerated infliximab well for 1 year. The latter had focal interstitial chronic inflammation on transbronchial biopsy. Infectious causes were carefully ruled out in both patients.
- An 84-year-old woman with rheumatoid arthritis who had taken leflunomide for 6 months developed severe interstitial pneumonitis 1 week after a second dose of infliximab (40). Infliximab was withdrawn and leflunomide was continued. The course of the disease was marked by rapidly progressive end-stage pulmonary fibrosis.
- A 35-year-old woman with severe Crohn's disease that had not responded to hydrocortisone, mercaptopurine, and mesalazine was given infliximab (41). Within 48 hours after a second dose she developed fever, a dry cough, and dyspnea, with severe respiratory distress and acute anemia. There was diffuse bilateral alveolar hemorrhage on a chest CT scan and she subsequently developed staphylococcal superinfection. There was full pulmonary recovery 6 months later.

In all cases a causal relation with infliximab treatment was based on a suggestive temporal association and reasonable exclusion of other causes. Possible leflunomide-associated interstitial pneumonitis, possibly aggravated by infliximab, could not be ruled out in the second report.

Exacerbation of pre-existing obstructive sleep apnea syndrome concomitant with infliximab infusion has been reported in a 62-year-old woman with rheumatoid arthritis (42).

Nervous system

Features of aseptic meningitis have been reported after multiple infliximab injections (43).

- A 53-year-old man with severe rheumatoid arthritis and mixed type III cryoglobulinemia received his first four injections of infliximab uneventfully, but 4 hours after the fifth injection had severe muscle pain in the lower limbs, which required morphine and abated within 3 days. Similar symptoms were observed after the sixth injection. There were no signs of meningitis, the cerebrospinal fluid contained lymphocytes and increased concentrations of protein and IgG. Cultures were negative and MRI scans of the brain and the spine were normal. The CSF was normal 1 month later.

The authors speculated that the most likely explanation for these observations was linked to the lack of transfer of high-molecular weight soluble receptors and IgG across the blood–brain barrier, implying that control of brain tumor necrosis factor alfa cannot be obtained with monoclonal antibodies. They thought that neurological complications in diseases other than multiple sclerosis might be related to control of tumor necrosis factor alfa in the periphery, resulting in an enhanced contribution of brain-derived tumor necrosis factor alfa or other cytokines, such as interleukin-1.

Neurological events suggestive of demyelinating disorders in patients treated with tumor necrosis factor alfa antagonists and reported to the FDA's Adverse Events Reporting System have been reviewed (44). These included 17 cases temporarily associated with etanercept and two with infliximab, but complete information was lacking in a number of cases. The various hypothetical mechanisms by which tumor necrosis factor alfa antagonists might produce demyelinating events have been discussed (45). Briefly, they cause an increase in peripheral T cell autoreactivity, and their inability to cross the blood–brain barrier may account for exacerbation of central demyelinating disorders.

- A 19-year-old woman taking azathioprine developed symptoms of multiple sclerosis 2 weeks after a second infusion of infliximab (46). An MRI scan confirmed a demyelinating process and there was clinical improvement without a further change in MRI examination.
- A 50-year-old woman developed visual loss and ocular pain in the left eye 3 weeks after her last infusion of infliximab (47). An MRI scan showed isolated retrobulbar optic neuritis. She recovered spontaneously after withdrawal of infliximab.

Whether these cases occurred by chance or reflected a true relation between infliximab and demyelinating disease is a matter of debate. As reviewed elsewhere, the actual number of reported cases does not appear to exceed the expected incidence in the untreated population (48).

A debatable case of rapidly progressive Parkinson's disease has been attributed to infliximab in a 72-year-old woman (49). Until more data are available, this report should be considered as anecdotal.

Several cases of peripheral nerve disorders have emerged.

- Two women aged 28 and 45 years had an acute, predominantly motor neuropathy after infliximab for Crohn's disease and collagenous colitis (50).
- Multifocal motor neuropathy occurred in a 34-year-old woman with rheumatoid arthritis (51).

The hallmark in these patients was the appearance of neurological symptoms after the fourth dose of infliximab and an electromyographic pattern of conduction block. Antiganglioside antibodies were detected in one patient and returned to normal within 6 months after withdrawal of infliximab. A possible autoimmune mechanism was suggested.

Sensory neuropathy has also been reported in two women with rheumatoid arthritis aged 41 and 48 years (52). The peripheral neuropathy was attributed to necrotizing vasculitis in one patient who first developed symptoms after her sixth infusion of infliximab, and to rapid exacerbation of pre-existing mononeuritis multiplex 8 hours after a first infusion of infliximab in the second patient.

Various other neurological abnormalities have been attributed to infliximab.

- A patient with rheumatoid arthritis developed the Miller Fisher syndrome variant of the Guillain–Barré syndrome while receiving infliximab. He had ataxia and dysarthria, which fluctuated in relation to each subsequent infliximab infusion and after 6 months culminated in areflexic flaccid quadriplegia (53).
- A 55-year-old man with a 27-year history of ankylosing spondylitis received infliximab and developed back pain and a paraparesis. Radiography showed rapid exacerbation of pre-existing spinal pseudoarthrosis at T11–12. Although the myelopathy could have developed over time and been unrelated to infliximab, the history and radiographic course suggested that suppression of inflammation by infliximab improved his activities of daily living, which paradoxically exacerbated pre-existing spinal pseudoarthrosis and hastened the onset of subsequent myelopathy (54).
- A 47-year-old man with rheumatoid arthritis received monthly infusions of infliximab 300 mg for 2 years (55). A brain MRI scan showed gadolinium enhancement of the cisternal segment of the right oculomotor nerve. There were no white matter lesions and no dural enhancement. After withdrawal of infliximab, the diplopia and ptosis gradually resolved over 3 months. The transient and isolated nature of the palsy described suggested demyelination. There was no evidence of infection, inflammation, or migraine.

Sensory systems

Optic neuropathy has been described in patients with rheumatoid arthritis taking infliximab. In three patients aged 54–62 years, blurred vision or visual field loss in one or both eyes occurred after the third dose (56).

- A 54-year-old man had blurred vision 34 days after a third dose of infliximab. Co-medication consisted of leflunomide, prednisone, naproxen, diazepam, fluoxetine, famotidine, metoprolol, and paracetamol or codeine. Fluorescein angiography showed capillary dilatation and vascular leakage in both optic nerve heads. He did not recover vision with glucocorticoid therapy.
- A 62-year-old woman had blurred vision 40 days after a third dose of infliximab. Co-medication consisted of atenolol, enalapril or hydrochlorothiazide, salicylic acid, terfenadine, and rofecoxib. Fluorescein angiography showed profuse vascular leakage. The left eye had a central scotoma and the optic nerve head was pale. A fourth dose of infliximab was given 7 weeks after the third dose, after which symptoms started in the right eye with a central scotoma. Methylprednisolone did not improve vision.
- A 54-year-old man developed loss of vision field 2 weeks after a third dose of infliximab. Co-medication consisted of prednisone, diclofenac, and omeprazole. Fluorescein angiography showed capillary dilatation and vascular leakage in the optic nerve heads.

All three patients had the toxic form of anterior optic neuropathy and MRI scanning ruled out demyelinating optic neuritis. Glucocorticoids, given to exclude external temporal arteritis, did not improve vision in any of the patients. Accumulation was speculated to be a factor in this adverse effect, because all three patients developed anterior optic neuropathy after the third dose of infliximab.

In one patient an additional infusion of infliximab produced similar symptoms in the previously unaffected eye; vision failed to improve despite infliximab withdrawal and steroid treatment.

- Retrobulbar optic neuritis was diagnosed after the ninth dose of infliximab in a 55-year-old woman (57). MRI scanning showed demyelination of the left optic nerve and the visual field defect improved after treatment with prednisone.

Psychiatric

A 30-year-old woman with evolving ileocolonic Crohn's disease received five intravenous infusions of infliximab 5 mg/kg over 2 years (58). About 2 hours after each infusion, she had *a panic attack* for 2–48 hours. After the fourth infusion, she needed paroxetine and bromazepam.

Metabolism

Body composition was assessed in patients with Crohn's disease before and after treatment with infliximab at 1 and 4 weeks (59). There were significant increases in body weight at 4 weeks and serum leptin concentrations at 1 and 4 weeks. The increase in serum leptin occurred at 1 week, when there were no significant changes in weight and fat mass, and was associated with down-regulation of TNF alfa-regulated mediators, solubleTNF receptor type II, and soluble intercellular antiadhesion molecule-1. Moreover, infliximab singificantly increased cholesterol concentrations at 1 week compared with the control patients, who received methylprednisolone.

Hematologic

A patient who had been treated for many years with classical therapy for rheumatoid arthritis developed a refractory anemia after treatment with infliximab + methotrexate (60).

Pancytopenia has been reported on several occasions in patients taking infliximab.

- A 45-year-old woman with underlying renal insufficiency developed pancytopenia 2 weeks after a single infusion of infliximab for scleroderma (61). There were no other suspected drug exposures and she later died from infectious complications.
- Neutropenia and thrombocytopenia occurred in a 60-year-old woman (62).
- Pancytopenia with bone marrow hypoplasia on biopsy occurred in a 66-year-old man (63).

The second and third cases were complicated by the use of concomitant drugs (methotrexate, leflunomide) known to be associated with hematological disorders. Additional data are therefore required before adding hematological toxicity to the adverse effects of infliximab.

A hemophagocytic syndrome was reported a patient with rheumatoid arthritis treated with infliximab (64).

- A 46-year-old woman with seropositive rheumatoid arthritis had active disease despite treatment with glucocorticoids, methotrexate, and sulfasalazine. Six weeks after the seventh infusion of infliximab 3 mg/kg she developed fever, dehydration, weight loss, profound lethargy, hepatomegaly, and pain in the right flank. She had thrombocytopenia (platelets 16×10^9/l), anemia, leukocytosis (15×10^9/l) lymphopenia (760×10^6/l), a low CD4 lymphocyte count (72×10^6/l), renal insufficiency, hyponatremia, hypoalbuminemia, and hypogammaglobulinemia. Liver enzymes were 20 times the upper end of the reference range, bilirubin 1.5 times, and lactate dehydrogenase five time. Urine and blood cultures grew *Escherichia coli*. Hemophagocytic syndrome was confirmed by bone marrow aspiration. Screening ruled out others possible causes than Escherichia coli and infliximab. Infliximab was withdrawn and the patient recovered with intravenous immunoglobulin and antibiotics.

The possible role of infliximab in the development of hypercoagulability disorders has been discussed in the context of a case of arterial thrombosis (65).

- A 72-year-old woman with refractory sarcoidosis developed venous thrombosis at a catheter site and extensive multiple thromboses in small arteries in her legs after receiving a third dose of infliximab for severe

enteropathy. Anticardiolipin antibodies were detected, but antinuclear and anti-double-stranded DNA antibodies were negative.

Although infliximab has been associated with autoantibody production, it is not known whether it contributed to hypercoagulability in this patient.

Liver

Acute hepatitis with infliximab has been described (66).

- A 44-year-old woman, who had used oral contraceptives for many years and had taken mesalazine, mercaptopurine, and prednisone for Crohn's disease for 7 years, developed clinical and biological signs of acute mixed hepatitis 19 days after a single dose of infliximab 5 mg/kg. There were no symptoms suggestive of hypersensitivity and liver histology showed cholestasis without inflammation or eosinophilia. Other causes, such as a recent viral infection (hepatitis A, B, C, cytomegalovirus, *Herpes simplex*) or gallstones, were ruled out. Among various autoantibodies, only antinuclear antibody titers were slightly raised. Complete normalization was observed 2 months later.

Although the patient took other potentially hepatotoxic drugs, the time-course suggested that infliximab was the cause.

- A 28-year-old man with refractory ulcerative colitis developed acute cholestatic liver damage after a single infusion of infliximab (67). The liver damage resolved spontaneously within 6 weeks.

Although a direct relation between infliximab and the acute liver damage could not be definitely established, this case suggests that infliximab can cause direct liver damage, the course of which is similar to acute cholestatic hepatitis and resolves after withdrawal of the drug.

Skin

Skin reactions, including erythema multiforme in three patients and a lichenoid eruption in one, were attributed to infliximab (68). One patient had similar lesions after etanercept. Patch tests with infliximab in three patients were negative, but produced a flare-up of lesions in one patient and recurrence of malaise and nausea in another patient, suggesting that infliximab is well absorbed percutaneously.

Other skin reactions have been described in patients treated with infliximab, including lichenoid dermatitis, a perniosis-like eruption, and superficial granuloma annulare (Table 2), but coincidental eruptions could not be ruled out and the authors provided no convincing evidence of causal relations (69). Other cases with recurrence or flare of the skin lesions on rechallenge gave more definitive evidence of the role of infliximab and included eczematous purpura of Doucas and Kapetenakis (70), eczema-like toxiderma (71) and an atopic dermatitis-like eruption (72).

Table 2 Infliximab-related adverse skin reactions

Age Sex	Disease	Medication	Adverse skin reaction	Outcome
30 F	Crohn's disease	Mesalazine 4 g/day Infliximab 1 x 5 mg/kg	Leukocytoclastic vasculitis	Infliximab withdrawn; improved with glucocorticoids
64 F	Rheumatoid arthritis	Methotrexate 10 mg/week Prednisolone 2 mg/day Infliximab 3 x 3 mg/kg	Lichenoid eruption	Improved with glucocorticoids; infliximab re-administered
68 F	Rheumatoid arthritis	Methotrexate 10 mg/week Infliximab 6 x 3 mg/kg	Perniosis	Infliximab withdrawn
46 M	Psoriasis	Infliximab 1 x 3 mg/kg	Superficial granuloma annulare	Infliximab continued; treated with glucocorticoids
38 F	Rheumatoid arthritis	Methotrexate 10 mg/week Infliximab 3 mg/kg	Perniosis	Infliximab withdrawn
36F	Psoriasis	Prednisolone 8 mg/day Infliximab 3 mg/kg	Acute folliculitis and dyshidrotic dermatitis	Topical erythromycin, glucocorticoids; infliximab continued

- A 36-year-old man developed a diffuse pruritic rash after treatment for 3 months with oral leflunomide and infliximab for palmoplantar pustular psoriasis (73). Withdrawal of both drugs resulted in improvement in the skin condition. Although patch tests to both leflunomide and infliximab were negative, rechallenge with infliximab resulted in recurrence of the eczematous rash.
- Alopecia areata occurred in a 51-year-old woman with rheumatoid arthritis and Sjögren's syndrome who received infliximab for 11 months (74). She developed non-scarring hair loss consistent with alopecia areata, which eventually evolved to 100% scalp involvement despite withdrawal of infliximab.
- A 23-year-old man with a history of Crohn's disease developed profuse warts on his penis and perianal region after two doses of infliximab (75). A diagnosis of genital condylomata acuminata was made.
- A 72-year-old man developed bullous skin lesions the day after receiving his fourth dose of infliximab for rheumatoid arthritis (76). Human antichimeric antibodies were positive, as were antinuclear antibodies, and he completely recovered after treatment with prednisone.

Four patients with no previous history of psoriasis experienced psoriasis or psoriasiform cutaneous eruptions (Table 3). As infliximab can improve severe psoriatic arthritis, a paradoxical adverse reaction to this agent was suggested.

Delayed onset of a short-lived maculopapular, urticarial rash has been reported in two children aged 10 and 16 years given infliximab for juvenile rheumatoid arthritis (80). They developed cutaneous lesions 13–18 days after the first or second injection, and later tolerated further infliximab administration well. There was no evidence of vasculitis on skin biopsy.

Two patients aged 20 and 56 years treated with infliximab for Behçet's disease developed multiple lesions of erythema nodosum 3 and 30 days after their third and fourth infusions respectively (81). Infliximab-induced exacerbation of previous erythema nodosum was suggested in the first patient. Because new lesions of erythema nodosum subsequently developed despite withdrawal of infliximab in this patient, and because no documentation of the outcome was provided in the other patient, any causal relation should be considered doubtful.

A typical nicotinic acid-like reaction, consisting of intense chest tightness and erythematous flushing, occurred within minutes of a first or subsequent infusion of infliximab in three children with refractory juvenile rheumatoid arthritis (82). Similar reactions were observed after further infusions despite various

Table 3 Reports of psoriatic eruptions associated with infliximab

Age Sex	Disease	Dosage	Time to onset	Outcome	Ref.
47 F	Seronegative rheumatoid arthritis	200 mg	2 months	Infliximab continued; limited improvement with topical steroids and salicylic acid	77
27 F	Ankylosing spondylitis	5 mg/kg	10 months	Infliximab continued; no further lesions after topical treatment	78
32 M	Ankylosing spondylitis	5 mg/kg	6 weeks	Infliximab withdrawn; partial improvement with systemic glucocorticoids	Haib
46 F	Crohn's disease	5 mg/kg	2 weeks	Lesions spontaneously cleared, recurred after 3rd injection, and cleared after infliximab withdrawn	79

prophylactic drug regimens, and only aspirin finally prevented recurrence.

Alopecia areata involving the scalp, eyebrows, and eyelashes has been reported in a 51-year-old woman who had received infliximab for 11 months for rheumatoid arthritis and Sjögren's syndrome (83).

Five patients developed erythematous annular plaques on the trunk and limbs while receiving four different TNF-α antagonists (84). One was taking lenalidomide for multiple myeloma, two were receiving infliximab, one was receiving etanercept for severe rheumatoid arthritis; and one was in a trial of adalimumab for psoriatic arthropathy. Skin biopsies showed diffuse interstitial granulomatous infiltration with lymphocytes, histiocytes, and eosinophils, and palisading degenerated collagen. Withdrawal of the medications led to complete resolution of the skin lesions.

Acute alopecia areata has been reported during treatment with infliximab in a subject who had never had it (cf. adalimumab above and efalizumab below) (85).

In three patients with severe Crohn's disease who required digestive surgery, infliximab before or immediately after surgery was discussed as an additional possible cause of postoperative poor wound healing with serious complications (86).

Musculoskeletal

Of three patients who received intravenous infliximab 5 mg/kg for peristomal pyoderma gangrenosum, one developed reactive arthritis and infliximab was withdrawn (87).

Immunologic

Antibodies to infliximab

Treatment with infliximab is associated with the formation of human antichimeric antibodies in about 10% of patients. Patients who are antibody positive are more likely to have an infusion reaction and potential loss of medication efficacy (88). Such antibodies were rarely detected in patients with rheumatoid arthritis who were also taking methotrexate, and low titers were detected in about 13% of patients with Crohn's disease. Their clinical relevance is unclear, although their presence has sometimes been associated with an increased risk of infusion reactions, the occurrence of serum sickness-like reactions after delayed re-treatment, and a shorter duration of response.

In a randomized, placebo-controlled trial in 573 patients with Crohn's disease, who responded to an initial infusion of infliximab and were then given repeated infusions, antibodies to infliximab were found in 14%; there was a trend toward a lower incidence of antibodies in patients taking concurrent glucocorticoids and immunosuppressive drugs (89). The incidence of infusion reactions was also higher in patients positive for antibodies to infliximab compared with patients without antibodies (16 versus 8%) and lower in patients who were taking both glucocorticoids and immunosuppressants compared with patients who were receiving neither (8 versus 32%).

The clinical significance of antibodies to infliximab has also been explored in 125 patients with Crohn's disease

who were given infliximab, of whom 61% had antibodies after the fifth infusion; however, there was no further increase in incidence after subsequent treatment (90). The presence of antibodies was associated with a 2.4-fold increase in the risk of infusion reactions, lower serum infliximab concentrations, and a shorter duration of clinical response, compared with patients with no infliximab antibodies. Patients who received concomitant immunosuppressive therapy had a lower incidence of infliximab antibodies, higher infliximab serum concentrations, and a longer duration of clinical response. Pretreatment with glucocorticoids may reduce the risk of antibody formation, but it is not known whether a pretreatment test for human antichimeric antibodies has a predictive value for adverse reactions (91). However, there were technical issues relating to the antibody assay and definition of clinically relevant antibody titers in this study.

Changes in antinuclear antibody (ANA) have been evaluated in 36 patients (mean age 30 years, range 12-59) with Crohn's disease treated with intravenous infliximab 5 mg/kg (92). Concomitant immunosuppressive drugs were given in 28 cases. At baseline, eight patients were ANA positive. At 6 weeks, no anti-double-stranded DNA antibodies were detectable. After retreatment, three of these eight patients had increasing ANA titers and two developed antibodies to dsDNA. Six of 28 ANA-negative patients changed their ANA status from baseline to 6 weeks. One re-treated patient had further increase in ANA titer and developed antibodies to dsDNA. None of the 36 patients developed a lupus-like syndrome.

In 62 adults with rheumatoid arthritis and 35 with spondylarthropathy, 32 and six respectively were ANA-positive (93). After infliximab, the numbers shifted to 51 and 31. At baseline, none of the patients had antibodies to dsDNA. After infliximab, seven and six patients respectively became anti-dsDNA positive, with IgM and IgA in seven and three. In some patients, there were antinucleosome antibodies, antihistone antibodies, or antibodies to extractable nuclear antigen after infliximab. Lupus-like syndrome was not observed.

Infusion reactions and the relation between antibodies to infliximab and the loss of response after infliximab have been studied in 53 patients with Crohn's disease who received 199 infusions of infliximab (5 mg/kg) (94). There were antibodies to infliximab in 19 of 53 patients (36%), including all seven patients with serious infusion reactions, and in 11 of 15 patients (73%) who lost their initial response compared with none of 21 continuous responders. Giving a second infusion within 8 weeks of the first or concurrent immunosuppressants significantly reduced the formation of antibodies to infliximab. In a subsequent randomized trial, 80 patients with Crohn's disease were randomized to intravenous hydrocortisone 200 mg or placebo immediately before their first and subsequent infliximab infusions. Titers of antibodies to infliximab were lower at week 16 among those who received hydrocortisone (1.6 versus 3.4 μg/ml), 26% of whom developed antibodies compared with 42% of placebo-treated patients. The authors concluded that loss of initial response and infusion reactions after infliximab is strongly related to the formation and titer of antibodies to infliximab. Giving a second infusion within 8 weeks of immunosuppressant therapy significantly reduces antibody formation. Intravenous hydrocortisone premedication significantly reduces the titers of antibodies to infliximab but does not eliminate their formation or infusion reactions.

Seven patients with Crohn's disease who had experienced immediate or delayed-hypersensitivity reactions to infliximab and one with infliximab-induced lupus were treated with adalimumab without any signs or symptoms of allergic reactions (95).

Antibody formation has been studied in patients with spondylarthropathy (n = 34) or rheumatoid arthritis (n = 59) who were treated with infliximab for 2 years and in 20 patients with spondylarthropathy who were treated with etanercept for 1 year (96). After 1 year, the infliximab-treated patients with spondylarthropathy or rheumatoid arthritis had new antinuclear antibodies in 41% and 62% respectively and anti-dsDNA antibodies in 49% and 71 %. Only 10% of etanercept-treated patients with spondylarthropathy developed antibodies. Isotyping showed almost exclusively IgM or IgM/IgA anti-dsDNA antibodies, which disappeared on withdrawal of treatment. Neither infliximab nor etanercept induced other lupus-related antibodies, such as anti-ENA antibodies, antihistone antibodies, or antinucleosome antibodies, and there was no clinical evidence of lupus-like syndrome. Similarly, infliximab, but not etanercept, selectively increased IgM but not IgG anticardiolipin antibody titers. Thus, the prominent antinuclear antibody and anti-dsDNA autoantibody response is not a pure class effect of TNF alfa blockers, is largely restricted to short-term IgM responses, and is not associated with other serological or clinical signs of lupus. Similar findings with anticardiolipin antibodies suggest that modulation of humoral immunity may be a more general feature of infliximab treatment.

Autoantibodies and autoimmunity

Infliximab may increase the risk of autoimmunity, but the presence of antibodies did not predict the risk of lupus-like syndrome. In trials, the incidence of infliximab-induced anti-double-stranded DNA antibodies ranged from 5 to 34% of patients, depending on the assay method used and the duration of exposure (97,98). However, these abnormalities were rarely associated with clinical manifestations. In two large randomized trials in more than 900 infliximab-treated patients, only three developed a lupus-like syndrome, with no evidence of systemic organ involvement (97,98). However, since then, several reports have detailed infliximab-induced, lupus-like syndrome in patients with Crohn's colitis or rheumatoid arthritis, with improvement on withdrawal of infliximab (99,100).

In 59 patients with rheumatoid arthritis a high incidence of autoimmunity, manifesting as an increased number of patients with antinuclear antibodies (69% versus 29% at baseline), anti-double-stranded DNA IgM antibodies (32% versus 0% at baseline), and antihistone IgM antibodies (79% versus 18% at baseline) after 30 weeks of infliximab treatment, has been confirmed (101). There were very similar findings in 39 patients with rheumatoid arthritis or ankylosing spondylitis after 2 years of follow-up; Antiphospholipid autoantibodies also occurred during treatment (23% of patients versus none at baseline), but vasculitis-associated autoantibodies or organ-specific autoantibodies against the thyroid or the liver were not detected (102). None of the patients included in these studies had lupus-like symptoms.

In a prospective study of autoimmunity in 125 patients treated with infliximab for Crohn's disease, the cumulative incidence of antinuclear antibodies during 24 months was 57%, and positivity was found after less than three infusions in almost 80% of patients (103). Among the antinuclear antibody-positive patients, about 30% were positive for double-stranded DNA and 21% for antihistone autoantibodies. Antinuclear antibodies were still present up to 1 year after the last infusion of infliximab. Two patients with high antinuclear antibody titers, both of whom were antihistone and double-stranded DNA autoantibody-positive, developed a lupus-like syndrome without any major organ involvement. One additional antinuclear antibody-positive patient had autoimmune hemolytic anemia 6 months after the first infusion of infliximab. There was a similar incidence of new autoantibodies after prolonged treatment in another study in 42 patients with rheumatic diseases, albeit that none developed clinical symptoms of autoimmunity (104). This study also suggested an increased risk of biological autoimmunity with the number of infusions or the total dose of infliximab.

Profound immunomodulation induced by TNF alfa inhibitors is associated with a relatively low incidence of immune-related complications, such as demyelinating disease and lupus-like syndrome. This contrasts sharply with the prominent induction of autoantibodies such as antinuclear antibodies (ANA) and anti–doublestranded DNA (anti-dsDNA) antibodies by TNF alfa blockers. This phenomenon has been recognized for several years, but the clinical and biological correlates of this antibody induction in autoimmune arthritis are not yet fully understood.

Lupus-like syndrome has been reported in seven patients (Table 4), all of whom had increased antinuclear antibody titers (new occurrences in six); six were positive for anti-double-stranded DNA and three for antihistone antibodies. In contrast, six other patients with moderately active lupus-like syndrome were successfully treated with infliximab without flares of lupus activity despite increased titers of anti-double-stranded DNA and anticardiolipin antibodies in four cases (105).

Polymyositis has been associated with infliximab (112).

- A 52-year-old woman with a 20-year history of inadequately controlled seropositive rheumatoid arthritis treated with non-steroidal anti-inflammatory drugs, prednisone 15 mg/day, and methotrexate 15 mg/week received intravenous infliximab 3 mg/kg after 0, 2, and 6 week and then every eighth week. After 14 months she had diffuse pain in the lower and upper limbs and

Table 4 Reports of lupus-like syndrome associated with infliximab

Age Sex	Disease	Time of onset	Main symptoms	Ref.
45 M	Rheumatoid arthritis	After 5th infusion	Fever, cough, eruption, arthralgia, pericardial and pleural effusions	(106)
61 F	Rheumatoid arthritis	10 days after 3rd injection	Fever, myalgia, arthralgia, eruption	(107)
54 F	Rheumatoid arthritis	2 weeks after 5th infusion	Fever, myalgia, polyarthritis	(Elkayam 502
37 F	Crohn's disease	After 5th infusion	Arthralgia, myalgia, pericarditis	(108)
53 F	Rheumatoid arthritis	4 weeks after 4th infusion	Photosensitive rash, acute polyarthritis, fever, pleural effusions	(109)
43 F	Rheumatoid arthritis	7 weeks after 4th infusion	Fever, synovitis, eruption, pleuritic chest pain	(110)
53 F	Rheumatoid arthritis	After 2nd, 3rd, and 4th infusions	Cutaneious lesions after each injection; cutaneous lupus later confirmed	(111)

progressive symmetrical proximal muscle weakness, accompanied by fever, dysphagia, dyspnea, and weight loss. Rheumatoid factor was 155 IU/ml, creatine kinase over 12 000 U/l, (MB fraction 529 U/l), aspartate transaminase 542 U/l, and lactate dehydrogenase 4533 U/l. Autoantibody tests were positive for antinuclear antibody 1:320, anti-dsDNA 1:20, pANCA 1:20, and double immunodiffusion for anti-Jo-1 antibody. Muscle biopsy showed diffuse fibre necrosis and inflammatory infiltrates. Infliximab-induced polymyositis was diagnosed and improved after intravenous methylprednisolone 1 g tds.

Infliximab-related vasculitis has rarely been described. Eight cases of vasculitis or vasculitic rash associated with infliximab (n=7) or etanercept (n=1) have been detailed in patients with rheumatoid arthritis, but only two were biopsy proven (113). Two patients had a concomitant rise in autoantibodies and the resolution of skin lesions was noted after withdrawal of the TNF alfa antagonist and/or treatment with prednisolone or cyclophosphamide. Although rheumatoid vasculitis could not be ruled out in several of these cases, the two patients who later received etanercept after developing lesions with infliximab had recurrent vasculitis or rash. Another case of biopsy-proven leukocytoclastic vasculitis has been reported after a single infusion of infliximab in a 24-year-old woman (114). This was probably a hypersensitivity reaction, as TNF alfa antagonists have sometimes been used to treat severe vasculitis.

Infliximab binds to tumor necrosis factor alfa on cell surfaces and produces apoptotic cell death, releasing the nucleosomal autoantigens that induce autoantibody formation (116).

- A 69-year-old woman with a 5-year history of rheumatoid arthritis developed drug-induced lupus after receiving infliximab for 23 weeks. She had initially been given methotrexate and prednisone for 4 years. Then, because of lack of efficacy, infliximab was introduced. After three infusions of infliximab and only partial remission the dose was increased to 5 mg/kg, with success. However, before the sixth infusion she developed fever, polyarthralgia, myalgia, and general malaise. Serology excluded viral infection. Autoantibody assessment was positive, confirming the diagnosis of drug-induced lupus.

Infusion reactions

The overall incidence of infusion reactions to infliximab is about 5%. Of 82 children with Crohn's disease who received 432 infusions, 12 (5.3% of 432 infusions and 15% of 82 patients) had infusion reactions (117). Eight received a total of 47 infusions after an infusion reaction; in 11 instances (23%), infusion reactions recurred. Thus, re-exposure to infliximab after an infusion reaction increases the risk of a further infusion reaction, but does not require withdrawal of infliximab.

The characteristics of infusion reactions to infliximab, defined as adverse events that occur during or within 1–2 hours after infusion, have been studied in 113 patients (1183 infusions) with rheumatoid arthritis (118). Although the rate of reactions per infusion was 8.8%, 60 (53%) patients had at least one reaction during treatment. Nearly half of these reactions occurred during the third and fourth infusions. The symptoms consisted of pruritus, urticaria, and/or facial or generalized swelling in 3.8% of all infusions, cardiopulmonary manifestations (hypotension, hypertension, tachycardia, or shortness of breath) in 3%, and miscellaneous signs (headache, nausea, and/or vomiting) in 2%. There was no increase in the frequency of infusion reactions after the dose of infliximab was increased from 3 to 5 mg/kg. Most of these reactions resolved promptly after discontinuation of the infusion, either spontaneously or after symptomatic treatment, and none was sufficiently severe to require hospitalization. Only three patients had to discontinue infliximab treatment because of infusion reactions. There was no clear benefit from the prophylactic use of diphenhydramine, which may in fact have increased the frequency of adverse reactions.

Severe infusion reactions have been observed (119).

- A 53-year-old woman with a 13-year history of rheumatoid arthritis received infliximab 3 mg/kg for 9 months, with a 20% improvement. Infliximab was replaced by methotrexate 12 mg/week but was restarted about 2 years later. She developed a fever and skin rush 10 days after the first infusion, which responded to hydrocortisone 100 mg. Before the next infusion she was given an antihistmaine, olopatadine hydrochloride 10 mg/day. The infusion rate of infliximab was lowered to less than half of the usual rate during the next infusion, but 15 minutes after the infusion, she had a skin rash and pruritis, followed by dyspnea and a swollen throat. The infusion was immediately stopped and she was given 50% oxygen, and intravenous hydrocortisone 200 mg and methylprednisolone 125 mg. Her symptoms resolved completely within 2 hours.

- A 49-year-old woman with a 16-year history of rheumatoid arthritis received infliximab for 10 months and then methotrexate 10.5 mg/week; 2 years later she was switched to infliximab again. During the first infusion, her body temperature rose from 35.6°C to 37.6°C and then steadily fell to baseline after the end of treatment. There were no adverse events during the second and third infusions, but 10 minutes after the start of the fourth infusion she started to sweat and looked pale. Her systolic blood pressure fell from 150 to 78 mmHg, but her heart rate was unchanged. There were no skin lesions or laryngeal swelling. The infusion was immediately stopped. She was given intravenous hydrocortisone 100 mg and recovered.

The mechanisms of the reactions in these patients were unclear. Development of a human antichimeric antibody against infliximab has been speculated. Antichimeric antibody titers are often not measured when infliximab is given at intervals of 8 weeks or less, because the antibody is undetectable when infliximab is present in the serum. However, an antichimeric antibody was detected retrospectively in the serum of both patients immediately before infliximab was resumed.

Hypersensitivity reactions

Both acute and delayed hypersensitivity reactions to infliximab have been reported in clinical trials (SEDA-24, 439).

Immediate infusion reactions to infliximab are usually defined by any significant adverse effect that occurs during or within 1–2 hours after the infusion. The symptoms mostly consist of flushing, rash, shortness of breath, wheeze, hotness, chest pain, vomiting, and abdominal pain.

Delayed reactions are defined by the occurrence of arthralgia and joint stiffness (that is a serum sickness-like reaction) in the days after infliximab administration; they have mostly been observed in patients with Crohn's disease who have received episodic treatment. In one patient the complication was associated with acute respiratory distress syndrome, which only became evident 10 days after re-treatment (91).

Incidence

Immediate hypersensitivity reactions to infliximab occur in 6–19% of adults.

In a retrospective evaluation of 165 patients (479 infliximab infusions) with Crohn's disease, the overall incidence of infusion reactions was 6.1% (29 episodes; 120). Acute infusion reactions within 24 hours of infusion were the most frequent (26 episodes) and delayed infusion reactions from 1 to 14 days after treatment were noted in three instances only. Prophylaxis with diphenhydramine and paracetamol and the use of a test dose of infliximab allowed additional infusions without consequences in patients with mild or moderate previous acute infusion reactions. Three of the four patients who had acute severe reactions received the same prophylaxis plus corticosteroids before re-treatment: one had a similar severe acute reaction, while the other two had no recurrences. This study also suggested that acute infusion reactions are probably not IgE-mediated, as tryptase and IgE serum concentrations were not raised.

Of 86 patients with Crohn's disease receiving infliximab 14% of patients experienced severe systemic reactions, with a significant difference between adults (21%) and children (3%), the reason for which was unclear (121).

There were severe infusion reactions, defined by any significant change in vital signs or the development of chest pain, wheeze, dyspnea, vomiting, abdominal pain, or rash, in 16 of 100 patients with refractory Crohn's disease (122). Half of them occurred during the first infusion, and the rate of infusion reactions was similar in patients taking concurrent immunosuppressants or glucocorticoids compared with those who were not. One patient had anaphylactic shock, five had significant hypotension, six had acute pulmonary symptoms, two had pruritus, flushing, or rash, and one had vomiting. The final patient, who had a previous history of chronic pancreatitis, had acute pancreatitis within 1 hour of treatment.

Immediate hypersensitivity reactions

Acute hypersensitivity reactions can mimic an anaphylactic reaction, but specific IgE antibodies have not so far been identified. A dose-escalation protocol has been proposed to desensitize patients who have had acute systemic reactions (123), but this has not always been successful (124). Although most reported anaphylactic reactions to infliximab have been mild, severe reactions can occur.

- A 36-year-old man with Crohn's disease became refractory to standard anti-inflammatory treatment (glucocorticoids, mercaptopurine, methotrexate, ciclosporin, tacrolimus; 124). Remission over 8 months was achieved with a single infusion of infliximab. With the onset of relapse he was given another infusion of infliximab and had an anaphylactic-like reaction within 1 minute.
- A 35-year-old woman with known hypersensitivity to mesalazine had severe symptoms, namely chest pain, dyspnea, productive cough, skin rash, and hypotension, during a third infusion of infliximab, and died 6 hours later from refractory hypotension and respiratory failure (125). Specific IgE or human antichimeric antibodies were not checked.

- A 33-year-old man with a 3-year history of Crohn's disease had previously received a well-tolerated single infusion of infliximab. When, 14 months later, he received a second infusion for exacerbation of the disease he had no immediate adverse effects, but complained of myalgia, arthralgia, nausea, and vomiting 7 days later and received diphenhydramine. After 3 days he had dyspnea, fever, and chills. An open lung biopsy showed features of eosinophilic pneumonia and no infections or other obvious causes were found. He subsequently worsened and required intubation and mechanical ventilation for 13 days. He was given glucocorticoids and quadruple antituberculosis drug therapy and recovered completely within 2 months. Human antichimeric antibodies were raised (13 times normal).
- A 73-year-old woman had three separate episodes of vascular purpura (with leukocytoclastic vasculitis during the third episode) during each sequence of treatment with etanercept; she later developed similar cutaneous lesions after a third injection of infliximab (126).
- A macrophage activation syndrome was reported in a 15 year old boy with a 9-year history of systemic polyarthritis (127). Less than 24 hours after a second infusion of infliximab he developed a high fever, chills, a rash, general malaise, and raised ESR, C-reactive protein, and transaminases, and pancytopenia. He recovered after 3 pulses of methylprednisolone 30 mg/kg.

Delayed hypersensitivity reactions

Delayed hypersensitivity reactions were mostly observed in patients with Crohn's disease who received episodic treatment. In one patient, this complication was associated with acute respiratory distress syndrome, which became evident only 10 days after retreatment (91).

Of 40 patients who had received multiple doses of an investigational liquid formulation of infliximab 2–4 years before, 10 had a severe delayed hypersensitivity reaction within 3–12 days after the first or the second re-infusion (115). This reaction mostly included myalgia, rash, fever, polyarthralgia, and pruritus. Although the six patients tested were negative for antibodies to infliximab before re-infusion, these antibodies were consistently raised after the reaction.

Susceptibility factors

Susceptibility factors for the development of severe systemic reactions after infliximab retreatment have been analysed in 52 adults and 34 children with Crohn's disease (121). Acute severe systemic reactions were defined by symptoms of anaphylactic reactions that required pharmacological treatment, and delayed severe systemic reactions were defined by the occurrence of arthralgia and joint stiffness (that is serum sickness-like symptoms) requiring glucocorticoids in the days after infliximab retreatment. According to these definitions, severe systemic reactions developed in 14% of patients (four acute and eight delayed) during retreatment. They were significantly more frequent in adults than in children (21 versus 3%), and delayed systemic reactions were observed exclusively in adults. These reactions mostly occurred during

the second infusion of infliximab, and particularly when retreatment was distant from the first infusion, that is beyond a 20-week interval. This suggested a higher potential for delayed hypersensitivity reactions when repeated doses are given within a longer time interval, and led the authors to recommend multiple early infusions if future infliximab retreatment is anticipated.

In a retrospective review of 361 infliximab infusions in 57 children with inflammatory bowel disease there were 35 episodes of infusion reactions (128). Female sex, previous episodes of infusion reactions, and the use of immunosuppressive therapy for less than 4 months were significant predictors of subsequent infusion reactions.

Infection risk

See also Adalimumab and Etanercept

Infliximab can increase the susceptibility of patients to severe infections, and in particular opportunistic infections (SEDA-26, 402). In patients who received repeated infusions of infliximab, infections requiring antimicrobial treatment occurred in about 30% of patients and severe infections in 4% (89).

Infectious complications associated with infliximab include tuberculosis, listeriosis, invasive aspergillosis, cutaneous nocardiosis, fatal Streptococcus pneumoniae sepsis with necrotizing fasciitis, fatal group A beta-hemolytic streptococcus sepsis with necrotizing fasciitis, *Pneumocystis jiroveci* pneumonia, histoplasmosis, coccidioidomycosis, and systemic candidiasis (129,130). The reported rates of opportunistic infections implicate a higher risk among patients treated with infliximab than with etanercept. This difference might be explained by the more common concurrent use of methotrexate with infliximab in patients with rheumatoid arthritis.

Bacterial infections

Blockade of tumor necrosis factor alfa impairs resistance to infections with intracellular pathogens such as mycobacteria, *Pneumocystis jiroveci*, *Listeria monocytogenes*, and *Legionella pneumophila* (131,132). Severe streptococcal and staphylococcal infections have also been observed. Case reports with very severe or fatal outcomes have usually been reported in patients taking concomitant immunosuppressants and have included:

- necrotizing fasciitis due to streptococcal infection (133)
- septicemia due to *Staphylococcus aureus* (134)
- *Listeria monocytogenes* infection (135)
- disseminated tuberculosis (136)
- listeriosis (131).

The safety and efficacy of infliximab have been assessed in 40 patients with severe active spondylarthropathy in a double-blind, randomized, placebo-controlled trial (137). One 65-year-old patient improved but 3 weeks after the third infusion developed a systemic illness. He had enlarged mediastinal lymph nodes and nodular lesion of the liver and spleen. Biopsy of the mediastinal lymph nodes showed tuberculosis, which was confirmed by culture. He was treated and recovered slowly.

Mycobacterium tuberculosis

In 2001, the FDA reported 70 cases of tuberculosis among 147 000 patients treated with infliximab worldwide. This number increased to 117 within 2 months of the report. Tuberculosis associated with TNF-α antagonists has an unusual presentation; more than half of the cases had extrapulmonary disease and a quarter had disseminated disease (138). Etanercept is also associated with tuberculosis and has a similar atypical presentation, with extrapulmonary disease in more than 50% of cases. Adalimumab has also been associated with tuberculosis during clinical trials, predominantly at high doses.

- Miliary tuberculosis occurred in a 43-year-old man only 6 weeks after starting infliximab for pyoderma gangrenosum and despite negative pre-treatment screening for latent tuberculosis (139).

As this patient originated from a country in which tuberculosis is highly endemic and also received glucocorticoids, the authors questioned whether systematic prophylaxis should be proposed in such cases.

Reactivation of latent tuberculosis is a major concern with infliximab (SEDA-26, 402), and accounts for about one-third of infections in these patients. According to data from the manufacturers, 130 cases of active tuberculosis were notified up to October 2001. Many of the cases were disseminated or extrapulmonary tuberculosis, and several patients died. Several case reports have provided detailed information in at least seven other patients, including three who developed miliary tuberculosis and one who developed *Mycobacterium tuberculosis* enteritis (140–144). A detailed analysis of 70 cases of tuberculosis reported to the FDA has been published (145). Two-thirds of the cases were noted after three or fewer infusions and 57% of the patients had extrapulmonary disease. There were 64 cases from countries with a low incidence of tuberculosis. From these reports and the number of patients treated with infliximab, the estimated rate of tuberculosis in patients with rheumatoid arthritis treated with infliximab was four times higher than the background rate. Patients with evidence of active infection should not receive infliximab until the infection is under control; all should be screened for tuberculosis before starting infliximab (146). From these and other data it has been estimated that the risk of tuberculosis in the first year of infliximab treatment is 0.035 in US citizens and 0.2% in non-US citizens. Further investigations, such as a chest X-ray and a Mantoux test, and prophylactic treatment with isoniazid, will show whether the incidence can be reduced in patients taking anti-TNF treatment (147).

The incidence rate of tuberculosis varies considerably according to several factors, such as race and country. In a recent US survey, the estimated incidence of tuberculosis among 6460 patients treated with infliximab was 62 cases per 100 000 patients compared with 6.2 in patients with rheumatoid arthritis before the widespread use of infliximab (148). The four cases reported in this survey occurred in patients without complete screening or prophylaxis for tuberculosis.

In 107 patients (191 patient-years) treated with infliximab for spondylarthropathy, severe infections occurred in eight (149). In particular, two patients developed disseminated tuberculosis and three had severe retropharyngeal abscesses. The development of tuberculosis has also been studied in 1540 patients, 86% of whom received infliximab and 14% etanercept, in a Spanish national database established for the long-term surveillance of patients with rheumatic diseases and treated with biological response modifiers (150). Tuberculosis was reported in 17 patients treated with infliximab (no case with etanercept), including four who had negative tuberculin tests and normal chest X-rays before treatment. Most cases involved extrapulmonary sites of infection and were diagnosed within 3 months of treatment. Two patients died from their infections. The estimated incidence of tuberculosis associated with infliximab ranged from 1113 to 1893 cases per 100 000 patients in the first 2 years of surveillance. Accordingly, the risk ratio for tuberculosis in infliximab-treated patients was 53-90 compared with the background rate, and 12-20 compared with a cohort of rheumatoid arthritis patients not treated with infliximab. The authors mentioned only one additional case of tuberculosis during the 10 months after the establishment of guidelines and recommendations by health authorities, but such reassuring data should be confirmed by further studies. Indeed, there have been reports of reactivation of latent tuberculosis in two patients after isoniazid prophylaxis for 6 months, suggesting that more prolonged prophylactic treatment should be completed before starting infliximab (151,152).

Testing for tuberculosis with the purified protein derivative test should be completed before starting therapy with infliximab (Scheinfeld 280). Caution should be exercised when considering the use of infliximab or any TNF-alfa antagonists in patients with chronic infections, a history of recurrent or latent infections, or an underlying condition that may predispose them to infections (153).

In a multicenter trial in 70 patients with ankylosing spondylitis given infliximab, treatment had to be withdrawn in three patients because of systemic tuberculosis, allergic granulomatosis of the lung, or mild leukopenia; after withdrawal all three recovered (32). However, the allergic granulomatosis of the lung was probably due to a hypersensitivity reaction.

Other bacterial organisms

There have been reports of severe opportunistic bacterial infections, including disseminated or cutaneous *Nocardia* infection (154,155), *Legionella pneumophila* pneumonia (156,157,158), and *Listeria monocytogenes* meningitis (159). In three of these six patients, the infection occurred only after the second or third infusion of infliximab, and infliximab was later restarted uneventfully in two cases. Although the incidence of listeriosis is probably very low, there was one case of life-threatening *Listeria meningitis* pneumonia in a population-based cohort study of 217 patients treated with infliximab for inflammatory bowel disease (160).

- Disseminated *Salmonella typhimurium* infection occurred after 28 weeks of infliximab and methotrexate treatment in a 29-year-old man with psoriatic arthropathy (161).
- *Moraxella catarrhalis* septic arthritis occurred 1 month after a fourth infusion of infliximab in a 45-year-old man with undifferentiated spondyloarthritis (162). He was taking no other immunosuppressive drugs at the time of diagnosis.
- Fatal staphylococcal sepsis due to adult respiratory distress syndrome has been reported in a 40-year-old woman after a sixth infusion of infliximab for Crohn's disease (163).
- An 18 year old man had Behçet's syndrome inadequately controlled by various immunosuppressive drugs (164). Mycophenolate mofetil was combined with infliximab 3 mg/kg at 0, 2, and 6 weeks. After the third infusion of infliximab, atraumatic pain and swelling of the right upper arm persisted for 3 days. An anechoic collection near the biceps muscle was detected by ultrasound and 2 ml of pus was aspirated, from which *Staphylococcus aureus* was isolated. The diagnosis was pyomyositis and infliximab was withdrawn. He recovered with flucloxacillin and gentamicin.
- A 40-year-old Caucasian man with rheumatoid arthritis received infliximab and 40 days after the tenth dose developed an acutely swollen, painful, erythematous left knee (165). Direct Gram stain showed Gram-negative pleomorphic coccobacilli in pairs or groups. The synovial fluid culture yielded a slow-growing Gram-negative coccobacillus, with pink pigmented mucoid colonies. The PCR product was sequenced as a strain of *Roseomonas mucosa*.
- A 42-year-old man with a 13-year history of ankylosing spondylitis was enrolled in a randomized controlled trial of the efficacy of infliximab. After four doses he developed an orbital cellulitis. Culture of a swab from the left eye grew a flucloxacillin-sensitive *Staphylococcus aureus* (166).
- An 11-year-old boy with Crohn's disease received infliximab and 3 days later developed fever, signs of cardiac failure, and *S. aureus* sepsis (167). At surgery an intramyocardial para-aortic abscess with destruction of the aortic valve was found, suggesting chronic infection, possibly activated by the use of infliximab.

Crohn's disease can lead to vasculitic changes of the aorta, which may have favored the development of the intramyocardial abscess in this case. The size of the abscess suggested persistence for several weeks.

Severe necrotizing fasciitis has been reported in a patient who was given infliximab (133).

- A 54-year-old man with rheumatoid arthritis for 12 years was given infliximab, with remission. He then developed a painful, confluent, erythematous, pustular rash over his trunk and limbs. Skin biopsy showed an acute pustular dermatitis. Five hours later he collapsed with a tachycardia (140/minute) and a blood pressure of 120/70 mmHg. He was apyrexial. His left leg was very tense, painful, and swollen, and he had a disseminated intravascular coagulopathy. There was marked necrosis

of his adductor compartment and fascia of his left thigh and necrotic muscles were debrided. Blood cultures and skin swabs grew group A hemolytic streptococci. He then became unstable and died, despite efforts at resuscitation.

Viral infections

Infliximab can compromise antiviral defence mechanisms. There have been detailed reports of cytomegalovirus retinitis (168) and life-threatening disseminated cytomegalovirus infection (169). Most of these patients were taking concomitant immunosuppressants at the time of diagnosis.

Cases of viral infections with TNF alfa antagonists are occasionally reported., including *Varicella* infection in a 45-year-old man (170) and disseminated *Herpes simplex* infection associated with the macrophage activation syndrome in an 8-year old girl (171).

The risk of infliximab treatment in carriers of hepatitis B surface antigen is also of concern, and there have been reports of hepatitis B reactivation in a chronic carrier (172), and fulminant hepatitis in a patient with a positive hepatitis B virus surface antigen before infliximab treatment (173). By contrast, infliximab or etanercept did not produce deleterious effects on liver function or viremia in 24 patients with hepatitis C virus infection (174).

In 500 consecutive patients treated with infliximab for Crohn's disease, viral infections were noted during the first six infusions in six patients and consisted of varicella zoster virus infections in three (primary varicella in one), genital *Herpes simplex* virus infection, infectious mononucleosis due to Epstein–Barr virus, or severe gastroenteritis (one case each) (18).

- Disseminated primary varicella infection with a fatal outcome has been reported 9 days after a first infusion of infliximab in a 26-year-old man who was also taking 6-mercaptopurine, glucocorticoids, and mesalazine for Crohn's disease (175).
- Genital condylomata acuminata occurred after a second dose of infliximab for Crohn's disease in a 23-year-old man who was also taking glucocorticoids and azathioprine (176).

In contrast to these reports, one study suggested that infliximab did not increase the load of Epstein–Barr virus in the short-term in patients with Crohn's disease (177).

- A 67-year-old woman with a 5-year history of rheumatoid arthritis, who had taken prednisone and methotrexate, was given infliximab (178). Her rheumatoid arthritis improved, but she developed multiple bilateral lesions of molluscum contagiosum on the upper and lower eyelids, despite normal CD4 and CD8 counts. She had had similar lesions during a previous course of infliximab. Excision biopsy confirmed the diagnosis.

Protozoal infections

There has been a detailed report of *P. jiroveci* pneumonia (179).

Two other cases have been reported (180,181), one of whom, aged 59 years, was also taking prednisone 40 mg/day, subsequently developed oral candidiasis and invasive aspergillosis. He died from progressive multiorgan failure. As he also had a low CD4 count, the authors wondered whether infliximab may have contributed to this anomaly.

In 217 patients treated with infliximab for inflammatory bowel disease, fatal *Pneumocystis jiroveci* pneumonia was noted once (19).

Fungal infections

In a review of 10 cases of histoplasmosis in patients treated with infliximab ($n = 9$) or etanercept ($n = 1$) the infection occurred within 1 week to 6 months after the first dose (182). Of these 10 patients, nine required treatment in an intensive care unit and one died. All lived in regions in which histoplasmosis was endemic. It was not possible to determine which patients had new infections or reactivation of previous infections.

In 41 patients with rheumatic disease who received a total of 300 infusions of infliximab over 9 months there were severe adverse effects in 15%, one of which was a case of histoplasmosis (183).

- A 28-year-old woman with unresponsive rheumatic disease developed histoplasmosis after a second infusion of infliximab. She had pet birds, and the authors thought that she had had reactivation of an infection rather than a new infection.

There have been other reports of histoplasmosis (184), invasive pulmonary aspergillosis (185), extensive pulmonary coccidioidomycosis (186), and one case of *Cryptococcus neoformans* pneumonia due to possible zoonotic transmission from a pet cockatiel (187).

Death

On the basis of so-called spontaneous capture, the Paul Ehrlich Institute was notified of 44 adverse drug reactions leading to the death of the patient after the use of infliximab in Germany (5). Sepsis or serious infections was reported in 24. According to the manufacturer, 20 000 patients have been treated in Germany with infliximab.

Health Canada received a total of 697 reports of suspected adverse reactions to infliximab over a $4\frac{1}{2}$ year period (188). Of these, 132 (19%) reports were considered serious and 14 (2%) resulted in death.

- A 64-year-old man without heart failure was found dead 18 hours after a single infusion of infliximab for rheumatoid arthritis (189). No obvious cause was found at autopsy, except that the patient was known to have had frequent intervention by a pacemaker that had been implanted for several years.

Long-Term Effects

Tumorigenicity

There is great concern about the potential development of malignancy after blockade of tumor necrosis factor alfa, and it is biologically plausible. However, it is unclear whether this is a drug-related or a disease-related phenomenon.

There have been several cases of lymphoproliferative disease (B cell non-Hodgkin's lymphoma and nodular sclerosing Hodgkin's disease) in the 9 months after infliximab infusion in patients with Crohn's disease (190). The FDA received reports of 26 cases of lymphoproliferative disorders in patients treated with etanercept ($n = 18$) or infliximab ($n = 8$) over 20 months (191). Although this reporting rate does not exceed the age-adjusted incidence of lymphomas in the USA, spontaneous reporting underestimates the true incidence. In addition, several findings were similar to those reported in patients taking immunosuppressive drugs after transplantation. For example, 81% of the reported cases were non-Hodgkin's lymphomas. Also, the median time to occurrence after the start of anti-TNF-alfa treatment was only 8 weeks. Finally, lymphoma regressed in two patients after withdrawal and without specific cytotoxic therapy. Although the actual incidence of neoplasia was low, additional long-term data that take into account concomitant or previous immunosuppressive treatment are needed before firm conclusions can be reached.

- A 47 year old man with erythrodermic psoriasis was treated with phototherapy, which was ineffective, and methotrexate 10 mg/week, which was withdrawn because of severe cytolytic hepatitis after the third dose (192). Ciclosporin 5 mg/kg, which he had taken for 5 years, was withdrawn because of renal impairment. Mycophenolate mofetil 2 mg/day over 6 weeks was ineffective. He was given infliximab 6 mg/kg at 0, 2, 6, 7 and 10 weeks and ciclosporin was reintroduced 3 months later. After 3 weeks, he developed a CD30+ T cell lymphoma. Epstein-Barr virus was negative. Ciclosporin was withdrawn and within 4 weeks the tumor regressed.

The authors cited a total of nine cases of lymphoid proliferation associated with TNF alfa therapies. Because of the short delay between ciclosporin reintroduction and the development of the tumor, infliximab was directly implicated as a co-factor that might have accelerated the development of the lymphoma.

The potential risk of lymphoma in patients treated with TNF-alfa antagonists has been discussed (193). Whether these agents are independently associated with an increased risk of lymphoma continues to be debated (194). This issue was analysed in two large cohorts of rheumatoid arthritis patients. From the data registered in the South Swedish Arthritis Treatment Group, which covered over 90% of arthritic patients treated with anti-TNF-alfa drugs in this area of Sweden, there were 11 cases of tumors and five of lymphomas among 757 patients treated with etanercept or infliximab (1603 person-years of risk) (195). Although there was no increase in the overall risk of total tumors, the relative risk of lymphoma was 11 times higher than that expected in the background population. More importantly, a direct comparison showed that the relative risk of lymphoma was five times higher in patients treated with anti-TNF-alfa drugs than in a community-based control group of 800 patients treated with conventional antirheumatic drugs and never exposed to biological agents. This difference persisted after adjustment with the Health Assessment Questionnaire, used as a marker of disease severity. The other cohort consisted of 18 572 patients and included 29 cases of lymphoma, with a standardized incidence ratio of 2.6 for infliximab, 3.8 for etanercept, 1.7 for methotrexate, and 1.0 for patients not receiving methotrexate or anti-TNF-alfa agents (196). Although both studies suggested an increased rate of lymphoma in patients treated with infliximab or etanercept, these results should be interpreted with caution, because of the very small number of cases and a possible role of higher disease activity in these patients.

Because of two additional case report of lymphoma and a brief review of 33 previously published cases with infliximab, the presence of Epstein–Barr virus infection was sought in four patients and was positive in three (197,198). Owing to the growing number of infections being reported in patients treated with anti-TNF-alfa drugs, triggering of Epstein–Barr virus-associated lymphoma by TNF-alfa antagonists should be considered. This is supported by the relatively short time interval between the start of treatment and the diagnosis of lymphoma in most reported cases.

Other reports of cancer putatively attributed to infliximab include one case of multiple keratoacanthomata and squamous cell cancers in a 76-year-old woman with a history of sun exposure and multiple non-melanoma skin cancers (199), a cutaneous T cell lymphoma in a 69-year-old man, and a systemic T cell lymphoma in an 81-year-old woman (200). The involvement of infliximab was suggested by rapid development of the cancer after starting infliximab and/or an aggressive course of disease in both of the patients with T cell lymphomas.

Since 2000, ADRAC has received 319 reports involving infliximab, etanercept, and adalimumab (201). The more serious reports were as follows: malignant melanoma (3 reports), tuberculosis (n = 4), lymphoma (n = 5), anaphylaxis (n = 9), sepsis (n = 10), lupus or lupus-like syndrome (n = 22), and pneumonia/lower respiratory tract infections (n = 23). The Australian Product Information has advised caution when considering these drugs in patients with a history of malignancy, or when considering continued treatment in those who develop a malignancy.

The extent to which TNF-α inhibitors increase the risk of serious malignancies has been assessed in patients with rheumatoid arthritis by meta-analysis to derive estimates of sparse harmful events occurring in randomized trials of TNF-α antagonists. From a systematic literature search (EMBASE, MEDLINE, Cochrane Library, and electronic abstract databases, annual scientific meetings of both the European League Against Rheumatism and the American College of Rheumatology, interviews of the manufacturers of the two licensed anti-TNF antibodies, and randomized placebo-controlled trials of infliximab and adalimumab), nine trials met the inclusion criteria; 3493 patients received anti-TNF antibody treatment and 1512 patients received placebo (202). The pooled odds ratio for malignancy was 3.3 (95% CI = 1.2, 9.1). Malignancies were significantly more common in

patients taking higher doses than in patients who received lower doses of TNF-α antibody antagonists. For patients treated with TNF-α antagonists in the included trials, the number needed to treat for harm (NNT$_H$) was 154 (95% CI = 91, 500) for one additional malignancy during 6–12 months.

In a multicenter matched-pairs study, the frequency of a new diagnosis of neoplasia in 404 patients with Crohn's disease receiving infliximab was comparable with 404 who had never received infliximab (203). There were nine patients with neoplasia (2.22%; one cholangiocarcinoma, three breast cancers, one skin cancer, one leukemia, one laryngeal cancer, and two anal carcinomas) among the former, compared with seven (1.73%; three intestinal adenocarcinomas, one basalioma, one spinalioma, one non-Hodgkin's lymphoma, and one breast cancer) among the latter.

.An unusual hepatocellular carcinoma and focal hepatic glycogenosis occurring in a non-cirrhotic patient with Crohn's disease who had received both azathioprine and infliximab (204). Whether infliximab directly or indirectly enhanced susceptibility to the development of hepatocellular carcinoma in this patient is not known.

Second-Generation Effects

Pregnancy

Of 131 pregnancies reported to a voluntary registry of adverse events during clinical trials, outcome data were available for 96 (191). There were live births in 67%, miscarriages in 15%, and therapeutic termination in 19%. These results are similar to those expected for the general population of pregnant women or pregnant women with Crohn's disease not exposed to infliximab. There was no increased risk of adverse outcomes.

Teratogenicity

The outcome of pregnancy after maternal exposure to infliximab immediately before conception or early in pregnancy has been detailed in two patients. One had a healthy baby (205) and the other, who had active disease and other drug exposure, delivered an extremely premature infant, who died 3 days later from intracerebral and intrapulmonary bleeding (206). In a brief report, the manufacturer mentioned 35 pregnancies with exposure to infliximab before and during pregnancy (207). There were miscarriages in five pregnancies, termination of pregnancy in four, and live births in 26; one infant had tetralogy of Fallot and one neonate died. However, the exact time of exposure was known in only 20 patients, and it occurred during the first trimester in 14. The data are therefore still insufficient to estimate the risk of inadvertent infliximab exposure during pregnancy.

The results of the manufacturer's post-marketing surveillance database, which included infliximab exposure before or during pregnancy, have been made available (191). Of 96 pregnancies with a prospectively documented outcome, exposure occurred exclusively before pregnancy in 32 patients or during the first trimester in 58. The time course of exposure was unknown in six. There were 63 live births (67 neonates), one preterm infant who died shortly after birth, 14 miscarriages, and 18 terminations of pregnancy. Three neonates had a congenital anomaly: tetralogy of Fallot, intestinal malrotation with a concomitant exposure to leflunomide, and hypothyroidism with delayed development. Follow-up of pregnancies after paternal exposure was also documented in 10 patients: there were nine healthy live births, and one miscarriage. There were no differences in outcome after maternal infliximab exposure compared with the general population of pregnant women or a historical cohort of patients with Crohn's disease. However, there were several limitations to this study, such as spontaneous reporting, lack of standardization of outcome ascertainment, a high rate of loss to follow-up, and the small number of patients exposed during the first trimester of pregnancy.

Susceptibility Factors

Genetic

Genetic studies have identified potential predictors of the response to infliximab. A –308 polymorphism in the promoter of the TNF alfa gene influences TNF alfa transcription. The association between the response to infliximab and the polymorphism in the TNF region at the lymphotoxin A locus is controversial. Allelic and genotype frequencies for the –308 TNF gene polymorphism have not been shown to be significantly different between responders and non-responders to infliximab, but non-responders tended to have a higher frequency of the rare TNF2 allele, which has been associated with increased production of TNF.

The NOD2 (or NOD2/CARD15) gene has recently been identified as a Crohn's disease susceptibility gene, and mutations in NOD2/CARD15 are associated with Crohn's disease. However, the hypothesis that mutations in NOD2/CARD15 indirectly alter TNF production and thereby influence differences in response to infliximab has not been substantiated.

The IgG Fc receptor gene, FCGR3A, encodes FcgRIIIa receptors expressed on macrophages and natural killer cells, and polymorphism in this gene is associated with varying affinity for IgG1 and potency in antibody-dependent cellular cytotoxicity, which has been implicated as one mechanism of action of infliximab in Crohn's disease. Therefore, polymorphism in FCGR3A has been suggested to predict the response to infliximab, which is an IgG1 antibody. Individuals with the FCGR3A genotype that is associated with a high affinity for IgG1 were more likely to have a biological and possibly a clinical response to infliximab (6).

Age

Special attention has been paid to the safety of infliximab and etanercept in children with juvenile idiopathic arthritis, in particular as regards to the possible risk of autoimmune disease and severe infectious disease, such as varicella zoster virus infection or tuberculosis (208). Whereas there were no cases of demyelination or lupus in these children, there were two cases of type I diabetes mellitus after etanercept treatment. A genetic predisposition was likely, but accelerated development of diabetes should be also considered, as suggested by experimental data that suggest an important role of TNF suppression in the progression of diabetes.

Older age was associated with reduced response to infliximab in patients with Crohn's disease in a European multicenter study, but a clear correlation between age and response could not be confirmed by other studies in the USA and UK (66). It is not clear why younger patients have a better response to infliximab.

Surgery

Severe postoperative complications in patients who have received infliximab before surgery have sometimes been mentioned in clinical trials or cohort studies. To assess this issue the rate of early and late (up to 3 months) major or minor surgical complications was retrospectively evaluated in patients treated with infliximab for Crohn's disease and compared with similar patients who had never received infliximab (208). Postoperative complications were not more frequent (19 complications) among 40 patients who received infliximab before intestinal resectional surgery compared with 15 complications in 39 patients who did not receive infliximab and who underwent similar surgery. The mean duration of hospital stay was similar in the two groups. The non significant increase in the early infection rate observed with infliximab (six cases versus one) was attributed to more frequent use of other immunosuppressive drugs in these patients.

Drug Administration

Drug dosage regimens

In carefully selected patients, infliximab infusion administered at home is safe and cost-effective. Infliximab infusion was performed at home in 10 children, who received 59 infusions of 7.5–10 mg/kg/dose. The calculated average savings per patient were $1335/100 mg infliximab (209). Home infusions lasted 2–5 hours. Infusions could be performed on any day of the week, and school absenteeism was reduced. The average patient satisfaction rating for home infusions was 9 on a scale from 1 to 10 (10 = most satisfied). Three patients had difficulty with intravenous access and required multiple attempts, but all were able to receive their infusions. One infusion was stopped because of arm pain above the infusion site. This patient had his next infusion in the hospital before returning to the home infusion program. There were no severe adverse events (palpitation, blood pressure instability, hyperemia, respiratory symptoms) during home infusion.

Drug-Drug Interactions

Azathioprine

Data from a study in 32 patients treated with azathioprine for Crohn's disease showed a significant increase in thioguanine nucleotide concentrations within 1-3 weeks after the first infusion of infliximab, suggesting an interaction between the two drugs (211). There were also a significant reduction in leukocyte count and a significant association between the increase in thioguanine nucleotide concentrations and the clinical response to infliximab. Whether these findings will also translate into an increased risk of azathioprine adverse effects has not been specifically investigated.

Drug-Smoking Interactions

A negative affect of smoking on the response to infliximab therapy has been reported in two studies from the USA and UK (66). Smokers with Crohn's disease had lower response rates to infliximab than non-smokers (22% versus 73%) and were more likely to relapse within 1 year of therapy. However, a large European study failed to confirm this association

References

1. Bell S, Kamm MA. Antibodies to tumour necrosis factor alpha as treatment for Crohn's disease. Lancet 2000;355(9207):858–60.
2. Wall GC, Heyneman C, Pfanner TP. Medical options for treating Crohn's disease in adults: focus on antitumor necrosis factor-alpha chimeric monoclonal antibody. Pharmacotherapy 1999;19(10):1138–52.
3. Maini R, St Clair EW, Breedveld F, Furst D, Kalden J, Weisman M, Smolen J, Emery P, Harriman G, Feldmann M, Lipsky P. Infliximab (chimeric anti-tumour necrosis factor alpha monoclonal antibody) versus placebo in rheumatoid arthritis patients receiving concomitant methotrexate: a randomised phase III trial. ATTRACT Study Group. Lancet 1999;354(9194):1932–9.
4. Keeling S, Oswald A, Russell AS, Maksymowych WP. Prospective observational analysis of the efficacy and safety of low-dose (3 mg/kg) infliximab in ankylosing spondylitis: 4-year follow up J Rheumatol 2006;33(3):558–61.
5. Andus T, Stange EF, Hoffler D, Keller-Stanislawski B. Suspected cases of severe side effects after infliximab (Remicade) in Germany. Med Klin (Munich) 2003;98:429–36.
6. Su C, Lichtenstein GR. Are there predictors of Remicade treatment success or failure? Adv Drug Deliv Rev 2005;57(2):237–45.
7. Bickston SJ, Lichtenstein GR, Arseneau KO, Cohen RB, Cominelli F. The relationship between infliximab treatment and lymphoma in Crohn's disease. Gastroenterology 1999;117(6):1433–7.
8. Morelli J, Wilson FA. Does administration of infliximab increase susceptibility to listeriosis? Am J Gastroenterol 2000;95(3):841–2.
9. Mikuls TR, Moreland LW. Benefit-risk assessment of infliximab in the treatment of rheumatoid arthritis. Drug Saf 2003;26:23–32.
10. Anonymous. Infliximab. Label to reflect haematological and neurological events. WHO Pharmaceutical Newslett 2004;5:2.
11. Gottlieb A, Chaudhari U, Mulcahy L, Li S, Dooley L, Baker D. Infliximab monotherapy provides rapid and sustained benefit for plaque type psoriasis. J Am Acad Dermatol 2003;48:829–35.
12. Drosou A, Kirsner R, Welsh E, Sullivan T, Kerdel F. Use of infliximab, an anti-tumor necrosis alpha antibody, for inflammatory dermatoses. J Cutan Med Surg 2003;7:382–86.
13. Sullivan T, Welsh E, Kerdel F, Burdick A, Kirsner R. Infliximab for hidradenitis suppurativa. Br J Dermatol 2003;149:1046–9.
14. Cabou C, Bagheri H, Cantagrel A, Mazieres B, Montastruc JL. Retrospective analysis of adverse effects of infliximab in a hospital rheumatology service. Therapie 2003;58:457–62.
15. Mookerjee RP, Sen S, Davies NA, Hodges SJ, Williams R, Jalan R. Tumour necrosis factor alpha is an important mediator of portal and systemic haemodynamic derangements in alcoholic hepatitis. Gut 2003;52:1182–7.
16. Suhler EB, Smith JR, Wertheim MS, Lauer AK, Kurz DE, Pickard TD, Rosenbaum JT. A prospective trial of infliximab therapy for refractory uveitis: preliminary safety and efficacy outcomes. Arch Ophthalmol 2005;123(7):903–12.
17. Oka H, Nishioka K, Togo M, Ochi T. The efficacy of infliximab for patients with rheumatoid arthritis in Japan: results of 5000 cases by post-marketing surveillance data. APLAR J Rheumatol 2006;9(2):142–5.
18. Colombel JF, Loftus EV Jr, Tremaine WJ, Egan LJ, Harmsen WS, Schleck CD, Zinsmeister AR, Sandborn WJ. The safety profile of infliximab in patients with Crohn's disease: the Mayo clinic experience in 500 patients. Gastroenterology 2004;126:19–31.
19. Ljung T, Karlen P, Schmidt D, Hellström PM, Lapidus A, Janczewska I, Sjöqvist U, Lofberg R. Infliximab in inflammatory bowel disease:clinical outcome in a population based cohort from Stockholm County. Gut 2004;53:849–53.
20. Seiderer J, Goke B, Ochsenkuhn T. Safety aspects of infliximab in inflammatory bowel disease patients. A retrospective cohort study in 100 patients of a German University Hospital. Digestion 2004;70:3–9.
21. Kinney T, Rawlins M, Kozarek R, France R, Patterson D. Immunomodulators and "on demand" therapy with infliximab in Crohn's disease: clinical experience with 400 infusions. Am J Gastroenterol 2003;98:608–12.
22. Weisman MH. What are the risks of biologic therapy in rheumatoid arthritis? An update on safety. J Rheumatol Suppl 2002;65:33–8.
23. Eklund KK, Peltomaa R, Leirisalo-Repo M. Occurrence of pulmonary thromboembolism during infliximab therapy. Clin Exp Rheumatol 2003;21:679.
24. Puli SR, Benage DD. Retinal vein thrombosis after infliximab (Remicade) treatment for Crohn's disease. Am J Gastroenterol 2003;98:939–40.
25. Grange L, Nissen MJ, Garambois K, Dumolard A, Duc C, Gaudin P, Juvin R. Infliximab-induced cerebral thrombophlebitis. Rheumatology 2005;44:260–1.
26. Ryan BM, Romberg M, Wolters F, Stockbrugger RW. Extensive forearm deep venous thrombosis following a severe infliximab infusion reaction. Eur J Gastroenterol Hepatol 2004;16:941–2.
27. Settergren M, Tornvall P. Does TNF-alpha blockade cause plaque rupture? Atherosclerosis 2004;173:149.
28. Shoukeir H, Awaida R, Gupta K, Kodsi R, Oswaldo B, Scileppi T, Tenner S. Myocardial infarction precipitated by infliximab infusion: report of case. Am J Gastroenterol 2004;Suppl:S165.
29. Sobkeng Goufack E, Mammou S, Scotto B, De Muret A, Maakaroun A, Socie G, Bacq Y. Thrombose des veines hépatiques au cours d'un traitement par infliximab (Remicade®) révélant une hémoglobinurie paroxystique nocturne. Gastroenterol Clin Biol 2004;28:596–9.

30. Cambien B, Bergmeier W, Saffaripour S, Mitchell HA, Wagner DD. Antithrombotic activity of TNF-alpha. J Clin Invest 2003;112:1589–96.

31. Gonzalez-Juanatey C, Testa A, Garcia-Castelo A, Garcia-Porrua C, Llorca J, Gonzalez-Gay MA. Active but transient improvement of endothelial function in rheumatoid arthritis patients undergoing long-term treatment with anti-tumor necrosis factor alpha antibody. Arthritis Rheum 2004;51:447–50.

32. Braun J, Brandt J, Listing J, Zink A, Alten R, Golder W, Gromnica-Ihle E, Kellner H, Krause A, Schneider M, Sorensen H, Zeidler H, Thriene W, Sieper J. Treatment of active ankylosing spondylitis with infliximab: a randomised controlled multicentre trial. Lancet 2002;359(9313):1187–93.

33. Baig I, Storch I, Katz S. Infliximab induced eosinophilic pleural effusion in inflammatory bowel disease. Am J Gastroenterol 2002;97(Suppl):177.

34. Weatherhead M, Masson S, Bourke SJ, Gunn MC, Burns GP. Interstitial pneumonitis after infliximab therapy for Crohn's disease. Inflamm Bowel Dis 2006;12(5):427–8.

35. Mori S, Imamura F, Kiyofuji C, Sugimoto M. Development of interstitial pneumonia in a rheumatoid arthritis patient treated with infliximab, an anti-tumor necrosis factor alpha-neutralizing antibody. Modern Rheumatol 2006;16:251–5.

36. Courtney PA, Alderdice J, Whitehead EM. Comment on methotrexate pneumonitis after initiation of infliximab therapy for rheumatoid arthritis. Arthritis Rheum 2003;49:617.

37. Kramer N, Chuzhin Y, Kaufman LD, Ritter JM, Rosenstein ED. Methotrexate pneumonitis after initiation of infliximab therapy for rheumatoid arthritis. Arthritis Rheum 2002;47:670–1.

38. Ostor AJ, Crisp AJ, Somerville MF, Scott DG. Fatal exacerbation of rheumatoid arthritis associated fibrosing alveolitis in patients given infliximab. BMJ 2004;329:1266.

39. Vesga L, Ghassemi K, Terdiman JP, Mahadevan U. Hypersensitivity pneumonitits associated with infliximab therapy. Am J Gastroenterol. 2004;99(Suppl):abstract 686.

40. Chatterjee S. Severe interstitial pneumonitis associated with infliximab therapy. Scand J Rheumatol 2004;33:276–7.

41. Panagi S, Palka W, Korelitz BI, Taskin M, Lessnau KD. Diffuse alveolar hemorrhage after infliximab treatment of Crohn's disease. Inflamm Bowel Dis 2004;10:274–7.

42. Zamarron C, Maceiras F, Gonzalez J, Gomez-Reino JJ. Worsening of obstructive sleep apnoeas in a patient with rheumatoid arthritis treated with anti-tumor necrosis factor. Respir Med 2004;98:123–5.

43. Marotte H, Charrin JE, Miossec P. Infliximab-induced aseptic meningitis. Lancet 2001;358(9295):1784.

44. Mohan N, Edwards ET, Cupps TR, Oliverio PJ, Sandberg G, Crayton H, Richert JR, Siegel JN. Demyelination occurring during anti-tumor necrosis factor alpha therapy for inflammatory arthritides. Arthritis Rheum 2001;44(12):2862–9.

45. Robinson WH, Genovese MC, Moreland LW. Demyelinating and neurologic events reported in association with tumor necrosis factor alpha antagonism: by what mechanisms could tumor necrosis factor alpha antagonists improve rheumatoid arthritis but exacerbate multiple sclerosis? Arthritis Rheum 2001;44(9):1977–83.

46. Thomas CW Jr, Weinshenker BG, Sandborn WJ. Demyelination during anti-tumor necrosis factor alpha therapy with infliximab for Crohn's disease. Inflamm Bowel Dis 2004;10:28–31.

47. Mejico LJ. Infliximab-associated retrobulbar optic neuritis. Arch Ophthalmol 2004;122:793–4.

48. Magnano MD, Robinson WH, Genovese MC. Demyelination and inhibition of tumor necrosis factor (TNF). Clin Exp Rheumatol 2004;22(Suppl 35):S134-40.

49. Hrycaj P, Korczowska I, Lacki JK. Severe Parkinson's disease in rheumatoid arthritis patient treated with infliximab. Rheumatology 2003;42:702–3.

50. Singer OC, Otto B, Steinmetz H, Ziemann U. Acute neuropathy with multiple conduction blocks after TNFalpha monoclonal antibody therapy. Neurology 2004;63:1754.

51. Rodriguez-Escalera C, Belzunegui J, Lopez-Dominguez L, Gonzalez C, Figueroa M. Multifocal motor neuropathy with conduction block in a patient with rheumatoid arthritis on infliximab therapy. Rheumatology 2005;44:132–3.

52. Richette P, Dieude P, Damiano J, Liote F, Orcel P, Bardin T. Sensory neuropathy revealing necrotizing vasculitis during infliximab therapy for rheumatoid arthritis. J Rheumatol 2004;31:2079–81.

53. In-Sook JS, Baer AN, Kwon HJ, Papadopoulos EJ, Siegel JN. Guillain–Barré and Miller Fisher syndromes occurring with tumor necrosis factor alpha antagonist therapy. Arthritis Rheum 2006;54(5):1429–34.

54. Sakaura H, Hosono N, Mukai Y, Fujii R, Yoshikawa H. Paraparesis due to exacerbation of preexisting spinal pseudoarthrosis following infliximab therapy for advanced ankylosing spondylitis. Spine J 2006;6(3):325–9.

55. Farukhi FI, Bollinger K, Ruggieri P, Lee MS. Infliximab-associated third nerve palsy. Arch Ophthalmol 2006;124:1055–7.

56. ten Tusscher MP, Jacobs PJ, Busch MJ, de Graaf L, Diemont WL. Bilateral anterior toxic optic neuropathy and the use of infliximab. BMJ 2003;326(7389):579.

57. Foroozan R, Buono LM, Sergott RC, Savino PJ. Retrobulbar optic neuritis associated with infliximab. Arch Ophthalmol 2002;120(7):985–7.

58. Roblin X, Oltean P, Heluwaert F, Bonaz B. Panic attack with suicide: an exceptional adverse effect of infliximab. Dig Dis Sci 2006;51(6):1056.

59. Franchimont D, Roland S, Gustot T, Quertinmont E, Toubouti Y, Gervy MC, Deviere J, Van Gossum A. Impact of infliximab on serum leptin levels in patients with Crohn's disease. J Clin Endocrinol Metab 2005;90(6):3510–6.

60. D'Alessandro G, Bianco MR, Politis S, Ferrandina C, Rossi G, Altomare E. Anemia refrattaria con eccesso di blasti (AREB) in paziente con artrite reumatoide in trattamento con methotrexate ed infliximab: descrizione di un caso clinico. [Refractory anemia with excess blasts (RAEB) in a patient with rheumatoid arthritis treated with methotrexate and infliximab.] Reumatismo 2006;58(1):59–61.

61. Menon Y, Cucurull E, Espinoza LR. Pancytopenia in a patient with scleroderma treated with infliximab. Rheumatology 2003;42:1273–4.

62. Vidal F, Fontova R, Richart C. Severe neutropenia and thrombocytopenia associated with infliximab. Ann Intern Med 2003;139:238–9.

63. Marchesoni A, Arreghini M, Panni B, Battafarano N, Uziel L. Life-threatening reversible bone marrow toxicity in a rheumatoid arthritis patient switched from leflunomide to infliximab. Rheumatology 2003;42:193–4.

64. Aouba A, De Bandt M, Aslangul E, Atkhen N, Patri B. Haemophagocytic syndrome in a rheumatoid arthritis patient treated with infliximab. Rheumatol (Oxf) 2003;42:800–2.

65. Yee AM, Pochapin MB. Treatment of complicated sarcoidosis with infliximab anti-tumor necrosis factor-alpha therapy. Ann Intern Med 2001;135(1):27–31.

66. Menghini VV, Arora AS. Infliximab-associated reversible cholestatic liver disease. Mayo Clin Proc 2001;76(1):84–6.

67. Ierardi E, Della Valle N, Cosimo N, M De Francesco, Stoppino V, Panella Carmine G. Onset of liver damage after a single administration of infliximab in a patient with refractory ulcerative colitis. Clin Drug Invest 2006;26(11):673–6.

68. Vergara G, Silvestre JF, Betlloch I, Vela P, Albares MP, Pascual JC. Cutaneous drug eruption to infliximab: report of 4 cases with an interface dermatitis pattern. Arch Dermatol 2002;138(9):1258–9.

69. Devos SA, Van Den Bossche N, De Vos M, Naeyaert JM. Adverse skin reactions to anti-TNF-alfa monoclonal antibody therapy. Dermatology 2003;206:388–90.

70. Wang LC, Medenica MM, Shea CR, Busbey S. Infliximab-induced eczematid-like purpura of Doucas and Kapetenakis. J Am Acad Dermatol 2003;49:157–8.

71. Dumont-Berset M, Laffitte E, Gerber C, Dudler J, Panizzon RG. Eczema-like toxidermia after infliximab. Dermatology 2003;207:240.

72. Wright RC. Atopic dermatitis-like eruption precipitated by infliximab. J Am Acad Dermatol 2003;49:160–1.

73. Dumont-Berset M, Laffitte E, Gerber C, Dudler J, Panizzon R. Eczematous drug eruption after infliximab. Br J Dermatol 2004;151:1272–3.

74. Ettefagh L, Nedorost S, Mirmirani P. Alopecia areata in a patient using infliximab: new insights into the role of tumor necrosis factor on human hair follicles. Arch Dermatol 2004;140:1012.

75. Somasekar A, R. Genital condylomata in a patient receiving infliximab for Crohn's disease. Postgrad Med 2004;80:358–9.

76. Kent PD, Davis JM 3rd, Davis MD, Matteson EL. Bullous skin lesions following infliximab infusion in a patient with rheumatoid arthritis. Arthritis Rheum 2002;46(8):2257–8.

77. Dereure O, Guillot B, Jorgensen C, Cohen JD, Combes B, Guilhou JJ. Psoriatic lesions induced by antitumour necrosis factor-alpha treatment: two cases. Br J Dermatol 2004;151:506–7.

78. Haibel H, Spiller I, Strasser C, Rudwaleit M, Dorner T, et al. Unexpected new onset or exacerbation of psoriasis in treatment of active ankylosing spondylitis with TNF-alpha blocking agents: four case reports. Ann Rheum Dis 2004;63 (Suppl 1):405.

79. Verea MM, Del Pozo J, Yebra-Pimentel MT, Porta A, Fonseca E. Psoriasiform eruption induced by infliximab. Ann Pharmacother 2004;38:54–7.

80. Tutar E, Ekici F, Nacar N, Arici S, Atalay S. Delayed maculopapular, urticarial rash due to infliximab in two children with systemic onset juvenile idiopathic arthritis. Rheumatology 2004;43:674–5.

81. Yucel AE, Kart-Koseoglu H, Akova YA, Demirhan B, Boyacioglu S. Failure of infliximab treatment and occurrence of erythema nodosum during therapy in two patients with Behçet's disease. Rheumatology 2004;43:394–6.

82. Becker M, Rose CD, McIlvain-Simpson G. Niacin-like reaction to infliximab infusion in systemic juvenile rheumatoid arthritis. J Rheumatol 2004;31:2529–30.

83. Ettefagh L, Nedorost S, Mirmirani P. Alopecia areata in a patient using infliximab: new insights into the role of tumor necrosis factor on human hair follicles. Arch Dermatol 2004;140:1012.

84. Deng A, Harvey V, Sina B, Strobel D, Badros A, Junkins-Hopkins JM, Samuels A, Oghilikhan M, Gaspari A. Interstitial granulomatous dermatitis associated with the use of tumor necrosis factor alpha inhibitors. Arch Dermatol 2006;142(2):198–202.

85. Tosti A, Pazzaglia M, Starace M, Bellavista S, Vincenzi C, Tonelli G. Alopecia areata during treatment with biologic agents. Arch Dermatol 2006;54(12):3782–9.

86. Griffin SP, Selby WS. Poor wound healing following surgery in three patients who received infliximab for Crohn's disease. J Gastroenterol Hepatol 2000;15(Suppl):78.

87. Mimouni D, Anhalt GJ, Kouba DJ, Nousari HC. Infliximab for peristomal pyoderma gangrenosum. Br J Dermatol 2003;148:813–6.

88. Scheinfeld N. A comprehensive review and evaluation of the side effects of the tumor necrosis factor alpha blockers etanercept, infliximab and adalimumab. J Dermatolog Treat 2004;15:280–94.

89. Hanauer SB, Feagan BG, Lichtenstein GR, Mayer LF, Schreiber S, Colombel JF, Rachmilewitz D, Wolf DC, Olson A, Bao W, Rutgeerts PACCENT I Study Group. Maintenance infliximab for Crohn's disease: the ACCENT I randomised trial. Lancet 2002;359(9317):1541–9.

90. Baert F, Noman M, Vermeire S, Van Assche G, D'Haens G, Carbonez A, Rutgeerts P. Influence of immunogenicity on the long-term efficacy of infliximab in Crohn's disease. N Engl J Med 2003;348(7):601–8.

91. Riegert-Johnson DL, Godfrey JA, Myers JL, Hubmayr RD, Sandborn WJ, Loftus EV Jr. Delayed hypersensitivity reaction and acute respiratory distress syndrome following infliximab infusion. Inflamm Bowel Dis 2002;8(3):186–91.

92. Garcia-Planella E, Doménech E, Esteve-Comas M, Bernal I, Cabré E, Boix J, Gassull MA. Development of antinuclear antibodies and its clinical impact in patients with Crohn's disease treated with chimeric monoclonal anti-TNFα antibodies (infliximab). Eur J Gastroenterol Hepatol 2003;15:351–4.

93. De Rycke L, Krutihof E, Van Damme N, et al. Antinuclear antibodies following infliximab treatment in patients with rheumatoid arthritis or spondylathropathy. Am Coll Rheumatol 2003;48:1015–23.

94. Farrell RJ, Alsahli M, Jeen YT, Falchuk KR, Peppercorn MA, Michetti P. Intravenous hydrocortisone premedication reduces antibodies to infliximab in Crohn's disease: a randomized controlled trial. Gastroenterology 2003;124:917–24.

95. Youdim A, Vasiliauskas EA, Targan SR, Papadakis KA, Ippoliti A, Dubinsky MC, Lechago J, Paavola J, Loane J, Lee SK, Gaiennie J, Smith K, Do J, Abreu MT. A pilot study of adalimumab in infliximab-allergic patients. Inflamm Bowel Dis 2004;10(4):333–8.

96. De Rycke L, Baeten D, Kruithof E, Van den BF, Veys EM, De Keyser F. Infliximab, but not etanercept, induces IgM anti-double-stranded DNA autoantibodies as main antinuclear reactivity: biologic and clinical implications in autoimmune arthritis. Arthritis Rheum 2005;52(7):2192–201.

97. Charles PJ, Smeenk RJ, De Jong J, Feldmann M, Maini RN. Assessment of antibodies to double-stranded DNA induced in rheumatoid arthritis patients following treatment with infliximab, a monoclonal antibody to tumor necrosis factor alpha: findings in open-label and randomized placebo-controlled trials. Arthritis Rheum 2000;43(11):2383–90.

98. Mikuls TR, Moreland LW. Benefit-risk assessment of infliximab in the treatment of rheumatoid arthritis. Drug Saf 2003;26(1):23–32.

99. Ali Y, Shah S. Infliximab-induced systemic lupus erythematosus. Ann Intern Med 2002;137(7):625–6.

100. Klapman JB, Ene-Stroescu D, Becker MA, Hanauer SB. A lupus-like syndrome associated with infliximab therapy. Inflamm Bowel Dis 2003;9(3):176–8.

101. Allanore Y, Sellam J, Batteux F, Job Deslandre C, Weill B, Kahan A. Induction of autoantibodies in refractory rheumatoid arthritis treated by infliximab. Clin Exp Rheumatol 2004;22:756–8.

102. Ferraro-Peyret C, Coury F, Tebib JG, Bienvenu J, Fabien N. Infliximab therapy in rheumatoid arthritis and ankylosing spondylitis-induced specific antinuclear and antiphospholipid autoantibodies without autoimmune clinical manifestations: a two-year prospective study. Arthritis Res Ther 2004;6:R535-43.

103. Vermeire S, Noman M, Van Assche G, Baert F, Van Steen K, Esters N, Joossens S, Bossuyt X, Rutgeerts P. Autoimmunity associated with anti-tumor necrosis factor alfa treatment in Crohn's disease: a prospective cohort study. Gastroenterology 2003;125:32–9.

104. Louis M, Rauch J, Armstrong M, Fitzcharles MA. Induction of autoantibodies during prolonged treatment with infliximab. J Rheumatol 2003;30:2557–62.

105. Aringer M, Graninger WB, Steiner G, Smolen JS. Safety and efficacy of tumor necrosis factor alpha blockade in systemic lupus erythematosus: an open-label study. Arthritis Rheum 2004;50:3161–9.

106. Benucci M, Li Gobbi F, Fossi F, Manfredi M, Del Rosso A. Drug-induced lupus after treatment with infliximab in rheumatoid arthritis. J Clin Rheumatol 2005;11:47–49.

107. Elkayam O, Caspi D. Infliximab induced lupus in patients with rheumatoid arthritis. Clin Exp Rheumatol 2004;22:502–3.

108. Kheterpal N, Patel S, Zawacki J, Wassef W. Infliximab-induced systemic lupus erythematosus in a patient with Crohn's colitis: a case report and review of the literature. Am J Gastroenterol 2004;99(Suppl):abstract 603.

109. Novak S, Cikes N. Infliximab-induced lupus or rheumatoid arthritis (RA) overlapping with systemic lupus erythematosus (SLE) unmasked by infliximab. Clin Exp Rheumatol 2004;22:268.

110. Russo PAJ, Tymms KE, Smith GR. Infliximab-induced systemic lupus erythematosus. APLAR J Rheumatol 2004;7:130–132.

111. Stratigos AJ, Antoniou C, Stamathioudaki S, Avgerinou G, Tsega A, Katsambas AD. Discoid lupus erythematosus-like eruption induced by infliximab. Clin Exp Dermatol 2004;29:150–3.

112. Musial J, Undas A, Celinska-Lowenhoff M. Polymyositis associated with infliximab treatment for rheumatoid arthritis. Rheumatol (Oxf) 2003;42:1566–8.

113. Jarrett SJ, Cunnane G, Conaghan PG, Bingham SJ, Buch MH, Quinn MA, Emery P. Anti-tumor necrosis factor-alfa therapy-induced vasculitis: case series. J Rheumatol 2003;30:2287–91.

114. McIlwain L, Carter JD, Bin-Sagheer S, Vasey FB, Nord J. Hypersensitivity vasculitis with leukocytoclastic vasculitis secondary to infliximab. J Clin Gastroenterol 2003;36:411–3.

115. Hanauer SB, Rutgeerts PJ, D'Haens G, Targan SR, Kam L, Present DH, Wagner C, LaSorda J, Sands B, Livingstone RA. Delayed hypersensitivity to infliximab (Remicade) re-infusion after a 2-4 year interval without treatment. Gastroenterology 1999;116:A731.

116. Favalli EG, Sinigaglia L, Varenna M, Arnoldi C. Drug-induced lupus following treatment with infliximab in rheumatoid arthritis. Lupus 2002;11(11):753–5.

117. Stephens MC, Shepanski MA, Mamula P, Markowitz JE, Brown KA, Baldassano RN. Safety and steroid-sparing experience using infliximab for Crohn's disease at a pediatric inflammatory bowel disease center. Am J Gastroenterol 2003;98:104–11.

118. Wasserman MJ, Weber DA, Guthrie JA, Bykerk VP, Lee P, Keystone EC. Infusion-related reactions to infliximab in patients with rheumatoid arthritis in a clinical practice setting: relationship to dose, antihistamine pretreatment, and infusion number. J Rheumatol 2004;31:1912–7.

119. Sugiura F, Kojima T, Oba M, Tsuchiya H, Ishiguro N. Anaphylactic reaction to infliximab in two rheumatoid arthritis patients who had previously received infliximab and resumed. Mod Rheumatol 2005;15(3):201–3.

120. Cheifetz A, Smedley M, Martin S, Reiter M, Leone G, Mayer L, Plevy S. The incidence and management of infusion reactions to infliximab: a large center experience. Am J Gastroenterol 2003;98(6):1315–24.

121. Kugathasan S, Levy MB, Saeian K, Vasilopoulos S, Kim JP, Prajapati D, Emmons J, Martinez A, Kelly KJ, Binion DG. Infliximab retreatment in adults and children with Crohn's disease: risk factors for the development of delayed severe systemic reaction. Am J Gastroenterol 2002;97(6):1408–14.

122. Farrell RJ, Shah SA, Lodhavia PJ, Alsahli M, Falchuk KR, Michetti P, Peppercorn MA. Clinical experience with infliximab therapy in 100 patients with Crohn's disease. Am J Gastroenterol 2000;95(12):3490–7.

123. Puchner TC, Kugathasan S, Kelly KJ, Binion DG. Successful desensitization and therapeutic use of infliximab in adult and pediatric Crohn's disease patients with prior anaphylactic reaction. Inflamm Bowel Dis 2001;7(1):34–7.

124. O'Connor M, Buchman A, Marshall G. Anaphylaxis-like reaction to infliximab in a patient with Crohn's disease. Dig Dis Sci 2002;47(6):1323–5.

125. Lankarani KB. Mortality associated with infliximab. J Clin Gastroenterol 2001;33(3):255–6.

126. McCain ME, Quinet RJ, Davis WE. Etanercept and infliximab associated with cutaneous vasculitis. Rheumatology (Oxford) 2002;41(1):116–7.

127. Lahdenne P, Vähäsalo P, Honkanen V. Infliximab or etanacerpt in the treatment of children with refractory juvenile idiopathic arthritis: an open label study. An Rheum Dis 2003;62:245–7.

128. Crandall WV, Mackner LM. Infusion reactions to infliximab in children and adolescents: frequency, outcome and a predictive model. Aliment Pharmacol Ther 2003;17(1):75–84.

129. Slifman NR, Gershon SK, Lee JH, Edwards ET, Braun MM. Listeria monocytogenes infection as a complication of treatment with tumor necrosis factor alfa-neutralizing agents. Arthritis Rheum 2003;48:319–24.

130. Mohan AK, Coté TR, Siegel JN, Braun MM. Infectious complications of biologic treatment of rheumatoid arthritis. Curr Opin Rheumatol 2003;15:179–84.

131. Kamath BM, Mamula P, Baldassano RN, Markowitz JE. *Listeria* meningitis after treatment with infliximab. J Pediatr Gastroenterol Nutr 2002;34(4):410–2.

132. Shanahan JC, St Clair W. Tumor necrosis factor-alpha blockade: a novel therapy for rheumatic disease. Clin Immunol 2002;103(3 Pt 1):231–42.

133. Chan AT, Cleeve V, Daymond TJ. Necrotising fasciitis in a patient receiving infliximab for rheumatoid arthritis. Postgrad Med J 2002;78(915):47–8.

134. Matzkies FG, Manger B, Schmitt-Haendle M, Nagel T, Kraetsch HG, Kalden JR, Schulze-Koops H. Severe septicaemia in a patient with polychondritis and Sweet's syndrome after initiation of treatment with infliximab. Ann Rheum Dis 2003;62(1):81–2.

135. Gluck T, Linde HJ, Scholmerich J, Muller-Ladner U, Fiehn C, Bohland P. Anti-tumor necrosis factor therapy and *Listeria monocytogenes* infection: report of two cases. Arthritis Rheum 2002;46(8):2255–7.

136. Liberopoulos EN, Drosos AA, Elisaf MS. Exacerbation of tuberculosis enteritis after treatment with infliximab. Am J Med 2002;113(7):615.

137. Van Den Bosch F, Kruithof E, Baeten D, Herssens A, de Keyser F, Mielants H, Veys EM. Randomized double-blind comparison of chimeric monoclonal antibody to tumor necrosis factor alpha (infliximab) versus placebo in active spondylarthropathy. Arthritis Rheum 2002;46(3):755–65.

138. Mutlu G, Mutlu E, Bellmeyer A, Rubinstein I. Pulmonary adverse events of anti-tumor necrosis factor-alpha antibody therapy. Am J Med 2006;119(8):639–46.

139. Uthman I, Kanj N, El-Sayad J, Bizri AR. Miliary tuberculosis after infliximab therapy in Lebanon. Clin Rheumatol 2004;23:279–80.

140. Mayordomo L, Marenco JL, Gomez-Mateos J, Rejon E. Pulmonary miliary tuberculosis in a patient with anti-TNF-alpha treatment. Scand J Rheumatol 2002;31(1):44–5.

141. Nunez Martinez O, Ripoll Noiseux C, Carneros Martin JA, Gonzalez Lara V, Gregorio Maranon HG. Reactivation tuberculosis in a patient with anti-TNF-alpha treatment. Am J Gastroenterol 2001;96(5):1665–6.

142. Roth S, Delmont E, Heudier P, Kaphan R, Cua E, Castela J, Verdier JM, Chichmanian RM, Fuzibet JG. Anticorps anti-TNF alpha (infliximab) et tuberculose: à propos de 3 cas. Rev Med Interne 2002;23(3):312–6.

143. Rovere Querini P, Vecellio M, Sabbadini MG, Ciboddo G. Miliary tuberculosis after biological therapy for rheumatoid arthritis. Rheumatology 2002;41(2):231.

144. Wagner TE, Huseby ES, Huseby JS. Exacerbation of *Mycobacterium tuberculosis* enteritis masquerading as Crohn's disease after treatment with a tumor necrosis factor-alpha inhibitor. Am J Med 2002;112(1):67–9.

145. Keane J, Gershon S, Wise RP, Mirabile-Levens E, Kasznica J, Schwieterman WD, Siegel JN, Braun MM. Tuberculosis associated with infliximab, a tumor necrosis factor alpha-neutralizing agent. N Engl J Med 2001; 345(15):1098–104.

146. Sandborn WJ, Hanauer SB. Infliximab in the treatment of Crohn's disease: a user's guide for clinicians. Am J Gastroenterol 2002;97(12):2962–72.

147. Antoni C, Braun J. Side effects of anti-TNF therapy: current knowledge. Clin Exp Rheumatol 2002;20(6 Suppl 28):S152–7.

148. Wolfe F, Michaud K, Anderson J, Urbansky K. Tuberculosis infection in patients with rheumatoid arthritis and the effect of infliximab therapy. Arthr Rheum 2004;50:372–9.

149. Baeten D, Kruithof E, Van den Bosch F, Van den Bossche N, Herssens A, Mielants H, De Keyser F, Veys EM. Systematic safety follow up in a cohort of 107 patients with spondyloarthropathy treated with infliximab: a new perspective on the role of host defence in the pathogenesis of the disease? Ann Rheum Dis 2003;62:829–34.

150. Gomez-Reino JJ, Carmona L, Valverde VR, Mola EM, Montero MD. Treatment of rheumatoid arthritis with tumor necrosis factor inhibitors may predispose to significant increase in tuberculosis risk: a multicenter active-surveillance report. Arthritis Rheum 2003;48:2122–7.

151. Parra Ruiz J, Ortego Centeno N, Raya Alvarez E. Development of tuberculosis in a patient treated with infliximab who had received prophylactic therapy with isoniazid. J Rheumatol 2003;30:1657–8.

152. Van der Klooster JM, Bosman RJ, Oudemans-van Straaten HM, van der Spoel JI, Wester JP, Zandstra DF. Disseminated tuberculosis, pulmonary aspergillosis and cutaneous Herpes simplex infection in a patient with infliximab and methotrexate. Intensive Care Med 2003;29:2327–9.

153. Dunlop H. Infliximab (Remicade) and etanercept (Enbrel): serious infections and tuberculosis. Can Med Assoc J 2004;171:992–3.

154. Singh SM, Rau NV, Cohen LB, Harris H. Cutaneous nocardiosis complicating management of Crohn's disease with infliximab and prednisone. Can Med Assoc J 2004;171:1063–4.

155. Smith SG, Bloomfeld RS. Disseminated Nocardia infection associated with Infliximab. Am J Gastroenterol 2004;99(Suppl):abstract 456.

156. Albert C, Vandenbos F, Brocq O, Carles D, Euller-Ziegler L. Légionellose chez une patiente sous infliximab. Rev Med Interne 2004;25:167–8.

157. Christidis DS, Liberopoulos EN, Tsiara SN, Drosos AA, Elisaf MS. Legionella pneumophila infection possibly related to treatment with infliximab. Infect Dis Clin Prac 2004;12:301–3.

158. Wondergem MJ, Voskuyl AE, van Agtmael MA. A case of legionellosis during treatment with a TNFalpha antagonist. Scand J Infect Dis 2004;36:310–1.

159. Bowie VL, Snella KA, Gopalachar AS, Bharadwaj P. Listeria meningitis associated with infliximab. Ann Pharmacother 2004;38:58–61.

160. Ljung T, Karlen P, Schmidt D, Hellström PM, Lapidus A, Janczewska I, Sjöqvist U, Lofberg R. Infliximab in inflammatory bowel disease: clinical outcome in a population based cohort from Stockholm County. Gut 2004;53:849–53.

161. Fu A, Bertouch JV, McNeil HP. Disseminated Salmonella typhimurium infection secondary to infliximab treatment. Arthritis Rheum 2004;50:3049–60.

162. Olivieri I, Padula A, Armignacco L, Sabatella V, Mancino M. Septic arthritis caused by Moraxella catarrhalis associated with infliximab treatment in a patient with undifferentiated spondarthritis. Ann Rheum Dis 2004;63:105–6.

163. Herrlinger KR, Borutta A, Meinhardt G, Stange EF, Fellermann K. Fatal staphylococcal sepsis in Crohn's disease after infliximab. Inflamm Bowel Dis 2004;10:655–6.

164. Kane D, Balint PV, Wood F, Sturrock RD. Early diagnosis of pyomyositis using clinic-based ultrasonography in a patient receiving infliximab therapy for Behcet's disease. Rheumatol (Oxf) 2003;42:1564–5.

165. Sipsas N, Papaparaskevas J, Stefanou I, Kalatzis K, Vlachoyiannopoulos P, Avlamis A. Septic arthritis due to *Roseomonas mucosa in a rheumatoid arthritis patient receiving infliximab therapy. Diag Microbiol Infect Dis* 2006;5(4):343–5.

166. Roos J, Ostor A. Orbital cellulitis in a patient receiving infliximab for ankylosing spondylitis. Am J Ophthalmol 2006;141(4):767–9.

167. Reichardt P, Dahnert I, Tiller G, Hausler HJ. Possible activation of an intramyocardial inflammatory process

(*Staphylococcus aureus*) after treatment with infliximab in a boy with Crohn disease. Eur J Pediatr 2002;161(5):281–3.

168. Haerter G, Manfras B, Schmitt M, Wendland T, Moch B. Severe CMV retinitis in a patient with HLA-B27 associated spondylarthropathy following immunosuppressive therapy with anti-TNF alpha (infliximab). Infection 2003;31(Suppl 1):150.

169. Helbling D, Breitbach TH, Krause M. Disseminated cytomegalovirus infection in Crohn's disease following antitumour necrosis factor therapy. Eur J Gastroenterol Hepatol 2002;14(12):1393–5.

170. Baumgart DC, Dignass AU. Shingles following infliximab infusion. Ann Rheum Dis 2002;61:661.

171. Skripak JM, Rodgers GL, Goldsmith DP. Disseminated herpes simplex virus infection associated with macrophage activation syndrome in a child with systemic juvenile idiopathic arthritis undergoing therapy with infliximab. Ped Res 2003;53:340–1.

172. Ostuni P, Botsios C, Punzi L, Sfriso P, Todesco S. Hepatitis B reactivation in a chronic hepatitis B surface antigen carrier with rheumatoid arthritis treated with infliximab and low dose methotrexate. Ann Rheum Dis 2003;62:686–7.

173. Michel M, Duvoux C, Hezode C, Cherqui D. Fulminant hepatitis after infliximab in a patient with hepatitis B virus treated for an adult onset still's disease. J Rheumatol 2003;30:1624–5.

174. Peterson JR, Hsu FC, Simkin PA, Wener MH. Effect of tumour necrosis factor alfa antagonists on serum transaminases and viraemia in patients with rheumatoid arthritis and chronic hepatitis C infection. Ann Rheum Dis 2003;62:1078–82.

175. Leung VS, Nguyen MT, Bush TM. Disseminated primary varicella after initiation of infliximab for Crohn's disease. Am J Gastroenterol 2004;99:2503–4.

176. Somasekar A, Alcolado R. Genital condylomata in a patient receiving infliximab for Crohn's disease. Postgrad Med J 2004;80:358–9.

177. Reijasse D, Le Pendeven C, Cosnes J, Dehee A, Gendre JP, Nicolas JC, Beaugerie L. Epstein–Barr virus viral load in Crohn's disease: effect of immunosuppressive therapy. Inflamm Bowel Dis 2004;10:85–90.

178. Cursiefen C, Grunke M, Dechant C, Antoni C, Junemann A, Holbach LM. Multiple bilateral eyelid molluscum contagiosum lesions associated with TNFalpha-antibody and methotrexate therapy. Am J Ophthalmol 2002;134(2):270–1.

179. Tai TL, O'Rourke KP, McWeeney M, Burke CM, Sheehan K, Barry M. *Pneumocystis carinii* pneumonia following a second infusion of infliximab. Rheumatology (Oxford) 2002;41(8):951–2.

180. Kaur N, Mahl TC. Pneumocystis carinii pneumonia with oral candidiasis after infliximab therapy for Crohn's disease. Dig Dis Sci 2004;49:1458–60.

181. Velayos FS, Sandborn WJ. Pneumocystis carinii pneumonia during maintenance anti-tumor necrosis factor-alpha therapy with infliximab for Crohn's disease. Inflamm Bowel Dis 2004;10:657–60.

182. Lee JH, Slifman NR, Gershon SK, Edwards ET, Schwieterman WD, Siegel JN, Wise RP, Brown SL, Udall JN Jr, Braun MM. Life-threatening histoplasmosis complicating immunotherapy with tumor necrosis factor alpha antagonists infliximab and etanercept. Arthritis Rheum 2002;46(10):2565–70.

183. Fitzcharles MA, Clayton D, Menard HA. The use of infliximab in academic rheumatology practice: an audit of early clinical experience. J Rheumatol 2002;29(12):2525–30.

184. Nakelchik M, Mangino JE. Reactivation of histoplasmosis after treatment with infliximab. Am J Med 2002;112(1):78.

185. Warris A, Bjorneklett A, Gaustad P. Invasive pulmonary aspergillosis associated with infliximab therapy. N Engl J Med 2001;344(14):1099–100.

186. Ramzan NN, Shapiro MS, Robinson E, Smilack JD. Use of infliximab leading to extensive pulmonary coccidioidomycosis. Am J Gastroenterol 2002;97(Suppl):157.

187. Shrestha RK, Stoller JK, Honari G, Procop GW, Gordon SM. Pneumonia due to Cryptococcus neoformans in a patient receiving infliximab: possible zoonotic transmission from a pet cockatiel. Respir Care 2004;49:606–8.

188. Katz J, Antoni C, Keenan G, Smith D, Jacobs S, Lichtenstein G. Outcome of pregnancy in women receiving infliximab for the treatment of Crohn's disease and rheumatoid arthritis. Am J Gastroenterol 2004;99:2385–92.

189. de' Clari F, Salani I, Safwan E, Giannacco A. Sudden death in a patient without heart failure after a single infusion of 200 mg infliximab: does TNF-alpha have protective effects on the failing heart, or does infliximab have direct harmful cardiovascular effects? Circulation 2002;105(21):E183.

190. Drewe E, Powell RJ. Clinically useful monoclonal antibodies in treatment. J Clin Pathol 2002;55(2):81–5.

191. Brown SL, Greene MH, Gershon SK, Edwards ET, Braun MM. Tumor necrosis factor antagonist therapy and lymphoma development: twenty-six cases reported to the Food and Drug Administration. Arthritis Rheum 2002;46(12):3151–8.

192. Mahe E, Descamps V, Grossin M, Fraitag S, Crickx B. CD30+ T-cell lymphoma in a patient with psoriasis treated with ciclosporin and infliximab. Br J Dermatol 2003;149:170–3.

193. van Vollenhoven RF. Benefits and risks of biological agents: lymphomas. Clin Exp Rheumatol 2004;22(Suppl 35):S122-5.

194. Symmons DP, Silman AJ. Anti-tumor necrosis factor alpha therapy and the risk of lymphoma in rheumatoid arthritis: no clear answer. Arthritis Rheum 2004;50:1703–6.

195. Geborek P, Bladstrom A, Turesson C, Gulfe A, Petersson IF, Saxne T, Olsson H, Jacobsson LT. Tumour necrosis factor blockers do not increase overall tumour risk in patients with rheumatoid arthritis, but may be associated with an increased risk of lymphomas. Ann Rheum Dis 2005;64:699–703.

196. Wolfe F, Michaud K. Lymphoma in rheumatoid arthritis: the effect of methotrexate and anti-tumor necrosis factor therapy in 18,572 patients. Arthritis Rheum 2004;50:1740–51.

197. Bucher C, Degen L, Dirnhofer S, Pless M, Herrmann R, Schraml P, Went P. Biologics in inflammatory disease: infliximab associated risk of lymphoma development. Gut 2005;54:732–3.

198. Losco A, Gianelli U, Cassani B, Baldini L, Conte D, Basilisco G. Epstein–Barr virus-associated lymphoma in Crohn's disease. Inflamm Bowel Dis 2004;10:425–9.

199. Esser AC, Abril A, Fayne S, Doyle JA. Acute development of multiple keratoacanthomas and squamous cell carcinomas after treatment with infliximab. J Am Acad Dermatol 2004;50:S75-7.

200. Adams AE, Zwicker J, Curiel C, Kadin ME, Falchuk KR, Drews R, Kupper TS. Aggressive cutaneous T-cell lymphomas after TNFalpha blockade. J Am Acad Dermatol 2004;51:660–2.

201. Anonymous. Tumor necrosis factor (TNF)-α inhibitors. Increased risk of malignancy. WHO Pharm Newslett 2007;1:5.

202. Bongartz T, Sutton AJ, Sweeting MJ, Buchan I, Matteson EL, Montori V. Anti-TNF antibody therapy in rheumatoid arthritis and the risk of serious infections and malignancies: systematic review and meta-analysis of rare harmful effects in randomized controlled trials. JAMA 2006;295(19):2275-85. Erratum: 2006;295(21):2482.

203. Biancone L, Orlando A, Kohn A, Colombo E, Sostegni R, Angelucci E, Rizzello F, Castiglione F, Benazzato L, Papi C, Meucci G, Regler G, Petruzziello C, Mocciaro F, Geremia A, CalabreseE, Cottone M, Pallone F .Infliximab and newly diagnosed neoplasia in Crohn's disease (CD). A multicentre matched pair study. Gut 2006;55:228-33.

204. Chen SC, Cummings OD, Hartley MP, Filomena CA, Cho WK. Hepatocellular carcinoma occurring in a patient with Crohn's disease treated with both azathioprine and infliximab. Dig Dis Sci 2006;51(5):952-5.

205. Burt MJ, Frizelle FA, Barbezat GO. Pregnancy and exposure to infliximab (anti-tumor necrosis factor-alfa monoclonal antibody). J Gastroenterol Hepatol 2003;18:465-6.

206. Srinivasan R. Infliximab treatment and pregnancy outcome in active Crohn's disease. Am J Gastroenterol 2001;96:2274-5.

207. Katz JA, Lichtenstein GR, Keenan GF, Jacobs SJ. Outcome of pregnancy in patients receiving Remicade (infliximab) for the treatment of Crohn's disease or rheumatoid arthritis. Gastroenterology 2001;120 Suppl 1:A69.

208. Dekker L, Armbrust W, Rademaker CM, Prakken B, Kuis W, Wulffraat NM. Safety of anti-TNFalpha therapy in children with juvenile idiopathic arthritis. Clin Exp Rheumatol 2004;22:252-8.

209. Marchal L, D'Haens G, Van Assche G, Vermeire S, Noman M, Ferrante M, Hiele M, Bueno De Mesquita M, D'Hoore A, Penninckx F, Rutgeerts P. The risk of postoperative complications associated with infliximab therapy for Crohn's disease: a controlled cohort study. Aliment Pharmacol Ther 2004;19:749-54.

210. Condino AA, Fidanza S, Hoffenberg EJ. A home infliximab infusion program. J Pediatr Gastroenterol Nutr 2005;40(1):67-9.

211. Roblin X, Serre-Debeauvais F, Phelip JM, Bessard G, Bonaz B. Drug interaction between infliximab and azathioprine in patients with Crohn's disease. Aliment Pharmacol Ther 2003;18:917-25.

Leflunomide

General Information

The prodrug leflunomide (N-(4'-trifluoromethylphenyl)-5-methylisoxazole-4-carboxamide) is an isoxazole derivative. Its main metabolite is the active compound, A77 1726 (1).

Mechanism of action

A77 1726 inhibits dihydro-rate dehydrogenase, the rate-limiting enzyme in pyrimidine synthesis. It inhibits the proliferation of T and B cells, and probably acts via the production and action of interleukin-2. Besides its immunomodulatory action, A77 1726 also has an anti-inflammatory action by inhibition of nuclear factor kappa B (NFκB), tumor necrosis factor alfa (TNF-α), and interleukin 1 beta (IL-1β), and increased production of transforming growth factor beta-1 (TGF-β1; 2–5).

Pharmacokinetics

After oral administration, leflunomide undergoes rapid metabolism in the gut wall, plasma, and liver to A77 1726 (M1), peak plasma concentrations of which are reached after 6–12 hours. A77 1726 is highly (99%) bound to plasma proteins. Its pharmacokinetics are not affected by food, and dosage requirements are not influenced by age or sex. Enterohepatic recirculation and biliary recycling contribute to the long half-life of 2 weeks. About 90% of a single dose of leflunomide is eliminated, 43% in the urine, primarily as leflunomide glucuronides and an oxalinic acid derivative of A77 1726, and 48% in the feces, primarily as A77 1726. Impaired renal function can result in increased plasma concentrations of A77 1726. Elimination of A77 1726 can be dramatically increased by using colestyramine or activated charcoal (6,7).

Indications and clinical efficacy

Leflunomide has anti-inflammatory, immunosuppressive, and virustatic effects. Its efficacy has been demonstrated in patients with rheumatoid arthritis and psoriatic arthritis and other conditions in randomized, double-blind, placebo-controlled trials and other studies (8–32), and it was approved for treatment of adult rheumatoid arthritis in August 1998 (Table 1; 33). In three large phase III trials (US301, $n = 482$; MN301, $n = 358$; MN302, $n = 999$), leflunomide was as effective and well tolerated as methotrexate and sulfasalazine and superior to placebo (34). These data were confirmed by a meta-analysis (35,36). Leflunomide is therefore indicated for patients with rheumatoid arthritis who have failed first-line disease modifying anti-rheumatic drug therapy on the basis of efficacy, safety, and costs (36). It is effective as monotherapy and in combination with methotrexate or infliximab (6).

Clinical experience with leflunomide in patients with other autoimmune diseases is limited. Extended indications for the use of leflunomide include treatment of Crohn's disease in patients who are intolerant of standard immunomodulator therapy (31), chronic sarcoidosis (32), maintenance therapy of complete or partial remission in Wegener's granulomatosis (30), and mild to moderate systemic lupus erythematosus (29) (Table 1).

Leflunomide has been used as an immunosuppressive agent in kidney and liver transplant recipients to spare calcineurin inhibitors and glucocorticoids and to slow progression of chronic kidney graft dysfunction (28,37) (Table 1).

In animals, leflunomide had excellent antiviral activity against cytomegalovirus (CMV). It is currently indicated as second-line therapy for CMV disease after solid organ transplantation and in recipients intolerant of ganciclovir (38). Leflunomide also reduces HIV replication by about 75% at concentrations that can be obtained with conventional dosing (39) and was intended for treatment of patients with HIV/AIDS refractory to HAART (40).

Table 1 Summary of the efficacy of leflunomide in controlled trials

Disease	Type of study; duration	Intervention	Outcome	References
Rheumatoid arthritis	Double-blind, randomized, controlled trial; 24 weeks	Leflunomide 50–100 mg/day for 1 day, then 5–25 mg/day (n = 300) versus placebo (n = 102)	Leflunomide 10 and 25 mg/day was significantly more effective than placebo	(8)
Rheumatoid arthritis	Double-blind, randomized, controlled trial; 12 months	Leflunomide 100 mg/day for 3 days, thereafter 20 mg/day (n = 182) versus methotrexate 7.5–15 mg/week (n = 180) versus placebo (n = 118)	American College of Rheumatology response and success rates were: leflunomide 52% and 41%, methotrexate 46% and 35%, and placebo 26% and 19%	(9)
Rheumatoid arthritis	Double-blind, randomized, controlled trial; 24 weeks	Leflunomide 100 mg/day for 3 days, then 20 mg/day (n = 133) versus sulfasalazine 2 g/day (n = 133) versus placebo (n = 92)	American College of Rheumatology 20 response rates were: leflunomide 55%, sulfasalazine 56%, and placebo 29%	(10,11)
Rheumatoid arthritis	Double-blind, randomized, controlled trial; 52 weeks	Leflunomide 100 mg/day for 3 days, then 20 mg/day (n = 501) versus methotrexate 7.5–15 mg/day (n = 498)	Both drugs effective, although methotrexate resulted in significantly greater improvement in tender and swollen joint counts compared with leflunomide	(12)
Rheumatoid arthritis	Double-blind, randomized, controlled trial; 6 months	Leflunomide 100 mg/day for 3 days, then 20 mg/day (n = 133) versus sulfasalazine 0.5–2 g/day (n = 133), versus placebo (n = 92)	Leflunomide slowed disease progression as early as 6 months, and there was continued retardation of radiographic progression at 2 years	(13)
Rheumatoid arthritis	Follow-up study; 2 years	Leflunomide (n = 98) versus methotrexate (n = 101)	American College of Rheumatology 20, 50, and 70 response rates for leflunomide versus methotrexate were 79 versus 67%, 56 versus 43%, and 26 versus 20%	(14)
Rheumatoid arthritis	Follow-up study; 2 years	Leflunomide 20 mg/day versus sulfasalazine 2 g/day	American College of Rheumatology 20 response rates were 82% leflunomide versus 60% sulfasalazine after 24 months	(15)
Rheumatoid arthritis	Follow-up study; 5 years	Leflunomide 10–20 mg/day (phase III) continued (n = 214)	American College of Rheumatology 20, 50, and 70 response rates after 1 year were maintained for up to 5 years	(16)
Rheumatoid arthritis	Single-center experience; 32 weeks	Leflunomide 100 mg/day for 3 days, then 20 mg/day plus infliximab 3 mg/kg at 2, 4, 8, 16, and 24 weeks (n = 20)	11/20 withdrawn (four infliximab infusion reactions, one Stevens-Johnson syndrome); the other patients achieved American College of Rheumatology 20 and 70 response rates in >80% and 46%	(17)
Rheumatoid arthritis	Double-blind randomized controlled trial; 24 weeks	Leflunomide 100 mg/day for 2 days, then 10 mg/day (n = 130) versus placebo (n = 133), both with methotrexate 10–25 mg/day	American College of Rheumatology 20 rates at 24 weeks: leflunomide + methotrexate 46% versus placebo + methotrexate 20%; similar drug withdrawal and adverse events rates	(18)
Rheumatoid arthritis	Multicenter experience; 24 weeks	Leflunomide 100 mg/day for 3 days, then 20 mg/day (n = 969)	191 withdrawn (107 adverse events, 26 lack of efficacy, 58 other reasons); 24% good and 45% moderate responses on the disease activity score, and 61%, 34%, and 9.6% achieved American College of Rheumatology 20, 50, and 70 response rates	(19)
Rheumatoid arthritis	Single-center experience; 3 months	Leflunomide 100 mg/day for 3 days, then 20 mg/day plus infliximab 3 mg/kg at 0, 6, and every 8 weeks (n = 17)	20 adverse effects in 13 patients; 8 discontinued	(20)
Rheumatoid arthritis	Single-center experience; 24 weeks,	Leflunomide 100 mg/day for 3 days, then 100 mg/week (n = 50)	American College of Rheumatology 20, 50, and 70 response rates at 24 weeks were 74%, 64%, and 28% (five withdrawn, six lost to follow-up)	(21)
Rheumatoid arthritis	Single-center experience; 6 months	Leflunomide 100 mg/day for 3 days, then 20 mg/day (n = 378)	American College of Rheumatology 20, 50, and 70 response rates at 6 months were 48%, 25%, and 12%	(22)

Table 1 Continued

Disease	Type of study; duration	Intervention	Outcome	References
Rheumatoid arthritis	Extension of double-blind, randomized, controlled trial; 48 weeks	Leflunomide + methotrexate continued (n = 96) and placebo + methotrexate switched to leflunomide 10 mg/day + methotrexate (n = 96)	American College of Rheumatology 20 response rate was 59% at 24 weeks and 55% at 48 weeks in patients maintained on leflunomide + methotrexate, and patients switched from placebo to leflunomide + methotrexate increased their American College of Rheumatology 20 response rates from 25% at 24 weeks to 57% at 48 weeks	(23)
Rheumatoid arthritis	Double-blind, randomized, controlled trial; 24 weeks	Leflunomide 10 mg/day and 100 mg on day 3 (n = 202) versus 20 mg/day and 100 mg on days 1–3 (n = 200)	American College of Rheumatology (20 response rates: leflunomide 10 mg 50% and 20 mg 57%; adverse events: leflunomide 10 mg 15% and 20 mg 12%	(24)
Rheumatoid arthritis	Multicenter experience; 11–911 days	Leflunomide 100 mg/day for 3 days, then 20 mg/day (n = 136)	76% clinical response after 12 months, but 76/136 (56%) leflunomide withdrawn (29% adverse drug reactions and 13% lack of efficacy)	(25)
Psoriatic arthropathy, psoriasis	Double-blind, randomized, controlled trial; 24 weeks	Leflunomide 100 mg/day for 3 days, then 20 mg/day (n = 95) versus placebo (n = 91)	Leflunomide 59% and placebo 30% were responders at 24 weeks according to the psoriatic arthritis response criteria	(26)
Psoriasis	Phase II study; 12 weeks	Leflunomide 20 mg/day (n = 8)	6/8 clinical effectiveness (psoriasis area and severity index score 20 at baseline versus 13 at 12 weeks)	(27)
Liver and kidney transplant recipients	Single-center experience	Leflunomide dosage adjusted to a trough concentration of 100 µg/ml (n = 53)	Immunosuppressive potency in liver and kidney transplant recipients, allowing dosage reduction of calcineurin inhibitors and glucocorticoids, but anemia might be dose-limiting after kidney transplantation	(28)
Systemic lupus erythematosus	Single-center experience, double-blind, randomized, controlled trial; 24 weeks	Leflunomide 100 mg/day for 3 days, then 100 mg/day (n = 6) versus placebo (n = 6)	Disease activity fell significantly in both groups after 6 months, and the reduction in SLE disease activity index from baseline to 24 weeks was significantly greater with leflunomide than with placebo	(29)
Wegener's granulomatosis	Phase II study; 52 weeks	Leflunomide 20–40 mg/day (n = 20)	Maintenance of complete or partial remission after cyclophosphamide + glucocorticoid therapy resulted in one major and eight minor relapses	(30)
Crohn's disease	Single-center experience; 3 years	Leflunomide 20 mg/day (n = 12)	8/12 clinical responses; seven continued maintenance therapy and one relapsed after follow-up of 6–78 weeks	(31)
Chronic sarcoidosis	Single-center experience; 1 year	Leflunomide 100 mg/day for 3 days, then 10–20 mg/day (n = 32; 17 leflunomide and 15 leflunomide + methotrexate)	Complete or partial responses in 13/17 leflunomide and in 12/15 leflunomide + methotrexate	(32)

Leflunomide is licensed in France for "active psoriatic rheumatism". Pharmacovigilance studies have confirmed some severe adverse effects (hepatic, cutaneous, and hematological) and have uncovered other previously unrecognized effects, such as interstitial pneumonia, hypertension, weight loss, and peripheral neuropathies. In France, leflunomide costs nearly 10 times more than methotrexate and it has been suggested that it should not be used to treat psoriatic arthropathy (41).

Comparative studies

In 285 patients with rheumatoid arthritis leflunomide was discontinued after 1 year in 57%, mainly because of adverse drug reactions (42%) (42). The discontinuation rate because of toxicity was higher for leflunomide than for other DMARDs studied, while discontinuation for inefficacy was similar.

General adverse drug reactions

The safety profile of leflunomide has been said to be excellent, with no myelosuppressive or nephrotoxic adverse effects (43,44). Its major adverse effects are gastrointestinal symptoms (diarrhea and nausea), abnormal liver function tests, skin rashes and pruritus, allergic reactions, alopecia, infections, weight loss, and hypertension (35,45–48). Minor adverse effects are musculoskeletal disorders. Rare adverse effects include sepsis, pancytopenia, interstitial lung disease, hypertriglyceridemia, vasculitis, aseptic meningitis, reversible neuropathy, and serious skin reactions (35,49–52).

In 3325 patients who took leflunomide, the rate of drug withdrawal was 42% within 33 months after approval by the US Food and Drugs Administration, and was more likely in patients who received a loading dose. The most common causes of discontinuation were inefficacy (30%), gastrointestinal symptoms (29%), non-adherence to therapy or loss to follow-up (14%), and raised liver enzymes (5%; 53).

However, the rate of adverse effects associated with leflunomide was significantly lower than with methotrexate and other disease-modifying antirheumatic drugs (DMARDs) in an analysis of 40 594 patients with rheumatoid arthritis (8,54). The incidences of adverse events per 1000 patient-years were as follows:

- no DMARDs: 383
- methotrexate: 145
- leflunomide monotherapy: 94
- methotrexate + other DMARDs: 70
- leflunomide + other DMARDs: 59
- leflunomide + methotrexate: 43
- other DMARDs: 143.

Leflunomide monotherapy also had the lowest rate of hepatic events in the DMARD monotherapy groups.

Further developments

Synthetic malononitrilamides (MNA) have been derived from A77 1726. FK778 is the most promising derivative, because of its much shorter half-life. It also blocks replication of herpesvirus in vitro and in vivo. It has therefore been used as part of an immunosuppressive regimen and as an antiviral agent after solid organ transplantation (55). FK778 is under investigation in a phase II trial after kidney transplantation (56).

Organs and Systems

Cardiovascular

The incidence of hypertension in patients with rheumatoid arthritis taking leflunomide 25 mg/day was 11% in a phase II trial (57). During phase III trials, there was new-onset hypertension in 2.1–3.7% (9,10). Increased sympathetic drive has been implicated in its pathogenesis, because leflunomide-induced hypertension is accompanied by an increased heart rate (58). However, this hypothesis remains to be tested.

Pulmonary hypertension has been described in association with leflunomide (59).

Respiratory

Respiratory symptoms in the MN301, US301, and MN302 trials in patients with rheumatoid arthritis included respiratory infections (21–27%), bronchitis (5–8%), increased cough (4–5%), rhinitis (2–5%), pharyngitis (2–3%), pneumonia (2–3%), and sinusitis (1–5%) (9,10,12).

In Japan, acute interstitial pneumonia due to leflunomide has been mentioned as a serious and severe adverse effect, with an incidence of 1.1% and a fatal outcome in 0.36% (60–62).

- A 75-year-old woman with rheumatoid arthritis developed rapidly progressive interstitial pneumonia 45 days after starting to take leflunomide and died of respiratory failure (63). Autopsy showed a mixed pattern of acute and organizing diffuse alveolar damage.
- A 77-year-old woman with rheumatoid arthritis and a history of methotrexate-induced pneumonitis suddenly developed dyspnea on exertion about 2 months after starting to take leflunomide and died (64). For more than 3 weeks after withdrawal of the drug she had a high concentration of an active metabolite of leflunomide.
- A 49-year-old man with rheumatoid arthritis taking methotrexate developed a skin eruption and a severe non-productive cough after taking leflunomide for 17 days (61). He died of respiratory failure 128 days after the diagnosis of acute interstitial pneumonia.
- A 54-year-old woman with rheumatoid arthritis developed an interstitial pneumonia 2 weeks after the end of a 6-week course of treatment with leflunomide (65). The onset of the pneumonia was preceded by raised serum

liver enzymes and hypertension. The acute respiratory failure improved with prednisolone and colestyramine.

However, clinical trials and subsequent observational studies outside Japan have not suggested that leflunomide causes an excess of pulmonary adverse effects (66).

Nevertheless, reports of lung damage atributed to leflunomide in patients outside Japan continue to appear For exmaple, the New Zealand Pharmacovigilance Centre (NZPhvC) and the Australian Adverse Drug Reactions Unit (ADRU) have received 14 reports of supposed pneumonitis in patients taking leflunomide, 12 in combination with methotrexate (67). In nine of these 12 patients pneumonitis occurred after leflunomide was added to methotrexate, usually within 12–20 weeks. One of two patients who died had possible previous methotrexate-induced pneumonitis. Leflunomide washout with colestyramine was used to treat three patients, one with life-threatening illness, with good results. This report suggests that prompt recognition is important to avoid life-threatening disease and supports the use of colestyramine to remove leflunomide, as has been reported in another case in which oral colestyramine was used (68).

- A 69-year-old woman with rheumatoid arthritis developed acute interstitial pneumonia 3 months after starting to take leflunomide. Methylprednisolone pulse therapy and colestyramine 24 g/day ameliorated her symptoms.

In 62 734 patients with rheumatoid arthritis who had used a DMARD there were 74 cases of serious interstitial lung disease, corresponding to a rate of 8.1 per 10 000 patients per year (107). Leflunomide increased the risk of interstitial lung disease (adjusted RR = 1.9; 95% CI = 1.1, 3.6). Among those who had not previously used methotrexate and without a history of interstitial lung disease, the risk associated with leflunomide was not increased (RR = 1.2; 95% CI = 0.4, 3.1), but it was increased among the others (RR = 2.6; 95% CI = 1.2, 5.6). Patients with a history of interstitial lung disease were twice as likely to have taken leflunomide as any other DMARD. Interstitial lung disease associated with the use of leflunomide is probably due to the fact that leflunomide is used in high-risk patients, particularly those who have used methotrexate or have pre-existing interstitial lung disease.

A pulmonary abscess occurred during leflunomide therapy in a patient with rheumatoid arthritis (69).

- A 43-year-old woman who had had rheumatoid arthritis for 5 years complained of fever, arthralgia/myalgia, and night sweating for 1 month. She had been taking only leflunomide 20 mg/day for 5 months. There was no evidence of active arthritis or vasculitic lesions. Her erythrocyte sedimentation rate was 145 mm/hour and C-reactive protein 1.6 g/l. All cultures were negative. A chest X-ray and CT scan showed a pulmonary abscess. *Staphylococcus aureus* was grown in the culture of a purulent sample obtained from the abscess under ultrasonography. The leflunomide was withdrawn, and sultamicillin 8 g/day was given for 6 weeks. Four weeks later, she had completely recovered and a CT scan showed significant improvement of the pulmonary abscess.

Rheumatoid lung nodulosis has been described during leflunomide therapy (70).

- A 77 year-old man with long-standing active seropositive nodular rheumatoid arthritis had a complete remission during 2 months of leflunomide therapy. After 10 months he developed limb pain associated with intensive bone uptake on a bone scan, consistent with hypertrophic pulmonary osteopathy. After 13 months progressive cavitary nodules, predominantly involving the basal segments of the right lung, were detected on a CT scan. A lung biopsy showed necrosis surrounded by epithelioid mononuclear inflammation with giant cells, consistent with rheumatoid disease.

- A 66 year-old man with long-standing active seropositive nodular rheumatoid arthritis achieved a complete remission during 2 months of leflunomide therapy. After 3 months he developed a productive cough. After 7 months a CT scan showed progressive cavitary nodules, predominantly involving the basal segments of the right lung. A lung biopsy showed necrosis surrounded by epithelioid mononuclear inflammation with giant cells, consistent with rheumatoid disease.

In both cases withdrawal of leflunomide was followed by arrest in the growth of the lung nodules, resolution of the limb pain, and gradual improvement in the bone scan. The authors suggested that monocytopenia was involved in the pathogenesis of this rare complication.

Pulmonary alveolar proteinosis is an uncommon disorder marked by abnormal accumulation of surfactant in the alveoli. Secondary pulmonary alveolar proteinosis can occur in patients who are immunosuppressed, usually with corticosteroids. Biopsy-proven pulmonary alveolar proteinosis has been reported in a patient taking leflunomide (71). Treatment with whole lung lavage and withdrawal of leflunomide produced a good result.

Imaging findings in 26 cases of leflunomide-related acute lung injury were similar to those caused by other drugs, including diffuse or widespread patchy ground-glass opacities and/or consolidation, often accompanied by septal thickening and intralobular reticular opacities (72). Of 23 cases 13 had pre-existing interstitial pulmonary disease on chest X-ray or CT scan. The imaging findings were classified into four patterns: diffuse alveolar damage, acute eosinophilic pneumonia, a hyper-reaction, and cryptogenic organizing pneumonia. Those with diffuse alveolar damage had a higher mortality rate, which did not reach conventional statistical significance.

Nervous system

Leflunomide can cause a peripheral reversible neuropathy (52,73–76). This neuropathy is usually axonal in nature, affecting multiple sensory or motor nerves of distal extremities. The mean time of onset of peripheral neuropathy was 6 months after the start of leflunomide therapy, with a range of 3 days to 3 years. Neurological improvement was more likely after drug withdrawal within 30 days after the onset of the symptoms of neuropathy compared with continuous administration (74).

Peripheral neuropathy attributed to leflunomide was observed in two patients (52).

- A 76-year-old man, with an 18-month history of seropositive rheumatoid arthritis, chronic emphysema, and pulmonary fibrosis, developed polymyalgia and was treated with glucocorticoids and azathioprine. Azathioprine was withdrawn after a rise in aspartate transaminase. He was then given leflunomide 100 mg over 3 days followed by 10 mg/day as a maintenance dosage. After 2 weeks, he developed a sensory neuropathy with a stocking distribution up to the malleoli and leflunomide was withdrawn 4 weeks later. During this time he had also been taking prednisolone, tramadol, disodium etidronate, indoramin, and celecoxib, none of which is known to cause neuropathy. Glucose, vitamin B12, serum folate, thyroid function, serum proteins, Bence–Jones protein electrophoresis, cryoglobulins, anti-neutrophil cytoplasmic antibodies, antinuclear antibodies, the Venereal Disease Research Laboratory test, and hepatitis B and C serology were all normal or negative. Nerve conduction was consistent with motor sensory axonal peripheral neuropathy of the lower limbs. On review 3 months after withdrawal of leflunomide, there was clear subjective and objective improvement of the neuropathy, confirmed by repeat nerve conduction studies.
- A 69-year-old woman with a 10-year history of seropositive erosive rheumatoid arthritis, previously treated with gold salts followed by methotrexate, started to take leflunomide and 3 months later reported numbness in the fingertips and feet bilaterally, with a glove-and-stocking sensory neuropathy involving all fingertips and extending to the mid-shins. Leflunomide was withdrawn. Other medications included prednisolone, lansoprazole, simvastatin, losartan, and amiodarone, which she had been taking for a long time without adverse effects. Screening tests for neuropathy, as in the previous case, were normal or negative. There was no cord or nerve root compression on magnetic resonance imaging of the cervical spine. Nerve conduction studies confirmed a sensory motor peripheral neuropathy. She reported marked improvement in her symptoms 3 months after withdrawal of treatment, and this was confirmed on clinical examination and repeat nerve conduction studies.

Two patients taking leflunomide developed severe sensorimotor axonal polyneuropathy starting 5 months after the start of leflunomide therapy; the symptoms rapidly improved after withdrawing leflunomide (77). Of 12 patients with leflunomide-related neuropathy 10 were older than 60 years. The mean delay to the onset of neuropathy was 9 months. The neuropathy improved after withdrawal in seven patients.

One case of leflunomide-induced aseptic meningitis has been reported (51).

Sensory systems

Leflunomide can cause cystoid macular edema (78).

Endophthalmitis associated with leflunomide and adalimumab has been reported (79).

- A 48-year-old woman taking leflunomide and adalimumab for rheumatoid arthritis developed endophthalmitis caused by *Propionibacterium acnes*. The diagnosis was confirmed by polymerase chain reaction and positive cultures. She underwent surgical treatment and was given intravitreal vancomycin, but developed retinal fibrosis and untreatable retinal detachment.

This report of endophthalmitis is consistent with previous reports associated with the use of TNF-α inhibitors. *Propionibacterium acnes* can cause pathological reactions in immunocompromised patients and can cause endophthalmitis, but only after ocular surgery or in intravenous drug users.

Metabolism

Life-threatening hypertriglyceridemia has been described during treatment with leflunomide (49).

Hematologic

Leflunomide-associated anemia has been reported in renal transplant recipients (30).

Pancytopenia, thrombocytopenia, and anemia can occur during leflunomide treatment (21,80–82). The risk of pancytopenia is increased when it is used in combination with methotrexate and in elderly patients. Its course can be fatal and the time of onset ranges from 11 days to 4 years (80). Anemia has been reported in renal transplant recipients (28).

Leflunomide-associated thrombocytosis and leukocytosis resolved after colestyramine washout and withdrawal of leflunomide (83).

Mouth

In the MN301, US301, and MN302 trials, mouth ulceration occurred in 3–5% (9,10,12).

Gastrointestinal

Leflunomide can cause gastrointestinal symptoms, such as diarrhea, dyspepsia, nausea, abdominal pain, and oral ulcers (19,84). They occur mostly during the first 6 months of treatment, are generally mild, and rarely require treatment withdrawal. Two patients with rheumatoid arthritis developed severe diarrhea and important weight loss more than 12 months after starting to take leflunomide. The symptoms were caused by colitis, but one had ulcerative colitis and the other microscopic colitis. The symptoms improved after withdrawal of leflunomide, making a causal relation probable. However, the heterogeneous histopathological findings did not allow any definitive conclusions about mechanism.

There was a higher rate of diarrhea in the leflunomide group in a double-blind, randomized, placebo-controlled trial in patients with active psoriatic arthropathy and psoriasis taking oral leflunomide. Leflunomide was given in a loading dose of 100 mg/day for 3 days followed by 20 mg/day for 24 weeks (26).

The combination of leflunomide 10 mg/day with methotrexate has been studied in a randomized, double-blind 24-week study in patients with rheumatoid arthritis (23). Patients who did not receive a loading dose of leflunomide had a lower incidence of diarrhea and nausea.

If leflunomide-associated persistent diarrhea or weight loss is serious, leflunomide should be withdrawn and colonic endoscopy is recommended. Given the long half-life of leflunomide a washout procedure with colestyramine should be considered whenever the problem is severe or persistent (70,84).

In the MN301, US301, and MN302 trials, gastrointestinal symptoms consisted of diarrhea (22–27%), nausea (13%), dyspepsia (6–10%), abdominal pain (6–8%), mouth ulceration (3–5%), vomiting (3–5%), anorexia (3%), and gastroenteritis (1–3%) (9,10,12). Diarrhea and nausea are more common in patients who receive a loading dose, but the onset of action can be delayed without the loading dose (36). Gastrointestinal symptoms occur mainly during the first 6 months after initiation of leflunomide. The severity of symptoms was mild. If there is severe diarrhea and/or weight loss, withdrawal of leflunomide and endoscopic examination is advised, since ulcerative and microscopic colitis have been detected under such circumstances (85). The pathophysiology of leflunomide-associated diarrhea and weight loss is unclear. Weight loss of 9–24 kg was observed in five of 70 patients who took leflunomide, despite normal concentrations of thyroid-stimulating hormone and no other gastrointestinal complaints (47).

Liver

Leflunomide can cause abnormal liver function tests, (35), and close monitoring of liver enzymes is important (88). However, the risk of serious and non-serious hepatic adverse events is not higher than with methotrexate (86).

The combination of leflunomide 10 mg/day with methotrexate has been studied in a randomized, double-blind 24-week study in patients with rheumatoid arthritis (23). Patients who were switched from placebo to leflunomide had a lower incidence of raised transaminases than patients who were initially treated with leflunomide.

Increased alanine transaminase activity was reported in the leflunomide group in a double-blind, randomized, placebo-controlled trial in 190 patients with active psoriatic arthropathy and psoriasis, who took a loading dose of 100 mg/day for 3 days followed by 20 mg/day orally for 24 weeks (26). However, serious liver toxicity did not occur.

In a randomized, double-blind, placebo-controlled pilot study over 24 weeks, six of 12 adults (11 women, 1 man; median age 41 years) with mild to moderate active systemic lupus erythematosus took oral leflunomide. Disease activity fell in both groups. Minor adverse events included transient rises in alanine transaminase, hypertension, and transient leukopenia (29).

In the MN301, US301, and MN302 trials, there were abnormal liver enzymes in 6–10% (9,10,12). The co-administration of methotrexate is a risk factor (18,87–89). According to the National Cancer Institute Common Toxicity Criteria, 8.9% of patients developed grade 2 or 3 hepatotoxicity within the first year, mainly within 6 months and in combination with methotrexate, after the start of leflunomide therapy based on liver enzyme determinations (72). The use of folate was also associated with less frequent changes in liver function tests (9,10,12). Nevertheless, leflunomide can cause severe liver injury (90–93), estimated at a rate of one in 200 users (94). Leflunomide is therefore not recommended in patients with significant liver impairment or evidence of infection with hepatitis B or C virus (95).

A CYP2C9 polymorphism has been implicated in the pathogenesis of leflunomide hepatotoxicity (92).

- A 67-year-old woman with rheumatoid arthritis developed diarrhea and raised liver enzymes after taking leflunomide for 15 days. Histologically, the liver showed acute hepatitis. She was homozygous for the CYP2C9*3 allele. The liver damage subsided within a few weeks.

Urinary tract

Interstitial nephritis occurred in one case of chronic overdose of leflunomide (96).

Skin

Adverse effects of leflunomide on the skin in patients with rheumatoid arthritis include alopecia (9–17%), rash (11–12%), pruritus (5–6%), dry skin (3%), and eczema (1–3%; 9,10,12). Single cases of exfoliative dermatitis (97), a lichenoid drug reaction (98), and skin ulceration (99) have been reported.

A photodistributed lichenoid drug eruption with rhabdomyolysis was observed in a patient taking leflunomide (100).

Leflunomide can cause toxic epidermal necrolysis (101).

- A woman with rheumatoid arthritis had taken glucocorticoids and methotrexate for 2 years when the methotrexate was replaced by leflunomide (102). Three weeks later she developed progressive generalized erythema with blisters, fever, chills, and erosive lesions on the lips and oral mucosa. The palmar and plantar surfaces had edema, erythema, and pulpitis with epidermolysis. Histology showed necrotic keratinocytes and epidermal spongiosis. After high-dose prednisolone and topical treatment she recovered within 14 days.

Leflunomide can cause skin ulceration. Two women, aged 59 and 63 years, were given leflunomide for rheumatoid arthritis and subsequently developed severe skin ulcers; after drug withdrawal the ulcers healed completely albeit very slowly (103).

Subacute cutaneous lupus erythematosus associated with leflunomide has been reported (104).

Hair

In 51 patients with proliferative lupus nephritis major adverse events in those who were taking leflunomide were infections (mainly herpes zoster) and alopecia (84).

Connective tissues

The risk of wound-healing complications after elective orthopedic surgery has been studied in 201 patients with rheumatoid arthritis or psoriatic arthropathy receiving methotrexate, etanercept, infliximab, adalimumab, anakinra, or leflunomide (105). Compared with patients who received methotrexate (n = 59), the risk of postoperative wound-healing complications in patients who received leflunomide (n = 32) was significantly increased: 14% versus 41% respectively. The authors recommended that leflunomide should be withdrawn preoperatively in patients with rheumatoid arthritis undergoing elective orthopedic surgical procedures, to reduce the risk of early wound-healing complications or infections.

Immunologic

In the treatment of rheumatoid arthritis leflunomide can cause a vasculitis, and acute necrotizing vasculitis is rare but serious (50,106).

Leflunomide caused severe skin reactions in five patients. All had taken leflunomide for rheumatoid arthritis 4–6 weeks before the onset of the reactions and had fever, rash, and generalized weakness (107). All had delayed onset, widespread and long lasting rashes, and internal organ involvement. These features suggest a drug hypersensitivity syndrome.

Infection risk

A total of 10 614 patients with rheumatoid arthritis and 1721 with musculoskeletal disorders were screened for *Herpes zoster* by semi-annual questionnaires (108). Patients with prior herpes zoster infection were excluded. The annualized incidence rate per 1000 patient-years was 13 (95% CI = 12, 15) in patients with rheumatoid arthritis and 15 (95% CI = 11, 18) in those with musculoskeletal disorders; there was no effect of age and sex. The following significant hazard ratios predictive of *Herpes zoster* were computed from multivariable analyses in patients with rheumatoid arthritis: cyclophosphamide 4.2 (95% CI = 1.6, 12), azathioprine 2.0 (1.2, 3.3), prednisone 1.5 (1.2, 1.8), leflunomide 1.4 (1.1,1.8), and COX-2 inhibitory NSAIDs 1.3 (1.1, 1.6).

Seven cases of tuberculosis have been reported in patients taking leflunomide (109,110).

Long-Term Effects

Mutagenicity

A minor metabolite of leflunomide, 4-Trifluoromethyl-aniline, was mutagenic in vitro (111).

Tumorigenicity

Male mice had an increased incidence of lymphoma at an oral leflunomide dose of 15 mg/kg, and female mice had a dose-related increased incidence of bronchoalveolar adenomas and carcinomas beginning at 1.5 mg/kg (111).

Second-Generation Effects

Fertility

Leflunomide did not affect fertility in rats (111).

Pregnancy

Leflunomide must be prophylactically withdrawn before a planned pregnancy (112).

Teratogenicity

In oral embryocytotoxicity and teratogenicity studies in rats and rabbits, leflunomide was embryocytotoxic (growth retardation, embryolethality) and teratogenic (malformations of the head, rump, vertebral column, ribs, and limbs; 111. Not only is leflunomide teratogenic and fetotoxic in animals, but its active metabolite is detectable in plasma up to 2 years after withdrawal. Therefore, the fetus could have in utero exposure to leflunomide up to 2 years after the end of treatment. Leflunomide has been classified as pregnancy category X by the Food and Drug Administration (111,113). However, experience in a very small group of pregnant women who took leflunomide and continued their pregnancy to term gave no indication of an increase in teratogenesis (114). Nevertheless, the majority of 30 pregnant women were elected to interrupt their pregnancies, except three patients (111). At present, withdrawal of leflunomide is mandatory before pregnancy, and colestyramine treatment is advised to wash out leflunomide (95,111,115,116). Both men and women who want to have a child should discontinue leflunomide and take colestyramine to wash it out. Leflunomide has not been studied in children, possibly because of its cytotoxic nature. In particular, its teratogenic potential may be a concern when treating adolescent girls (117).

Leflunomide is classified in category X of fetal risk (Table 1) (118). A wash-out regimen may reduce the risk of fetal harm. Conception scheduling or early pregnancy detection is required for better clinical counselling and the avoidance of unnecessary risk.

Lactation

Breast feeding by nursing mothers is not recommended, because it is unknown if leflunomide is excreted in human milk (95,111).

Drug Administration

Drug dosage regimens

Leflunomide is taken orally. In most regimens it is begun with a loading dose of 100 mg/day over 3 days followed by a maintenance dosage of 10–20 mg/day. Leflunomide 100 mg/week had similar effectiveness and less toxicity in open trials compared with daily dosing (21,119).

The efficacy and safety profile of leflunomide 10 mg (n = 202; loading dose on day 3, 100 mg/day) and 20 mg (n = 200; loading dose on days 1–3, 100 mg/day) have been investigated in patients with active rheumatoid arthritis over 24 weeks (24). There was no significant difference between the groups regarding the American College of Rheumatology 20% criteria (50 versus 57%). The lower leflunomide dosage regimen resulted in more adverse events requiring withdrawal (15 versus 12%) and a higher rate of serious adverse events (13 versus 10%).

Drug overdose

Two cases of leflunomide overdose have been reported.

- A 70-year-old man with chronic active rheumatoid arthritis was given leflunomide in a loading dose of 100 mg/day followed by 10 mg/day (96). The initial response was modest and the dose was increased to 20 mg/day, but the patient actually took 100 mg/week plus 20 mg/day. The serum creatinine concentration increased from 140 μmol/l to 287 μmol/l over 2 years. A renal biopsy showed tubulointerstitial nephritis. Leflunomide was withdrawn immediately and prednisolone 20 mg/day was started. The creatinine returned to 160 μmol/l within 1 month.
- A 40-year-old woman with rheumatoid arthritis took leflunomide 100 mg/day for 3 days and 20 mg/day thereafter (120). After 28 days it was realized that she had continued to take the 100 mg tablets, resulting in a dosage of 120 mg/day. She was immediately hospitalized and colestyramine washout procedure was performed. She had no adverse effects.

Drug–Drug Interactions

Infliximab
The administration of infliximab after or simultaneously with leflunomide seems to be safe and effective in patients with rheumatoid arthritis (20,121,122).

Rifampicin
Multiple doses of rifampicin increase leflunomide concentrations (123).

Warfarin
Interactions of leflunomide with warfarin have been reported (124).

- A 49-year-old man with resistant rheumatoid arthritis took leflunomide 100 mg/day for 3 days. His international normalized ratio (INR) had been stable for 1 year while he was taking warfarin, and 2 days before starting treatment with leflunomide it was 3.4. After he took the second dose of leflunomide, he developed gross hematuria. His INR had risen to 11, and warfarin was withdrawn. The hematuria resolved spontaneously several hours later, but his INR remained raised for the next 2 days, even though he had stopped taking warfarin. He was given intravenous vitamin K 1 mg on the third day, and 12 hours later the INR fell to 1.9. Subsequently he began taking warfarin again, but at a lower dose of 1 mg/day, which was sufficient to maintain his INR within the target range.
- A 61-year-old Caucasian woman taking long-term warfarin for recurrent thromboembolism and atrial fibrillation had a raised international normalized ratio (INR) after she started taking leflunomide for rheumatoid arthritis (125). Her INR had been stable for 4 months before this. She patient required an overall 22% reduction in her weekly warfarin dose to maintain the INR within the target range of 2.0–3.0 after adding leflunomide.

The frequency of INR monitoring should be increased in patients receiving leflunomide and warfarin.

As to mechanism, A77 1726 inhibits CYP2C9 and might increase the systemic availability of CYP2C9 substrates, such as warfarin and phenytoin (124,126).

Management of Adverse Drug Reactions

Usually, overdosage and adverse events can be managed by dosage reduction, the addition of colestyramine, and symptomatic therapy (36). However, in one study in patients with rheumatoid arthritis, leflunomide 10 mg/day compared with 20 mg/day was associated with less efficacy and more adverse events leading to treatment withdrawal (24). Colestyramine 3×8 g/day for 11 days is recommended to wash out leflunomide, if A77 1726 plasma concentrations do not fall to 0.02 mg/l or less, additional colestyramine is advised. Without this washout procedure, it can take up to 2 years to reach A77 1726 plasma concentrations of 0.02 mg/l. Oral activated charcoal 50 g every 6 hours for 24 hours also reduced plasma A77 1726 concentrations (95).

Plasma A77 1726 concentrations can be measured by high-performance liquid chromatography (127,128). Monitoring of platelets, white blood cells, hemoglobin, and alanine transaminase activity is advised at baseline, monthly for 6 months, and every 6–8 weeks thereafter. Leflunomide should be withdrawn if pulmonary symptoms such as cough and dyspnea start or worsen (95).

References

1. Bartlett RR, Schleyerbach R. Immunopharmacological profile of a novel isoxazol derivative, HWA 486, with potential antirheumatic activity—I. Disease modifying action on adjuvant arthritis of the rat. Int J Immunopharmacol 1985;7(1):7–18.
2. Imose M, Nagaki M, Kimura K, Takai S, Imao M, Naiki T, Osawa Y, Asano T, Hayashi H, Moriwaki H. Leflunomide protects from T-cell-mediated liver injury in mice through inhibition of nuclear factor kappaB. Hepatology 2004;40(5):1160–9.
3. Manna SK, Mukhopadhyay A, Aggarwal BB. Leflunomide suppresses TNF-induced cellular responses: effects on NF-kappa B, activator protein-1, c-Jun N-terminal protein kinase, and apoptosis. J Immunol 2000;165(10):5962–9.
4. Breedveld FC, Dayer JM. Leflunomide: mode of action in the treatment of rheumatoid arthritis. Ann Rheum Dis 2000;59(11):841–9.

5. Manna SK, Aggarwal BB. Immunosuppressive leflunomide metabolite (A77 1726) blocks TNF-dependent nuclear factor-kappa B activation and gene expression. J Immunol 1999;162(4):2095–102.

6. Kremer JM. What I would like to know about leflunomide. J Rheumatol 2004;31(6):1029–31.

7. Rozman B. Clinical pharmacokinetics of leflunomide. Clin Pharmacokinet 2002;41(6):421–30.

8. Mladenovic V, Domljan Z, Rozman B, Jajic I, Mihajlovic D, Dordevic J, Popovic M, Dimitrijevic M, Zivkovic M, Campion G, et al. Safety and effectiveness of leflunomide in the treatment of patients with active rheumatoid arthritis. Results of a randomized, placebo-controlled, phase II study. Arthritis Rheum 1995;38(11):1595–603.

9. Strand V, Cohen S, Schiff M, Weaver A, Fleischmann R, Cannon G, Fox R, Moreland L, Olsen N, Furst D, Caldwell J, Kaine J, Sharp J, Hurley F, Loew-Friedrich I. Treatment of active rheumatoid arthritis with leflunomide compared with placebo and methotrexate. Leflunomide Rheumatoid Arthritis Investigators Group. Arch Intern Med 1999;159(21):2542–50.

10. Smolen JS, Kalden JR, Scott DL, Rozman B, Kvien TK, Larsen A, Loew-Friedrich I, Oed C, Rosenburg R. Efficacy and safety of leflunomide compared with placebo and sulphasalazine in active rheumatoid arthritis: a double-blind, randomised, multicentre trial. European Leflunomide Study Group. Lancet 1999;353(9149):259–66.

11. Smolen JS. Efficacy and safety of the new DMARD leflunomide: comparison to placebo and sulfasalazine in active rheumatoid arthritis. Scand J Rheumatol Suppl 1999;112:15–21.

12. Emery P, Breedveld FC, Lemmel EM, Kaltwasser JP, Dawes PT, Gomor B, Van Den Bosch F, Nordstrom D, Bjorneboe O, Dahl R, Horslev-Petersen K, Rodriguez De La Serna A, Molloy M, Tikly M, Oed C, Rosenburg R, Loew-Friedrich I. A comparison of the efficacy and safety of leflunomide and methotrexate for the treatment of rheumatoid arthritis. Rheumatology (Oxford) 2000;39(6):655–65.

13. Larsen A, Kvien TK, Schattenkirchner M, Rau R, Scott DL, Smolen JS, Rozman B, Westhovens R, Tikly M, Oed C, Rosenburg REuropean Leflunomide Study Group. Slowing of disease progression in rheumatoid arthritis patients during long-term treatment with leflunomide or sulfasalazine. Scand J Rheumatol 2001;30(3):135–42.

14. Cohen S, Cannon GW, Schiff M, Weaver A, Fox R, Olsen N, Furst D, Sharp J, Moreland L, Caldwell J, Kaine J, Strand V. Two-year, blinded, randomized, controlled trial of treatment of active rheumatoid arthritis with leflunomide compared with methotrexate. Utilization of Leflunomide in the Treatment of Rheumatoid Arthritis Trial Investigator Group. Arthritis Rheum 2001;44(9):1984–92.

15. Scott DL, Smolen JS, Kalden JR, van de Putte LB, Larsen A, Kvien TK, Schattenkirchner M, Nash P, Oed C, Loew-Friedrich IEuropean Leflunomide Study Group. Treatment of active rheumatoid arthritis with leflunomide: two year follow up of a double blind, placebo controlled trial versus sulfasalazine. Ann Rheum Dis 2001;60(10):913–23.

16. Kalden JR, Schattenkirchner M, Sorensen H, Emery P, Deighton C, Rozman B, Breedveld F. The efficacy and safety of leflunomide in patients with active rheumatoid arthritis: a five-year followup study. Arthritis Rheum 2003;48(6):1513–20.

17. Kiely PD, Johnson DM. Infliximab and leflunomide combination therapy in rheumatoid arthritis: an open-label study. Rheumatology (Oxford) 2002;41(6):631–7.

18. Kremer JM, Genovese MC, Cannon GW, Caldwell JR, Cush JJ, Furst DE, Luggen ME, Keystone E, Weisman MH, Bensen WM, Kaine JL, Ruderman EM, Coleman P, Curtis DL, Kopp EJ, Kantor SM, Waltuck J, Lindsley HB, Markenson JA, Strand V, Crawford B, Fernando I, Simpson K, Bathon JM. Concomitant leflunomide therapy in patients with active rheumatoid arthritis despite stable doses of methotrexate. A randomized, double-blind, placebo-controlled trial. Ann Intern Med 2002;137(9):726–33.

19. Dougados M, Emery P, Lemmel EM, de la Serna R, Zerbini CA, Brin S, van Riel P. Efficacy and safety of leflunomide and predisposing factors for treatment response in patients with active rheumatoid arthritis: RELIEF 6-month data. J Rheumatol 2003;30(12):2572–9.

20. Godinho F, Godfrin B, El Mahou S, Navaux F, Zabranieski L, Cantagrel A. Safety of leflunomide plus infliximab combination therapy in rheumatoid arthritis. Clin Exp Rheumatol 2004;22(3):328–30.

21. Jaimes-Hernandez J, Robles-San Roman M, Suarez-Otero R, Davalos-Zugasti ME, Arroyo-Borrego S. Rheumatoid arthritis treatment with weekly leflunomide: an open-label study. J Rheumatol 2004;31(2):235–7.

22. Nyugen M, Kabir M, Ravaud P. Short-term efficacy and safety of leflunomide in the treatment of active rheumatoid arthritis in everyday clinical use. Clin Drug Invest 2004;24(2):103–12.

23. Kremer J, Genovese M, Cannon GW, Caldwell J, Cush J, Furst DE, Luggen M, Keystone E, Bathon J, Kavanaugh A, Ruderman E, Coleman P, Curtis D, Kopp E, Kantor S, Weisman M, Waltuck J, Lindsley HB, Markenson J, Crawford B, Fernando I, Simpson K, Strand V. Combination leflunomide and methotrexate (MTX) therapy for patients with active rheumatoid arthritis failing MTX monotherapy: open-label extension of a randomized, double-blind, placebo controlled trial. J Rheumatol 2004;31(8):1521–31.

24. Poor G, Strand VLeflunomide Multinational Study Group. Efficacy and safety of leflunomide 10 mg versus 20 mg once daily in patients with active rheumatoid arthritis: multinational double-blind, randomized trial Rheumatology (Oxford) 2004;43(6):744–9.

25. Van Roon EN, Jansen TL, Mourad L, Houtman PM, Bruyn GA, Griep EN, Wilffert B, Tobi H, Brouwers JR. Leflunomide in active rheumatoid arthritis: a prospective study in daily practice. Br J Clin Pharmacol 2004;58(2):201–8.

26. Kaltwasser JP, Nash P, Gladman D, Rosen CF, Behrens F, Jones P, Wollenhaupt J, Falk FG, Mease PTreatment of Psoriatic Arthritis Study Group. Efficacy and safety of leflunomide in the treatment of psoriatic arthritis and psoriasis: a multinational, double-blind, randomized, placebo-controlled clinical trial. Arthritis Rheum 2004;50(6):1939–50.

27. Tlacuilo-Parra JA, Guevara-Gutierrez E, Rodriguez-Castellanos MA, Ornelas-Aguirre JM, Barba-Gomez JF, Salazar-Paramo M. Leflunomide in the treatment of psoriasis: results of a phase II open trial. Br J Dermatol 2004;150(5):970–6.

28. Williams JW, Mital D, Chong A, Kottayil A, Millis M, Longstreth J, Huang W, Brady L, Jensik S. Experiences with leflunomide in solid organ transplantation. Transplantation 2002;73(3):358–66.

29. Tam LS, Li EK, Wong CK, Lam CW, Szeto CC. Double-blind, randomized, placebo-controlled pilot study of leflunomide in systemic lupus erythematosus. Lupus 2004;13(8):601–4.

30. Metzler C, Fink C, Lamprecht P, Gross WL, Reinhold-Keller E. Maintenance of remission with leflunomide in Wegener's granulomatosis. Rheumatology (Oxford) 2004;43(3):315–20.

31. Prajapati DN, Knox JF, Emmons J, Saeian K, Csuka ME, Binion DG. Leflunomide treatment of Crohn's disease patients intolerant to standard immunomodulator therapy. J Clin Gastroenterol 2003;37(2):125–8.

32. Baughman RP, Lower EE. Leflunomide for chronic sarcoidosis. Sarcoidosis Vasc Diffuse Lung Dis 2004;21(1):43–8.

33. Kaltwasser JP, Behrens F. Leflunomide: long-term clinical experience and new uses. Expert Opin Pharmacother 2005;6(5):787–801.

34. Li EK, Tam LS, Tomlinson B. Leflunomide in the treatment of rheumatoid arthritis. Clin Ther 2004;26(4):447–59.

35. Osiri M, Shea B, Robinson V, Suarez-Almazor M, Strand V, Tugwell P, Wells G. Leflunomide for the treatment of rheumatoid arthritis: a systematic review and metaanalysis. J Rheumatol 2003;30(6):1182–90.

36. Maddison P, Kiely P, Kirkham B, Lawson T, Moots R, Proudfoot D, Reece R, Scott D, Sword R, Taggart A, Thwaites C, Williams E. Leflunomide in rheumatoid arthritis: recommendations through a process of consensus. Rheumatology (Oxford) 2005;44(3):280–6.

37. Hardinger KL, Wang CD, Schnitzler MA, Miller BW, Jendrisak MD, Shenoy S, Lowell JA, Brennan DC. Prospective, pilot, open-label, short-term study of conversion to leflunomide reverses chronic renal allograft dysfunction. Am J Transplant 2002;2(9):867–71.

38. John GT, Manivannan J, Chandy S, Peter S, Jacob CK. Leflunomide therapy for cytomegalovirus disease in renal allograft recepients. Transplantation 2004;77(9):1460–1.

39. Schlapfer E, Fischer M, Ott P, Speck RF. Anti-HIV-1 activity of leflunomide: a comparison with mycophenolic acid and hydroxyurea. AIDS 2003;17(11):1613–20.

40. Kelly LM, Lisziewicz J, Lori F. "Virostatics" as a potential new class of HIV drugs. Curr Pharm Des 2004;10(32):4103–20.

41. Anonymous. Leflunomide: new indication. In psoriatic rheumatism: too many risks, too little efficacy. Prescrire Int 2005;14(78):123–6.

42. Bettembourg-Brault I, Gossec L, Pham T, Gottenberg JE, Damiano J, Dougados M. Leflunomide in rheumatoid arthritis in daily practice: treatment discontinuation rates in comparison with other DMARDs. Clin Exp Rheumatol 2006;24(2):168–71.

43. First MR. An update on new immunosuppressive drugs undergoing preclinical and clinical trials: potential applications in organ transplantation. Am J Kidney Dis 1997;29(2):303–17.

44. Shoker AS. Immunopharmacologic therapy in renal transplantation. Pharmacotherapy 1996;16(4):562–75.

45. van Riel PL, Smolen JS, Emery P, Kalden JR, Dougados M, Strand CV, Breedveld FC. Leflunomide: a manageable safety profile. J Rheumatol Suppl 2004;71:21–4.

46. Hoi A, Littlejohn GO. Aminotransferase levels during treatment of rheumatoid arthritis with leflunomide in clinical practice. Ann Rheum Dis 2003;62(4):379.

47. Coblyn JS, Shadick N, Helfgott S. Leflunomide-associated weight loss in rheumatoid arthritis. Arthritis Rheum 2001;44(5):1048–51.

48. Hewitson PJ, Debroe S, McBride A, Milne R. Leflunomide and rheumatoid arthritis: a systematic review of effectiveness, safety and cost implications. J Clin Pharm Ther 2000;25(4):295–302.

49. Laborde F, Loeuille D, Chary-Valckenaere I. Life-threatening hypertriglyceridemia during leflunomide therapy in a patient with rheumatoid arthritis. Arthritis Rheum 2004;50(10):3398.

50. Macdonald J, Zhong T, Lazarescu A, Gan BS, Harth M. Vasculitis associated with the use of leflunomide. J Rheumatol 2004;31(10):2076–8.

51. Cohen JD, Jorgensen C, Sany J. Leflunomide-induced aseptic meningitis. Joint Bone Spine 2004;71(3):243–5.

52. Carulli MT, Davies UM. Peripheral neuropathy: an unwanted effect of leflunomide? Rheumatology (Oxford) 2002;41(8):952–3.

53. Siva C, Eisen SA, Shepherd R, Cunningham F, Fang MA, Finch W, Salisbury D, Singh JA, Stern R, Zarabadi SA. Leflunomide use during the first 33 months after food and drug administration approval: experience with a national cohort of 3,325 patients. Arthritis Rheum 2003;49(6):745–51.

54. Cannon GW, Holden WL, Juhaeri J, Dai W, Scarazzini L, Stang P. Adverse events with disease modifying antirheumatic drugs (DMARD): a cohort study of leflunomide compared with other DMARD. J Rheumatol 2004;31(10):1906–11.

55. Fitzsimmons WE, First MR. FK778, a synthetic malononitrilamide. Yonsei Med J 2004;45(6):1132–5.

56. Vanrenterghem Y, van Hooff JP, Klinger M, Wlodarczyk Z, Squifflet JP, Mourad G, Neuhaus P, Jurewicz A, Rostaing L, Charpentier B, Paczek L, Kreis H, Chang R, Paul LC, Grinyo JM, Short C. The effects of FK778 in combination with tacrolimus and steroids: a phase II multicenter study in renal transplant patients. Transplantation 2004;78(1):9–14.

57. Rozman B. Clinical experience with leflunomide in rheumatoid arthritis. Leflunomide Investigators' Group. J Rheumatol Suppl 1998;53:27–32.

58. Rozman B, Praprotnik S, Logar D, Tomsic M, Hojnik M, Kos-Golja M, Accetto R, Dolenc P. Leflunomide and hypertension. Ann Rheum Dis 2002;61(6):567–9.

59. Martinez-Taboada VM, Rodriguez-Valverde V, Gonzalez-Vilchez F, Armijo JA. Pulmonary hypertension in a patient with rheumatoid arthritis treated with leflunomide. Rheumatology (Oxford) 2004;43(11):1451–3.

60. McCurry J. Japan deaths spark concerns over arthritis drug. Lancet 2004;363(9407):461.

61. Kamata Y, Nara H, Kamimura T, Haneda K, Iwamoto M, Masuyama J, Okazaki H, Minota S. Rheumatoid arthritis complicated with acute interstitial pneumonia induced by leflunomide as an adverse reaction. Intern Med 2004;43(12):1201–4.

62. Ito S, Sumida T. Interstitial lung disease associated with leflunomide. Intern Med 2004;43(12):1103–4.

63. Ochi S, Harigai M, Mizoguchi F, Iwai H, Hagiyama H, Oka T, Miyasaka N. Leflunomide-related acute interstitial pneumonia in two patients with rheumatoid arthritis: autopsy findings with a mosaic pattern of acute and organizing diffuse alveolar damage. Mod Rheumatol 2006;16(5):316–20.

64. Hirabayashi Y, Shimizu H, Kobayashi N, Kudo K. Leflunomide-induced pneumonitis in a patient with rheumatoid arthritis. Intern Med 2006;45(10):689–91.

65. Takeishi M, Akiyama Y, Akiba H, Adachi D, Hirano M, Mimura T. Leflunomide induced acute interstitial pneumonia. J Rheumatol 2005;32(6):1160–3.

66. Scott DL. Interstitial lung disease and disease modifying anti-rheumatic drugs. Lancet 2004;363(9416):1239–40.

67. Savage RL, Highton J, Boyd IW, Chapman P. Pneumonitis associated with leflunomide: a profile of New Zealand and Australian reports. Intern Med J 2006;36(3):162–9.

68. Suissa S, Hudson M, Ernst P. Leflunomide use and the risk of interstitial lung disease in rheumatoid arthritis. Arthritis Rheum 2006;54(5):1435–9.

69. Ulusoy H, Bilgici A, Kuru O, Celenk C. Pulmonary abscess due to leflunomide use in rheumatoid arthritis: a case report. Rheumatol Int 2005;25(2):139–42.

70. Rozin A, Yigla M, Guralnik L, Keidar Z, Vlodavsky E, Rozenbaum M, Nahir AM, Balbir-Gurman A. Rheumatoid lung nodulosis and osteopathy associated with leflunomide therapy. Clin Rheumatol 2006;25(3):384–8.

71. Wardwell NR, Jr., Miller R, Ware LB. Pulmonary alveolar proteinosis associated with a disease-modifying antirheumatoid arthritis drug. Respirology 2006;11(5):663–5.

72. Sakai F, Noma S, Kurihara Y, Yamada H, Azuma A, Kudoh S, Ichikawa Y. Leflunomide-related lung injury in patients with rheumatoid arthritis: imaging features. Mod Rheumatol 2005;15(3):173–9.

73. Bharadwaj A, Haroon N. Peripheral neuropathy in patients on leflunomide. Rheumatology (Oxford) 2004;43(7):934.

74. Bonnel RA, Graham DJ. Peripheral neuropathy in patients treated with leflunomide. Clin Pharmacol Ther 2004;75(6):580–5.

75. Kopp HG, Moerike K, Kanz L, Hartmann JT. Leflunomide and peripheral neuropathy: a potential interaction between uracil/tegafur and leflunomide. Clin Pharmacol Ther 2005;78(1):89–90.

76. Martin K, Bentaberry F, Dumoulin C, Longy-Boursier M, Lifermann F, Haramburu F, Dehais J, Schaeverbeke T, Begaud B, Moore N. Neuropathy associated with leflunomide: a case series. Ann Rheum Dis 2005;64(4):649–50.

77. Gabelle A, Antoine JC, Hillaire-Buys D, Coudeyre E, Camu W. Neuropathie axonale sévère et léflunomide. Rev Neurol (Paris) 2005;161(11):1106–9.

78. Barak A, Morse LS, Schwab I. Leflunomide (Arava)-induced cystoid macular oedema. Rheumatology (Oxford) 2004;43(2):246–8.

79. Montero JA, Ruiz-Moreno JM, Rodriguez AE, Ferrer C, Sanchis E, Alio JL. Endogenous endophthalmitis by *Propionibacterium acnes associated with leflunomide and adalimumab therapy. Eur J Ophthalmol 2006;16(2):343–5.*

80. Chan J, Sanders DC, Du L, Pillans PI. Leflunomide-associated pancytopenia with or without methotrexate. Ann Pharmacother 2004;38(7–8):1206–11.

81. Hill RL, Topliss DJ, Purcell PM. Pancytopenia associated with leflunomide and methotrexate. Ann Pharmacother 2003;37(1):149.

82. Auer J, Hinterreiter M, Allinger S, Kirchgatterer A, Knoflach P. Severe pancytopenia after leflunomide in rheumatoid arthritis. Acta Med Austriaca 2000;27(4):131–2.

83. Koenig AS, Abruzzo JL. Leflunomide induced fevers, thrombocytosis, and leukocytosis in a patient with relapsing polychondritis. J Rheumatol 2002;29(1):192–4.

84. Cui TG, Hou FF, Ni ZH, Chen XM, Zhang FS, Zhu TY, Zhao XZ, Bao CD, Zhao MH, Wang GB, Qian JQ, Cai GY, Li YN, Lu FM, Mei CL, Zou WZ, Wang H. [Treatment of proliferative lupus nephritis with leflunomide and steroid: a prospective multi-center controlled clinical trial]. Zhonghua Nei Ke Za Zhi 2005;44(9):672–6.

85. Verschueren P, Vandooren AK, Westhovens R. Debilitating diarrhoea and weight loss due to colitis in two RA patients treated with leflunomide. Clin Rheumatol 2005;24(1):87–90.

86. Suissa S, Ernst P, Hudson M, Bitton A, Kezouh A. Newer disease-modifying antirheumatic drugs and the risk of serious hepatic adverse events in patients with rheumatoid arthritis. Am J Med 2004;117(2):87–92.

87. van Roon EN, Jansen TL, Houtman NM, Spoelstra P, Brouwers JR. Leflunomide for the treatment of rheumatoid arthritis in clinical practice: incidence and severity of hepatotoxicity. Drug Saf 2004;27(5):345–52.

88. Cannon GW, Kremer JM. Leflunomide. Rheum Dis Clin North Am 2004;30(2):295–309.

89. Gao JS, Wu H, Tian J. [Treatment of patients with juvenile rheumatoid arthritis with combination of leflunomide and methotrexate.]Zhonghua Er Ke Za Zhi 2003;41(6):435–8.

90. Schiemann U, Kellner H. Gastrointestinale Nebenwirkungen der Therapie rheumatischer Erkrankungen. [Gastrointestinal side effects in the therapy of rheumatologic diseases.] Z Gastroenterol 2002; 40(11):937–43.

91. Anonymous. Severe liver damage with leflunomide. Prescrire Int 2001;10(55):149.

92. Sevilla-Mantilla C, Ortega L, Agundez JA, Fernandez-Gutierrez B, Ladero JM, Diaz-Rubio M. Leflunomide-induced acute hepatitis. Dig Liver Dis 2004;36(1):82–4.

93. Thomasset SC, Ong SL, Large SR. Post-coronary artery bypass graft liver failure: a possible association with leflunomide. Ann Thorac Surg 2005;79(2):698–9.

94. Moynihan R. FDA officials argue over safety of new arthritis drug. BMJ 2003;326(7389):565.

95. Aventis Pharmaceuticals Inc. Arava Tablets (leflunomide) 10 mg, 20 mg, 100 mg Product information. 2005.

96. Haydar AA, Hujairi N, Kirkham B, Hangartner R, Goldsmith DJ. Chronic overdose of leflunomide inducing interstitial nephritis. Nephrol Dial Transplant 2004;19(5): 1334–5.

97. Bandyopadhyay D. Exfoliative dermatitis induced by leflunomide therapy. J Dermatol 2003;30(11):845–6.

98. Canonne-Courivaud D, Carpentier O, Dejobert Y, Hachulla E, Delaporte E. Toxidermie lichenoïde au léflunomide (Arava). [Lichenoid drug reaction to leflunomide.] Ann Dermatol Venereol 2003;130(4):435–7.

99. McCoy CM. Leflunomide-associated skin ulceration. Ann Pharmacother 2002;36(6):1009–11.

100. Rivarola de Gutierrez E, Abaca H. Photodistributed lichenoid drug eruption with rhabdomyolysis occurring during leflunomide therapy. Dermatology 2004;208(3):232–3.

101. Teraki Y, Hitomi K, Sato Y, Hamamatsu Y, Izaki S. Leflunomide-induced toxic epidermal necrolysis. Int J Dermatol 2006;45(11):1370–1.

102. Fischer TW, Bauer HI, Graefe T, Barta U, Elsner P. Erythema multiforme-like drug eruption with oral involvement after intake of leflunomide. Dermatology 2003; 207(4):386–9.

103. Jakob A, Porstmann R, Rompel R. Hautulzerationen nach Leflunomid Therapie bei zwei Patienten mit rheumatoider Arthritis. [Skin ulceration after leflunomide treatment in two patients with rheumatoid arthritis.] J Dtsch Dermatol Ges 2006;4(4):324–7.

104. Kerr OA, Murray CS, Tidman MJ. Subacute cutaneous lupus erythematosus associated with leflunomide. Clin Exp Dermatol 2004;29(3):319–20.

105. Fuerst M, Mohl H, Baumgartel K, Ruther W. Leflunomide increases the risk of early healing complications in patients with rheumatoid arthritis undergoing elective orthopedic surgery. Rheumatol Int 2006;26(12):1138–42.

106. Holm EA, Balslev E, Jemec GB. Vasculitis occurring during leflunomide therapy. Dermatology 2001;203(3):258–9.

107. Shastri V, Betkerur J, Kushalappa PA, Savita TG, Parthasarathi G. Severe cutaneous adverse drug reaction to leflunomide: a report of five cases. Indian J Dermatol Venereol Leprol 2006;72(4):286–9.

108. Wolfe F, Michaud K, Chakravarty EF. Rates and predictors of herpes zoster in patients with rheumatoid arthritis and non-inflammatory musculoskeletal disorders. Rheumatology (Oxford) 2006;45(11):1370–5.

109. Hocevar A, Rozman B, Praprotnik S, Lestan B, Erzen D, Petric V, Tomsic M. Leflunomide-associated tuberculosis? Rheumatology 2006;45(2):228–9.

110. Grover R, Dhir V, Aneja R, Arya V, Galle A, Marwaha V, Kumar A. Severe infections following leflunomide therapy for rheumatoid arthritis. Rheumatol (Oxf) 2006;45(7):918–20.

111. Brent RL. Teratogen update: reproductive risks of leflunomide (Arava); a pyrimidine synthesis inhibitor: counseling women taking leflunomide before or during pregnancy and men taking leflunomide who are contemplating fathering a child. Teratology 2001;63(2):106–12.

112. Ostensen M. Antirheumatische Therapie und Reproduktion. Einfluss auf Fertilitat, Schwangerschaft und Stillzeit. [Antirheumatic therapy and reproduction. The influence on fertility, pregnancy and breast feeding]. Z Rheumatol 2006;65(3):217–4.

113. De Santis M, Straface G, Cavaliere A, Carducci B, Caruso A. Paternal and maternal exposure to leflunomide: pregnancy and neonatal outcome. Ann Rheum Dis 2005;64(7):1096–7.

114. Brent RL. Utilization of animal studies to determine the effects and human risks of environmental toxicants (drugs, chemicals, and physical agents). Pediatrics 2004;113(Suppl 4):984–95.

115. Kaplan MJ. Leflunomide Aventis Pharma. Curr Opin Investig Drugs 2001;2(2):222–30.

116. Ostensen M. Disease specific problems related to drug therapy in pregnancy. Lupus 2004;13(9):746–50.

117. Ilowite NT. Current treatment of juvenile rheumatoid arthritis. Pediatrics 2002;109(1):109–15.

118. Casanova Sorní C, Romá Sánchez E, Pelufo Pellicer A, Poveda Andrés JL. Leflunomida: valoración del riesgo teratógeno en el primer trimestre de embarazo. Farm Hosp 2005;29(4):265–8.

119. Jakez-Ocampo J, Richaud-Patin Y, Granados J, Sanchez-Guerrero J, Llorente L. Weekly leflunomide as monotherapy for recent-onset rheumatoid arthritis. Arthritis Rheum 2004;51(1):147–8.

120. Kamali S, Kasapoglu E, Uysal M, Inanc M, Gul A. An unusual overdose of leflunomide in a patient with rheumatoid arthritis. Ann Pharmacother 2004;38(7-8):1320–1.

121. Flendrie M, Creemers MC, Welsing PM, van Riel PL. The influence of previous and concomitant leflunomide on the efficacy and safety of infliximab therapy in patients with rheumatoid arthritis; a longitudinal observational study. Rheumatology (Oxford) 2005;44(4):472–8.

122. Hansen KE, Cush J, Singhal A, Cooley DA, Cohen S, Patel SR, Genovese M, Sundaramurthy S, Schiff M. The safety and efficacy of leflunomide in combination with infliximab in rheumatoid arthritis. Arthritis Rheum 2004;51(2):228–32.

123. Kale VP, Bichile LS. Leflunomide: a novel disease modifying anti-rheumatic drug. J Postgrad Med 2004;50(2):154–7.

124. Lim V, Pande I. Leflunomide can potentiate the anticoagulant effect of warfarin. BMJ 2002;325(7376):1333.

125. Chonlahan J, Halloran MA, Hammonds A. Leflunomide and warfarin interaction: case report and review of the literature. Pharmacotherapy 2006;26(6):868–71.

126. Rettie AE, Jones JP. Clinical and toxicological relevance of CYP2C9: drug-drug interactions and pharmacogenetics. Annu Rev Pharmacol Toxicol 2005;45:477–94.

127. Chan V, Charles BG, Tett SE. Rapid determination of the active leflunomide metabolite A77 1726 in human plasma by high-performance liquid chromatography. J Chromatogr B Analyt Technol Biomed Life Sci 2004;803(2):331–5.

128. Schmidt A, Schwind B, Gillich M, Brune K, Hinz B. Simultaneous determination of leflunomide and its active metabolite, A77 1726, in human plasma by high-performance liquid chromatography. Biomed Chromatogr 2003;17(4):276–81.

Methotrexate

General Information

Methotrexate is a folic acid antagonist that acts by inhibiting dihydrofolate reductase. Owing to its immunosuppressive and anti-inflammatory properties, low-dosage methotrexate (7.5–15 mg/week) has been extensively investigated for other therapeutic purposes characterized by inflammation or cellular proliferation. Since the mid-1980s, methotrexate has become one of the most widely used disease-modifying anti-rheumatic drugs (DMARDs) in rheumatoid arthritis. It also has a significant degree of efficacy in psoriasis, asthma, and inflammatory bowel disease, and may also be effective in systemic lupus erythematosus, giant cell arteritis, and Wegener's granulomatosis. The exact mechanisms by which methotrexate affects these diseases are still uncertain, and its clinical effects probably result from multiple biochemical events at a variety of cellular sites (1).

General adverse effects

Most of the experience regarding the adverse effects of low-dose methotrexate has accumulated in patients with rheumatoid arthritis. Adverse effects are very common during the first year of treatment and reach an incidence of 60–70%. However, they are rarely severe enough to require permanent drug withdrawal, even after very long-term treatment. Based on a cohort study of 152 patients with rheumatoid arthritis, the probability of methotrexate continuation was 30% at 10 years, and adverse effects were the most frequent reason (50%) for drug withdrawal (2). Even though the overall withdrawal rate for methotrexate-induced adverse effects is 7–16%, long-term methotrexate treatment required drug withdrawal because of adverse effects less often than several other second-line DMARDs (SEDA-22, 416). In a retrospective analysis of 437 rheumatoid arthritis patients treated for 3–106 months (mean = 35 months), the most common adverse effects were gastrointestinal disorders (20%), raised liver function tests (13%), respiratory disorders (6.4%), hematological abnormalities (4.4%), weakness (3.4%), central nervous system disorders (2.8%), infections (2.3%), mucocutaneous disorders (2.3%), and arthralgia (1.8%; 3). A Ritchie's index of 10 or less, a low polymorphonuclear leukocyte count, and the absence of rheumatoid factor predicted the occurrence of adverse effects.

In one study, 10 patients (of an original 29) were still taking methotrexate after a mean of 13 years and a mean cumulative dose of 9.7 g (4). The overall drug withdrawal rate was 48%, and the rate of adverse effects, particularly on the gut and central nervous system, fell with time (85% at baseline, 90% at 90 months, 62% at 160 months). It was felt that routine folate supplementation might have contributed to the observed reduction in toxicity, except for mouth ulcers or soreness. Very similar findings were found in another long-term (132 months) prospective study (5).

Raised methotrexate serum concentrations (over 100 nmol/l at 36–42 hours after ingestion) are expected to increase the likelihood of several adverse effects, that is, gastrointestinal and hematological effects, but similar adverse effects can be found even with low methotrexate serum concentrations. Reduced red cell folate concentrations during methotrexate treatment also related to adverse effects and rises in liver enzymes, and red cell folate concentrations above 800 nmol/l protected against common adverse effects and treatment withdrawal (6). Several investigators now advocate the concomitant use of folic acid (5–7 mg/week and up to 27.5 mg/week) to reduce some of methotrexate-associated adverse effects without reducing its efficacy (7).

Prevention of adverse effects

It is possible to reduce the incidence of several adverse effects of methotrexate by using folic or folinic acid. The usual practice is to give weekly folic acid in patients who are taking weekly methotrexate (on a different day) and daily folinic acid in those who are taking daily methotrexate. Folic acid supplementation is now commonly given to reduce the adverse effects of methotrexate, in particular its mucosal and gastrointestinal toxic effects (SED-14, 1297; SEDA-23, 406), but less is known about how long this should be continued in patients taking long-term treatment.

In a meta-analysis of 307 patients with rheumatoid arthritis from seven randomized clinical trials, of whom 147 took folate supplementation, hematological adverse effects were not significantly reduced in the folate group (8). However, there was a 79% reduction in mucosal and gastrointestinal adverse effects in patients taking folic acid and a non-significant trend toward a reduction (42%) in patients taking folinic acid. Disease activity was not modified by low doses of folate. Finally, the authors noted that folinic acid is more expensive.

In 75 patients with rheumatoid arthritis taking methotrexate (up to 20 mg/week) and folic acid (5 mg/day), folic acid was withdrawn and the patients were randomized to restart folic acid (n = 38) or to take placebo (n = 37) double-blind, and were regularly assessed for 1 year (9). There were more withdrawals with placebo (46%) than with folic acid (21%) and more nausea. There were no obvious differences in efficacy. This suggests that folic acid supplementation is still helpful in the long term.

Organs and Systems

Cardiovascular

Cardiovascular adverse effects of methotrexate are extremely rare.

- There has been one detailed report of ventricular dysrhythmias and myocardial infarction, with recurrence of frequent ventricular extra beats on each readministration of methotrexate in a 36-year-old man (10).

It has been suggested that methotrexate increases mortality in patients with rheumatoid arthritis with cardiovascular co-morbidity (11). This assumption was based on a retrospective analysis of 632 patients with rheumatoid arthritis, of whom 73 died. The simultaneous presence of methotrexate and evidence of cardiovascular disease was an independent predictor of mortality. There was no such association with other DMARDs. The authors suggested that this effect may result from a methotrexate-induced increase in serum homocysteine, encouraging atherosclerosis.

Respiratory

Isolated and sustained cough is an unusual adverse effect of methotrexate. Among 13 patients who had a cough, only three met the criteria for methotrexate-induced pneumonitis (12). An irritant effect of methotrexate on the airways was therefore suggested.

Pneumonitis
Acute or subacute interstitial pneumonitis is an important but unpredictable and potentially life-threatening adverse effect of low-dose methotrexate (13–16).

Presentation
In patients with definite or probable methotrexate-induced lung injury, the predominant clinical features include shortness of breath, cough, and fever (13). Pathological examination usually shows an interstitial inflammatory cell infiltrate (sometimes granulomatous or with alveolar damage), and variable degrees of interstitial fibrosis. Unfortunately, confirmatory evidence is sometimes hard to obtain, particularly in patients with rheumatoid arthritis in whom rheumatoid interstitial lung disease can also occur. Infectious pneumonias, particularly viral or *Pneumocystis jiroveci* pneumonia, which resemble methotrexate pneumonitis and can occur as a result of immunosuppression, should also be carefully excluded.

- Pulmonary endoalveolar hemorrhage was a possible complication of pneumonitis in a 57-year-old woman who voluntarily increased her dosage of methotrexate from 7.5 mg once a week to 7.5 mg/day for 15 days (17).

The potential severity of methotrexate pneumonitis was finally exemplified in a careful retrospective multicenter study of 29 patients with definite or probable criteria for methotrexate-induced lung injury (13). Overall, five patients (17%) died, two of them after methotrexate rechallenge.

Frequency

The prevalence of methotrexate pneumonitis has been variably estimated from 0.3 to 18%, with a mean estimated prevalence of 3.3% (14,16). In a review of the respiratory complications of methotrexate, the authors concluded that pneumonitis occurs in 7% of patients, in 25% of whom it is fatal as a result of respiratory failure (18). This can occur with any dose of methotrexate, given via any route; it has occurred after the intrathecal administration of 12 mg given for central nervous system prophylaxis (19). In a review of 194 patients with rheumatoid arthritis and 38 with psoriatic arthritis, the prevalences of pneumonitis were 2.1 and 0.03% respectively (14), which is similar to the 3.2% incidence in a prospective study of 124 patients with rheumatoid arthritis (20). Another analysis performed over 5 years showed that the estimated prevalence of definite or probable pneumonitis was only 0.86% in 1162 patients (10 patients, of whom three died), but this conclusion was based on a limited retrospective identification of cases (21).

Mechanism

Even though methotrexate pneumonitis was first described about 30 years ago, very little is known about the mechanism, and whether it is due to direct cumulative toxicity, hypersensitivity, or an idiosyncratic reaction. In one case, interleukin-8 was speculated to play an important role in the pathogenesis (22).

Susceptibility factors

Susceptibility factors for methotrexate pneumonitis are still poorly understood. In one study, no risk factors were identified and periodic pulmonary function tests were not predictive (20). In contrast, advanced age, diabetes, pre-existing rheumatoid pleuropulmonary involvement or previous lung disease, previous use of DMARDs, and hypoalbuminemia were suggested as the most reliable predictors of methotrexate-induced pneumonitis in a large historical case-control study (15,23). The weekly dose, the cumulative dose, and the duration of treatment were not related to its occurrence. A history of drug-induced pulmonary disorders was also thought to favor methotrexate pneumonitis, but this was based on a single case report in a patient who previously had aminorex-induced primary pulmonary hypertension (SEDA-22, 416).

Management

The management of methotrexate pneumonitis primarily requires methotrexate withdrawal and supportive care. Although glucocorticoids are commonly used, there is as yet no evidence that they positively influence the outcome. Any readministration of methotrexate is dangerous, and four of six patients treated again with methotrexate developed recurrent lung toxicity, of whom two died (13).

Based on a report of 9 cases and a careful reanalysis of 123 previously published cases, the clinical spectrum and histopathology of methotrexate-induced pneumonitis have been reviewed (24). The authors stressed that methotrexate pneumonitis should be promptly recognized to avoid a severe outcome, although no specific features could be identified compared with other drug-induced adverse lung effects and no definite pathological findings compared with rheumatoid lung. Diagnostic criteria therefore mostly included a history of exposure, the exclusion of other pulmonary diseases, especially infections, and the presence of pulmonary infiltrates on the chest X-ray. Once methotrexate pneumonitis developed, 13% of the patients died from respiratory failure, clearly underlining the fact that methotrexate pneumonitis is potentially life-threatening. Methotrexate reintroduction should also be strongly discouraged in such cases, because about 25% of patients experience recurrence.

Nervous system

Reports of necrotizing leukoencephalopathy in association with methotrexate have been verified by biopsy or autopsy (25,26). Serial electroencephalography can predict this, since slow-wave activity develops during the administration of high-dose methotrexate. Autopsy has shown widespread necrosis and spongiosis in the cerebral and cerebellar white matter in such cases (25).

Chronic brain edema, multifocal white matter necrosis, and deep brain atrophy have been reported in patients who received high-dose methotrexate therapy, with an incidence of 4% (27). All patients received methotrexate 8–9 g/m^2 intravenously over 4 hours. The encephalopathy began abruptly, an average of 6 days after the second or third weekly treatment, presenting with behavioral abnormalities. These ranged from laughter to lethargy or unresponsiveness. In some patients, there were focal sensorimotor or reflex signs and generalized seizures. The disorder lasted from 15 minutes to 72 hours, and it disappeared as abruptly as it began, without specific treatment.

A rare case of a reversible neurological disturbance associated with focal subcortical white matter pathology has been described after administration of methotrexate 3 g/m^2. In patients who received 8–12.5 g/m^2, the incidence of neurological abnormalities was 4%. All of these patients were also receiving methotrexate intrathecally as well, but the relevance of this is not known (28).

In one case, low-dose methotrexate was implicated in leukoencephalopathy (29).

Treatment with intrathecal methotrexate of children under 5 years of age with acute lymphoblastic leukemia (irrespective of other drugs) has structural and functional effects on the developing neocerebellar–frontal subsystem (30).

Acute dysarthria has been attributed to methotrexate (31).

- A 71-year-old man was given oral methotrexate (15 mg/week) for a cutaneous T cell lymphoma. Within 3 weeks he developed progressive dysarthria and incoordination, and neurological examination showed mild buccofacial dyskinesia. Complete examination was otherwise normal, and he fully recovered 6–8 weeks after methotrexate withdrawal.

This case is reminiscent of other previously reported neurological abnormalities with low-dose methotrexate.

Psychological, psychiatric

There was a significantly higher risk of late cognitive impairment (concentration and memory) in patients (n = 39) taking adjuvant cyclophosphamide, fluorouracil, and methotrexate than in controls matched for age, disease, surgery, and radiation dose (32).

In studies of the neurotoxic effects of low-dose methotrexate treatment, dizziness, headache, visual disturbances or hallucinations, lack of concentration, cognitive dysfunction, and depression-like symptoms were detected in 1–35% of patients (33,34). Advanced age and mild renal insufficiency were possible susceptibility factors (34).

Nutrition

Of patients receiving high-dose methotrexate (5–8 g/m^2), 95% developed a significant increase in serum phenylalanine concentrations, probably due to inhibition of dihydropteridine reductase (35). The clinical significance of this is not obvious, although it is possible that it may contribute to the transient neurological disturbance observed in some patients taking high-dose methotrexate.

Hematologic

Significant hematological abnormalities occur in 10–24% of patients who take methotrexate. Mild to moderate leukopenia is the most frequent, followed by thrombocytopenia. Isolated thrombocytopenia and anemia are uncommon (SEDA-22, 416; 36). In a retrospective study in 315 patients, 13 had thrombocytopenia, two of whom also had pancytopenia (37). Thrombocytopenia correlated with the weekly dosage of methotrexate administered on the same day as NSAIDs, and methotrexate was safely reintroduced in patients who developed thrombocytopenia as a result of concomitant administration of both drugs, provided that NSAIDs were withheld at least on the day of methotrexate administration.

Pancytopenia is a rare but potentially fatal complication, and numerous reports have been published. The characteristics and incidence of pancytopenia have been carefully re-evaluated from case reports and clinical trials published from 1980 to 1995 (38). Of 70 reported cases, 12 patients died (17%). Impaired renal function was the most important contributing factor (54%), particularly in fatal cases (10/12). Other important susceptibility factors included advanced age (over 65 years), hypoalbuminemia, concurrent infection, and/or concomitant multiple medications (particularly co-trimoxazole). The mean cumulative dosage was 675 (10–4800) mg, and the minimal cumulative methotrexate dose leading to fatal pancytopenia was 10 mg. This confirms that pancytopenia can occur at any time during treatment, even in the absence of known susceptibility factors. Bone marrow biopsy showed megaloblastosis and hypocellularity. Eosinophilia and increased mean corpuscular volume were rarely observed. In an overall review of five long-term prospective studies

(511 patients), the calculated incidence of methotrexate-induced pancytopenia was 1.4%. Although severe myelosuppression sometimes required folinic acid, there are as yet no data to determine whether prophylactic folate supplementation can reduce the incidence of pancytopenia.

In a double-blind, placebo-controlled study of the safety and efficacy of methotrexate therapy combined with glucocorticoids in patients with giant cell arteritis over 24 months, adverse events were defined as a new diagnosis of any condition during treatment (39). The combination of methotrexate plus prednisolone reduced the number of relapses and improved the course of the disease. Methotrexate was withdrawn in three patients who had adverse events that were clearly drug-related. One had leukopenia, anemia, and mucositis, one developed pancytopenia, and one oral ulcers. These patients were not taking folic acid or folinic acid supplements.

Gastrointestinal

Gastrointestinal adverse effects (stomatitis, anorexia, abdominal pain, dyspepsia, nausea, vomiting, diarrhea, and weight loss) are very common, particularly after oral administration of methotrexate (up to 50%), and often require dosage adjustment (3). Folic acid supplementation reduces the incidence of several gastrointestinal adverse effects.

Stomatitis can sometimes be particularly harmful and has been reported as the cause of transient or permanent treatment withdrawal in 4.5 and 1.1% of 1539 patients respectively (40). However, one study did not show significant differences in the number of oral lesions or the duration or frequency of stomatitis between patients with rheumatoid arthritis taking methotrexate and those not taking methotrexate (19/51 versus 9/46), although the prevalence of ulceration was higher in the methotrexate group (41).

Liver

Cytolytic hepatitis has been reported in a 58-year-old man being treated with intramuscular methotrexate 10 mg/week (total dose over the previous 4 years 2.3 g); it resolved within 2 weeks of stopping therapy (42).

There has been a report of 14 cases of hepatotoxicity in 68 patients when methotrexate 10 mg/week was given chronically. Liver biopsies showed hepatic changes after about 1 g of cumulative treatment given over 2 years (43).

Hepatic fibrosis and cirrhosis

The main concern over long-term treatment with methotrexate is hepatic fibrosis and cirrhosis. Methotrexate hepatotoxicity was initially reported in children given high daily dose methotrexate for leukemia. After its introduction for the treatment of psoriasis, several papers published in the late 1960s pointed out the possible risk of severe hepatic fibrosis and cirrhosis in patients taking moderate daily doses. Since then many studies have focused on the extent of long-term methotrexate hepatotoxicity in patients taking low-dose methotrexate for psoriasis and rheumatoid arthritis. However, the evidence on

Table 1 Susceptibility factors for hepatotoxicity of methotrexate

Strong association	Previous or concurrent heavy alcohol use
	Pre-existing liver disease
	Daily methotrexate administration
	Renal insufficiency
Probable association	Duration of methotrexate treatment (over 2 years)
	Cumulative methotrexate dose (over 1500 mg)
	Prior treatment with arsenicals
	Obesity with diabetes mellitus
Possible or potential association	Maximum weekly dose over 25 mg
	Obesity alone
	Diabetes mellitus alone
	Heterozygous alpha$_1$-antitrypsin deficiency
	Felty's syndrome
	Prior treatment with vitamin A
	Concurrent NSAID use
	Concurrent treatment with ciclosporin
	Concurrent PUVA treatment
No association	Sex
	HLA phenotype
	Extent of psoriatic skin involvement
	Duration of rheumatoid arthritis
	Glucocorticoid therapy
Negative association	Concurrent folate supplementation
	Concurrent hydroxychloroquine use

the frequency and severity of severe liver disease in these patients is still highly controversial, since there may be liver histological changes before methotrexate treatment, particularly in patients with psoriasis. Furthermore, there are numerous confounding factors (Table 1) which can contribute to histological liver changes, leading several authors to suggest as early as 1990 that methotrexate-induced hepatic fibrosis and cirrhosis is uncommon and only occurs in patients with other susceptibility factors (44).

Frequency

The incidence of liver cirrhosis after a mean dose of 2 g is 7–10%. Once 1.5 g has been administered (45), or 2 years after starting long-term treatment, biopsy should be discussed (46).

Liver failure or cirrhosis were identified among 24 patients in a retrospective survey of more than 16 600 patients with rheumatoid arthritis who had taken methotrexate for at least 5 years, giving an estimated 5-year frequency of one in 1000 (47).

No morphological features of methotrexate hepatotoxicity were demonstrated after 2 years of methotrexate treatment in 48 patients with primary biliary cirrhosis (48).

Collectively, the available data suggest that methotrexate rarely causes significant serious liver damage in patients who have been otherwise carefully selected, who present no risk factors for methotrexate-induced hepatotoxicity, and who have received lower weekly dosages with strict monitoring of liver function (for example transaminases) in order to reduce methotrexate doses when liver enzymes are persistently raised (49).

Diagnosis and monitoring

Routine liver function tests do not reliably indicate liver damage, and they may not become abnormal until there is already considerable liver damage. It is therefore common practice to monitor patients by conducting annual liver biopsies. Measurement of the serum amino-terminal propeptide of type III procollagen (PIII PI) has been used as an alternative to liver biopsy; high concentrations correlate with fibrosis on liver biopsy (50). No patient with a normal serum concentration had an abnormal biopsy. An increase in the plasma phenylalanine/tyrosine ratio in children and adolescents can provide clinical evidence of liver damage before the appearance of symptoms in patients who have taken high doses of methotrexate (51).

Methods of monitoring patients for possible methotrexate hepatotoxicity and guidelines have been reviewed (49,52,53). It should be mentioned that the frequent rise in serum transaminases (involving 30–80% of patients) after the start of treatment is transient and does not predict liver damage; only persistently abnormal transaminases are potential indicators of methotrexate hepatotoxicity.

Mechanism

Folate depletion may be a factor in the pathogenesis of methotrexate-induced liver disease. In 30 patients on long-term methotrexate therapy, aimed at determining whether erythrocyte concentrations of folate and methotrexate might provide an indication for liver biopsy, there was no difference between red cell folate concentrations in patients with cirrhosis or progressive liver fibrosis and patients without fibrosis or with non-progressive hepatic fibrosis. Erythrocyte methotrexate concentrations were higher in patients with progressive hepatic disease, but cumulative dose and length of treatment were stronger predictors. In individual cases, erythrocyte folate and methotrexate concentrations were not a reliable guide (54).

Pathology

In patients with rheumatoid arthritis, baseline histological liver abnormalities were less common, with mild fibrosis only in 0–15% of patients. In retrospective studies with no pre-methotrexate liver biopsies, mild fibrosis was found in 3–35% of patients taking methotrexate, moderate or severe fibrosis in 0–10%, and cirrhosis in 0–2%. However, no case of cirrhosis was identified in studies which compared pre- and postmethotrexate biopsies or sequential biopsies while on long-term methotrexate, that is, a mean cumulative dose of 1200–5000 mg (53). Again, both worsening and improvement of histological lesions occurred. The application of guidelines to prevent methotrexate hepatotoxicity may account for these reassuring results. Liver biopsy changes were moderate or absent in patients with juvenile rheumatoid arthritis who took a cumulative dose of over 3000 mg (SEDA-21, 388; 52).

In 22 of 29 patients (76%) who were treated with low-pulse doses of methotrexate for rheumatoid arthritis, liver biopsy specimens showed variability in liver cell nuclear size, glycogenated nuclei, and fatty change. Occasionally there was mild portal infiltration with lymphocytes. There were no significant differences in age, duration of treatment, or cumulative dose amongst the cases. Serial increases in serum transaminases and/or alkaline phosphatase activity and development of hypoalbuminemia during treatment were indicators of development of liver disease (55).

In another study, the pathological lesions found in liver biopsies from patients treated with methotrexate were non-specific, consisting usually of macrovesicular steatosis, nuclear pleomorphism, chronic inflammatory infiltrates in the portal tracts, focal liver cell necrosis, fibrosis, and cirrhosis (53).

The pathological features of methotrexate-induced liver damage have been comprehensively reviewed (53). In patients with psoriasis, baseline liver biopsies were often abnormal, with mild fibrosis, moderate or severe fibrosis, and cirrhosis in 0–30, 0–7, and 0–1.5% respectively. These figures increased after methotrexate use, with fibrosis and cirrhosis in 14–34 and 0–21% respectively.

Ultrastructural studies have sometimes identified Ito cell prominence and collagen deposition in the perisinusoidal space of Disse during the first months of treatment and before the appearance of any signs of fibrosis, but these findings have been disputed in rheumatoid arthritis patients. Using immunohistochemical quantification, increased matrix proteins, collagen and transforming growth factor alpha were also found as possible early markers of methotrexate hepatotoxicity (56).

Susceptibility factors

The susceptibility factors for methotrexate-induced hepatotoxicity are listed in Table 1.

In a meta-analysis of 636 patients from 15 studies, who took chronic low-dose methotrexate for rheumatoid arthritis or psoriasis, the risk of liver toxicity increased with cumulative dose and heavy alcohol intake (57).

In one study, the risk of developing cirrhosis progressively increased with the total cumulative dose of methotrexate, from 13% at 2200 mg to 26% at 4000 mg (58). However, studies that compared sequential liver biopsies in patients on treatment and included specific recommendations for patient selection and the monitoring of methotrexate hepatotoxicity, gave contrasting results, with a lower incidence of cirrhosis even after high cumulative methotrexate doses (up to 5100 mg; 53). In addition, although histological lesions can worsen during treatment, improvement or absence of progression of prior fibrosis/cirrhosis has been found in very long-term follow-up of patients still taking methotrexate after 10 years (59).

The incidence and susceptibility factors of rises in serum transaminases have been detailed from a retrospective analysis of 66 patients with rheumatoid arthritis (60). There was an asymptomatic increase in serum transaminases in 42 and 49% of patients respectively, an incidence 4–5 times greater than that found in 21 patients taking other DMARDs. Although most of the rises in transaminases were transient and spontaneously reversible, 14 patients had sustained rises. There was a close relation between the incidence of high transaminases and the weight-adjusted dose of methotrexate. In a multivariate regression analysis, only obesity, methotrexate dose (over 0.15 mg/kg/week), and the concomitant presence of gastrointestinal adverse effects were significantly and independently associated with the likelihood of a rise in alanine transaminase. In the 14 patients who had persistently high transaminases, weekly folic acid 5 mg produced a sustained fall in serum alanine transaminase within 3 months, but three patients had to be withdrawn because of exacerbation of rheumatoid arthritis.

Urinary tract

Low-dose methotrexate is usually not regarded as nephrotoxic, and one report of nephrotic syndrome with minimal change disease on renal biopsy should be regarded with caution, since there was recovery after glucocorticoid treatment and withdrawal of concomitant NSAIDs (SEDA-22, 416).

However, renal toxicity occurs with high-dose methotrexate and more likely to occur with concomitant administration of other nephrotoxic agents, such as aminoglycosides, cephalosporins, NSAIDs, and diuretics (61).

The pathogenesis of methotrexate-induced nephrotoxicity is not understood, but it is thought to result from crystallization of methotrexate in the renal tubules. Adequate hydration and urinary alkalinization are necessary to minimize this effect (62). Urinary beta$_2$

microglobulin may be a useful marker of methotrexate nephrotoxicity (63).

When serum methotrexate concentrations are high, leucovorin (folinic acid) rescue may protect against renal damage. Methotrexate concentrations are only transiently lowered by hemoperfusion, and they are unaffected by peritoneal dialysis once there is acute renal insufficiency. Sustained reductions in drug concentrations and recovery of renal function have been reported after charcoal hemoperfusion followed by hemodialysis (64,65).

Co-administration of methotrexate and procarbazine in the treatment of medulloblastomas increases the risk of methotrexate nephrotoxicity. Delayed administration of methotrexate until 72 hours after procarbazine therapy has been given may reduce this risk (66).

Skin

Since the first descriptions of the rapid development of a large number of nodules, also termed "accelerated nodulosis," in methotrexate-treated patients, a number of such reports have accumulated in patients with rheumatoid arthritis or, more rarely, psoriatic arthritis (67–69). Nodulosis is characterized by the development of small, painful, multiple nodules, sometimes disseminated; pulmonary, meningeal, or pericardial nodulosis has also been reported in a few patients (SEDA-21, 387; 68,70,71). Four cases of nodulosis and four of cutaneous vasculitis were noted during a long-term follow-up of 437 rheumatoid arthritis patients (3), but the estimated incidence of accelerated nodulosis was found to be higher in other studies: that is, 8–12% (5,67,71).

The nodules can appear at any time during treatment, with or without concomitant cutaneous vasculitis, and are usually found in patients with erosive disease and a high titer of rheumatoid factor. This has raised the question as to whether they are a reason to modify treatment, and whether they are rheumatic or represent a true adverse effect of methotrexate; certainly, methotrexate-associated nodulosis is very similar to idiopathic rheumatoid arthritis nodulosis and sometimes disappears despite continuation of methotrexate. However, prompt regression on methotrexate withdrawal and recurrence on rechallenge in several patients strongly argue for a causal drug-related effect.

There was a characteristic clinical and histopathological spectrum of skin lesions, distinct from rheumatoid papules, in four patients who took low-dose methotrexate for acute flares of collagen vascular disease (72). These so-called methotrexate-induced rheumatoid papules developed shortly after methotrexate administration consisted of erythematous indurated papules mostly affecting the proximal limbs, and disappeared after methotrexate was withdrawn or tapered. Histology showed inflammatory infiltrates of interstitially arranged histiocytes and a few neutrophils, but no features of leukocytoclastic vasculitis.

Isolated cutaneous leukocytoclastic vasculitis occurs infrequently in patients taking methotrexate, and an immediate-type hypersensitivity reaction has been thought to be involved, in view of prompt recurrence

after drug readministration or a positive mast cell degranulation test as recorded in several patients (SEDA-21, 388; SEDA-22, 417; 73).

Other isolated reports included the occurrence of skin ulceration (SEDA-22, 388) and one fatal case of toxic epidermal necrolysis (SEDA-21, 388).

Persistent hyperpigmentation is an unusual manifestation of weekly administration of methotrexate (74).

- Severely ulcerated psoriatic plaques and acute extensive exfoliative dermatitis occurred in a 37-year-old man who had taken methotrexate for 5 years for psoriasis (75).

In the context of a case of severe reactivation of recent sunburn after a single injection of methotrexate for ectopic pregnancy in a 40-year-old woman, the authors reviewed the literature on methotrexate photosensitivity (76). Photodermatitis reactivation is the only well-documented type of photosensitivity associated with methotrexate. It can occur if methotrexate is given at 2–5 days after excessive exposure to ultraviolet or X-radiation.

A previously unreported skin reaction mimicking Stevens–Johnson syndrome has been reported (77).

- A 61-year-old woman inadvertently took a high dose of methotrexate (10 mg/day) for psoriasis, and developed mucosal ulcers after 3 months. One month later, methotrexate (20 mg/week) was restarted, but she developed painful oral ulceration and burning skin lesions 3 days later. She had an erythema multiform-like rash and several buccal ulcers. There was a moderate pancytopenia. Histological examination of the skin showed features consistent with an acute graft-versus-host reaction. All medications except aspirin were withdrawn, and she recovered fully after treatment with calcium folinate and prednisolone.

The authors speculated that concomitant aspirin may have contributed to this severe reaction.

Hair

Mild alopecia is common in patients taking methotrexate (78,79).

Nails

Yellow nail pigmentation without paronychia has been noted in a patient with psoriasis taking methotrexate (80).

Musculoskeletal

Arthralgia and myalgia sometimes occur within 24 hours of methotrexate injections in patients with rheumatoid arthritis. These transient effects, which can be accompanied by fatigue, malaise, and various neuropsychological disorders, have escaped recognition, but they occurred in 10% of patients over 18 months and sometimes resulted in treatment withdrawal (81).

Leg pain and spontaneous fractures attributed to prolonged high-dose methotrexate therapy in pediatric oncology have been recognized since the 1970s, but there have been some cases in patients taking low-dose methotrexate

(82,83). All the same, it is still controversial as to whether methotrexate can actually cause changes in bone metabolism (84). There was a significant reduction in bone mineral density in 11 postmenopausal women taking methotrexate for primary biliary cirrhosis compared with 11 matched controls not taking methotrexate (85). Among 133 patients with rheumatoid arthritis, methotrexate without glucocorticoids was not associated with changes in the bone mineral density after 3 years of treatment, but methotrexate plus prednisone (over 5 mg/day) produced greater bone loss than prednisone alone (86). In contrast, another study failed to show accelerated bone loss in methotrexate users compared with non-users, but the study was limited to 10 patients in each group (87).

The possible effects of methotrexate on bone metabolism and bone loss have been discussed in the context of two adults (88) and in relation to a study in children with juvenile rheumatoid arthritis (89) who had delayed bone healing after surgery. The two adults, aged 52 and 62 years, had been taking methotrexate (7.5 and 15 mg/week) for 14 and 15 months when they underwent metatarsal and tibial osteotomy. Because X-ray examination 5 and 6 months after surgery showed non-union, methotrexate was withdrawn; the bone healed promptly in both patients within 2 months. The authors thought that the outcome in these patients without risk factors for bone fragility suggested that temporary methotrexate withdrawal should be considered in cases of delayed bone healing after surgery.

In contrast, in a longitudinal study of 32 patients with juvenile rheumatoid arthritis, there was no evidence of deleterious effects of long-term, low-dose methotrexate on bone mass density (89). The cumulative dose of glucocorticoids, weight, and height were the main determinants of bone mass changes.

Furthermore, there is evidence that it is disease activity rather than methotrexate that accounts for changes in bone mass (90). This 2-year longitudinal study involved 22 patients taking methotrexate and 18 patients taking other DMARDs; it was strictly controlled for the use of glucocorticoids. There were significant and equal reductions in trabecular bone mineral density in both groups. Bone loss was most marked in patients with active disease.

Sexual function

Impotence has very rarely been attributed to methotrexate (91).

Reproductive system

Although the occurrence of gynecomastia requiring surgical excision in two patients might have been coincidental (92), in another patient it disappeared after methotrexate withdrawal and recurred on rechallenge (93).

Immunologic

Immediate hypersensitivity reactions are rare after low-dose methotrexate.

- A 53-year-old woman had three episodes of angioedema while taking methotrexate, with no recurrence after withdrawal (94).

Vasculitis has been infrequently reported in patients taking low-dose methotrexate (SEDA-21, 388; SEDA-22, 417; 95). Although most cases have been observed in patients with rheumatoid arthritis, suggesting that the underlying disease plays a part, vasculitis has also been described in a patient with ankylosing spondylitis (96). Methotrexate was also reported to have exacerbated pre-existing urticarial vasculitis in a 32-year-old woman; the lesions recurred after rechallenge (97).

Autacoids

Tumor lysis syndrome has been attributed to methotrexate.

- A 14-year-old girl receiving large-dose methotrexate for Burkitt's lymphoma developed tumor lysis syndrome, which progressed to renal insufficiency and cutaneous vasculitis of the palms and soles (98).

Infection risk

Methotrexate-related immunosuppression can be expected to increase the likelihood of infections. The infection rate reported in patients taking low-dose methotrexate has varied from one study to another. In a literature review focusing on patients with rheumatoid arthritis taking methotrexate, the mean infection rate was 1.8% in retrospective studies, 4.6% in open studies, and 11.6% in double-blind studies (99). Infections usually occurred within 1.5 years of starting treatment and mostly comprised common respiratory or cutaneous bacterial infections, *Herpes zoster*, and, more rarely, opportunistic infections. In one comparative study, the overall risk of infections was considered to be low and similar in patients taking methotrexate and azathioprine (99), but others have found a higher prevalence of infections and an increase in antibiotic use in patients with rheumatoid arthritis taking methotrexate as compared to other DMARDs, except cyclophosphamide (100,101).

An accumulating series of case reports has focused on the possible more frequent occurrence of opportunistic infections despite normal leukocyte counts in patients treated for rheumatoid arthritis or, less often, psoriasis (99,102,103). Various bacterial, fungal, and viral opportunistic infections have been described, with *Pneumocystis jiroveci* pneumonia as the most frequently reported (SEDA-21, 389; SEDA-22, 417). Although the most severe, sometimes fatal, infectious diseases were usually observed in patients also taking glucocorticoids (SEDA-22, 417; 104,105), severe infections can also occur in occasional patients not taking concomitant glucocorticoids (SEDA-21, 389) 103,(106–109).

Acute reactivation of a presumed quiescent chronic hepatitis B infection in one reported case after methotrexate withdrawal suggests that T cell-mediated immunological rebound might lead to rapid destruction of infected hepatocytes (110).

Long-Term Effects

Tumorigenicity

The evidence that methotrexate is carcinogenic is inconclusive and mostly based on case reports or analyses of cohort studies without control groups (102,111). For example, malignant neoplasms (urothelial carcinoma of the bladder, a malignant teratoma, and a dermal squamous cell carcinoma) have been described in three patients taking prolonged courses of methotrexate 7.5–15 mg/week (112).

From a retrospective study in more than 16 000 rheumatoid arthritis patients, the risk of hematological malignancy in methotrexate-treated patients was thought to be very small and not different from that observed in patients who used other DMARDs (113). In 426 patients with rheumatoid arthritis who took methotrexate for a mean of 37 months (follow-up period 4.6 years), the incidence rate of new cancers (4 cases/1000 person-years) was similar to that found in the general population (2.8 cases/1000 person-years; 114). Another preliminary study did not show an excess in the risk of lymphoproliferative disorders in patients with rheumatoid arthritis receiving long-term methotrexate maintenance (115). Earlier studies in patients with psoriasis did not show a higher incidence of cancers in patients on methotrexate compared with the general population (102,116).

In contrast, there have been several isolated reports of methotrexate-induced lymphomas (SEDA-21, 388; SEDA-22, 417; 117,118). The pathological features in these cases have ranged from benign lymphoid hyperplasia to non-Hodgkin's lymphoma, and more rarely Hodgkin's disease (117), and patients usually had the typical features of lymphoproliferative disorders as found in immunosuppressed patients, that is, transplant patients or patients with congenital or acquired immune deficiency syndromes. Exceptionally, cases of pseudolymphoma have also been reported (SEDA-21, 389).

- Two patients developed lymphomas within 3 years of methotrexate treatment, and the authors suggested that an increase in serum IgE concentrations might anticipate the development of lymphoma in patients with rheumatoid arthritis treated with methotrexate (119).
- A cutaneous B cell lymphoma occurred in a 58-year-old man who had been treated with intramuscular methotrexate 10 mg/week for 4 years (total dose 2.3 g); the lymphoma resolved spontaneously 2 weeks after withdrawal of therapy (120).

A convincing argument implicating methotrexate as the cause of lymphomas is the possible spontaneous remission of lymphoproliferation after methotrexate withdrawal, as reported in several cases (SEDA-22, 389; 117,118). However, the putative pathophysiological mechanisms of methotrexate-induced lymphomas are unclear, and the drug's precise role, as well as that of the underlying disease as a confounding factor, needs to be investigated. The risk of a lymphoma in rheumatoid arthritis probably has more to do with the disease and its activity than with methotrexate treatment (115,121).

Low-dosage methotrexate is also a possible factor in the development of Epstein–Barr virus-associated lymphoproliferative disease, but the role of the Epstein–Barr virus in these cases is unclear. Epstein–Barr virus infection does not appear to be mandatory for the development of lymphoproliferation in patients taking methotrexate, but it was nevertheless found in about one-half of patients who developed lymphomas (SEDA-22, 389; 117,122).

Lymphoproliferative disorders have been observed during treatment of sarcoidosis and connective tissue diseases with low-dose methotrexate.

- A 51-year-old man with systemic sarcoidosis took methotrexate for 36 months and developed a large anal fissure with a diffuse polymorphic infiltrate containing large Epstein–Barr virus-positive lymphoid cells, similar to the classical B cell lymphoproliferative disorders that occur in immunosuppressed transplant recipients of solid organs (123).

This case supports the hypothesis that immunosuppressant therapy may contribute to an increased risk of Epstein–Barr virus-associated lymphoproliferative disorders.

Some of the mechanisms and risk factors of methotrexate-associated non-Hodgkin's lymphoma in patients with rheumatoid arthritis have been reviewed, including an analysis of the characteristic features of 25 detailed published cases (124). Although the epidemiological evidence is limited, several reports of spontaneous remission of lymphomas after methotrexate withdrawal strongly support a cause-and-effect relation.

A second malignancy in a patient taking methotrexate for chronic lymphatic leukemia has been described (125).

- A 55-year-old man with chronic lymphocytic leukemia and rheumatoid arthritis took methotrexate for 4 years and developed a B cell non-Hodgkin's lymphoma in the shoulder and axillary lymph nodes; he had Epstein–Barr viral antigens in the serum. After radiation and chemotherapy had failed, complete remission was achieved with a combination of rituximab and EPOCH (etoposide + prednisone + vincristine + cyclophosphamide + doxorubicin).

The authors thought that T cell deficiency induced by methotrexate, chronic lymphatic leukemia, and rheumatoid arthritis may have contributed to the development of the B cell lymphoma.

Other malignancies, such as malignant melanoma, multiple myeloma, leukemia or solid cancers, have been seldom reported (SEDA-21, 389; SEDA-22, 389; 91,126), and the association with methotrexate therapy is uncertain.

Second-Generation Effects

Teratogenicity

Owing to its known teratogenic effects, methotrexate is usually considered to be contraindicated in pregnancy, and several authors have recommended withdrawing methotrexate at least 3 months before a planned pregnancy. Most of our knowledge on the consequences of in utero exposure to methotrexate is derived from oncology patients. In this setting, the fetal methotrexate syndrome mimics the aminopterin syndrome, with central nervous system abnormalities, skeletal defects, and more rarely cardiac abnormalities. The critical period of exposure is 6–8 weeks after conception and the minimal weekly dose is 10 mg (127), but one report suggested that the critical period may extend to week 11 in patients exposed to high-dose methotrexate (SEDA-22, 417).

- A 3-year-old infant born to a woman who had taken methotrexate 37.5 mg/week throughout the first 8 weeks after conception had significant developmental delay with mental retardation, which might therefore be a feature of the fetal methotrexate syndrome (128).

The developmental effects of in utero exposure to methotrexate have been reviewed, including a brief mention of three original cases (129), and a series of pregnancy outcomes in four patients exposed to low-dose methotrexate during early pregnancy has been reported more extensively (130). Of 24 patients available for evaluation, who took 2.5–35 mg/week and were accidentally exposed from the beginning of pregnancy up to 19 weeks gestation, pregnancy ended in spontaneous abortion in four and elective abortion in three (including one case of major malformation). Of the 17 neonates, three had major malformations. The malformations mostly consisted of central nervous system or craniofacial abnormalities and skeletal defects. Three patients had been exposed up to 8 weeks of gestation and one from 8 to 10 weeks, and the methotrexate doses were 12.5–35 mg/week. This is consistent with the threshold dose of 10 mg/week and the timing of exposure previously suggested for fetal methotrexate syndrome.

Susceptibility Factors

Age

Children with Down's syndrome have a significantly increased risk of leukemia and an increased risk of methotrexate-associated toxicity. Hyperdiploid lymphoblasts with extra copies of chromosome 21 generate higher concentrations of the active methotrexate metabolite. This is because of increased intracellular transport of methotrexate via the reduced folate carrier, whose gene is localized to chromosome 21 and may also account for the increased methotrexate-associated toxicity in patients with Down's syndrome and acute lymphoblastic leukemia (131).

Renal disease

Impaired renal function is a susceptibility factor for methotrexate-induced pancytopenia.

- A 57-year-old man who had been on hemodialysis for the past 5 years developed severe pancytopenia 12 days after a single dose of methotrexate 5 mg (132).
- Severe complications, mostly bone marrow suppression and related complications, occurred in three patients on regular hemodialysis for end-stage renal disease (133).

Osteosarcoma

Patients with osteosarcoma treated with methotrexate, vincristine, and doxorubicin are at risk of late adverse effects. Of 106 chemotherapy-treated patients with osteosarcoma, 24 died, nine relapsed, and three developed a second malignancy during follow-up of at least 20 years (134). Event-free survival and overall survival were significantly lower than in a previous study with a 3-year follow up period (event-free survival 38% versus 53%; overall survival 44% versus 67%).

Drug Administration

Drug dosage regimens

Of 106 medication errors reported to the FDA associated with methotrexate there were 25 deaths and 48 other serious outcomes (135). The most common types of errors involved confusion about the once-weekly dosage schedule (30%) and other dosage errors (22%). The most frequent indication for use was rheumatoid arthritis (42%). Of the errors, 39 were attributable to the prescriber, 21 to the patient, 20 to dispensing, and 18 to administration by a health-care professional.

Drug–Drug Interactions

Aspirin

Aspirin and methotrexate compete for renal tubular secretion, and aspirin alters the systemic and renal clearances of intravenous methotrexate (136). However, the clinical relevance of this interaction is not clear. In one study, aspirin (mean dose 4.5 g) in 12 patients did not cause more toxicity than other NSAIDs taken by 22 other patients (137).

Benzimidazoles

Methotrexate is transported by breast cancer resistance protein (BCRP; ABCG2) and multidrug resistance-associated protein1–4 (MRP1–4; ABCC1–4). In patients with cancer, co-administration of benzimidazoles and methotrexate can result in profound methotrexate-induced toxicity coinciding with an increase in the serum concentrations of methotrexate and its main metabolite 7-hydroxymethotrexate (138). Benzimidazoles differentially affect transport of methotrexate mediated by BCRP and MRP2 and competition for BCRP may explain the clinical interaction between methotrexate and benzimidazoles.

Carboxypeptidase G2

Carboxypeptidase G2 is used when unexpected toxicity or renal insufficiency occurs during high-dose methotrexate therapy. Leucovorin is used to antagonize the effects of methotrexate on purine metabolism, but its protective effect is antagonized by carboxypeptidase G2. Carboxypeptidase G2 should therefore be administered to patients with caution (139)

Co-trimoxazole

Drugs that inhibit folate metabolism increase the likelihood of serious adverse reactions to methotrexate, particularly hematological toxicity. The additional risk of myelosuppression and subsequent severe pancytopenia has been particularly exemplified by the combination of methotrexate and co-trimoxazole (trimethoprim plus sulfamethoxazole; 140). This should also be taken into account in patients taking trimethoprim alone (SEDA-22, 418).

Even low-dose short-course methotrexate therapy can cause a fatal outcome. A patient with rheumatoid arthritis who had taken a low-dose short course of methotrexate developed severe pancytopenia followed by bacterial and monilial sepsis after taking co-trimoxazole for an intercurrent infection (141). The proposed mechanisms of this interaction are either protein binding displacement of methotrexate by co-trimoxazole or competition between the two drugs for renal tubular excretion. It has also been postulated that methotrexate and co-trimoxazole act synergistically to produce significant folate deficiency, which leads to megaloblastic changes. Co-trimoxazole rarely causes megaloblastic anemia alone; however, this effect is more likely to occur in patients with pre-existing folate deficiency. If this drug combination cannot be avoided, the patient should be closely monitored for signs of hematological toxicity. Calcium leucovorin may be necessary to treat megaloblastic anemia and neutropenia resulting from folic acid deficiency.

Etanercept

The pharmacokinetics of etanercept 25 mg subcutaneously twice weekly were not altered by concurrent methotrexate 20 mg oral weekly in 682 patients with rheumatoid arthritis in a phase IIIb trial (142). Thus, no etanercept dosage adjustment is needed for patients taking concurrent methotrexate.

Etretinate

A case of severe hepatitis has been attributed to the combination of methotrexate with etretinate (143), a finding that was not explained by a pharmacokinetic interaction between the two drugs (144).

Fluorouracil

There is sequence-dependent synergy between fluorouracil and methotrexate. Pre-treatment with methotrexate enhances the formation of fluorouridine monophosphate and hence fluorouridine triphosphate; this enhances RNA-directed toxicity. In studies in which methotrexate has been given 1 hour before fluorouracil, response rates did not differ significantly. However, when it was given 4 hours or more before, there were significantly better response rates (145).

Glucocorticoids

Dexamethasone increased the hepatotoxicity of methotrexate in 57 children with brain tumors (146). The hepatotoxicity was not related to differences in serum concentrations and was independent of bone marrow toxicity or mucositis.

There have been conflicting studies on the interaction between low-dose methotrexate and long-term glucocorticoids. In one study, there was a significantly increased AUC and a reduction in methotrexate clearance compared with patients not taking glucocorticoids (147), and in another there was no change (148). Collectively, the data suggest that the interaction, if any, is of little clinical significance.

NSAIDs

Theoretically, NSAIDs can increase methotrexate serum concentrations by competition for renal tubular secretion (149), which is mediated by the human organic anion transporters hOAT1 (SLC22A6) and hOAT3 (SLC22A8). Delayed methotrexate elimination occurred in a patient with Hodgkin's disease who took the NSAID loxoprofen (150). Loxoprofen and its trans-hydroxylated metabolite, an active major metabolite, markedly inhibited methotrexate transport by hOAT1 and hOAT3.

Since the publication of case histories reporting severe toxic effects in patients taking methotrexate and NSAIDs, there has been much concern among patients taking low-dose methotrexate (SEDA-20, 89; SEDA-21, 100). However, most of the reports related to patients taking doses of methotrexate higher than those recommended in rheumatoid arthritis. From often mutually contradictory data, it appears that co-administration of most NSAIDs and stable low-dose methotrexate is relatively safe and that the supposed risks have little clinical significance in patients with normal renal function who are regularly monitored for hepatic, hematological, and renal toxicity (151).

In one study there was a significant reduction in renal methotrexate clearance and creatinine clearance in patients who took NSAIDs plus a high maintenance dose of methotrexate (16.6 mg/week), but no change in either variable in patients taking a stable maintenance dose of 7.5 mg/week (152). This suggests that patients taking higher doses should be more closely monitored for early signs of renal impairment that could predispose them to methotrexate toxicity.

Co-administration of methotrexate with lumiracoxib, a novel cyclo-oxygenase-2 selective inhibitor, was well tolerated in 18 patients (mean age 49 years) with stable rheumatoid arthritis and had no significant effect on methotrexate pharmacokinetics, protein binding, or urinary excretion (153).

Penicillin

Concomitant penicillin administration has been reported to exacerbate the hematological toxicity of low-dose methotrexate (154). This could have been due to inhibition of the tubular secretion of methotrexate.

Probenecid

Probenecid competes with methotrexate for renal tubular secretion, and can cause severe hematological toxicity.

- Severe pancytopenia occurred in an elderly patient taking low-dose methotrexate and probenecid (155).

Sulfasalazine

Interaction of sulfasalazine with reduced folate carrier, the dominant cell membrane transporter for natural folates and methotrexate, may limit the efficacy of combination therapy in patients with rheumatoid arthritis. Studies of cellular transport kinetics have shown that sulfasalazine is a potent non-competitive inhibitor of reduced folate carrier-mediated cellular uptake of methotrexate and leucovorin (156). There was marked loss of methotrexate efficacy when methotrexate was co-administered with sulfasalazine. Along with diminished efficacy of methotrexate, there was evidence of cellular folate depletion by the demonstration of a sulfasalazine dose-dependent reduction in leucovorin accumulation. At clinically relevant plasma concentrations, interactions of sulfasalazine with the reduced folate carrier provide a biochemical rationale for folate deficiency during sulfasalazine treatment as well as the lack of additivity/synergism of the combination of sulfasalazine and methotrexate when these disease-modifying antirheumatic drugs are given simultaneously. These results provide a rationale for the use of folate supplementation and for staggering the administration of these drugs over time.

Triamterene

Drugs that inhibit folate metabolism increase the likelihood of serious adverse reactions to methotrexate, particularly hematological toxicity. Bone marrow suppression and reduced plasma folate concentrations resulted from the concomitant administration of triamterene with methotrexate (157).

References

1. Cronstein BN. Molecular therapeutics. Methotrexate and its mechanism of action. Arthritis Rheum 1996;39(12):1951–60.
2. Alarcon GS, Tracy IC, Strand GM, Singh K, Macaluso M. Survival and drug discontinuation analyses in a large cohort of methotrexate treated rheumatoid arthritis patients. Ann Rheum Dis 1995;54(9):708–12.
3. Bologna C, Viu P, Picot MC, Jorgensen C, Sany J. Long-term follow-up of 453 rheumatoid arthritis patients treated with methotrexate: an open, retrospective, observational study. Br J Rheumatol 1997;36(5):535–40.
4. Kremer JM. Safety, efficacy, and mortality in a long-term cohort of patients with rheumatoid arthritis taking methotrexate: followup after a mean of 13.3 years Arthritis Rheum 1997;40(5):984–5.
5. Weinblatt ME, Maier AL, Fraser PA, Coblyn JS. Longterm prospective study of methotrexate in rheumatoid arthritis: conclusion after 132 months of therapy. J Rheumatol 1998;25(2):238–42.
6. Andersen LS, Hansen EL, Knudsen JB, Wester JU, Hansen GV, Hansen TM. Prospectively measured red cell folate levels in methotrexate treated patients with rheumatoid arthritis: relation to withdrawal and side effects. J Rheumatol 1997;24(5):830–7.
7. Morgan SL, Baggott JE, Vaughn WH, Austin JS, Veitch TA, Lee JY, Koopman WJ, Krumdieck CL, Alarcon GS. Supplementation with folic acid during methotrexate therapy for rheumatoid arthritis. A double-blind, placebo-controlled trial. Ann Intern Med 1994;121(11):833–41.
8. Ortiz Z, Shea B, Suarez-Almazor ME, Moher D, Wells GA, Tugwell P. The efficacy of folic acid and folinic acid in reducing methotrexate gastrointestinal toxicity in rheumatoid arthritis. A metaanalysis of randomized controlled trials. J Rheumatol 1998;25(1):36–43.
9. Griffith SM, Fisher J, Clarke S, Montgomery B, Jones PW, Saklatvala J, Dawes PT, Shadforth MF, Hothersall TE, Hassell AB, Hay EM. Do patients with rheumatoid arthritis established on methotrexate and folic acid 5 mg daily need to continue folic acid supplements long term? Rheumatology (Oxford) 2000;39(10):1102–9.
10. Kettunen R, Huikuri HV, Oikarinen A, Takkunen JT. Methotrexate-linked ventricular arrhythmias. Acta Derm Venereol 1995;75(5):391–2.
11. Landewe RB, van den Borne BE, Breedveld FC, Dijkmans BA. Methotrexate effects in patients with rheumatoid arthritis with cardiovascular comorbidity. Lancet 2000;355(9215):1616–7.
12. Schnabel A, Dalhoff K, Bauerfeind S, Barth J, Gross WL. Sustained cough in methotrexate therapy for rheumatoid arthritis. Clin Rheumatol 1996;15(3):277–82.
13. Kremer JM, Alarcon GS, Weinblatt ME, Kaymakcian MV, Macaluso M, Cannon GW, Palmer WR, Sundy JS, St Clair EW, Alexander RW, Smith GJ, Axiotis CA. Clinical, laboratory, radiographic, and histopathologic features of methotrexate-associated lung injury in patients with rheumatoid arthritis: a multicenter study with literature review. Arthritis Rheum 1997;40(10):1829–37.
14. Salaffi F, Manganelli P, Carotti M, Subiaco S, Lamanna G, Cervini C. Methotrexate-induced pneumonitis in patients with rheumatoid arthritis and psoriatic arthritis: report of five cases and review of the literature. Clin Rheumatol 1997;16(3):296–304.
15. Golden MR, Katz RS, Balk RA, Golden HE. The relationship of pre-existing lung disease to the development of methotrexate pneumonitis in patients with rheumatoid arthritis. J Rheumatol 1995;22(6):1043–7.
16. Barrera P, Laan RF, van Riel PL, Dekhuijzen PN, Boerbooms AM, van de Putte LB. Methotrexate-related pulmonary complications in rheumatoid arthritis. Ann Rheum Dis 1994;53(7):434–9.
17. Kokelj F, Plozzer C, Muzzi A, Ciani F. Endoalveolar haemorrhage due to methotrexate overdosage in a patient treated for psoriatic arthritis. J Dermatol Treat 1999;10:67–9.
18. Massin F, Coudert B, Marot JP, Foucher P, Camus P, Jeannin L. La pneumopathie du methotrexate. [Pneumopathy caused by methotrexate.] Rev Mal Respir 1990;7(1):5–15.
19. Martins da Cunha AC, Bartsch CH, Gadner H. Acute respiratory failure after intrathecal methotrexate administration. Pediatr Hematol Oncol 1990;7(2):189–92.
20. Cottin V, Tebib J, Massonnet B, Souquet PJ, Bernard JP. Pulmonary function in patients receiving long-term low-dose methotrexate. Chest 1996;109(4):933–8.
21. Bartram SA. Experience with methotrexate-associated pneumonitis in northeastern England: comment on the article by Kremer et al. Arthritis Rheum 1998;41(7):1327–8.

22. Yoshida S, Onuma K, Akahori K, Sakamoto H, Yamawaki Y, Shoji T, Nakagawa H, Hasegawa H, Amayasu H. Elevated levels of IL-8 in interstitial pneumonia induced by low-dose methotrexate. J Allergy Clin Immunol 1999;103(5 Pt 1):952–4.

23. Alarcon GS, Kremer JM, Macaluso M, Weinblatt ME, Cannon GW, Palmer WR, St Clair EW, Sundy JS, Alexander RW, Smith GJ, Axiotis CA. Risk factors for methotrexate-induced lung injury in patients with rheumatoid arthritis. A multicenter, case-control study. Methotrexate-Lung Study Group. Ann Intern Med 1997;127(5):356–64.

24. Imokawa S, Colby TV, Leslie KO, Helmers RA. Methotrexate pneumonitis: review of the literature and histopathological findings in nine patients. Eur Respir J 2000;15(2):373–81.

25. Fujii Y, Mizuno Y, Hongo T, Igarashi Y, Arai T, Kino I, Okamoto K. [Serial spectral EEG analysis in a patient with non-Hodgkin's lymphoma complicated by leukoencephalopathy induced by high-dose methotrexate.]Gan To Kagaku Ryoho 1988;15(4 Pt 1):713–7.

26. Poskitt KJ, Steinbok P, Flodmark O. Methotrexate leukoencephalopathy mimicking cerebral abscess on CT brain scan. Childs Nerv Syst 1988;4(2):119–21.

27. Ebner F, Ranner G, Slavc I, Urban C, Kleinert R, Radner H, Einspieler R, Justich E. MR findings in methotrexate-induced CNS abnormalities. Am J Neuroradiol 1989;10(5):959–64.

28. Borgna-Pignatti C, Battisti L, Marradi P, Balter R, Caudana R. Transient neurologic disturbances in a child treated with moderate-dose methotrexate. Br J Haematol 1992;81(3):448.

29. Worthley SG, McNeil JD. Leukoencephalopathy in a patient taking low dose oral methotrexate therapy for rheumatoid arthritis. J Rheumatol 1995;22(2):335–7.

30. Lesnik PG, Ciesielski KT, Hart BL, Benzel EC, Sanders JA. Evidence for cerebellar–frontal subsystem changes in children treated with intrathecal chemotherapy for leukemia: enhanced data analysis using an effect size model. Arch Neurol 1998;55(12):1561–8.

31. Aplin CG, Russell-Jones R. Acute dysarthria induced by low dose methotrexate therapy in a patient with erythrodermic cutaneous T cell lymphoma: an unusual manifestation of neurotoxicity. Clin Exp Dermatol 1999;24(1):23–4.

32. Schagen SB, van Dam FS, Muller MJ, Boogerd W, Lindeboom J, Bruning PF. Cognitive deficits after postoperative adjuvant chemotherapy for breast carcinoma. Cancer 1999;85(3):640–50.

33. Rau R, Schleusser B, Herborn G, Karger T. Longterm combination therapy of refractory and destructive rheumatoid arthritis with methotrexate (MTX) and intramuscular gold or other disease modifying antirheumatic drugs compared to MTX monotherapy. J Rheumatol 1998;25(8):1485–92.

34. Wernick R, Smith DL. Central nervous system toxicity associated with weekly low-dose methotrexate treatment. Arthritis Rheum 1989;32(6):770–5.

35. Dhondt JL, Farriaux JP, Millot F, Taret S, Hayte JM, Mazingue F. Methotrexate a haute close et hyperphenylalaninennie. [High-dose methotrexate and hyperphenylalaninemia.] Arch Fr Pediatr 1991;48(4):249–51.

36. Lapadula G, De Bari C, Acquista CA, Dell'Accio F, Covelli M, Iannone F. Isolated thrombocytopenia associated with low dose methotrexate therapy. Clin Rheumatol 1997;16(4):429–30.

37. Franck H, Rau R, Herborn G. Thrombocytopenia in patients with rheumatoid arthritis on long-term treatment with low dose methotrexate. Clin Rheumatol 1996;15(3):266–70.

38. Gutierrez-Urena S, Molina JF, Garcia CO, Cuellar ML, Espinoza LR. Pancytopenia secondary to methotrexate therapy in rheumatoid arthritis. Arthritis Rheum 1996;39(2):272–6.

39. Jover JA, Hernandez-Garcia C, Morado IC, Vargas E, Banares A, Fernandez-Gutierrez B. Combined treatment of giant-cell arteritis with methotrexate and prednisone. a randomized, double-blind, placebo-controlled trial. Ann Intern Med 2001;134(2):106–14.

40. Carpenter EH, Plant MJ, Hassell AB, Shadforth MF, Fisher J, Clarke S, Hothersall TE, Dawes PT. Management of oral complications of disease-modifying drugs in rheumatoid arthritis. Br J Rheumatol 1997;36(4):473–8.

41. Ince A, Yazici Y, Hamuryudan V, Yazici H. The frequency and clinical characteristics of methotrexate (MTX) oral toxicity in rheumatoid arthritis (RA): a masked and controlled study. Clin Rheumatol 1996;15(5):491–4.

42. Fisher A, Mor E, Hytiroglou P, Emre S, Boccagni P, Chodoff L, Sheiner P, Schwartz M, Thung SN, Miller C. FK506 hepatotoxicity in liver allograft recipients. Transplantation 1995;59(11):1631–2.

43. Baughman RP, Koehler A, Bejarano PA, Lower EE, Weber FL Jr. Role of liver function tests in detecting methotrexate-induced liver damage in sarcoidosis. Arch Intern Med 2003;163:615–20.

44. Kaplan MM. Methotrexate hepatotoxicity and the premature reporting of Mark Twain's death: both greatly exaggerated. Hepatology 1990;12(4 Pt 1):784–6.

45. Lin Y, Huang Y, Lee S, Wu J, Chang C, Chen C, Hwang S. [Clinical study of methotrexate-induced hepatic injury in patients with psoriasis.]Chin J Gastroenterol 1991;8:277–81.

46. Cunliffe RN, Scott BB. Review article: monitoring for drug side-effects in inflammatory bowel disease. Aliment Pharmacol Ther 2002;16(4):647–62.

47. Walker AM, Funch D, Dreyer NA, Tolman KG, Kremer JM, Alarcon GS, Lee RG, Weinblatt ME. Determinants of serious liver disease among patients receiving low-dose methotrexate for rheumatoid arthritis. Arthritis Rheum 1993;36(3):329–35.

48. Bach N, Thung SN, Schaffner F. The histologic effects of low-dose methotrexate therapy for primary biliary cirrhosis. Arch Pathol Lab Med 1998;122(4):342–5.

49. Kremer JM, Alarcon GS, Lightfoot RW Jr, Willkens RF, Furst DE, Williams HJ, Dent PB, Weinblatt ME. Methotrexate for rheumatoid arthritis. Suggested guidelines for monitoring liver toxicity. American College of Rheumatology. Arthritis Rheum 1994;37(3):316–28.

50. Risteli J, Sogaard H, Oikarinen A, Risteli L, Karvonen J, Zachariae H. Aminoterminal propeptide of type III procollagen in methotrexate-induced liver fibrosis and cirrhosis. Br J Dermatol 1988;119(3):321–5.

51. Hilton MA, Bertolone S, Patel CC. Daily profiles of plasma phenylalanine and tyrosine in patients with osteogenic sarcoma during treatment with high-dose methotrexate-citrovorum rescue. Med Pediatr Oncol 1989;17(4):265–70.

52. Roenigk HH Jr, Auerbach R, Maibach HI, Weinstein GD. Methotrexate in psoriasis: revised guidelines. J Am Acad Dermatol 1988;19(1 Pt 1):145–56.

53. West SG. Methotrexate hepatotoxicity. Rheum Dis Clin North Am 1997;23(4):883–915.

54. Zachariae H, Schroder H, Foged E, Sogaard H. Methotrexate hepatotoxicity and concentrations of methotrexate and folate in erythrocytes—relation to liver fibrosis and cirrhosis. Acta Dermatol Venereol 1987;67(4):336–40.

55. Tolman KG, Clegg DO, Lee RG, Ward JR. Methotrexate and the liver. J Rheumatol Suppl 1985;12(Suppl 12):29–34.

56. Jaskiewicz K, Voigt H, Blakolmer K. Increased matrix proteins, collagen and transforming growth factor are early markers of hepatotoxicity in patients on long-term methotrexate therapy. J Toxicol Clin Toxicol 1996;34(3):301–5.

57. Whiting-O'Keefe QE, Fye KH, Sack KD. Methotrexate and histologic hepatic abnormalities: a meta-analysis. Am J Med 1991;90(6):711–6.

58. Zachariae H, Kragballe K, Sogaard H. Methotrexate induced liver cirrhosis. Studies including serial liver biopsies during continued treatment. Br J Dermatol 1980;102(4):407–12.

59. Zachariae H, Sogaard H, Heickendorff L. Methotrexate-induced liver cirrhosis. Clinical, histological and serological studies—a further 10-year follow-up. Dermatology 1996;192(4):343–6.

60. Suzuki Y, Uehara R, Tajima C, Noguchi A, Ide M, Ichikawa Y, Mizushima Y. Elevation of serum hepatic aminotransferases during treatment of rheumatoid arthritis with low-dose methotrexate. Risk factors and response to folic acid. Scand J Rheumatol 1999;28(5):273–81.

61. Maiche AG, Lappalainen K, Teerenhovi L. Renal insufficiency in patients treated with high dose methotrexate. Acta Oncol 1988;27(1):73–4.

62. Christensen ML, Rivera GK, Crom WR, Hancock ML, Evans WE. Effect of hydration on methotrexate plasma concentrations in children with acute lymphocytic leukemia. J Clin Oncol 1988;6(5):797–801.

63. Amino K, Kawaguchi N, Matsumoto S, Manabe J, Ishii Y, Tabata D, Machida M. [Urinary beta 2-microglobulin as an indicator for impaired excretion of methotrexate.]Gan To Kagaku Ryoho 1988;15(11):3103–7.

64. Molina R, Fabian C, Cowley B Jr. Use of charcoal hemoperfusion with sequential hemodialysis to reduce serum methotrexate levels in a patient with acute renal insufficiency. Am J Med 1987;82(2):350–2.

65. Relling MV, Stapleton FB, Ochs J, Jones DP, Meyer W, Wainer IW, Crom WR, McKay CP, Evans WE. Removal of methotrexate, leucovorin, and their metabolites by combined hemodialysis and hemoperfusion. Cancer 1988;62(5):884–8.

66. Price P, Thompson H, Bessell EM, Bloom HJ. Renal impairment following the combined use of high-dose methotrexate and procarbazine. Cancer Chemother Pharmacol 1988;21(3):265–7.

67. Kerstens PJ, Boerbooms AM, Jeurissen ME, Fast JH, Assmann KJ, van de Putte LB. Accelerated nodulosis during low dose methotrexate therapy for rheumatoid arthritis. An analysis of ten cases. J Rheumatol 1992;19(6):867–71.

68. Falcini F, Taccetti G, Ermini M, Trapani S, Calzolari A, Franchi A, Cerinic MM. Methotrexate-associated appearance and rapid progression of rheumatoid nodules in systemic-onset juvenile rheumatoid arthritis. Arthritis Rheum 1997;40(1):175–8.

69. Muzaffer MA, Schneider R, Cameron BJ, Silverman ED, Laxer RM. Accelerated nodulosis during methotrexate therapy for juvenile rheumatoid arthritis. J Pediatr 1996;128(5 Pt 1):698–700.

70. Alarcon GS, Koopman WJ, McCarty MJ. Nonperipheral accelerated nodulosis in a methotrexate-treated rheumatoid arthritis patient. Arthritis Rheum 1993;36(1):132–3.

71. Combe B, Didry C, Gutierrez M, Anaya JM, Sany J. Accelerated nodulosis and systemic manifestations during methotrexate therapy for rheumatoid arthritis. Eur J Med 1993;2(3):153–6.

72. Goerttler E, Kutzner H, Peter HH, Requena L. Methotrexate-induced papular eruption in patients with rheumatic diseases: a distinctive adverse cutaneous reaction produced by methotrexate in patients with collagen vascular diseases. J Am Acad Dermatol 1999;40(5 Pt 1):702–7.

73. Halevy S, Giryes H, Avinoach I, Livni E, Sukenik S. Leukocytoclastic vasculitis induced by low-dose methotrexate: in vitro evidence for an immunologic mechanism. J Eur Acad Dermatol Venereol 1998;10(1):81–5.

74. Toussirot E, Wendling D. Methotrexate-induced hyperpigmentation in a rheumatoid arthritis patient. Clin Exp Rheumatol 1999;17(6):751.

75. Peters T, Theile-Ochel S, Chemnitz J, Sohngen D, Hunzelmann N, Scharffetter-Kochanek K. Exfoliative dermatitis after long-term methotrexate treatment of severe psoriasis. Acta Derm Venereol 1999;79(5):391–2.

76. Khan AJ, Brook S, Marghoob AA, Prestia AE, Spector IJ. Methotrexate and the photodermatitis reactivation reaction: a case report and review of the literature. Cutis 2000;66(5):379–82.

77. Hani N, Casper C, Groth W, Krieg T, Hunzelmann N. Stevens–Johnson syndrome-like exanthema secondary to methotrexate histologically simulating acute graft-versus-host disease. Eur J Dermatol 2000;10(7):548–50.

78. Basu TK, Williams DC, Raven RW. Methotrexate and alopecia. Lancet 1973;2(7824):331.

79. Weinblatt ME. Toxicity of low dose methotrexate in rheumatoid arthritis. J Rheumatol Suppl 1985;12(Suppl 12):35–9.

80. Malka N, Reichert S, Trechot P, Barbaud A, Schmutz JL. Yellow nail pigmentation due to methotrexate. Dermatology 1998;197(3):276.

81. Halla JT, Hardin JG. Underrecognized postdosing reactions to methotrexate in patients with rheumatoid arthritis. J Rheumatol 1994;21(7):1224–6.

82. Singwe M, Le Gars L, Karneff A, Prier A, Kaplan G. Multiple stress fractures in a scleroderma patient on methotrexate therapy. Rev Rhum Engl Ed 1998;65(7–9):508–10.

83. Zonneveld IM, Bakker WK, Dijkstra PF, Bos JD, van Soesbergen RM, Dinant HJ. Methotrexate osteopathy in long-term, low-dose methotrexate treatment for psoriasis and rheumatoid arthritis. Arch Dermatol 1996;132(2):184–7.

84. Mazzantini M, Di Munno O. Methotrexate and bone mass. Clin Exp Rheumatol 2000;18(Suppl 1):S87–92.

85. Blum M, Wallenstein S, Clark J, et al. Effect of methotrexate treatment on bone in postmenopausal women with primary biliary cirrhosis. J Bone Min Res 1996;11:S436.

86. Buckley LM, Leib ES, Cartularo KS, Vacek PM, Cooper SM. Effects of low dose methotrexate on the bone mineral density of patients with rheumatoid arthritis. J Rheumatol 1997;24(8):1489–94.

87. Carbone LD, Kaeley G, McKown KM, Cremer M, Palmieri G, Kaplan S. Effects of long-term administration of methotrexate on bone mineral density in rheumatoid arthritis. Calcif Tissue Int 1999;64(2):100–1.

88. Gerster JC, Bossy R, Dudler J. Bone non-union after osteotomy in patients treated with methotrexate. J Rheumatol 1999;26(12):2695–7.

89. Bianchi ML, Cimaz R, Galbiati E, Corona F, Cherubini R, Bardare M. Bone mass change during methotrexate treatment in patients with juvenile rheumatoid arthritis. Osteoporos Int 1999;10(1):20–5.

90. Mazzantini M, Di Munno O, Incerti-Vecchi L, Pasero G. Vertebral bone mineral density changes in female rheumatoid arthritis patients treated with low-dose methotrexate. Clin Exp Rheumatol 2000;18(3):327–31.

91. Blackburn WD Jr, Alarcon GS. Impotence in three rheumatoid arthritis patients treated with methotrexate. Arthritis Rheum 1989;32(10):1341–2.

92. Thomas E, Leroux JL, Blotman F. Gynecomastia in patients with rheumatoid arthritis treated with methotrexate. J Rheumatol 1994;21(9):1777–8.

93. Del Paine DW, Leek JC, Jakle C, Robbins DL. Gynecomastia associated with low dose methotrexate therapy. Arthritis Rheum 1983;26(5):691–2.

94. Freeman AM, Dasgupta B. Angio-neurotic oedema associated with methotrexate treatment in rheumatoid arthritis. Rheumatology (Oxford) 1999;38(9):908.

95. Fondevila Carlos G, Milone Gustavo A, Santiago P. Cutaneous vasculitis after intermediate dose of methotrexate (IDMTX). Br J Haematol 1989;72(4):591–2.

96. Borman P, Bodur H, Gulec AT, Ucan H, Seckin U, Mocan G. Atypical methotrexate dermatitis and vasculitis in a patient with ankylosing spondylitis. Rheumatol Int 2000;19(5):191–3.

97. Borcea A, Greaves MW. Methotrexate-induced exacerbation of urticarial vasculitis: an unusual adverse reaction. Br J Dermatol 2000;143(1):203–4.

98. Suresh S, Lozono S, Hall SC. Large-dose intravenous methotrexate-induced cutaneous toxicity: can oral magnesium oxide reduce pain? Anesth Analg 2003;96:1413–4.

99. Boerbooms AM, Kerstens PJ, van Loenhout JW, Mulder J, van de Putte LB. Infections during low-dose methotrexate treatment in rheumatoid arthritis. Semin Arthritis Rheum 1995;24(6):411–21.

100. Singh G, Fries JF, Williams CA, Zatarain E, Spitz P, Bloch DA. Toxicity profiles of disease modifying antirheumatic drugs in rheumatoid arthritis. J Rheumatol 1991;18(2):188–94.

101. van der Veen MJ, van der Heide A, Kruize AA, Bijlsma JW. Infection rate and use of antibiotics in patients with rheumatoid arthritis treated with methotrexate. Ann Rheum Dis 1994;53(4):224–8.

102. Kanik KS, Cash JM. Does methotrexate increase the risk of infection or malignancy? Rheum Dis Clin North Am 1997;23(4):955–67.

103. LeMense GP, Sahn SA. Opportunistic infection during treatment with low dose methotrexate. Am J Respir Crit Care Med 1994;150(1):258–60.

104. Gatnash AA, Connolly CK. Fatal chickenpox pneumonia in an asthmatic patient on oral steroids and methotrexate. Thorax 1995;50(4):422–3.

105. Wallace JR, Luchi M. Fatal cytomegalovirus pneumonia in a patient receiving corticosteroids and methotrexate for mixed connective tissue disease. South Med J 1996;89(7):726–8.

106. Hayem G, Meyer O, Kahn MF. *Listeria monocytogenes* infection in a patient treated with methotrexate for rheumatoid arthritis. J Rheumatol 1996;23(1):198–9.

107. Krebs S, Gibbons RB. Low-dose methotrexate as a risk factor for *Pneumocystis carinii* pneumonia. Mil Med 1996;161(1):58–60.

108. Lyon CC, Thompson D. *Herpes zoster* encephalomyelitis associated with low dose methotrexate for rheumatoid arthritis. J Rheumatol 1997;24(3):589–91.

109. Roux N, Flipo RM, Cortet B, Lafitte JJ, Tonnel AB, Duquesnoy B, Delcambre B. *Pneumocystis carinii* pneumonia in rheumatoid arthritis patients treated with methotrexate. A report of two cases. Rev Rhum Engl Ed 1996;63(6):453–6.

110. Narvaez J, Rodriguez-Moreno J, Martinez-Aguila MD, Clavaguera MT. Severe hepatitis linked to B virus infection after withdrawal of low dose methotrexate therapy. J Rheumatol 1998;25(10):2037–8.

111. Beauparlant P, Papp K, Haraoui B. The incidence of cancer associated with the treatment of rheumatoid arthritis. Semin Arthritis Rheum 1999;29(3):148–58.

112. Trenkwalder P, Eisenlohr H, Prechtel K, Lydtin H. Three cases of malignant neoplasm, pneumonitis, and pancytopenia during treatment with low-dose methotrexate. Clin Investig 1992;70(10):951–5.

113. Moder KG, Tefferi A, Cohen MD, Menke DM, Luthra HS. Hematologic malignancies and the use of methotrexate in rheumatoid arthritis: a retrospective study. Am J Med 1995;99(3):276–81.

114. Bologna C, Picot MC, Jorgensen C, Viu P, Verdier R, Sany J. Study of eight cases of cancer in 426 rheumatoid arthritis patients treated with methotrexate. Ann Rheum Dis 1997;56(2):97–102.

115. Wolfe F. Inflammatory activity, but not methotrexate or prednisone use predicts non-Hodgkin's lymphoma in rheumatoid arthritis: a 25-year study of 1767 RA patients. Arthritis Rheum 1998;41(Suppl):S188.

116. Bailin PL, Tindall JP, Roenigk HH Jr, Hogan MD. Is methotrexate therapy for psoriasis carcinogenic? A modified retrospective–prospective analysis. JAMA 1975;232(4):359–62.

117. Georgescu L, Quinn GC, Schwartzman S, Paget SA. Lymphoma in patients with rheumatoid arthritis: association with the disease state or methotrexate treatment. Semin Arthritis Rheum 1997;26(6):794–804.

118. Salloum E, Cooper DL, Howe G, Lacy J, Tallini G, Crouch J, Schultz M, Murren J. Spontaneous regression of lymphoproliferative disorders in patients treated with methotrexate for rheumatoid arthritis and other rheumatic diseases. J Clin Oncol 1996;14(6):1943–9.

119. Kono H, Inokuma S, Matsuzaki Y, Nakayama H, Yamazaki J, Hishima T, Maeda Y. Two cases of methotrexate induced lymphomas in rheumatoid arthritis: an association with increased serum IgE. J Rheumatol 1999;26(10):2249–53.

120. Viraben R, Brousse P, Lamant L. Reversible cutaneous lymphoma occurring during methotrexate therapy. Br J Dermatol 1996;135(1):116–8.

121. Baecklund E, Ekbom A, Sparen P, Feltelius N, Klareskog L. Disease activity and risk of lymphoma in patients with rheumatoid arthritis: nested case-control study. BMJ 1998;317(7152):180–1.

122. Kamel OW, van de Rijn M, LeBrun DP, Weiss LM, Warnke RA, Dorfman RF. Lymphoid neoplasms in patients with rheumatoid arthritis and dermatomyositis: frequency of Epstein–Barr virus and other features associated with immunosuppression. Hum Pathol 1994;25(7):638–43.

123. Theate I, Michaux L, Dardenne S, Guiot Y, Briere J, Emile FJ, Fabiani B, Detry R, Gaulard P. Groupe d'Etude des Lymphomes de l'Adulte (GELA). Epstein-Barr virus-associated lymphoproliferative disease occurring in a patient with sarcoidosis treated by methotrexate and methylprednisolone. Eur J Haematol 2002;69(4):248–53.

124. Georgescu L, Paget SA. Lymphoma in patients with rheumatoid arthritis: what is the evidence of a link with methotrexate? Drug Saf 1999;20(6):475–87.

125. Stewart M, Malkovska V, Krishnan J, Lessin L, Barth W. Lymphoma in a patient with rheumatoid arthritis receiving methotrexate treatment: successful treatment with rituximab. Ann Rheum Dis 2001;60(9):892–3.

126. Dubin Kerr L, Troy K, Isola L. Temporal association between the use of methotrexate and development of leukemia in 2 patients with rheumatoid arthritis. J Rheumatol 1995;22(12):2356–8.

127. Ostensen M, Ramsey-Goldman R. Treatment of inflammatory rheumatic disorders in pregnancy: what are the safest treatment options? Drug Saf 1998;19(5):389–410.

128. Del Campo M, Kosaki K, Bennett FC, Jones KL. Developmental delay in fetal aminopterin/methotrexate syndrome. Teratology 1999;60(1):10–2.

129. Lloyd ME, Carr M, McElhatton P, Hall GM, Hughes RA. The effects of methotrexate on pregnancy, fertility and lactation. QJM 1999;92(10):551–63.

130. Ostensen M, Hartmann H, Salvesen K. Low dose weekly methotrexate in early pregnancy. A case series and review of the literature. J Rheumatol 2000;27(8):1872–5.

131. Taub JW, Ge Y. Down syndrome, drug metabolism and chromosome 21. Pediatr Blood Cancer 2005;44(1):33–9.

132. Nakamura M, Sakemi T, Nagasawa K. Severe pancytopenia caused by a single administration of low dose methotrexate in a patient undergoing hemodialysis. J Rheumatol 1999;26(6):1424–5.

133. Chatham WW, Morgan SL, Alarcon GS. Renal failure: a risk factor for methotrexate toxicity. Arthritis Rheum 2000;43(5):1185–6.

134. Longhi A, Pasini E, Bertoni F, Pignotti E, Ferrari C, Bacci G. Twenty-year follow-up of osteosarcoma of the extremity treated with adjuvant chemotherapy. J Chemother 2004;16(6):582–8.

135. Moore TJ, Walsh CS, Cohen MR. Reported medication errors associated with methotrexate. Am J Health Syst Pharm 2004;61(13):1380–4.

136. Stewart CF, Fleming RA, Germain BF, Seleznick MJ, Evans WE. Aspirin alters methotrexate disposition in rheumatoid arthritis patients. Arthritis Rheum 1991;34(12):1514–20.

137. Rooney TW, Furst DE, Koehnke R, Burmeister L. Aspirin is not associated with more toxicity than other nonsteroidal antiinflammatory drugs in patients with rheumatoid arthritis treated with methotrexate. J Rheumatol 1993;20(8):1297–302.

138. Breedveld P, Zelcer N, Pluim D, Sonmezer O, Tibben MM, Beijnen JH, Schinkel AH, van Tellingen O, Borst P, Schellens JH. Mechanism of the pharmacokinetic interaction between methotrexate and benzimidazoles: potential role for breast cancer resistance protein in clinical drug–drug interactions. Cancer Res 2004;64(16):5804–11.

139. Hempel G, Lingg R, Boos J. Interactions of carboxypeptidase G2 with 6S-leucovorin and 6R-leucovorin in vitro: implications for the application in case of methotrexate intoxications. Cancer Chemother Pharmacol 2005;55(4):347–53.

140. Jeurissen ME, Boerbooms AM, van de Putte LB. Pancytopenia and methotrexate with trimethoprim–sulfamethoxazole. Ann Intern Med 1989;111(3):261.

141. Bartha P, Bron R, Levy Y. [Fatal pancytopenia and methotrexate-trimethoprim-sulfamethoxazole interaction.] Harefuah 2004;143(6):398-400, 464.

142. Zhou H, Mayer PR, Wajdula J, Fatenejad S. Unaltered etanercept pharmacokinetics with concurrent methotrexate in patients with rheumatoid arthritis. J Clin Pharmacol 2004;44(11):1235–43.

143. Beck HI, Foged EK. Toxic hepatitis due to combination therapy with methotrexate and etretinate in psoriasis. Dermatologica 1983;167(2):94–6.

144. Larsen FG, Nielsen-Kudsk F, Jakobsen P, Schroder H, Kragballe K. Interaction of etretinate with methotrexate pharmacokinetics in psoriatic patients. J Clin Pharmacol 1990;30(9):802–7.

145. Damon LE, Cadman E, Benz C. Enhancement of 5-fluorouracil antitumor effects by the prior administration of methotrexate. Pharmacol Ther 1989;43(2):155–85.

146. Wolff JE, Hauch H, Kuhl J, Egeler RM, Jurgens H. Dexamethasone increases hepatotoxicity of MTX in children with brain tumors. Anticancer Res 1998;18(4B):2895–9.

147. Lafforgue P, Monjanel-Mouterde S, Durand A, Catalin J, Acquaviva PC. Is there an interaction between low doses of corticosteroids and methotrexate in patients with rheumatoid arthritis? A pharmacokinetic study in 33 patients. J Rheumatol 1993;20(2):263–7.

148. Koerber H, Gross WL, Iven H. Do steroids influence low dose methotrexate pharmacokinetics? J Rheumatol 1994;21(6):1170–2.

149. van Meerten E, Verweij J, Schellens JH. Antineoplastic agents. Drug interactions of clinical significance. Drug Saf 1995;12(3):168–82.

150. Uwai Y, Taniguchi R, Motohashi H, Saito H, Okuda M, Inui K. Methotrexate-loxoprofen interaction: involvement of human organic anion transporters hOAT1 and hOAT3. Drug Metab Pharmacokinet 2004;19(5):369–74.

151. Miles SM, Bird HA. Clinical signifiance of drug interactions with antirheumatic agents. Clin Immunother 1996;5:205–13.

152. Kremer JM, Hamilton RA. The effects of nonsteroidal antiinflammatory drugs on methotrexate (MTX) pharmacokinetics: impairment of renal clearance of MTX at weekly maintenance doses but not at 7.5 mg J Rheumatol 1995;22(11):2072–7.

153. Hartmann SN, Rordorf CM, Milosavljev S, Branson JM, Chales GH, Juvin RR, Lafforgue P, Le Parc JM, Tavernier CG, Meyer OC. Lumiracoxib does not affect methotrexate pharmacokinetics in rheumatoid arthritis patients. Ann Pharmacother 2004;38(10):1582–7.

154. Mayall B, Poggi G, Parkin JD. Neutropenia due to low-dose methotrexate therapy for psoriasis and rheumatoid arthritis may be fatal. Med J Aust 1991;155(7):480–4.

155. Basin KS, Escalante A, Beardmore TD. Severe pancytopenia in a patient taking low dose methotrexate and probenecid. J Rheumatol 1991;81(4):609–10.

156. Jansen G, van der HJ, Oerlemans R, Lems WF, Ifergan I, Scheper RJ, Assaraf YG, Dijkmans BA. Sulfasalazine is a potent inhibitor of the reduced folate carrier: implications for combination therapies with methotrexate in rheumatoid arthritis. Arthritis Rheum 2004;50(7):2130–9.

157. Richmond R, McRorie ER, Ogden DA, Lambert CM. Methotrexate and triamterene—a potentially fatal combination? Ann Rheum Dis 1997;56(3):209–10.

Monoclonal antibodies

General Information

Human monoclonal antibody immunotherapy in clinical medicine has been an exciting prospect for some time, and increasing numbers of such antibodies have gradually become available (1,2).

An illustration of the potential of human monoclonal antibodies was provided by the HA-1A antibody, a human monoclonal IgM specific for the core/lipid A part of endotoxin. Among 291 patients with Gram-negative bacteremia treated with this antibody there was a significant reduction in mortality (3). Since then other patient groups have been treated, and apart from local urticaria, flushing, and mild transient hypotension, no adverse reactions were noted (4,5). No patient has developed antibodies to HA-1A. Although the initial results seem promising, more trials are needed to substantiate the therapeutic efficacy of HA-1A.

Numerous investigators have reported and reviewed the clinical application of monoclonal antibodies in various areas, including organ transplantation, neoplastic diseases, severe sepsis, and chronic inflammatory diseases. Collectively, these antibodies generally did not produce major adverse effects. The rapid development of antibodies against murine monoclonal antibodies is one of the most important clinical limitations to their therapeutic use, but the development of humanized (chimeric human/murine) monoclonal antibodies has improved their safety. Monoclonal antibodies have also been used in non-immune mediated diseases, such as cancer, septic shock, reperfusion, and as antiplatelet drugs. Treatment of neoplastic diseases with monoclonal antibodies is theoretically attractive. Unfortunately none of the monoclonal antibodies available at present has been demonstrated to be strictly tumor-specific, and binding of antibody to normal cells has been shown to be the major unknown factor for toxicity (6).

Monoclonal antibodies that are dealt with in separate monographs are abciximab, alemtuzumab, anti-CD4 antibody, basiliximab, daclizumab, edrecolomab, gemtuzumab ozogamicin, ibritumomab, muromonab-CD3, omalizumab, palivizumab, rituximab, and trastuzumab.

Nomenclature

Modern international non-proprietary drug names have two parts. The suffix, or stem, tells you what group the drug belongs to, ideally chosen to reflect its pharmacological action. For instance, -vastatin denotes HMG Co-A reductase inhibitors (-stat- often being used for enzyme inhibitors); -olol denotes beta-blockers (but beware stanozolol); and -mycins are antibiotics. The prefix is chosen at will. It might reflect the structure or source of the drug (for example diclofenac, virginiamycin), the inventor's love of opera or the cinema (for example mimimycin, rifampicin (7)), or just whimsy.

The monoclonal antibodies have a prefix and three substems. All, with one exception (muromonab), end in-

mab for monoclonal antibody. The penultimate syllable (or substem) indicates the animal source and the prepenultimate syllable indicates the target (Table 1). The prefix (one or two syllables) is chosen at random. Finally, if the antibody is conjugated to a toxin, an extra word is added; aritox, for example, denotes the A chain of ricin.

For example, trastuzumab can be parsed as follows: tras-tu-zu-mab. The -zu- denotes a humanized antibody and the -tu- a tumor target. If you wanted to show that it targets the breast specifically, you could call it tramazumab.

Uses

The uses of some monoclonal antibodies are listed in Table 2.

Several anti-human T cell monoclonal antibodies have undergone preliminary trials in the treatment of renal allograft rejection. Most of these monoclonal antibodies were not effective than muromonab (1). T10B9, an anti-human pan-T lymphocyte monoclonal antibody, had similar efficacy but caused less fever, severe infection, respiratory, gastrointestinal, or neurological symptoms than muromonab (SEDA-22, 409). Other monoclonal antibodies, such as chimeric anti-CD7 and murine anti-ICAM-1 (CD54; enlimomab), were devoid of adverse effects or produced only minimal and transient adverse effects (SED-13, 1134).

Anti-CD4 monoclonal antibodies, for example OKT4A, BF-5, cM-T412 (clenoliximab, keliximab), are continuously being investigated, although in small numbers of patients, after transplantation or in chronic inflammatory diseases, such as rheumatoid arthritis (SEDA-20, 340; SEDA-21, 379; 2,8,9). Significant clinical immunomodulation has sometimes been obtained, with only transient and self-limiting, first-dose effects, namely headache, fever and chills, gastrointestinal disorders, hypotension, and tachycardia (SEDA-21, 379). Whereas most other adverse effects were not specifically associated with these monoclonal antibodies, mild skin eruptions and transient increases in hepatic enzymes, with one reversible case of liver failure, have been attributed to B-F5, a murine IgG1 CD4 monoclonal antibody (10).

Various monoclonal antibodies have been developed to be used as carrier molecules or as immunoconjugates to target drugs, enzymes, isotopes, or toxins to tumor cells. Some of the available data have been summarized (11), but there is still insufficient evidence of clinical benefit.

Rodent monoclonal antibodies

Compared with the therapeutic use of human monoclonal antibodies, the use of rodent (mouse or rat) monoclonal antibodies in vivo is disadvantageous because the xenogeneic antibody can induce immune responses that will mitigate the effectiveness of the antibody and/or cause adverse reactions in the recipient. Thus, the authors of one report concluded that antimouse immunoglobulin responses in human patients have limited the usefulness of murine monoclonal antibodies in more than half of

Table 1 The components of the names of monoclonal antibodies

Prepenultimate syllable (general target)	Prepenultimate syllable (specific tumor target)	Penultimate syllable (species source)
-ba(c)- = bacterium	-co(l)- = colon	-a- = rat
-ci(r)- = cardiovascular	-go(t)- = gonad (testis)	-e- = hamster
-le(s)- = infectious lesions	-go(v)- = gonad (ovary)	-i- = primate
-li(m)- = immunomodulation	-ma(r)- = mammary	-o- = mouse
-vi(r)- = virus	-me(l)- = melanoma	-u- = human
-pr(o) = prostate		-abo- = rat-mouse hybrid
-tu(m)- = tumor (unspecified)		-xi- = chimeric
		-zu- = humanized

Table 2 Some monoclonal antibodies and their uses

Monoclonal antibody	Uses
Abciximab	Prevention of ischemic cardiac complications during percutaneous coronary interventions; short-term prevention of myocardial infarction
Adalimumab	Rheumatoid arthritis Crohn's disease, psoriasis
Afelimomab	Treatment of sepsis
Alemtuzumab	Chronic lymphocytic leukemia
Apolizumab	Chronic lymphocytic leukemia
Basiliximab	Prevention of acute renal allograft rejection
Bevacizumab	Metastatic breast and colorecta cancer
Clenoliximab	Rheumatoid arthritis
Daclizumab	Prevention of acute renal allograft rejection
Edrecolomab	Adjuvant therapy for cancer after colorectal surgery
Efalizumab	Treatment of severe plaque psoriasis
Enlimomab	Burns; stroke; prevention of acute rejection and delayed onset of graft function in cadaveric renal transplantation
Epratuzumab	Non-Hodgkin's lymphoma
Gemtuzumab	CD33-positive acute myelogenous leukemia
Infliximab	Rheumatoid arthritis; ankylosing spondylitis; Crohn's disease
Inolimomab	Prevention of graft rejection
Keliximab	Rheumatoid arthritis
Muromonab	Prevention of acute renal allograft rejection
Natalizumab	Acute relapse in multiple sclerosis; Crohn's disease
Odulimomab	Prevention of ischemic renal damage during kidney transplantation
Omalizumab	Prevention of allergic asthma and seasonal rhinitis
Palivizumab	Prevention of respiratory syncytial virus infection
Ranibizumab	Age-related molecular degeneration
Rituximab	Chemotherapy-resistant advanced follicular lymphoma; diffuse non-Hodgkin's lymphoma
Trastuzumab	HER2 receptor-positive breast cancer
Visilizumab	Treatment of glucocorticoid-refractory acute graft-versus-host disease

those treated (12). The formation of human antimouse antibodies has been described both when murine monoclonal antibodies are used as a diagnostic tool in vivo and when they are used therapeutically (13–16).

Common adverse effects of treatment with murine monoclonal antibodies include fever, chills, and malaise in 21–23% of cases and urticaria and pruritus in 15–18% (17).

The murine monoclonal antibody muromonab directed against the CD3 structure on T lymphocytes has proved to be an important therapeutic agent with potent immunosuppressive actions, and its extensive use provides examples of the adverse effects of rodent monoclonal antibodies. It is used to reverse acute rejection episodes

in kidney, heart, liver, or pancreas allografts and for graft-versus-host disease in bone marrow transplant recipients, when glucocorticoids have failed, or to avoid ciclosporin nephrotoxicity and the inconvenience of polyclonal antilymphocyte globulins (18). Despite its efficacy in over 90% of cases, muromonab causes a number of adverse effects, such as fluid retention and acute pulmonary edema (19), while marked early adverse effects include fever, chills, nausea, vomiting, headache, and hypotension, the last being attributed to systemic vasodilatation.

Other rodent monoclonal antibodies against cell membrane markers (CD molecules) have been described. The adverse effects of such antibodies can be ascribed to the general adverse effects of a heterologous protein, or to effects of the cell-targeting mechanisms (for example cell lysis).

General adverse effects

Although the adverse effects of most monoclonal antibodies were very few or benign, the possibility of more severe or unusual late complications should be considered, as illustrated by several case reports. In one patient, both immediate and delayed injection site reactions were noted after injections of a type I recombinant human interleukin-1 receptor (rhu IL-1RI), and positive cutaneous tests and specific IgE antibodies strongly suggested an immune-mediated allergic reaction (20).

Severe migratory polyarthritis with fever, an urticarial rash, and renal involvement have been reported after the first dose of CAMPATH-1G, a rat antihuman monoclonal antibody reactive against CDw52 antigens, used before marrow transplantation in a 25-year-old patient (21). In patients with renal transplants or rheumatoid arthritis, alemtuzumab, a humanized monoclonal antibody directed against the CDw52 antigen found on lymphocytes, produced only mild to moderate first-dose symptoms, such as fever and rigors, nausea and vomiting, bone pain, dyspnea, and headache (SED-13, 1134; SEDA-20, 380). By contrast, there was a high incidence of severe lymphopenia associated with infectious complications during the intravenous administration for low-grade lymphoma (22). Finally, several patients with rheumatoid arthritis treated with infliximab (a chimeric monoclonal anti-TNF-alfa antibody) or CDP-571 (a human anti-TNF-alfa antibody) developed various autoantibodies (23). Although there were no clinical consequences in these patients, the possible delayed development of overt autoimmune diseases should still be considered.

The mechanisms of adverse effects of monoclonal antibodies include sensitization due to the xenogeneic nature of the product, specific suppression of physiological functions, and secondary activation of inflammatory cells or mediators, which might be characterized by the cytokine release syndrome, as observed with muromonab-CD3 or rituximab (24). Although sensitization may be frequent, its clinical relevance is still limited, with only rare cases of allergic reactions. Although this has been strongly debated with muromonab-CD3 (orthoclone; SED-14, 1309), the available information on the risk of infections or cancers with other monoclonal antibodies is still limited, but does not suggest an increased risk.

References

1. Cosimi AB. Future of monoclonal antibodies in solid organ transplantation. Dig Dis Sci 1995;40(1):65–72.
2. Delmonico FL, Cosimi AB. Anti-CD4 monoclonal antibody therapy. Clin Transplant 1996;10(5):397–403.
3. Ziegler EJ, Fisher CJ Jr, Sprung CL, Straube RC, Sadoff JC, Foulke GE, Wortel CH, Fink MP, Dellinger RP, Teng NN, et al. Treatment of gram-negative bacteremia and septic shock with HA-1A human monoclonal antibody against endotoxin. A randomized, double-blind, placebo-controlled trial. The HA-1A Sepsis Study Group. N Engl J Med 1991;324(7):429–36.
4. Fisher CJ Jr, Zimmerman J, Khazaeli MB, Albertson TE, Dellinger RP, Panacek EA, Foulke GE, Dating C, Smith CR, LoBuglio AF. Initial evaluation of human monoclonal anti-lipid A antibody (HA-1A) in patients with sepsis syndrome. Crit Care Med 1990;18(12):1311–5.
5. Kappos L, Polman C, Pozzilli C, et alEuropean Study Group on interferon beta-1b in secondary progressive MS. Placebo-controlled multicentre randomised trial of interferon beta-1b in treatment of secondary progressive multiple sclerosis. Lancet 1998;352(9139):1491–7.
6. Lightner DJ, Vessella RL, Chiou RK, Palme DF, Lange PH. Immunotherapy for renal cell carcinoma: recent results. World J Urol 1986;4:222.
7. Aronson J. That's show business. BMJ 1999;319(7215):972.
8. Delmonico FL, Cosimi AB, Covlin R, et al. Murine OKT4A immunosuppression in cadaver donor renal allograft recipients: a Cooperative Clinical Trials in Transplantation pilot study. Transplantation 1997;63(8):1087–95.
9. Perosa F, Scudeletti M, Imro MA, Dammacco F, Luccarelli G, Indiveri F. Anti-CD4 monoclonal antibody (mAb) and anti-idiotypic mAb to anti-CD4 in the therapy of autoimmune diseases. Clin Exp Rheumatol 1997;15(2):201–10.
10. Dantal J, Ninin E, Hourmant M, Boeffard F, Cantarovich D, Giral M, Wijdenes J, Soulillou JP, Le Mauff B. Anti-CD4 MoAb therapy in kidney transplantation—a pilot study in early prophylaxis of rejection. Transplantation 1996;62(10):1502–6.
11. Panousis C, Pietersz GA. Monoclonal antibody-directed cytotoxic therapy: potential in malignant diseases of aging. Drugs Aging 1999;15(1):1–13.
12. Larrick JW, Bourla JM. Prospects for the therapeutic use of human monoclonal antibodies. J Biol Response Mod 1986;5(5):379–93.
13. Courtenay-Luck NS, Epenetos AA, Moore R, Larche M, Pectasides D, Dhokia B, Ritter MA. Development of primary and secondary immune responses to mouse monoclonal antibodies used in the diagnosis and therapy of malignant neoplasms. Cancer Res 1986;46(12 Pt 1):6489–93.
14. Reynolds JC, Vecchio SD, Sakara H, et al. Antimurine antibody response to mouse monoclonal antibodies: clinical findings and implications. Nucl Med Biol 1989;16:121.
15. Schroff RW, Foon KA, Beatty SM, Oldham RK, Morgan AC Jr. Human anti-murine immunoglobulin responses in patients receiving monoclonal antibody therapy. Cancer Res 1985;45(2):879–85.
16. Shawler DL, Bartholomew RM, Smith LM, Dillman RO. Human immune response to multiple injections of murine monoclonal IgG. J Immunol 1985;135(2):1530–5.
17. Dillman RO, Beauregard JC, Halpern SE, Clutter M. Toxicities and side effects associated with intravenous infusions of murine monoclonal antibodies. J Biol Response Mod 1986;5(1):73–84.
18. Burke GW 3rd, Vercellotti GM, Simmons RL, Howe RB, Canafax DM, Najarian JS. Reversible pancytopenia following OKT3. Use in the context of multidrug immunosuppression for kidney allografting. Transplantation 1989;48(3):403–8.
19. Lee CW, Logan JL, Zukoski CF. Cardiovascular collapse following orthoclone OKT3 administration: a case report. Am J Kidney Dis 1991;17(1):73–5.
20. Grammer LC, Roberts M. Cutaneous allergy to recombinant human type I IL-1 receptor (rhu IL-1RI). J Allergy Clin Immunol 1997;99(5):714–5.

21. Varadi G, Or R, Rund D, Orbach H, Slavin S, Nagler A. Severe migratory polyarthritis following in vivo CAMPATH-1G. Bone Marrow Transplant 1995;16(6):843–5.
22. Tang SC, Hewitt K, Reis MD, Berinstein NL. Immunosuppressive toxicity of CAMPATH1H monoclonal antibody in the treatment of patients with recurrent low grade lymphoma. Leuk Lymphoma 1996;24(1–2):93–101.
23. Rankin ECC, Isenberg DA. Monoclonal antibody therapy in rheumatoid arthritis. An update on recent progress. Clin Immunother 1996;6:143–53.
24. Breedveld FC. Therapeutic monoclonal antibodies. Lancet 2000;355(9205):735–40.

Penicillamine

General Information

Penicillamine is dimethylcysteine or 2-amino-3-mercapto-3-methylbutyric acid, a sulfur-containing amino acid. It has three functional groups: an alpha-amine, a carboxyl, and a sulfhydryl, which largely determine its pharmacological effects. Because the levorotatory isomer, L-penicillamine, is a pyridoxine antagonist and toxic, the racemic mixture has been replaced for medicinal purposes by purified D-penicillamine. Here "penicillamine" refers to the D-isomer unless otherwise specified.

Acetylpenicillamine is a weaker chelating agent than penicillamine, has no effect on collagen cross-links, and is not effective in rheumatoid arthritis. It has been used in the treatment of mercury poisoning (1).

As its name suggests, penicillamine is a degradation product of penicillin. There have been several reviews of the chemistry, pharmacokinetics, and pharmacology of penicillamine (SED-12, 537; (2). After oral administration about two-thirds (50–70%) of a dose of penicillamine is absorbed. As much as 33% can be degraded in the gut before absorption can take place. With a half-life of less than 1 hour, penicillamine is rapidly cleared after oral administration, largely by formation of disulfides with plasma albumin and with low-molecular weight thiols, such as cysteine and glutathione. Low-molecular weight disulfides constitute the major urinary metabolites. The penicillamine-albumin disulfide, on the other hand, has a long half-life. The consequence of this is slow accumulation: in healthy volunteers pseudo-steady-state plasma concentrations of penicillamine-albumin disulfide are not reached until the second week of daily administration. Peak plasma concentrations of penicillamine occur at 1.5–4 hours after ingestion and range from 5 μmol/l after 150 mg to 28 μmol/l after 800 mg (when conventional-release oral formulations are used). About 80% of penicillamine is protein-bound; about 7% occurs as L-cysteine-D-penicillamine disulfide, 5% as penicillamine disulfide, and 6% as free penicillamine. A large proportion is rapidly excreted in the urine, mainly as the disulfide or as the disulfide metabolite conjugated with cysteine; formation and excretion of the latter can cause cysteine depletion. Some penicillamine is converted to S-methyl-penicillamine and is either excreted by the kidneys or metabolized in the liver. Although S-methylation is a quantitatively minor elimination pathway, S-methyl-penicillamine is a potential substrate for sulfoxide formation, and patients with rheumatoid arthritis who form the sulfoxide at a reduced rate are at greater risk of adverse effects (3). The concentrations of penicillamine and its metabolites within cells and at the cell surface are largely unknown, but may be relevant to variability in response in regard to cellular sites of action.

Uses

Penicillamine have been used in the treatment of rheumatoid arthritis, Wilson's disease, and cystinuria. Although penicillamine and gold compounds were both originally used in rheumatoid arthritis on the basis of erroneous pharmacological hypotheses, they have been strongholds in the treatment of debilitating rheumatoid arthritis for more than a quarter of a century (4). Whereas they do not have much effect on the progression of joint damage, they have unexpectedly been found to be associated with a remarkable diversity of serious adverse reactions. In hindsight, they have played central roles in improvements in the understanding of the pathology of rheumatoid arthritis and of the methods of studying the benefits and harms of therapeutic strategies in rheumatoid arthritis and other chronic progressive diseases.

However, there is now less interest in penicillamine for the treatment of rheumatoid arthritis has been illustrated in recent reviews, in which little or no reference is made to penicillamine as a DMARD (5,6). Nor does it have a place in the management of pulmonary fibrosis (7) or biliary cirrhosis (8). On the other hand, in the treatment of Wilson's disease and various forms of acute and chronic metal poisoning, penicillamine is still being used.

In a study in the Department of Clinical Effectiveness and Audit in the Freeman Hospital in Newcastle-upon-Tyne, UK, on adherence to treatment guidelines for disease-modifying antirheumatic drugs (DMARDs), only a small proportion of patients used penicillamine (less than 40 of 1250 patients); today the most commonly used DMARDs are methotrexate and sulfasalazine (9). Penicillamine was the drug with the highest rate of non-adherence. This may simply be an artefact secondary to the small number of patients or, given that penicillamine is rarely used these days, could reflect complacency with treatment already taken for many years.

General trends in the treatment of rheumatoid arthritis in the past decade have been more aggressive treatment in early disease with disease-modulating antirheumatic drugs (DMARDs; (10) and the use of combinations of DMARDs (11). Strategies for improving the long-term outcome in rheumatoid arthritis include early specialist referral for DMARD treatment and the avoidance of NSAID-induced gastrointestinal and renal toxicity (12). However, a 28-year observational study in Austria of the patterns of use of DMARDs has illustrated how penicillamine has given way to other drugs, in particular methotrexate and sulfasalazine (13,14). The advent of novel drugs with different mechanisms of action, such as cytokine antagonists, has empowered rheumatologists with effective new instruments (15–17).

Some believe that early, aggressive, and continuous use of DMARDs and of combinations thereof slows joint destruction, modifies the natural course of the disease, and improves outcome (18,19). On closer inspection, however, the evidence still seems thin. Schemes for treatment and monitoring are variable and complex, and none is demonstrably superior to any other. It is in any case always important to tailor treatment to the needs of the individual patient rather than following rigid guidelines.

In other reviews, the conclusion has again been reached that the long-term use of DMARDs, including penicillamine, is limited by both frequent loss of response and serious adverse reactions, and that the advantages of combination DMARDs treatments remain controversial (SEDA-19, 229; SEDA-20, 219; SEDA-25, 266; 20,21). In particular, the treatment of juvenile rheumatoid arthritis is difficult, since DMARDs are often poorly active in children and some (gold compounds, sulfasalazine) cause special adverse reactions, such as the macrophage activation syndrome (which in turn can lead to severe infections; (22). There is still much to be achieved and improved. As Fries has put it (21): "Determining the most clinically useful DMARD combinations and the optimal sequence of DMARD use requires effectiveness studies, Bayesian approaches and analyses of long-term outcomes. Such approaches will allow optimization of multiple drug therapies in rheumatoid arthritis, and should substantially improve the long-term outcome for many patients." In the same paper it was emphasized that patients taking penicillamine should have blood cell counts and urine protein measurements every 2 weeks during drug titration and then about monthly for as long as treatment lasts.

Since the recognition of the superior effectiveness of methotrexate and the publications of the Pediatric Rheumatology Collaborative Study Group, penicillamine has been used infrequently in juvenile rheumatoid arthritis. The maximum daily dose is about 10 mg/kg (750 mg/day; (23). This dosage is reached in three equal steps, each of 6–8 weeks' duration. Perhaps more than gold, penicillamine acts slowly, taking 9 months to 3 years for maximum effectiveness.

In a small trial, penicillamine together with metacycline was not effective in progressive multiple sclerosis (24).

Observational studies

In an Austrian study, patients with rheumatoid arthritis were followed for a mean of 10 years (25). Of 27 courses of penicillamine, 13 were discontinued because of adverse effects, 12 because of lack of effectiveness, and two because of remission. Furthermore, an analysis of the reasons for DMARD withdrawal in patients in the Czech and Slovak Republics has underlined the fact that lack of effectiveness is, in addition to adverse effects, an important reason for stopping penicillamine (26).

Long-term follow-up data in 88 children with Wilson's disease, including 43 taking penicillamine, have been reported (27). The drug was withdrawn in seven cases because of adverse effects: bone marrow suppression in three, hematuria in two, a rash in one, and hemolytic anemia in one. Hemolytic anemia is a poorly documented adverse effect of penicillamine and it is unfortunate that in this case no details were given. In three more children with adverse effects the drug was continued; two had a rash and one drowsiness.

Comparative studies

Penicillamine 600–1800 mg/day (n = 23) and zinc sulfate (n = 12) have been compared in Wilson's disease (28). Neuropsychiatric symptoms became worse or remained unchanged in 75% of the patients who received penicillamine, whereas zinc sulfate improved these symptoms in 90% of patients. In six patients penicillamine was withdrawn because of adverse reactions: proteinuria and microhematuria in two, high titers of antinuclear antibodies or a lupus-like syndrome in three, and amenorrhea in one. The drugs were equally effective in improving liver involvement and there were no differences in follow-up hepatic copper contents.

Systematic reviews

The Cochrane Hepato-Biliary Group in Copenhagen have reported a meta-analysis of the benefit to harm balance of penicillamine in primary biliary cirrhosis, encompassing seven clinical trials and 706 patients (29). In the penicillamine group there was a four-fold increase in adverse events, often serious adverse reactions characteristic of penicillamine, while there was no beneficial effect on hard end-points.

General adverse effects

In clinical trials about 50% of patients experienced one or more adverse effects and withdrawal was necessary in about one-third (30–34). A mucocutaneous reaction (for example a rash or stomatitis) is the most frequent reason for discontinuing the drug (35). Long-term follow-up studies have shown that many patients (up to 80%) stop taking penicillamine, either because of adverse effects or lack of efficacy (35–39).

Adverse effects are less common when small doses are used, when increments are made only slowly, when patients are closely monitored, and when penicillamine has been tolerated for some years. However, in a meta-analysis of a large series of clinical trials, dose was not a strong determinant of the risk of adverse effects (dose range 500–1250 mg/day; 31). With regard to the safe use of penicillamine the words of Huskisson (1981) are still true (40): "Perhaps the most important aspect of the surveillance of patients receiving penicillamine is the need for the physician and patient to be able to contact each other. The physician must find the patient if his blood count changes. The patient must find the physician if he becomes ill. Disasters have occurred when patients consulted physicians who were unaware of the problems of penicillamine and instituted unwise therapy for them. Penicillamine can only be used by those who know how to use it and skilful management [of its adverse effects] is a most important aspect, perhaps the most important aspect of the treatment."

In patients with rheumatoid arthritis, delayed disease complications or serious intercurrent disorders can be mistaken for complications of treatment with penicillamine or other drugs (SEDA-21, 252). Anyone responsible for a patient taking penicillamine must bear in mind that serious adverse reactions can occur suddenly and at any time during treatment, even with very small doses (as low as 125 mg/day) and after many years. Penicillamine can be the unexpected cause of serious adverse reactions as an additive to Chinese herbs (41).

Early effects are gastrointestinal upsets and, more characteristically, loss of taste. Although a fall in the number of platelets is common, serious thrombocytopenia is less frequent. After long-term use of high doses, skin collagen and elastin are impaired, resulting in increased friability and sometimes in disorders such as perforating elastoma or cutis laxa; the latter has also been observed in neonates.

Hypersensitivity reactions are frequent early in a course of penicillamine, with urticarial or maculopapular rashes, fever, and lymphadenopathy. Cross-allergy to penicillin can occur. In addition, the use of penicillamine can be complicated by a unique variety of often serious autoimmune reactions, involving the skin, kidneys, liver, lungs, muscles, or other organs. Proteinuria is found in more than 10% of patients and sometimes develops into the nephrotic syndrome. Pemphigus, myasthenia gravis, polymyositis, or a lupus-like syndrome occur in smaller percentages. Reactions such as aplastic anemia, Goodpasture's syndrome, or thrombotic thrombocytopenic purpura (Moschcowitz's syndrome) are rare but serious.

Although lymphatic malignancies have been described in a few patients using penicillamine (SEDA-11, 212; SEDA-8, 237), a causal relation is considered unlikely.

Combinations with other drugs used in rheumatoid arthritis

Adding chloroquine or hydroxychloroquine to penicillamine in the management of rheumatoid arthritis probably offers no therapeutic advantages, produces more adverse effects, and may even be less effective (SEDA-10, 223; 42–45). A combination of penicillamine and sulfasalazine seems to be more effective, although the extent of the advantage is uncertain, and adverse effects may be more frequent (42). In one study penicillamine and intramuscular gold together produced much earlier improvement, but efficacy and adverse effects did not differ significantly compared with either drug alone. In an open, uncontrolled study, the combination of penicillamine and intramuscular gold yielded the highest proportion of remissions in patients with refractory rheumatoid arthritis (42). The possible consequences of previous intolerance to gold compounds in association with adverse reactions to penicillamine administration have been reviewed (SEDA-8, 236); at present no firm conclusions can be made. Penicillamine does not chelate gold stores in the body.

Comparisons with other drugs used in rheumatoid arthritis

In an outpatient study in New Zealand, the changing patterns were studied in the use of "slow-acting" antirheumatic drugs (46). There were increases in the use of methotrexate and of drugs in combination, whereas there was a marked reduction in the use of auranofin. Penicillamine had the highest "average toxicity" score. However, despite the increased popularity of sulfasalazine and immunosuppressive drugs, drugs such as penicillamine continue to be used worldwide. In a long-term follow-up study, the proportion of patients who continued to take their first DMARD or who were in remission at 5 years was 53% for penicillamine, compared with 34% for aurothiomalate, 31% for auranofin, and 30% for hydroxychloroquine (47). Of the 179 patients who used penicillamine, 36 stopped taking it because of adverse effects (see Table 1). In an open, randomized, follow-up study of patients with rheumatoid arthritis, 98 were allocated to penicillamine (median daily dose 750 mg, range 375–1000 mg) and 102 to sulfasalazine (48). Over follow-up for 12 years as many as 95 patients (48%) died, four from peptic ulcer disease complications, illustrating the prevalence of premature mortality in patients with rheumatoid arthritis. Only four of the 98 patients continued to take penicillamine. Major reasons for withdrawal of penicillamine, other than death, were adverse effects ($n = 47$) and lack or loss of effect ($n = 36$) (see Table 1). In neither study was any of the deaths thought to have been related to penicillamine. The picture given in Table 1 illustrates the remarkable diversity and seriousness of the adverse reactions pattern of penicillamine.

A diagnostic and monitoring database program called DIAMOND runs across a network of personal computers throughout the Staffordshire Rheumatology Centre (49). For about 10 years, drug histories, blood test results, and clinical correspondence files for about 2000 patients have been accessible, and the system is linked to the main hospital pathology database. The DIAMOND system has been used to study adverse reactions and durations of treatment for commonly prescribed DMARDs, including penicillamine (combination treatments excluded). With a median survival time of 34 months, penicillamine held an intermediate position, between methotrexate (< 96 months) and azathioprine (13 months) at the extremes; 38% of the patients continued to take penicillamine after 5 years. There were strong associations between penicillamine and both proteinuria and thrombocytopenia, both well-established adverse effects of penicillamine. Myasthenia gravis occurred in eight of 582 penicillamine users (1.4%) and not in patients using other DMARDs.

Prevention

Some 15 years ago, a more aggressive "sawtooth" strategy (early continual serial use) for the treatment of rheumatoid with disease-modifying drugs (DMARDs) was

Table 1 Adverse effects leading to the withdrawal of penicillamine in two studies

Reference	(40)	(39)
Total number of patients	98	179
Patients with adverse effects	47 (48%)	37 (20%)
Proteinuria	17	8
Rash, pruritus, or mouth ulcers		16
Nausea/vomiting	7	2
Rash	9	
Abdominal pain/dyspepsia	2	4
Thrombocytopenia	4	1
Leukopenia	2	2
Mouth ulcers	4	
Malaise	1	1
Exacerbation of joint pains		1
Myasthenia gravis		1
Pemphigus		1
Lupus-like syndrome	1	

advocated (SEDA-19, 229). There is now evidence that DMARDs, when carefully monitored, are both less toxic and less effective than previously thought (50). Apparently, the sawtooth strategy has not changed the balance of benefit and harm of these drugs. No single DMARD or combination of DMARDs stood out favorably with respect to efficacy, toxicity, or survival. Ineffectiveness, rather than toxicity, was the main reason for drug withdrawal. A Canadian study has added to the evidence that the long-term results of treatment with DMARDs, such as penicillamine and gold, are disappointing, as well as in patients treated early in the course of their disease (51). After 3 years, only 30% were still taking penicillamine. After 6 years only 20% of patients had not been withdrawn, and there were no substantial differences between the drugs.

The effect of a patient education program, taught by rheumatology nurse practitioners, on adherence of patients to treatment with penicillamine has been studied (52). The program significantly and persistently increased adherence over a period of 6 months in 51 patients compared with 49 controls (who used penicillamine without the educational program). Most of the patients (in both groups) had adverse effects, including thrombocytopenia in two and myasthenia gravis in one. The number of patients who asked to have penicillamine withdrawn was far higher in the control group ($n = 12$) compared with the patient education group ($n = 2$). Taste disturbances, for example, led to self-withdrawal in four patients, all in the control group. On the other hand, the patients in the patient education group were much more reluctant to withdraw, even in the event of serious adverse effects.

Dose relation

In a comparison of high doses (750–1000 mg/day) and low doses (125 mg every other day) of penicillamine in the treatment of early diffuse systemic sclerosis, there were no differences in efficacy (53). However, 16 of the 20

adverse event-related withdrawals were in the high-dose group. Seven of the 34 patients in the high-dose group had proteinuria (over 1 g/day) compared with only one of the 32 patients in the low-dose group. On the other hand, and in accordance with previous experience (SED-14, 723), other recorded adverse reactions, including myasthenia gravis, flu-like illness, thrombocytopenia, stomatitis, and rash, were only slightly more common in the high-dose group.

Time-course

Certain adverse effects occur predominantly during the first few months of treatment, for example taste alterations and non-specific hypersensitivity reactions, whereas others are more frequent during the second half-year of treatment (thrombocytopenia, proteinuria) or become apparent even later (for example collagen insufficiency). However, almost the entire spectrum of possible adverse reactions can occur at any time and without warning throughout a course of treatment with penicillamine. Although different schemes may be used, the monitoring of penicillamine treatment usually includes regular testing of platelet and white cell counts, a blood smear, proteinuria, and hematuria.

Organs and Systems

Cardiovascular

Penicillamine has no direct effect on the cardiovascular system. However, penicillamine-associated polymyositis can involve cardiac muscle and cause dysrhythmias, Adams–Stokes attacks, and death. Necrotizing vasculitis can occur as an immunological reaction to penicillamine (54). The effect of penicillamine on collagen and elastin fibers, which causes characteristic skin lesions, also includes the vascular wall, but effects of vascular insufficiency have not been reported.

Respiratory

Although penicillamine has no direct effects on the lungs (55), its use is associated with a spectrum of pulmonary injury: interstitial and alveolar reactions, pulmonary fibrosis, bronchiolitis obliterans, and pulmonary/renal syndromes (56–60). However, the differentiation between drug reactions and pulmonary disorders secondary to rheumatic or other underlying diseases is often difficult. The clinical presentation of bronchiolitis obliterans is acute, with cough, shortness of breath, and other non-specific respiratory complaints. The prognosis is often poor. Two separable but overlapping groups have been described: acute and chronic cellular bronchiolitis with less conspicuous scarring, and constrictive bronchiolitis, with histology varying from fibrotic and inflammatory lesions to complete small airway obliteration (SED-12, 539; 59,61–63).

In addition, several autoimmune reactions to penicillamine can secondarily affect pulmonary function. Penicillamine-induced polymyositis (64) or myasthenia gravis can cause respiratory failure, even requiring ventilatory support (65). The diagnosis and management of lupus-induced pleurisy have been reviewed (66).

Alveolar hemorrhage can occur with penicillamine, usually as part of a life-threatening pulmonary-renal syndrome resembling Goodpasture's syndrome (67,68).

Rhinitis, bronchospasm, and asthma can occur as a manifestation of hypersensitivity to penicillamine (SEDA-5, 248; 69–71) and rarely of the Churg–Strauss syndrome (72). Rhinitis can also be a symptom of penicillamine-induced pemphigus (73). In one patient a large pulmonary cyst developed concomitantly with skin lesions characteristic of the use of large doses of penicillamine (74). Microscopic derangement of the elastic fibers predominated. Although the frequency is uncertain, penicillamine can be associated with recurrent respiratory tract infections, that is secondary to IgA deficiency (75,76) or as part of the "yellow nail syndrome" (SEDA-9, 223).

Nervous system

Penicillamine, both L-penicillamine and the racemic mixture, strongly inhibit pyridoxal-dependent enzymes, cause pyridoxine deficiency in animal experiments, and are neurotoxic. Although this effect is much weaker with D-penicillamine, a few case reports have shown that D-penicillamine can also occasionally cause a polyneuropathy, as either a toxic or an allergic reaction (77–80). Rarely, an optic neuropathy (81) or a polyradiculoneuropathy (Guillain–Barré syndrome; 82,83) can occur.

When penicillamine is started in patients with Wilson's disease, pre-existing neurological involvement can acutely worsen; convulsions, muscle spasms, and coma can occur and death can follow (84–89). Worsening of neurological symptoms after starting therapy with penicillamine can occur in up to 50% of neurologically affected patients with Wilson's disease (87,88) and penicillamine can precipitate serious neurological injury in previously asymptomatic patients (90,91). It is uncertain if this results from alterations of copper distribution at submolecular, subcellular, transcellular, or transorganic levels, or whether it results from some other property of penicillamine (for example its capacity to donate sulfhydryl groups). Since the initial damage may be caused by copper decompartmentalization, it has been suggested that pretreatment with lipid-soluble antioxidants, such as vitamin E, may be useful (85), whereas at least some of these effects may reflect secondary pyridoxine deficiency. Supplementary oral pyridoxine may be advisable (88).

Two patients have been described with the internuclear ophthalmoplegia syndrome, probably induced by penicillamine. In one it was secondary to serious progressive intracerebral necrotizing vasculitis (54), in the other the underlying condition was a myasthenic reaction (92). Isolated cases have been described of neuromyotonia (93) and diffuse fasciculations (94), attributed to penicillamine.

In 18 patients treated with Wilson's disease penicillamine 600-3000 mg/day was gradually introduced over a period of 2-3 weeks, adjusted to urinary copper excretion, and after clinical improvement a maintenance dose of 600-900 mg/day was given (95). There was initial neurological deterioration, in particular of tremor and dysarthria, in 10 of the patients, but it reversed within 2-4 months. One patient had a hypersensitivity reaction (rash with leukopenia) and another developed cutaneous elastosis of the neck, characteristic of high doses of penicillamine.

In one case acute neurological deterioration in a young child after high doses of penicillamine had a fatal outcome (96).

- A seriously ill 8-year-old girl, weight 22 kg, with progressive jaundice, hepatomegaly, bilious vomiting, abdominal distension, coagulopathy, swelling of the feet, low-grade fever, drowsiness, and Kayser–Fleischer rings, was given fresh frozen plasma. After a challenge test with penicillamine 1 g plus pyridoxine 25 mg she developed jerky movements of the limbs, titubation of the head, and dysarthria. Since these symptoms were suspected to be due to penicillamine, oral zinc sulfate was begun and 3 days later penicillamine was resumed in a dose of 62.5 mg/day, increasing the dose by doubling every 2 days. When a dose of 500 mg/day (22.7 mg/kg/day) was reached there was recurrence of the neurological symptoms and penicillamine was withdrawn. Subsequently there was worsening of liver failure, gastrointestinal bleeding, peritonitis, and hepatic encephalopathy, and the child died.

Myasthenia

Penicillamine can induce a myasthenia gravis-like reaction, indistinguishable from idiopathic myasthenia gravis (41,65,90,108,97–111). It develops in up to 4% of patients using penicillamine, is most often described in patients with rheumatoid arthritis, but can also occur with other indications (for example biliary cirrhosis (112) or eosinophilic fasciitis (113)). However, it reportedly does not occur in Wilson's disease (114). The reaction often starts with involvement of ocular muscles, but any striated muscle can become involved. In contrast to other drug causes, it is characteristic of penicillamine-related myasthenia that about 90% of patients have antiacetylcholine receptor antibodies (111). The antigenic properties of circulating acetylcholine receptor antibodies in penicillamine-induced and idiopathic myasthenia are similar to those in recent-onset cases of spontaneous myasthenia gravis (102,109). Antistriational and antinuclear antibodies (115) can be present, and a sensitive immunoassay for striational autoantibodies can be used to monitor patients taking penicillamine for the development of myasthenia (104). In one study, measurement of acetylcholine receptor antibodies was considered to be of little or no use in routine monitoring of patients using penicillamine, because in 20% of patients antibodies were detected at least on one occasion, although none of the patients had signs or symptoms of myasthenia, and the antibody tests returned to normal despite continuation of the drug (116). Others have advised annual monitoring of every patient taking penicillamine, to detect subclinical changes in neuromuscular transmission and by acetylcholine receptor antibody testing (117,118).

- A 68-year-old woman, with HLA type DR1+, had been taking penicillamine (dose not specified) for 9 months for erosive seropositive rheumatoid arthritis (119). T cell clones were highly specific for D-penicillamine, but not for L-penicillamine or D-cysteine, and were restricted to HLA DR1. They responded well to blood mononuclear cells prepulsed with D-penicillamine but not to autologous B cell lines pulsed with D-penicillamine.

Apparently, penicillamine can couple directly to distinctive peptides resident in surface DR1 molecules on circulating macrophages or dendritic cells. In another article, apparently concerning the same patient, the same group described the selection of T cell clones specific for the ε (rather than the α or γ) subunit, responding to peptide ε 201–219 (120). They were restricted to HLA-DR52a (a member of the strongly predisposing HLA A1-B8-DR3 haplotype). Since these T cells had a pathogenic Th1 phenotype with the potential to induce complement-activating antibodies, they could be important targets for selective immunotherapy. In another patient, penicillamine-related myasthenia gravis developed simultaneously with polymyositis and pemphigus (121).

In spite of the similarities, there are some differences between spontaneous and penicillamine-induced myasthenia in respect to genetics. Myasthenic reactions to penicillamine appear to occur in a special genetic subgroup of patients, in whom there is a higher prevalence of the HLA antigens DRI and Bw35, and a lower prevalence of the antigens DR3 (which is associated with idiopathic myasthenia) and DR4 (which is increased in rheumatoid arthritis; 122,123).

Myasthenia usually improves rapidly after withdrawal of penicillamine, but it may have a protracted course. Fatal cases have occurred. Unrecognized myasthenia can present with prolonged paralysis after general anesthesia. For this reason, for patients taking penicillamine undergoing anesthesia the same precautions are advisable as for patients known to have myasthenia gravis (124).

Penicillamine unexpectedly caused myasthenia gravis when present as an unrecognized adulterant in Chinese herbs (41).

Sensory systems

Taste

Alteration or loss of taste is a characteristic adverse effect of penicillamine. Depending on the dose used, taste impairment (dysgeusia) occurs in 10–25% of patients and when daily doses in excess of 900 mg are used this increases to over 50% (SED-11, 466; 28,125). It usually develops in about the sixth week of treatment. Patients complain of requiring increasing amounts of sugar and spices. Food does not taste normal, but salty or metallic, or like cotton wool or blotting paper. Identification of certain foods becomes difficult. Absolute taste loss can ensue but the sense of smell is unaltered. Spontaneous recovery usually follows within 6–8 weeks, despite continuation of the drug. Dysgeusia can occur at any time and can be persistent (126).

In a review of drug-induced olfactory disorders, penicillamine was mentioned as a cause of abnormal smell (127). However, there may have been confusion with its effect on taste.

In patients with Wilson's disease, penicillamine is rapidly attached to copper and, although higher doses are used, taste disturbances develop in a lower frequency, about 4% (SED-8, 536). It has been suggested that dysgeusia is related to deficiency of copper or zinc, but a strong connection between taste impairment and urinary copper excretion has not been demonstrated (128). Serum copper concentrations remained within normal limits and copper supplements were not effective in prevention (129).

In another study, there was an association with reduced serum zinc concentrations, and taste recovered after zinc supplements were given, although it should be remembered that spontaneous recovery occurs in most patients (130).

Taste alterations have been reported with other sulfhydryl compounds, including pyritinol, captopril, and propylthiouracil (131), suggesting that the thiol moiety is involved. However, dysgeusia has not been observed in many studies on the use of penicillamine in children (SEDA-7, 258; 132).

Eyes

In a study of the feasibility of giving penicillamine to five neonates with extremely low birth weights, there were no signs of immediate intolerance (133). Against an incidence of retinopathy of prematurity of 54% in a historical cohort, only one of the children had mild transient retinopathy.

Optic neuropathy has only rarely been reported in association with penicillamine (81). In one patient, blurred vision occurred as a result of the development of bilateral choroidal hemorrhage complicating penicillamine-induced thrombocytopenia (134).

Ocular pseudotumor has been described in one patient as part of an ANCA-positive vasculitis (135).

Endocrine

A few patients are on record with suspected penicillamine-induced thyroiditis, one case being associated with a myasthenic reaction (136,137).

Metabolism

Penicillamine had a small effect on urinary glucaric acid excretion in patients with rheumatoid arthritis (138). This effect was thought to be the result of an indirect effect on hepatic metabolism and not to be related to disease activity.

Anti-insulin antibodies and hypoglycemia

One of the remarkable autoimmune phenomena that penicillamine can cause is the induction of anti-insulin antibodies, with resultant hypoglycemia (autoimmune hypoglycemia; 139,140). In these patients, there are high concentrations of immunoreactive insulin, despite undetectable free insulin. When penicillamine is withdrawn antibody titers fall sharply. The occurrence of hypoglycemia rather than hyperglycemia is not fully understood (141).

In two previously well-controlled diabetic patients taking penicillamine who developed hypoglycaemia, no reference was made to anti-insulin antibodies (142).

In a study using a competitive radiobinding assay, as many as 43% of patients with rheumatoid arthritis using penicillamine had autoantibodies against insulin (143). These antibodies did not appear to affect pancreatic beta-cells, as the response to intravenous glucose was normal and there were no episodes of hypoglycemia. Other sulfhydryl compounds that have occasionally been reported to cause autoimmune hypoglycemia are tiopronin, pyritinol, and thiamazole (methimazole; 144).

Enzyme inhibition

In in vitro studies penicillamine inhibited angiotensin-converting enzyme (ACE) and carboxypeptidase (145). Penicillamine interferes with the functions of the copper-containing enzyme ceruloplasmin, and some of the penicillamine- and copper-containing complexes formed in vivo have a superoxide dismutase effect (2). In patients with scleroderma, penicillamine normalized collagen metabolism, by inhibiting beta-galactosidase activity (146).

Nutrition

L-penicillamine strongly inhibits pyridoxal-dependent enzymes and causes pyridoxine deficiency in animals. Although D-penicillamine is much less active in this respect, there is some reduction in pyridoxine, and in a report of penicillamine-associated polyneuropathy, pyridoxine supplements for patients receiving D-penicillamine were advised (77).

Metal metabolism

Penicillamine is a potent chelator of metals. The stability of complexes of metals with penicillamine varies in the following order (from highest to lowest): mercury, lead, nickel, copper, zinc, cadmium, cobalt, iron, manganese (147–149). Most human data refer to copper, lead, and mercury.

Because of the strong affinity of penicillamine for copper and other metals, it is used in the treatment of Wilson's disease and lead poisoning. In other patients, however, this effect may sometimes cause deficiencies (SED-8, 531), especially of copper (SEDA-10, 223). Copper deficiency has been thought to play a role in the occasionally reported alopecia and in the loss of taste that is often experienced by patients with rheumatoid arthritis taking penicillamine (but rarely in Wilson's disease), but this could not be confirmed (128).

Penicillamine-induced deficiency of both copper and iron has been held responsible for the development of anemia (150), but serum iron concentrations do not usually change in patients using penicillamine (SED-8, 535).

The influence on metals such as copper and zinc may be difficult to assess, since penicillamine not only increases the excretion but also the absorption of these metals (151). A zinc deficiency syndrome, with skin lesions, alopecia, granulocytopenia, and eye damage, has been described in association with penicillamine (152).

Hematologic

The pathogenesis of hematological reactions to penicillamine is uncertain, but the available evidence suggests that pharmacological as well as immunological processes may be involved (153–155).

Of 29 Indian patients with severe Wilson's disease, all using penicillamine (full dose 750 mg/day) who were followed for 2 years to evaluate prognostic factors, 14 had progressive deterioration (group A) and 15 consistent improvement (group B) (156). In 13 patients (8 in group A and 5 in group B) penicillamine was withdrawn on 26 occasions. In two patients penicillamine was permanently withdrawn because of persistent hematological adverse effects (not specified). In the remainder the drug was temporarily withdrawn for a variety of reasons, notably hematological events and paradoxical worsening of the symptoms of Wilson's disease, but also financial constraints or poor understanding of the need for regular life-long use. When the full dose of penicillamine was given initially, there was paradoxical worsening in four patients (three in group A, one in group B). Two patients in group A died during the study, both of septicemia (organism not specified).

In the ARAMIS PMS Program, hematological events regarded as adverse effects of penicillamine, calculated per 1000 person-years, were as follows: pancytopenia 10, low white blood cell count 8, low platelet count 18, and polycythemia 2 (157). Serious blood dyscrasias, although rare, are among the most important adverse effects of penicillamine (SED-12, 541; 158,159). The assessment of the frequency of penicillamine-related hematological reactions can be hindered by the use of other potentially hemotoxic drugs, such as analgesics or gold compounds.

Eosinophilia can occur in up to 25% of patients using penicillamine, but is of little value in predicting serious hypersensitivity reactions (160).

Thrombocytopenia occurs in about 10–16% of patients and requires withdrawal in up to 10% (27,28,125), but these percentages vary considerably, presumably reflecting the use of different doses of penicillamine and different definitions of thrombocytopenia. In a series of 309 spontaneous case reports of drug-related thrombocytopenia, penicillamine was the fifth most common cause (18 cases, 6%; 161). The fall in platelet count is usually transient, but it is occasionally a warning of impending profound and dangerous thrombocytopenia or other serious hematological reactions, such as aplastic anemia or thrombotic thrombocytopenic purpura. Thrombocytopenia mainly develops during the first 6 months of penicillamine administration and appears to be associated with certain HLA antigens (DRA4, A1, C4BQO). Platelet counts fall to some extent in about 75% of patients taking penicillamine and it can be difficult to decide when to withdraw it. Platelet counts are recommended initially at 2-weekly intervals and subsequently each month, in addition to clear instructions to the patient. Weekly checks are needed when counts fall to between 100 and $70 \times 10^9/l$, and daily checks when below 70. If the platelet count falls progressively or falls below $70 \times 10^9/l$ penicillamine should be immediately withdrawn (162).

In all but one of 26 children with Wilson's disease who were treated with penicillamine 20 mg/kg/day, there were fewer adverse reactions than expected: two patients developed a rash, one patient had to stop taking the drug because of a lupus-like syndrome, and another had thrombocytopenia, which resolved after treatment with prednisone (163).

Concurrent thrombocytopenia and anemia have been attributed to penicillamine (164).

- A 66-year-old woman had taken penicillamine 200 mg/day for 8 months for long-standing systemic sclerosis, together with erythromycin (800 mg/day) for prophylaxis of pulmonary infection. Her platelet count was $39 \times 10^9/l$ and her hemoglobin concentration 7.3 g/dl. The leukocyte count was $3 \times 10^9/l$ with a normal differential count. There was no hemolysis. A bone marrow aspirate showed mild hypoplasia and reduced megakaryopoiesis. Incubation with penicillamine produced inhibition of erythroid and megokaryocyte burst-forming units, but not of granulocyte/macrophage colony-forming units, suggesting a selective effect of penicillamine on erythropoiesis and megakaryopoiesis. The blood cell counts recovered gradually on withdrawal of both penicillamine and erythromycin, treatment with corticosteroids, and a blood transfusion.

The authors did not make reference to the effects of incubating the bone marrow with erythromycin.

There have been several cases of thrombotic thrombocytopenic purpura or Moschcowitz's syndrome, characterized by intravascular coagulation, thrombocytopenia, and hemolysis, as a rare but life-threatening complication of penicillamine (165–168). There is one case report of Evans' syndrome, thrombocytopenic purpura in combination with autoimmune hemolytic anemia, in suspected association with penicillamine (169). In this patient antiplatelet antibodies as well as antibodies against erythrocytes were detected.

Penicillamine can cause other serious hematological reactions such as agranulocytosis and aplastic anemia (35,155,157,170–179).

- A 35-year-old woman with Wilson's disease had to stop taking penicillamine (250 mg/day) after 3 weeks because of leukopenia and fever (180).
- Pure red-cell aplasia developed in a 40-year-old woman as a rare idiosyncratic hematological reaction to penicillamine (115). Withdrawal of the drug, which had been taken in a daily dose of 500 mg for rheumatoid arthritis, and a short course of glucocorticoids was followed by permanent recovery.

Sideroblastic anemia has been attributed to penicillamine (181).

Because of its effect on ceruloplasmin and, in turn, the utilization of stored iron, penicillamine is considered to be able to cause iron deficiency anemia (150,182,183).

Penicillamine can also cause hemolytic anemia (SEDA-8, 535; 184), although good clinical evidence of this is lacking. A positive Coomb's test can occur as part of a lupus-like syndrome (185).

Polycythemia (156), leukocytosis, and thrombocytosis have been mentioned in association with penicillamine, but data are lacking.

Mouth

Stomatitis is a troublesome adverse effect of DMARDs. Ulcers of the oral mucosa are not uncommon in patients taking penicillamine (201,186) and lead to withdrawal in 3.1% of patients (187). However, stomatitis may be a consequence of multiple factors, including hematinic deficiency, virus or Candida infection, recurrent aphthous ulceration, or Sjögren's syndrome. Moreover, aphthous stomatitis often occurs in users of non-steroidal anti-inflammatory drugs (188).

When high doses are used, stomatitis may reflect impaired collagen synthesis. In one patient, mucosal ulcers were associated with leiomyomatosis in the peripheral serosa, which in turn caused intestinal obstruction (189). In another patient taking penicillamine for Wilson's disease, the removal of an impacted maxillary third molar was followed by the development of an oroantral fistula, presumably as a result of impaired collagen synthesis and disturbed wound healing (190). Furthermore, oral ulcers may be an important warning sign of penicillamine-induced agranulocytosis.

Cheilosis has also been reported (191). Oral lesions in patients using penicillamine may be due to pemphigus, cicatricial pemphigoid, or lichen planus, even in the absence of lesions outside the oral cavity. In 56 consecutive patients taking penicillamine, oral lichen planus was found in as many as seven (192). Penicillamine-induced cicatricial pemphigoid can be associated with oral ulcers as well as lesions of the esophagus, and stenosis can develop.

Gastrointestinal

Gastrointestinal complaints, including nausea, vomiting, heartburn, abdominal distress, and diarrhea, occur in up to one-third of patients starting penicillamine and may account for up to half of the withdrawals in the first 3 months of treatment (SED-12, 541; 27,28,185). However, penicillamine is not known to be ulcerogenic (SED-8, 535; SEDA-2, 217; 193), and the nature of gastrointestinal effects is not clear. Gastrointestinal symptoms are less frequent with initially low doses that are slowly increased. Taking penicillamine with food improves tolerance but reduces its absorption.

- A woman taking penicillamine developed dysphagia, heartburn, and weight loss; numerous large aphthoid ulcers were found in the esophagus (194).

Sulfhydryl compounds can damage the gut mucosa, but examination of the mucosa of cysteinuric patients who reported gastrointestinal upsets while taking penicillamine showed no evidence of structural damage (195).

Although less well documented than with gold, penicillamine can also occasionally cause life-threatening colitis (196).

Liver

Several case reports have demonstrated that penicillamine can cause liver damage (SEDA-13, 199; 197), mainly cholestatic hepatitis, often associated with other signs of hypersensitivity such as fever, rash (198), and pulmonary (171,199) or hematological reactions (174). In two children with Wilson's disease, penicillamine was thought to have caused persistence of a pre-existing increase in aminotransferase activity (200).

- A 30-year-old Japanese man with polyarthritis, in whom sodium aurothiomalate for 3 years had been ineffective, was given penicillamine 200 mg/day (201). After 10 days he became febrile and 2 days later jaundiced. A lymphocyte stimulation test against penicillamine was positive, suggesting type IV hypersensitivity. Later on he had a good response to tiopronin, without further adverse reactions.

In 29 Chinese patients, there was evidence in one that DMARDs and chronic viral hepatitis have synergistic hepatotoxic effects (202). However, the relevance of this anecdotal observation is uncertain.

Copper and iron are both capable of electron exchange and play a complex role in oxygen utilization. Copper proteins are critical in the transfer and transport of iron (203). In four patients with Wilson's disease, the fall in serum ceruloplasmin concentrations after treatment with penicillamine was associated with increased hepatic iron content; in two of these patients serum ferritin was increased (204). In another patient a liver biopsy taken after 15 years of treatment with penicillamine and zinc showed iron-laden hepatocytes, whereas histochemically detectable iron had been absent from an initial biopsy (205). The copper-containing protein ceruloplasmin and its membrane-bound homolog hephaestin are pivotal in iron metabolism. In addition there are intracellular transfer proteins ("chaperones") that deliver copper to ferroxidase proteins. Intracellular ferroxidase proteins accelerate the efflux of iron through stimulating the conversion of Fe^{2+} to Fe^{3+} and subsequent binding to transferrin. Presumably, excess loss of copper due to penicillamine or penicillamine plus zinc can reduce ferroxidase activity and cause intracellular iron deposition and paradoxical deterioration in liver function. Therefore, during treatment of Wilson's disease when the non-ceruloplasmin-bound copper falls to within the reference range (< 150 ng/ml), the maintenance dose of penicillamine should be reduced to the minimum needed; temporary withdrawal of penicillamine may even be indicated (203).

Pancreas

There have been three poorly documented cases of pancreatitis attributed to penicillamine (SED-8, 385; SEDA-2, 217).

Urinary tract

Penicillamine is often associated with renal damage. Proteinuria occurs in about 10–25% of patients taking penicillamine (SED-11, 464; 27,28,125,156,206–209) and occurs in 50% of patients with cysteinuria (SEDA-8, 236). However, microalbuminuria is common in patients with rheumatoid arthritis and may reflect either rheumatoid nephropathy or renal injury caused by penicillamine (or other drugs, such as gold compounds; 210). In about 5% of patients, proteinuria is the reason for withdrawing penicillamine. To avoid renal damage, response-dependent prescribing is recommended in rheumatoid arthritis, starting with a low dose and making increments at intervals of at least 1–2 months. Frequent urine testing is necessary, particularly during the first 18 months. Mild proteinuria (< 1 g/day) occurs most frequently, is often transient, and may be coincidental. Moderate proteinuria may be penicillamine-induced but need not be progressive or clinically harmful; close monitoring is indicated in such cases, and a temporary reduction in dose is advisable, although withdrawal of penicillamine may not be needed. When proteinuria increases, nephrotic syndrome can develop, necessitating withdrawal (211). In cysteinuria it is advisable to withdraw penicillamine when proteinuria exceeds 5 g/day (212), but in rheumatoid arthritis a lower limit of 2 g/day has been proposed (213). Nephropathy mainly develops during the second 6 months of treatment with penicillamine (213). It is more frequent in patients with a low sulfoxidation capacity (3,214) and with the HLA antigens DR3 and B8 (SEDA-11, 212; 215). Although nephropathy is thought to be rare in Japanese people (SEDA-8, 235; 30), it has been encountered in Japan (216).

In a comparison of high doses (750–1000 mg/day) and low doses (125 mg every other day) of penicillamine in the treatment of early diffuse systemic sclerosis, seven of the 34 patients in the high-dose group had proteinuria (over 1 g/day) compared with only one of the 32 in the low-dose group (53). Rheumatoid arthritis is a risk factor for renal disease, and the distinction from adverse drug reactions can be difficult in these patients (SED-14, 729).

On the basis of experience in one patient and 10 published case histories, the "scleroderma-pulmonary-renal syndrome," a rare and usually fatal complication of systemic sclerosis, characterized by fulminant alveolar hemorrhage and rapidly progressive renal insufficiency, has been reviewed (217). In their patient penicillamine was continued, and the disease progressed. Five of the 11 patients in their review had been using penicillamine.

In a prospective study of renal disease in 235 patients with early rheumatoid arthritis, persistent proteinuria and a raised serum creatinine concentration were predominantly related to drugs, including penicillamine and other DMARDs, whereas isolated hematuria was more directly associated with the activity of the disease process (218). Risk factors for drug-induced proteinuria were raised C-reactive protein, raised erythrocyte sedimentation rate, and age over 50 years.

Of 44 patients with rheumatoid arthritis, 24 had proteinuria (219). Two of these had drug-related nephropathy (penicillamine and gold, respectively); both had nonselective tubuloglomerular proteinuria, type V.

The principal renal lesion associated with proteinuria is membranous glomerulopathy or minimal-change glomerulopathy (209,214,220,221), characterized by minor thickening of the basement membrane or no change on light microscopy, but striking disturbances of the glomerular structures on electron microscopy (fusion of epithelial cell foot processes, subepithelial electron-dense deposits, and mesangial cell hyperactivity). Immunofluorescence microscopy shows granular deposits that contain IgG and C3 (222). These immunoglobulin deposits are not the result of precipitation of circulating immune complexes, as was previously thought. The available evidence suggests that the nephritogenic antigen, although still not identified, is expressed in the glomerulus and the immune complexes are formed in situ (220,223). Although proteinuria may be profound, serum creatinine is usually unaltered and penicillamine glomerulopathy usually has a good prognosis. Proteinuria can nevertheless continue for longer than 12 months after withdrawal and microscopic lesions can persist for longer. Although penicillamine nephropathy is more frequent when high doses are taken, it can also occur with small doses (for example 125 mg/day). On rechallenge, nephropathy does not necessarily relapse (SEDA-10, 218), and a history of previous gold nephropathy is not thought to be a risk factor (216). In one study, titers of antigalactosyl antibodies were correlated with the prior development of penicillamine (or gold) nephropathy (224).

Occasionally, penicillamine-associated renal injury is proliferative and progressive, extending beyond the basement membrane, with crescent formation in the glomeruli, and encompassing other renal structures, for example in the case of renal vasculitis, IgM nephropathy (225), or as part of a more general reaction; persistent renal insufficiency can develop and death can follow (209,226–231).

Penicillamine-induced lupus-like syndrome can be associated with proliferating glomerulonephritis with mesangial involvement and interstitial infiltrates (226,232). In such cases antibodies to native DNA can be found.

A rare but life-threatening complication of penicillamine is the development of a Goodpasture's syndrome-like reaction, characterized by alveolar hemorrhage, crescentic glomerulonephritis, and fever (67,233–237). In contrast to genuine Goodpasture's syndrome, circulating antiglomerular basement membrane antibodies are not detected (235), perhaps because the antigen concerned is not present in the test extracts used (236). Patients who have taken immunosuppressive therapy have a comparatively good outcome, but plasmapheresis and hemodialysis may be needed (233).

- A 65-year-old man with systemic sclerosis was given penicillamine, slowly increasing from an initial dose of 250 mg/day to a maintenance dose of 1000 mg/day (238). Over 2.5 years his skin lesions improved markedly. However, he developed atrial fibrillation and impaired renal function (serum creatinine 186 µmol/l, proteinuria, red cell casts, and an abnormal sediment with 50-100 red cells and 20-50 white cells per high-power field). He was given a beta-blocker, an anticoagulant, and an antianginal drug, and soon after had severe hemoptysis; the anticoagulant was withdrawn. His renal insufficiency and hemoptysis worsened and chest X-rays showed increasing alveolar infiltrates, suggesting continued hemorrhage. A diagnosis of Goodpasture's syndrome was made, penicillamine was withdrawn and plasmapheresis begun. Serological studies for anti-dsDNA and antiglomerular basement membrane antibodies were negative (ANCA not done). Nine days after hospitalization a ventricular septum defect developed and he died 36 days after admission. At autopsy there was focal segmental sclerosing glomerulopathy with periglomerular inflammatory infiltrates in some sections and mesangial thickening due to an increase in the mesangial matrix. Immunofluorescence showed diffuse global granular deposits in the glomeruli; staining for IgG, IgM, IgA, or C3 was negative. Electron microscopy showed diffuse thickening of the glomerular basement membrane. In the lungs there were interstitial fibrosis and severe hemorrhages. Pulmonary artery plexiform lesions suggested pulmonary hypertension. There was a pattern of cystic transformation of the lung parenchyma in the lower lobes, and metaplasia of the alveolar lining. The alveolar capillary membrane was replaced by interstitial fibrosis. There was profound intra-alveolar hemorrhage, diffusely distributed throughout the lung. In addition to severe coronary artery disease, there was a recent anterior wall infarct, leading to rupture of the ventricular septum.

The authors commented that anti-glomerular basement membrane antibodies had been present in only one of the previously published cases and that in three of these patients no immunoglobulins or C3 deposits were found on immunofluorescence examination. Presumably penicillamine sensitizes against basement membrane epitopes that are somewhat different from those in genuine Goodpasture's syndrome. They did not comment on the mixed nature of the pulmonary pathology and hemorrhages in this patient and the link with Goodpasture's syndrome.

Serious renal injury can develop as a late complication of pre-existing benign penicillamine nephropathy (233,239). Unfortunately, microscopic hematuria has limited predictive value for imminent serious renal injury, since in most patients who take penicillamine it is a transient or coincidental finding (SEDA-7, 260). The diagnosis of penicillamine-induced renal injury is often difficult because of the frequent association of rheumatoid arthritis with renal disorders (211,217,240–242), including spontaneous membranous glomerulopathy (243), or with injury caused by concomitant analgesics (244).

In a comprehensive study of 158 Japanese patients with rheumatoid arthritis, there was an obvious relation between membranous nephropathy and exposure to disease-modifying antirheumatic drugs (DMARDs) in 40 of 49 patients (245). In this study penicillamine (15%), bucillamine (67%), and gold compounds (17%) clearly predominated.

Penicillamine-induced nephrotic syndrome in published reports of 63 patients has been reviewed (246). The mean duration of penicillamine use before detection of proteinuria was 7.6 months and the mean duration of use until the diagnosis of nephrotic syndrome was 11.9 months. The mean dose at the time of diagnosis was 1 g/day and the peak amount of proteinuria was 11 g/day. Proteinuria usually improved or recovered within 7 months after withdrawal of penicillamine; treatment with corticosteroids in 12 patients produced a faster response. Five patients died with sepsis; two had received corticosteroids. There was minimal change disease in 27% of the patients and 55% had membranous glomerulonephritis. However, because of the literature search strategy this study may not represent the full picture of penicillamine nephropathy.

- A 12-year-old boy with a history of a generalized pruritic rash after penicillin took penicillamine up to 500 mg/day for Wilson's disease (247). He had a rash after using penicillamine for 1 week. The penicillamine was stopped for 3 days. He developed nephrotic syndrome 2 weeks after restarting penicillamine. On electron microscopy, there was the typical picture of minimal change disease with extensive foot process effacement.

In rare cases penicillamine can cause extracapillary glomerulonephritis with more extensive and serious glomerular injury leading to progressive and persistent renal insufficiency. One such patient has been described with a review of 26 similar published cases (248).

- A 51-year-old woman, who used penicillamine, maximum dose 600 mg/day, for systemic sclerosis, developed microscopic hematuria after 11 months. The penicillamine was withdrawn. Three months later she had progressive renal insufficiency. A biopsy showed extracapillary glomerulonephritis, with central fibrinoid necrosis and segmental mesangial proliferation, and

marked tubulointerstitial lesions. After treatment with glucocorticoids, cyclophosphamide, and 12 plasma exchanges her renal function improved slightly.

In half of the 26 patients renal damage was associated with alveolar hemorrhage (248). In eight patients plasma exchange treatment was performed. Seven patients died, including four with alveolar hemorrhage; 12 ended up with more or less chronic renal insufficiency. Only seven patients regained normal renal function; five of these had had plasma exchange.

- Acute renal insufficiency together with diffuse alveolar hemorrhage and bilateral pulmonary infiltrates was suspected to have been caused by penicillamine (500 mg/day for 6 months) in a 34-year-old white woman, who took penicillamine for progressive systemic sclerosis (249). Because of disseminated intravascular coagulation, a biopsy was not made and the role of penicillamine remained uncertain.

Hemolytic–uremic syndrome has been described in a patient with paradoxical rapid progression of systemic sclerosis (250).

- A 58-year-old man with a complex history of Hashimoto's thyroiditis and mixed cellularity Hodgkin's disease in complete remission developed systemic sclerosis involving the skin and the lungs but not the kidneys. He was given penicillamine 250 mg/day and prednisone 60 mg/day. After a few weeks there was rapidly progressive skin thickening, spreading from the hands to the trunk. However, his treatment was not altered, and 4 months later he developed hemolytic–uremic syndrome with microangiopathic hemolytic changes, thrombocytopenia, and acute renal insufficiency, with proteinuria, hematuria, and granular casts in the urine. The renal insufficiency persisted and he died with fulminant sepsis.

Three case reports from Belgium and France have illustrated the fact that rarely proliferative crescent-forming extracapillary glomerulonephritis and renal insufficiency can also occur (251,252). All three patients had taken penicillamine for systemic sclerosis. Antimyeloperoxidase antineutrophil cytoplasm antibodies were found in all three; one patient also had alveolar hemorrhage (that is Goodpasture's syndrome).

A clinical algorithm for the management of hematuria, for example in patients taking penicillamine or NSAIDs, has been published (253). It should be borne in mind that in such patients hematuria may be symptomatic of underlying pathology (for example a tumor of the urinary tract).

In one study in children with low-level lead poisoning, urinary incontinence was mentioned as a suspected adverse effect of penicillamine (254).

Skin

There is probably no other medicine that causes skin reactions with such a high frequency and of such striking diversity as penicillamine (see Table 2).

Table 2 Penicillamine-associated skin disorders

Maculopapular or urticarial rashes
Seborrheic dermatitis
Lichen planus-like eruptions
Psoriasiform eruptions
Erythema annulare
Photosensitivity
Pemphigus (erythematosus, foliaceus, vulgaris)
Bullous pemphigoid
Cicatricial pemphigoid
Dermatomyositis
Graft-versus-host reactions
Systemic lupus-like syndrome
Discoid lupus; subacute cutaneous lupus
Erythema multiforme and toxic epidermal necrolysis
Tardive dermopathy (friability, miliary papules, hemorrhagic   bullae)
Elastosis perforans serpiginosa
Pseudoxanthoma elasticum
Cutis laxa (hyperelastica)
Cutaneous pseudolymphoma
Acantholytic dermatosis (Grover's disease)

During the first few weeks of treatment, allergic reactions occur in about one patient in five (SED-11, 465; 30).

Maculopapular or urticarial rashes are frequent and can be associated with pruritus, edema, lymphadenopathy, arthralgia, fever, and eosinophilia. Patients with previous hypersensitivity to penicillin are more likely to experience a rash when taking penicillamine. Cross-allergy to penicillin can occur, but the risk of a severe allergic reaction to penicillamine in penicillin-allergic patients is thought to be low (255,256). Skin reactions may be more common in the presence of the HLA antigen DRw6 (257), and rashes and febrile reactions were more frequent in patients with anti-Ro(SSA) antibodies (258). Early allergic reactions do not usually necessitate permanent withdrawal of penicillamine, and can often be overcome by lowering the dose or by timely withdrawal of the drug and the use of a glucocorticoid. On the other hand, a non-specific eruption can be the first sign of a serious penicillamine-induced skin disorder, for example pemphigus.

There were no serious adverse reactions in 55 children who received 66 courses of low-dose penicillamine (about 15 mg/kg/day for a mean period of 77 days) for mild to moderate lead poisoning (259). However, in three children penicillamine was withdrawn because of a transient rash.

Paradoxically, penicillamine is occasionally involved in the development of rare diseases for which it is also sometimes used, such as systemic sclerosis-like lesions (260) and circumscribed scleroderma (or morphea; 261,262).Penicillamine can cause localized scleroderma (also known as morphea), which has been reviewed (271).

A rash or photosensitivity can also occur as part of the penicillamine-induced lupus-like syndrome (263–265). Type II bullous systemic lupus erythematosus (266) and necrotizing vasculitis (54) have been attributed to penicillamine. In one report, a hypersensitivity reaction to penicillamine with a skin rash and fever was associated with low back pain (267).

Erythema multiforme and toxic epidermal necrolysis are considered to occur as adverse reactions to penicillamine (SEDA-12, 465; 179).

Various other skin lesions have been described.

- In one inconclusive case report acantholytic dermatosis (Grover's disease) was described as a suspected adverse reaction to penicillamine (268). This is a papulovesicular eruption in elderly people, characterized histologically by focal acantholytic dyskeratosis.
- In a female patient acne and hirsutism developed in association with breast enlargement, probably induced by penicillamine (269).
- In a 31-year-old Korean woman with Wilson's disease, high doses (1–2 g/day) of penicillamine led to the development of a dermopathy, with mildly itchy, matchhead-sized, cream-colored papules on top of dark reddish plaques on both knees and elbows (270).

Bullous lesions can occur in scleroderma (localized, generalized, or systemic), and this highlights the diagnostic problems in such patients (272). In one of the four case histories presented in this paper, the bullous eruption, in a patient taking penicillamine for systemic sclerosis, was diagnosed as penicillamine-induced pemphigus foliaceus.

- A man with a history of penicillin allergy developed a hypersensitivity reaction of the penis when his wife was taking penicillamine (273).

Pseudomycosis fungoides, a subset of the pseudolymphoma syndrome, is a rare skin disease that has been associated with a variety of drugs, notably carbamazepine, but also penicillamine (274).

Effects on collagen and elastin

When penicillamine is administered for a long time and in high doses (for example for Wilson's disease) it can cause a characteristic delayed skin eruption, with increased friability, hemorrhagic bullous lesions, and miliary papules (74,276–282). The lesions develop predominantly in those parts of the skin that are often exposed to trauma. This disorder is a manifestation of the effects of penicillamine on collagen and elastin. Occasionally, these eruptions imitate other rare dermatological diseases and take the shape of elastosis perforans serpiginosa, cutis hyperelastica (cutis laxa; 283), or pseudoxanthoma elasticum (284–286); however, the histological and ultrastructural characteristics of the penicillamine variants differ from those of the spontaneous disorders.

In delayed penicillamine skin disorders, abnormal elastic tissue also exists in non-lesional skin, and has occasionally been documented in other organs (lungs, blood vessels, ileum, visceral adventitia, joint tissue), but the clinical implications of these findings are uncertain. In one study, multiple lymphangiectases and bloodvessel-lymphatic anastomoses were observed (278). Clinically manifest impairment of collagen and elastin has been reported in association with much lower penicillamine doses than had previously been recognized (287–289). In five of eight patients receiving penicillamine for rheumatoid arthritis, there was elastic fiber damage in joint capsules, suggesting that penicillamine-associated collagen injury may be common (289), although in only one case there was also elastic fiber damage in a skin biopsy. The fact that the lesions in delayed penicillamine skin disorders concentrate in flexural areas (neck, axillae, antecubital fossae, and buttocks) may reflect the accelerated turnover rate of elastin in these areas, secondary to shearing stresses and stretching. Perhaps impairment of collagen interferes with wound healing.

Presumably, the mechanism underlying penicillamine dermopathy is inhibition by penicillamine of cross-linkage of collagen fibers. In addition, the enzyme lysyl oxidase, required for the cross-linking of collagen fibers, is copper-dependent and may be inhibited by copper chelation by penicillamine. Another argument for a possible role of copper deficiency is the fact that cutis laxa is common in Menke's disease, a rare genetically determined disturbance of copper metabolism. Perforating elastoma occurs when abnormal elastic fibers accumulate, cause a foreign body reaction, and are transepidermally eliminated. Although the patient was also thought to have elastolytic involvement of the lining of the upper respiratory tract, there was no objective evidence of this.

Elastosis perforans serpiginosa, cutis laxa, and pseudoxanthoma elasticum

In rare cases, penicillamine dermopathy mimics elastosis perforans serpiginosa, cutis laxa, or pseudoxanthoma elasticum.

Elastosis perforans serpiginosa

Elastosis perforans serpiginosa starts as red umbilicated papules that coalesce to form annular (serpiginous or arcuate) lesions with clear centres. There are microscopically thickened coarse elastic fibers, extruding through narrow epidermal channels.

- A 37-year-old Japanese woman, who was taking penicillamine (500 mg/day) for systemic sclerosis, developed papules distributed in characteristic arcuate patterns of the skin of her neck (290). Histologically there was transepidermal elimination of degenerative elastic particles.

The typical high-dose degenerative dermatosis associated with penicillamine, characterized by elastosis perforans serpiginosa and pseudo-pseudoxanthoma elasticum, has been described in two other patients (291).

- A 25-year-old woman who had taken penicillamine (dose unspecified) for Wilson's disease for 14 years and developed pseudoxanthoma elasticum-like lesions. There were hyperkeratotic reddish brown papules in a semicircle of about 5 cm around a central area of atrophic skin in the in the neck and yellow "plucked chicken" lesions in the neck and axillae. A biopsy showed elastosis perforans serpiginosa, with focal acanthosis, parakeratosis, and transepidermal elimination of elastotic material in the epidermis. The dermis contained thickened elastic fibers with small lateral projections with a toothbrush-like aspect, surrounded by a granulomatous infiltrate with giant cells, some engulfing elastic fibers. Ultrastructural histology showed altered elastic fibers with an electron-lucent core and branching protrusions, and collagen fibres with uneven calibres and sometimes fragmentation. Topical glucocorticoids and tretinoin were ineffective, and penicillamine was replaced by zinc, after which a few new smaller lesions developed for up to 3 months.
- A 25-year-old woman with Wilson's disease, who had taken penicillamine 1.2 g/day for 16 years, developed an asymptomatic plaque in the neck, with red keratotic papules suggestive of elastosis perforans serpiginosa. A biopsy showed increased amounts of enlarged and fragmented elastic fibers in the upper reticular dermis and a mild polymorphous infiltrate with lymphocytes, histiocytes, and neutrophils. Ultrastructural examination showed elastic fibers with abnormal electron-lucent cores and angular branches with lateral budding. Penicillamine was replaced by zinc, but no outcome information was given.

The long delay before proper management of the disorder in these cases illustrates a lack of awareness of the possible effects on the skin of the long-term treatment with penicillamine.

- A 10-year-old girl started taking penicillamine 1 g daily for Wilson's disease (292). After about 20 years she developed skin laxity in the axillae, groins, and abdomen, multiple yellowish 2-3 mm papules with a "plucked skin" appearance in her neck, and denuded nodules in the perianal area. A biopsy showed transepidermal elimination of thickened elastic fibers with prominent lateral protrusions and the typical "lumpy-bumpy" or "bramble bush" appearance. No follow-up information was given.

Cutis laxa

Cutis laxa presents with loose redundant skin folds, reduced elasticity of the skin, and connective tissue involvement.

- An 84-year-old woman, who had been taking penicillamine 1.2 g/day for 50 years for Wilson's disease, developed generalized, rapidly progressive, acquired cutis laxa (293). Faulty production of collagen and elastin fibers lead to gross folding of the skin, giving it an appearance reminiscent of the folds of the cerebral cortex.

In one patient the characteristic features of both of elastosis perforans serpiginosa and cutis laxa developed (294).

- A 36-year-old man, who had had Wilson's disease since the age of 4 years, had used penicillamine for about 13 years in a dosage of 2–3 g/day. He developed an itching papular eruption, which initially resolved after withdrawal of the drug but recurred and progressed 6 months later. Generalized cutis laxa developed, with perforating elastolytic nodules on the neck and elastosis perforans serpiginosa over the shoulders. A biopsy showed perforating channels from the dermis through the epidermis, with a surrounding inflammatory infiltrate and horseshoe-shaped multinuclear giant cells phagocytosing abnormal elastic fibers. Van Giesen staining showed a lumpy-bumpy appearance of elastin fibers, typical of penicillamine dermopathy, as originally described by Bardach et al. (SED-14, 730).

Pseudoxanthoma elasticum

Pseudoxanthoma elasticum is characterized by coalescent yellow waxy papules with a "plucked chicken" appearance (because of the prominence of follicular orifices in the papules) and a marked laxity and wrinkling of the skin, resulting in redundant skin folds. In delayed penicillamine skin disorders gross abnormalities of elastic and collagen fibers are seen on electron microscopy. Elastic fibers have "moth-eaten," "saw-toothed," or "bramble bush thorns" appearances. Collagen fibers show large differences in thickness. Elastic tissue stains show an increase in the number of elastic fibers and irregular serrated fibers. The elastin content of lesional skin is three times greater than normal, whereas the number of elastin cross-links is only 15% of normal. In electron photomicrographs, dermal elastic fibers are studded with multiple perpendicular buds of different sizes and shapes, described as "lumpy-bumpy" and show varying degrees of fragmentation. Aggregations of granular elastinophilic material surround the central core of normal mature elastic tissue. In contrast to spontaneous pseudoxanthoma elasticum there is no calcium deposition in elastic fibers.

- A 47-year-old man had been using penicillamine 1.5 mg/day for 18 years for Wilson's disease. He developed pseudo-pseudoxanthoma combined with dysphagia and dyspnea. Biopsy specimens showed systemic involvement of elastic fibers, including skin, lung, esophageal muscle, gum, and pharyngeal and cervical connective tissue. All biopsies showed abnormal elastic fibers, consisting of a central core of uneven thickness with many lateral arborizations. There were branches at right angles to the main fibers, with perpendicular lateral arborizations off these, producing a stag-horn or fractal appearance. On the other hand, the adjacent collagen fibers were normal in structure.

Pseudo-pseudoxanthoma elasticum, caused by the use of high doses of penicillamine, has also been described (295).

Wound healing

In the past, penicillamine, because of its effects on collagen synthesis, has been suspected of interfering with normal wound healing. Experience of 217 operations in 150 patients did not show such effects, and consequently, there does not seem to be a need for stopping penicillamine before surgery (296). On the other hand, a few reports have suggested that penicillamine can, at least in some patients, have deleterious effects on wound healing (189,297).

Pemphigus

Pemphigus is a bullous autoimmune disorder of the skin, characteristically associated with antidesmoglein antibodies. Although many different drugs have been described as a cause of pemphigus, there is a remarkably strong predominance of penicillamine (and other sulfhydryl compounds; 298–301). Three groups of pemphigus-inducing drugs can be distinguished (302):

1. thiol drugs (for example penicillamine);
2. "masked thiol drugs" (sulfur-containing drugs that undergo metabolic changes to form thiol groups, for example piroxicam, beta-lactam compounds);
3. drugs with an active amide group (for example dipyrone, enalapril).

Thiol-related pemphigus usually presents as the foliaceus variant, with comparatively few immunofluorescence findings and a good prognosis, whereas drugs with an active amide group can provoke pemphigus vulgaris with a less favorable prognosis on drug withdrawal. A pemphigus-like eruption (303–315) develops in 1–2% of the users of penicillamine (SEDA-11, 213). Penicillamine is by far the most frequent cause of the drug-related variant.

- A 71-year-old woman taking penicillamine (dosage not specified) developed pemphigus vulgaris rather than pemphigus foliaceus, which is the usual form of pemphigus that penicillamine causes (316). She presented with pustular bullae (due to secondary infection with *Pseudomonas aeruginosa*), and the indication for penicillamine was not rheumatoid arthritis but systemic sclerosis.
- A 64-year-old woman, who had used penicillamine 500 mg/day for 3 years for rheumatoid arthritis, developed a bullous skin eruption affecting her neck and limbs (317). After treatment with prednisolone (dose not specified) she improved, but relapsed when the dose was reduced below 10 mg. Eleven months after the onset of blistering, penicillamine was discontinued and within 2 months the prednisolone was also stopped, with no recurrence of the eruption during 12 months follow-up. Direct immunofluorescence was positive for

immunoglobulin G and complement component C3, and indirect immunofluorescence was positive on the roof of the NaCl split skin preparation.

- A Japanese patient with systemic sclerosis developed pemphigus foliaceus while taking penicillamine (dose not specified) and prednisolone (318). A direct immunofluorescence test showed intercellular space deposits of IgG, and the ELISA index to anti-desmoglein 1 antibodies was raised to 115 (reference range <20). Withdrawal of penicillamine resulted in improvement of the skin lesions and a remarkably rapid fall in the titer of Dsg 1 antibodies, suggesting that the production of these antibodies required constant exposure to the drug.

A case report of typical penicillamine dermopathy in a woman with Wilson's disease was of particular interest because of its resemblance to pemphigus (319).

- A 49-year-old Chinese woman, who had been taking penicillamine 1.5 g/day for Wilson's disease for 5 years (cumulative dose about 3 kg), developed skin fragility, easy bruising, and over both elbows recurrent hemorrhagic blisters and multiple tiny white papules with underlying cutaneous atrophy and purpura; there were no intact vesicles or bullae (320). A skin biopsy showed a milium cyst containing laminated keratin, consistent with milia secondary to a healed hemorrhagic blister. There was paucity of elastic fibers in the dermis; direct and indirect immunofluorescence tests were negative. Other manifestations of penicillamine dermopathy (elastosis perforans serpiginosa, pseudoxanthoma elasticum, and cutis laxa) were absent. Reducing the dose of penicillamine to 500 mg/day was followed by marked improvement.

In this patient the negative immunohistochemical findings excluded pemphigus.

There has been a detailed report of histopathology and immunomorphology in three patients with superficial pemphigus, in one possibly related to previous use of penicillamine (321). The findings suggested that pemphigus erythematosus and pemphigus foliaceus are respectively localized and generalized variants of superficial pemphigus. The patients had antibodies against desmoglein 1 (but not desmoglein 2) and against a 230 kDa and a 190 kDa protein. Although the co-existence of pemphigus and bullous pemphigoid is considered to be extremely rare, all three patients also had bullous pemphigoid antigen BP230-specific antibodies.

A consultation of the database of the Committee on Safety of Medicines in London showed that 41 cases of bullous pemphigoid have been reported in suspected connection with penicillamine, suggesting that this adverse reaction is less rare that the published literature suggests.

Pemphigus usually recedes when penicillamine is stopped, but can persist for many years (322,324), and recur on rechallenge (322); fatal cases have occurred (323,324). Pemphigus that continues after drug withdrawal is referred to as triggered pemphigus, whereas a reaction that clears soon after withdrawal is called induced pemphigus (301).

Although it is usually rapidly reversible, penicillamine-induced pemphigus can run a protracted course (SED-14, 730). In a report from the Netherlands, penicillamine-related pemphigus foliaceus was highly resistant to treatment for 7 years (325). Eventually the intravenous administration of low doses of normal human immunoglobulin (40 mg/kg/day for 5 days in cycles of 3 weeks), together with dexamethasone pulse therapy, led to remission.

The entire clinical and pathological spectrum of pemphigus can occur in association with penicillamine, that is pemphigus erythematosus, pemphigus foliaceus, pemphigus vulgaris, and bullous pemphigoid (315). In this order of sequence the level of blister formation descends from the superficial layers to the deeper layers of the epidermis toward the basement membrane and subepidermal tissue. Penicillamine-induced pemphigus is predominantly of the foliaceus type. As in spontaneous pemphigus, antidesmoglein antibodies are present, although they may not be found in early stages. In pemphigus vulgaris antibodies react with desmoglein 3 and in pemphigus foliaceus with desmoglein 1, suggesting that different antigens are involved (326,327). The antibody reactivity of patients with idiopathic and penicillamine-related pemphigus appeared to be the same (300), which is suggestive of a similar basic molecular mechanism. Sometimes the characteristic lesions of different eruptions, for example pemphigus, bullous or cicatricial pemphigoid, lupus erythematosus, discoid lupus, or seborrheic dermatitis, can be seen in one and the same patient taking penicillamine (SEDA-11, 213; SEDA-15, 239; 318). This suggests differences in the pathogenic process rather than the simultaneous occurrence of different reactions.

Penicillamine has epidermotropic properties and accumulates in the skin. There are several possible mechanisms involved in penicillamine-induced pemphigus (SED-12, 544):

- penicillamine may cause acantholysis by direct destruction of epidermal intercellular attachment (without pemphigus antibodies; 328–330);
- the drug may induce autoantigens through modification of epidermal differentiation or interaction with epidermal tissues;
- penicillamine may change immunological tolerance, influence T-suppressor cells, and elicit autoimmune responses (296,297).

There is still uncertainty about the precise underlying processes. Apart from a reduced frequency of the rheumatoid arthritis-associated antigen B15, penicillamine-induced pemphigus does not appear to be strongly associated with a characteristic HLA antigen pattern (331,332).

Penicillamine-induced pemphigus can pose diagnostic difficulties, for example because it can present as a nonspecific rash, seborrheic dermatitis, erythema annulare (333), isolated stomatitis, or even rhinitis (73). Because of the friability of the superficial blisters, the bullous nature of pemphigus erythematosus and pemphigus foliaceus may be overlooked.

Since beta-lactam antibiotics also appear to be associated with pemphigus, especially ampicillin and amoxicillin, an earlier hypothesis (SEDA-5, 244) that this (and perhaps other reactions) to beta-lactam antibiotics may in fact be induced by the hydrolytic metabolite penicillamine has received attention (296,299).

A rare but potentially serious skin reaction to penicillamine is cicatricial pemphigoid (334,335). These patients can have symblepharon and entropion of the eyes, ulcers in the mouth, and blistering lesions on the trunk, extremities, and perineum (336). Involvement of the esophageal or vaginal epithelium can cause stenosis.

Ulcerative lesions of the vagina can occur in patients taking penicillamine, as a manifestation of pemphigus or cicatricial pemphigoid, or following impaired collagen synthesis (SED-8, 533; 337).

Graft-versus-host-like eruptions

Although rarely described, skin reactions that mimic graft-versus-host disease are an established complication of penicillamine (SED-14, 731). The similarity of the pathology of these drug-induced eruptions to those that occur after bone marrow transplantation has been reviewed (338). The drug-related eruptions may have different manifestations and can, for example, resemble smallpox, lichen planus (339), eczema, or other eruptions (340). However, their histological features are similar to those seen in cutaneous graft-versus-host disease, in particular eruptions in which liquefactive necrosis is seen at the interface between the epidermis and the cutis. One of the possible mechanisms involved in hypersensitivity reactions to sulfhydryl-containing drugs is based on the immune response of T cells to the sulfhydryl group, which arises when binding of IL-2 to the IL-2 receptor induces autoreactive T cells (341). The concentrations of IL-2 and IL-2 receptor were closely associated with the onset and severity of cutaneous graft-versus-host disease, suggesting an etiological similarity between the disease and skin eruptions induced by sulfhydryl-containing drugs. Proliferation of autoreactive T cells is induced by the binding of IL-2 to its receptor in these patients.

With seven cases in 56 consecutive patients taking penicillamine in one study, oral lichen planus may be fairly frequent (191). Most patients have erosive oral lichen planus, but bullous, plaque-like, or "classic" lichen planus can occur. Rarely a psoriasiform eruption has been reported with penicillamine (342).

Hair

Alopecia has occasionally been reported in association with penicillamine (156), but is ill-understood; hair loss can occur in association with polymyositis (343).

Nails

The peculiar yellow nail syndrome (SEDA-9, 223), characterized by dystrophy of the nails, lymphedema, pleural effusion, and bronchial involvement, has occasionally been reported in association with penicillamine and also with bucillamine (SEDA-9, 223; SED-13, 612; 344–347). It

has been suggested that penicillamine and bucillamine, because of their structural similarity to cysteine, might disturb nail growth by interfering with keratin synthesis. Although the nail changes and injury to other organs probably develop by different mechanisms, in patients with nail changes a careful search for possible systemic disorders is needed.

Monosymptomatic nail changes, with longitudinal ridging, transverse or longitudinal defects of the nail plate, absence of lunulae, and a tendency toward onychoschizia, can also occur as adverse effects of penicillamine (348).

Musculoskeletal

Joint symptoms in patients taking penicillamine vary from "creaking" and subjective discomfort and worsening of joint pain to severe arthralgia (349–351). Paradoxical acute severe exacerbation of rheumatoid arthritis has been reported in three patients, probably induced by penicillamine (352). Arthritis can also be a manifestation of penicillamine-induced systemic lupus erythematosus.

Although rare, Wilson's disease may itself be associated with a polyarthritis resembling rheumatoid arthritis and when it develops during the use of penicillamine it can be mistaken for an adverse reaction to the drug (353). Demineralization osteopathy has been reported in a study on the use of D-penicillamine in Wilson's disease (SED-8, 536).

- Progressive eosinophilic fasciitis with muscular involvement in a 35-year-old Brazil woman has been attributed to penicillamine (250 mg/day; 354).

In a prospective analysis of 74 women with systemic sclerosis, low bone mineral density and densitometric osteoporosis were related to the menopause and not to the previous use of penicillamine or other drugs (355).

Reproductive system

Gigantism of the breasts (macromastia) can occur in patients using penicillamine (SEDA-8, 238; 270,356–360). It usually develops in women and very rarely as gynecomastia in men (359,361). There is resemblance to the pubertal form of massive breast enlargement. It can be painful and has been encountered in pre- and postmenopausal women, with normal and increased prolactin concentrations. Histological examination mainly shows increased connective tissue and no changes in the glandular tissue.

- In one patient, the breasts were tender and grew progressively larger during each menstrual period.
- A 55-year-old premenopausal woman took penicillamine 1 g/day for 2 years for localized scleroderma (362). She used no other drugs. She noticed a gradual enlargement of her breasts, from a size B to size D+ bra cup. There were no palpable masses or tenderness. The only abnormal laboratory test finding was a positive test for homogeneous antinuclear antibodies (titer < 1:80), which is often found in patients with scleroderma. Serum prolactin was normal. Penicillamine was

withdrawn and the breast enlargement regressed over 3 months; the bra cup size reverted to B.

- In a 25-year-old woman with Wilson's disease, treatment with penicillamine (1.5 g/day) was first followed by the development of hirsutism, mainly of the face (270). After she started to use an oral contraceptive, her breasts enlarged rapidly and she experienced cyclic mastodynia; in addition, gingival hyperplasia developed. All symptoms improved on withdrawal of penicillamine, but additional mammoplasty was needed.

The sequence of events in the last patient suggested that the use of the oral contraceptive contributed to the development of macromastia.

In one case breast enlargement was accompanied by systemic lupus erythematosus (363).

- A 37-year-old woman with a 7-year history of rheumatoid arthritis had taken penicillamine for about 1–2 years (dose not specified). When she presented at the Cambridge Breast Unit she had had rapidly increasing painful enlargement of the breasts for 7 months. The breasts were symmetrically enlarged (from an A cup to DD) and had thickened and erythematous skin. There were several palpable masses; mammography showed no evidence of malignancy and an ultrasound scan showed large hypo-echoic nodules with engorged vessels. Histology of a large lump in the left breast showed a fibroadenoma. Immunohistochemistry for estrogen receptors showed 50% nuclear staining. She had stopped taking penicillamine 2 months before because of a lupus-like syndrome with thrombocytopenia, lymphopenia, and positive ANA and DNA antibodies (whether single-stranded or double-stranded was not stated).

Although breast gigantism is a rare manifestation of idiopathic SLE, in this case autoimmune substances could have stimulated mammary duct proliferation or mimicked estrogen or other growth factors in the breast.

Immunologic

Several experimental studies in humoral and cell-mediated immune systems have demonstrated numerous effects of penicillamine on the immune system; these findings are in keeping with a reduction in the overactivity of helper T lymphocyte that is found in rheumatoid arthritis (2,364). There is a fall in the numbers of immunoglobulin-secreting cells, and cultured mononuclear cells produce less IgA, IgG, and IgM. There is suppression of the autologous mixed lymphocyte reaction (365) and reduced hydroxyl radical generation from polymorphonuclear leukocytes (366). Penicillamine reduces the clearance of immune complexes and inhibits the complement cascade (367).

Penicillamine is uniquely likely among therapeutic drugs to cause autoimmune reactions (see Table 3).

Clinically and pathologically these variants of autoimmune disorders are closely similar to or indistinguishable from the spontaneous diseases. A major difference is that the patients usually recover when penicillamine is withdrawn. Differences in HLA configurations also suggest

Table 3 Autoimmune-like reactions reported in suspected association with penicillamine

Pemphigus (erythematosus, foliaceus, vulgaris)
Bullous pemphigoid, cicatricial pemphigoid
Graft-versus-host-like skin eruptions
Myasthenia gravis
Dermatomyositis/polymyositis
Glomerulonephritis
Lupus-like syndrome
Goodpasture's syndrome
Autoimmune hypoglycemia
Thyroiditis
Sjögren's syndrome
Aplastic anemia
Thrombocytopenia
Agranulocytosis
Thrombotic thrombocytopenic purpura (Moschcowitz's syndrome)
Evans' syndrome
Churg–Strauss syndrome
Necrotizing vasculitis
Guillain–Barré syndrome

that penicillamine-induced and spontaneous autoimmune disorders occur in different populations.

During penicillamine treatment autoantibodies develop in a high proportion of patients without clinical disease (368). For example, penicillamine can be associated with the development of anticentromere antibodies (369,370). Although these are usually a marker of serious autoimmune diseases, in association with penicillamine, the phenomenon was not accompanied by clinical symptoms and disappeared after stopping the drug.

In the serum of three patients with acute hypersensitivity reactions to penicillamine, complement-binding antibodies against penicillamine were detected (371). Patients with Wilson's disease are not known to have an abnormal immune status. The striking variability of penicillamine-induced pathology, including autoimmune reactions such as SLE, is also seen in patients with Wilson's disease, but the proportion of these patients in whom withdrawal is necessary is smaller, about 2–8% (80,87,88,372).

An unusual case report showed that low back pain can be a manifestation of drug hypersensitivity (268).

Anaphylaxis
Although hypersensitivity reactions are frequent, systemic anaphylaxis has only been reported rarely (373).

ANCA-positive vasculitis
Various vasculitic diseases, including Wegener's granulomatosis, microscopic polyangiitis, Churg–Strauss syndrome, and crescentic glomerulonephritis, are associated with antineutrophil cytoplasmic antibodies (ANCA) or leukocytoclastic vasculitis. In drug-induced ANCA-positive vasculitis antimyeloperoxidase antibodies are most often found; they produce a perinuclear pattern of staining by indirect immunofluorescence (pANCA), but anti-proteinase 3 (anti-PR3) antibodies can also occur (cANCA).

The possible drug causes of ANCA-positive vasculitis with high titers of antimyeloperoxidase antibodies in 30 new patients have been reviewed (134). The findings illustrate that this type of vasculitis is a predominantly drug-induced disorder. Only 12 of the 30 cases were not related to a drug. The most frequently implicated drug was hydralazine (10 cases); the rest involved propylthiouracil (three cases), penicillamine (two cases), allopurinol (two cases), and sulfasalazine.

- A 49-year-old woman with systemic sclerosis, taking penicillamine 750 mg/day, developed a vasculitis, with an orbital pseudotumor and, 2 months later, fatal alveolar hemorrhage. She also had antinuclear antibodies with a homogeneous pattern.
- A 56-year-old woman with systemic sclerosis taking penicillamine 750 mg/day had homogeneous antinuclear antibodies and antibodies to native DNA. Her manifestations of vasculitis were glomerulonephritis with renal insufficiency, pulmonary hemorrhage, and bilateral hemothorax (that is similar to Goodpasture's syndrome).

As the authors pointed out, practically all drugs known to cause ANCA-positive vasculitis (including penicillamine) have also been associated with a lupus-like syndrome, suggesting the possibility of a similar underlying mechanism. However, the presence of discriminating markers (such as anti-elastase and antilactoferrin antibodies) in drug-induced ANCA-positive vasculitis, but not in idiopathic cases, is suggestive of different pathways in these conditions.

In three Japanese patients with penicillamine-associated glomerulonephritis, antimyeloperoxidase ANCA assays were strongly positive (374). These patients had been taking penicillamine for rheumatoid arthritis in daily doses of 100, 200, and 300 mg for 32, 42, and 39 months respectively. All three had proteinuria, hematuria, anemia, and rapidly progressive renal insufficiency. Histological examination showed crescentic glomerulonephritis with granular deposits of IgG, IgM, IgA, C1q, and C3 in the mesangium. Penicillamine was withdrawn and the patients were given steroid pulse therapy, warfarin, and in two cases cyclophosphamide. Renal function gradually improved and the antineutrophil cytoplasmic antibodies disappeared.

- In a 69-year-old man with penicillamine-induced crescentic glomerulonephritis ANCA tests were repeatedly negative (375). He had been taking penicillamine up to 750 mg/day for systemic sclerosis.

Churg–Strauss syndrome

The Churg–Strauss syndrome is a rare disease, with eosinophilia, vasculitis, and granulomas, involving many organ systems (skin, lungs, kidneys, gastrointestinal tract, joints, heart, and central nervous system); rhinitis and asthma are often early manifestations. In one of two patients with the syndrome, penicillamine might have triggered its development (72); however, withdrawing the drug had no effect on the course of the disease and the relation was therefore uncertain.

Dermatomyositis and polymyositis

Penicillamine can cause other serious autoimmune reactions involving the muscles: dermatomyositis, with its characteristic facial rash (376), and polymyositis (64,105,106,343,377–388). Effects vary from only biochemical abnormalities, through moderate muscular weakness, to severe polymyositis with myolysis and sometimes myocarditis. There can be dysrhythmias, heart block, and Adams–Stokes attacks (384) and deaths have occurred (106). Muscle weakness can cause secondary respiratory failure (64,343). The clinical, pathological, and electromyographic features are similar to those of idiopathic polymyositis.

Antinuclear antibodies are found in about 90% of cases of penicillamine-induced polymyositis, a finding that may be helpful in distinguishing this condition from true polymyositis (379). In one patient anti-Jo-1 antibodies were found, which was thought to be an epiphenomenon and not pathogenic (86). Myositis occurs in about 1% of patients taking penicillamine and appears to be relatively common in Japanese and Indian patients (SEDA-15, 240; 28,377,385). HLA investigations showed that the antigens DR2 and DQw1 are increased in patients with penicillamine-induced myositis, suggesting that myositis occurs in a specific genetic subgroup (385). Of interest is the report of a patient with penicillamine-associated polymyositis who had a relapse after administration of ampicillin (380).

In penicillamine-induced polymyositis, weakness can be the presenting symptom and it may at first be mistaken for myasthenia (64).

The diagnostic pitfalls of penicillamine-induced polymyositis have been reviewed in the light of a report of a patient in whom postural changes were at first mistaken for possible ankylosing spondylitis (387).

IgA deficiency

IgA deficiency is a rare penicillamine-induced immune disorder, which can be accompanied by recurrent upper respiratory tract infections (75,76,390). IgA deficiency is more likely to develop when there is improved rheumatic disease activity, together with other adverse effects (for example rash, thrombocytopenia, proteinuria).

Lupus-like syndrome

Serological features of systemic lupus erythematosus develop in about 7% of patients taking penicillamine (184,240,264–266,391). A clinical lupus-like syndrome is less frequent (about 2%) and is as frequent in rheumatoid arthritis as in Wilson's disease. Characteristic phenomena are polyarthropathy, rash, pleurisy, fever, leukopenia, thrombocytopenia, antinuclear antibodies, and LE cells. The syndrome can be associated with antibodies to native DNA, renal damage, and neurological symptoms. The disorder usually improves in a few weeks or months after stopping penicillamine, but serological tests may remain abnormal for a longer period. Also, type II bullous systemic lupus erythematosus has been attributed to penicillamine (267). Penicillamine is no longer used in juvenile rheumatoid arthritis, in particular because of lack of effect and the possibility of inducing a lupus-like syndrome (392).

- A 6-year-old Taiwanese girl, who had taken penicillamine (dosage not specified) for Wilson's disease for 17 months, developed arthralgia, fever, and oral ulcers (393). She had antinuclear antibodies with a homogeneous pattern at a dilution of 1/5120, and a direct Coombs' test was positive. On the other hand, anti-DNA antibodies were within the reference range and antibodies against non-histone nuclear antigens (Sm, RNP, SS-A/Ro, SS-B/La, Scl-70) were all negative. She improved with prednisolone, and penicillamine was continued in a lower dosage.

Sjögren's syndrome

There have been two reports of Sjögren's syndrome (keratoconjunctivitis sicca, xerostomia, swelling of the parotids) in suspected association with penicillamine (394,395). In one study, reference was made to a patient with a Henoch–Schönlein-like syndrome as a suspected adverse reaction to penicillamine, but no details were given (396).

Multiple autoimmune reactions

Penicillamine often elicits multiple adverse reactions in the same patient, illustrating its immunomodulatory actions. Examples are listed in Table 4.

In a long-term prospective study of 69 patients taking penicillamine (750 mg/day) for progressive systemic sclerosis, 27 had adverse effects requiring either temporary reduction or complete withdrawal of therapy. Five of these had two, or, in one case, three different reactions (125).

- A 47-year-old woman developed concurrent pemphigus and myasthenia gravis (with ptosis and diplopia), apparently induced by penicillamine (500 mg/day for rheumatoid arthritis; 398).

In another patient, pemphigus, polymyositis, and myasthenia gravis developed simultaneously (121).

- A 67-year-old patient with rheumatoid arthritis had taken penicillamine 600 mg/day for 15 months when a skin eruption developed. Although no intercellular substance or basement membrane antibodies were found, a biopsy showed characteristic intraepidermal blistering. Direct immunofluorescence showed anti-IgG and anti-C3 antibodies, and desmoglein immunolabelling

(32–2B) favored drug-induced pemphigus. In addition, acetylcholine receptor antibodies were found. After the withdrawal of penicillamine there was rapid improvement of pemphigus and myasthenia. However, polymyositis was progressive, required high doses of corticosteroids for about 18 months, and improved only slowly.

Desensitization

The National Taiwan University Hospital has reported successful desensitization with prednisolone in a patient with hypersensitivity to penicillamine (399).

- A 14-year-old boy with Wilson's disease had a rash, fever, and angioedema repeatedly after the administration of penicillamine (600 mg/day). He was given prednisolone 30 mg/day for 2 days and then 20 mg/day. He was given penicillamine in an initial dose of 300 mg/day, which was increased to 600 mg/day in increments of 150 mg over 3 days and subsequently to 900 mg/day. Prednisolone was gradually discontinued over a 4-week interval, and penicillamine was increased to 1.2 g/day without further problems.

Infection risk

In a nested case-control study in Mexican patients with rheumatoid arthritis encompassing 1274 patient years, the risk factors were determined for acquiring infectious diseases (400). In addition to the cumulative doses of methotrexate and the duration of corticosteroids use, the mean daily dose of penicillamine was a risk factor. In one patient the infection was secondary to neutropenia. Tests for a possible immunoglobulin deficiency were not performed.

Long-Term Effects

Mutagenicity

In one experimental study it has been suggested that penicillamine may be mutagenic (401).

Tumorigenicity

There are a few case reports of lymphatic malignancies in patients using penicillamine, but epidemiological data in support of the association are lacking (SEDA-7, 259; 402–404).

Table 4 Examples of simultaneous multiple reactions reported with penicillamine

Pulmonary alveolitis, pancytopenia, cholestatic hepatitis, stomatitis, proctitis, skin rash, proteinuria, renal insufficiency (60)
Cholestatic hepatitis with allergic pneumonitis (199)
Pemphigus and nephrosis (minimal change nephropathy) (397)
Pemphigus and myasthenia gravis (398)
Thyroiditis and myasthenia gravis (135)
Polyradiculopathy and nephrosis (78)
Aplastic anemia and cholestatic hepatitis (174)
Gingival hyperplasia, acne, hirsutism, breast gigantism (270)
Agranulocytosis and toxic epidermal necrolysis (179)

Second-Generation Effects

Teratogenicity

Since the original case report of Mjølnerød et al (405), prenatal exposure to penicillamine has also been known to cause congenital cutis laxa and other malformations., although in 18 patients taking penicillamine (mean dosage 1000 mg/day), three women had five neonates, none of whom had teratogenic effects (95).

- A 35-year-old woman with Wilson's disease took penicillamine 1 g/day during the first 20 weeks of gestation and 500 mg/day afterwards (406). An ultrasound at 16 weeks showed arthrogryposis, bowed femurs, and a single umbilical artery. Because of oligohydramnios vaginal delivery was induced after 37 weeks. The male child had normal chromosomes. He had a low body weight (2190 g), a head circumference of only 31.5 cm, generalized cutis laxa, severe micrognathia, contractures of all limbs, internally rotated shoulders, flexed elbows, wrists, knees, and hips, camptodactyly, clubfeet, flat posteriorly rotated ears, bridged palmar creases, and undescended testes. The reflexes were brisk but muscle bulk and tone were normal. A chest radiograph showed hooked clavicles and a bell-shaped thorax, and a brain MRI showed agenesis of the corpus callosum and colpocephaly. At age 8 months there was a near full resolution of the cutis laxa but there was profound developmental delay and cortical blindness. Auditory brainstem-evoked potentials were abnormal at 5 months and at about 1 year partial complex seizures developed. A CT scan showed reduced brain volume, enlarged ventricles, corpus callosum agenesis, and bilateral subdural hygromas. The neonatal blood copper concentration at 24 hours was 400 (reference range 600–1900) µg/l.

A 5-year-old maternal half-brother, who had been exposed to penicillamine 1 g/day throughout gestation, had partial agenesis of the corpus callosum but was developmentally normal; there was no history of cutis laxa or contractures. The findings in this child were reminiscent of those in an earlier case, a boy with cutis laxa who also had growth retardation, facial abnormalities (a broad nasal bridge and low-set ears), contractures of the hips and knees, and simian creases (407). His mother had taken penicillamine 900 mg/day for rheumatoid arthritis. Of 11 children with probable penicillamine embryopathy six had cutis laxa, five had joint abnormalities, four had central nervous system malformations, and four of seven boys had inguinal hernias (406). The nervous system abnormalities in the other three children were hydrocephalus in two and congenital blindness and cerebral palsy in one.

Penicillamine should be withdrawn during pregnancy in patients with rheumatoid arthritis (408–410). It should be added, however, that in Wilson's disease it is also worth considering if it is possible to control copper metabolism with less penicillamine or without it altogether.

- A baby with a bilateral cleft lip with total cleft palate was born at 41 weeks to a 22-year-old mother who had taken penicillamine (dosage not specified) throughout an uncomplicated pregnancy for Wilson's disease (411). The child did not have a lax skin.

This case was found as part of a case-control study of 24 696 mothers of malformed infants. It was the only case of penicillamine exposure in the entire series. However, cleft lip has not previously been observed in association with maternal use of penicillamine, and there is little reason for suspecting the drug.

Fetotoxicity

Neonatal neutropenia has been reported in connection with maternal use of penicillamine (412).

- A 22–year-old woman, who had been taking penicillamine (600 mg/day) and zinc sulfate (600 mg/day) for Wilson's disease diagnosed at age 9, gave birth after 29-30 weeks gestation to a boy of 1.3 kg after elective cesarean section because of premature rupture of the membranes and uterine contractions. The baby had respiratory distress syndrome despite antenatal betametasone and was treated with mechanical ventilation, exogenous surfactant (Survanta 100 mg/kg), sultamicillin, and amikacin. During the 24 hours after birth, neutropenia developed (1.47×10^9/l; leukocytes 387×10^6/l). Neutropenia resolved spontaneously during the next 4 days.

Although penicillamine was the suspected cause, a possible role of other drugs, notably the surfactant and antibiotics, was difficult to rule out.

Susceptibility Factors

Genetic factors

Several studies have shown an increased frequency of penicillamine adverse effects in patients with low sulfoxidation activity, especially with regard to proteinuria and probably thrombocytopenia and myasthenia gravis (SED-12, 547; 3,209,413,414). The sulfoxidation capacity is expressed as the sulfoxidation index, calculated as the percentage of administered S-carboxymethyl-L-cysteine (750 mg), excreted as sulfoxides in the urine in 8 hours. A sulfoxidation index above 6% is taken as indicative of relative impairment of sulfoxidation capacity.

Certain adverse reactions to penicillamine are associated with increased or decreased frequencies of HLA antigens (SEDA-8, 235; SEDA-11, 212; 27,415–422). Most consistently reported are the associations between proteinuria and the antigens B8 and DR3 and between thrombocytopenia and DR4. These associations are not strong enough to include HLA typing into the routine of treatment with penicillamine. The relative risk of toxicity for patients possessing either HLA-DR3 or poor sulfoxidation appeared to be 25 as compared with those possessing neither; if these tests could be simplified, a valuable opportunity would become available for identifying patients at risk (215,409). Racial factors may be involved: proteinuria is less frequent in Japanese people, whereas polymyositis occurs at an increased frequency in India and Japan (215,352).

Age

Although published experience in children is limited, penicillamine has the same pattern of adverse effects as in adults. However, an interesting difference is that taste dysfunction has so far not been reported in children (SED-10, 221; SEDA-14, 198). In two children with Wilson's disease, penicillamine was thought to have caused persistence of a pre-existing increase in amintransase activity (200).

Other features of the patient

Patients with previous hypersensitivity to penicillin are more likely to experience a rash when taking penicillamine. Cross-allergy to penicillin can occur, but the risk of a severe allergic reaction to penicillamine in penicillin-allergic patients is thought to be low. An important measure to reduce the frequency of adverse reactions of penicillamine is to start with a small dosage (for example 125 mg/day in rheumatoid arthritis), to increase the dosage only slowly, and to maintain treatment with the lowest effective dosage. Nevertheless, serious complications such as nephrosis, pemphigus, alveolitis, and polymyositis have occurred while only 250 mg/day or less was used (SEDA-8, 235; 58,195,377).

The absorption of penicillamine can be significantly altered by alimentary factors. Changing habits, for example taking penicillamine between meals instead of with food, or stopping iron supplements, can precipitate adverse reactions by increased absorption.

Early hypersensitivity reactions are usually transient, and although there is undoubtedly an increased risk, in patients with a history of previous adverse reactions to penicillamine (or gold), re-exposure may not be followed by a relapse (SEDA-10, 218). In the case of serious complications, such as agranulocytosis, profound thrombocytopenia, polymyositis, or Goodpasture's syndrome, the repeated use of penicillamine carries unacceptable risks. Commencing penicillamine in patients with Wilson's disease can aggravate or even precipitate neurological involvement.

Antibodies to the Ro(SSA) cellular antigen (258,423) and circulating cryoglobulins (258) are risk factors for adverse reactions to penicillamine. AntiRo (SSA) antibodies characterize a distinct group of patients with rheumatoid arthritis who are almost exclusively female, express more activated B cell function, have a high prevalence of Sjögren's features, and commonly develop adverse reactions to penicillamine. Rashes and febrile reactions were especially associated with anti-Ro(SSA) antibodies, and renal pathology was more frequent in men (258).

Drug–Drug Interactions

Antacids

Antacids that contain aluminium or magnesium can reduce the absorption of penicillamine by up to 45%, presumably because increased gastric pH favors oxidation to the poorly absorbed disulfide (195,424,425).

Iron compounds

Iron compounds reduce the systemic availability of penicillamine to about 35% and copper excretion to about 28%, probably as a result of catalysis of the oxidation of penicillamine to its disulfide (2,420,426). Even the iron present in certain multivitamin formulations can be sufficient to cause interference, and when a patient who has regularly taken iron stops taking it, increased absorption of penicillamine and adverse effects can ensue (427,428).

Probenecid

When probenecid is co-administered with penicillamine in cystinuria, the efficacy of the penicillamine is significantly reduced (429).

Interference with Diagnostic Tests

Alpha-1 antitrypsin

Penicillamine can cause an artificially abnormal alpha-1 antitrypsin protein pattern, which can result in diagnostic errors (430).

Diagnosis of Adverse Drug Reactions

Reporting adverse reactions

The organization and preliminary results of an intensified voluntary reporting system for rheumatologists in the UK West Midlands for studying the safety of DMARDs have been described (431).

References

1. Florentine MJ, Sanfilippo DJ 2nd. Elemental mercury poisoning. Clin Pharm 1991;10(3):213–21.
2. Joyce DA. D-penicillamine pharmacokinetics and pharmacodynamics in man. Pharmacol Ther 1989;42(3):405–27.
3. Madhok R, Zoma A, Torley HI, Capell HA, Waring R, Hunter JA. The relationship of sulfoxidation status to efficacy and toxicity of penicillamine in the treatment of rheumatoid arthritis. Arthritis Rheum 1990;33(4):574–7.
4. Moreland LW, Russell AS, Paulus HE. Management of rheumatoid arthritis: the historical context. J Rheumatol 2001;28(6):1431–52.
5. Sokka T, Hannonen P, Mottonen T. Conventional disease-modifying antirheumatic drugs in early arthritis. Rheum Dis Clin N Am 2005;31:729-44.
6. Choy EHS, Smith C, Dore CJ, Scott DL. A meta-analysis of the efficacy and toxicity of combining disease-modifying anti-rheumatic drugs in rheumatoid arthritis based on patient withdrawal. Rheumatology 2005;44:1414-21.
7. Bouros D, Antoniou KM. Current and future therapeutic approaches in idiopathic pulmonary fibrosis. Eur Respir J 2005;26:693-702.
8. Kaplan MM, Gershwin ME. Primary biliary cirrhosis. N Engl J Med 2005;353:126-73.
9. Kay LJ, Lapworth K. Safety monitoring for disease-modifying anti-rheumatic drugs in primary and secondary care:

adherence to local and national guidelines and patient's views. Rheumatology (Oxford) 2004;43(1):105.

10. Parkinson S, Alldred A. Drug regimens for rheumatoid arthritis. Hosp Pharm 2002;9:11–5.

11. Sibilia J. Combinaison de traitements de fond dans la polyarthrite rhumatoïde. [Combination therapy for rheumatoid arthritis.] Ann Med Interne (Paris) 2002; 153(1):41–52.

12. Capell H, McCarey D, Madhok R, Hampson R. "5D" outcome in 52 patients with rheumatoid arthritis surviving 20 years after initial disease modifying antirheumatic drug therapy. J Rheumatol 2002;29(10):2099–105.

13. Aletaha D, Smolen JS. Laboratory testing in rheumatoid arthritis patients taking disease-modifying antirheumatic drugs: clinical evaluation and cost analysis. Arthritis Rheum 2002;47(2):181–8.

14. Furst DE. The combination of methotrexate, sulfasalazine and hydroxychloroquine is highly effective in rheumatoid arthritis. Clin Exp Rheumatol 1999;17(1):39–40.

15. Blumberg SN, Fox DA. Rheumatoid arthritis: guidelines for emerging therapies. Am J Manag Care 2001;7(6):617–26.

16. Menninger H. Combination therapy for rheumatoid arthritis: update 2001. Aktuel Rheumatol 2001;26:146–58.

17. Russell A, Haraoui B, Keystone E, Klinkhoff A. Current and emerging therapies for rheumatoid arthritis, with a focus on infliximab: clinical impact on joint damage and cost of care in canada. Clin Ther 2001;23(11):1824–38.

18. Lacaille D. Rheumatology: 8. Advanced therapy. CMAJ 2000;163(6):721–8.

19. Madhok R, Kerr H, Capell HA. Recent advances: rheumatology. BMJ 2000;321(7265):882–5.

20. Simon LS. DMARDs in the treatment of rheumatoid arthritis: current agents and future developments. Int J Clin Pract 2000;54(4):243–9.

21. Fries JF. Current treatment paradigms in rheumatoid arthritis. Rheumatology (Oxford) 2000;39(Suppl 1):30–5.

22. Prieur AM, Quartier P. Comparative tolerability of treatments for juvenile idiopathic arthritis. Biodrugs 2000;14:159–83.

23. Cassidy JT. Medical management of children with juvenile rheumatoid arthritis. Drugs 1999;58(5):831–50.

24. Dubois B, D'Hooghe MB, De Lepeleire K, Ketelaer P, Opdenakker G, Carton H. Toxicity in a double-blind, placebo-controlled pilot trial with D-penicillamine and metacycline in secondary progressive multiple sclerosis. Mult Scler 1998;4(2):74–8.

25. Skoumal M, Wottawa A. Long-term observation study of Austrian patients with rheumatoid arthritis. Acta Med Austriaca 2002;29(2):52–6.

26. Pavelka K, Forejtova S, Pavelkova A, Zvarova J, Rovensky J, Tuchynova A. Analysis of the reasons for DMARD therapy discontinuation in patients with rheumatoid arthritis in the Czech and Slovak republics. Clin Rheumatol 2002;21(3):220–6.

27. Dhawan A, Taylor RM, Cheeseman P, De Silva P, Katsiyiannakis L, Mieli-Vergani G. Wilson's disease in children: 37-year experience and revised King's score for liver transplantation. Liver Transplant 2005;11:441–8.

28. Medici V, Trevisan CP, D'Inca R, Barollo M, Zancan L, Fagiuoli S, Martines D, Irato P, Sturniolo GC. Diagnosis and management of Wilson's disease: results of a single center experience. J Clin Gastroenterol 2006;40(10):936–41.

29. Gong Y, Klingenberg SL, Gluud C. Systematic review and meta-analysis: D-penicillamine vs. placebo/no intervention in patients with primary biliary cirrhosis—Cochrane Hepato-Biliary Group. Aliment Pharmacol Ther 2006;24(11):1535–44.

30. Moens HJ, Ament BJ, Feltkamp BW, van der Korst JK. Longterm followup of treatment with D-penicillamine for rheumatoid arthritis: effectivity and toxicity in relation to HLA antigens. J Rheumatol 1987;14(6):1115–9.

31. Cooperative Systematic Studies of Rheumatic Disease Group. Toxicity of longterm low dose D-penicillamine therapy in rheumatoid arthritis. J Rheumatol 1987;14(1):67–73.

32. Kutsuna T, Maeda K, Okamoto T. [Long-term results of D-penicillamine treatment in rheumatoid arthritis.]Ryumachi 1986;26(4):270–7.

33. Kashiwazaki S. Current status of D-penicillamine therapy in Japan. Z Rheumatol 1988;47(Suppl 1):38–40.

34. Felson DT, Anderson JJ, Meenan RF. The comparative efficacy and toxicity of second-line drugs in rheumatoid arthritis. Results of two metaanalyses. Arthritis Rheum 1990;33(10):1449–61.

35. De La Mata J, Blanco FJ, Gomez-Reino JJ. Survival analysis of disease modifying antirheumatic drugs in Spanish rheumatoid arthritis patients. Ann Rheum Dis 1995;54(11):881–5.

36. Wolfe F, Hawley DJ, Cathey MA. Termination of slow acting antirheumatic therapy in rheumatoid arthritis: a 14-year prospective evaluation of 1017 consecutive starts. J Rheumatol 1990;17(8):994–1002.

37. Taylor HG, Samanta A. Penicillamine in rheumatoid arthritis. A problem of toxicity. Drug Saf 1992;7(1):46–53.

38. Pincus T, Marcum SB, Callahan LF. Longterm drug therapy for rheumatoid arthritis in seven rheumatology private practices: II. Second line drugs and prednisone. J Rheumatol 1992;19(12):1885–94.

39. Conaghan PG, Brooks P. Disease-modifying antirheumatic drugs, including methotrexate, gold, antimalarials, and D-penicillamine. Curr Opin Rheumatol 1995;7(3):167–73.

40. Huskisson EC. The side effects of penicillamine therapy in rheumatoid arthritis. J Rheumatol Suppl 1981;7:146–8.

41. Raynauld JP, Lee YS, Kornfeld P, Fries JF. Unilateral ptosis as an initial manifestation of D-penicillamine induced myasthenia gravis. J Rheumatol 1993;20(9):1592–3.

42. Jaffe IA. Combination therapy of rheumatoid arthritis—rationale and overview. J Rheumatol Suppl 1990;25:24–7.

43. Bunch TW, O'Duffy JD, Tompkins RB, O'Fallon WM. Controlled trial of hydroxychloroquine and D-penicillamine singly and in combination in the treatment of rheumatoid arthritis. Arthritis Rheum 1984;27(3):267–76.

44. Gibson T, Emery P, Armstrong RD, Crisp AJ, Panayi GS. Combined D-penicillamine and chloroquine treatment of rheumatoid arthritis—a comparative study. Br J Rheumatol 1987;26(4):279–84.

45. Dijkmans BA, de Vries E, de Vreede TM. Synergistic and additive effects of disease modifying anti-rheumatic drugs combined with chloroquine on the mitogen-driven stimulation of mononuclear cells. Clin Exp Rheumatol 1990;8(5):455–9.

46. Horsfall MW, Shaw JP, Highton J, Cranch PJ. Changing patterns in the use of slow acting antirheumatic drugs for the treatment of rheumatoid arthritis. NZ Med J 1998;111(1067):200–3.

47. Jessop JD, O'Sullivan MM, Lewis PA, Williams LA, Camilleri JP, Plant MJ, Coles EC. A long-term five-year randomized controlled trial of hydroxychloroquine, sodium aurothiomalate, auranofin and penicillamine in the treatment of patients with rheumatoid arthritis. Br J Rheumatol 1998;37(9):992–1002.

48. Capell HA, Maiden N, Madhok R, Hampson R, Thomson EA. Intention-to-treat analysis of 200 patients with rheumatoid arthritis 12 years after random allocation to either sulfasalazine or penicillamine. J Rheumatol 1998;25(10):1880–6.

49. Hill J, Bird H, Johnson S. Effect of patient education on adherence to drug treatment for rheumatoid arthritis: a randomised controlled trial. Ann Rheum Dis 2001;60(9):869–75.

50. Sokka T, Hannonen P. Utility of disease modifying antirheumatic drugs in "sawtooth" strategy. A prospective study of early rheumatoid arthritis patients up to 15 years. Ann Rheum Dis 1999;58(10):618–22.

51. Galindo-Rodriguez G, Avina-Zubieta JA, Russell AS, Suarez-Almazor ME. Disappointing longterm results with disease modifying antirheumatic drugs. A practice based study. J Rheumatol 1999;26(11):337–2343.

52. Grove ML, Hassell AB, Hay EM, Shadforth MF. Adverse reactions to disease-modifying anti-rheumatic drugs in clinical practice. QJM 2001;94(6):309–19.

53. Clements PJ, Furst DE, Wong WK, Mayes M, White B, Wigley F, Weisman MH, Barr W, Moreland LW, Medsger TA Jr, Steen V, Martin RW, Collier D, Weinstein A, Lally E, Varga J, Weiner S, Andrews B, Abeles M, Seibold JR. High-dose versus low-dose D-penicillamine in early diffuse systemic sclerosis: analysis of a two-year, double-blind, randomized, controlled clinical trial. Arthritis Rheum 1999;42(6):1194–203.

54. Pless M, Sandson T. Chronic internuclear ophthalmoplegia. A manifestation of D-penicillamine cerebral vasculitis. J Neuroophthalmol 1997;17(1):44–6.

55. Haerden J, Coolen L, Dequeker J. The effect of D-penicillamine on lung function parameters (diffusion capacity) in rheumatoid arthritis. Clin Exp Rheumatol 1993;11(5):509–13.

56. Turner-Warwick M. Adverse reactions affecting the lung: possible association with D-penicillamine. J Rheumatol Suppl 1981;7:166–8.

57. Camus P. Manifestations respiratoires associées aux traitements par la D-pénicillamine. [The respiratory complications of D-pénicillamine therapy.] Rev Fr Mal Respir 1982;10(1):7–20.

58. Shettar SP, Chattopadhyay C, Wolstenholme RJ, Swinson DR. Diffuse alveolitis on a small dose of penicillamine. Br J Rheumatol 1984;23(3):220–4.

59. Cannon GW. Antirheumatic drug reactions in the lung. Baillieres Clin Rheumatol 1993;7(1):147–71.

60. Bauer P, Bollaert P, Dopff C, Vignaud JM, Lambert H, Larcan A. Syndrome de détresse respiratoire aiguë d'évolution fatale au cours d'un traitement par D-pénicillamine. [Syndrome of acute respiratory distress with a fatal development in a treatment with D-pénicillamine.] Presse Méd 1988;17(19):961–2.

61. Padley SP, Adler BD, Hansell DM, Muller NL. Bronchiolitis obliterans: high resolution CT findings and correlation with pulmonary function tests. Clin Radiol 1993;47(4):236–40.

62. Honda T, Hachiya T, Hayasaka M, Morita M, Nakagawa S, Kusama Y, Kubo K, Sekiguchi M, Kobayashi O. [A case of rheumatoid arthritis with obstructive bronchiolitis appearing after D-penicillamine therapy.]Nihon Kyobu Shikkan Gakkai Zasshi 1993;31(9):1195–200.

63. Anaya JM, Diethelm L, Ortiz LA, Gutierrez M, Citera G, Welsh RA, Espinoza LR. Pulmonary involvement in rheumatoid arthritis. Semin Arthritis Rheum 1995;24(4):242–254.

64. Jenkins EA, Hull RG, Thomas AL. D-penicillamine and polymyositis: the significance of the anti-Jo-1 antibody. Br J Rheumatol 1993;32(12):1109–10.

65. Drosos AA, Christou L, Galanopoulou V, Tzioufas AG, Tsiakou EK. D-pénicillamine induced myasthenia gravis: clinical, serological and genetic findings. Clin Exp Rheumatol 1993;11(4):387–91.

66. Wang DY. Diagnosis and management of lupus pleuritis. Curr Opin Pulm Med 2002;8(4):312–6.

67. Lauque D, Courtin JP, Fournie B, Oksman F, Pourrat J, Carles P. Syndrome pneumo-rénal induit par la d-pénicillamine: syndrome de Goodpasture ou polyartérite microscopique?. [Pneumorenal syndrome induced by d-penicillamine: Goodpasture's syndrome or microscopic polyarteritis?.] Rev Med Interne 1990;11(2):168–71.

68. Vazquez-Del Mercado M, Mendoza-Topete A, Best-Aguilera CR, Garcia-De La Torre I. Diffuse alveolar hemorrhage in limited cutaneous systemic sclerosis with positive perinuclear antineutrophil cytoplasmic antibodies. J Rheumatol 1996;23(10):1821–3.

69. Storch W. Seltene immunologisch bedingte Asthmaformen. Atemw-Lungenkrkh 1990;16:271–2.

70. Lagier F, Cartier A, Dolovich J, Malo JL. Occupational asthma in a pharmaceutical worker exposed to penicillamine. Thorax 1989;44(2):157–8.

71. Grobbelaar J, Meyers OL. Penicillamine therapy in rheumatoid arthritis. S Afr Med J 1984;65(18):715–7.

72. Stockmann G. Die Stellung des Churg–Strauss-Syndrome zwischen anderen hypereosinophilen, granulomatösen und vaskulitischen Erkrankungen. [The status of Churg–Strauss syndrome among other hypereosinophilic, granulomatous and vasculitic diseases.] Z Rheumatol 1988;47(6):388–96.

73. Presley AP. Penicillamine induced rhinitis. BMJ (Clin Res Ed) 1988;296(6632):1332.

74. Bardach H, Gebhart W, Niebauer G. "Lumpy-bumpy" elastic fibers in the skin and lungs of a patient with a penicillamine-induced elastosis perforans serpiginosa. J Cutan Pathol 1979;6(4):243–52.

75. Stanworth DR. d-Penicillamine-induced immunodeficiency. In: Dawkins RL, Christiansen FT, Zilko PJ, editors. Immunogenetics in Rheumatology: Musculoskeletal Disease and d-Penicillamine. Amsterdam: Excerpta Medica, 1982:358.

76. Negishi M, Kobayashi K, Ide H, et al. A case report of selective IgA deficiency in rheumatoid arthritis treated with d-penicillamine. J Showa Med Assoc 1990;50:205–9.

77. Pool KD, Feit H, Kirkpatrick J. Penicillamine-induced neuropathy in rheumatoid arthritis. Ann Intern Med 1981;95(4):457–8.

78. Pedersen PB, Hogenhaven H. Penicillamin-induced neuropathy in rheumatoid arthritis. Acta Neurol Scand 1990;81(2):188–90.

79. Mayr N, Graninger W, Wessely P. Polyneuropathie bei chronischer Polyarthritis unter d-Penicillamin: medikamentös induziert?. [A chemically induced polyneuropathy in chronic polyarthritis treated with D-penicillamine?.] Wien Klin Wochenschr 1983;95(3):86–8.

80. Stremmel W, Meyerrose KW, Niederau C, Hefter H, Kreuzpaintner G, Strohmeyer G. Wilson disease: clinical presentation, treatment, and survival. Ann Intern Med 1991;115(9):720–6.

81. Klingele TG, Burde RM. Optic neuropathy associated with penicillamine therapy in a patient with rheumatoid arthritis. J Clin Neuroophthalmol 1984;4(2):75–8.

82. Knezevic W, Mastaglia FL, Quintner J, Zilko PJ. Guillain–Barré syndrome and pemphigus foliaceus associated with D-penicillamine therapy. Aust NZ J Med 1984;14(1):50–2.

83. Matsubara K, Noda T, Nakano I, Shikano Y, Maeda M, Mori S. A case of progressive systemic sclerosis with acute polyradiculoneuropathy during d-penicillamine therapy. Nishinihon J Dermatol 1990;52:1120–6.

84. Hilz MJ, Druschky KF, Bauer J, Neundorfer B, Schuierer G. Morbus Wilson—kritische Verschlechterung unter hochdosierter parenteraler Penicillamin-Therapie. [Wilson's disease—critical deterioration under high-dose parenteral penicillamine therapy.] Dtsch Med Wochenschr 1990;115(3):93–7.

85. Pall HS, Williams AC, Blake DR. Deterioration of Wilson's disease following the start of penicillamine therapy. Arch Neurol 1989;46(4):359–61.

86. Veen C, van den Hamer CJ, de Leeuw PW. Zinc sulphate therapy for Wilson's disease after acute deterioration during treatment with low-dose D-penicillamine. J Intern Med 1991;229(6):549–52.

87. Barbosa ER, Scaff M, Canelas HM. Degenera ção hepatolenticular. Avaliação da evolução neurologica em 76 casos tratados. [Hepatolenticular degeneration: evaluation of neurological course in 76 treated cases.] Arq Neuropsiquiatr 1991;49(4):399–404.

88. Tankanow RM. Pathophysiology and treatment of Wilson's disease. Clin Pharm 1991;10(11):839–49.

89. Kher A, Bharucha BA, Kumta NB. Wilson's disease: initial worsening of neurologic syndrome with penicillamine therapy. Indian Pediatr 1992;29(7):927–9.

90. Glass JD, Reich SG, Mahlon R, DeLong MR. Wilson's disease. Development of neurological disease after beginning penicillamine therapy. Arch Neurol 1990;47(5):595–6.

91. Porzio S, Iorio R, Vajro P, Pensati P, Vegnente A. Penicillamine-related neurologic syndrome in a child affected by Wilson disease with hepatic presentation. Arch Neurol 1997;54(9):1166–8.

92. George J, Spokes EG. Myasthenic pseudo-internuclear ophthalmoplegia due to penicillamine. J Neurol Neurosurg Psychiatry 1984;47(9):1044.

93. Reeback J, Benton S, Swash M, Schwartz MS. Penicillamine-induced neuromyotonia. BMJ 1979;1(6176):1464–5.

94. Pinals RS. Diffuse fasciculations induced by D-penicillamine. J Rheumatol 1983;10(5):809–10.

95. Pellecchia MT, Criscuolo C, Longo K, Campanella G, Filla A, Barone P. Clinical presentation and treatment of Wilson's disease: a single-centre experience. Eur Neurol 2003;50:48–52.

96. Paul AC, Varkki S, Yohannan NB, Eapen CE, Chandy G, Raghupathy P. Neurologic deterioration in a child with Wilson's disease on penicillamine therapy. J Gastroenterol 2003;22:104–5.

97. Liu GT, Bienfang DC. Penicillamine-induced ocular gravis in rheumatoid arthritis. J Clin Neuroophthalmol 1990;10(3):201–5.

98. Katz LJ, Lesser RL, Merikangas JR, Silverman JP. Ocular myasthenia gravis after D-penicillamine administration. Br J Ophthalmol 1989;73(12):1015–8.

99. Ferbert A. D-Penicillamin-induzierte okuläre Myasthenie bei Psoriasisarthritis. [D-penicillamine-induced ocular myasthenia in psoriatic arthritis.] Nervenarzt 1989; 60(9):576–9.

100. Chapat-Jolivet F, Wendling D, Moulin T, et al. Myasthénie induite par la d-pénicillamine au cours du traitement de la polyarthrite rhumatoïde. Rhumatologic 1989;41:181–8.

101. Zakarian H, Viallet F, Acquaviva PC, Khalil R. Syndrome myasthénique induit par la d-pénicillamine au cours de la polyarthrite rhumatoïde. Sem Hop Paris 1989;65:2052–6.

102. Tzartos SJ, Morel E, Efthimiadis A, Bustarret AF, D'Anglejan J, Drosos AA, Moutsopoulos HA. Fine antigenic specificities of antibodies in sera from patients with D-penicillamine-induced myasthenia gravis. Clin Exp Immunol 1988;74(1):80–6.

103. Paladini G, Mazzanti G, Mysco G, et al. La sindrome miastenica indotta da d-penicillamina nell'artrite reumatoide: caraterri clinici e genetici. Reumatismo 1988; 40:139–44.

104. Cikes N, Momoi MY, Williams CL, Howard FM Jr, Hoagland HC, Whittingham S, Lennon VA. Striational autoantibodies: quantitative detection by enzyme immunoassay in myasthenia gravis, thymoma, and recipients of D-penicillamine or allogeneic bone marrow. Mayo Clin Proc 1988;63(5):474–81.

105. Derman H, Theron HP. A propos de trois observations de syndrome myasthénique induit par la D-pénicillamine. [3 cases of myasthenic syndrome induced by D-penicillamine.] Bull Soc Ophtalmol Fr 1987;87(11):1235–43.

106. Dubost JJ, Soubrier M, Bouchet F, Kemeny JL, Lhopitaux R, Bussiere JL, Sauvezie B. Complications neuromusculaires de la D-pénicillamine dans la polyarthrite rhumatoide. [Neuromuscular complications of D-penicillamine in rheumatoid arthritis.] Rev Neurol (Paris) 1992; 148(3):207–11.

107. Norscini N, Lancman M, Doctorovich D, Poeraniec C, Bauso Toselli L, Granillo R. Miastenia gravis inducida por d-penicilamina. Presentacion de un caso y revision de la literatura. Rev Neurol Argent 1990;15:59–62.

108. Kuriyama S, Hosoya T, Sakai O. [D-penicillamine induced myasthenia gravis in a patient with rheumatoid arthritis.]Ryumachi 1991;31(3):298–302.

109. Voltz R, Hohlfeld R, Fateh-Moghadam A, Witt TN, Wick M, Reimers C, Siegele B, Wekerle H. Myasthenia gravis: measurement of anti-AChR autoantibodies using cell line TE671. Neurology 1991;41(11):1836–8.

110. Hanabusa K, Ohtsuki H, Watanabe S, Okano M, Hasebe S, Tadokoro Y. d-Penicillamine-induced ocular myasthenia gravis in rheumatoid arthritis. Folia Ophthalmol Jpn 1993;44:1306–10.

111. Wittbrodt ET. Drugs and myasthenia gravis. An update. Arch Intern Med 1997;157(4):399–408.

112. Chuah SY, Wong NW, Goh KL. Lethargy in a patient with cirrhosis. Postgrad Med J 1997;73(857):177–9.

113. Kato Y, Naito Y, Narita Y, Kuzuhara S. D-penicillamine-induced myasthenia gravis in a case of eosinophilic fasciitis. J Neurol Sci 1997;146(1):85–6.

114. Komal Kumar RN, Patil SA, Taly AB, Nirmala M, Sinha S, Arunodaya GR. Effect of D-penicillamine on neuromuscular junction in patients with Wilson disease. Neurology 2004;63(5):935–6.

115. Morel E, Feuillet-Fieux MN, Vernet-der Garabedian B, Raimond F, D'Anglejan J, Bataille R, Sany J, Bach JF. Autoantibodies in D-penicillamine-induced myasthenia gravis: a comparison with idiopathic myasthenia and rheumatoid arthritis. Clin Immunol Immunopathol 1991; 58(3):318–30.

116. Kolarz G, El-Shohoumi M, Maida EM, Scherak O. Azetylcholin rezeptor-Antikorper unter d-Penicillamin-Therapie. Ther Oesterr 1991;6:735–42.

117. Dominkus M, Chlud K, Maida EM, Grisold W. Monitoring of patients with rheumatoid arthritis in longterm administration of D-penicillamine. J Rheumatol 1992; 19(10):1648–50.

118. Dominkus M, Grisold W, Albrecht G. Stimulation single fiber EMG study in patients receiving a long-term D-

penicillamine treatment for rheumatoid arthritis. Muscle Nerve 1992;15(11):1300–1.

119. Hill M, Beeson D, Moss P, Jacobson L, Bond A, Corlett L, Newsom-Davis J, Vincent A, Willcox N. Early-onset myasthenia gravis: a recurring T-cell epitope in the adult-specific acetylcholine receptor epsilon subunit presented by the susceptibility allele HLA-DR52a. Ann Neurol 1999;45(2):224–31.

120. Hill M, Moss P, Wordsworth P, Newsom-Davis J, Willcox N. T cell responses to D-penicillamine in drug-induced myasthenia gravis: recognition of modified DR1: peptide complexes. J Neuroimmunol 1999;97(1–2):146–53.

121. Jan V, Callens A, Machet L, Machet MC, Lorette G, Vaillant L. Pemphigus polymyosite et myasthénie induites par la D-pénicillamine. [D-penicillamine-induced pemphigus, polymyositis and myasthenia.] Ann Dermatol Venereol 1999;126(2):153–6.

122. Garlepp MI, Dawkins RL, Christiansen FT. HLA antigens and acetylcholine receptor antibodies in penicillamine induced myasthenia gravis. BMJ (Clin Res Ed) 1983;286(6375):1442–3.

123. Andonopoulos AP, Terzis E, Tsibri E, Papasteriades CA, Papapetropoulos T. D-penicillamine induced myasthenia gravis in rheumatoid arthritis: an unpredictable common occurrence? Clin Rheumatol 1994;13(4):586–8.

124. Fried MJ, Protheroe DT. D-penicillamine induced myasthenia gravis. Its relevance for the anaesthetist. Br J Anaesth 1986;58(10):1191–3.

125. Jimenez SA, Sigal SH. A 15-year prospective study of treatment of rapidly progressive systemic sclerosis with D-penicillamine. J Rheumatol 1991;18(10):1496–503.

126. Gabutti V. Current therapy for thalassemia in Italy. Ann NY Acad Sci 1990;612:268–74.

127. Nores JM, Biacabe B, Bonfils P. Troubles olfactifs d'origine médicamenteuse: analyse et revue de la littérature. [Olfactory disorders due to medications: analysis and review of the literature.] Rev Med Interne 2000;21(11):972–7.

128. Knudsen L, Weismann K. Taste dysfunction and changes in zinc and copper metabolism during penicillamine therapy for generalized scleroderma. Acta Med Scand 1978;204(1–2):75–9.

129. Tausch G, Broll H, Eberl R. D-Penicillamin (Artamin) als Basistherapie bei chronischer Polyarthritis. [D-penicillamine (Artamin) as basic therapeutic agent in the treatment of chronic rheumatoid arthritis.] Wien Klin Wochenschr 1973;85(4):59–63.

130. Gutierrez Fuentes JA, Vazquez Gallego MC, Fernandez Remis JE, Arroyo Vicente M, Schuller Perez A. Ageusia como manifestacion secundaria del tratiamento con D-penicillamina. [Ageusia as a secondary manifestation of treatment with D-penicillamine.] Rev Clin Esp 1984;172(3):149–51.

131. Schiffman SS. Taste and smell in disease (first of two parts). N Engl J Med 1983;308(21):1275–9.

132. Prieur AM, Piussan C, Manigne P, Bordigoni P, Griscelli C, Reinert P, de Goujon F, Lefur JM, Garnier JM. Arthrite chronique juvénile. Etude en double insu de l'efficacité et de la tolérance de la D-pénicillamine. [Juvenile chronic arthritis. Double-blind study of the efficacy and tolerance of D-penicillamine.] Arch Fr Pediatr 1985;42(2):91–6.

133. Christensen RD, Alder SC, Richards SC, Horn JT, Lambert DK, Baer VL. A pilot trial testing the feasibility of administering D-penicillamine to extremely low birth weight neonates. J Perinatol 2006;26(2):120–4.

134. Klepach GL, Wray SH. Bilateral serous retinal detachment with thrombocytopenia during penicillamine therapy. Ann Ophthalmol 1981;13(2):201–3.

135. Choi HK, Merkel PA, Walker AM, Niles JL. Drug-associated antineutrophil cytoplasmic antibody-positive vasculitis: prevalence among patients with high titers of antimyeloperoxidase antibodies. Arthritis Rheum 2000;43(2):405–13.

136. Delrieu F, Menkes CJ, Sainte-Croix A, Babinet P, Chesneau AM, Delbarre F. Myasthénie et thyroidite auto-immune au course du traitements de la polyarthrite rhumatoïde par la D-pénicillamine. Etude anatomo-clinique d'un cas. [Myasthenia gravis and autoimmune thyroiditis during the treatment of rheumatoid polyarthritis with D-penicillamine. Anatomoclinical study of 1 case.] Ann Med Interne (Paris) 1976;127(10):739–43.

137. Bertrand JL, Rousset H, Queneau P, Ollagnier M. Thyroïdite auto-immune, une complication rare du traitement à la D-pénicillamine. [Autoimmune thyroiditis. A rare complication of treatment with D-penicillamine.] Therapie 1981;36(3):333–6.

138. Addyman R, Beyeler C, Astbury C, Bird HA. Urinary glucaric acid excretion in rheumatoid arthritis: influence of disease activity and disease modifying drugs. Ann Rheum Dis 1996;55(7):478–81.

139. Benson EA, Healey LA, Barron EJ. Insulin antibodies in patients receiving penicillamine. Am J Med 1985;78(5):857–60.

140. Herranz L, Rovira A, Grande C, Suarez A, Martinez-Ara J, Pallardo LF, Gomez-Pan A. Autoimmune insulin syndrome in a patient with progressive systemic sclerosis receiving penicillamine. Horm Res 1992;37(1–2):78–80.

141. Becker RC, Martin RG. Penicillamine-induced insulin antibodies. Ann Intern Med 1986;104(1):127–8.

142. Elling P, Elling H. Penicillamine, captopril, and hypoglycemia. Ann Intern Med 1985;103(4):644–5.

143. Vardi P, Brik R, Barzilai D, Lorber M, Scharf Y. Frequent induction of insulin autoantibodies by D-penicillamine in patients with rheumatoid arthritis. J Rheumatol 1992;19(10):1527–30.

144. Faguer de Moustier B, Burgard M, Boitard C, Desplanque N, Fanjoux J, Tchobroutsky G. Syndrome hypoglycémique auto-immun induit par le pyritinol. [Auto-immune hypoglycemic syndrome induced by pyritinol.] Diabete Metab 1988;14(4):423–9.

145. Sheikh IA, Kaplan AP. Assessment of kininases in rheumatic diseases and the effect of therapeutic agents. Arthritis Rheum 1987;30(2):138–45.

146. Schulze E, Herrmann K, Haustein UF, Krusche U, Rothenburger I. Einfluss von Penicillin und D-Penicillamin auf die Betagalactosidaseaktivität bei Patienten met progressiver Sklerodermie. [Effect of penicillin and D-penicillamine on beta-galactosidase activity in patients with progressive scleroderma.] Dermatol Monatsschr 1988;174(11):661–6.

147. Doornbos DA, Faber JS. Studies on metal complexes of drugs. D-penicillamine and N-acetyl-D-penicillamine. Pharm Weekbl 1964;99:289–309.

148. Doornbos DA. Stability constants of metal complexes of L-cysteine, D-penicillamine, N-acetyl-D-penicillamine and some biguanides. Determination of stoichiometric stability constants by an accurate method for pH measurement. Pharm Weekbl 1968;103(45):1213–27.

149. Kuchinskas EJ, Rosen Y. Metal chelates of DL-penicillamine. Arch Biochem Biophys 1962;97:370–2.

150. Cutolo M, Accardo S, Cimmino MA, Rovetta G, Bianchi G, Bianchi V. Hypocupremia-related hypochromic anemia during D-penicillamine treatment. Arthritis Rheum 1982;25(1):119–20.

151. Dastych M, Jezek P, Richtrova M. Der Einfluss einer Penicillamintherapie auf die Konzentration von Zink, Kupfer, Eisen, Kalzium und Magnesium in Serum und auf deren Ausscheidung in Urin. [Effect of penicillamine therapy on the concentration of zinc, copper, iron, calcium and magnesium in the serum and their excretion in urine.] Z Gastroenterol 1986;24(3):157–60.

152. Klingberg WG, Prasad AS, Oberleas D. Zinc deficiency following penicillamine therapy. In: Prasad AS, editor. Trace Elements in Human Health and Disease. New York: Academic Press, 1979:358.

153. Hammond WP, Miller JE, Starkebaum G, Zweerink HJ, Rosenthal AS, Dale DC. Suppression of in vitro granulocytopoiesis by captopril and penicillamine. Exp Hematol 1988;16(8):674–80.

154. Hamilton JA, Williams N. In vitro inhibition of myelopoiesis by gold salts and D-penicillamine. J Rheumatol 1985;12(5):892–6.

155. Thomas D, Gallus AS, Brooks PM, Tampi R, Geddes R, Hill W. Thrombokinetics in patients with rheumatoid arthritis treated with D-penicillamine. Ann Rheum Dis 1984;43(3):402–6.

156. Prashanth LK, Taly AB, Sinha S, Ravishankar S, Arunodaya GR, Vasudev MK Swamy HS. Prognostic factors in patients presenting with severe neurological forms of Wilson's disease. Q J Med 2005;98:557–63.

157. Singh G, Fries JF, Williams CA, Zatarain E, Spitz P, Bloch DA. Toxicity profiles of disease modifying antirheumatic drugs in rheumatoid arthritis. J Rheumatol 1991;18(2):188–94.

158. Kay AG. Myelotoxicity of D-penicillamine. Ann Rheum Dis 1979;38(3):232–6.

159. Netter P, Trechot P, Bannwarth B, Faure G, Royer RJ. Effets secondaires de la D-Pénicillamine et du pyritinol. Etude Coopérative des centres de pharmacovigilance hospitalière français. [Side effects of D-penicillamine and pyritinol. Cooperative study among French hospital drug surveillance centers.] Therapie 1985;40(6):475–9.

160. Edelman J, Maguire KF, Owen ET. Eosinophilia in rheumatoid patients treated with D-penicillamine. J Rheumatol 1984;11(5):624–5.

161. Pedersen-Bjergaard U, Andersen M, Hansen PB. Drug-induced thrombocytopenia: clinical data on 309 cases and the effect of corticosteroid therapy. Eur J Clin Pharmacol 1997;52(3):183–9.

162. Hill HF. Treatment of rheumatoid arthritis with penicillamine. Semin Arthritis Rheum 1977;6(4):361–88.

163. Sanchez-Albisua I, Garde T, Hierro L, Camarena C, Frauca E, de la Vega A, Diaz MC, Larrauri J, Jara P. A high index of suspicion: the key to an early diagnosis of Wilson's disease in childhood. J Pediatr Gastroenterol Nutr 1999;28(2):186–90.

164. Katayama Y, Kohriyama K, Matsui T. In vitro inhibition of hematopoiesis in a patient with systemic sclerosis treated with D-penicillamine. J Rheumatol 1999;26(11):2493–5.

165. Trice JM, Pinals RS, Plitman GI. Thrombotic thrombocytopenic purpura during penicillamine therapy in rheumatoid arthritis. Arch Intern Med 1983;143(7):1487–8.

166. Holdrinet RS, Namdar Z, Haanen C. Thrombotic thrombocytopenic purpura: clinical course and response to therapy in twelve patients. Neth J Med 1988;33(3–4):113–32.

167. Ahmed F, Sumalnop V, Spain DM, Tobin MS. Thrombohemolytic thrombocytopenic purpura during penicillamine therapy. Arch Intern Med 1978;138(8):1292–3.

168. Speth PA, Boerbooms AM, Holdrinet RS, Van de Putte LB, Meyer JW. Thrombotic thrombocytopenic purpura associated with D-penicillamine treatment in rheumatoid arthritis. J Rheumatol 1982;9(5):812–3.

169. Masson C, Bregeon C, Ifrah N, Berton V, Housseau F, Renier JC. Syndrome d'Evans sous D-pénicillamine au cours d'une polyarthrite rhumatoïde. Intérêt de l'association corticoïdes–danazol. [Evans' syndrome caused by D-penicillamine in rheumatoid arthritis. Value of the corticoids–danazol combination.] Rev Rhum Mal Osteoartic 1991;58(7):519–22.

170. Henzgen M, Hein G. Agranulozytose und andere Nebenwirkungen. Erfahrungen mit der d-Penicillamintherapie bei der Rheumatoidarthritis. Z Klin Med 1985;40:521.

171. Umeki S, Konishi Y, Yasuda T, Morimoto K, Terao A. D-penicillamine and neutrophilic agranulocytosis. Arch Intern Med 1985;145(12):2271–2.

172. Ramselaar AC, Dekker AW, Huber-Bruning O, Bijlsma JW. Acquired sideroblastic anaemia after aplastic anaemia caused by D-penicillamine therapy for rheumatoid arthritis. Ann Rheum Dis 1987;46(2):156–8.

173. Ehrlich JC, Van Paasen HC. Een dodelijke bijwerking van penicillamine. Ned Tijdschr Geneeskd 1984;128:1790.

174. Fishel B, Tishler M, Caspi D, Yaron M. Fatal aplastic anaemia and liver toxicity caused by D-penicillamine treatment of rheumatoid arthritis. Ann Rheum Dis 1989;48(7):609–10.

175. Petrides PE, Gerhartz HH. D-penicillamine-induced agranulocytosis: hematological remission upon treatment with recombinant GM-CSF. Z Rheumatol 1991;50(5):328–9.

176. Lowenthal RM, Cohen ML, Atkinson K, Biggs JC. Apparent cure of rheumatoid arthritis by bone marrow transplantation. J Rheumatol 1993;20(1):137–40.

177. Kaufman DW, Kelly JP, Jurgelon JM, Anderson T, Issaragrisil S, Wiholm BE, Young NS, Leaverton P, Levy M, Shapiro S. Drugs in the aetiology of agranulocytosis and aplastic anaemia. Eur J Haematol Suppl 1996;60:23–30.

178. Mary JY, Guiguet M, Baumelou E. Drug use and aplastic anaemia: the French experience. French Cooperative Group for the Epidemiological Study of Aplastic Anaemia. Eur J Haematol Suppl 1996;60:35–41.

179. Ward K, Weir DG. Life threatening agranulocytosis and toxic epidermal necrolysis during low dose penicillamine therapy. Ir J Med Sci 1981;150(8):252–3.

180. Chan KH, Cheung RTF, Au-Yeung KM, Mak W, Cheng TS, Ho SL. Wilson's disease with depression and parkinsonism. J Clin Neurosci 2005;12:303–5.

181. Kandola L, Swannell AJ, Hunter A. Acquired sideroblastic anaemia associated with penicillamine therapy for rheumatoid arthritis. Ann Rheum Dis 1995;54(6):529–30.

182. Williams DM. Copper deficiency in humans. Semin Hematol 1983;20(2):118–28.

183. Frieden E. The copper connection. Semin Hematol 1983;20(2):114–7.

184. LaRusso NF, Wiesner RH, Ludwig J, MacCarty RL, Beaver SJ, Zinsmeister AR. Prospective trial of penicillamine in primary sclerosing cholangitis. Gastroenterology 1988;95(4):1036–42.

185. Demelia L, Vallebona E, Perpignano G, Pitzus F. Positivizzazione di sierologia lupica in corso di morbo di

Wilson in trattamento con penicillamina. Reumatismo 1991;43:119–24.

186. Capell HA, Marabani M, Madhok R, Torley H, Hunter JA. Degree and extent of response to sulphasalazine or penicillamine therapy for rheumatoid arthritis: results from a routine clinical environment over a two-year period. Q J Med 1990;75(276):335–44.

187. Carpenter EH, Plant MJ, Hassell AB, Shadforth MF, Fisher J, Clarke S, Hothersall TE, Dawes PT. Management of oral complications of disease-modifying drugs in rheumatoid arthritis. Br J Rheumatol 1997;36(4):473–8.

188. Fenton DA, Young ER, Wilkinson JD. Recurrent aphthous ulceration. BMJ (Clin Res Ed) 1983;286:1062.

189. Wassef M, Galian A, Pepin B, Haguenau M, Vassel P, Hautefeuille P, Brazy J. Unusual digestive lesions in a patient with Wilson's disease treated with long-term penicillamine. N Engl J Med 1985;313(1):49.

190. Greene MW, King RC, Alley RS. Management of an oroantral fistula in a patient with Wilson's disease: case report and review of the literature. Oral Surg Oral Med Oral Pathol 1988;66(3):293–6.

191. Rajendran N, Koteeswaran A, Kala M. Penicillamine-induced cheilosis. Indian J Dermatol Venereol Leprol 1985;51:50.

192. Blasberg B, Dorey JL, Stein HB, Chalmers A, Conklin RJ. Lichenoid lesions of the oral mucosa in rheumatoid arthritis patients treated with penicillamine. J Rheumatol 1984;11(3):348–51.

193. Lyle WH. Letter: Peptic ulceration and D-penicillamine. Lancet 1974;2(7875):285.

194. Ramboer C, Verhamme M. D-penicillamine-induced oesophageal ulcers. Acta Clin Belg 1989;44(3):189–91.

195. Perrett D. The metabolism and pharmacology of D-penicillamine in man. J Rheumatol Suppl 1981;7:41–50.

196. Houghton AD, Nadel S, Stringer MD. Penicillamine-associated total colitis. Hepatogastroenterology 1989;36(4):198.

197. Roux H, Bonnefoy-Cudraz M, Antipoff GM. Les complications hépatiques de la d-pénicillamine. Rhumatologie 1984;36:233.

198. Gefel D, Harats N, Lijovetsky G, Eliakim M. Cholestatic jaundice associated with D-penicillamine therapy. Scand J Rheumatol 1985;14(3):303–6.

199. Kumar A, Bhat A, Gupta DK, Goel A, Malaviya AN. D-penicillamine-induced acute hypersensitivity pneumonitis and cholestatic hepatitis in a patient with rheumatoid arthritis. Clin Exp Rheumatol 1985;3(4):337–9.

200. Menara M, Zancan L, Sturniolo GC. Penicillamine hepatotoxicity in the treatment of Wilson's disease. J Pediatr Gastroenterol Nutr 1992;14(3):353–4.

201. Matsukawa Y, Saito N, Nishinarita S, Horie T, Ryu J. Therapeutic effect of tiopronin following D-penicillamine toxicity in a patient with rheumatoid arthritis. Clin Rheumatol 1998;17(1):73–4.

202. Mok MY, Ng WL, Yuen MF, Wong RW, Lau CS. Safety of disease modifying anti-rheumatic agents in rheumatoid arthritis patients with chronic viral hepatitis. Clin Exp Rheumatol 2000;18(3):363–8.

203. Schilsky ML. The irony of treating Wilson's disease. Am J Gastroenterol 2001;96(11):3055–7.

204. Shiono Y, Wakusawa S, Hayashi H, Takikawa T, Yano M, Okada T, Mabuchi H, Kono S, Miyajima H. Iron accumulation in the liver of male patients with Wilson's disease. Am J Gastroenterol 2001;96(11):3147–51.

205. Luca P, Demelia L, Lecca S, Ambu R, Faa G. Massive hepatic haemosiderosis in Wilson's disease. Histopathology 2000;37(2):187–9.

206. Rook AH, Freundlich B, Jegasothy BV, Perez MI, Barr WG, Jimenez SA, Rietschel RL, Wintroub B, Kahaleh MB, Varga J, Heald PW, Steen V, Massa MC, Murphy GF, Perniciaro C, Istfan M, Ballas SK, Edelson RL. Treatment of systemic sclerosis with extracorporeal photochemotherapy. Results of a multicenter trial. Arch Dermatol 1992;128(3):337–46.

207. Stein HB, Schroeder ML, Dillon AM. Penicillamine-induced proteinuria: risk factors. Semin Arthritis Rheum 1986;15(4):282–7.

208. Hall CL, Jawad S, Harrison PR, MacKenzie JC, Bacon PA, Klouda PT, MacIver AG. Natural course of penicillamine nephropathy: a long term study of 33 patients. BMJ (Clin Res Ed) 1988;296(6629):1083–6.

209. Combe C, Deforges-Lasseur C, Chehab Z, De Precigout, Aparicio M. La lithiase cystinique et son traitement par la d-pénicillamine. Semin Hop 1992;68:746–50.

210. Pedersen LM, Nordin H, Svensson B, Bliddal H. Microalbuminuria in patients with rheumatoid arthritis. Ann Rheum Dis 1995;54(3):189–92.

211. DeSilva RN, Eastmond CJ. Management of proteinuria secondary to penicillamine therapy in rheumatoid arthritis. Clin Rheumatol 1992;11(2):216–9.

212. Stephens AD. Cystinuria and its treatment: 25 years experience at St. Bartholomew's Hospital. J Inherit Metab Dis 1989;12(2):197–209.

213. Hill GS. Drug-associated glomerulopathies. Toxicol Pathol 1986;14(1):37–44.

214. Emery P, Panayi G. Penicillamine nephropathy. BMJ (Clin Res Ed) 1988;296(6635):1538.

215. Speerstra F, van de Putte LB, Rasker JJ, Reekers P, Vandenbroucke JP. The relationship between aurothioglucose- and D-penicillamine-induced proteinuria. Scand J Rheumatol 1984;13(4):363–8.

216. Yoshida A, Morozumi K, Suganuma T, Aoki J, Sugito K, Koyama K, Oikawa T, Fujinimi T, Matsumoto Y. [Clinicopathological study of nephropathy in patients with rheumatoid arthritis.]Ryumachi 1991;31(1):14–21.

217. Bar J, Ehrenfeld M, Rozenman J, Perelman M, Sidi Y, Gur H. Pulmonary-renal syndrome in systemic sclerosis. Semin Arthritis Rheum 2001;30(6):403–10.

218. Koseki Y, Terai C, Moriguchi M, Uesato M, Kamatani N. A prospective study of renal disease in patients with early rheumatoid arthritis. Ann Rheum Dis 2001;60(4):327–31.

219. Niederstadt C, Happ T, Tatsis E, Schnabel A, Steinhoff J. Glomerular and tubular proteinuria as markers of nephropathy in rheumatoid arthritis. Rheumatology (Oxford) 1999;38(1):28–33.

220. Verroust PJ. Kinetics of immune deposits in membranous nephropathy. Kidney Int 1989;35(6):1418–28.

221. Isenring P, de Cotret PR, Delage C, Kingma I, Lebel M. d-Penicillamine induced reversible minimal change nephropathy in rheumatoid arthritis. J Nephrol 1991;4:245–8.

222. Dische FE, Swinson DR, Hamilton EB, Parsons V. Immunopathology of penicillamine-induced glomerular disease. J Rheumatol 1984;11(5):584–5.

223. Druet P, Kleinknecht D. Les néphropathies glomérulaires d'origine toxique. [Toxic glomerulonephritis.] Presse Méd 1989;18(37):1840–5.

224. Malaise MG, Davin JC, Mahieu PR, Franchimont P. Elevated antigalactosyl antibody titers reflect renal injury after gold or D-penicillamine in rheumatoid arthritis. Clin Immunol Immunopathol 1986;40(2):356–64.

225. Rehan A, Johnson K. IgM nephropathy associated with penicillamine. Am J Nephrol 1986;6(1):71–4.

226. Ntoso KA, Tomaszewski JE, Jimenez SA, Neilson EG. Penicillamine-induced rapidly progressive glomerulonephritis in patients with progressive systemic sclerosis: successful treatment of two patients and a review of the literature. Am J Kidney Dis 1986;8(3):159–63.

227. Williams AJ, Fordham JN, Barnes CG, Goodwin FJ. Progressive proliferative glomerulonephritis in a patient with rheumatoid arthritis treated with D-penicillamine. Ann Rheum Dis 1986;45(1):82–4.

228. Suda M, Yoshikawa Y, Suzuki T, Dohi Y, Shibata T. [A case report of rheumatoid arthritis which showed acute renal failure, nephrotic syndrome and drug-related lupus-like syndrome caused by D-penicillamine.]Nippon Jinzo Gakkai Shi 1990;32(11):1235–41.

229. Donnelly S, Levison DA, Doyle DV. Systemic lupus erythematosus-like syndrome with focal proliferative glomerulonephritis during D-penicillamine therapy. Br J Rheumatol 1993;32(3):251–3.

230. Rejchrt S, Hrncir Z, Pinterova E. [Rheumatoid arthritis developing into systemic lupus erythematosus during long-term treatment with penicillamine and sulfasalazine.]Vnitr Lek 1991;37(6):597–603.

231. Almirall J, Alcorta I, Botey A, Revert L. Penicillamine-induced rapidly progressive glomerulonephritis in a patient with rheumatoid arthritis. Am J Nephrol 1993;13(4):286–8.

232. Gaertner HV. Drug-associated nephropathy. In: Grundman E, editor. Drug-induced Pathology. Vol. 69. Current Topics in Pathology. Berlin: Springer-Verlag, 1980:358.

233. Karpinski J, Jothy S, Radoux V, Levy M, Baran D. D-penicillamine-induced crescentic glomerulonephritis and antimyeloperoxidase antibodies in a patient with scleroderma. Case report and review of the literature. Am J Nephrol 1997;17(6):528–32.

234. Sadjadi SA, Seelig MS, Berger AR, Milstoc M. Rapidly progressive glomerulonephritis in a patient with rheumatoid arthritis during treatment with high dosage d-penicillamine. Ann Rheum Dis 1985;45:82.

235. Devogelaer JP, Pirson Y, Vandenbroucke JM, Cosyns JP, Brichard S, Nagant de Deuxchaisnes C. D-penicillamine induced crescentic glomerulonephritis: report and review of the literature. J Rheumatol 1987;14(5):1036–41.

236. Leatherman JW, Davies SF, Hoidal JR. Alveolar hemorrhage syndromes: diffuse microvascular lung hemorrhage in immune and idiopathic disorders. Medicine (Baltimore) 1984;63(6):343–61.

237. Macarron P, Garcia Diaz JE, Azofra JA, Martin de Francisco J, Gonzalez E, Fernandez G, Sampedro J. D-penicillamine therapy associated with rapidly progressive glomerulonephritis. Nephrol Dial Transplant 1992;7(2):161–4.

238. Derk CT, Jimenez SA. Goodpasture-like syndrome induced by D-penicillamine in a patient with systemic sclerosis: report and review of the literature. J Rheumatol 2003;30:1616–20.

239. Bindi P, Gilson B, Aymard B, Noel LH, Wieslander J. Antiglomerular basement membrane glomerulonephritis following D-penicillamine-associated nephrotic syndrome. Nephrol Dial Transplant 1997;12(2):325–7.

240. Scherberig JE, Sniehotta KP, Miehlke K, Schoeppe W. Nierenbeteiligung bei rheumatoider Arthritis. Nieren Hochdrukkr 1987;16:69.

241. Boers M, Croonen AM, Dijkmans BA, Breedveld FC, Eulderink F, Cats A, Weening JJ. Renal findings in rheumatoid arthritis: clinical aspects of 132 necropsies. Ann Rheum Dis 1987;46(9):658–63.

242. Cantagrel A, Fournie B, Pourrat J, Conte JJ, Fournie A. Hématurie microscopique d'origine rénale au cours de la polyarthrite rhumatoïde. [Renal microscopic hematuria in rheumatoid polyarthritis.] Rev Med Interne 1991; 12(1):31–6.

243. Honkanen E, Tornroth T, Pettersson E, Skrifvars B. Membranous glomerulonephritis in rheumatoid arthritis not related to gold or D-penicillamine therapy: a report of four cases and review of the literature. Clin Nephrol 1987;27(2):87–93.

244. Feehally J, Wheeler DC, Mackay EH, Oldham R, Walls J. Recurrent acute renal failure with interstitial nephritis due to D-penicillamine. Ren Fail 1987;10(1):55–7.

245. Nakano M, Ueno M, Nishi S, Shimada H, Hasegawa H, Watanabe T, Kuroda T, Sato T, Maruyama Y, Arakawa M. Analysis of renal pathology and drug history in 158 Japanese patients with rheumatoid arthritis. Clin Nephrol 1998;50(3):154–60.

246. Habib GS, Saliba W, Nashashibi M, Armali Z. Penicillamine and nephrotic syndrome. Eur J Intern Med 2006;17(5):343–8.

247. Siafakas CG, Jonas MM, Alexander S, Herrin J, Furuta GT. Early onset of nephrotic syndrome after treatment with D-penicillamine in a patient with Wilson's disease. Am J Gastroenterol 1998;93(12):2544–6.

248. Marchand-Courville S, Dhib M, Fillastre JP, Godin M. Glomerulonéphrites extracapillaires secondaires à la D-pénicillamine. A propos d'une observation et revue de la littérature. [Extracapillary glomerulonephritis secondary to D-penicillamine. Apropos of 1 case and review of the literature.] Nephrologie 1998;19(1):25–32.

249. Phillips D, Phillips B, Mannino D. A case study and national database report of progressive systemic sclerosis and associated conditions. J Womens Health 1998;7(9):1099–104.

250. Haviv YS, Safadi R. Rapid progression of scleroderma possibly associated with penicillamine therapy. Clin Drug Invest 1998;15:61–3.

251. Kyndt X, Ducq P, Bridoux F, Reumaux D, Makdassi R, Gheerbrant JD, Vanhille P. Glomerulonéphrite extracapillaire avec anticorps anti-myeloperoxydase chez 2 malades ayant une sclérodermie systémique traitée par D-pénicillamine. [Extracapillary glomerulonephritis with anti-myeloperoxidase antibodies in 2 patients with systemic scleroderma treated with penicillamine D.] Presse Méd 1999;28(2):67–70.

252. Marlier S, Gisserot O, Yao N, Hecht M, Paris JF, Carli P, Chagnon A. Glomerulonéphrite extracapillaire lors d'un traitement par D-pénicillamine. [Extra-capillary glomerulonephritis induced by D-penicillamine therapy.] Presse Méd 1999;28(13):689–90.

253. Mazhari R, Kimmel PL. Hematuria: an algorithmic approach to finding the cause. Cleve Clin J Med 2002;69(11):870–6.

254. Shannon M, Graef J, Lovejoy FH Jr. Efficacy and toxicity of D-penicillamine in low-level lead poisoning. J Pediatr 1988;112(5):799–804.

255. Bell CL, Graziano FM. The safety of administration of penicillamine to penicillin-sensitive individuals. Arthritis Rheum 1983;26(6):801–3.

256. Oliver I, Liberman UA, DeVries A. Lupus-like syndrome induced by penicillamine in cystinuria. JAMA 1972;220(4):588.

257. Pachoula-Papasteriades C, Boki K, Varla-Leftherioti M, Kappos-Rigatou I, Fostiropoulos G, Economidou J. HLA-A,-B, and -DR antigens in relation to gold and D-

penicillamine toxicity in Greek patients with RA. Dis Markers 1986;4(1–2):35–41.

258. Vlachoyiannopoulos PG, Zerva LV, Skopouli FN, Drosos AA, Moutsopoulos HM. D-penicillamine toxicity in Greek patients with rheumatoid arthritis: anti-Ro(SSA) antibodies and cryoglobulinemia are predictive factors. J Rheumatol 1991;18(1):44–9.

259. Shannon MW, Townsend MK. Adverse effects of reduced-dose d-penicillamine in children with mild-to-moderate lead poisoning. Ann Pharmacother 2000;34(1):15–8.

260. Miyagawa S, Yoshioka A, Hatoko M, Okuchi T, Sakamoto K. Systemic sclerosis-like lesions during long-term penicillamine therapy for Wilson's disease. Br J Dermatol 1987;116(1):95–100.

261. Liddle BJ. Development of morphoea in rheumatoid arthritis treated with penicillamine. Ann Rheum Dis 1989;48(11):963–4.

262. Schachter RK. Localized scleroderma. Curr Opin Rheumatol 1990;2(6):947–55.

263. Enzenauer RJ, West SG, Rubin RL. D-penicillamine-induced lupus erythematosus. Arthritis Rheum 1990; 33(10):1582–5.

264. Chin GL, Kong NC, Lee BC, Rose IM. Penicillamine induced lupus-like syndrome in a patient with classical rheumatoid arthritis. J Rheumatol 1991;18(6):947–8.

265. Tsankov NK, Lazarova AZ, Vasileva SG, Obreshkova EV. Lupus erythematosus-like eruption due to D-penicillamine in progressive systemic sclerosis. Int J Dermatol 1990;29(8):571–4.

266. Condon C, Phelan M, Lyons JF. Penicillamine-induced type II bullous systemic lupus erythematosus. Br J Dermatol 1997;136(3):474–5.

267. Bannwarth B, Schaeverbeke T, Dehais J. Low back pain associated with penicillamine. BMJ 1991;303(6801):525.

268. Zvulunov A, Grunwald MH, Avinoach I, Halevy S. Transient acantholytic dermatosis (Grover's disease) in a patient with progressive systemic sclerosis treated with D-penicillamine. Int J Dermatol 1997;36(6):476–7.

269. Rose BI, LeMaire WJ, Jeffers LJ. Macromastia in a woman treated with penicillamine and oral contraceptives. A case report. J Reprod Med 1990;35(1):43–5.

270. Pyo JY, Lee WJ, Koo DW. A case of penicillamine dermatopathy. Korean J Dermatol 2001;39:341–3.

271. Melani L, Caproni M, Cardinali C, Antiga E, Bernacchi E, Schincaglia E, Fabbri P. A case of nodular scleroderma. J Dermatol 2005;32(12):1028–31.

272. Sehgal VN, Srivastava G, Aggarwal AK, Behl PN, Choudhary M, Bajaj P. Localized scleroderma/morphea. Int J Dermatol 2002;41(8):467–75.

273. Rencic A, Goyal S, Mofid M, Wigley F, Nousari HC. Bullous lesions in scleroderma. Int J Dermatol 2002;41(6):335–9.

274. Newbold PC. Contact reaction to penicillamine in vaginal secretions. Lancet 1979;1(8130):1344.

275. Gül Ü, Kiliç A, Dursun A. Carbamazepine-induced pseudo mycosis fungoides. Ann Pharmacother 2003;37:1441–3.

276. Iozumi K, Nakagawa H, Tamaki K. Penicillamine-induced degenerative dermatoses: report of a case and brief review of such dermatoses. J Dermatol 1997;24(7):458–65.

277. Dootson G, Sarkany I. D-penicillamine induced dermopathy in Wilson's disease. Clin Exp Dermatol 1987; 12(1):66–8.

278. Pasquali Ronchetti I, Quaglino D Jr, Baccarani Contri M, Hayek J, Galassi G. Dermal alterations in patients with Wilson's disease treated with D-penicillamine. J Submicrosc Cytol Pathol 1989;21(1):131–9.

279. Goldstein JB, McNutt NS, Hambrick GW Jr, Hsu A. Penicillamine dermatopathy with lymphangiectases. A clinical, immunohistologic, and ultrastructural study. Arch Dermatol 1989;125(1):92–7.

280. Light N, Meyrick Thomas RH, Stephens A, Kirby JD, Fryer PR, Avery NC. Collagen and elastin changes in D-penicillamine-induced pseudoxanthoma elasticum-like skin. Br J Dermatol 1986;114(3):381–8.

281. Camus JP, Koeger AC. D-Pénicillamine et collagène. [D-penicillamine and collagen.] Ann Biol Clin (Paris) 1986;44(3):296–9.

282. Nimni ME. Penicillamine and collagen metabolism. Scand J Rheumatol Suppl 1979;(28):71–8.

283. Buckley C, Sankey EA, Harris D, Wright S. Case update—progressive skin laxity secondary to penicillamine treatment. Clin Exp Dermatol 1991;16(4):310–1.

284. Narron GH, Zec N, Neves RI, Manders EK, Sexton FM Jr. Penicillamine-induced pseudoxanthoma elasticum-like skin changes requiring rhytidectomy. Ann Plast Surg 1992;29(4):367–70.

285. Bolognia JL, Braverman I. Pseudoxanthoma-elasticum-like skin changes induced by penicillamine. Dermatology 1992;184(1):12–8.

286. Layton AM, Cunliffe WJ. Electrocautery as a successful treatment for penicillamine-induced elastosis perforans serpiginosa. J Dermatol Treat 1991;2:111–2.

287. Dalziel KL, Burge SM, Frith PA, Ryan TJ, Mowat A. Elastic fibre damage induced by low-dose D-penicillamine. Br J Dermatol 1990;123(3):305–12.

288. Sahn EE, Maize JC, Garen PD, Mullins SC, Silver RM. D-penicillamine-induced elastosis perforans serpiginosa in a child with juvenile rheumatoid arthritis. Report of a case and review of the literature. J Am Acad Dermatol 1989;20(5 Pt 2):979–88.

289. Price RG, Prentice RS. Penicillamine-induced elastosis perforans serpiginosa. Tip of the iceberg? Am J Dermatopathol 1986;8(4):314–20.

290. Matsushita A, Hiruma M, Ogawa H, Watanabe S, Saeki T. A case of D-penicillamine-induced elastosis perforans serpiginosa in a women with systemic sclerosis. Nishinihon J Dermatol 1999;61:451–4.

291. Bécuwe C, Dalle S, Ronger-Savlé S, Skowron F, Balme B, Kanitakis J, Thomas L. Elastosis perforans serpiginosa associated with pseudo-pseudoxanthoma elasticum during treatment of Wilson's disease with penicillamine. Dermatology 2005;210:60–3.

292. Choi H-J, Lee D-K, Chang S-E, Lee M-W, Choi J-H, Moon K-C, Koh J-K. An iatrogenic dermatosis with ulceration. Clin Exp Dermatol 2005;30:463–4.

293. Fraysse T, De Wazieres B. Maladie de Wilson et "vieille peau". Pract Med Ther 2001;15:38–9.

294. Hill VA, Seymour CA, Mortimer PS. Pencillamine-induced elastosis perforans serpiginosa and cutis laxa in Wilson's disease. Br J Dermatol 2000;142(3):560–1.

295. Coatesworth AP, Darnton SJ, Green RM, Cayton RM, Antonakopoulos GN. A case of systemic pseudo-pseudoxanthoma elasticum with diverse symptomatology caused by long-term penicillamine use. J Clin Pathol 1998;51(2):169–71.

296. Zacher J, Spath S, Wessinghage D, Waertel G. Basistherapie der chronisch-entzündlichem Gelenkerkrankungen met D-penicillamin und Wundheilungsstörungen bei rheumaorthopädischen

Eingriffen. [Basic therapy of chronic inflammatory joint diseases with D-penicillamine and disorders of wound healing in rheumatoid orthopedic interventions.] Z Rheumatol 1988;47(Suppl 1):41–3.

297. Burry HC. Penicillamine and wound healing—a potential hazard? Postgrad Med J 1974;50(Suppl 2):75–6.

298. Mutasim DF, Pelc NJ, Anhalt GJ. Drug-induced pemphigus. Dermatol Clin 1993;11(3):463–71.

299. Brenner S, Halevy S, Livni E, Schewach-Millet M, Sandbank M, Wolf R. Macrophage migration inhibition test in patients with drug-induced pemphigus. Isr J Med Sci 1993;29(1):44–6.

300. Wolf R, Brenner S. Arzneimittelbedingter Pemphigus-Uebersicht. Z Hautkrankh 1991;66:289–93.

301. Zillikens D, Zentner A, Burger M, Hartmann AA, Burg G. Pemphigus foliaceus durch Penicillamin. [Pemphigus foliaceus caused by penicillamine.] Hautarzt 1993;44(3):167–71.

302. Brenner S, Bialy-Golan A, Anhalt GJ. Recognition of pemphigus antigens in drug-induced pemphigus vulgaris and pemphigus foliaceus. J Am Acad Dermatol 1997;36(6 Pt 1):919–23.

303. Penas PF, Buezo GF, Carvajal I, Dauden E, Lopez A, Diaz LA. D-penicillamine-induced pemphigus foliaceus with autoantibodies to desmoglein-1 in a patient with mixed connective tissue disease. J Am Acad Dermatol 1997;37(1):121–3.

304. McGovern TW, Bennion SD. Diffuse blisters and erosions in a patient with limited scleroderma. Penicillamine-induced pemphigus foliaceus (PIPF). Arch Dermatol 1997;133(4):501.

305. Verret JL, Avene IM, Smulevici A, Esparbes M. Les pemphigus induits par la pénicillamine: á propos de trois cas. J Agregres 1983;16:209.

306. Hashimoto K, Shafran KM, Webber PS, Lazarus GS, Singer KH. Anti-cell surface pemphigus autoantibody stimulates plasminogen activator activity of human epidermal cells. A mechanism for the loss of epidermal cohesion and blister formation. J Exp Med 1983;157(1):259–72.

307. Hashimoto K, Singer K, Lazarus GS. Penicillamine-induced pemphigus. Immunoglobulin from this patient induces plasminogen activator synthesis by human epidermal cells in culture: mechanism for acantholysis in pemphigus. Arch Dermatol 1984;120(6):762–4.

308. Bahmer FA, Bambauer R, Stenger D. Penicillamine-induced pemphigus foliaceus-like dermatosis. A case with unusual features, successfully treated by plasmapheresis. Arch Dermatol 1985;121(5):665–8.

309. Tholen S. Arzneimittelbedingter Pemphigus. [Drug-induced pemphigus.] Z Hautkr 1986;61(10):719–23.

310. Walton S, Keczkes K, Robinson AE. A case of penicillamine-induced pemphigus, successfully treated by plasma exchange. Clin Exp Dermatol 1987;12(4):275–6.

311. Kind P, Goerz G, Gleichmann E, Plewig G. Penicillamin induzierter Pemphigus. [Penicillamine-induced pemphigus.] Hautarzt 1987;38(9):548–52.

312. Buckley C, Barry C, Woods R, Dervan P, O'Loughlin S. Penicillamine induced pemphigus—a report of 2 cases. Ir J Med Sci 1988;157(8):267–8.

313. Civatte J. Durch Medikamente induzierte Pemphigus-Erkrankungen. [Drug-induced pemphigus diseases.] Dermatol Monatsschr 1989;175(1):1–7.

314. Willemsen MJ, De Coninck AL, De Raeve LE, Roseeuw DI. Penicillamine-induced pemphigus erythematosus. Int J Dermatol 1990;29(3):193–7.

315. Rasmussen HB, Jepsen LV, Brandrup F. Penicillamine-induced bullous pemphigoid with pemphigus-like antibodies. J Cutan Pathol 1989;16(3):154–7.

316. Shapiro M, Jimenez S, Werth VP. Pemphigus vulgaris induced by D-penicillamine therapy in a patient with systemic sclerosis. J Am Acad Dermatol 2000;42(2 Pt 1):297–9.

317. Weller R, White MI. Penicillamine in the etiology of bullous pemphigoid. Ann Pharmacother 1998;32(12):1368.

318. Nagao K, Tanikawa A, Yamamoto N, Amagai M. Decline of anti-desmoglein 1 IgG ELISA scores by withdrawal of D-penicillamine in drug-induced pemphigus foliaceus. Clin Exp Dermatol 2005;30:43–5.

319. Tang MBY, Chin TM, Yap CK, Ng SK. A case of penicillamine-induced dermopathy. Ann Acad Med Singapore 2003;32:703–5.

320. Choi H-J, Lee D-K, Chang S-E, Lee M-W, Choi J-H, Moon K-C, Koh J-K. An iatrogenic dermatosis with ulceration. Clin Exp Dermatol 2005;30:463–4.

321. Karlhofer FM, Hashimoto T, Slupetzky K, Kiss M, Liu Y, Amagai M, Pieczkowski F, Foedinger D, Kirnbauer R, Stingl G. 230-kDa and 190-kDa proteins in addition to desmoglein 1 as immunological targets in a subset of pemphigus foliaceus with a combined cell-surface and basement membrane zone immune staining pattern. Exp Dermatol 2003;12:646–54.

322. Verma KK, Pasricha JS. Pemphigus foliaceous induced by penicillamine. Indian J Dermatol Venereol Leprol 1990;56:234–5.

323. Piette-Brion B, de Bast C, Chamoun E, de Dobbeleer G, Andre J, Huybrechts A, Ledoux M, Achten G. Pemphigus superficial apparu lors du traitement d'une polyarthrite rhumatoïde par D-pénicillamine et piroxicam. [Superficial pemphigus during the treatment of rheumatoid polyarthritis with D-penicillamine and piroxicam (Feldene).] Dermatologica 1985;170(6):297–301.

324. Kohn SR. Fatal penicillamine-induced pemphigus foliaceus-like dermatosis. Arch Dermatol 1986;122(1):17.

325. Toth GG, Jonkman MF. Successful treatment of recalcitrant penicillamine-induced pemphigus foliaceus by low-dose intravenous immunoglobulins. Br J Dermatol 1999;141(3):583–5.

326. Korman NJ, Eyre RW, Zone J, Stanley JR. Drug-induced pemphigus: autoantibodies directed against the pemphigus antigen complexes are present in penicillamine and captopril-induced pemphigus. J Invest Dermatol 1991;96(2):273–4.

327. Bedane C, Bernard P, Dang PM, Amici JM, Catanzano G, Bonnetblanc JM. Étude ultrastructurale des antigènes-cibles du pemphigus foliacé et du pemphigus vulgaire. A propos de deux observations. [Ultrastructural study of pemphigus foliaceus and pemphigus vulgaris antigens. Apropos of 2 cases.] Ann Dermatol Venereol 1991;118(11):888–90.

328. Ruocco V, de Angelis E, Lombardi ML, Pisani M. In vitro acantholysis by captopril and thiopronine. Dermatologica 1988;176(3):115–23.

329. Yokel BK, Hood AF, Anhalt GJ. Induction of acantholysis in organ explant culture by penicillamine and captopril. Arch Dermatol 1989;125(10):1367–70.

330. Lombardi ML, de Angelis E, Rossano F, Ruocco V. Imbalance between plasminogen activator and its inhibitors in thiol-induced acantholysis. Dermatology 1993;186(2):118–22.

331. Bauer-Vinassac D, Menkes CJ, Muller JY, Escande JP. HLA system and penicillamine induced pemphigus in nine cases of rheumatoid arthritis. Scand J Rheumatol 1992;21(1):17–9.

332. Wilkinson SM, Smith AG, Davis MJ, Hollowood K, Dawes PT. Rheumatoid arthritis: an association with pemphigus foliaceous. Acta Derm Venereol 1992;72(4):289–91.

333. Aydemir EH, Is imen A, Aksoy F. d-Penisilamin'e bagli eritem anuler benzeri pemfigus. Deri Hast Frengi Ars 1988;22:247–50.

334. Shuttleworth D, Graham-Brown RA, Hutchinson PE, Jolliffe DS. Cicatricial pemphigoid in D-penicillamine treated patients with rheumatoid arthritis—a report of three cases. Clin Exp Dermatol 1985;10(4):392–7.

335. Peyri J, Servitje O, Ribera M, Henkes J, Ferrandiz C. Cicatricial pemphigoid in a patient with rheumatoid arthritis treated with D-penicillamine. J Am Acad Dermatol 1986;14(4):681.

336. Marti-Huguet T, Quintana M, Cabiro I. Cicatricial pemphigoid associated with D-penicillamine treatment. Arch Ophthalmol 1989;107(8):1115.

337. Hallauer W, Gartner HV, Kronenberg KH, Manz G. Immunkomplexnephritis mit nephrotischem Syndrom unter Therapie mit D-Penizillamin. [Immune complex nephritis with nephrotic syndrome following D-penicillamine therapy.] Schweiz Med Wochenschr 1974;104(12):434–8.

338. Takatsuka H, Takemoto Y, Yamada S, Mori A, Wada H, Fujimori Y, Okamoto T, Kanamaru A, Kakishita E. Similarity between eruptions induced by sulfhydryl drugs and acute cutaneous graft-versus-host disease after bone marrow transplantation. Hematology 2002;7(1):55–7.

339. Powell FC, Rogers RS, Dickson ER. Lichen planus, primary biliary cirrhosis and penicillamine. Br J Dermatol 1982;107(5):616.

340. Kitamura K, Aihara M, Osawa J, Naito S, Ikezawa Z. Sulfhydryl drug-induced eruption: a clinical and histological study. J Dermatol 1990;17(1):44–51.

341. Kitamura K, Aihara M, Osawa J, Naito S, Ikezawa Z. Clinical histological study of drug eruptions induced by sulfhydryl drugs. Proc Jpn Soc Investig Dermatol 1988;12:136–7.

342. Forgie JC, Highet AS. Psoriasiform eruptions associated with penicillamine. BMJ (Clin Res Ed) 1987;294:1101.

343. Jimenez-Balderas FJ, Rangel J, Mintz G. Penicillamine induced myositis: correlation between urinary zinc excretion and serum creatine. J Rheumatol 1991;18(6):945–7.

344. Garcia-Nieto AV, Fernandez Roldan JC, Martinez-Sanchez F, Gonzalez Gomez J, Moreno Gimenez JC. Yellow nail syndrome by d-penicillamine. Actas Dermo-Sifiliogr 1997;88:191–5.

345. Ilchyshyn A, Vickers CF. Yellow nail syndrome associated with penicillamine therapy. Acta Derm Venereol 1983;63(6):554–5.

346. Dubost JJ, Fraysse P, Ristori JM, Rampon S. Syndrome des ongles jaunes avec dilatation des bronches après traitement d'une polyarthrite rhumatoïde par la d-pénicillamine. Semin Hop Paris 1988;64:1548–51.

347. Ichikawa Y, Shimizu H, Arimori S. "Yellow nail syndrome" and rheumatoid arthritis. Tokai J Exp Clin Med 1991;16(5–6):203–9.

348. Bjellerup M. Nail-changes induced by penicillamine. Acta Derm Venereol 1989;69(4):339–41.

349. Sturrock RD, Brooks PM. Penicillamine and creaking joints. BMJ 1974;3(5930):575.

350. Stein HB, Patterson AC, Offer RC, Atkins CJ, Teufel A, Robinson HS. Adverse effects of D-penicillamine in rheumatoid arthritis. Ann Intern Med 1980;92(1):24–9.

351. Halperin EC, Thier SO, Rosenberg LE. The use of D-penicillamine in cystinuria: efficacy and untoward reactions. Yale J Biol Med 1981;54(6):439–46.

352. Butler D, Tiliakos NA. Penicillamine-induced exacerbation of rheumatoid arthritis. South Med J 1986;79(6):778–9.

353. Narvaez J, Alegre-Sancho JJ, Juanola X, Roig-Escofet D. Arthropathy of Wilson's disease presenting as noninflammatory polyarthritis. J Rheumatol 1997;24(12):2494.

354. Dulcine M, Borges C, Vianna MADAG, Neto EFB. Eosinophilic fasciitis with subclinical myopathy with exacerbated myositis after using the d-penicillamine. Rev Bras Reumatol 1999;39:303–6.

355. Sampaio-Barros PD, De Paiva Magalhaes E, Sachetto Z, Samara AM, Marques Neto JF. Bone mineral density in systemic sclerosis. Rev Bras Reumatol 2000;40:153–8.

356. Kahl LE, Medsger TA Jr, Klein I. Massive breast enlargement in a patient receiving D-penicillamine for systemic sclerosis. J Rheumatol 1985;12(5):990–1.

357. Craig HR. Penicillamine induced mammary hyperplasia: report of a case and review of the literature. J Rheumatol 1988;15(8):1294–7.

358. Spaeth M, Berkl M, Miehle W. Mammahyperplasie und d-Penicillamin. Aktuel Rheumatol 1991;16:214–6.

359. Caballeria J, Caballeria L, Cabre J, Bruguera M, Rodes J. Mammary hyperplasia secondary to treatment with d-penicillamine in a patient with Wilson's disease. Gastroenterol Hepatol 1993;16:607–9.

360. O'Hare PM, Frieden IJ. Virginal breast hypertrophy. Pediatr Dermatol 2000;17(4):277–81.

361. Salliere D, Clerc D, Bisson M, Massias P. Gynécomastie transitoire an course d'un traitement par la D-pénicillamine. [Transient gynecomastia during treatment with D-penicillamine.] Presse Méd 1984;13(37):2265.

362. Tchebiner JZ. Breast enlargement induced by D-penicillamine. Ann Pharmacother 2002;36(3):444–5.

363. Upponi SS, Jadav AM, Bobrow L, Purushotham AD. Breast hypertrophy related to D-penicillamine? Breast 2001;10:349–50.

364. Rosada M, Fiocco U, De Silvestro G, Doria A, Cozzi L, Favaretto M, Todesco S. Effect of D-pénicillamine on the T cell phenotype in scleroderma. Comparison between treated and untreated patients. Clin Exp Rheumatol 1993;11(2):143–8.

365. Panayi GS, Mills MM. Second-line drug treatment in rheumatoid arthritis associated with depressed autologous mixed lymphocyte reaction. Rheumatol Int 1986;6(1):25–9.

366. Miyachi Y, Yoshioka A, Imamura S, Niwa Y. Decreased hydroxyl radical generation from polymorphonuclear leucocytes in the presence of D-penicillamine and thiopronine. J Clin Lab Immunol 1987;22(2):81–4.

367. Sim E, Dodds AW, Goldin A. Inhibition of the covalent binding reaction of complement component C4 by penicillamine, an anti-rheumatic agent. Biochem J 1989;259(2):415–9.

368. Price EJ, Venables PJ. Drug-induced lupus. Drug Saf 1995;12(4):283–90.

369. Haberhauer G, Broll H. Drug-induced anticentromere antibody? Z Rheumatol 1989;48(2):99–100.

370. Haberhauer G. D-penicillamine (DPA)-induced anticentromere antibody (ACA). Clin Exp Rheumatol 1989;7(3):332–4.

371. Storch W. Antikörper gegen D-penicillamin bei primär biliärer Zirrhose. [Antibodies against D-penicillamine in primary biliary cirrhosis.] Immun Infekt 1990;18(1):22–3.

372. Yarze JC, Martin P, Munoz SJ, Friedman LS. Wilson's disease: current status. Am J Med 1992;92(6):643–54.

373. Tanphaichitr K. D-penicillamine-induced bronchial spasm. South Med J 1980;73(6):788–90.

374. Nanke Y, Akama H, Terai C, Kamatani N. Rapidly progressive glomerulonephritis with D-penicillamine. Am J Med Sci 2000;320(6):398–402.

375. Garcia-Porrua C, Gonzalez-Gay MA, Bouza P. D-penicillamine-induced crescentic glomerulonephritis in a patient with scleroderma. Nephron 2000;84(1):101–2.

376. Kolsi R, Bahloul Z, Hachicha J, Gouiaa R, Jarraya A. Dermatopolymyosite induite par la D-pénicillamine au cours de la polyarthrite rhumatoïde. A propos d'un cas avec revue de la littérature. [Dermatopolymyositis induced by D-penicillamine in rheumatoid polyarthritis. Apropos of 1 case with review of the literature.] Rev Rhum Mal Osteoartic 1992;59(5):341–4.

377. Takahashi K, Ogita T, Okudaira H, Yoshinoya S, Yoshizawa H, Miyamoto T. D-penicillamine-induced polymyositis in patients with rheumatoid arthritis. Arthritis Rheum 1986;29(4):560–4.

378. Matsumura T, Yuhara T, Yamane K, Kono I, Kabashima T, Kashiwagi H. D-penicillamine-induced polymyositis occurring in patients with rheumatoid arthritis: a report of two cases and demonstration of a positive lymphocyte stimulation test to D-penicillamine. Henry Ford Hosp Med J 1986;34(2):123–6.

379. Masson CJ, Menard HA, Audran M, Renier JC, Lussier A, Myhal DM. Polymyosite induite par la D-pénicillamine lors d'arthrite rhumatoïde: à propos de deux cas avec des anticorps antinucléaire. [Polymyositis induced by D-penicillamine treatment of rheumatoid arthritis: apropos of 2 cases with antinuclear antibodies.] Union Med Can 1986;115(12):855–9.

380. Ostensen M, Husby G, Aarli J. Polymyositis with acute myolysis in a patient with rheumatoid arthritis treated with penicillamine and ampicillin. Arthritis Rheum 1980;23(3):375–7.

381. Car J, Lorette G, Jacob C. Dermatomyosite induite par la d-pénicillamine. Semin Hop 1987;63:399.

382. Leden I, Libelius R. Penicillamine-induced polymyositis. Scand J Rheumatol 1985;14(1):90–3.

383. Carroll GJ, Will RK, Peter JB, Garlepp MJ, Dawkins RL. Penicillamine induced polymyositis and dermatomyositis. J Rheumatol 1987;14(5):995–1001.

384. Christensen PD, Sorensen KE. Penicillamine-induced polymyositis with complete heart block. Eur Heart J 1989;10(11):1041–4.

385. Taneja V, Mehra N, Singh YN, Kumar A, Malaviya A, Singh RR. HLA-D region genes and susceptibility to D-penicillamine-induced myositis. Arthritis Rheum 1990;33(9):1445–7.

386. Santos JC, Velasco JA. Polymyositis due to D-penicillamine in a patient with systemic sclerosis. Clin Exp Dermatol 1991;16(1):76.

387. Fukuda S, Murata Y, Takahashi T, Hatada Y, Tsushima Y, Takemori H, Yoshida Y, Okushima T. d-Penicillamine-induced polymyositis in a patient with rheumatoid arthritis. Saishin-Igaku 1990;45:1854–9.

388. Larbre JP, Perret P, Collet P, Llorca G. Antinuclear antibodies during pyrithioxine treatment. Br J Rheumatol 1990;29(6):496–7.

389. Barrera P, den Broeder AA, van den Hoogen FH, van Engelen BG, van de Putte LB. Postural changes, dysphagia, and systemic sclerosis. Ann Rheum Dis 1998; 57(6):331–8.

390. Ibel H, Feist D, Endres W, Belohradsky BH. D-Penicillamin-induzierter IgA-Mangel bei der Therapie der Wilsonschen Erkrankung. [D-penicillamine-induced IgA deficiency in the therapy of Wilson's disease.] Klin Padiatr 1990;202(6):427–9.

391. Chalmers A, Thompson D, Stein HE, Reid G, Patterson AC. Systemic lupus erythematosus during penicillamine therapy for rheumatoid arthritis. Ann Intern Med 1982;97(5):659–63.

392. Chikanza IC. Juvenile rheumatoid arthritis: therapeutic perspectives. Paediatr Drugs 2002;4(5):335–48.

393. Lin HC, Hwang KC, Lee HJ, Tsai MJ, Ni YH, Chiang BL. Penicillamine induced lupus-like syndrome: a case report. J Microbiol Immunol Infect 2000;33(3):202–4.

394. May V, Aristoff H, Lecoq G. Syndrome de Gougerot–sjögren induit par la D-pénicillamine. A propos d'un cas. [Gougerot–Sjögren syndrome induced by D-penicillamine. Apropos of a case.] Rev Rhum Mal Osteoartic 1977;44(7–9):497–501.

395. Proceedings. International Symposium on Penicillamine, Miami, 1980. Pruzanski, E editor. J Rheumatol 1981; 8(Suppl 7):181.

396. Dubois RS, Rodgerson DO, Hambidge KM. Treatment of Wilson's disease with triethylene tetramine hydrochloride (Trientine). J Pediatr Gastroenterol Nutr 1990;10(1):77–81.

397. Savill JS, Chia Y, Pusey CD. Minimal change nephropathy and pemphigus vulgaris associated with penicillamine treatment of rheumatoid arthritis. Clin Nephrol 1988;29(5):267–70.

398. Jones E, Sobkowski WW, Murray SJ, Walsh NM. Concurrent pemphigus and myasthenia gravis as manifestations of penicillamine toxicity. J Am Acad Dermatol 1993;28(4):655–6.

399. Hsu HL, Huang FC, Ni YH, Chang MH. Steroids used to desensitize penicillamine allergy in Wilson disease. Acta Paediatr Taiwan 1999;40(6):448–50.

400. Hernandez-Cruz B, Cardiel MH, Villa AR, Alcocer-Varela J. Development, recurrence, and severity of infections in Mexican patients with rheumatoid arthritis. A nested case-control study. J Rheumatol 1998;25(10):1900–7.

401. Speit G, Haupter S. Cytogenetic effects of penicillamine. Mutat Res 1987;190(3):197–203.

402. Gilman PA, Holtzman NA. Acute lymphoblastic leukemia in a patient receiving penicillamine for Wilson's disease. JAMA 1982;248(4):467–8.

403. Sheldon P, Wood JK. Remission of arthritis and radiological improvement after combination therapy for non-Hodgkin's lymphoma in a patient with rheumatoid arthritis undergoing treatment with D-penicillamine. Ann Rheum Dis 1985;44(8):556–8.

404. Anonymous. Neoplasms in rheumatoid arthritis: update on clinical and epidemiologic data. Am J Med 1985; 78(1A):1–83.

405. Mjolnerod OK, Dommerud SA, Rasmussen K, Gjeruldsen ST. Congenital connective-tissue defect probably due to D-penicillamine treatment in pregnancy. Lancet 1971;1(7701):673–5.

406. Pinter R, Hogge WA, McPherson E. Infant with severe penicillamine embryopathy born to a woman with Wilson disease. Am J Med Genet 2004;128:294–8.

407. Solomon L, Abrams G, Dinner M, Berman L. Neonatal abnormalities associated with D-penicillamine treatment during pregnancy. N Engl J Med 1977;296(1):54–5.

408. Miehle W. Aktuelles zu D-Penicillamin and Schwangerschaft. [Current aspects of D-penicillamine and pregnancy.] Z Rheumatol 1988;47(Suppl 1):20–3.

409. Rosa FW. Teratogen update: penicillamine. Teratology 1986;33(1):127–31.

410. Frishman WH. Chelation therapy for coronary artery disease: panacea or quackery? Am J Med 2001;111(9):729–30.

411. Martinez-Frias ML, Rodriguez-Pinilla E, Bermejo E, Blanco M. Prenatal exposure to penicillamine and oral clefts: case report. Am J Med Genet 1998;76(3):274–5.

413. Emery P, Panayi GS, Huston G, Welsh KI, Mitchell SC, Shah RR, Idle JR, Smith RL, Waring RH. D-Penicillamine induced toxicity in rheumatoid arthritis: the role of sulphoxidation status and HLA-DR3. J Rheumatol 1984;11(5):626–32.

414. Seideman P, Ayesh R. Reduced sulphoxidation capacity in D-penicillamine induced myasthenia gravis. Clin Rheumatol 1994;13(3):435–7.

415. In: Dawkins RL, Christiansen FT, Zilko PJ, editors. Immunogenetics in Rheumatology: Musculoskeletal Disease and d-Penicillamine. Amsterdam: Excerpta Medica, 1982:358.

416. Speerstra F, Reekers P, van de Putte LB, Vandenbroucke JP. HLA associations in aurothioglucose- and D-penicillamine-induced haematotoxic reactions in rheumatoid arthritis. Tissue Antigens 1985;26(1):35–40.

417. Welsh KI, Black CM. The major histocompatibility system and its relevance to rheumatological disorders. In: Carson DW, Moll JMH, editors. Recent Advances in Rheumatology. Edinburgh: Churchill Livingstone, 1983:147.

418. Scherak O, Smolen JS, Mayr WR, Mayrhofer F, Kolarz G, Thumb NJ. HLA antigens and toxicity to gold and penicillamine in rheumatoid arthritis. J Rheumatol 1984;11(5):610–4.

419. Dequeker J, Van Wanghe P, Verdickt W. A systematic survey of HLA-A,B,C and D antigens and drug toxicity in rheumatoid arthritis. J Rheumatol 1984;11(3):282–6.

420. Ford PM. HLA antigens and drug toxicity in rheumatoid arthritis. J Rheumatol 1984;11(3):259–61.

421. Bardin T, Dryll A, Ryckewaert A. Système HLA et accidents du traitement de la polyarthrite rhumatoïde par la D-pénicillamine. [HLA system and complications of the treatment of rheumatoid polyarthritis with D-penicillamine.] Rev Rhum Mal Osteoartic 1986;53(1):27–9.

422. Perrier P, Raffoux C, Thomas P, Tamisier JN, Busson M, Gaucher A, Streiff F. HLA antigens and toxic reactions to sodium aurothiopropanol sulphonate and D-penicillamine in patients with rheumatoid arthritis. Ann Rheum Dis 1985;44(9):621–4.

423. Skopouli FN, Andonopoulos AP, Moutsopoulos HM. Clinical implications of the presence of anti-Ro (SSA) antibodies in patients with rheumatoid arthritis. J Autoimmun 1988;1(4):381–8.

424. Osman MA, Patel RB, Schuna A, Sundstrom WR, Welling PG. Reduction in oral penicillamine absorption by food, antacid, and ferrous sulfate. Clin Pharmacol Ther 1983;33(4):465–70.

425. Ifan A, Welling PG. Pharmacokinetics of oral 500-mg penicillamine: effect of antacids on absorption. Biopharm Drug Dispos 1986;7(4):401–5.

426. Lyle WH, Pearcey DF, Hui M. Inhibition of penicillamine-induced cupruresis by oral iron. Proc R Soc Med 1977;70(Suppl 3):48–9.

427. Harkness JA, Blake DR. Penicillamine nephropathy and iron. Lancet 1982;2(8312):1368–9.

428. Muijsers AO, van de Stadt RJ, Henrichs AM, Ament HJ, van der Korst JK. D-penicillamine in patients with rheumatoid arthritis. Serum levels, pharmacokinetic aspects, and correlation with clinical course and side effects. Arthritis Rheum 1984;27(12):1362–9.

429. Yu TF, Roboz J, Johnson S, Kaung C. Studies on the metabolism of D-penicillamine and its interaction with

probenecid in cystinuria and rheumatoid arthritis. J Rheumatol 1984;11(4):467–70.

430. Whitehouse DB, Lovegrove JU, Hopkinson DA. Variation in alpha-1-antitrypsin phenotypes associated with penicillamine therapy. Clin Chim Acta 1989; 179(1):109–15.

431. Jobanputra P, Maggs F, Homer D, Bevan J. Monitoring and assessing the safety of disease-modifying antirheumatic drugs: a West Midlands experience. Drug Saf 2002;25(15):1099–105.

432. Yalaz M, Aydogdu S, Ozgenc F, Akisu M, Kultursay N, Yagci RV. Transient fetal myelosuppressive effect of D-penicillamine when used in pregnancy Minerva Pediatr 2003;55:625–8.

Rituximab

See also Monoclonal antibodies

General Information

Rituximab, a chimeric monoclonal antibody directed against the CD20 antigen of normal and malignant B lymphocytes, produces prolonged depletion of B lymphocytes. It has been used to treat refractory or relapsing follicular non-Hodgkin's lymphoma and has been tried in other B cell malignancies, including low-grade non-Hodgkin's lymphoma and diffuse large B cell lymphoma. There has also been interest in its use to treat autoimmune diseases (1–3) and in reducing anti-HLA antibodies in patients awaiting renal transplantation (4).

A wide range of adverse events has been reported in most patients (5), and most adverse events are associated with infusions, including chills and fever, related to cytokine release, allergic reactions, cardiopulmonary syndrome, and tumor lysis syndrome (6,7). A transient flu-like syndrome is very common (50–90%), particularly after the first infusion of rituximab, and is often associated with various hypersensitivity-like symptoms (5–20%). In the most severe cases, patients had life-threatening cytokine release syndrome with dyspnea, bronchospasm, hypoxia, hypotension, urticaria, and angioedema. Deaths have been reported in eight of 12 000–14 000 patients after drug launch.

Severe reactions to rituximab are rare, but are seen in patients with bulky tumors or with leukemic involvement with high numbers of CD20 positive cells (8,9) and were ascribed to a rapid tumor lysis syndrome (8,10,11). In 11 patients with malignant B cell leukemia, first-dose reactions were significantly more severe in patients whose baseline lymphocyte count was higher than $50 \times 10^6/l$ and were also associated with raised peak serum concentrations of tumor necrosis factor alfa and interleukin-6 (12).

Organs and Systems

Cardiovascular

Cardiac dysrhythmias have been reported in 8% of patients treated with rituximab in patients with lymphomas (13).

Acute coronary syndrome has been reported during rituximab therapy. It was speculated that release of cytokines during rituximab infusion caused vasoconstriction, platelet activation, or rupture of an atherosclerotic plaque (14).

- A 71-year-old man, with a history of type II diabetes mellitus, hypertension, a myocardial infarction 12 years before, and percutaneous transluminal coronary angioplasty 11 years before, was given chlorambucil for B cell chronic lymphocytic leukemia without a response (14). Rituximab 375 mg/m^2 was therefore, started at a rate of 50 mg/hour intravenously after premedication with paracetamol, diphenhydramine, and methylprednisolone. Four hours later he developed substernal pain radiating to the neck and left arm with a sinus tachycardia; the pain responded to glyceryl trinitrate; the cardiac enzymes were not raised. Rituximab 30 mg/hour was restarted after an interval of 2 hours. He developed identical symptoms and rituximab was withdrawn.

Respiratory

Desquamative alveolitis has been reported in a 55-year-old woman with mantle-cell lymphoma given rituximab (15).

Interstitial pneumonitis has been reported after rituximab therapy for immune thrombocytopenic purpura (16).

- A 77-year-old woman with a 2 year history of immune thrombocytopenic purpura did not respond with a rise in platelet count during a 4-week course of rituximab 375 mg/m^2 once weekly. Co-medication consisted of prednisolone 60 mg/day, danazol 600 mg/day, and warfarin (INR 2–3) because of a mechanical aortic valve. Two weeks after the last infusion of rituximab, elective splenectomy was cancelled because of interstitial pneumonitis. Her pulmonary symptoms improved after the dose of prednisolone was tapered and withdrawn over 2 months.

A patient with non-Hodgkin's lymphoma received rituximab and developed symptomatic, biopsy-proven multinodular bronchiolitis obliterans with organizing pneumonia (BOOP) (17).

Nervous system

A fatal central nervous system lesion was reported during therapy with rituximab for an Epstein Barr virus-linked lymphoma after transplantation (18).

Reversible posterior leucoencephalopathy has been reported after rituximab infusion (19).

- A 38-year-old woman with a 13-year history of systemic lupus erythematosus and a small brain infarct with an episode of diplopia and blurring of vision had recurrent occipital headaches, blurring of vision, seizures, and hypertension (210/120 mmHg) after receiving a second weekly course of intravenous rituximab 375 mg/m^2. Concomitant treatment consisted of quarterly infusions of cyclophosphamide and oral anticoagulation (INR 2.5–3.0). Thrombotic microangiopathy and increased lupus activity were diagnosed. Her kidney function deteriorated and she required hemodialysis. After 6 days a third infusion of rituximab was given and she developed an occipital headache, blurring of vision, and seizures 6 hours later. An MRI scan showed high-intensity signals in the cortical and subcortical white matter of the parietal lobes and the lateral posterior and lateral portions of the temporal lobes, consistent with reversible posterior leucoencephalopathy. Hypertensive and anticonvulsant therapy resolved the symptoms within 24 hours. Plasmapheresis, intravenous cyclophosphamide, and methylprednisolone were started. Six weeks later the MRI scan was normal and renal function had improved.

The authors speculated that an interaction with anti-CD20 expressed on activated endothelial cells or systemic lupus erythematosus itself had contributed to the occurrence of reversible posterior leucoencephalopathy.

Sensory systems

A variety of ocular adverse effects, including conjunctivitis, transient ocular edema, and visual changes, occurred in 7% of patients receiving rituximab (13).

- A 60-year-old man with heavily pretreated and refractory mucosa-associated lymphoid tissue (MALT) lymphoma developed bilateral orbital swelling and lymphadenopathy (20). Given the lack of standard chemotherapy for refractory MALT lymphoma, he was given rituximab 375 mg/m^2 (25 mg/hour increasing to 100 mg/hour) plus cladribine and was given intravenous diphenhydramine 50 mg and oral paracetamol 650 mg 30 minutes before the rituximab infusion. Within 2 hours he developed painful bilateral edema of the eyelids and sclerae. Therapy was interrupted, and he was given intravenous hydrocortisone. Rituximab was restarted at a rate of 25 mg/hour after the edema had subsided, and he was given the total dose. One week later, the treatment was repeated, again with diphenhydramine and paracetamol prophylaxis, and was well tolerated. He received six additional doses of rituximab without any adverse events.

Gradual tumor destruction by immune effector cells, leading to local cytokine release and accumulation may have resulted in local edema in this patient.

Hematologic

The factors associated with toxicity in patients with B cell lymphoma receiving rituximab have been studied in Japan (21). By univariate analysis overall non-hematological toxic effects (grade 2 or greater) were more frequent in patients with extranodal disease and especially in those with bone marrow involvement. Fever was more frequent in patients with raised LDH activity, whereas chills/rigors and vomiting were more frequent in patients with extranodal disease. Patients with raised LDH activity or extranodal disease may therefore require closer monitoring. Hematological toxic effects of grade 3 or worse were more common in women.

B cell depletion

- A 26-year-old woman with a diffuse large B cell lymphoma received CHOP (cyclophosphamide, hydroxydaunomycin, Oncovin, and prednisone), rituximab, and radiotherapy (22). She developed a transfusion-dependent anemia. Bone marrow biopsy confirmed pure red cell aplasia and parvovirus infection. She had no antibodies to parvovirus, suggesting that she never had a previous exposure. Intravenous immunoglobulin resulted in a reticulocytosis and recovery of her hemoglobin.

The authors suggested that rituximab had depleted her primary B cells, resulting in an inability to mount a primary immune response to parvovirus infection. Parvovirus is pathogenic to red cell precursors, causing their destruction before release from the bone marrow.

Persistent B-cell depletion has been reported after the use of rituximab for thrombocytopenic purpura (23).

Depletion of B lymphocytes by rituximab was suggested as a likely explanation for the occurrence of chronic parvovirus B19 infection complicated by pure red cell aplasia in a 45-year-old patient (24).

- A 14-year-old girl with autoimmune thrombocytopenic purpura unresponsive to intravenous immunoglobulin and high-dose steroids developed an intracranial hemorrhage and was given four weekly doses of rituximab 375 mg/m^2. Her CD19+ cells became undetectable after the second dose and her platelet count rapidly increased. She recovered completely.

Neutropenia

Severe delayed neutropenia after rituximab was evaluated in 53 consecutively treated patients with non-Hodgkin's lymphoma (25). There were eight episodes of grade 4 neutropenia at 1-5 months after rituximab, including three occasions in combination with chemotherapy. Sepsis occurred in three cases. All the episodes developed after a period of either normal or mildly depressed neutrophil counts after treatment with rituximab. Episodes of neutropenia were associated with disordered immune status, manifested by lymphopenia and hypogammaglobulinemia, raising the possibility that either a disturbance of the balance of lymphocyte subsets or an immune dyscrasia induced by rituximab resulted in the development of this type of neutropenia.

Agranulocytosis unresponsive to growth factors was reported after rituximab therapy (26).

- A 46 year old man with lymphocyte-predominant Hodgkin disease stage IV achieved a partial response after standard chemotherapy. When the diagnosis was modified to diffuse large B cell lymphoma, standard CHOP chemotherapy resulted in another brief partial response. After disease progression, he responded to two cycles of ifosfamide, mesna, carboplatin, and etoposide. After CD34 cell transplantation he was given rituximab on days 30 and 37. From day 77 to day 122, his white blood cell count fell from 5 x 10^9/l to 1 x 10^9/l and his neutrophils from 86% to 0%. The bone marrow was hypocellular with little maturation of the myeloid series and no evidence of relapse. Screening for infection and autoantibodies was negative. Despite drug withdrawal and administration of GCSF/GM-CSF, the neutropenia persisted for 2 months. Ciclosporin was started and the neutrophil count recovered within 5 days.

Neutropenia in rituximab-treated patients with lymphomas can be considered as one end of a spectrum of immunohematological sequelae due to autoimmune myelopathy, often associated with rituximab-induced T cell large granular lymphocytes. Patients treated with rituximab were divided into four groups by peripheral blood morphology and flow cytometry:

1. those with peripheral blood T-LGL lymphocytosis (n=11), including profound neutropenia (n=10) of 1-5 months duration or thrombocytopenia (n=1); eight patients developed neutropenia after transplantation;
2. those with neutropenia without T-LGL lymphocytosis (n=4);
3. those with T-LGL lymphocytosis without cytopenias (n=2);
4. those with neither cytopenias nor T-LGL lymphocytosis (n=17).

After a median follow-up of 13 months the patients with neutropenia did not have an increased risk of infection (27).

Late-onset neutropenia occurred in six patients who were given rituximab after stem cell transplantation; it can last for up to 1 year (28).

- A 30 year-old man with intestinal CD20-positive Burkitt's lymphoma and retroperitoneal lymphadenopathy was treated with hyper-CVAD chemotherapy (cyclophosphamide, vincristine, doxorubicin, dexamethasone, high-dose methotrexate, and cytarabine) combined with rituximab for eight courses over 5 months (29). Four weeks after the end of treatment he developed marked neutropenia and hypogammaglobulinemia, which persisted for 1 year. However, he did not develop any severe infections.

Of 107 patients who received rituximab-containing chemotherapy as primary treatment for CD20-positive B-cell lymphomas, 23 developed late-onset neutropenia after a median of 411 days (neutrophil count 1.0 x 10^9/l or less) at a median of 106 days after the last course of chemotherapy (30). The median neutrophil count nadir was 0.61 x 10^9/l. These episodes were generally self-limiting; one patient was given filgrastim. There were no serious infectious episodes.

Late-onset grade 4 neutropenia occurred in three of 54 patients with non-Hodgkin's lymphoma treated with rituximab between September 2001 and March 2004 (31). The neutropenia occurred after 5–25 weeks and recurred 4 and 17 weeks after first onset in two patients. There were five episodes in a total of 332 cycles of rituximab therapy. The bone marrow showed neutrophil maturation arrest with or without reversible myeloid dysplasia in three episodes and selective depletion of the myeloid series in one. Neither circulating immune complexes nor antineutrophil antibodies were detected.

All cases of unexplained delayed-onset peripheral blood cytopenias of WHO grades II–IV in an unselected series of patients receiving rituximab have been analysed (32). There were 77 courses of rituximab (corresponding to 317 rituximab infusions) given to 72 consecutive patients with non-Hodgkin's lymphoma; nine received rituximab alone, 50 were associated with chemotherapy or with chemotherapy, and 18 with autologous stem cell transplantation. There were 23 cases of cytopenias: neutropenia in 21 cases, thrombocytopenia in eight, and anemia in four. There were multiple cytopenias in nine cases. Neutropenia developed after a median of 10 weeks after the last dose of rituximab, anemia after 5 weeks, and thrombocytopenia after 4 weeks. There were severe infections in four of 21 neutropenic patients compared with two of 56 controls. The cytopenias eventually resolved in nine of 18 evaluable cases after a median of 10 (range 1–23) weeks. Of age, sex, histology, bone marrow infiltration, hypogammaglobulinemia, previous chemotherapy, autologous stem cell transplantation, and the dosage regimen of rituximab, only previous treatment with chemotherapy and more than four doses of rituximab were significantly associated with a higher risk of cytopenias.

Thrombocytopenia

In a phase II study, rituximab 375 mg/m^2, fludarabine 100 mg/m^2, and cyclophosphamide 750 mg/m^2 were evaluated in the treatment of relapsed follicular lymphoma. Unexpected severe hematological toxicity with significant prolonged thrombocytopenia WHO grade 3/4 occurred in six of 17 patients and led to early termination of the trial (33). Cytology and serology suggested a direct toxic effect. Older patients (mean age 65 versus 57 years) were significantly more likely to develop this toxic effect; no other clinical or hematological parameters differed statistically between those with thrombocytopenia and those without. The addition of rituximab to fludarabine/cyclophosphamide in relapsed follicular lymphoma may have led to this increase in the risk of thrombocytopenia. Caution should therefore be exercised when combining these drugs in patients with relapsed follicular lymphoma, especially older patients.

Rituximab-induced thrombocytopenia occurred in a patient with mantle cell lymphoma (34).

- A 57-year-old man with mantle cell lymphoma stage IV and massive splenomegaly received rituximab 375 mg/m^2 as part of induction chemotherapy. The white cell count was 10.8 x 10^9/l, hemoglobin 9.4 g/dl, and platelets 151 x 10^9/l. After the first infusion of rituximab 638 mg

over 4 hours, he developed fever and rigors and was given paracetamol and pethidine. On the next day his white cell count was 6 x 10^9/l, hemoglobin 7.7 g/dl, and platelets 8 x 10^9/l. After a platelet transfusion, the platelet count increased to 39 x 10^9/l. He was given CHOP (cyclophosphamide, hydroxydaunomycin, vincristine, prednisolone) 3 days after the rituximab infusion and the platelet count rose to 82 x 10^9/l. After a second cycle of chemotherapy 3 weeks later, the platelet count fell within hours after rituximab infusion from 133 x 10^9/l to 8 x 10^9/l. Serum sickness was ruled out by C1q and C3d assays within the reference ranges.

The pathophysiology of rituximab-induced thrombocytopenia is unclear. The authors speculated that it was due to a soluble CD20 antigen–antibody reaction and immune-mediated cell lysis by complement activation or CD20 antigen on the platelets themselves, leading to antibody-mediated cell destruction.

Rituximab caused hemorrhagic thrombocytopenia in a patient with hairy cell leukemia (35).

- A 44-year-old man with hairy cell leukemia developed an abscess in the right erector spinae muscle and was given intravenous antibiotics for *Staphylococcus aureus* infection and granulocyte colony-stimulating factor. His neutropenia persisted and was given rituximab. Some hours later he developed severe knee-pain, hemorrhagic blisters in the mouth, petechiae on the legs, and gastrointestinal bleeding. The platelet count fell from 31 to 6 x 10^9/l. He developed raises D-dimer concentrations, which normalized within 6 days of treatment with interferon.

Thrombocytopenia leading to gastrointestinal bleeding has been attributed to rituximab (36).

Combined neutropenia and thrombocytopenia

Transient severe acute thrombocytopenia and neutropenia occurred a few days after rituximab infusion in two children with autoimmune hemolytic anemia (37). In both cases, the cytopenia resolved within a few days.

Liver

Fatal adenoviral hepatitis has been reported in a patient with Waldenstrom's macroglobulinemia treated with rituximab (38). This case demonstrates the emerging association between rituximab and fatal viral reactivation. Other cases have been reported with hepatitis viruses.

- A woman with relapsed cutaneous follicular center B-cell lymphoma and secondary lymph-node involvement had a complete remission with rituximab alone. However, 1 year later she had fatal hepatitis B virus reactivation (39).
- A 59-year-old man developed fatal acute hepatitis with reactivated hepatitis B virus after receiving rituximab for a malignant lymphoma; he developed a positive HBsAg titer (40).
- A patient with a diffuse large B-cell lymphoma and hepatitis C virus-related hepatic cirrhosis developed a mass in her left breast (41). She was given rituximab

monotherapy on 3 consecutive weeks, but treatment had to be withdrawn because of hematological toxicity. The hepatitis C viral load increased, but then fell gradually after rituximab was stopped.

Skin

Stevens–Johnson syndrome has been attributed to rituximab (42).

- A 33-year-old man with a follicular non-Hodgkin lymphoma entered a phase II trial of rituximab. The first two cycles were given without infusion-related toxicity, but during the second cycle mucositis was noticed. Before the third cycle he developed a pruritic rash on the trunk, grade 2 mucositis, and weight loss. He was given oral fluconazole, aciclovir, and antihistamines, which led to improvement. One week after the third infusion of rituximab he had grade 3 orogenital mucositis and the maculopapular rash on the trunk worsened, with areas of ulceration. Rituximab was withdrawn. Stevens–Johnson syndrome was confirmed by biopsy.

An urticarial reaction occurred in a patient with primary cutaneous B-cell lymphoma receiving rituximab (43).

- A 37-year-old man with a primary cutaneous B-cell lymphoma was treated with 8 intravenous doses of weekly rituximab and developed an urticarial reaction at the site of the tumor patches and excision scars 1 hour after the first dose. The lesions disappeared spontaneously after withdrawal of rituximab temporarily for 1 hour. Rituximab was then given uneventfully.

Immunologic

Infusion reactions with rituximab are generally well tolerated, as with most monoclonal antibodies. Most reactions are limited to the first infusion, including nausea, chills, and fever. They occur in over 90% of patients. More serious is the cytokine-release syndrome, which occurs within 60–90 minutes and is characterized by fever, chills, rigors, bronchospasm, hypoxia, hypotension, urticaria, and angioedema. Infusion must be discontinued, and the patient carefully monitored with chest radiography and fluid and electrolyte assessment and treated with oxygen and bronchodilators.

Delayed hypersensitivity or serum sickness has been reported after rituximab (44). In a phase II trial of the German Hodgkin Lymphoma Study Group, 14 patients were treated with rituximab 375 mg/m^2 once a week for 4 weeks (45). Paracetamol and antihistamines were given 1 hour before rituximab infusion that was started at 50 mg/hour during the first hour and gradually increased to a maximum of 400 mg/hour. There were infusion-related adverse effects in 11 patients. The most common adverse effects were chills in 71%, fever (50%), rhinitis (21%), nausea (21%), pruritus (21%), leukopenia (14%), and dizziness (14%). The adverse effects occurred mainly during the first infusion and resolved within 1 hour after the end of the infusion. In addition, one patient died 5 months after treatment from a pneumonia related to a tracheoesophageal fistula and one patient developed a lung adenocarcinoma 11 months after treatment.

Drug-induced hypersensitivity pneumonia has been attributed to rituximab. Few similar reactions have been described. Two were fatal, but none was associated with pulmonary hemorrhage. A 2.5:1 ratio between the interstitial alveolar T4/T8 lymphocytes in the reported case was similar to the findings in methotrexate-induced pneumonitis and farmers' lung (46).

- A 65-year-old man developed a progressive dry cough and digital clubbing after starting rituximab + CHOP chemotherapy for non-Hodgkin's lymphoma. Lung biopsy showed loose non-necrotic granulomas on a background of mild fibrosis and rare eosinophils, compatible with drug-induced hypersensitivity pneumonia. Associated manifestations were a high eosinophil count, raised serum concentrations of IgE, and a skin rash consistent with pigmented purpuric dermatitis. Glucocorticoids were marginally efficacious in treating this reaction.

Rituximab can cause a leukocytoclastic vasculitis (47).

- A 67-year-old woman with follicular non-Hodgkin's lymphoma received a standard course of rituximab. After the third dose she developed increasingly severe pruritus and a generalized rash. There were grouped hemorrhagic vesicles and bullae on the upper thighs and backs of the legs. A skin biopsy showed a leukocytoclastic vasculitis. Rituximab was withdrawn and she received a single dose of intravenous dexamethasone. The lesions regressed over 1 week.

Autacoids

Cytokine release syndrome has been attributed to rituximab (48).

- A 14-year-old boy with acute lymphoblastic leukemia had an anaplastic astrocytoma subtotally resected and was then treated with irradiation and chemotherapy. A leukemic relapse was refractory to salvage therapy and he was given rituximab. After a small fraction of the standard dose (375 mg/m^2) the infusion had to be interrupted because of acute lumbar pain. Two days later, after rituximab had been restarted, he developed a fatal systemic inflammatory response syndrome and died, possibly because of uncontrollable cytokine release syndrome associated with sepsis.

A rapid tumor clearance syndrome can occur within 30–60 minutes, with similar symptoms. Lymphocytes rapidly disappear from the peripheral blood and uric acid and lactate dehydrogenase increase markedly. Treatment includes interruption of the infusion, hydration, allopurinol, oxygen, and bronchodilators. It mainly occurs in patients with high white blood cell counts, such as those with chronic lymphatic leukemia.

Infection risk

There have been isolated reports of viral infections and hepatitis B virus reactivation in carriers of hepatitis B surface antigen (HbsAg) (49,50). Hepatitis B virus escape mutants can be essential for reactivation after rituximab.

- A 73 year old man with a history of hepatitis B was treated with five courses of CHOP and then with rituximab for a diffuse large-cell lymphoma (49). After complete resolution, he had anti-HBs antibodies over 1000 IU/l and HbsAg was negative. He subsequently had acute hepatitis (anti-HBs 868 IU/l, HbsAg positive, HBV-DNA 8.6×10^8 copies/ml). Lamivudine reduced the viral load (HBV-DNA 2.4×10^5 copies/ml) within 2 weeks, but he did not recover hepatic function and died after 19 days. Hepatitis B virus sequence analysis showed five mutations in the major antigenic region (L110R, R122K, Y/F134S, P142L, and D144A), compatible with escape of an endogenous strain from the patient's own anti-HBs, which was non-pathogenic until rituximab therapy.

Severe viral infections/reactivation that have been reported in patients given rituximab have included fulminant hepatitis B (51), parvovirus-induced red cell aplasia (24), and fatal *Varicella zoster* infection (52). There was a high incidence of reactivation of cytomegalovirus and *V. zoster* virus when rituximab was combined with high-dose chemotherapy in high-risk patients with non-Hodgkin's lymphoma (53).

Treatment with the chimeric anti-CD20 monoclonal antibody rituximab induces rapid and long-lasting depletion of circulating B cells (see Hematologic above). Enteroviral meningoencephalitis after rituximab occurred in a child with immune thrombocytopenia and in an adult with relapsed B cell lymphoma.

- A boy with severe autoimmune thrombocytopenia was treated from 4 to 10 years of age with intensive immunosuppression and hemopoietic stem cell transplantation when he was 8 (54). Twenty months after transplantation, he was given four courses of rituximab 375 mg/m²/week in combination with prednisone 0.4 mg/kg/day and dapsone 3mg/kg/day. After 6 months, the prednisone was tapered to 0.15 mg/kg/day and he relapsed. A second course of four infusions of rituximab were given, resulting in resolution of thrombocytopenia. Eleven months later, he developed progressive alteration in cognitive function, aphasia, sensorimotor deafness, a mild fever, and an extrapyramidal syndrome. A brain MRI scan showed diffuse white matter abnormalities, and enteroviral protein was detected by PCR in plasma and cerebrospinal fluid. The leukocyte count in the cerebrospinal fluid was $27-33 \times 10^6/l$. He was given intravenous immunoglobulin and pleconaril, and dapsone was withdrawn. Seven months later he recovered from the enteroviral meningoencephalitis, with negative PCR but unchanged brain MRI abnormalities.
- A 53 year old man with a follicular lymphoma Ann Arbor stage IIIA responded to low-dose chemotherapy

but relapsed 28 months later (54). Rituximab 375 mg/m²/week over 4 weeks induced a second complete remission. He developed a fever, headache, diffuse paresthesia, difficulty in concentrating, sensorimotor deafness, diplopia, ataxia, and a pyramidal syndrome 6 months after the last infusion of rituximab. A brain MRI scan showed evidence of myelitis and asymmetric signal enhancement in the right parietal meninges. In the cerebrospinal fluid the lymphocyte count was $300 \times 10^6/l$ and echovirus 13 was isolated. The duodenal wall was thickened on a CT scan and duodenal biopsy showed a second lymphoma. After high-dose glucocorticoids, and polychemotherapy the neurological symptoms partially improved and hemopoietic stem cell transplantation was performed. Two months after transplantation the neurological symptoms and mild fever returned. Enterovirus was detected by PCR in the cerebrospinal fluid. He recovered with residual effects after high-dose intravenous immunoglobulin and pleconaril.

Mixed cryoglobinemia is a chronic immune-complex mediated disease, often associated with vascular, renal, and neurological lesions and hepatitis C. Almost 10% of patients progress to frank B-cell non-Hodgkin's lymphoma. Rituximab 375 mg/m²/week was given intravenously for 4 consecutive weeks to 20 patients with mixed cryoglobinemia and hepatitis C virus-positive chronic active liver disease resistant to interferon alfa (55). There was a complete response in 16. Rituximab caused an increase in HCV-RNA to about twice baseline without significant variation in serum transaminases or deterioration of liver disease.

Rituximab can cause reactivation of hepatitis B virus infection (56,57).

- A woman with non-Hodgkin's lymphoma developed hepatitis B virus reactivation after rituximab treatment. HBs antigens and HBs, HBe, and HBc antibodies were positive, but HBe antigens were negative (57). She was treated with three courses of rituximab plus anticancer drugs and one course of anticancer drugs. Prednisolone was not given. After the fourth course of chemotherapy with the third dose of rituximab she developed hepatic dysfunction, and the serum titers of HBs and HBc antibodies suddenly fell. After administration of lamivudine she gradually recovered from liver failure.

The use of rituximab in immunosuppressed patients can cause life-threatening infection (58,59), among which fatal enteroviral meningoencephalitis has been reported (60)

- A 75-year-old man with a long history of recurrent lymphoplasmacytoid lymphoma developed a diffuse large-cell lymphoma affecting the adrenal glands and causing severe hypoadrenalism. It responded to rituximab, cyclophosphamide, doxorubicin, vincristine, and prednisolone (R-CHOP) chemotherapy. Seven months later he developed signs of gastroenteritis, septicemia, and coma. PCR testing of the cerebrospinal fluid suggested enteroviral encephalitis and he initially responded to intravenous immunoglobulins but died after 14 weeks.

Cytomegalovirus gastritis has also been attributed to rituximab (61).

- A 65-year old woman was treated for a diffuse large cell type non-Hodgkin's lymphoma with six courses of cyclophosphamide, doxorubicin, vincristine, and prednisone (CHOP) plus rituximab, with a good partial response. Two weeks after radiotherapy (3000 cGy) to the para-iliac and inguinal regions, she developed epigastric pain and diarrhea without blood and mucus. Upper gastrointestinal endoscopy showed multiple linear exudative gastric ulcers containing hyperchromatic epithelial cells with nuclear viral inclusions (owl's eye), which were positive for monoclonal antibodies against cytomegalovirus. She responded to intravenous ganciclovir.

Caution may be needed when using rituximab in patients with a history of endocarditis (62).

- A 54 year old woman with cerebral lupus was treated successfully with rituximab, but developed a *Streptococcus intermedius* infection on valves that had been damaged by Libman–Sacks endocarditis more than 20 years before.

Long-Term Effects

Tumorigenicity

A second cancer is possible when treating a tumor by mutagenicity or immunosuppression. There may be a link between the therapy given and the development of Merkel cell carcinoma (63).

- A 54-year-old man with stage I follicular lymphocytic lymphoma with cervical lymph nodes underwent splenectomy followed by chemotherapy with chlorambucil and had a partial response. Five months later, when he developed generalized lymphadenopathy and bone marrow involvement, he received fludarabine, cyclophosphamide, and rituximab, with complete remission. Ten months later he developed a Merkel cell carcinoma involving the liver and lymph nodes. The disseminated tumor was chemoresistant and he died. His lymphoma remained in complete clinical remission throughout this time.

Two patients developed a peripheral T cell non-Hodgkin's lymphoma after rituximab therapy, one after 15 months and the other after 18 months (64).

Rituximab was suggested as a possible cause of aggressive peripheral T cell lymphoma in two patients 15 and 18 months after the use of rituximab for low-grade B cell non-Hodgkin's lymphoma (65,66).

Merkel cell carcinoma, an uncommon neuroendocrine carcinoma of the skin, has been reported after therapy with rituximab and cladribine (67).

- A 51-year-old woman with chronic lymphatic leukemia received 4 courses of cladribine and then another four courses in combination with rituximab. She developed a

red lump on the right cheek 2 months after the last course. A Merkel cell carcinoma was diagnosed hsitologically and immunohistologically. It was treated by surgically resection followed by local adjuvant radio-chemotherapy.

Another patient developed a rapidly growing Merkel cell carcinoma after receiving rituximab for an acquired factor VIII inhibitor (68).

Three cases of cutaneous squamous-cell carcinoma occurred during prolonged treatment with rituximab (69).

- An 80-year-old woman was treated with rituximab 375 mg/m^2 weekly after a second relapse of non-Hodgkin's lymphoma. She had a history of a squamous cell carcinoma on the middle finger, which had been treated with surgery and radiotherapy. After a sixth cycle of rituximab, the carcinoma recurred, with multiple subcutaneous deposits on the back of the hand. Radiotherapy produced a complete response.
- A 56-year-old man was treated at the time of a third relapse with rituximab 375 mg/m^2 weekly for 4 weeks followed by maintenance therapy. After a fifth cycle he developed a rapidly growing area of unstable skin on his scalp. Histopathology showed a poorly differentiated squamous cell carcinoma.
- A 64-year-old woman with follicular non-Hodgkin's lymphoma was given with rituximab 375 mg/m» on three occasions. During the third course she developed a rapidly enlarging skin lesion on her nose requiring excision. Histopathology showed a moderately differentiated squamous cell carcinoma.

Second-Generation Effects

Pregnancy

Very few cases of rituximab administration during pregnancy have been described.

- A woman with autoimmune hemolytic anemia received rituximab during her first trimester; there were no significant effects on B cell counts or the immune status of the neonate (70).
- A pregnant woman with relapsed follicular non-Hodgkin's lymphoma took rituximab unintentionally during the first trimester (71). The disease stabilized and following an uncomplicated pregnancy a healthy child was born at full term. Careful hematological and immunological monitoring showed no adverse effects from exposure to rituximab.

Monitoring Therapy

Infusion of immunotherapeutic monoclonal antibodies against normal or tumor cells can lead to loss of targeted epitopes, a phenomenon called antigenic modulation. In patients with chronic lymphocytic leukemia rituximab caused substantial loss of CD20 on B cells in the circulation, when rituximab plasma concentrations were high (72). Such antigenic modulation can severely compromise therapeutic efficacy, and the authors postulated that the B cells had been stripped of the rituximab/CD20 complex by monocytes or macrophages in a reaction mediated by FcγR. An in vitro model based on reacting rituximab-opsonized CD20(+) cells with acceptor THP-1 monocytes demonstrated this mechanism. After 45 minutes rituximab and CD20 were removed from opsonized cells and both were demonstrable on acceptor THP-1 cells. The reaction occurred equally well in the presence and absence of normal human serum, and monocytes isolated from peripheral blood also promoted the stripping of CD20 from rituximab-opsonized cells. The transfer of rituximab/CD20 complexes to THP-1 cells was mediated by FcγR.

Management of Adverse Drug Reactions

Accurate determination of rituximab plasma concentrations is important for proper dosing of patients and for correlating rituximab concentrations with clinical responses. However, there is currently no assay available that uses easily obtainable commercial reagents. One assay is based on flow cytometry and quantifies immunologically active rituximab based on its ability to bind to CD20 on Raji cells. Two other methods are based on flow cytometry and ELISA and measure rituximab based on its antigenic properties. The assays are accurate, in good agreement with one another, and can all measure rituximab concentrations as low as about 1 µg/ml in both serum and plasma. Patients with chronic lymphocytic leukemia receiving rituximab had lower plasma rituximab concentrations than patients with other B cell lymphomas at all times over the usual 4-week course of therapy. The rituximab plasma concentration in patients with chronic lymphocytic leukemia often falls to below 1 µg/ml 1 week after each infusion, substantially lower than the values found in comparable patient without chronic lymphocytic leukemia. In patients with chronic lymphocytic leukemia who have not previously received rituximab the concentrations of non-cell associated CD20 are not sufficient either to interfere with an in vitro assay of rituximab or to block the potential therapeutic action of rituximab in vivo (73).

Pregnancy

The optimal treatment of non-Hodgkin's lymphoma during pregnancy has not been well defined. The potential teratogenic effects of conventional chemotherapeutic drugs preclude their use during the first trimester. Data on the use of rituximab during pregnancy are scarce.

- A pregnant woman with relapsed indolent follicular non-Hodgkin's lymphoma was unintentionally treated with rituximab during the first trimester. The treatment stabilized the disease. Following an uncomplicated pregnancy, a healthy child was born at full term and careful hematological and immunological monitoring showed no adverse effects resulting from exposure to rituximab (74).

This case suggests that rituximab may be one option for treatment of non-Hodgkin's lymphoma in early pregnancy.

Susceptibility factors

Genetic Japanese patients (n = 68) with relapsed or refractory aggressive B cell lymphoma were treated with an infusion of rituximab 375 mg/m2 on 8 consecutive weeks (75). Mild to moderate infusion-related toxic effects were common after the first infusion, but all were reversible. Raised lactate dehydrogenase activity and refractoriness to prior chemotherapy were unfavorable factors that affected the overall response rate and progression-free survival. Serum trough concentrations and AUC of rituximab in responders were significantly higher than in non-responders.

References

1. Levine TD. Rituximab in the treatment of dermatomyositis: an open-label pilot study. Arthritis Rheum 2005;52(2):601–7.
2. Keogh KA, Wylam ME, Stone JH, Specks U. Induction of remission by B lymphocyte depletion in eleven patients with refractory antineutrophil cytoplasmic antibody-associated vasculitis. Arthritis Rheum 2005;52(1):262–8.
3. Gottenberg JE, Guillevin L, Lambotte O, Combe B, Allanore Y, Cantagrel A, Larroche C, Soubrier M, Bouillet L, Dougados M, Fain O, Farge D, Kyndt X, Lortholary O, Masson C, Moura B, Remy P, Thomas T, Wendling D, Anaya JM, Sibilia J, Mariette X. Club Rheumatismes et Inflammation (CRI). Tolerance and short term efficacy of rituximab in 43 patients with systemic autoimmune diseases. Ann Rheum Dis 2005;64(6):913–20.
4. Vieira CA, Agarwal A, Book BK, Sidner RA, Bearden CM, Gebel HM, Roggero AL, Fineberg NS, Taber T, Kraus MA, Pescovitz MD. Rituximab for reduction of anti-HLA antibodies in patients awaiting renal transplantation: 1. Safety, pharmacodynamics, and pharmacokinetics. Transplantation 2004;77(4):542–8.
5. Onrust SV, Lamb HM, Balfour JA. Rituximab. Drugs 1999;58(1):79–88.
6. Boye J, Elter T, Engert A. An overview of the current clinical use of the anti-CD20 monoclonal antibody rituximab. Ann Oncol 2003;14:520–35.
7. Ozguroglu M, Turna H. Rituximab-induced tumor progression: does it really happen? Med Oncol 2004;21(2):205–6.
8. Byrd JC, Waselenko JK, Maneatis TJ, Murphy T, Ward FT, Monahan BP, Sipe MA, Donegan S, White CA. Rituximab therapy in hematologic malignancy patients with circulating blood tumor cells: association with increased infusion-related side effects and rapid blood tumor clearance. J Clin Oncol 1999;17(3):791–5.
9. Davis TA, White CA, Grillo-Lopez AJ, Velasquez WS, Link B, Maloney DG, Dillman RO, Williams ME, Mohrbacher A, Weaver R, Dowden S, Levy R. Single-agent monoclonal antibody efficacy in bulky non-Hodgkin's lymphoma: results of a phase II trial of rituximab. J Clin Oncol 1999;17(6):1851–7.
10. Yang H, Rosove MH, Figlin RA. Tumor lysis syndrome occurring after the administration of rituximab in lymphoproliferative disorders: high-grade non-Hodgkin's lymphoma and chronic lymphocytic leukemia. Am J Hematol 1999;62(4):247–50.
11. van der Kolk LE, Grillo-Lopez AJ, Baars JW, Hack CE, van Oers MH. Complement activation plays a key role in the side-effects of rituximab treatment. Br J Haematol 2001;115(4):807–11.
12. Winkler U, Jensen M, Manzke O, Schulz H, Diehl V, Engert A. Cytokine-release syndrome in patients with B-

cell chronic lymphocytic leukemia and high lymphocyte counts after treatment with an anti-CD20 monoclonal antibody (rituximab, IDEC-C2B8). Blood 1999;94(7):2217–24.

13. Foran JM, Rohatiner AZ, Cunningham D, Popescu RA, Solal-Celigny P, Ghielmini M, Coiffier B, Johnson PW, Gisselbrecht C, Reyes F, Radford JA, Bessell EM, Souleau B, Benzohra A, Lister TA. European phase II study of rituximab (chimeric anti-CD20 monoclonal antibody) for patients with newly diagnosed mantle-cell lymphoma and previously treated mantle-cell lymphoma, immunocytoma, and small B cell lymphocytic lymphoma. J Clin Oncol 2000;18(2):317–24.

14. Garypidou V, Perifanis V, Tziomalos K, Theodoridou S. Cardiac toxicity during rituximab administration. Leuk Lymphoma 2004;45(1):203–4.

15. Zerga M, Cerchetti L, Cicco J, Constantini P, De Riz M. Desquamative alveolitis: an unusual complication of treatment with Mabthera. Blood 1999;94(Suppl 1):271.

16. Swords R, Power D, Fay M, O'Donnell R, Murphy PT. Interstitial pneumonitis following rituximab therapy for immune thrombocytopenic purpura (ITP). Am J Hematol 2004;77(1):103–4.

17. Biehn SE, Kirk D, Rivera MP, Martinez AE, Khandani AH, Orlowski RZ. Bronchiolitis obliterans with organizing pneumonia after rituximab therapy for non-Hodgkin's lymphoma. Hematol Oncol 2006;24(4):234–7.

18. Sirvent-Von Bueltzingsloewen A, Sirvent N, Morand P, Cassuto JP. Fatal central nervous system lesions emerging during anti-CD20 monoclonal antibody therapy (Rituximab) for a post transplantation Epstein Barr virus-linked lymphoma. Med Pediatr Oncol 2003;40:408–9.

19. Mavragani CP, Vlachoyiannopoulos PG, Kosmas N, Boletis I, Tzioufas AG, Voulgarelis M. A case of reversible posterior leucoencephalopathy syndrome after rituximab infusion. Rheumatology (Oxford) 2004;43(11):1450–1.

20. Oribe N, Tanimoto TE, Shimoda K, Hikiji W, Mitsugi K, Takase K, Henzan H, Numata A, Miyamoto T, Fukuda T, Nagafuji K, Harada M. Edema of the eyelids and sclera after rituximab infusion for orbital MALT lymphoma. Haematologica 2004;89(6 Suppl):EIM14.

21. Igarashi T, Kobayashi Y, Ogura M, Kinoshita T, Ohtsu T, Sasaki Y, Morishima Y, Murate T, Kasai M, Uike N, Taniwaki M, Kano Y, Ohnishi K, Matsuno Y, Nakamura S, Mori S, Ohashi Y, Tobinai K. IDEC-C2B8 Study Group in Japan. Factors affecting toxicity, response and progression-free survival in relapsed patients with indolent B-cell lymphoma and mantle cell lymphoma treated with rituximab: a Japanese phase II study. Ann Oncol 2002;13(6):928–43.

22. Song KW, Mollee P, Patterson B, Brien W, Crump M. Pure red cell aplasia due to parvovirus following treatment with CHOP and rituximab for B-cell lymphoma. Br J Haematol 2002;119(1):125–7.

23. Bisogno G. Persistent B-cell depletion after rituximab for thrombocytopenic purpura. Eur J Pediatr 2007;166(1):85–6.

24. Sharma VR, Fleming DR, Slone SP. Pure red cell aplasia due to parvovirus B19 in a patient treated with rituximab. Blood 2000;96(3):1184–6.

25. Chaiwatanatorn K, Lee N, Grigg A, Filshie R, Firkin F. Delayed-onset neutropenia associated with rituximab therapy. Br J Haematol 2003;121:913–8.

26. Rose AL, Forsythe AM, Maloney DG. Agranulocytosis unresponsive to growth factors following rituximab in vivo purging. Blood 2003;101:4225–6.

27. Papadaki T, Stamatopoulos K, Anagnostopoulos A, Fassas A. Rituximab-associated immune myelopathy. Blood 2003;102:1557–8.

28. Lemieux B, Tartas S, Traulle C, Espinouse D, Thieblemont C, Bouafia F, Alhusein Q, Antal D, Salles G, Coiffier B. Rituximab-related late-onset neutropenia after autologous stem cell transplantation for aggressive non-Hodgkin's lymphoma. Bone Marrow Transplant 2004;33(9):921–3.

29. Hofer S, Viollier R, Ludwig C. Delayed-onset and long-lasting severe neutropenia due to rituximab. Swiss Med Wkly 2004;134(5-6):79–80.

30. Nitta E, Izutsu K, Sato T, Ota Y, Takeuchi K, Kamijo A, Takahashi K, Oshima K, Kanda Y, Chiba S, Motokura T, Kurokawa M. A high incidence of late-onset neutropenia following rituximab-containing chemotherapy as a primary treatment of CD20-positive B-cell lymphoma: a single-institution study. Ann Oncol 2007;18(2):364–9.

31. Fukuno K, Tsurumi H, Ando N, Kanemura N, Goto H, Tanabashi S, Okamoto K, Moriwaki H. Late-onset neutropenia in patients treated with rituximab for non-Hodgkin's lymphoma. Int J Hematol 2006;84(3):242–7.

32. Cattaneo C, Spedini P, Casari S, Re A, Tucci A, Borlenghi E, Ungari M, Ruggeri G, Rossi G. Delayed-onset peripheral blood cytopenia after rituximab: frequency and risk factor assessment in a consecutive series of 77 treatments. Leuk Lymphoma 2006;47(6):1013–7.

33. Leo E, Scheuer L, Schmidt-Wolf IG, Kerowgan M, Schmitt C, Leo A, Baumbach T, Kraemer A, Mey U, Benner A, Parwaresch R, Ho AD. Significant thrombocytopenia associated with the addition of rituximab to a combination of fludarabine and cyclophosphamide in the treatment of relapsed follicular lymphoma. Eur J Haematol 2004;73(4):251–7.

34. Shah C, Grethlein SJ. Case report of rituximab-induced thrombocytopenia. Am J Hematol 2004;75(4):263.

35. Thachil J, Mukherje K, Woodcock B. Rituximab-induced haemorrhagic thrombocytopenia in a patient with hairy cell leukaemia. Br J Haematol 2006;135(2):273–4.

36. Hagberg H, Lundholm L. Rituximab, a chimaeric anti-CD20 monoclonal antibody, in the treatment of hairy cell leukaemia. Br J Haematol 2001;115(3):609–11.

37. Larrar S, Guitton C, Willems M, Bader-Meunier B. Severe hematological side effects following rituximab therapy in children. Haematologica 2006;91(8 Suppl):ECR36.

38. Iyer A, Mathur R, Deepak BV, Sinard J. Fatal adenoviral hepatitis after rituximab therapy. Arch Pathol Lab Med 2006;130(10):1557–60.

39. Perceau G, Diris N, Estines O, Derancourt C, Lévy S, Bernard P. Late lethal hepatitis B virus reactivation after rituximab treatment of low-grade cutaneous B-cell lymphoma. Br J Dermatol 2006;155(5):1053–6.

40. Sera T, Hiasa Y, Michitaka K, Konishi I, Matsuura K, Tokumoto Y, Matsuura B, Kajiwara T, Masumoto T, Horiike N, Onji M. Anti-HBs-positive liver failure due to hepatitis B virus reactivation induced by rituximab. Intern Med 2006;45(11):721–4.

41. Aksoy S, Abali H, Kilickap S, Erman M, Kars A. Accelerated hepatitis C virus replication with rituximab treatment in a non-Hodgkin's lymphoma patient. Clin Lab Haematol 2006;28(3):211–4.

42. Lowndes S, Darby A, Mead G, Lister A. Stevens–Johnson syndrome after treatment with rituximab. Ann Oncol 2002;13(12):1948–50.

43. Errante D, Bernardi D, Bianco A, De Nardi S, Salvagno L. Rituximab-related urticarial reaction in a patient treated for primary cutaneous B-cell lymphoma. Ann Oncol 2006;17(11):1720–1.

44. Hellerstedt B, Ahmed A. Delayed-type hypersensitivity reaction or serum sickness after rituximab treatment. Ann Oncol 2003;14:1792.

45. Rehwald U, Schulz H, Reiser M, et al. Treatment of relapsed CD20+ Hodgkin lymphoma with the monoclonal antibody rituximab is effective and well tolerated: results of a phase 2 trial of the German Hodgkin Lyphoma Study Group. Blood 2003;101:420–4.

46. Alexandrescu DT, Dutcher JP, O'Boyle K, Albulak M, Oiseth S, Wiernik PH. Fatal intra-alveolar hemorrhage after rituximab in a patient with non-Hodgkin lymphoma. Leuk Lymphoma 2004;45(11):2321–5.

47. Kandula P, Kouides PA. Rituximab-induced leukocytoclastic vasculitis: a case report. Arch Dermatol 2006;142(2):246–7.

48. Seifert G, Reindl T, Lobitz S, Seeger K, Henze G. Fatal course after administration of rituximab in a boy with relapsed all: a case report and review of literature. Haematologica 2006;91(6 Suppl):ECR23.

49. Westhoff TH, Jochimsen F, Schmittel A, Stoffler-Meilicke M, Schafer JH, Zidek W, Gerlich WH, Thiel E. Fatal hepatitis B virus reactivation by an escape mutant following rituximab therapy. Blood 2003;102:1930.

50. Hernandez JA, Diloy R, Salat D, del Rio N, Martinez X, Castellvi JM. Fulminant hepatitis subsequent to reactivation of precore mutant hepatitis B virus in a patient with lymphoma treated with chemotherapy and rituximab. Haematologica 2003;88:ECR22.

51. Dervite I, Hober D, Morel P. Acute hepatitis B in a patient with antibodies to hepatitis B surface antigen who was receiving rituximab. N Engl J Med 2001;344(1):68–9.

52. Bermudez A, Marco F, Conde E, Mazo E, Recio M, Zubizarrcta A. Fatal visceral varicella-zoster infection following rituximab and chemotherapy treatment in a patient with follicular lymphoma. Haematologica 2000;85(8):894–5.

53. Ladetto M, Zallio F, Vallet S, Ricca I, Cuttica A, Caracciolo D, Corradini P, Astolfi M, Sametti S, Volpato F, Bondesan P, Vitolo U, Boccadoro M, Pileri A, Gianni AM, Tarella C. Concurrent administration of high-dose chemotherapy and rituximab is a feasible and effective chemo/immunotherapy for patients with high-risk non-Hodgkin's lymphoma. Leukemia 2001;15(12):1941–9.

54. Quartier P, Tournilhac O, Archimbaud C, Lazaro L, Chaleteix C, Millet P, Peigue-Lafeuille H, Blanche S, Fischer A, Casanova JL, Travade P, Tardieu M. Enteroviral meningoencephalitis after anti-CD20 (rituximab) treatment. Clin Infect Dis 2003;36:e47-9.

55. Sansonno D, De Re Valli, Lauletta G, Tucci FA, Boiocchi M, Dammacco F. Monoclonal antibody treatment of mixed cryoglobulinemia resistant to interferon a with an anti-CD20. Blood 2003;101:3818–26.

56. Soong YL, Lee KM, Lui HF, Chow WC, Tao M, Li Er LS. Hepatitis B reactivation in a patient receiving radiolabeled rituximab. Ann Hematol 2005;84(1):61–2.

57. Tsutsumi Y, Kawamura T, Saitoh S, Yamada M, Obara S, Miura T, Kanamori H, Tanaka J, Asaka M, Imamura M, Masauzi N. Hepatitis B virus reactivation in a case of non-Hodgkin's lymphoma treated with chemotherapy and rituximab: necessity of prophylaxis for hepatitis B virus reactivation in rituximab therapy. Leuk Lymphoma 2004;45(3):627–9.

58. Basse G, Ribes D, Kamar N, Esposito L, Rostaing L. Life-threatening infections following rituximab therapy in renal transplant patients with mixed cryoglobulinemia. Clin Nephrol 2006;66(5):395–6.

59. van der Velden WJ, Blijlevens NM, Klont RR, Donnelly JP, Verweij PE. Primary hepatic invasive aspergillosis with progression after rituximab therapy for a post transplantation lymphoproliferative disorder. Ann Hematol 2006;85(9):621–3.

60. Padate BP, Keidan J. Enteroviral meningoencephalitis in a patient with non-Hodgkin's lymphoma treated previously with rituximab. Clin Lab Haematol 2006;28(1):69–71.

61. Unluturk U, Aksoy S, Yonem O, Bayraktar Y, Tekuzman G. Cytomegalovirus gastritis after rituximab treatment in a non-Hodgkin's lymphoma patient. World J Gastroenterol 2006;12(12):1978–9.

62. Armstrong D, Wright S, McVeigh C, Finch M. Infective endocarditis complicating rituximab (anti-CD20 monoclonal antibody) treatment in an SLE patient with a past history of Libman-Sacks endocarditis: a case for antibiotic prophylaxis? Clin Rheumatol 2006;25(4):583–4.

63. Cohen Y, Amir G, Polliack A. Development and rapid dissemination of Merkel-cell carcinomatosis following therapy with fludarabine and rituximab for relapsing follicular lymphoma. Eur J Haematol 2002;68(2):117–9.

64. Cheson BD. Rituximab: clinical development and future directions. Expert Opin Biol Ther 2002;2(1):97–110.

65. Micallef IN, Kirk A, Norton A, Foran JM, Rohatiner AZ, Lister TA. Peripheral T-cell lymphoma following rituximab therapy for B-cell lymphoma. Blood 1999;93(7):2427–8.

66. Tetreault S, Abler SL, Robbins B, Saven A. Peripheral T-cell lymphoma after anti-CD20 antibody therapy. J Clin Oncol 1998;16(4):1635–7.

67. Robak E, Biernat W, Krykowski E, Jeziorski A, Robak T. Merkel cell carcinoma in a patient with B-cell chronic lymphocytic leukemia treated with cladribine and rituximab. Leuk Lymphoma 2005;46(6):909–14.

68. Wirges ML, Saporito F, Smith J. Rapid growth of Merkel cell carcinoma after treatment with rituximab. J Drugs Dermatol 2006;5(2):180–1.

69. Fogarty GB, Bayne M, Bedford P, Bond R, Kannourakis G. Three cases of activation of cutaneous squamous-cell carcinoma during treatment with prolonged administration of rituximab. Clin Oncol (R Coll Radiol) 2006;18(2):155–6.

70. Ojeda-Uribe M, Gilliot C, Jung G, Drenou B, Brunot A. Administration of rituximab during the first trimester of pregnancy without consequences for the newborn. J Perinatol 2006;26(4):252–5.

71. Kimby E, Sverrisdottir A, Elinder G. Safety of rituximab therapy during the first trimester of pregnancy: a case history. Eur J Haematol 2004;72(4):292–5.

72. Beum PV, Kennedy AD, Williams ME, Lindorfer MA, Taylor RP. The shaving reaction: rituximab/CD20 complexes are removed from mantle cell lymphoma and chronic lymphocytic leukemia cells by THP-1 monocytes. J Immunol 2006;176(4):2600–9.

73. Beum PV, Kennedy AD, Taylor RP. Three new assays for rituximab based on its immunological activity or antigenic properties: analyses of sera and plasmas of RTX-treated patients with chronic lymphocytic leukemia and other B cell lymphomas. J Immunol Methods 2004;289(1-2):97–109.

74. Kimby E, Sverrisdottir A, Elinder G. Safety of rituximab therapy during the first trimester of pregnancy: a case history. Eur J Haematol 2004;72(4):292–5.

75. Tobinai K, Igarashi T, Itoh K, Kobayashi Y, Taniwaki M, Ogura M, Kinoshita T, Hotta T, Aikawa K, Tsushita K, Hiraoka A, Matsuno Y, Nakamura S, Mori S, Ohashi Y;IDEC-C2B8 Japan Study Group. Japanese multicenter phase II and pharmacokinetic study of rituximab in relapsed or refractory patients with aggressive B-cell lymphoma. Ann Oncol 2004;15(5):821–30.

Sulfasalazine

General Information

Sulfasalazine is a sulfonamide derivative. The term "sulfonamide" is generic for derivatives of para-amino-benzenesulfonamide (sulfanilamide), which is similar in structure to para-aminobenzoic acid (PABA), a co-factor required by bacteria for folic acid synthesis. The sulfonamides act by competitive inhibition of the incorporation of PABA into tetrahydropteroic acid. Sulfonamides have a higher affinity for the microbial enzyme tetrahydropteroic acid synthetase than the natural substrate PABA. Sulfonamides have a wide range of antimicrobial activity against both Gram-positive and Gram-negative organisms (1). In therapeutic dosages they have only a bacteriostatic effect, and as single agents therefore have a limited role in drug therapy (1). Sulfonamides have been combined with trimethoprim or trimethoprim analogues, since such combinations result in a bactericidal effect (2). Adverse reactions during the administration of sulfamethoxazole + trimethoprim (co-trimoxazole, BAN) can be due to either compound. Although sulfonamides are thought to cause adverse reactions more often than trimethoprim, the culprit in the individual patient can only be determined by re-exposure to the individual agents.

Based on their pharmacological properties and clinical uses, sulfonamides can be classified into four groups (1):

1. short- or medium-acting sulfonamides;
2. long-acting sulfonamides;
3. topical sulfonamides;
4. sulfonamide derivatives used for inflammatory bowel disease and thermatoid arthritis.

Short- or medium-acting sulfonamides include the earliest varieties of azosulfonamides (Prontosil, Neoprontosil), sulfapyridine (Dagenan), sulfathiazole (Cibazol), sulfanilamide, and sulfadiazine. With the exception of sulfadiazine, these compounds are no longer used. Sulfadiazine and more recent compounds, including sulfafurazole (sulfisoxazole), sulfamethoxazole, sulfametrole, sulfacitine, and sulfamethizole, are rapidly absorbed and rapidly eliminated. Compared with the older generation they are more soluble, less toxic, and probably less allergenic. Sulfamethoxazole is a medium-acting sulfonamide that is often combined with trimethoprim (as co-trimoxazole). Long-acting sulfonamides include sulfametoxydiazine, sulfadimethoxine, and other compounds, of which many are no longer available, as they were associated with severe hypersensitivity reactions. Although these compounds have the advantage of long administration intervals, their long half-lives (over 100 hours) can be deleterious in case of adverse reactions. A long-acting drug that is still widely used is sulfadoxine (N-(5,6-dimethoxy-4-pyrimidinyl)-sulfanilamide). It is primarily used in combination with pyrimethamine (Fansidar) for the treatment and prophylaxis of malaria.

The topical use of sulfonamides has been discouraged, because of the high risk of sensitization. Nevertheless, sulfacetamide and sulfadicramide are still used topically for eye infections. Topical silver sulfadiazine (see monograph on Silver) is widely and successfully used in treating burns and leg ulcers (3,4). Since sulfonamides are easily absorbed through skin lesions, the same adverse reactions can occur as after systemic use.

Sulfasalazine (salicylazosulfapyridine) has been widely used to treat ulcerative colitis and regional ileitis (Crohn's disease). It is a compound of sulfapyridine and 5-aminosalicylate, linked by a diazo bond. Sulfasalazine is broken down in the large bowel to sulfapyridine, which is absorbed systemically, and 5-aminosalicylate, which reaches high concentrations in the feces (5). Sulfasalazine is not used for the antibacterial properties of the sulfapyridine, but for the local anti-inflammatory effect of 5-aminosalicylate in the gut. Because most of the adverse reactions are thought to be due to the absorbed sulfapyridine, the combination has largely been replaced in clinical practice by newer drugs that contain only 5-aminosalicylic acid (mesalazine), such as mesalazine itself and diazosalicylate (olsalazine; 5). However, sulfasalazine is also used to heat thermotoid arthritis.

General adverse effects

The frequency and severity of the adverse effects of sulfonamides correspond to those seen with other antibacterial agents (2–5%). Dose-related effects, which tend to be more troublesome than serious, include gastrointestinal symptoms, headache, and drowsiness. Crystalluria can occur, but urinary obstruction is rare. Hematological adverse effects due to folic acid antagonism occur primarily in combination with trimethoprim. Hemolytic anemia occurs in patients with enzyme deficiencies and abnormal hemoglobins. Hypersensitivity is thought to be the mechanism of many adverse effects of the sulfonamides. They can be life-threatening, and immediate withdrawal is recommended. The most important reactions include anaphylactic shock, a serum sickness-like syndrome, systemic vasculitis, severe skin reactions (Stevens–Johnson syndrome and toxic epidermal necrolysis), pneumonitis, hepatitis, and pancytopenia. Sulfonamides should not be used in the third trimester of pregnancy. In premature infants, they displace bilirubin from plasma albumin and can cause kernicterus. Carcinogenicity has not been reported with the use of sulfonamides.

Sulfanilamide and the history of adverse drug reactions

The first major drug catastrophe in the 20th century history of the public control of drugs occurred in 1937 in the USA. A pharmacist introduced Elixir Sulfanilamide, which consisted of sulfanilamide dissolved in diethylene glycol. It had been tested for flavor, appearance, and fragrance, but not for safety. After taking the drug, over 100 patients died in severe pain; many were children, who were given Elixir Sulfanilamide for sore throats and coughs. Public outrage created support for proposed legislation to reinforce the public control of drugs that was pending in the US Congress (6). This led to the US 1938 Food, Drug, and Cosmetic Act, which is still the country's legal foundation for the public control of drugs and devices intended for use in the diagnosis, cure, mitigation, treatment, or prevention of disease in humans or animals. It has been a model for similar legislation in many other countries.

The 1938 Food, Drug, and Cosmetic Act prohibited traffic in new drugs, unless they were safe for use under the conditions of use prescribed on their labels. The Act also explicitly required the labeling of drug products with adequate directions for use.

The burden of proof of harm of new drugs was laid on the Federal Food and Drug Agency (FDA). Companies that wanted to manufacture and sell new drugs in interstate commerce had to investigate their safety and report to the FDA. Unless the FDA, within a specified period of time, found that the safety of a drug had not been established, the company could proceed with its marketing. The FDA was also authorized to remove from the market any drug it could prove to be unsafe (7).

The US Supreme Court also established in 1941, in a legal case over drug adulteration, that responsible individuals in a company can be held personally accountable for the quality of the products manufactured by the company, and that distributors of pharmaceuticals are responsible for the quality of their products, even if they are manufactured elsewhere (8).

After World War II, the pharmaceuticals market changed radically, as many companies started industrial production of drugs that had previously been manufactured in pharmacies. Announcements of new industrially produced drugs were hailed as part of technological advancement, as significant a sign of progress as the launching of satellites and putting a man on the moon. However, public safeguards against the risks of drugs remained unchanged in most countries. Thus, control of the effects of drugs largely lay in the hands of the manufacturers, even though the responsibility for taking precautions rested with pharmacists and doctors.

Organs and Systems

Cardiovascular

Sulfonamide myocarditis has been described in relation to earlier sulfonamides and occurs in combination with other hypersensitivity reactions (9).

Respiratory

Respiratory reactions to sulfonamides include migratory pulmonary infiltrates, chronic pneumonia, asthma, and pulmonary angiitis. These reactions are thought to be mainly due to hypersensitivity, although the precise mechanisms are not well understood (10–12). The link to the drug has been proven in most cases by recurrence after re-exposure to the same sulfonamide or to co-trimoxazole.

The sulfapyridine moiety of sulfasalazine, used in inflammatory bowel disease, can produce adverse pulmonary reactions (13).

The time between the last exposure to a sulfonamine and the first clinical symptoms varies from hours to a few days, and the lung pathology disappears in most patients within a few days after withdrawal. Most commonly, pulmonary involvement presents with fever, dyspnea, cough, and shortness of breath. Clinical examination reveals râles in the lungs, and there may be pulmonary infiltrates in the chest X-ray. Pulmonary function tests may show bronchial obstruction (14), and arterial blood gases show hypoxemia (13). Whereas bronchial obstruction is probably an immediate reaction (type I), pulmonary infiltrates may correspond to a type III reaction, similar to the mechanism responsible for extrinsic allergic alveolitis (13,14). Eosinophilia is present in 8–58% of cases (11,12,14,15). Histologically, the lung tissue is infiltrated by inflammatory cells, and in most cases the alveoli contain numerous macrophages and eosinophils in a protein-rich edema fluid.

Based on the predominant symptoms and their duration, four categories of sulfonamide-related pulmonary hypersensitivity reactions can be distinguished (16–18):

1. transient or migratory pulmonary infiltrations associated with eosinophilia (Loeffler's syndrome; 15,19–21)
2. chronic eosinophilic pneumonia (16,20)
3. asthma with pulmonary eosinophilia (10–12,14)
4. allergic angiitis with pulmonary involvement (18).

In the first three of these, the adverse reaction is limited to the lung, whereas in the fourth the lung involvement is part of a systemic reaction. Syndromes such as allergic granulomatosis and angiitis (Churg–Strauss syndrome) or Wegener's granulomatosis are not associated with the use of sulfonamides (18).

A 68-year-old woman who had taken sulfasalazine for rheumatoid arthritis. for 6 months developed bronchiolitis obliterans organizing pneumonia (BOOP) associated with an eosinophilia of $970 \times 10^6/l$ (22).

Nervous system

Neurological disturbances that have been attributed to sulfonamides include polyneuritis, neuritis, and optic neuritis (23,24).

Sensory systems

Eyes

Drug induced uveitis is rare. Antibiotics that have been implicated include rifabutin and sulfonamides. Furthermore, nearly all antibiotics injected intracamerally have been reported to produce uveitis (25). Topical administration of a corticosteroid and a cycloplegic (such as atropine) is suitable as initial treatment. Withdrawal of causative drugs is not always necessary (26).

Transient myopia can be caused by topical or systematic sulfonamides (27–29).

Psychological, psychiatric

Headache, drowsiness, lowered mental acuity, and other psychiatric effects can be caused by sulfonamides (30).

However, these adverse effects are rare, and the causative role of the drug is usually not clearly established.

Metabolism

Several sulfonamides, including co-trimoxazole in high doses, can produce hyperchloremic metabolic acidosis.

Hematologic

Sulfonamides have adverse effects on all bone marrow–derived cell lines. The resulting disturbances include hemolytic anemia, folate deficiency anemia, neutropenia, thrombocytopenia, and pancytopenia. While adverse effects on erythrocytes are rare, the rates of leukopenia, neutropenia, and thrombocytopenia are highly variable. In a hospital drug monitoring program, leukopenia or neutropenia occurred in 0.4% of 1809 patients treated with co-trimoxazole (31), and thrombocytopenia of mild-to-moderate degree in 0.1% (31,32), similar to figures recorded in other studies (33,34). Pancytopenia is an extremely rare form of adverse reaction to sulfonamides (35).

Erythrocytes

Sulfonamides rarely have adverse effects on erythrocytes. However, there are various mechanisms by which sulfonamide-induced hemolytic anemia can occur (36):

- abnormally high blood concentrations, due to large doses or reduced excretion of the drug in patients with renal disease (37)
- acquired hypersusceptibility, as reflected by the development of a positive Coombs' test (38,39)
- genetically determined abnormalities of erythrocyte metabolism, for example deficiency of glucose-6-phosphate dehydrogenase or of diaphorase (40,41)
- the presence of an abnormal, so-called "unstable", hemoglobin in the erythrocyte, for example hemoglobin Zürich (42,43), hemoglobin Torino (44), hemoglobin Hasharon (45), and hemoglobins H and M (41).

Simple and readily available in vitro methods have been used to demonstrate the pathogenetic mechanisms, including Coombs' test, Harris's test (46), a quantitative assay or screening for glucose-6-phosphate dehydrogenase activity after recovery (47,48), a test for Heinz bodies, the buffered isopropanol technique (49) to detect abnormal hemoglobins, and hemoglobin electrophoresis (36,41). The direct antiglobulin (Coombs') test can be negative in spite of an immune mechanism. If such a mechanism is suspected and the direct Coombs' test is negative, the indirect Coombs' test on the patient's serum with the addition of the suspected sensitizing agent can be of diagnostic value (50). Heinz bodies in the erythrocytes can be important for early differentiation of a sulfonamide-induced reaction, which could further progress to hemolytic anemia (51). This result can also be of help in distinguishing this from other kinds of anemia.

Sulfonamides are not directly associated with folate deficiency and megaloblastic anemias. Sulfasalazine can affect the absorption of folates, but inflammatory bowel disease can also be responsible for reduced folate absorption. Only in combination with trimethoprim are sulfonamides thought to deplete folate stores in patients with pre-existing deficiency of folate or vitamin B_{12} (52).

Leukocytes

Since the days when chloramphenicol was more commonly used, it has been recognized that many antimicrobial drug are associated with severe blood dyscrasias, such as aplastic anemia, neutropenia, agranulocytosis, thrombocytopenia, and hemolytic anemia. Information on this association has come predominantly from case series and hospital surveys (53–55). Some evidence can be extracted from population-based studies that have focused on aplastic anemia and agranulocytosis and their association with many drugs, including antimicrobial drugs (56,57). The incidence rates of blood dyscrasias in the general population have been estimated in a cohort study with a nested case-control analysis, using data from a General Practice Research Database in Spain (58). The study population consisted of 822 048 patients aged 5–69 years who received at least one prescription (in all 1 507 307 prescriptions) for an antimicrobial drug during January 1994 to September 1998. The main outcome measure was a diagnosis of neutropenia, agranulocytosis, hemolytic anemia, thrombocytopenia, pancytopenia, or aplastic anemia. The incidence was 3.3 per 100 000 person-years in the general population. Users of antimicrobial drugs had a relative risk (RR), adjusted for age and sex, of 4.4, and patients who took more than one class of antimicrobial drug had a relative risk of 29. Among individual antimicrobial drugs, the greatest risk was with cephalosporins (RR = 14), followed by the sulfonamides (RR = 7.6) and penicillins (RR = 3.1).

Agranulocytosis was not infrequent in the early sulfonamide era. The first cases were observed in association with sulfanilamide (59,60), Prontosil (59), sulfapyridine (60,61), sulfathiazole (62), sulfadiazine (62), and sulfasalazine (63). Even with topical silver sulfadiazine, agranulocytosis as a consequence of systemic absorption has been reported (64).

Special observations in patients with agranulocytosis favor an immunological/allergic mechanism rather than a toxic one. Several points justify this view:

1. the sulfonamide is well tolerated by most patients during the initial phase of treatment
2. sulfonamide concentrations in the serum, when determined, are not particularly high in patients with hematological complications
3. in some patients, skin rash, fever, and arthritis start concomitantly with or even before the appearance of leukopenia or agranulocytosis
4. re-exposure to a single dose can be followed by a second episode of severe agranulocytosis
5. an agglutinin for leukocytes has been identified in patients' serum shortly after withdrawal of the drug (61)
6. using in vitro techniques, positive reactions to the drug with the lymphocyte transformation test or inhibition

of colony growth in bone marrow have been found (65,66); however, the results of lymphocyte transformation tests must be interpreted with caution—sometimes they are positive in patients who have been exposed to the drug without any evidence of a hypersensitivity reaction.

Gastrointestinal

Nausea, vomiting, and anorexia occur in a few patients taking sulfonamides (1). They are usually related to dosage, the disposition of the individual patient, and how the question concerning adverse effects is asked.

Liver

Three forms of liver injury may be related to sulfonamides:

1. hepatitis of the hepatocellular type (67–71)
2. hepatitis of the mixed hepatocellular type accompanied by cholestatic features (72)
3. chronic active hepatitis, possibly leading to cirrhosis (73).

The number of cases of sulfonamide hepatitis published annually fell markedly after 1947, with the introduction of the newer short-acting derivatives (72).

Hitherto, the connection with a sulfonamide has always been investigated by administering a test dose. Immunological in vitro methods that show sensitization to the drug, for example the lymphocyte transformation test, are of limited value. In some patients the hepatic injury develops in connection with a general reaction, such as serum sickness-like syndrome, generalized vasculitis, or rash (74,75). In patients with hypersensitivity, re-exposure can result in generalized malaise, nausea, back pain, and chills within one to several hours (69,73). However, symptoms can be delayed for as long as several days (72). Daily monitoring of liver function on re-exposure seems to be important, since subjective signs can be absent despite rising activities of serum transaminases and alkaline phosphatase (68).

Even in patients with chronic active hepatitis, the histopathology of the liver damage was indistinguishable from non-drug-induced pathology. The degree of piecemeal necrosis usually varies from one area to another. Antinuclear factor and lupus erythematosus factor were positive in some cases (73). Early recognition of drug-induced liver disease is of great importance, since liver injury can be completely reversible after withdrawal.

Pancreas

Pancreatitis has been attributed to sulfonamides. Sulfasalazine (76) has been implicated by re-exposure. The 5-aminosalicylic acid moiety of sulfasalazine may be responsible (77,78).

In a survey of 1590 cases of acute pancreatitis in Denmark from 1991 to 2002 and 15 913 age- and sex-matched controls there was an increased risk of acute pancreatitis in patients with Crohn's disease (OR = 3.7; 95% CI = 1.9, 7.6) and a non-significant 1.5-fold increased risk of ulcerative colitis (79). The use of 5-aminosalicylic acid or sulfasalazine was not associated with an increased risk of acute pancreatitis. In all patients taking 5-aminosalicylic acid and sulfasalazine the adjusted odds ratios for acute pancreatitis were 0.7 (95% CI = 0.4, 2.2) and 1.5 (95% CI = 0.4, 5.2) respectively. Restricted to patients with inflammatory bowel diseases only, the respective adjusted odds ratios for acute pancreatitis were 0.7 (95% CI = 0.1, 3.8) and 0.6 (95% CI = 0.1-6.7).

Urinary tract

Renal complications that occur in relation to sulfonamide administration include crystalluria, tubular necrosis, interstitial nephritis, and glomerular lesions as part of a vasculitis syndrome.

Sulfonamides and their metabolites are excreted in large amounts in the urine. They are relatively insoluble in the acid environment and tend to precipitate in the collecting tubules, calyces, and pelvis of the kidney, and possibly in the ureters. The course is typically benign but adequate hydration and alkalinization may be required (80). Nephrocalcinosis can cause hematuria, renal colic, or acute renal insufficiency (81). Urinary obstruction with anuria/oliguria was seen primarily with the earlier, less soluble sulfonamides. With the newer and more soluble sulfonamides crystal formation is rare, as is acute renal insufficiency due to other mechanisms. During recent years renal complications have been seen more often in patients with AIDS, because of the use of large doses of sulfonamides combined with trimethoprim against infection with *Pneumocystis jiroveci* (formerly *Pneumocystis carinii*) or *Toxoplasma* encephalitis. Reduced fluid intake and low urinary pH favor crystal formation, and so both adequate fluid intake (about 2 l/day for adults) and urine alkalinization are encouraged when larger doses of sulfonamides are used (81–86). For the diagnosis of sulfonamide crystalluria, the Lignin test is recommended. At room temperature crystals can even be found in the urine of patients taking sulfamethoxazole, which is readily soluble (87).

Other renal complications reported with sulfonamides are:

- acute tubular necrosis or tubulointerstitial nephritis (83,88);
- interstitial nephritis (89), in some cases combined with granulomatous lesions (90,91);
- acute vasculitis (92);
- acute renal insufficiency in association with a serum sickness-like syndrome, generalized vasculitis, or rashes in combination with hepatic damage (74).

Acute anuria or oliguria is often the first symptom, not only in patients with tubular necrosis or tubulointerstitial nephritis, but also in those with allergic vasculitis. Non-oliguric renal insufficiency can also occur. It is not yet clear whether tubular necrosis in association with sulfonamides is a toxic, collateral, or hypersusceptibility reaction. The unstable hydroxylamine metabolites of some sulfonamides can act as direct renal toxins.

In a French analysis of 22 510 urinary calculi performed by infrared spectroscopy, drug-induced urolithiasis was divided into two categories: first, stones with drugs physically embedded ($n = 238$; 1.0%), notably indinavir monohydrate ($n = 126$; 53%), followed by triamterene ($n = 43$; 18%), sulfonamides ($n = 29$; 12%), and amorphous silica ($n = 24$; 10%); secondly, metabolic nephrolithiasis induced by drugs ($n = 140$; 0.6%), involving mainly calcium/vitamin D supplementation ($n = 56$; 40%) and carbonic anhydrase inhibitors ($n = 33$; 24%) (93). Drug-induced stones are responsible for about 1.6% of all calculi in France. Physical analysis and a thorough drug history are important elements in the diagnosis.

Skin

Rashes are common during sulfonamide administration, and the rate increases with duration of therapy. Maculopapular reactions are most common and occur in about 1–3% of patients (94–98). In a survey of 5923 pediatric records, 3.46% of prescriptions for sulfonamides were followed by the development of a rash, although none was severe enough to require hospitalization (99).

Urticaria, fixed drug eruptions (97,100–103), erythema nodosum (104), photosensitivity reactions (105), and generalized skin reactions involving light-exposed areas (105–107) are less common.

Other skin eruptions seen with sulfonamides include erythema multiforme, vesicular and bullous rashes, and exfoliative dermatitis (148). In erythema multiforme, linear depositions of IgA at the dermoepidermal junction have been suggested to play a pathogenic role (98).

The most severe skin reactions associated with sulfonamides are the severe forms of erythema multiforme, Stevens–Johnson syndrome, and toxic epidermal necrolysis (108–116).

Mortality in drug-induced toxic epidermal necrolysis has been estimated to be about 20–30% (117,118), and in Stevens–Johnson syndrome 1–10% (110–112,115). Some severe skin reactions start with a maculopapular rash or generalized erythema. The culprit drug is often either a long-acting formulation or a short-acting drug that has been continued over a long period. In both toxic epidermal necrolysis and Stevens–Johnson syndrome immediate withdrawal of the sulfonamide and all other non-essential drugs is required, as well as adequate supportive therapy with fluids, proteins, and electrolytes, in order to prevent renal insufficiency and respiratory distress syndrome (117,118). Occasionally, toxic epidermal necrolysis must be distinguished from staphylococcal scalded skin syndrome (Lyell's syndrome) by histology. In toxic epidermal necrolysis, there is subepidermal cleavage of the skin at the level of the basal cells, resulting in full-thickness denudation, whereas in scalded skin syndrome the split occurs in the upper epidermis near the granular layer just beneath the stratum corneum (119).

The role of sulfonamides as an etiological factor in the Stevens–Johnson syndrome is extremely difficult to evaluate, except for patients with re-exposure or in situations where the drug was given prophylactically for meningitis

(109) or pneumonia (111,112,114,115). In the first epidemiological study in 1968, 100 000 individuals were given prophylactic sulfadoxine (Fanasil) and 997 (1.0%) had skin reactions (107). Of these, about 100 had severe reactions, such as erythroderma with jaundice, Stevens–Johnson syndrome, or toxic epidermal necrolysis; 11 died from these complications, that is about one in 10 000 patients treated with the probably causative drug. It is not known how many would have had similar skin reactions unrelated to the drug. However, the benefit to risk balance of meningitis prophylaxis clearly favored the use of sulfonamides (110). A second report (111) showed an incidence of three cases of Stevens–Johnson syndrome in 480 healthy, newly recruited Bantu mineworkers treated prophylactically with sulfadimethoxine. In a third epidemiological study in Mozambique in 1981, 149 000 inhabitants in one town were given a single dose of sulfadoxine as mass prophylaxis in an attempt to stem an outbreak of cholera (110); 22 patients with typical Stevens–Johnson syndrome were admitted to hospital over 18 days; three died.

In one case toxic epidermal necrolysis caused by co-trimoxazole improved with high-dose methylprednisolone (120). However, previous studies of the use of glucocorticoids in toxic epidermal necrolysis have given contradictory results.

Most of the cutaneous adverse reactions to sulfonamides are associated with increased in vitro reactivity to sulfonamide metabolites, such as unstable hydroxylamines (121,122). In some cases glutathione deficiency has been proposed as a major mechanism. This seems to be important in patients with AIDS, in whom glutathione deficiency is frequent, and in whom skin rashes are much more common than in other patients (121,122). A predominance of slow acetylator phenotype has also been observed among patients with sulfonamide hypersensitivity reactions, and an association with the phenotypes HLA-A29, B-12, and DR-7 in patients with bullous cutaneous reactions (121,124–126).

Immunologic

Sulfa allergy refers to a specific hypersensitivity response to a group of chemicals containing a sulfonamide moiety covalently bound to a benzene ring; drugs structurally similar to sulfonamides may cross-react, for example sulfonylureas, thiazides, and furosemide (127). Sulfa allergy is most consistent with an immune-mediated reaction with delayed onset, 7–14 days after the start of therapy, characterized by fever, rash, and eosinophilia. IgG antibodies may be present and directed against proteins in the endoplasmic reticulum (about 80% of patients) or against the drug covalently bound to protein (about 5% of patients). High-dose methylprednisolone sodium succinate (250 mg every 6 hours for 48 hours) may not only alleviate the signs but also markedly attenuate the antibody response, as reported in a 19-year-old man (128).

Hypersusceptibility to sulfonamides has been proposed to be the mechanism for many adverse reactions, including anaphylactic shock, serum sickness-like syndrome, systemic allergic vasculitis, drug fever (up to 1–2% in some series), lupus-like syndrome, myocarditis, pulmonary infiltrates, interstitial nephritis, aseptic meningitis, hepatotoxicity, blood dyscrasias (agranulocytosis, thrombocytopenia, eosinophilia, pancytopenia), and a wide variety of skin reactions (urticaria, erythema nodosum, erythema multiforme, erythroderma, toxic epidermal necrolysis, and photosensitivity).

Urticarial and maculopapular rashes are the most frequent adverse reactions to sulfonamides after gastrointestinal symptoms. Although hypersusceptibility is suspected to be the mechanism for these adverse effects, type I allergic reactions, which are induced by IgE antibodies, have been confirmed only rarely. It appears that with the older sulfonamides severe reactions were more frequent. In some patients who have immediate hypersensitivity reactions to sulfonamides, IgE has been found that can bind to an N4-sulfonamidoyl determinant (N4-SM; 127).

- A 34-year-old man with a history of occasional mild episodes of presumed Crohn's disease developed a perirectal abscess and was given sulfasalazine 1 g qds (129). After stopping medication for a few weeks he started again and a day later developed a macular rash over his arms, later spreading to his trunk and lower extremities. He subsequently developed recurrent fevers of 103–104°F, moderate diarrhea, and diffuse abdominal pain. His liver function tests were abnormal and his white cell count was raised at 15.4 x 10^9/l. The sulfasalazine was withdrawn and he was given broad-spectrum antibiotics. Hepatitis serologies, a Monospot test, and blood cultures were all negative, but Epstein Barr virus serology showed a positive viral capsid IgG and negative IgM. An abdominal CT scan showed enlarged mesenteric and inguinal lymph nodes and a slightly enlarged spleen. Over the next 4 days he progressively worsened with worse liver function tests, leukocytosis, and a prolonged prothrombin time. He developed bloody diarrhea and needed transfusions. He became confused and had episodes of hallucinations. He rapidly improved with methylprednisolone 40 mg bd.

The authors proposed that this illness was due to a sulfonamide hypersensitivity reaction exacerbated by Epstein–Barr virus infection.

Prediction

It is desirable to predict hypersusceptibility reactions to sulfonamides. IgE-induced in vitro reactions to sulfonamides have mainly been studied in the last 15 years (130–132). A lymphocyte toxicity assay showed a positive result in about 70% of patients with a maculopapular rash, an urticarial reaction, or erythema multiforme (132). This biochemical test determines the percent of cell death due to toxic metabolites. The same in vitro reaction using the hydroxylamine metabolite of sulfamethoxazole gave significantly different results in six patients with fever and skin rash with or without hepatitis than in control patients (120). Unfortunately, in most adverse reactions it is not known whether the reaction is dose-related or allergic. Individual differences in metabolism predispose to idiosyncratic reactions, for example sulfonamides

are metabolized by *N*-acetylation (mediated by a genetically determined polymorphic enzyme) and oxidation to potentially toxic metabolites (124,125). Fever and rash were observed significantly more often in slow than in fast acetylators (124,125). Systemic glutathione deficiency, with a consequently reduced capacity to scavenge such toxic metabolites, might contribute to these adverse reactions, particularly in patients with AIDS (134,135). Unfortunately, there are no reliable in vitro tests to predict idiosyncratic reactions in vivo (120,121,124,125,135).

Cross-reactivity

The immunogenicity of sulfonamide antimicrobials may be due to the presence of an arylamine group at the N4 position of the sulfonamide molecule. Thus, allergic cross-reactions between different sulfonamides can occur. Therefore, in cases of known hypersusceptibility to a specific sulfonamide exposure to other sulfonamides should be avoided. Cross-reactions can even occur with *para*-aminosalicylic acid and local anesthetics of the procaine type; however, the real frequency of these cross-sensitivities is not known and their significance is undetermined. It should be noted that as many as 50% of patients with rash have recovered in spite of continued treatment with the same drug (137), and even agranulocytosis did not occur after later re-exposures to the causative agent (122).

Susceptibility factors

In an in vitro study, plasma from HIV-positive patients was less able to detoxify nitrososulfamethoxazole than control plasma, suggesting that a disturbance in redox balance in HIV-positive patients may alter metabolic detoxification capacity, thereby predisposing to sulfonamide hypersensitivity (138).

Types of reaction
Type I reactions
Anaphylactic shock occurs rarely with sulfonamides (121,130,136,139,140).

Type III reactions
A serum sickness-like syndrome has been observed during sulfonamide administration. This diagnosis should be limited to patients with at least three of the symptoms of classical serum sickness, that is fever, rash, allergic arthritis, lymphadenopathy, and possibly leukopenia or neutropenia. Histologically, severe serum sickness-like syndrome seems to correspond to an allergic vasculitis (93,141). Most of the descriptions of serum sickness-like syndrome with histopathological documentation have been associated with older sulfonamides that are no longer used (142). In some severe forms of serum sickness-like syndrome, the reaction can be complicated by a number of unusual organ manifestations, including plasmacytosis, lymphocytosis, monoclonal gammopathy (143,144), interstitial myocarditis (9), allergic pneumonitis, nephropathy, liver damage, and nervous system disorders (93,139).

Lupus-like syndromes

Sulfonamides can cause three different clinical and biological syndromes similar or identical to systemic lupus erythematosus (145,146):

1. exacerbation of pre-existing lupus erythematosus
2. triggering of lupus erythematosus in a susceptible patient
3. serum sickness-like syndrome resembling lupus erythematosus clinically and serologically.

There may be positive LE cells and antinuclear factors. In exacerbation or triggering of lupus erythematosus, two pathogenetic mechanisms may be involved:

1. a reaction to the pharmacological properties of the drug, such as occurs with other drugs, such as hydralazine, diphenylhydantoin, procainamide, isoniazid, and practolol (145–150);
2. a hypersensitivity reaction (146,151,152).

In type I reactions, exposure time, and especially re-exposure time, are usually longer than 1–2 months. In type II reactions, exposure is more variable, lasting from hours to days or up to 1–2 months (185–187). Some patients with ulcerative colitis have developed arthropathy, possibly polyserositis, hematological abnormalities, and even loss of consciousness with positive LE cell and antinuclear antibody tests during treatment with sulfasalazine (144,146).

Diagnosis

No diagnostic tests are available to confirm sulfonamide hypersensitivity, and while avoidance of the drug is generally appropriate when a previous hypersensitivity reaction is suspected, desensitization protocols are available for use in HIV patients in whom *Pneumocystis jiroveci* pneumonia prophylaxis or treatment is indicated (153).

Desensitization

Desensitization has been tried with sulfonamides and especially co-trimoxazole. Desensitization with the combination seems to be essential in patients with AIDS, since co-trimoxazole is the first choice against *Pneumocystis jiroveci* pneumonia and toxoplasmosis. Desensitization is successful in 75% of patients with AIDS (154–156). However, the procedure is not completely safe and even anaphylactic shock can occur (131).

Body temperature

Drug fever due to sulfonamides is usually accompanied by a skin reaction; however, fever without other manifestations can occur (125,126).

Long-Term Effects

Drug resistance

Salmonella typhimurium DT104 is usually resistant to ampicillin, chloramphenicol, streptomycin, sulfonamides, and tetracycline. An outbreak of 25 culture-confirmed cases of multidrug-resistant *S. typhimurium* DT104 has been identified in Denmark (157). The strain was resistant to the abovementioned antibiotics and nalidixic acid and had reduced susceptibility to fluoroquinolones. A swineherd was identified as the primary source (155). The DT104 strain was also found in cases of salmonellosis in Washington State, and soft cheese made with unpasteurized milk was identified as an important vehicle of its transmission (158).

Second-Generation Effects

Fertility

Male infertility with oligospermia has been reported during treatment with sulfasalazine (159,160). However, inflammatory bowel disease can also affect the maturation of spermatozoa (161).

Teratogenicity

The sulfonamides appear to have little if any effect on early human development. This is indicated by the absence of case reports or epidemiological survey data during pregnancy. In one study of 50 282 mother–child pairs, 1455 were exposed to sulfonamides during the first 4 months; there was no increase in the relative risk of any malformation (162,163).

Fetotoxicity

Sulfonamides should not be given to pregnant women in the third trimester of pregnancy. They can displace bilirubin from plasma albumin and cause kernicterus (bilirubin encephalopathy) (164–167). For the same reason, the administration of sulfonamides to lactating women or premature infants should be avoided. Successful treatment of neonatal hyperbilirubinemia with higher bilirubin concentrations has been established using exchange transfusion and phototherapy.

Susceptibility Factors

Genetic factors

The acetylator phenotype of a patient can affect the frequency and severity of adverse reactions to drugs that are metabolized by acetylation (42,124,125).

In patients with porphyria, sulfonamides should not be used (168).

Other features of the patient

Although patients with HIV infection are more likely to develop generalized skin reactions to sulfonamides, they can be used for prophylaxis and therapy.

Relative contraindications to sulfonamides are systemic lupus erythematosus and a known predisposition to lupus-like reactions. Allergic reactions to antimicrobials are frequent in patients with Sjögren's syndrome. They are especially susceptible to reactions to penicillins, cephalosporins, and sulfonamides, but reactions to macrolides and tetracyclines also seem to be over-represented in these patients (169).

Drug–Drug Interactions

Alkalis

Urine alkalinization increases the urinary excretion of sulfonamides (170,171).

References

1. Zinner SH, Mayer KH. Basic principles in the diagnosis and management of infectious diseases: sulfonamides and trimethoprim. In: Mandell GL, Douglas RG, Bennett JE, editors. Principles and Practice of Infectious Diseases. 4th ed.. Edinburgh: Churchill Livingstone, 1996:354.

2. Bushby SR, Hitchings GH. Trimethoprim, a sulphonamide potentiator. Br J Pharmacol Chemother 1968;33(1):72–90.

3. Ballin JC. Evaluation of a new topical agent for burn therapy. Silver sulfadiazine (silvadene). JAMA 1974;230(8):1184–5.

4. Lowbury EJ, Babb JR, Bridges K, Jackson DM. Topical chemoprophylaxis with silver sulphadiazine and silver nitrate chlorhexidine creams: emergence of sulphonamide-resistant Gram-negative bacilli. BMJ 1976;1(6008): 493–6.

5. Sutherland LR, May GR, Shaffer EA. Sulfasalazine revisited: a meta-analysis of 5-aminosalicylic acid in the treatment of ulcerative colitis. Ann Intern Med 1993;118(7):540–9.

6. US Congress. House Committee on Interstate and Foreign Commerce and Its Subcommittee on Public Health and Environment, 1974. In: A Brief Legislative History of the Food, Drug, and Cosmetic Act. Committee Print No. 14. Washington DC: US Government Printing Offices, 1974:1–4.

7. USA, 52 Stat. 1040, 75th Congress, 3rd session, 25 June, 1938.

8. USA vs Dotterweich, 1941.

9. French AJ, Weller CV. Interstitial myocarditis following the clinical and experimental use of sulfonamide drugs. Am J Pathol 1942;18:109.

10. Jones GR, Malone DN. Sulphasalazine induced lung disease. Thorax 1972;27(6):713–7.

11. Thomas P, Seaton A, Edwards J. Respiratory disease due to sulphasalazine. Clin Allergy 1974;4(1):41–7.

12. Scherpenisse J, van der Valk PD, van den Bosch JM, van Hees PA, Nadorp JH. Olsalazine as an alternative therapy in a patient with sulfasalazine-induced eosinophilic pneumonia. J Clin Gastroenterol 1988;10(2):218–20.

13. Wang KK, Bowyer BA, Fleming CR, Schroeder KW. Pulmonary infiltrates and eosinophilia associated with sulfasalazine. Mayo Clin Proc 1984;59(5):343–6.

14. Klinghoffer JF. Löffler's syndrome following use of a vaginal cream. Ann Intern Med 1954;40(2):343–50.

15. Fiegenberg DS, Weiss H, Kirshman H. Migratory pneumonia with eosinophilia associated with sulfonamide administration. Arch Intern Med 1967;120(1):85–9.

16. Crofton JW, Livingstone JL, Oswald NC, Roberts AT. Pulmonary eosinophilia. Thorax 1952;7(1):1–35.

17. Reeder WH, Goodrich BE. Pulmonary infiltration with eosinophilia (PIE syndrome). Ann Intern Med 1952; 36(5):1217–40.

18. Chumbley LC, Harrison EG Jr, DeRemee RA. Allergic granulomatosis and angiitis (Churg–Strauss syndrome).

Report and analysis of 30 cases. Mayo Clin Proc 1977; 52(8):477–84.

19. Loeffler W. Ueber flüchtige Lungenilfiltrate (mit Eosinophilie). Beitr Klin Tuberk 1932;79:368.

20. Ellis RV, McKinlay CA. Allergic pneumonia. J Lab Clin Med 1941;26:1427.

21. Von Meyenburg H. Das eosinophile Lungenilfilträt: pathologische Anatomie und Pathogenese. Schweiz Med Wochenschr 1942;72:809.

22. Ulubaş B, Sahin G, Ozer C, Aydin O, Ozgür E, Apaydin D. Bronchiolitis obliterans organizing pneumonia associated with sulfasalazine in a patient with rheumatoid arthritis. Clin Rheumatol 2004;23(3):249–51.

23. Plogge H. Ueber zentrale und periphere nervöse Schäden nach Eubasinummedikation. Dtsch Z Nervenheilkd 1940;151:205.

24. Bucy PC. Toxic optic neuritis resulting from sulfanilamide. JAMA 1937;109:1007.

25. Moorthy RS, Valluri S, Jampol LM. Drug-induced uveitis. Surv Ophthalmol 1998;42(6):557–70.

26. Anonymous. Drug-induced uveitis can usually be easily managed. Drugs Ther Perspect 1998;11:11–4.

27. Bovino JA, Marcus DF. The mechanism of transient myopia induced by sulfonamide therapy. Am J Ophthalmol 1982;94(1):99–102.

28. Hook SR, Holladay JT, Prager TC, Goosey JD. Transient myopia induced by sulfonamides. Am J Ophthalmol 1986;101(4):495–6.

29. Carlberg O. Zur Genese der Sulfonamidmyopie. Acta Ophthalmol 1942;20:275.

30. Wade A, Reynolds JE. In: Sulfonamides. London: The Pharmaceutical Press, 1982:1457.

31. Baumgartner A, Hoigné R, Müller U, et al. Medikamentöse Schäden des Blutbildes: Erfahrungen aus dem Komprehensiven Spital-Drug-Monitoring Bern, 1974–1979. Schweiz Med Wochenschr 1982;112:1530.

32. Muller U. Hämatologische Nebenwirkungen von Medikamenten. [Hematologic side effects of drugs.] Ther Umsch 1987;44(12):942–8.

33. Havas L, Fernex M, Lenox-Smith I. The clinical efficacy and tolerance of co-trimoxazole (Bactrim; Septrim). Clin Trials J 1973;3:81.

34. Hoigne R, Klein U, Muller U. Results of four-week course of therapy of urinary tract infections: a comparative study using trimethoprim with sulfamethoxazole (Bactrim; Roche) and trimethoprim alone. In: Hejzlar M, Semonsky M, Masak S, editors. Advances in Antimicrobial and Antineoplastic Chemotherapy. Munchen-Berlin-Wien: Urban and Schwarzenberg, 1972:1283.

35. Scott JL, Cartwright GE, Wintrobe MM. Acquired aplastic anemia: an analysis of thirty-nine cases and review of the pertinent literature. Medicine (Baltimore) 1959;38(2):119–72.

36. Zinkham WH. Unstable hemoglobins and the selective hemolytic action of sulfonamides. Arch Intern Med 1977;137(10):1365–6.

37. De Leeuw N, Shapiro L, Lowenstein L. Drug-induced hemolytic anemia. Ann Intern Med 1963;58:592–607.

38. Worlledge SM. Immune drug-induced haemolytic anemias. Semin Hematol 1969;6(2):181–200.

39. Fishman FL, Baron JM, Orlina A. Non-oxidative hemolysis due to salicylazosulfapyridine: evidence for an immune mechanism. Gastroenterology 1973;64:727.

40. Cohen SM, Rosenthal DS, Karp PJ. Ulcerative colitis and erythrocyte G6PD deficiency. Salicylazosulfapyridine-provoked hemolysis. JAMA 1968;205(7):528–30.

41. Meyer UA. Drugs in special patient groups: Clinical importance of genetics in drug effects. In: Melmon KL,

Morelli HF, Hoffman BB, Nierenberg DW, editors. Nelmon and Morelli's Clinical Pharmacology, Basic Principles in Therapeutics. 3rd ed.. New York-St Louis-San Francisco, etc: McGraw-Hill, 1992:875.

42. Frick PG, Hitzig WH, Stauffer U. Das Hämoglobin Zürich-Syndrom. [Hemoglobin-Zurich syndrome.] Schweiz Med Wochenschr 1961;91:1203–5.

43. Hitzig WH, Frick PG, Betke K, Huisman TH. Hämoglobin Zürich: eine neue Hämoglobinanomalie mit Sulfonamid-induzierter Innenkörperanämie. [Hemoglobin Zurich: a new hemoglobin anomaly with sulfonamide-induced inclusion body anemia.] Helv Paediatr Acta 1960;15:499–514.

44. Beretta A, Prato V, Gallo E, Lehmann H. Haemoglobin Torino—alpha-43 (CD1) phenylalanine replaced by valine. Nature 1968;217(133):1016–8.

45. Adams JG, Heller P, Abramson RK, Vaithianathan T. Sulfonamide-induced hemolytic anemia and hemoglobin Hasharon. Arch Intern Med 1977;137(10):1449–51.

46. Harris JW. Studies on the mechanism of a drug-induced hemolytic anemia. J Lab Clin Med 1956;47(5):760–75.

47. Beutler E. In: Red cell metabolism. Edinburgh/London: Churchill-Livingstone, 1986:16.

48. Gaetani GD, Mareni C, Ravazzolo R, Salvidio E. Haemolytic effect of two sulphonamides evaluated by a new method. Br J Haematol 1976;32(2):183–91.

49. Huisman TH. In: Hemoglobinopathies. Edinburgh/London: Churchill-Livingstone, 1986:15.

50. Shinton NK, Wilson C. Autoimmune haemolytic anaemia due to phenacetin and p-aminosalicylic acid. Lancet 1960;1:226.

51. Lyonnais J. Production de corps de Heinz associée à la prise de salicylazosulfapyridine. [Production of Heinz bodies after administration of salicylaszosulfapyridine.] Union Med Can 1976;105(2):203–5.

52. Streeter AM, Shum HY, O'Neill BJ. The effect of drugs on the microbiological assay of serum folic acid and vitamin B12 levels. Med J Aust 1970;1(18):900–1.

53. George JN, Raskob GE, Shah SR, Rizvi MA, Hamilton SA, Osborne S, Vondracek T. Drug-induced thrombocytopenia: a systematic review of published case reports. Ann Intern Med 1998;129(11):886–90.

54. Wright MS. Drug-induced hemolytic anemias: increasing complications to therapeutic interventions. Clin Lab Sci 1999;12(2):115–8.

55. Arneborn P, Palmblad J. Drug-induced neutropenia—a survey for Stockholm 1973–1978. Acta Med Scand 1982;212(5):289–92.

56. Baumelou E, Guiguet M, Mary JY. Epidemiology of aplastic anemia in France: a case-control study. I. Medical history and medication use. The French Cooperative Group for Epidemiological Study of Aplastic Anemia. Blood 1993;81(6):1471–8.

57. Anonymous. Anti-infective drug use in relation to the risk of agranulocytosis and aplastic anemia. A report from the International Agranulocytosis and Aplastic Anemia Study. Arch Intern Med 1989;149(5):1036–40.

58. Huerta C, Garcia Rodriguez LA. Risk of clinical blood dyscrasia in a cohort of antibiotic users. Pharmacotherapy 2002;22(5):630–6.

59. Johnston FD. Granulocytopenia following the administration of sulphanilamide compounds. Lancet 1938;2:1044.

60. Rinkoff SS, Spring M. Toxic depression of the myeloid elements following therapy with the sulfonamides: report of 8 cases. Ann Intern Med 1941;15:89.

61. Moeschlin S. Immunological granulocytopenia and agranulocytosis; clinical aspects. Sang 1955;26(1):32–51.

62. Rios Sanchez I, Duarte L, Sanchez Medal L. Agramulocitosis. Analisis de 29 episodes en 19 pacientes. [Agranulocytosis. Analysis of 29 episodes in 19 patients.] Rev Invest Clin 1971;23(1):29–42.

63. Ritz ND, Fisher MJ. Agranulocytosis due to administration of salicylazosulfapyridine (azulfidine). JAMA 1960;172:237.

64. Jarrett F, Ellerbe S, Demling R. Acute leukopenia during topical burn therapy with silver sulfadiazine. Am J Surg 1978;135(6):818–9.

65. Maurer LH, Andrews P, Rueckert F, McIntyre OR. Lymphocyte transformation observed in Sulfamylon agranulocytosis. Plast Reconstr Surg 1970;46(5):458–62.

66. Rhodes EG, Ball J, Franklin IM. Amodiaquine induced agranulocytosis: inhibition of colony growth in bone marrow by antimalarial agents. BMJ (Clin Res Ed) 1986;292(6522):717–8.

67. Fries J, Siragenian R. Sulfonamide hepatitis. Report of a case due to sulfamethoxazole and sulfisoxazole. N Engl J Med 1966;274(2):95–7.

68. Kaufman SF. A rare complication of sulfadimethoxine (Madribon) therapy. Calif Med 1967;107(4):344–5.

69. Konttinen A, Perasalo JO, Eisalo A. Sulfonamide hepatitis. Acta Med Scand 1972;191(5):389–91.

70. Konttinen A. Hepatotoxicity of sulphamethoxyridazine. BMJ 1972;2(806):168.

71. Sotolongo RP, Neefe LI, Rudzki C, Ishak KG. Hypersensitivity reaction to sulfasalazine with severe hepatotoxicity. Gastroenterology 1978;75(1):95–9.

72. Dujovne CA, Chan CH, Zimmerman HJ. Sulfonamide hepatic injury. Review of the literature and report of a case due to sulfamethoxazole. N Engl J Med 1967;277(15):785–8.

73. Tonder M, Nordoy A, Elgjo. Sulfonamide-induced chronic liver disease. Scand J Gastroenterol 1974;9(1):93–6.

74. Chester AC, Diamond LH, Schreiner GE. Hypersensitivity to salicylazosulfapyridine: renal and hepatic toxic reactions. Arch Intern Med 1978;138(7):1138–9.

75. Shaw DJ, Jacobs RP. Simultaneous occurrence of toxic hepatitis and Stevens–Johnson syndrome following therapy with sulfisoxazole and sulfamethoxazole. Johns Hopkins Med J 1970;126(3):130–3.

76. Block MB, Genant HK, Kirsner JB. Pancreatitis as an adverse reaction to salicylazosulfapyridine. N Engl J Med 1970;282(7):380–2.

77. Suryapranata H, De Vries H, et al. Pancreatitis associated with sulphasalazine. BMJ 1986;292:732.

78. Deprez P, Descamps C, Fiasse R. Pancreatitis induced by 5-aminosalicylic acid. Lancet 1989;2(8660):445–6.

79. Munk EM, Pedersen L, Floyd A, Nørgård B, Rasmussen HH, Sørensen HT. Inflammatory bowel diseases, 5-aminosalicylic acid and sulfasalazine treatment and risk of acute pancreatitis: a population-based case-control study. Am J Gastroenterol 2004;99(5):884–8.

80. Crespo M, Quereda C, Pascual J, Rivera M, Clemente L, Cano T. Patterns of sulfadiazine acute nephrotoxicity. Clin Nephrol 2000;54(1):68–72.

81. Perazella MA. Crystal-induced acute renal failure. Am J Med 1999;106(4):459–65.

82. Christin S, Baumelou A, Bahri S, Ben Hmida M, Deray G, Jacobs C. Acute renal failure due to sulfadiazine in patients with AIDS. Nephron 1990;55(2):233–4.

83. Miller MA, Gallicano K, Dascal A, Mendelson J. Sulfadiazine urolithiasis during antitoxoplasma therapy. Drug Invest 1993;5:334.

84. Simon DI, Brosius FC 3rd, Rothstein DM. Sulfadiazine crystalluria revisited. The treatment of *Toxoplasma*

encephalitis in patients with acquired immunodeficiency syndrome. Arch Intern Med 1990;150(11):2379–84.

85. Furrer H, von Overbeck J, Jaeger P, Hess B. Sulfadiazin-Nephrolithiasis und Nephropathie. [Sulfadiazine nephrolithiasis and nephropathy.] Schweiz Med Wochenschr 1994;124(46):2100–5.

86. Craig WA, Kunin CM. Trimethoprim–sulfamethoxazole: pharmacodynamic effects of urinary pH and impaired renal function. Studies in humans. Ann Intern Med 1973;78(4):491–7.

87. Carbone LG, Bendixen B, Appel GB. Sulfadiazine-associated obstructive nephropathy occurring in a patient with the acquired immunodeficiency syndrome. Am J Kidney Dis 1988;12(1):72–5.

88. Robson M, Levi J, Dolberg L, Rosenfeld JB. Acute tubulo-interstitial nephritis following sulfadiazine therapy. Isr J Med Sci 1970;6(4):561–6.

89. Baker SB, Williams RT. Acute interstitial nephritis due to drug sensitivity. BMJ 1963;5346:1655–8.

90. Pusey CD, Saltissi D, Bloodworth L, Rainford DJ, Christie JL. Drug associated acute interstitial nephritis: clinical and pathological features and the response to high dose steroid therapy. Q J Med 1983;52(206):194–211.

91. Cryst C, Hammar SP. Acute granulomatous interstitial nephritis due to co-trimoxazole. Am J Nephrol 1988;8(6):483–8.

92. Van Rijssel TG, Meyler L. Necrotizing generalized arteritis due to the use of sulfonamide drugs. Acta Med Scand 1948;132:251.

93. Cohen-Solal F, Abdelmoula J, Hoarau MP, Jungers P, Lacour B, Daudon M. Les lithiases urinaires d'origine medicamenteuse. [Urinary lithiasis of medical origin.] Therapie 2001;56(6):743–50.

94. Bigby M, Jick S, Jick H, Arndt K. Drug-induced cutaneous reactions. A report from the Boston Collaborative Drug Surveillance Program on 15,438 consecutive inpatients, 1975 to 1982. JAMA 1986;256(24):3358–63.

95. Sonntag MR, Zoppi M, Fritschy D, Maibach R, Stocker F, Sollberger J, Buchli W, Hess T, Hoigne R. Exantheme unter häufig angewandten Antibiotika und anti-bakteriellen Chemotherapeutika (Penicilline, speziell Aminopenicilline, Cephalosporine und Cotrimoxazol) sowie Allopurinol. [Exanthema during frequent use of antibiotics and antibacterial drugs (penicillin, especially aminopenicillin, cephalosporin and cotrimoxazole) as well as allopurinol. Results of The Berne Comprehensive Hospital Drug Monitoring Program.] Schweiz Med Wochenschr 1986;116(5):142–5.

96. Hunziker T, Braunschweig S, Zehnder D, Hoigné R, Kunzi UP. Comprehensive Hospital Drug Monitoring (CHDM) adverse skin reactions, a 20-year survey. Allergy 1997;52(4):388–93.

97. Arndt KA, Jick H. Rates of cutaneous reactions to drugs. A report from the Boston Collaborative Drug Surveillance Program. JAMA 1976;235(9):918–23.

98. Gomez B, Sastre J, Azofra J, Sastre A. Fixed drug eruption. Allergol Immunopathol (Madr) 1985;13(2):87–91.

99. Ibia EO, Schwartz RH, Wiedermann BL. Antibiotic rashes in children: a survey in a private practice setting. Arch Dermatol 2000;136(7):849–54.

100. Tonev S, Vasileva S, Kadurina M. Depot sulfonamid associated linear IgA bullous dermatosis with erythema multiforme-like clinical features. J Eur Acad Dermatol Venereol 1998;11(2):165–8.

101. Kauppinen K, Stubb S. Fixed eruptions: causative drugs and challenge tests. Br J Dermatol 1985;112(5):575–8.

102. Pasricha JS. Drugs causing fixed eruptions. Br J Dermatol 1979;100(2):183–5.

103. Sehgal VN, Rege VL, Kharangate VN. Fixed drug eruptions caused by medications: a report from India. Int J Dermatol 1978;17(1):78–81.

104. Rollof SI. Erythema nodosum in association with sulphathiazole in children; a clinical investigation with special reference to primary tuberculosis. Acta Tuberc Scand Suppl 1950;24:1–215.

105. Kuokkanen K. Drug eruptions. A series of 464 cases in the Department of Dermatology, University of Turku, Finland, during 1966–1970. Acta Allergol 1972;27(5):407–38.

106. Epstein JH. Photoallergy. A review. Arch Dermatol 1972;106(5):741–8.

107. Harber LC, Bickers DR, Armstrong RB, et al. Drug photosensitivity: phototoxic and photoallergic mechanisms. Semin Dermatol 1982;1:183.

108. Connor EE. Sulfonamide antibiotics. Prim Care Update Ob Gyns 1998;5:32–5.

109. Bottiger LE, Strandberg I, Westerholm B. Drug-induced febrile mucocutaneous syndrome with a survey of the literature. Acta Med Scand 1975;198(3):229–33.

110. Bergoend H, Loffler A, Amar R, Maleville J. Réactions cutanées survenues au cours de la prophylaxie de masse de la méningite cérébrospinale par un sulfamide long-rétard (à propos de 997 cas). [Cutaneous reactions appearing during the mass prophylaxis of cerebrospinal meningitis with a long-delayed action sulfonamide (apropos of 997 cases).] Ann Dermatol Syphiligr (Paris) 1968;95(5):481–90.

111. Taylor GM. Stevens–Johnson syndrome following the use of an ultra-long-acting sulphonamide. S Afr Med J 1968;42(20):501–3.

112. Hernborg A. Stevens–Johnson syndrome after mass prophylaxis with sulfadoxine for cholera in Mozambique. Lancet 1985;2(8463):1072–3.

113. Lyell A. A review of toxic epidermal necrolysis in Britain. Br J Dermatol 1967;79(12):662–71.

114. Bjornberg A. Fifteen cases of toxic epidermal necrolysis (Lyell). Acta Dermatol Venereol 1973;53(2):149–52.

115. Cohlan SQ. Erythema multiforme exudativum associated with use of sulfamethoxypyridazine. JAMA 1960;173:799–800.

116. Gottschalk HR, Stone OJ. Stevens–Johnson syndrome from ophthalmic sulfonamide. Arch Dermatol 1976;112(4):513–4.

117. Hoigne R. Interne Manifestationen und Labor-befunde beim Lyell-Syndrom. In: Braun-Falco O, Bandmann HJ, editors. Das Lyell-Syndrom. Bern-Stuttgart-Wien: Verlag H Huber, 1970:27.

118. Revuz J, Roujeau JC, Guillaume JC, Penso D, Touraine R. Treatment of toxic epidermal necrolysis. Creteil's experience. Arch Dermatol 1987;123(9):1156–8.

119. Amon RB, Dimond RL. Toxic epidermal necrolysis. Rapid differentiation between staphylococcal- and drug-induced disease. Arch Dermatol 1975;111(11):1433–7.

120. Soylu H, Akkol N, Erduran E, Aslan Y, Gunes Z, Yildiran A. Co-trimoxazole-induced toxic epidermal necrolysis treated with high dose methylprednisolone. Ann Med Sci 2000;9:38–40.

121. Shear NH, Rieder MJ, Spielberg SP, et al. Hypersensitivity reactions to sulfonamide antibiotics are mediated by a hydroxylamine metabolite. Clin Res 1987;35:717.

122. Shear NH, Spielberg SP. In vitro evaluation of a toxic metabolite of sulfadiazine. Can J Physiol Pharmacol 1985;63(11):1370–2.

123. Nixon N, Eckert JF, Holmesk B. The treatment of agranulocytosis with sulfadiazine. Am J Med Sci 1943;206:713.

124. Roujeau JC, Bracq C, Huyn NT, Chaussalet E, Raffin C, Duedari N. HLA phenotypes and bullous cutaneous reactions to drugs. Tissue Antigens 1986;28(4):251–4.

125. Shear NH, Spielberg SP, Grant DM, Tang BK, Kalow W. Differences in metabolism of sulfonamides predisposing to idiosyncratic toxicity. Ann Intern Med 1986;105(2):179–84.

126. Rieder MJ, Shear NH, Kanee A, Tang BK, Spielberg SP. Prominence of slow acetylator phenotype among patients with sulfonamide hypersensitivity reactions. Clin Pharmacol Ther 1991;49(1):13–7.

127. Dwenger CS. 'Sulpha' hypersensitivity. Anaesthesia 2000;55(2):200–1.

128. Bedard K, Smith S, Cribb A. Sequential assessment of an antidrug antibody response in a patient with a systemic delayed-onset sulphonamide hypersensitivity syndrome reaction. Br J Dermatol 2000;142(2):253–8.

129. Halmos B, Anastopoulos HT, Schnipper LE, Ballesteros E. Extreme lymphoplasmacytosis and hepatic failure associated with sulfasalazine hypersensitivity reaction and a concurrent EBV infection—case report and review of the literature. Ann Hematol 2004;83(4):242–6.

130. Carrington DM, Earl HS, Sullivan TJ. Studies of human IgE to a sulfonamide determinant. J Allergy Clin Immunol 1987;79(3):442–7.

131. Sher MR, Suchar C, Lockey RF. Anaphylactic shock induced by oral desensitization to trimethoprim/sulfmethoxazole. J Allergy Immunol 1986;77:133.

132. Gruchalla RS, Sullivan TJ. Detection of human IgE to sulfamethoxazole by skin testing with sulfamethoxazoyl-poly-L-tyrosine. J Allergy Clin Immunol 1991;88(5):784–92.

133. Ghajar BM, Naranjo CA, Shear NH, Lanctot KL. Improving the accuracy of the differential diagnosis of idiosyncratic adverse drug reactions (IADRs): skin eruptions and sulfonamides. Clin Pharmacol Ther 1990;47(2):127.

134. Delomenie C, Mathelier-Fusade P, Longuemaux S, Rozenbaum W, Leynadier F, Krishnamoorthy R, Dupret JM. Glutathione S-transferase (GSTM1) null genotype and sulphonamide intolerance in acquired immunodeficiency syndrome. Pharmacogenetics 1997;7(6):519–20.

135. Coopman SA, Johnson RA, Platt R, Stern RS. Cutaneous disease and drug reactions in HIV infection. N Engl J Med 1993;328(23):1670–4.

136. Woody RC, Brewster MA. Adverse effects of trimethoprim–sulfamethoxazole in a child with dihydropteridine reductase deficiency. Dev Med Child Neurol 1990;32(7):639–42.

137. Kreuz W, Gungor T, Lotz C, Funk M, Kornhuber B. "Treating through" hypersensitivity to cotrimoxazole in children with HIV infection. Lancet 1990;336(8713):508–9.

138. Naisbitt DJ, Vilar FJ, Stalford AC, Wilkins EG, Pirmohamed M, Park BK. Plasma cysteine deficiency and decreased reduction of nitrososulfamethoxazole with HIV infection. AIDS Res Hum Retroviruses 2000;16(18):1929–38.

139. Binns PM. Anaphylaxis after oral sulphadiazine; two reactions in the same patient within eight days. Lancet 1958;1(7013):194–5.

140. Reichmann J. Anaphylaktischer Schock durch intravenöse Sulfonamidapplikation mit letalem Ausgang. [Anaphylactic shock caused by intravenous sulfonamide application with fatal outcome.] Dtsch Gesundheitsw 1960;15:1139–41.

141. Rich AR. Additional evidence of the role of hypersensitivity in the etiology of periarteritis nodosa. Bull Johns Hopkins Hosp 1942;71:375.

142. Zeek PM, Smith CC, Weeter JC. Studies on periarteritis nodosa. III. Differentiation between vascular lesions of periarteritis nodosa and of hypersensitivity. Am J Pathol 1948;24:889.

143. Delage C, Lagace R. Maladie sérique avec hyperplasie ganglionnaire pseudo-lymphomateuse secondaire à la prise de salicylazosulfapyridine. [Serum sickness with pseudolymphomatous lymph node hyperplasia caused by salicylazosulfapyridine.] Union Med Can 1975;104(4):579–84.

144. Han T, Chawla PL, Sokal JE. Sulfapyridine-induced serum-sickness-like syndrome associated with plasmacytosis, lymphocytosis and multiclonal gamma-globulinopathy. N Engl J Med 1969;280(10):547–8.

145. Lee SL, Rivero I, Siegel M. Activation of systemic lupus erythematosus by drugs. Arch Intern Med 1966;117(5):620–6.

146. Hoigne R, Biedermann HP, Naegeli HR. INH-induzierter systemischer Lupus erythematodes: 2. Beobachtungen mit Reexposition. Schweiz Med Wochenschr 1975;105:1726.

147. Clementz GL, Dolin BJ. Sulfasalazine-induced lupus erythematosus. Am J Med 1988;84(3 Pt 1):535–8.

148. Alarcon-Segovia D. Drug-induced lupus syndromes. Mayo Clin Proc 1969;44(9):664–81.

149. Griffiths ID, Kane SP. Sulphasalazine-induced lupus syndrome in ulcerative colitis. BMJ 1977;2(6096):1188–9.

150. Hess E. Drug-related lupus. N Engl J Med 1988;318(22):1460–2.

151. Cohen P, Gardner FH. Sulfonamide reactions in systemic lupus erythematosus. JAMA 1966;197(10):817–9.

152. Honey M. Systemic lupus erythematosus presenting with sulphonamide hypersensitivity reaction. BMJ 1956;(4978):1272–5.

153. Tilles SA. Practical issues in the management of hypersensitivity reactions: sulfonamides. South Med J 2001;94(8):817–24.

154. Torgovnick J, Arsura E. Desensitization to sulfonamides in patients with HIV infection. Am J Med 1990;88(5):548–9.

155. Finegold I. Oral desensitization to trimethoprim–sulfamethoxazole in a patient with acquired immunodeficiency syndrome. J Allergy Clin Immunol 1986;78(5 Pt 1):905–8.

156. Papakonstantinou G, Fuessl H, Hehlmann R. Trimethoprim-sulfamethoxazole desensitization in AIDS. Klin Wochenschr 1988;66(8):351–3.

157. Villar RG, Macek MD, Simons S, Hayes PS, Goldoft MJ, Lewis JH, Rowan LL, Hursh D, Patnode M, Mead PS. Investigation of multidrug-resistant *Salmonella* serotype typhimurium DT104 infections linked to raw-milk cheese in Washington State. JAMA 1999;281(19):1811–6.

158. Molbak K, Baggesen DL, Aarestrup FM, Ebbesen JM, Engberg J, Frydendahl K, Gerner-Smidt P, Petersen AM, Wegener HC. An outbreak of multidrug-resistant, quinolone-resistant *Salmonella enterica* serotype typhimurium DT104. N Engl J Med 1999;341(19):1420–5.

159. Levi AJ, Toovey S, Hudson E. Male infertility due to sulphasalazine. Gastroenterology 1981;80:1208.

160. Tobias R, Sapire KE, Coetzee T, Marks IN. Male infertility due to sulphasalazine. Postgrad Med J 1982;58(676):102–3.

161. Karbach U, Ewe K, Schramm P. Samenqualität bei Patienten mit Morbus Crohn. [Quality of semen in patients with Crohn's disease.] Z Gastroenterol 1982;20(6):314–20.

162. Heinonen OP, Slone D, Shapiro S. Antimicrobial and antiparasitic agents. In: Heinonen OP, Slone D, Shapiro S, editors. Birth Defects and Drugs in Pregnancy. 4th ed.. Boston-Bristol-London: John Wright PSG Inc, 1982:296.

163. Karkinen-Jaaskelainen, Saxen L. Maternal influenza, drug consumption, and congenital defects of the central nervous system. Am J Obstet Gynecol 1974;118(6):815–8.

164. Brodersen R. Prevention of kernicterus, based on recent progress in bilirubin chemistry. Acta Paediatr Scand 1977;66(5):625–34.

165. Diamond I, Schmid R. Experimental bilirubin encephalopathy. The mode of entry of bilirubin-14C into the central nervous system. J Clin Invest 1966;45(5):678–89.
166. Andersen DH, Blanc WA, Crozier DN, Silverman WA. A difference in mortality rate and incidence of kernicterus among premature infants allotted to two prophylactic antibacterial regimens. Pediatrics 1956;18(4):614–25.
167. Wadsworth SJ, Suh B. In vitro displacement of bilirubin by antibiotics and 2-hydroxybenzoylglycine in newborns. Antimicrob Agents Chemother 1988;32(10):1571–5.
168. Peterkin GA, Khan SA. Iatrogenic skin disease. Practitioner 1969;202(207):117–26.
169. Antonen JA, Markula KP, Pertovaara MI, Pasternack AI. Adverse drug reactions in Sjögren's syndrome. Frequent allergic reaction and a specific trimethoption associated systemic reaction. Scand J Pheumatol 1999;28(3):157–9.
170. Hartshorn EA. Drug interaction. Drug Intell 1968;2:174.
171. Kabins SA. Interactions among antibiotics and other drugs. JAMA 1972;219(2):206–12.

Thioguanine

See also Azathioprine

General Information

Thioguanine (6-thioguanine) is a thiopurine closely related to mercaptopurine and azathioprine. It is a metabolic product after the administration of both those drugs. It is being increasingly used as an alternative in patients with inflammatory bowel disease who are intolerant of or refractory to azathioprine, 6-mercaptopurine, or methotrexate.

Observational studies

Thioguanine 40 mg /day for 24 weeks was evaluated in 37 patients with chronic active Crohn's disease (1). Adverse events included headache (n = 17), minor infections (n = 11), nausea (n = 10), eczema (n = 4), pruritus (n = 3), arthralgia (n = 3), alopecia (n = 3), leukopenia (n = 2), vomiting (n = 2), photoallergic reactions (n = 2), rashes (n = 2), raised transaminases (n = 2), dysesthesia (n = 1), erythema nodosum (n = 1), rotavirus infection (n = 1), anemia (n = 1), thrombocytopenia (n = 1), and pancreatitis (n = 1). Treatment with withdrawn in six patients because of leukopenia (n = 2), headache (n = 2), mild pancreatitis (n = 1), or pneumonia (n = 1). Thioguanine was more effective in azathioprine-intolerant than in azathioprine-refractory patients.

In 32 patients with inflammatory bowel disease intolerant of azathioprine/mercaptopurine, thioguanine 20 mg/day (n = 19) or 40 mg/day (n = 13) had to be withdrawn in six because of adverse effects, including nausea, diarrhea, malaise, fever, arthralgia, stomach cramps, and rigid fingers (2). Two patients taking thioguanine 40 mg/day developed joint pains that resolved after dosage reduction.

Organs and Systems

Liver

Thioguanine caused laboratory abnormalities in 29 of 111 patients with inflammatory bowel disease (3). Raised liver enzymes and reduced platelet counts (below 200 x 10^9/l) were most commonly observed. Male sex (OR = 2.9; 95%CI = 1.1, 7.3) and preferential 6-methylmercaptopurine production after the administration of mercaptopurine/azathioprine (OR = 3.0; 95%CI = 1.2, 7.4) were independently associated with laboratory abnormalities. There was no association with duration of thioguanine treatment, cumulative dose, or thioguanine nucleotide concentrations. The median increases in transaminase and alkaline phosphatase activity were 39, 30, and 75 U/L respectively and the median reduction in platelet count was 115 x 10^9/l. Nodular regenerative hyperplasia occurred in 76% of the patients with abnormal liver function tests who underwent biopsy compared with and 33% of those who did not have abnormal liver function tests. Nodular regenerative hyperplasia is therefore common in thioguanine-treated patients with inflammatory bowel disease and its progression and reversibility are unknown. Thioguanine should therefore not be used in patients with inflammatory bowel disease.

A patient taking thioguanine for a flare of Crohn's disease developed abnormal liver function tests in the absence of other offending agents (4).

- A 27 year old man with a 10-year history of Crohn's disease, intolerance of azathioprine and infliximab, and failure to respond to methotrexate and prednisone was given thioguanine 40 mg/day. After 2 weeks, he complained lower abdominal pain. The erythrocyte thioguanine nucleotide concentration was 1.156 pmol/8 x 10^8 cells and 6-methylmercaptopurine was undetectable. After 4 weeks the alanine transaminase activity peaked at 803 IU/l and thioguanine was withdrawn. The alanine transaminase returned to normal within 1 month. The TPMT activity was 7.9 U/ml of erythrocytes, consistent with a heterozygote genotype for TPMT.

Out of 95 patients with inflammatory bowel disease who were intolerant of azathioprine or 6-mercaptopurine 20 stopped taking low-dose 6-thioguanine maintenance therapy (mean 25 mg) [5]. The reasons for withdrawal of 6- thioguanine were gastrointestinal complaints (31%), malaise (15%), and hepatotoxicity (15%). Of 75 patients who continued to take 6-thioguanine, seven had hepatotoxicity. Therefore, 6-thioguanine should be administered only in prospective trials.

Immunologic

Thioguanine hypersensitivity occurred in four of 21 patients with inflammatory bowel disease and azathioprine/mercaptopurine intolerance, including two with gastroenteritis-like syndromes and two with nausea and flu-like symptoms (6).

Long-Term Effects

Tumorigenicity

The risk of lymphoma may be increased by about fourfold in patients with inflammatory bowel disease taking thiopurines, as a result of the medications, the severity of the underlying disease, or a combination of the two [7].

Increased chemical reactivity of DNA 6-thioguanine is an important contributor to its antileukemic effects. The same enhanced reactivity may contribute to the increased risk of acute myeloid leukaemia and skin cancer in thiopurine-treated organ transplant patients [8].

Second-Generation Effects

Pregnancy

Data on the use of 6-thioguanine in pregnancy are rare and controversial. Two patients with Crohn's disease took low doses of 6-thioguanine throughout their pregnancies [9]. The two infants were healthy, without congenital abnormalities and or laboratory signs of myelosuppression or hepatocellular injury. The infants had significantly lower concentrations of 6-thioguanine nucleotides in their erythrocytes (ratio 1:12) than the mothers.

Susceptibility Factors

Genetic

See azathioprine.

References

1. Herrlinger KR, Kreisel W, Schwab M, Schoelmerich J, Fleig WE, Ruhl A, Reinshagen M, Deibert P, Fellermann K, Greinwald R, Stange EF. 6-Thioguanine – efficacy and safety in chronic active Crohn's disease. Aliment Pharmacol Ther 2003;17:503-8.
2. Derijks LJJ, de Jong DJ, Glissen LPL, Engels LGJB, Hooymans PM, Jansen JMBJ, Mulder CJJ. 6-Thioguanine seems promising in azathioprine- or 6-mercaptopurine-intolerant inflammatory bowel disease patients: a short-term saftey assessment. Eur J Gastroenterol Hepatol 2003;15:63-7.
3. Dubinsky MC, Vasiliauskas EA, Singh H, Abreu MT, Papadakis KA, Tran T, Martin P, Vierling JM, Geller SA, Targan SR, Poordad FF. 6-thioguanine can cause serious liver injury in inflammatory bowel disease patients. Gastroenterology 2003;125:298-303.
4. Rulyak SJ, Saunders MD, Lee SD. Hepatotoxicity associated with 6-thioguanine therapy for Crohn's disease. J Clin Gastroenterol 2003;36:234-7.
5. de Boer NK, Derijks LJ, Gilissen LP, Hommes DW, Engels LG, de Boer SY et al. On tolerability and safety of a maintenance treatment with 6-thioguanine in azathioprine or 6-mercaptopurine intolerant IBD patients. World J Gastroenterol 2005;11(35):5540-4.
6. Dubinsky MC, Feldman EJ, Abreu MT, Targam SR, Vasiliauskas EA. Thioguanine: a potential alternate thiopurine for IBD patients allergic to 6-mercaptopurine or azathioprine. Am J Gastroenterol 2003;98:1058-63.
7. McGovern DP, Jewell DP. Risks and benefits of azathioprine therapy. Gut 2005;54(8):1055-9.
8. Karran P. Thiopurines, DNA damage, DNA repair and therapy-related cancer. Br Med Bull 2006;79-80:153-70.
9. de Boer NK, Van Elburg RM, Wilhelm AJ, Remmink AJ, Van Vugt JM, Mulder CJ, Van Bodegraven AA. 6-Thioguanine for Crohn's disease during pregnancy: thiopurine metabolite measurements in both mother and child. Scand J Gastroenterol 2005;40(11):1374-7.

DRUGS USED IN THE TREATMENT OF GOUT

Allopurinol

General Information

Allopurinol is an inhibitor of xanthine oxidase, used to lower serum uric acid concentrations in the long-term treatment of gout and in the prevention of acute gout in people who are susceptible to hyperuricemia. Allopurinol is itself metabolized to its active metabolite, oxipurinol, by xanthine oxidase.

Comparisons with antimonials in leishmaniasis

Allopurinol has an antileishmanial effect in vitro and in animals, its effect being strongly increased by the addition of antimonial compounds. Allopurinol alone as well as in combination with meglumine antimoniate has been used in clinical studies. In a small study in patients with leishmaniasis and HIV infection, clinical and parasitological cure was achieved in four of five cases treated for 4 weeks, but in only one of the six treated for 3 weeks (1).

Allopurinol and meglumine antimoniate (Glucantime) have been evaluated in a randomized controlled trial in 150 patients with cutaneous leishmaniasis (2). They received oral allopurinol (15 mg/kg/day) for 3 weeks or intramuscular meglumine antimoniate (30 mg/kg/day, corresponding to 8 mg/kg/day of pentavalent antimony, for 2 weeks), or combined therapy. There were a few adverse effects in those who used allopurinol: nausea, heartburn ($n = 3$), and mild increases in transaminases ($n = 2$). These symptoms subsided on drug withdrawal.

In an open study, 72 patients each received meglumine antimoniate (60 mg/kg/day) or allopurinol (20 mg/kg/day) plus low-dose meglumine antimoniate (30 mg/kg/day) for 20 days, and each was followed for 30 days after the end of treatment (3). Only six patients in the combined treatment group complained of mild abdominal pain and nausea; however, one patient who received meglumine antimoniate developed a skin eruption. Generalized muscle pain and weakness occurred in four patients.

Organs and Systems

Nervous system

Apart from headache and vertigo, adverse effects of allopurinol involving the nervous system are rare. Transient peripheral neuropathy has been reported (SEDA-18, 107).

Seizures, which were unresponsive to standard anticonvulsive therapy, disappeared when allopurinol was withdrawn in a patient with a primary neurological disorder (4).

In contrast, occasional reports that allopurinol may have an anticonvulsive effect prompted its use in therapy-resistant epileptic patients. Withdrawal in one of these patients precipitated a convulsive status epilepticus (SEDA-16, 114).

- A 60-year-old man developed aseptic meningitis after taking allopurinol on two separate occasions (5).

Sensory systems

Allopurinol can reportedly cause cataracts (6), but in one study there was no evidence to confirm this risk (SEDA-15, 104).

Hematologic

Eosinophilia and leukocytosis are part of a general hypersensitivity reaction to allopurinol. Leukopenia and neutropenia are sometimes associated with allopurinol. Patients taking cytostatic therapy are more susceptible to bone marrow depression if they take allopurinol as well (SED-9, 155); however, this has not been confirmed in other reports (7). Agranulocytosis is extremely rare.

Cases of aplastic anemia, some in patients with renal insufficiency, have been reported (SEDA-13, 84; 8–10), confirming the need to reduce the dose of allopurinol in patients with renal insufficiency and to monitor toxicity (SEDA-16, 114).

- Pure red cell aplasia occurred in a 79-year-old man taking allopurinol (dosage not stated) (11). The anemia promptly resolved after withdrawal, strongly supporting a drug effect.

Liver

Hepatitis can be part of a generalized hypersensitivity reaction. Hepatotoxicity ranges from mild granulomatous hepatitis to severe hepatocellular necrosis (SED-5, 155; SEDA-4, 70). Renal impairment seems to be a prerequisite for a severe hepatic reaction.

Urinary tract

Vasculitis due to a general hypersensitivity reaction can cause renal insufficiency and oliguria. Histological findings are vasculitis and tubular necrosis with fibrinoid deposits. Acute renal insufficiency due to xanthine crystals in the kidney tubules during antineoplastic chemotherapy has been reported (12).

Since allopurinol blocks xanthine conversion to uric acid, urinary xanthine excretion is increased, creating a risk of xanthine crystal formation in the urinary system or even in muscles; this can result in nephrolithiasis (13). It is still an open question whether a predisposition to renal disease or renal disease itself is required to precipitate these adverse effects. It is also not known whether increased excretion of orotic acid, due to an interaction of allopurinol with pyrimidine formation, has any consequences for these adverse effects or for its role in reducing glucose tolerance.

Granulomatous interstitial nephritis (SEDA-12, 94) and two cases of interstitial cystitis have been described during long-term treatment with allopurinol (SEDA-21, 108).

- A 79-year-old man without a history of allergies; developed a granulomatous interstitial nephritis after he had taken allopurinol for 10 years (14).

Skin

Skin reactions to allopurinol have a general incidence of 10%, are more common in patients with renal disorders and in those taking thiazide diuretics, and are closely correlated with persistently high serum concentrations of oxipurinol (15). The positive association of severe skin reactions with HLA haplotypes AW33 and B17 suggests a genetic predisposition to these reactions (16).

Rash, urticaria, erythematous eruptions, papulovesicular reactions, and pruritus may be the only signs of hypersensitivity or may be part of a generalized reaction.

Dangerous reactions such as exfoliative dermatitis and Lyell's syndrome rarely develop (SEDA-5, 108).

Unusual skin lesions with a benign lymphocyte infiltration have been documented (SEDA-14, 96). Toxic pustuloderma can be added to the list (SEDA-18, 108).

An allopurinol-induced fixed drug eruption was successfully treated by desensitization (SEDA-21, 108).

Allopurinol can uncover latent lichen planus (17).

- A 59-year-old man, who had taken Zyloric® tablets 100 mg (allopurinol, lactose, povidone, magnesium stearate, corn starch; Laboratoires Glaxo Wellcome, Marly-le-Roy, France) for 15 years developed a maculopapular rash 3 days after switching to a generic substitute, Allopurinol Ge® (allopurinol, yellow beeswax, hydrogenated soy, vegetable oils, peanut oil, soy lecithin, polysorbate 80, ethylparahydroxybenzoate, gelatine, glycerol, sorbitol, sorbitan, yellow iron oxide, titanium dioxide; Laboratoires Eurogenerics, Boulogne Billancourt, France) (18). This was withdrawn, and 4 days later the rash resolved spontaneously. Histology showed perivascular lymphohistiocytic infiltration with polymorphonuclear eosinophils. Two months later he took Zyloric again and 3 days later developed generalized itchy eczematous plaques, with more severe involvement in flexures. Three months later Zyloric was withdrawn and the rash resolved in 3 days. Patch tests with the standard series of excipients and preservatives, allopurinol 10% in petrolatum, water, and alcohol, Allopurinol Ge 30% in petrolatum, water, and alcohol, Zyloric 30% in petrolatum, water, and alcohol, and the excipients of two commercial formulations (glycerol, sorbitol 10% in water, titanium dioxide 10% in water, hydrogenated soy, peanut oil, soy lecithin, gelatine, methylparahydroxybenzoate, ethylparahydroxybenzoate, and propylparahydroxybenzoate), and pricks tests with allopurinol, Zyloric, Allopurinol Ge, and their excipients were all negative.

The authors suggested that something about the generic allopurinol formulation may have sensitized this patient to allopurinol.

Generalized eosinophilic pustular folliculitis has been reported in a 71-year-old Cambodian man who took allopurinol for 8 weeks; the rash resolved over 8 weeks after withdrawal of allopurinol and treatment with oral and topical corticosteroids (19).

Musculoskeletal

Myositis and rhabdomyolysis have been attributed to allopurinol (20).

- A 73-year-old woman with chronic renal insufficiency developed generalized muscular weakness and pain 6 days after starting to take allopurinol 200 mg/day. Her serum creatine kinase activity was increased and the diagnosis was rhabdomyolysis, attributed to severe myositis. The serum concentration of oxipurinol was also high. The muscle weakness resolved in 7 weeks with intermittent hemodiafiltration.

Fever, myalgia, and arthralgia have been reported in a patient taking captopril and allopurinol (21).

Acute gout can be exacerbated at the beginning of allopurinol treatment unless the drug is combined with colchicine or an anti-inflammatory drug (22).

Immunologic

Hypersensitivity reactions to allopurinol occur in about 10–15% of patients. Desensitization with both oral and intravenous allopurinol has been successful (SEDA-17, 114). In the allopurinol hypersensitivity syndrome, the skin is most prominently involved (23). Symptoms develop after 2–5 weeks of treatment. Hepatic involvement is present in 40% and renal involvement in 45%; 25% of patients have combined renal and hepatic lesions. The hypersensitivity syndrome has been estimated to occur in 1 in 1000 hospitalized patients. A major complication is an extensive cutaneous staphylococcal infection with septicemia and endocarditis. Gastrointestinal hemorrhage, disseminated intravascular coagulation, adult respiratory distress syndrome, cerebral vasculitis, and peripheral axonal neuropathy have also been described (SEDA-21, 109). Death occurs in 20–30% of patients with severe hypersensitivity syndrome.

There are reports of a possible association between severe drug-induced erythema multiforme and reactivation of infection with human herpesvirus 6. The reactivation is thought to have contributed in some way to the development of allopurinol hypersensitivity reactions (24,25). Epstein-Barr virus has also been implicated (26).

Allopurinol has been associated, albeit rarely, with pANCA (antineutrophil cytoplasmic antibodies with a peripheral pattern) positivity. A generalized cutaneous vasculitis has been associated with the presence in the serum of pANCA and antimyeloperoxidase antibodies (27). A skin biopsy of a lesion showed leukocytoclastic vasculitis with eosinophilic infiltration. Allopurinol was withdrawn and the symptoms resolved completely. The possible drug causes of ANCA-positive vasculitis with high titers of antimyeloperoxidase antibodies in 30 new patients have been reviewed (28). The findings illustrate that this type of vasculitis is a predominantly drug-induced disorder. Only 12 of the 30 cases were not related to a drug. Allopurinol was implicated in two of the other 18 cases.

Treatment of the allopurinol hypersensitivity syndrome includes drug withdrawal and the administration of systemic corticosteroids (prednisone 40–200 mg/day) for several months. Desensitization strategies allow some patients to resume allopurinol therapy later without any further problem (29–31). The standard desensitization protocol consists of an initial allopurinol dosage of 50 μg/day, increasing every 3 days to a target of 50–100 mg/day. The interval between dosage increases can be extended to 5 days or more in elderly patients with multiple co-morbidity. Using this protocol, desensitization was successful in 25 out of 32 patients (78%); 28 patients completed the desensitization protocol and 21 did so without requiring deviation from the standard dosage schedule and without adverse effects. During the follow-up for 902 patient-months, seven of the 28 patients had recurrent skin eruptions after completing the desensitization protocol and after rechallenge with allopurinol. Desensitization to allopurinol is not recommended for all patients, but it can be useful in selected patients who have had a pruritic maculopapular eruption during treatment with allopurinol and who cannot be treated with other drugs.

Susceptibility Factors

Renal disease

Renal impairment and diuretic therapy predispose to an increased frequency of adverse effects. The exact mechanisms have still to be elucidated. The active metabolite, oxipurinol or alloxanthine, accumulates in renal insufficiency and also in patients taking a low protein diet (15).

Drug–Drug Interactions

Aluminium hydroxide

When aluminium hydroxide is given with allopurinol, the serum uric acid concentration can increase, probably because the antacid reduces the absorption of allopurinol (SEDA-13, 84).

Ampicillin

Concomitant administration of allopurinol with ampicillin may increase the incidence of adverse skin reactions. In one study, these occurred in 22% of patients taking the combination (32). However, this interaction was not confirmed in a later investigation (33).

Ciclosporin

Two well-documented reports have described a marked increase in ciclosporin serum concentrations when allopurinol was co-administered (SEDA-18, 108).

Cytostatic drugs

The risk of bone marrow depression by cytostatic drugs is potentiated by allopurinol, which also appears to potentiate the therapeutic effect of purine cytostatic drugs, since it competitively inhibits their metabolic breakdown. Studies in animals suggest that this reaction occurs only with oral mercaptopurine (34), although there is older evidence that the toxicity of cyclophosphamide and other cytostatic drugs can be increased by allopurinol (SED-9, 156). The danger of combining allopurinol with azathioprine has been confirmed by cases of bone marrow suppression, particularly in patients with impaired renal function (SEDA-16, 114).

Fluorouracil

Concurrent administration of allopurinol with fluorouracil inhibits the intracellular formation of fluorouridine monophosphate from fluorouracil in normal tissues. In tumor cells that activate fluorouracil by alternative pathways, antitumor responses are still seen (35). Allopurinol increased the half-life of high-dose fluorouracil when it was given by intravenous bolus but not when it was given by 5-day continuous infusion (35).

Allopurinol ameliorates fluorouracil-induced granulocytopenia and possibly lessens the severity of mucositis (36). Allopurinol mouthwash (450 mg total in methylcellulose) given immediately and 1, 2, and 3 hours after fluorouracil reduced the incidence and severity of mucositis in six patients (37) and in another study of 42 patients there was significant reduction of oral toxicity and prolonged pain relief (38). In a randomized, double-blind, placebo-controlled trial, in 44 patients, allopurinol mouthwashes resolved stomatitis in nine of 22 treated patients, and diminished its intensity in 10 (39). However, in another randomized, double-blind, crossover study of allopurinol, mouthwash in 77 patients did not ameliorate fluorouracil-induced mucositis (40), nor did allopurinol reduce the toxicity of intravenously administered fluorouracil (41). Allopurinol is not currently recommended in the prophylaxis of fluorouracil-induced mucositis.

Furosemide

Interstitial nephritis with granulomatous hepatitis has been attributed to an interaction of furosemide with allopurinol (42). As in previous reports (SEDA-11, 198) the evidence for this interaction is not convincing. The role of allopurinol in causing the illness is credible, but the role of furosemide is doubtful.

Penicillins

The risk of rashes caused by aminopenicillins does not seem to be increased by parallel treatment with allopurinol (43), as had been suggested before (44).

Thiazides

Thiazides enhance the excretion of orotic acid, which is already increased during allopurinol treatment, but the implications for the frequency of adverse effects are not known.

References

1. Laguna F, Lopez-Velez R, Soriano V, Montilla P, Alvar J, Gonzalez-Lahoz JM. Assessment of allopurinol plus meglumine antimoniate in the treatment of visceral leishmaniasis in patients infected with HIV. J Infect 1994;28(3):255–9.
2. Esfandiarpour I, Alavi A. Evaluating the efficacy of allopurinol and meglumine antimoniate (Glucantime) in the treatment of cutaneous leishmaniasis. Int J Dermatol 2002;41(8):521–4.
3. Momeni AZ, Reiszadae MR, Aminjavaheri M. Treatment of cutaneous leishmaniasis with a combination of allopurinol and low-dose meglumine antimoniate. Int J Dermatol 2002;41(7):441–3.
4. Weiss EB, Forman P, Rosenthal IM. Allopurinol-induced arteritis in partial HGPRTase deficiency. Atypical seizure manifestation. Arch Intern Med 1978;138(11):1743–4.
5. Greenberg LE, Nguyen T, Miller SM. Suspected allopurinol-induced aseptic meningitis. Pharmacotherapy 2001;21(8):1007–9.
6. Lerman S, Megaw J, Fraunfelder FT. Further studies on allopurinol therapy and human cataractogenesis. Am J Ophthalmol 1984;97(2):205–9.
7. Boston Collaborative Drug Surveillance Program. Allopurinol and cytotoxic drugs. Interaction in relation to bone marrow depression. JAMA 1974;227(9):1036–40.
8. Stolbach L, Begg C, Bennett JM, Silverstein M, Falkson G, Harris DT, Glick J. Evaluation of bone marrow toxic reaction in patients treated with allopurinol. JAMA 1982;247(3):334–6.
9. Ohno I, Ishida Y, Hosoya T, Kobayashi M, Sakai O. [Allopurinol induced aplastic anemia in a patient with chronic renal failure.]Ryumachi 1990;30(4):281–6.
10. Okafuji K, Shinohara K. [Aplastic anemia probably induced by allopurinol in a patient with renal insufficiency.]Rinsho Ketsueki 1990;31(1):85–8.
11. Shankar P, Aish L, Hassoun H. Allopurinol-induced pure red cell aplasia. Am J Hematol 2003;73:69.
12. Gomez GA, Stutzman L, Chu TM. Xanthine nephropathy during chemotherapy in deficiency of hypoxanthine-guanine phosphoribosyltransferase. Arch Intern Med 1978;138(6):1017–9.
13. Stote RM, Smith LH, Dubb JW, Moyer TP, Alexander F, Roth JL. Oxypurinol nephrolithiasis in regional enteritis secondary to allopurinol therapy. Ann Intern Med 1980;92(3):384–5.
14. Almirall J, Orellana R, Martínez Ocaña JC, Esteve V, Andreu X. Nefritis intersticial granulomatosa crónica por alopurinol. [Allopurinol-induced chronic granulomatous interstitial nephritis.] Nefrologia 2006;26(6):741–4.
15. Hande KR, Noone RM, Stone WJ. Severe allopurinol toxicity. Description and guidelines for prevention in patients with renal insufficiency. Am J Med 1984;76(1):47–56.
16. Chan SH, Tan T. HLA and allopurinol drug eruption. Dermatologica 1989;179(1):32–3.
17. Chau NY, Reade PC, Rich AM, Hay KD. Allopurinol-amplified lichenoid reactions of the oral mucosa. Oral Surg Oral Med Oral Pathol 1984;58(4):397–400.
18. Chandeclerc ML, Tréchot P, Martin S, Weber-Muller F, Schmutz JL, Barbaud A. Cutaneous adverse drug reaction induced by a generic substitute of Zyloric® with a residual sensitization to allopurinol. Allergy 2006;61(12):1492–3.
19. Ooi CG, Walker P, Sidhu SK, Gordon LA, Marshman G. Allopurinol induced generalized eosinophilic pustular folliculitis. Australas J Dermatol 2006;47(4):270-3. Allopurinol induced generalized eosinophilic pustular folliculitis.
20. Terawaki H, Suzuki T, Yoshimura K, Hasegawa T, Takase H, Nemoto T, Hosoya T. [A case of allopurinol-induced muscular damage in a chronic renal failure patient.]Nippon Jinzo Gakkai Shi 2002;44(1):50–3.
21. Samanta A, Burden AC. Fever, myalgia, and arthralgia in a patient on captopril and allopurinol. Lancet 1984;1(8378):679.
22. Kot TV, Day RO, Brooks PM. Preventing acute gout when starting allopurinol therapy. Colchicine or NSAIDs? Med J Aust 1993;159(3):182–4.
23. Lupton GP, Odom RB. The allopurinol hypersensitivity syndrome. J Am Acad Dermatol 1979;1(4):365–74.
24. Suzuki Y, Inagi R, Aono T, Yamanishi K, Shiohara T. Human herpesvirus 6 infection as a risk factor for the development of severe drug-induced hypersensitivity syndrome. Arch Dermatol 1998;134(9):1108–12.
25. Masaki T, Fukunaga A, Tohyama M, Koda Y, Okuda S, Maeda N, Kanda F, Yasu Kawa M, Hashimoto K, Horikawa T, Ueda M. Human herpes virus 6 encephalitis in alloprurinol-induced hypersensitivity syndrome. Acta Dermatol Venereol 2003;83:128–31.
26. Descamps V, Mahe E, Houhou N, Abaramowitz L, Rozenberg F, Ranger-Rogez S, Crickx B. Drug-induced hypersensitivity syndrome associated with Epstein-Barr virus infection. Br J Dermatol 2003;148:1032–4.
27. Choi HK, Merkel PA, Niles JL. ANCA-positive vasculitis associated with allopurinol therapy. Clin Exp Rheumatol 1998;16(6):743–4.
28. Choi HK, Merkel PA, Walker AM, Niles JL. Drug-associated antineutrophil cytoplasmic antibody-positive vasculitis: prevalence among patients with high titers of antimyeloperoxidase antibodies. Arthritis Rheum 2000;43(2):405–13.
29. Tanna SB, Barnes JF, Seth SK. Desensitization to allopurinol in a patient with previous failed desensitization. Ann Pharmacother 1999;33(11):1180–3.
30. Vazquez-Mellado J, Guzman Vazquez S, Cazarin Barrientos J, Gomez Rios V, Burgos-Vargas R. Desensitisation to allopurinol after allopurinol hypersensitivity syndrome with renal involvement in gout. J Clin Rheumatol 2000;6:266–8.
31. Fam AG, Dunne SM, Iazzetta J, Paton TW. Efficacy and safety of desensitization to allopurinol following cutaneous reactions. Arthritis Rheum 2001;44(1):231–8.
32. Boston Collaborative Drug Surveillance Program. Excess of amphicillin rashes associated with allopurinol or hyperuricemia. A report from the Boston Collaborative Drug Surveillance Program, Boston University Medical Center. N Engl J Med 1972;286(10):505–7.
33. Sonntag MR, Zoppi M, Fritschy D, Maibach R, Stocker F, Sollberger J, Buchli W, Hess T, Hoigne R. Exantheme unter haufig angewandten Antibiotika und antibakteriellen Chemotherapeutika (Penicilline, speziell Aminopenicilline, Cephalosporine und Cotrimoxazol) sowie Allopurinol. [Exanthema during frequent use of antibiotics and antibacterial drugs (penicillin, especially aminopenicillin, cephalosporin and cotrimoxazole) as well as allopurinol. Results of The Berne Comprehensive Hospital Drug Monitoring Program.] Schweiz Med Wochenschr 1986;116(5):142–5.
34. Zimm S, Narang PK, Ricardi R, et al. The effect of allopurinol on the pharmacokinetics of oral and parenteral (i.v.) 6-mercaptopurine Proc Am Assoc Cancer Res 1982;23:210.

35. Chabner BA, Myers CE. Clinical pharmacology of cancer chemotherapy. In: Devita VT, Hellman S, Rosenberg SA, editors. Cancer: Principles and Practice of Oncology. 3rd ed.. Philadelphia: Lippincoft, 1990:349–95.

36. Woolley PV, Ayoob MJ, Smith FP, Lokey JL, DeGreen P, Marantz A, Schein PS. A controlled trial of the effect of 4-hydroxypyrazolopyrimidine (allopurinol) on the toxicity of a single bolus dose of 5-fluorouracil. J Clin Oncol 1985;3(1):103–9.

37. Clark PI, Slevin ML. Allopurinol mouthwashes and 5-fluorouracil induced oral toxicity. Eur J Surg Oncol 1985;11(3):267–8.

38. Tsavaris NB, Komitsopoulou P, Tzannou I, Loucatou P, Tsaroucha-Noutsou A, Kilafis G, Kosmidis P. Decreased oral toxicity with the local use of allopurinol in patients who received high dose 5-fluorouracil. Sel Cancer Ther 1991;7(3):113–7.

39. Porta C, Moroni M, Nastasi G. Allopurinol mouthwashes in the treatment of 5-fluorouracil-induced stomatitis. Am J Clin Oncol 1994;17(3):246–7.

40. Loprinzi CL, Cianflone SG, Dose AM, Etzell PS, Burnham NL, Therneau TM, Hagen L, Gainey DK, Cross M, Athmann LM, et al. A controlled evaluation of an allopurinol mouthwash as prophylaxis against 5-fluorouracil-induced stomatitis. Cancer 1990;65(8):1879–82.

41. Howell SB, Pfeifle CE, Wung WE. Effect of allopurinol on the toxicity of high-dose 5-fluorouracil administered by intermittent bolus injection. Cancer 1983;51(2):220–5.

42. Mousson C, Justrabo E, Tanter Y, Chalopin JM, Rifle G. Néphrite interstitielle et hépatite aiguës granulomateuses d'origine médicamenteuse: rôle possible de l'association allopurinol–furosémide. [Acute granulomatous interstitial nephritis and hepatitis caused by drugs. Possible role of an allopurinol–furosemide combination.] Nephrologie 1986;7(5):199–203.

43. Hoigné R, Sonntag MR, Zoppi M, Hess T, Maibach R, Fritschy D. Occurrence of exanthema in relation to aminopenicillin preparations and allopurinol. N Engl J Med 1987;316(19):1217.

44. Jick H, Porter JB. Potentiation of ampicillin skin reactions by allopurinol or hyperuricemia. J Clin Pharmacol 1981;21(10):456–8.

Benzbromarone

General Information

Benzbromarone is a benzofuran derivative chemically related to amiodarone. It increases uric acid excretion by non-specifically inhibiting its tubular reabsorption.

It was introduced in the 1970s, but in 2003 was withdrawn by Sanofi-Synthélabo after reports of serious hepatotoxicity, although it is still marketed in several countries by other drug companies.

It has also been used in patients with venous disorders to prevent, retard, or reverse varicose degenerative changes in the vessel wall.

The half-life of benzbromarone is about 3 hours, but it has a uricosuric metabolite, 6-hydroxybenzbromarone, with a much longer half-life (up to 30 hours). It is metabolized by CYP2C9 in the liver.

Benzbromarone causes diarrhea (3–4% of patients), urate and oxalate stones, urinary sand, renal colic, and allergy in a small number of patients (1). Liver damage, which reverses after withdrawal, has been described (SEDA-18, 108).

The benefit to harm balance of benzbromarone has been assessed in the light of its clinical benefits, the efficacy of alternatives, such as allopurinol and probenecid, particularly in patients with renal impairment, the risk of hepatotoxicity from benzbromarone, and the risk of adverse reactions to allopurinol and probenecid (2). The authors gave recommendations on the use of benzbromarone.

Organs and Systems

Liver

Four cases of benzbromarone-induced hepatotoxicity were identified from the literature and 11 have been reported by Sanofi-Synthélabo. Only one of the four published cases showed a clear relation between the drug and liver injury as demonstrated by rechallenge. The other three lacked incontrovertible evidence to support an association. Even if all the reported cases were assumed to be due to benzbromarone, the estimated risk of hepatotoxicity in Europe was approximately 1 in 17 000 patients, although it may be higher in Japan.

The authors thought it likely that the risks of hepatotoxicity could be ameliorated by using a graded dosage increase, together with regular monitoring of liver function and that the withdrawal of benzbromarone had not been in the best interests of patients with gout.

Liver damage reportedly reverses after withdrawal (SEDA-18, 108)

Drug–Drug Interactions

Anticoagulants

As benzbromarone is a coumarin derivative, it can potentiate the effects of anticoagulants, which act as vitamin K antagonists.

References

1. Masbernard A, Giudicelli CP. Ten years' experience with benzbromarone in the management of gout and hyperuricaemia. S Afr Med J 1981;59(20):701–6.

2. Lee MH, Graham GG, Williams KM, Day RO. A benefit-risk assessment of benzbromarone in the treatment of gout. Was its withdrawal from the market in the best interest of patients? Drug Saf 2008;31(8):643–65.

Colchicine

General Information

Colchicine is an antimitotic agent, highly effective in the treatment of gout, but associated with considerable toxicity. Diarrhea is used as a criterion for adequate dosage. Accidental overdosage occurs relatively often and can be dangerous. For these reasons, NSAIDs (except aspirin) are often used in acute gout instead of colchicine.

There is controversy about the long-term toxicity of colchicine. In familial Mediterranean fever, low dosages of colchicine (1–2 mg/day) for 15–18 years have been well tolerated, even by young patients (SEDA-16, 114).

Prescribers have been reminded by New Zealand's Medsafe Pharmacovigilance Team of the revised dosage advice for colchicine, which is now second-line therapy for acute gout, because of the risk of serious adverse effects (1,2). Colchicine is very toxic in overdose, and deaths have occurred. The use of high doses in acute gout is not appropriate, especially in patients who are elderly, have impaired renal or hepatic function, or weigh less than 50 kg. Medsafe has advised that:

- colchicine should be considered a second-line treatment for acute gout, when NSAIDs are contraindicated, inefficacious, or poorly tolerated;
- the dosage interval should be increased to 6 hours;
- the maximum daily dose in the first 24 hours should be 2.5 mg;
- the maximum cumulative dose over 4 days should not exceed 6 mg or 3 mg in elderly people;
- colchicine is contraindicated in severe renal or hepatic impairment and the dose should be reduced in patients with less severe impairment.

In addition, continued dosing until adverse gastrointestinal events occur "is no longer considered safe or appropriate". Medsafe has urged prescribers to write clear dosage advice on the prescription, to inform patients of the revised dosage advice, to stress how important it is not to exceed the maximum doses, to warn patients of the symptoms of colchicine toxicity, and to advise them to stop taking the drug immediately and see a doctor if symptoms such as nausea, vomiting, and diarrhea occur.

Organs and Systems

Nervous system

Neuropathy, polyneuritis, toxic encephalitis, delirium, and coma have occurred only in severe colchicine intoxication. During prolonged treatment, neuritis, muscular weakness and myopathy occur more commonly than was previously thought in patients with impaired renal function. In some cases the neuromyopathy was part of multi-organ system failure, but in others the syndrome was not accompanied by other features of colchicine toxicity. Patients taking long-term colchicine should take low dosages (probably no more than 0.6 mg/day) and have their serum creatine kinase monitored (SEDA-12, 94).

Psychological

Despite that fact that studies in animals have suggested that colchicine may adversely affect cognitive function, in 55 patients, mean age 74 years, with familial Mediterranean fever colchicine for an average of 25 years had no adverse effects on cognitive function (3).

Metabolism

Transient diabetes and hyperlipidemia have been reported. Metabolic acidosis is probably a consequence of heavy, cholera-like diarrhea. Progressive reduction of libido was attributed to colchicine in patients with familial Mediterranean fever (4).

Electrolyte balance

Water and electrolyte disturbances, including inappropriate antidiuresis, can occur in patients who have taken high doses of colchicine (5,6), including hypernatremia and polyuria (7).

Hematologic

Bone marrow depression is common after colchicine overdose and intoxication and less common in therapeutic doses. Fatal cases of agranulocytosis are more often associated with bone marrow aplasia (SEDA-4, 70; 8). Bone marrow depression usually occurs between the third and sixth days of acute intoxication. Cytoplasmic inclusions in neutrophils and megaloblastic anemia have been described. Administration of therapeutic doses intravenously and orally to two patients with reduced renal function caused profound prolonged neutropenia complicated by septicemia, which ended in death (SEDA-13, 84).

Gastrointestinal

Gastrointestinal symptoms often develop after therapeutic doses and are even used for dose titration. Diarrhea is often followed by nausea, vomiting, and abdominal pain. Long-term therapy can provoke steatorrhea, malabsorption, and defects in intestinal enzyme activity (9).

Urinary tract

Acute renal insufficiency has been associated with colchicine intoxication (10).

Skin

Blood dyscrasias are associated with ecchymosis and purpura. Allergic skin changes are rare. Alopecia is common after acute intoxication and prolonged treatment (SEDA-5, 109). A fixed drug eruption has been reported (SEDA-21, 109).

Colchicine toxicity in a patient presenting with altered mental function caused a diffuse, blanchable, violaceous, morbilliform rash on the trunk and proximal limbs; metaphase-arrested keratinocytes with underlying basal vacuolization were typical of colchicine toxicity (11).

Musculoskeletal

Acute rhabdomyolysis with fever, muscle cramps, rises in creatine phosphokinase and lactic acid dehydrogenase activity, phlebitis at the injection site, and transitory leukopenia and thrombocytopenia have been reported (12).

Colchicine-induced myopathy generally causes painless subacute muscle weakness but can cause pain (13).

- A 76-year-old man with chronic renal failure and gout who was taking colchicine 0.5 mg tds for 3 days each month developed bilateral lower leg weakness and severe myalgia. His serum creatinine concentration was 681 µmol/l and creatinine kinase 959 IU/l. There were reduced amplitudes of motor and sensory nerve conduction velocities and electromyography showed small-amplitude, short-duration, polyphasic waves over the right biceps. A muscle biopsy showed vacuolar changes in the cytoplasm, all consistent with colchicine neuromyopathy. After withdrawal of colchicine, the creatinine kinase activity fell by about 50% in 6 days, the myalgia abated, and the muscle weakness improved gradually over the next 2 weeks.

Colchicine-induced myopathy with associated myotonia has rarely been reported (14). Colchicine myopathy with or without neuropathy can occur more often than has previously been thought, especially in elderly patients with chronic renal insufficiency taking long-term low doses of colchicine (SEDA-12, 94). Acute rhabdomyolysis can occur (see also Drug-drug interactions below).

Second-Generation Effects

Fertility

Reversible azoospermia (later not confirmed) was observed after long-term treatment with colchicines (15).

Pregnancy

Owing to its antimitotic properties, colchicine should not be given during pregnancy (SED-9, 158; 16).

Susceptibility Factors

Renal disease

There have been single case reports of severe colchicine-induced myopathy in which impaired renal function caused insufficient elimination of colchicine (17). The dosage of colchicine should be adjusted according to creatinine clearance during long-term use to avoid the risk of myoneuropathy (SEDA-16, 114). Colchicine should not be used in patients undergoing hemodialysis, since it cannot be removed by either dialysis or exchange transfusion (18).

Drug Administration

Drug dosage regimens

It has been suggested that the dosages of colchicine recommended by the *British National Formulary* in patients with gout should be revised; lower doses are probably better tolerated and equally efficacious (19).

Drug administration route

Intravenous administration is potentially much more toxic than oral administration; because of its unfavorable benefit to harm, balance and the availability of less dangerous treatments, colchicine should not be given intravenously (SEDA-5, 109; SEDA-13, 84; SEDA-16, 115).

Drug overdose

Acute intoxication with colchicine occurs relatively often, because the therapeutic dose is close to the toxic dose. Gastrointestinal, hematological, and neurological reactions are the most frequent effects (SEDA-7, 118). An accidental overdose of colchicine by nasal insufflation has been reported in a young male drug abuser who had mistaken it for metamfetamine. The effects included gastrointestinal distress, myalgia, thrombocytopenia, hypocalcemia, and hypophosphatemia (20). Electrolyte disturbances can occur (5–7). Deaths have been reported (6).

Drug–Drug Interactions

The pharmacokinetics and drug interactions of colchicine have been reviewed (21). Three proteins are important:

- tubulin, the pharmacological receptor (target) for colchicine; colchicine binds to tubulin, preventing polymerization and thereby disrupting microtubule function; the dissociation half-life of the tubulin–colchicine complex is 20–30 hours and this determines the half-life of colchicine;
- intestinal and hepatic CYP3A4, by which colchicine is metabolized; drug interactions can occur when colchicine is combined with other drugs that are CYP3A4 substrates;
- P-glycoprotein, which affects its tissue distribution and excretion via the biliary tract and kidneys; drug interactions can occur when colchicine is combined with other drugs that are P-glycoprotein substrates.

The combination of colchicine with other myotoxic drugs (for example statins and gemfibrozil) can cause acute rhabdomyolysis. This potential interaction has clinical relevance, as these classes of drugs are often prescribed together for patients with renal insufficiency. In two cases simvastatin (22) and atorvastatin (23) were blamed and in the third, gemfibrozil (24) was thought to have contributed to colchicine-induced rhabdomyolysis. The rhabdomyolysis that occurs when simvastatin is combined with colchicine may be due to inhibition of CYP3A4.

While these single case reports require confirmation, and although the interaction is probably rare, it would be wise to avoid such combinations if possible, or to monitor susceptible patients carefully.

Ciclosporin

Acute reversible ciclosporin toxicity occurred in a renal transplant patient a few days after colchicine was administered for an acute attack of gout (SEDA-16, 115). Other potential adverse effects of combining colchicine with ciclosporin include diarrhea, increases in serum liver enzymes, bilirubin, and creatinine, and less often severe myalgia (SEDA-19, 101). Acute myopathy, associated with neuropathy in one case, has been observed in two young renal transplant recipients (SEDA-22, 119).

Clarithromycin

Concomitant treatment with clarithromycin can increase the effect of colchicine (25) and fatal colchicine toxicity has been reported (13).

- Fatal colchicine intoxication occurred in a 67-year-old man who had taken clarithromycin 500 mg bd for 4 days (26).

Clarithromycin may have inhibited colchicine metabolism and caused a rise in colchicine concentration.

In a retrospective case-control study of 116 patients who took clarithromycin and colchicine, nine of the 88 patients who took the two drugs concomitantly died, compared with only one of the 28 patients who took the two drugs sequentially (27). Multivariate analysis of the 88 patients showed that longer overlapping therapy, baseline renal function impairment, and pancytopenia were independently associated with death. This study had several limitations but it cannot be dismissed, as further reports have been published that document severe adverse reactions after co-administration of colchicine with clarithromycin (28,29).

- A 68-year-old man with acute gouty arthritis and a community-acquired pneumonia was given colchicine 0.5 mg every 6 hours and clarithromycin 500 mg tds. On day 5 the dose of colchicine was reduced to 0.5 mg every 8 hours because of diarrhea. On day 11 both drugs were withdrawn and the next day he developed a paralytic ileus, recurrence of fever, hypotension, pancytopenia, and acute renal and hepatic insufficiency. He died on day 13 and post-mortem examination showed agranulocytosis and massive hepatic necrosis.
- A 55-year-old woman with acute gout and pneumonia was given colchicine 0.5 mg tds and clarithromycin 250 mg bd. After five doses of colchicine and three of clarithromycin she developed severe leukopenia and thrombocytopenia. Bone marrow biopsy showed marked hypocellularity. She developed a febrile neutropenia and died after 12 days.

- A 71-year-old man taking colchicine 1.5 mg/day for Familial Mediterranean Fever was given clarithromycin, amoxicillin and omeprazole for 7 days for *Helicobacter pylori* eradication. After 3 days he developed fever, abdominal pain, and bloody diarrhea, and after 8 days pancytopenia, dehydration, and metabolic acidosis. The dosage of colchicine was reduced to 0.5 mg/day. He was rehydrated and recovered fully. The previous dosage of colchicine was gradually reinstituted without adverse effects.

Fibrates

Rhabdomyolysis due to the combination of colchicine with gemfibrozil has been reported in a 40-year-old man with amyloidosis and chronic liver disease (30).

HMG coenzyme A reductase inhibitors (statins)

Concomitant treatment with statins can cause myopathy or rhabdomyolysis. There have also been single case reports of rhabdomyolysis with simvastatin, atorvastatin, and possibly gemfibrozil (SEDA-28, 133). The combination of colchicine with other potentially myotoxic drugs, such as gemfibrozil and other statins, has clinical relevance, as these classes of drugs are often co-prescribed in patients with renal insufficiency.

- A 70-year-old man, who had taken fluvastatin for 2 years for dyslipidemia, developed rhabdomyolysis and acute renal insufficiency 10 days after starting to take colchicine 1.5 mg/day (31). He had raised creatine kinase and aspartate transaminase activities, and serum myoglobin and creatinine concentrations. Colchicine and fluvastatin were withdrawn and his gout was treated with intraarticular glucocorticoid injections. The laboratory findings normalized over about 10 days. Fluvastatin was subsequently restarted without problems and 2 months later his renal function was normal.
- A 65-year-old woman, who was taking pravastatin 20 mg/day and losartan, diuretics, and aspirin for ischemic heart disease, was given colchicine 1.5 mg/day for gout, and 20 days later developed symmetrical proximal muscle weakness in the legs with reduced tendon reflexes and electromyography consistent with muscle disease (32). She had raised creatine kinase, aspartate transaminase, and lactate dehydrogenase activities. Blood urea nitrogen and serum creatinine concentrations were slightly raised. Colchicine and pravastatin were withdrawn and within 7 days her clinical and laboratory findings normalized. She had another attack of gout 12 days later and was given colchicine 1.0 mg/day without adverse effects.
- A 74-year old Asian man who was taking prophylactic colchicine for gout developed proximal muscle weakness 2 weeks after starting to take lovastatin (33). The deep tendon reflexes were symmetrical and reduced in both arms and legs. Serum creatine kinase was 8370 U/l (0–130 U/l), and electromyography showed a myopathic pattern. Lovastatin and colchicine were withdrawn and after several weeks the creatine kinase activity gradually returned to normal, with normal muscle strength.

- A 45-year-old man with nephrotic syndrome took colchicine 1.5 mg/day for amyloidosis for 3 years without adverse effects (34). He then took atorvastatin 10 mg/day for hypercholesterolemia and after 2 weeks developed dyspnea, altered thinking, severe fatigue, myalgia, and reduced muscle strength. The creatinine concentration was 714 μmol/l, the creatine kinase activity 9035 U/l, and there was myoglobinuria and acute renal failure. His muscle strength improved after withdrawal of atorvastatin and colchicine.

Colchicine and most of the statins are biotransformed in the liver, primarily by CYP3A4, which may explain the increased risk of myopathy during concurrent therapy. However, pravastatin and fluvastatin are not primarily metabolized by cytochrome P450 isoenzymes (35) and in such cases the interaction may be mediated by P glycoprotein.

Verapamil

An interaction of colchicine with verapamil has been described (36).

- An 83-year-old man taking verapamil developed a flaccid tetraparesis after taking colchicine 2 mg over 2 days for acute gout. He developed severe muscle weakness in his legs and arms, and electrophysiology showed axonal damage. Five days after taking colchicine he had raised serum and cerebrospinal fluid colchicine concentrations. Serum verapamil and norverapamil concentrations were normal, as was renal function.

The authors suggested that inhibition of P glycoprotein in the blood–brain barrier by verapamil and its metabolite norverapamil had led to accumulation of colchicine in the nervous system, causing the acute neurological damage.

References

1 Anonymous. Colchicine. Toxic in overdose: reminder. WHO Newslett 2006;4:5–6.

2 Australian Adverse Drug Reactions Advisory Committee. Medsafe Pharmacovigilace Team. Colchicine–safe use is critical. Prescriber Update 2006;27(1):2.

3. Leibovitz A, Lidar M, Baumoehl Y, Livneh A, Segal R. Colchicine therapy and the cognitive status of elderly patients with familial Mediterranean fever. Isr Med Assoc J 2006;8(7):469–72.

4. Peters RS, Lehman TJ, Schwabe AD. Colchicine use for familial Mediterranean fever. Observations associated with long-term treatment. West J Med 1983;138(1):43–6.

5. Gaultier M, Bismuth C, Autret A, Pillon M. Anti-diurèse inappropriée après intoxication aiguë par la colchicine. 2 cas. [Inappropriate antidiuresis after acute colchicine poisoning. 2 cases.] Nouv Presse Méd 1975;4(44):3132–4.

6. Milne ST, Meek PD. Fatal colchicine overdose: report of a case and review of the literature. Am J Emerg Med 1998;16(6):603–8.

7. Usalan C, Altun B, Ulusoy S, Erdem Y, Yasavul U, Turgan C, Caglar S. Hypernatraemia and polyuria due to high-dose colchicine in a suicidal patient. Nephrol Dial Transplant 1999;14(6):1556–7.

8. Liu YK, Hymowitz R, Carroll MG. Marrow aplasia induced by colchicine. A case report. Arthritis Rheum 1978;21(6):731–5.

9. Ben-Chetrit E, Levy M. Colchicine: 1998 update. Semin Arthritis Rheum 1998;28(1):48–59.

10. Rosset L, Descombes E, Fellay G, Regamey C. Toxicité multisystèmique de la colchicine et insuffisance rènale à propos d'un cas. [Multi-systemic toxicity of colchicine and renal failure: apropos of a case.] Schweiz Med Wochenschr 1998;128(49):1953–7.

11. Mason SE, Smoller BR, Wilkerson AE. Colchicine intoxication diagnosed in a skin biopsy: a case report. J Cutan Pathol 2006;33(4):309–11.

12. Letellier P, Langeard M, Agullo M. Rhabdomyolise secondaire à une série d'injections intraveineuses de colchicine. J Med Caen 1979;14:157.

13. Lai IC, Cheng CY, Chen HH, Chen WY, Chen PY. Colchicine myoneuropathy in chronic renal failure patients with gout. Nephrology (Carlton) 2006;11(2):147–50.

14. Caglar K, Odabasi Z, Safali M, Yenicesu M. Colchicine-induced myopathy with myotonia in a patient with chronic renal failure. Clin Neurol Neurosurg 2003;105:274–6.

15. Merlin HE. Azoospermia caused by colchicine—a case report. Fertil Steril 1972;23(3):180–1.

16. Wallace SL, Ertel NH. Colchicine: current problems. Bull Rheum Dis 1969;20(4):582–7.

17 Wilbur K, Makowsky M. Colchicine myotoxicity: case reports and literature review. Pharmacotherapy 2004;24:1784–92.

18. Rieger EH, Halasz NA, Wahlstrom HE. Colchicine neuromyopathy after renal transplantation. Transplantation 1990;49(6):1196–8.

19. Morris I, Varughese G, Mattingly P. Colchicine in acute gout. BMJ 2003;327:1275–6.

20. Baldwin LR, Talbert RL, Samples R. Accidental overdose of insufflated colchicine. Drug Saf 1990;5(4):305–12.

21. Niel E, Scherrmann JM. Colchicine today. Joint Bone Spine 2006;73(6):672–8.

22. Hsu WC, Chen WH, Chang MT, Chiu HC. Colchicine-induced acute myopathy in a patient with concomitant use of simvastatin. Clin Neuropharmacol 2002;25:266–8.

23. Phanish MK, Krishnamurthy S, Bloodworth LL. Colchicine-induced rhabdomyolysis. Am J Med 2003;114:166–7.

24. Atmaca H, Sayarlioglu H, Kulah E, Demircan N, Akpolat T. Rhabdomyolysis associated with gemfibrozil–colchicine therapy. Ann Pharmacother 2002;36:1719–21.

25. Akdag I, Ersoy A, Kahvecioglu S, Gullulu M, Dilek K. Acute colchicine intoxication during clarithromycin administration in patients with chronic renal failure. J Nephrol 2006;19(4):515–7.

26. Dandekar SS, Laidlaw DA. Suprachoroidal haemorrhage after addition of clarithromycin to warfarin. J R Soc Med 2001;94(11):583–4.

27 Hung IF, Wu AK, Cheng VC, Tang BS, To KW, Yeung CK, Woo PC, Lau SK, Cheung BM, Yuen KY. Fatal interaction between clarithromycin and colchicine in patients with renal insufficiency: a retrospective study. Clin Infect Dis 2005;41:291–300.

28 Cheng VCC, Ho PL, Yuen KY. Two probable cases of serious drug interaction between clarithromycin and colchicine. South Med J 2005;98:811–3.

29 Rollot F, Pajot O, Chauvelot-Moachon L, Nazal EM, Kélaïdi C, Blache P. Acute colchicines intoxication during clarithromycin administration. Ann Pharmacother 2004;38:2074–7.

30. Atmaca H, Sayarlioglu H, Kulah E, Demircan N, Akpolat T. Rhabdomyolysis associated with gemfibrozil–colchicine therapy. Ann Pharmacother 2002;36(11):1719–21.

31 Atasoyu EM, Evrenkaya TR, Solmazgul E. Possible colchicine rhabdomyolysis in a fluvastatin-treated patient. Ann Pharmacother 2005;39:1368–9.

32 Alayli G, Cengiz K, Cantürk F, Durmus D, Akyol Y, Menekse EB. Acute myopathy in a patient with concomitant use of pravastatin and colchicine. Ann Pharmacother 2005;39:1358–61.

33. Torgovnick J, Sethi N, Arsura E. Colchicine and HMG Co-A reductase inhibitors induced myopathy—a case report. Neurotoxicology 2006;27(6):1126–7.

34. Tufan A, Dede DS, Cavus S, Altintas ND, Iskit AB, Topeli A. Rhabdomyolysis in a patient treated with colchicine and atorvastatin. Ann Pharmacother 2006;40(7-8):1466–9.

35 Hsu WC, Chen WH, Chang MT, Chiu HC. Colchicine-induced acute myopathy in a patient with concomitant use of simvastatin. Clin Neuropharmacol 2002;25:266–8.

36. Tröger U, Lins H, Scherrmann JM, Wallesch CW, Bode-Boger SM. Tetraparesis associated with colchicine is probably due to inhibition by verapamil of the P-glycoprotein efflux pump in the blood-brain barrier. BMJ 2005;331(7517):613.

Febuxostat

General Information

Febuxostat is a non-purine xanthine oxidase inhibitor (1,2,3,4,5).Its pharmacology, efficacy, and safety has been the subject of a systematic review (6).It most common adverse effects include liver function test abnormalities, diarrhea, headache, nausea, vomiting, abdominal pain, and dizziness (7).

Pharmacokinetics

In a phase I study of oral febuxostat 10, 20, 30, 40, 50, 70, 90, 120, 160, 180, and 240 mg/day in 12 subjects at each dose (10 febuxostat plus 2 placebo), absorption was rapid, with a median t_{max} of 0.5–1.3 hours (8). The pharmacokinetics were not time dependent and were linear in the 10–120 mg/day dose range but non-linear at higher doses. The mean apparent total clearance was 10–12 l/hour and the apparent volume of distribution at steady state was 33–64 l. The half-life was 1.3–16 hours. Febuxostat was metabolized by glucuronidation (22–44% of the dose) and oxidation (2–8%); only 1–6% of the dose was excreted unchanged via the kidneys.

Comparative studies

In 760 patients with gout and with serum urate concentrations of at least 480 µmol/l (8.0 mg/dl) febuxostat 80 or 120 mg/day or allopurinol 300 mg/day were given for 52 weeks (9).More of those who took high-dose febuxostat withdrew than those who took allopurinol or low-dose febuxostat. Four of the 507 patients in the two febuxostat groups (0.8 percent) and none of the 253 patients in the allopurinol group died; all deaths were from causes that the investigators (while still blinded to treatment) judged to be unrelated to the study drugs.

In two double-blind randomized trials in 762 and 1072 patients in which various doses of febuxostat were compared with a standard dose of allopurinol, febuxostat was associated with more attacks of gout during the first two months of treatment, despite preventive measures (30–35% versus 22%) (10). At 3–6 months of treatment neither drug reduced the incidence of attacks of gout more effectively than placebo. In the short term, severe cardiac disorders were 4–5 times more frequent with febuxostat than with allopurinol. Treatment withdrawals due to hepatic disorders were more frequent with febuxostat than with allopurinol (2.8% versus 0.4%). The authors concluded that patients with hyperuricemia should continue to take allopurinol as first-line treatment and probenecid as second-line treatment if allopurinol is ineffective.

Placebo-controlled studies

Febuxostat, allopurinol, and placebo have been compared for 28 weeks in 1072 subjects with hyperuricaemia and gout, including some with impaired renal function (11). Febuxostat was used in one of three doses (80, 120, or 240 mg/day) and allopurinol in one of two does (300 or 100 mg/day, based on renal function). The proportions of subjects who had any adverse event or serious adverse event were similar across the groups, although diarrhea and dizziness were more frequent in those who took febuxostat 240 mg/day. The primary reasons for withdrawal were similar across the groups except for gout flares, which were more frequent with febuxostat.

Susceptibility Factors

Age and sex

Age and sex had no clinically important effects on the pharmacokinetics, pharmacodynamics, and safety of once-daily oral febuxostat 80 mg in healthy men and women aged 18–40 years and over 65 years after 7 days (12). Following multiple dosing with febuxostat, there were no statistically significant differences in the plasma or urinary pharmacokinetic or pharmacodynamic parameters between subjects.

References

1. Hoskison TK, Wortmann RL. Advances in the management of gout and hyperuricaemia. Scand J Rheumatol 2006;35(4):251-60.

2. Okamoto K. [Inhibitors of xanthine oxidoreductase.] Nippon Rinsho 2008;66(4):748-53.

3. Ichida K. [New antihyperuricemic medicine: febuxostat, Puricase, etc.] Nippon Rinsho. 2008;66(4):759-65.

4. Anonymous. Febuxostat (Uloric) for chronic treatment of gout. Med Lett Drugs Ther 2009;51(1312):37-8.

5. Keenan RT, Pillinger MH. Febuxostat: a new agent for lowering serum urate. Drugs Today (Barc) 2009;45(4):247-60.

6. Yu KH. Febuxostat: a novel non-purine selective inhibitor of xanthine oxidase for the treatment of hyperuricemia in

gout. Recent Pat Inflamm Allergy Drug Discov 2007;1(1):69-75.

7. Pohar S, Murphy G. Febuxostat for prevention of gout attacks. Issues Emerg Health Technol 2006;(87):1-4.

8. Khosravan R, Grabowski BA, Wu JT, Joseph-Ridge N, Vernillet L. Pharmacokinetics, pharmacodynamics and safety of febuxostat, a non-purine selective inhibitor of xanthine oxidase, in a dose escalation study in healthy subjects. Clin Pharmacokinet 2006;45(8):821-41.

9. Becker MA, Schumacher HR Jr, Wortmann RL, MacDonald PA, Eustace D, Palo WA, Streit J, Joseph-Ridge N. Febuxostat compared with allopurinol in patients with hyperuricemia and gout. N Engl J Med 2005;353(23):2450–61.

10. Anonymous. Febuxostat: new drug. Hyperuricaemia: risk of gout attacks. Prescrire Int. 2009;18(100):63–5.

11. Schumacher HR Jr, Becker MA, Wortmann RL, Macdonald PA, Hunt B, Streit J, Lademacher C, Joseph-Ridge N. Effects of febuxostat versus allopurinol and placebo in reducing serum urate in subjects with hyperuricemia and gout: a 28-week, phase III, randomized, double-blind, parallel-group trial. Arthritis Rheum 2008;59(11):1540–8.

12. Khosravan R, Kukulka MJ, Wu JT, Joseph-Ridge N, Vernillet L. The effect of age and gender on pharmacokinetics, pharmacodynamics, and safety of febuxostat, a novel nonpurine selective inhibitor of xanthine oxidase. J Clin Pharmacol 2008;48(9):1014–24.

Probenecid

General Information

Probenecid is a uricosuric agent. It is generally well tolerated. Soreness of the gums, gastrointestinal irritation, skin rashes, pyrexia, and the nephrotic syndrome have been reported (1).

Drug interactions with probenecid arise, because it is an inhibitor of the renal tubular secretion of acids and bases (2).

Second-Generation Effects

Lactation

Probenecid can enter breast milk (3).

- A breast-fed infant of a 30-year-old woman taking oral probenecid and cefalexin for a breast infection developed severe diarrhea. The average concentrations of probenecid and cefalexin in the milk were 964 and 745 µg/l respectively, corresponding to infant doses of 145 micrograms/kg/day of probenecid and 112 micrograms/kg/day of cefalexin.

The infant's adverse effects were rated as possible for probenecid and probable for cefalexin based on the Naranjo probability scale.

Drug–Drug Interactions

Antibiotics

Probenecid inhibits the renal tubular secretion of various penicillins (4–7) and many cephalosporins (7–21). Ceforanide is not affected (22).

Aspirin

In low dosages (up to 2 g/day), aspirin reduces urate excretion and blocks the effects of probenecid and other uricosuric agents (23,24). However, in 11 patients with gout, aspirin 325 mg/day had no effect on the uricosuric action of probenecid (23). In higher dosages (over 5 g/day), salicylates increase urate excretion and inhibit the effects of spironolactone, but it is not clear whether these phenomena are of importance.

Beta-lactam antibiotics

Probenecid inhibits the tubular resorption of anions and inhibits the renal excretion of most beta-lactam antibiotics (35,36).

Chloroquine

Probenecid may increase the risk of chloroquine-induced retinal damage (25).

Ciprofloxacin

The renal excretion of ciprofloxacin was reduced and plasma concentrations increased by probenecid (37).

Dapsone

Probenecid increases plasma dapsone concentrations by inhibiting its renal clearance (26).

Fluoroquinolones

Probenecid increases the serum concentrations of cinoxacin (38), enoxacin (39), and nalidixic acid (40) probably by inhibiting their renal tubular secretion.

Indometacin

Interactions with indometacin have been documented through inhibition of renal tubular excretion (27,28). In 17 patients with rheumatoid arthritis, probenecid 500 mg bd improved the therapeutic response to indometacin 25 mg tds over 3 weeks (29). There were changes in the pharmacokinetics of indometacin, which the authors attributed to a reduction in the non-renal clearance of indometacin, possibly because of reduced biliary clearance.

Methotrexate

Probenecid reduces the renal tubular secretion of methotrexate, enhancing its effect (30) and may reduce its plasma protein binding (31).

Probenecid competes with methotrexate for renal tubular secretion, and can cause severe hematological toxicity.

- Severe pancytopenia occurred in an elderly patient taking low-dose methotrexate and probenecid (41).

Moxifloxacin

Concomitant administration of probenecid did not affect the elimination of moxifloxacin (42).

Neuraminidase inhibitors

In healthy subjects probenecid completely blocked the renal secretion of the active metabolite of oseltamivir after oral administration, increasing its AUC 2.5 times (43). In vitro studies of the metabolite on the human renal organic anionic transporter I (hOAT1) were investigated in Chinese hamster ovary cells stably transfected with the transporter. The metabolite was a low-efficiency substrate for hOAT1 and a very weak inhibitor of hOAT1-mediated transport of *para*-aminohippuric acid. Probenecid inhibited the transport of the metabolite, *para*-aminohippuric acid, and amoxicillin via hOAT1.

Rifamycins

Probenecid can increase the serum concentration of rifampicin; this can reduce costs and hepatotoxicity in long-term therapy (44). Interactions of rifampicin with probenecid have been reviewed (45).

Sevoflurane

The effect of the uricosuric agent probenecid in prolonged sevoflurane anesthesia has been examined in 64 patients randomized to receive high-flow or low-flow anesthesia with sevoflurane with or without preoperative oral probenecid (46). There were no differences in urea, creatinine, or creatinine clearance among the treatments. However, patients who received low-flow sevoflurane had some evidence of renal tubular injury (raised urinary markers) compared with those who received either high-flow anesthesia or probenecid.

Sulfinpyrazone

Probenecid reduces the renal tubular secretion of sulfinpyrazone but there is no change in the uricosuric effect (32).

Torasemide

Probenecid blocks the natriuretic effect of torasemide (SEDA-21, 229).

Valaciclovir

In an open, single-dose study of the effects of probenecid and cimetidine on the pharmacokinetics of valaciclovir and its metabolite aciclovir in 12 healthy men, valaciclovir 1 g, valaciclovir plus probenecid 1 g, valaciclovir plus cimetidine 800 mg, and valaciclovir with a combination of probenecid and cimetidine were studied (47). At three subsequent administrations, drug regimens were alternated among groups so that each group received each regimen. Probenecid and cimetidine respectively increased the mean C_{max} of valaciclovir by 23 and 53%

and its AUC by 22 and 73%. Probenecid and cimetidine also respectively increased the mean aciclovir C_{max} by 22 and 8% and its AUC by 48 and 27%. The combination had a greater effect than either drug alone. Neither cimetidine nor probenecid affected the absorption of valaciclovir.

Zidovudine

Probenecid reduces the renal tubular secretion of zidovudine (33,34).

In two healthy volunteers, co-administration of probenecid 500 mg every 6 hours altered the pharmacokinetics of a single oral dose of zidovudine 200 mg (33). There was an increase in the average AUC, with a corresponding reduction in oral clearance, attributed to an inhibitory effect of probenecid on the glucuronidation and renal excretion of zidovudine.

Eight subjects took zidovudine for 3 days with and without probenecid 500 mg every 8 hours for 3 days, and then additional quinine sulfate 260 mg every 8 hours (48). Probenecid increased the AUC of zidovudine by 80%. Quinine prevented the probenecid effect but had no effect on zidovudine kinetics when it was taken without probenecid by four other subjects. All of the effects were secondary to changes in zidovudine metabolism, since neither probenecid nor quinine changed the renal elimination of zidovudine.

References

1. Scott JT, O'Brien PK. Probenecid, nephrotic syndrome, and renal failure. Ann Rheum Dis 1968;27(3):249–52.
2. Cunningham RF, Israili ZH, Dayton PG. Clinical pharmacokinetics of probenecid. Clin Pharmacokinet 1981;6(2):135–51.
3. Ilett KF, Hackett LP, Ingle B, Bretz PJ. Transfer of probenecid and cephalexin into breast milk. Ann Pharmacother 2006;40(5):986–9.
4. Waller ES, Sharanevych MA, Yakatan GJ. The effect of probenecid on nafcillin disposition. J Clin Pharmacol 1982;22(10):482–9.
5. Allen MB, Fitzpatrick RW, Barratt A, Cole RB. The use of probenecid to increase the serum amoxycillin levels in patients with bronchiectasis. Respir Med 1990;84(2):143–6.
6. Krogsgaard MR, Hansen BA, Slotsbjerg T, Jensen P. Should probenecid be used to reduce the dicloxacillin dosage in orthopaedic infections? A study of the dicloxacillin-saving effect of probenecid. Pharmacol Toxicol 1994;74(3):181–4.
7. Tuano SB, Brodie JL, Kirby WM. Cephaloridine versus cephalothin: relation of the kidney to blood level differences after parenteral administration. Antimicrobial Agents Chemother (Bethesda) 1966;6:101–6.
8. Kaplan K, Reisberg BE, Weinstein L. Cephaloridine: antimicrobial activity and pharmacologic behavior. Am J Med Sci 1967;253(6):667–74.
9. Applestein JM, Crosby EB, Johnson WD, Kaye D. In vitro antimicrobial activity and human pharmacology of cephaloglycin. Appl Microbiol 1968;16(7):1006–10.
10. Taylor WA, Holloway WJ. Cephalexin in the treatment of gonorrhea. Int J Clin Pharmacol 1972;6(1):7–9.
11. Duncan WC. Treatment of gonorrhea with cefazolin plus probenecid. J Infect Dis 1974;130(4):398–401.

12. Mischler TW, Sugerman AA, Willard DA, Brannick LJ, Neiss ES. Influence of probenecid and food on the bioavailability of cephradine in normal male subjects. J Clin Pharmacol 1974;14(11–12):604–11.

13. Wise R, Reeves DS. Pharmacological studies on cephacetrile in human volunteers. Curr Med Res Opin 1974;2(5):249–55.

14. Griffith RS, Black HR, Brier GL, Wolny JD. Effects of probenecid on the blood levels and urinary excretion of cefamandole. Antimicrob Agents Chemother 1977;11(5):809–12.

15. Welling PG, Dean S, Selen A, Kendall MJ, Wise R. Probenecid: an unexplained effect on cephalosporin pharmacology. Br J Clin Pharmacol 1979;8(5):491–5.

16. Reeves DS, Bullock DW, Bywater MJ, Holt HA, White LO, Thornhill DP. The effect of probenecid on the pharmacokinetics and distribution of cefoxitin in healthy volunteers. Br J Clin Pharmacol 1981;11(4):353–9.

17. LeBel M, Paone RP, Lewis GP. Effect of probenecid on the pharmacokinetics of ceftriaxone. J Antimicrob Chemother 1983;12(2):147–55.

18. Stoeckel K, Trueb V, Dubach UC, McNamara PJ. Effect of probenecid on the elimination and protein binding of ceftriaxone. Eur J Clin Pharmacol 1988;34(2):151–6.

19. Ko H, Cathcart KS, Griffith DL, Peters GR, Adams WJ. Pharmacokinetics of intravenously administered cefmetazole and cefoxitin and effects of probenecid on cefmetazole elimination. Antimicrob Agents Chemother 1989; 33(3):356–61.

20. Corvaia L, Li SC, Ioannides-Demos LL, Bowes G, Spicer WJ, Spelman DW, Tong N, McLean AJ. A prospective study of the effects of oral probenecid on the pharmacokinetics of intravenous ticarcillin in patients with cystic fibrosis. J Antimicrob Chemother 1992;30(6):875–8.

21. Shukla UA, Pittman KA, Barbhaiya RH. Pharmacokinetic interactions of cefprozil with food, propantheline, metoclopramide, and probenecid in healthy volunteers. J Clin Pharmacol 1992;32(8):725–31.

22. Jovanovich JF, Saravolatz LD, Burch K, Pohlod DJ. Failure of probenecid to alter the pharmacokinetics of ceforanide. Antimicrob Agents Chemother 1981;20(4):530–2.

23. Harris M, Bryant LR, Danaher P, Alloway J. Effect of low dose daily aspirin on serum urate levels and urinary excretion in patients receiving probenecid for gouty arthritis. J Rheumatol 2000;27(12):2873–6.

24. Brooks CD, Ulrich JE. Effect of ibuprofen or aspirin on probenecid-induced uricosuria. J Int Med Res 1980;8(4):283–5.

25. Frankel EB. Visual defect from chloroquine phosphate. Arch Dermatol 1975;111(8):1069.

26. Goodwin CS, Sparell G. Inhibition of dapsone excretion by probenecid. Lancet 1969;2(7626):884–5.

27. Brooks PM, Bell MA, Sturrock RD, Famaey JP, Dick WC. The clinical significance of indomethacin–probenecid interaction. Br J Clin Pharmacol 1974;1:287.

28. Sinclair H, Gibson T. Interaction between probenecid and indomethacin. Br J Rheumatol 1986;25(3):316–7.

29. Baber N, Halliday L, Sibeon R, Littler T, Orme ML. The interaction between indomethacin and probenecid. A clinical and pharmacokinetic study. Clin Pharmacol Ther 1978;24(3):298–307.

30. Liegler DG, Henderson ES, Hahn MA, Oliverio VT. The effect of organic acids on renal clearance of methotrexate in man. Clin Pharmacol Ther 1969;10(6):849–57.

31. Evans WE, Christensen ML. Drug interactions with methotrexate. J Rheumatol Suppl 1985;12(Suppl 12):15–20.

32. Perel JM, Dayton PG, Snell MM, Yu TF, Gutman AB. Studies of interactions among drugs in man at the renal level: probenecid and sulfinpyrazone. Clin Pharmacol Ther 1969;10(6):834–40.

33. Hedaya MA, Elmquist WF, Sawchuk RJ. Probenecid inhibits the metabolic and renal clearances of zidovudine (AZT) in human volunteers. Pharm Res 1990;7(4):411–7.

34. Veal GJ, Back DJ. Metabolism of Zidovudine. Gen Pharmacol 1995;26(7):1469–75.

35. Young DS. Effects of Drugs on Clinical Laboratory Tests. 3rd ed.. Washington: AACC Press;. 1990.

36. Garton AM, Rennie RP, Gilpin J, Marrelli M, Shafran SD. Comparison of dose doubling with probenecid for sustaining serum cefuroxime levels. J Antimicrob Chemother 1997;40(6):903–6.

37. Jaehde U, Sorgel F, Reiter A, Sigl G, Naber KG, Schunack W. Effect of probenecid on the distribution and elimination of ciprofloxacin in humans. Clin Pharmacol Ther 1995;58(5):532–41.

38. Rodriguez N, Madsen PO, Welling PG. Influence of probenecid on serum levels and urinary excertion of cinoxacin. Antimicrob Agents Chemother 1979;15(3):465–9.

39. Wijnands WJ, Vree TB, Baars AM, van Herwaarden CL. Pharmacokinetics of enoxacin and its penetration into bronchial secretions and lung tissue. J Antimicrob Chemother 1988;21(Suppl B):67–77.

40. Vree TB, Van den Biggelaar-Martea M, Van Ewijk-Beneken Kolmer EW, Hekster YA. Probenecid inhibits the renal clearance and renal glucuronidation of nalidixic acid. A pilot experiment. Pharm World Sci 1993; 15(4):165–70.

41. Basin KS, Escalante A, Beardmore TD. Severe pancytopenia in a patient taking low dose methotrexate and probenecid. J Rheumatol 1991;81(4):609–10.

42. Stass H, Kubitza D. Profile of moxifloxacin drug interactions. Clin Infect Dis 2001;32(Suppl 1):S47–50.

43. Hill G, Cihlar T, Oo C, Ho ES, Prior K, Wiltshire H, Barrett J, Liu B, Ward P. The anti-influenza drug oseltamivir exhibits low potential to induce pharmacokinetic drug interactions via renal secretion-correlation of in vivo and in vitro studies. Drug Metab Dispos 2002;30(1):13–9.

44. Pankaj R, Lal S, Rao RS. Effect of probenecid on serum rifampicin levels. Indian J Lepr 1985;57(2):329–33.

45. Baciewicz AM, Self TH. Rifampin drug interactions. Arch Intern Med 1984;144(8):1667–71.

46. Higuchi H, Wada H, Usui Y, Goto K, Kanno M, Satoh T. Effects of probenecid on renal function in surgical patients anesthetized with low-flow sevoflurane. Anesthesiology 2001;94(1):21–31.

47. De Bony F, Tod M, Bidault R, On NT, Posner J, Rolan P. Multiple interactions of cimetidine and probenecid with valaciclovir and its metabolite acyclovir. Antimicrob Agents Chemother 2002;46(2):458–63.

48. Kornhauser DM, Petty BG, Hendrix CW, Woods AS, Nerhood LJ, Bartlett JG, Lietman PS. Probenecid and zidovudine metabolism. Lancet 1989;2(8661):473–5.

Rasburicase

General information

Rasburicase is recombinant urate oxidase, which causes the breakdown of uric acid to 5-hydroxyisourate, which is further broken down to allantoin. Although there is a gene for urate oxidase in human, it is non-functional, and purine catabolism therefore ends with uric acid. This may be advantageous, because uric acid is an antioxidant. In the root nodules of legumes urate oxidase is necessary for nitrogen fixation.

Rasburicase is used in the prevention and treatment of chemotherapy-induced hyperuricemia in patients with hematological malignancies [1,2,3,4,5,6,7,8,9]. In early clinical trials in patients who had received cancer chemotherapy rasburicase significantly reduced plasma uric acid concentrations from baseline by 2–4 times more than oral allopurinol 10 mg/kg/day. In these trials there was no evidence of renal impairment; rashes occurred in about 2% of patients, and bronchospasm, nausea and vomiting, and hemolysis less often.

Rasburicase has also been used to treat acute gout in a patient who developed severe urticaria/angioedema after receiving allopurinol, did not tolerate colchicine, and responded poorly to other treatments [10]

Observational studies

In 173 children and 72 adults with malignancy who were treated with intravenous rasburicase 0.20 mg/kg/day for 1–7 days there was a dramatic reduction in uric acid concentrations in all patients whether they received it for prophylaxis (n = 79) or treatment (n = 166) [11]. The median post-treatment concentrations were 30–42 µmol/l. Repeated administrations were also effective in 11 patients. Four children and five adults had mild adverse reactions that were drug related or of unknown cause; in two children, the adverse events occurred during the second course.

In eight patients who received rasburicase, a single dose produced rapid sustained reduction of plasma uric acid concentrations, and the effect was sustained for up to 96 hours; no adverse events were reported [12].

In a prospective study in 37 Korean children with hematological malignancies intravenous rasburicase 0.2 mg/kg/day was given for 3–5 days [13]. Drug-related adverse effects were mild and reversible and there were no grade 4 or serious adverse events.

Rasburicase was ineffective in controlling tumor lysis syndrome in a 4-day-old neonate with congenital precursor B cell acute lymphoblastic leukemia, despite several intravenous doses (two doses of 0.1 mg/kg and four doses of 0.2 mg/kg) and aggressive supportive therapy [14]. The authors suggested that in the presence of immature renal function other interventions and alternative antitumor strategies may be needed.

Comparative studies

In a multicenter randomized comparison of allopurinol and rasburicase in 52 children with leukemia or lymphoma at high risk of tumor lysis syndrome, the drugs were given for 5–7 days during induction chemotherapy [15]. The mean uric acid $AUC_{0 \rightarrow 96}$ was 7.6 hours.mmol/l with rasburicase and 19.7 hours.mmol/l with allopurinol. In this study, an 11-year-old boy with pre-B precursor acute lymphoblastic leukemia receiving rasburicase developed hemolysis and disseminated intravascular coagulopathy, which resolved after withdrawal; he did not have G6PD deficiency and the relation of this event to the treatment was not clear. No patients had anaphylactic reactions and there was no evidence of antibodies to rasburicase.

Organs and Systems

Respiratory

Two cases of fatal respiratory arrest have been reported in patient who received rasburicase [16].

- A 51-year-old woman with a history of allergy to codeine developed acute myelogenous leukemia and was given allopurinol and hydroxycarbamide, followed 12 hours later by intravenous rasburicase 0.20 mg/kg/day infusion; during the infusion she developed progressive dyspnea and cardiopulmonary arrest and died, despite cardiopulmonary resuscitation.
- A 51-year-old man developed leukemia and was given allopurinol, prednisone, and hydroxycarbamide; he was given rasburicase 18 hours later and a second dose on the next morning; during the infusion his dyspnea increased and he had a cardiopulmonary arrest resulting in anoxic brain damage.

The authors attributed these reactions to acute severe bronchospasm, secondary to an anaphylactic reaction to rasburicase, probably associated with tobacco-induced bronchial damage, since both patients were smokers.

Nervous system

An acute myoclonic reaction has been attributed to rasburicase [17].

- A 35-year-old woman with non-Hodgkin's lymphoma was given rasburicase 0.20 mg/kg in advance of chemotherapy and within 2 hours became confused, agitated, and mute, with generalized myoclonus and muscular spasticity, with neck extension and protracted deviation of the mouth to the left followed by decorticate positioning of the arms and legs. She was given intravenous diphenhydramine 25 mg, which produced immediate relaxation of the myoclonus and muscle spasticity but did not affect the mutism. Over the next 24 hours she had several episodes of myoclonus and muscle spasticity, which responded to intravenous diphenhydramine. She recovered completely after 36 hours.

Mineral metabolism

Of 25 patients treated with rasburicase and urine alkalinization, eight had hypocalcemia and hyperphosphatemia and 10 had hypophosphatemia; the last of these was more common in children with B-cell lymphomas [18]. The authors suggested that alkalinization should be avoided during treatment with rasburicase.

Hematologic

Hemolytic anemia and methemoglobinemia has been attributed to rasburicase in a patient with glucose-6-phosphate dehydrogenase (G6PD) deficiency [19].

- A 50-year-old African–American man was given a single dose of intravenous rasburicase 22.5 mg for acute renal failure secondary to hyperuricemia. He developed methemoglobinemia of 15% and a hemolytic anemia; the hemoglobin fell from 14.8 to 5.3 g/dl. He made a full recovery after aggressive fluid therapy, blood transfusions, and respiratory support. G6PD deficiency was subsequently confirmed.

Rasburicase is contraindicated in patients with G6PD deficiency, in whom it can cause hemolytic anemia and methemoglobinemia.

Other cases of methemoglobinemia have been reported [20].

References

1. Easton J, Noble S, Jarvis B. Rasburicase. Paediatr Drugs 2001;3(6):433-7.
2. Goldman SC. Rasburicase: potential role in managing tumor lysis in patients with hematological malignancies. Expert Rev Anticancer Ther 2003;3(4):429-33.
3. Yim BT, Sims-McCallum RP, Chong PH. Rasburicase for the treatment and prevention of hyperuricemia. Ann Pharmacother 2003;37(7-8):1047-54.
4. Bessmertny O, Robitaille LM, Cairo MS. Rasburicase: a new approach for preventing and/or treating tumor lysis syndrome. Curr Pharm Des 2005;11(32):4177-85.
5. Cheson BD, Dutcher BS. Managing malignancy-associated hyperuricemia with rasburicase. J Support Oncol 2005;3(2):117-24.
6. Jeha S, Pui CH. Recombinant urate oxidase (rasburicase) in the prophylaxis and treatment of tumor lysis syndrome. Contrib Nephrol 2005;147:69–79.
7. Ueng S. Rasburicase (Elitek): a novel agent for tumor lysis syndrome. Proc (Bayl Univ Med Cent) 2005;18(3):275–9.
8. Oldfield V, Perry CM. Rasburicase: a review of its use in the management of anticancer therapy-induced hyperuricaemia. Drugs 2006;66(4):529–45.
9. Oldfield V, Perry CM. Spotlight on rasburicase in anticancer therapy-induced hyperuricemia. BioDrugs 2006;20(3):197–9.
10. Richette P, Bardin T. Successful treatment with rasburicase of a tophaceous gout in a patient allergic to allopurinol. Nat Clin Pract Rheumatol 2006;2(6):338–42.
11. Pui CH, Jeha S, Irwin D, Camitta B. Recombinant urate oxidase (rasburicase) in the prevention and treatment of malignancy-associated hyperuricemia in pediatric and adult patients: results of a compassionate-use trial. Leukemia 2001;15(10):1505–9.
12. Liu CY, Sims-McCallum RP, Schiffer CA. A single dose of rasburicase is sufficient for the treatment of hyperuricemia in patients receiving chemotherapy. Leuk Res 2005;29(4):463–5.
13. Shin HY, Kang HJ, Park ES, Choi HS, Ahn HS, Kim SY, Chung NG, Kim HK, Kim SY, Kook H, Hwang TJ, Lee KC, Lee SM, Lee KS, Yoo KH, Koo HH, Lee MJ, Seo JJ, Moon HN, Ghim T, Lyu CJ, Lee WS, Choi YM. Recombinant urate oxidase (rasburicase) for the treatment of hyperuricemia in pediatric patients with hematologic malignancies: results of a compassionate prospective multicenter study in Korea. Pediatr Blood Cancer 2006;46(4):439–45.
14. McNutt DM, Holdsworth MT, Wong C, Hanrahan JD, Winter SS. Rasburicase for the management of tumor lysis syndrome in neonates. Ann Pharmacother 2006;40(7-8):1445–50.
15. Goldman SC, Holcenberg JS, Finklestein JZ, Hutchinson R, Kreissman S, Johnson FL, Tou C, Harvey E, Morris E, Cairo MS. A randomized comparison between rasburicase and allopurinol in children with lymphoma or leukemia at high risk for tumor lysis. Blood 2001;97(10):2998–3003.
16. Trujillo M, Morales M. Rasburicase-induced fatal respiratory arrest? Ann Oncol 2007;18(2):399–400.
17. Pitini V, Bramanti P, Arrigo C, Sessa E, La Gattuta G, Amata C. Acute neurotoxicity as a serious adverse event related to rasburicase in a non-Hodgkin's lymphoma patient. Ann Oncol 2004;15(9):1446.
18. van den Berg H, Reintsema AM. Renal tubular damage in rasburicase: risks of alkalinisation. Ann Oncol 2004;15(1):175–6.
19. Browning LA, Kruse JA. Hemolysis and methemoglobinemia secondary to rasburicase administration. Ann Pharmacother 2005;39(11):1932–5.
20. Kizer N, Martinez E, Powell M. Report of two cases of rasburicase-induced methemoglobinemia. Leuk Lymphoma 2006;47(12):2648–50.

Sulfinpyrazone

General Information

Sulfinpyrazone, a pyrazolone derivative, is used both as a uricosuric agent and as an anti-platelet drug. It has similar adverse effects to those of phenylbutazone when taken for long term (SEDA-6, 104). In a large number of patients who took the drug for secondary prevention of myocardial infarction (an indication that was not subsequently accepted), the incidence of adverse effects was not high (1).

Organs and Systems

Respiratory

Sulfinpyrazone can precipitate bronchoconstriction in some aspirin-sensitive patients (2). There is no cross-sensitivity with dipyrone.

Hematologic

Prolonged treatment with sulfinpyrazone produces a high incidence of thrombocytopenia and granulocytopenia. After withdrawal, these effects are completely reversible (SED-9, 157; 3). Sulfinpyrazone also inhibits platelet aggregation (4).

Sulfinpyrazone has been implicated in the development of myelomonocytic leukemia and multiple myeloma when given with colchicine (3).

Urinary tract

Impairment of renal function and even acute renal insufficiency can follow sulfinpyrazone treatment, by various mechanisms: immunoallergic-induced acute interstitial nephritis, inhibition of renal prostaglandins, and precipitation of uric acid stones. These changes are probably reversible, since there have been cases in which renal impairment spontaneously normalized on withdrawal (5).

Susceptibility Factors

The antinatriuretic effects of sulfinpyrazone could be dangerous in patients with impaired cardiac function (6).

Drug–Drug Interactions

Aspirin

In low dosages (up to 2 g/day), aspirin reduces urate excretion and blocks the effects of sulfinpyrazone. In higher dosages (over 5 g/day), salicylates increase urate excretion.

Beta-blockers

Sulfinpyrazone interferes with the antihypertensive action of beta-blockers (7).

Phenylbutazone

Sulfinpyrazone has a biphasic interaction with phenylbutazone (enhancement followed by antagonism).

Probenecid

Probenecid reduces the renal tubular secretion of sulfinpyrazone but there is no change in the uricosuric effect (9).

Warfarin

By reducing the metabolic clearance of warfarin, sulfinpyrazone enhances its hypoprothrombinemic effect, with life-threatening consequences (8).

References

1. Sherry S. The Anturan reinfarction trial. New Engl J Med 1980;303:50.
2. Szczeklik A, Czerniawska-Mysik G, Nizankowska E. Sulfinpyrazone and aspirin-induced asthma. N Engl J Med 1980;303(12):702–3.
3. Witwer MW, Schmid FR, Tesar JT. Acute myelomonocytic leukaemia and multiple myeloma after sulphinpyrazone and colchicine treatment of gout. BMJ 1976;2(6027):89.
4. Schwartz AD, Pearson HA. Aspirin, platelets, and bleeding. J Pediatr 1971;78(3):558–60.
5. Durham DS, Ibels LS. Sulphinpyrazone-induced acute renal failure. BMJ (Clin Res Ed) 1981;282(6264):609.
6. Hauselmann HJ, Studer H. Antinatriuretische Wirkung von Sulphinpyrazon. [Antinatriuretic effect of sulfinpyrazone.] Schweiz Med Wochenschr 1981;111(27–28):1030.
7. Brater DC. Drug–drug and drug–disease interactions with nonsteroidal anti-inflammatory drugs. Am J Med 1986;80(1A):62–77.
8. Bailey RR, Reddy J. Potentiation of warfarin action by sulphinpyrazone. Lancet 1980;1(8162):254.
9. Perel JM, Dayton PG, Snell MM, Yu TF, Gutman AB. Studies of interactions among drugs in man at the renal level: probenecid and sulfinpyrazone. Clin Pharmacol Ther 1969;10(6):834–40.

Index of drug names

Note: Locators followed by 't' refer to tables illustrated in that page.

Printed in the United States
By Bookmasters